examination
PAEDIATRICS

5th edition

A guide to paediatric training

examination
PAEDIATRICS

5th edition

A guide to paediatric training

Wayne Harris
MBBS, MRCP (UK), FRACP
Senior Staff Specialist in Paediatrics,
West Moreton South Burnett Health Service District
Senior Lecturer, Department of Paediatrics and Child Health,
University of Queensland, Brisbane, Australia

ELSEVIER

ELSEVIER

Elsevier Australia. ACN 001 002 357
(a division of Reed International Books Australia Pty Ltd)
Tower 1, 475 Victoria Avenue, Chatswood, NSW 2067

Notice

Practitioners and researchers must always rely on their own experience and knowledge in evaluating and using any information, methods, compounds or experiments described herein. Because of rapid advances in the medical sciences, in particular, independent verification of diagnoses and drug dosages should be made. To the fullest extent of the law, no responsibility is assumed by Elsevier, authors, editors or contributors for any injury and/or damage to persons or property as a matter of products liability, negligence or otherwise, or from any use or operation of any methods, products, instructions, or ideas contained in the material herein.

Although all advertising material is expected to conform to ethical (medical) standards, inclusion in this publication does not constitute a guarantee or endorsement of the quality or the value of such product or the claims made of it by its manufacturer.

National Library of Australia Cataloguing-in-Publication Data

---

Harris, Wayne, 1958- author.

Examination paediatrics: a guide to paediatric training / Wayne Harris.

5th Edition.

9780729542517 (paperback)

Includes index.

Pediatrics.
Pediatrics–Examinations, questions, etc.

Senior Content Strategist: Larissa Norrie
Content Development Specialist: Vanessa Ridehalgh
Project Manager: Devendran Kannan
Edited by Leanne Poll
Proofread by Jon Forsyth
Design by Stan Lamond
Index by Innodata Indexing
Typeset by Toppan Best-set Premedia Limited
Printed in China

Dedication

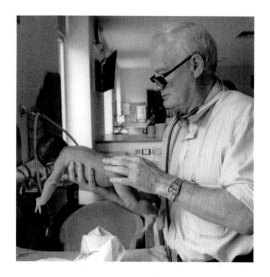

To Dr Tors Clothier MBChB, FACRRM, FRACP (Hon)

The complete paediatrician; part Albert Schweitzer, part Mahatma Gandhi, part Indiana Jones

Tors Clothier has had a remarkably rich and diverse peripatetic career, guided by, in his words, 'an almost sacred calling to serve children and their parents, especially the dispossessed, the sore and afflicted, spurred on by the vulnerability of sick and hurt children and the pathos of their parents'. This arose out of his exposure to the iniquities of apartheid in the country of his birth.

Tors was born in Johannesburg in 1946, graduated MBChB from the University of Cape Town in 1972, did his internship in Cape Town in 1973 and left South Africa permanently for South America in 1974. There he had jobs as a river doctor on the Amazon in Peru, and a fiord doctor in the Bismarck Archipelago in Southern Chile. This was truncated by the rise of Pinochet. Then he enjoyed a stint as a children's medical officer and army doctor in Rhodesia, before going to New Zealand to catch up with his future wife, June, whom he had met at the Hospital Amazonico in Peru. He arrived in Australia at the end of 1976 and had various medical officer jobs in Tasmania. He then worked as a general practitioner in Tasmania, Cairns and Darwin, before doing 4 years at Princess Margaret Hospital in Perth as a paediatric registrar, followed by 6 years at Royal Alexandra Hospital for Children in Sydney, where I first met Tors in 1986. He was the consummate clinician, his knowledge base astounding, his experience far-reaching. He was (and remains) a superb diagnostician, a brilliant teacher, humble, compassionate; the ideal role model for an aspiring paediatric doctor. He always put the child front and centre. He treated everyone with respect. He became my mentor. I suggested that his vast experience perhaps could be better utilised in Alice Springs, where I had worked the previous year. I felt that Tors 'belonged' in Alice Springs, there being a paucity of senior paediatric doctors of his calibre.

Tors went to Alice Springs in 1989. He became a figure of legend, his clinical acumen unsurpassed. In 1992, during a 6-month locum consultant post at Alice Springs Hospital, I got to work with Tors again. It remains the most rewarding clinical attachment of my career: third-world medicine in a first-world hospital, working alongside the best general paediatrician I have ever met.

Tors stayed in Alice Springs for 25 years. He left in 2014. In those years he acquired, in his words, 'a modest expertise in Indigenous Child Health, and an abiding love and respect for one of the oldest continuous cultures on Earth, while being appalled by their plight'. He also 'learned to love the shimmering light, wide open blue skies, ochre and grey and marching hills of central Australia'. Along the way Tors obtained a FACRRM, and was awarded an Honorary FRACP. In his own words, 'I have been fortunate to have worked for and with many special people in the Caring professions who have enriched my life with their friendship insights and expertise. I have been blessed by the love and support of an amazing woman'.

Tors has pursued his career with dedication, compassion and humility, working alongside like-minded able colleagues. I have met scores of doctors, including many professors, whom Tors has taught and guided, who concur with my impression of him. Tors has inspired countless residents and registrars by being the 'complete' paediatrician. He continues to inspire.

Contents

Foreword to the fifth edition

The adult and paediatric examinations for entry to advanced training for the Fellowship of the Royal Australasian College of Physicians (FRACP) are recognised as ranking among the most difficult specialty examinations in the world. Since 1992, Wayne Harris's *Examination Paediatrics* has helped candidates prepare for their clinical examination day. It has become important reading for FRACP candidates and those preparing for similar examinations in many parts of the world. The book has even been spotted in the briefcases of College examiners who feel the need to revise their own approach before they examine.

The first edition of *Examination Paediatrics* was written at a time when most of the information about the examination was handed down to candidates from senior registrars who had recently sat for it. Some were inclined to tell terrifying stories about the ordeal, perhaps in part for their own amusement. This book clarified and demystified the examination by explaining it in detail and outlining ways to conquer it. Over the years the adult and paediatric exams have become fairer but remain rigorous and challenging. There have been changes in the examination format and in paediatrics itself. The fifth edition of this book for examination candidates is right up to date with paediatrics and changes to the testing format.

For many years, we as examiners for the adult FRACP clinical exams have had the opportunity to watch videos of paediatric exam candidates performing short-case examinations at their annual exam calibration sessions. We observe in amazement as the candidate entertains and examines the small patient at the same time, often chasing the child around the room, all of this while being watched by both examiners and parents. It makes the adult short-case examination seem very tame.

Wayne Harris's book is full of helpful advice to assist candidates in managing this complicated process. As well as the factual knowledge needed to pass the exam, techniques for managing the patient, the parents and the examiners as well as the candidate's own fears and anxieties are explored in a most comforting way. The new edition contains more detailed sections on cardiology and congenital heart disease—a much-feared exam problem. New long and short cases, including six new neurology cases, are included.

Examination Paediatrics remains essential reading for FRACP candidates and those undertaking similar examinations. Don't underestimate the importance of reading widely, learning and practicing your own system of examination until it is second nature for every system, and being prepared for surprises. We wish all candidates the very best of luck, and remember as you prepare never give up or give in.

Nicholas J Talley,
MBBS (Hons) (NSW), MD (NSW), PhD (Syd), MMedSci (Clin Epi)
(Newcastle), FRACP, FAFPHM, FAHMS, FRCP (London & Edinburgh),
FACP, FACG, AGAF, FAMS, FRCPI (Hons)
Laureate Professor and Pro Vice-Chancellor, Global Research,
University of Newcastle, NSW, Australia
Senior Staff Specialist, John Hunter Hospital, Newcastle, NSW, Australia

Simon O'Connor,
FRACP, DDU, FCSANZ
Cardiologist, The Canberra Hospital; Clinical Senior Lecturer, Australian National
University Medical School, Canberra, ACT, Australia

Preface

'Tomorrow's battle is won during today's practice.'
SAMURAI MAXIM

The first edition of this book was written 25 years ago, to assist candidates preparing for the Fellowship of the Royal Australasian College of Physicians (Part 1) Examination in Paediatrics, or for the Membership of the Royal College of Physicians (Part 2) Examination in Paediatrics (now the MRCPCH), inspired by Talley and O'Connor's book *Examination Medicine*. Back in 1992 there was no limit to the number of attempts one could have to pass the FRACP examination. Several of my senior colleagues had passed the clinical exam on their tenth attempt; clinically they were all exceptional. Over the years the format of the exam has changed, and in 2017 the number of attempts is now limited to three for the clinical exam, increasing the focus on passing the first time. This book is designed for that goal.

This edition has been extensively expanded to try to keep up with the advances in medical knowledge, which accelerate each year. Each previous long case has been updated, five new ones added, including three neurocutaneous syndromes (NF1, TSC and SWS), hypopituitarism and Rett syndrome. Each previous short case has been updated, and eight new ones added including lymphadenopathy, ataxia, nystagmus, proptosis, and body asymmetry. There are new expanded sections of previous chapters; in particular the cardiology chapter has been improved and now is profusely illustrated with over 50 colour images. There are many new mnemonics. In each edition I have stressed this is not the 'Einstein Encyclopaedia of Paediatrics'; its purpose is to make the hurdle of any paediatric examination easier to clear.

In the words of Sir Karl Popper, the great philosopher of science: **'All life is problem solving'**.

Don't panic! Good luck!

Wayne Harris
July 2017

Preface to the first edition

'Don't panic.'
THE HITCHHIKER'S GUIDE TO THE GALAXY, DOUGLAS ADAMS

This book has been written to assist candidates preparing for the Fellowship of the Royal Australasian College of Physicians (Part 1) Examination in Paediatrics. It is also intended to assist candidates preparing for the Membership of the Royal College of Physicians (Part 2) Examination in Paediatrics. It was inspired by Talley and O'Connor's book Examination Medicine, written to assist in the preparation for the Royal Australasian College of Physicians' Internal Medicine (Part I) Examination.

We have tried to present a structured and comprehensive approach to the clinical examination of the paediatric patient in a way that is particularly relevant for the postgraduate degrees of the FRACP (Part 1) and the MRCP (Part 2). Approaches are presented for most of the common-examination long and short cases.

This book is not designed to be the 'Einstein Encyclopaedia of Paediatrics'. As a supplement to the major texts and journal articles, it aims to demonstrate approaches that the authors have found successful.

Our combined experience of the FRACP examination comprises six written examinations, and six clinical examinations (including two 'extra time' cases), and for the MRCP, one clinical examination. This broad coverage of most conceivable contingencies ensures that many of the approaches have been tested (successfully) in the actual examination settings by the authors, while others have been tested by our peers in their examinations.

We hope that this book will be useful for examination candidates, and also helpful to paediatric residents/house officers, senior medical students and general practitioners who deal with children.

While every effort has been made to ensure the accuracy of the information herein, especially with regard to drug selection and dosage, appropriate information sources should be consulted, particularly for new or uncommon drugs. It is the clinician's responsibility to check the appropriateness of an opinion in relation to acute clinical situations and new developments. Any comments or suggestions will be gratefully and humbly received, so that future editions of this book may prove to be more useful.

Good luck!

Wayne Harris
Brian Timms
Robin Choong
1992

Acknowledgements/ Special thanks ...

To my family for supporting me throughout the months spent producing this edition.

To my friends and colleagues, Dr Brian Timms and Dr Robin Choong, two of my favourite people, for supporting me as co-authors over the first and second editions of this book, and for encouraging me to complete the third and fourth editions, and this edition.

To the following wonderful people, for your unwavering support, and encouragement: Mr Charles Waterstreet, Dr Ian Shellshear, Dr Bheem Rajpal, Dr Bernadette Panlaque, Dr Kirsten Zahnow, Dr Fauzia Mohammed, Dr Ryan Wellington, Dr Steven Liew, Dr Jim Pelekanos, Dr Li Chuen Wong, Dr Sunday Pan, Dr Anand Ramineni and Dr Smriti Joshi.

Reviewers

I would like to thank the following specialists who were kind enough to review different sections of the book. Their comments were invaluable. However, the book does not necessarily reflect the opinions of these specialists.

Geoffrey Ambler FRACP
Paediatric Endocrinologist, The Children's Hospital at Westmead (CHW)

Chris Barnes FRACP
Paediatric Haematologist, The Royal Children's Hospital (RCH), Parkville

John Burke FRACP
Paediatric Nephrologist, Lady Cilento Children's Hospital (LCCH), Brisbane

Anita Cairns FRACP
Paediatric Neurologist, LCCH

Sophie Calvert FRACP
Paediatric Neurologist, LCCH

Anthony Catto-Smith FRACP
Director, Department of Gastroenterology, LCCH

John Christodoulou FRACP, AM
Chair in Genomic Medicine, Melbourne Children's Campus, Murdoch Children's Research Institute, University of Melbourne Department of Paediatrics

Robin Choong FRACP, AIMM
Senior Staff Specialist, Paediatric Intensive Care and Paediatric Emergency Medicine,
CHW

Louise Conwell FRACP
Paediatric Endocrinologist, LCCH

Andrew Cotterill FRACP
Director, Department of Endocrinology, LCCH

Luciano Dalla-Pozza FRACP
Department Head, Oncology Unit, CHW

David Dossetor FRANZCP
Consultant Psychiatrist, Head of Developmental Psychiatry, CHW

Peter Downie FRACP
Head of Children's Cancer Centre, Monash Health, Victoria

Geoff Kewley FRACP
Consultant Paediatrician, Sydney

Sloane Madden FRANZCP
Paediatric Psychiatrist, Director of Eating Disorders Service, Sydney Children's
Hospital Network, CHW

Edward O'Loughlin MD, FRACP
Head of Gastroenterology Services, CHW

Peter Procopis FRACP, AM
Paediatric Neurologist, Adjunct Professor Paediatrics and Child Health, CHW

Hugo Sampaio FRACP
Paediatric Neurologist, Sydney Children's Hospital, Randwick

Hiran Selvadurai FRACP
Head of Respiratory Medicine, Kids Research Institute, CHW

Brian Timms FRACP
Consultant Paediatrician, Consultant Neonatologist, Melbourne

Claire Wainwright FRACP
Paediatric Respiratory Physician, LCCH

Chris Whight FRACP
Paediatric Cardiologist, Prince Charles Hospital, Brisbane

Ben Whitehead FRACP
Director, Rheumatology Service, LCCH

Abbreviations

1,25(OH)2 D3	calcitriol
3β-HSD	3 beta-hydroxysteroid dehydrogenase
3D	three-dimensional
3DE	three-dimensional echocardiography
5-ASA	5-aminosalicylate
6-MP	6-mercaptopurine
6-MMP	6-methylmercaptopurine
6MWT	6-minute walking test
6-TG	6-thioguanine
7vPCV	heptavalent conjugated pneumococcal vaccine
21OHD-CAH	congenital adrenal hyperplasia due to 21-hydroxylase deficiency
11OHD-CAH	congenital adrenal hyperplasia due to 11-beta hydroxylase deficiency
17OHD-CAH	congenital adrenal hyperplasia due to 17-hydroxylase deficiency
17OHP	1-hydroxyprogesterone
AAI	atlanto-axial instability
AAN	American Academy of Neurology
AAP	American Academy of Pediatrics
AAVC	accessory atrioventricular connection
ABC	airway, breathing, circulation
ABPA	allergic bronchopulmonary aspergillosis
ACA	anterior cerebral artery
ACCP	American College of Chest Physicians
ACE	angiotensin-converting enzyme
AChR	acetylcholine receptor
ACM	Arnold–Chiari malformation
ACR	acute cellular rejection *and/or* American College of Rheumatology
ACS	acute chest syndrome (in sickle cell disease)
ACTH	adrenocorticotropic hormone
AD	autosomal dominant
ADD	attention deficit disorder
ADEM	acute disseminated encephalomyelitis
a-DGP	anti-deamidated gliadin-related peptide
ADH	antidiuretic hormone
ADHD	attention deficit hyperactivity disorder
ADI-R	Autism Diagnostic Interview—Revised
ADL	activities of daily living
ADLTLE	autosomal-dominant lateral temporal lobe epilepsy (aka ADPEAF)
ADNFLE	autosomal-dominant nocturnal frontal lobe epilepsy (aka ENFL)
ADOS	Autism Diagnostic Observation Schedule
ADPEAF	autosomal-dominant partial epilepsy + auditory features (aka ADLTLE)
ADR	Adriamycin
AED	anti-epileptic drug

AFO	ankle-foot orthosis
AGC	aspartate glutamate carrier
AGS	Alagille syndrome
AGV	Ahmed Glaucoma Valve
AHA	American Heart Association
AHCDO	Australian Haemophilia Centre Directors' Organisation
AHI	apnoea hypoxic index
AIDs	anti-inflammatory drugs
AIDS	acquired immune deficiency syndrome
AIR	anaesthesia-induced rhabdomyolysis
aka	also known as
ALL	acute lymphoblastic leukaemia
ALP	alkaline phosphatase
ALT	alanine aminotransferase
ALTE	apparent life-threatening event
AMH/MIS	anti-Müllerian hormone/Müllerian-inhibiting substance
AML	acute myeloid leukaemia
AN	anorexia nervosa
ANA	antinuclear antibody
ANC	absolute neutrophil count
ANLL	acute non-lymphoblastic leukaemia
AP	anteroposterior
APCC	activated prothrombin complex concentrate
APD	automated peritoneal dialysis
aPTT	activated partial thromboplastin time
AR	autosomal recessive
ARB	angiotensin II receptor blocker
AS	aortic stenosis
ASCA	anti-Saccharomyces cerevisiae antibodies
ASD	atrial septal defect *and/or* autism spectrum disorder
ASQ	Ages and Stages Questionnaire
AST	aspartate aminotransferase
AT	alpha-1-antitrypsin *and/or* ataxia telangiectasia
ATG	anti-thymocyte globulin
AT-III	antithrombin 3
ATN	acute tubular necrosis
ATNR	asymmetric tonic neck reflex
ATZ	alpha-1-antitrypsin Z
AV	atrioventricular
AVM	arteriovenous malformation
AVN	atrioventricular node *and/or* avascular necrosis
AVNRT	atrioventricular node re-entry tachycardia
AZA	azathioprine
BAV	bicuspid aortic valve
B–B	Bardet–Biedl syndrome
BDP-HFA	beclomethasone dipropionate
BDZ	benzodiazepine
BECTS	benign epilepsy with centrotemporal spikes
BFNS	benign familial neonatal seizures
BiPAP	bilevel positive airways pressure

BMD	bone mineral density *and/or* Becker muscular dystrophy
BMI	body mass index
BMTx	bone marrow transplantation
BN	bulimia nervosa
BPD	bronchopulmonary dysplasia
BsAbs	bispecific T-cell engager antibodies
BSL	blood sugar level (commonly used term for plasma glucose level)
BSS	Bernard–Soulier syndrome
BTX-A	botulinum toxin A
BUD	budesonide
B-W	Beckwith-Wiedemann syndrome
C1	atlas; first cervical vertebra
C2	axis; second cervical vertebra
CAB	chlorambucil
CACN	calcium channel
CAE	childhood absence epilepsy
CAH	congenital adrenal hyperplasia *and/or* chronic active hepatitis
CAI	central adrenal insufficiency
CAL	café-au-lait
CALM	café-au-lait macules
CAPD	continuous ambulatory peritoneal dialysis
CAR	Central Africa Republic
CAR-T-cells	chimeric antigen receptors
CARS	Childhood Autism Rating Scale
CAS	Child Assessment Schedule
CATCH-22	cardiac defects, abnormal facies, thymic hypoplasia (and T cell deficiency), cleft palate, hypoparathyroidism (and hypocalcaemia), chromosome 22 microdeletions (22q11)
CBAVD	congenital bilateral absence of the vas deferens
CBCL	child behaviour checklist
CB-SCT	cord-blood-derived stem cell transplantation
CBZ	carbamazepine
CCF	congestive cardiac failure
CCP	citrullinated cyclic peptide
CCPD	continuous cycling peritoneal dialysis
CCPT	Connors continuous performance test
CD	Crohn's disease and/or cadaveric donor
CDA	Child Disability Allowance
CDH	congenital dislocation of the hip
CDI	Child Development Inventories
CDP	constitutional delayed puberty (and growth)
CF	cystic fibrosis
CFC	cardio-facial-cutaneous syndrome and/or chlorinated fluorocarbons
CFCS	communication function classification system
CFLD	cystic fibrosis-associated liver disease
CFR-BD	cystic fibrosis-related bone disease
CFRD	cystic fibrosis-related diabetes
CFTR	cystic fibrosis transmembrane conductance regulator
CGH	comparative genomic hybridization (array same as CMA)
CGMS	continuous glucose monitoring system

CH	congenital hemihypertrophy
CHAQ	Childhood Health Assessment Questionnaire
CHARGE	colobomatous malformation of eye, heart, atresia choanae, retardation (cognitive and somatic), genital anomalies, ear anomalies +/− deafness
CHAT	Checklist for Autism in Toddlers
CHD	congenital heart disease
CHILD	congenital hemidysplasia, ichthyosiform (erythroderma), limb defects
CHO	carbohydrate
CHQ	Child Health Questionnaire
CHR	cholinergic receptor *and/or* carbohydrate ratio
CI	cochlear implantation
CIC	ciclesonide
CKD	chronic kidney disease
CKD-MBD	chronic kidney disease mineral bone disease
CLCN	chloride channel
CLD	chronic liver disease *and/or* chronic lung disease
CLZ	clonazepam
CMA	chromosomal microarray analysis (same as CGH)
CMC	capillary malformation, congenital
CML	chronic myeloid leukaemia
CMP	cow's milk protein
CMT	Charcot-Marie-Tooth disease
CMV	cytomegalovirus
CNF1	congenital nephrotic syndrome of the Finnish type
CNI	calcineurin inhibitor
CNS	central nervous system
CNV	copy-number variant
CO	cerebral oedema
CO2	carbon dioxide
COFS	cerebro-oculo-facial-skeletal syndrome
COG	children's oncology group
COX-2	cyclo-oxygenase 2
CP	cerebral palsy
CPA	cyclophosphamide *and/or* CP Alliance
CPAP	continuous positive airways pressure
CPHD	combined pituitary hormone deficiency
CPL	choice passion life
CPR	cardiopulmonary resuscitation
CRF	chronic renal failure
CRH	corticotrophin-releasing hormone
CRINS	corticosteroid-resistant idiopathic nephrotic syndrome
CRP	C-reactive protein
CS	corticosteroid
CSA	cyclosporine A
CSF	cerebrospinal fluid
CSINS	corticosteroid-sensitive idiopathic nephrotic syndrome
CSWS	epileptic encephalopathy with continuous spike-and-wave during sleep
CT	computed tomography

CTAF	conotruncal anomaly face syndrome
CTE	CT enterography
CTS	centrotemporal spikes
CVA	cerebrovascular accident
CVAD	central venous access device
CVS	cardiovascular system *and/or* chorionic villus sampling
CXR	chest X-ray
CYP17A1	cytochrome P450 enzyme 17-hydroxylase
CYP21A2	cytochrome P450 enzyme 21-hydroxylase
DAPC	dystrophin-associated protein complex
DAT	dopamine transporter
dB	decibel
DBCL	Developmental Behaviour Checklist
DBS	deep brain stimulation
DCCT	Diabetes Control and Complications Trial
DCD	developmental coordination disorder (clumsiness)
DCH	diffuse choroidal haemangioma
DCM	dilated cardiomyopathy
DDAVP	desmopressin (1-deamino 8-D arginine vasopressin)
DDH	developmental dysplasia of the hip
DDST	Denver developmental screening test
DDST-II	Denver developmental screening test—II (revised)
DEXA or DXA	dual x-ray absorptiometry
DFO	desferrioxamine
DFP	deferiprone
DFS	deferasirox
DFT	deferitrin
DFZ	deflazacort
DGGE	denaturing gradient gel electrophoresis
DGS	DiGeorge syndrome
DHEA	dehydroepiandrosterone
DHEAS	dehydroepiandrosterone sulphate
DHT	dihydrotestosterone
DHTR	delayed haemolytic transfusion reaction
DIC	disseminated intravascular coagulation
DICA	Diagnostic Interview for Children and Adolescents
DIDMOAD	diabetes insipidus-diabetes mellitus-optic atrophy-deafness (Wolfram)
DIOS	distal intestinal obstruction syndrome
DISC	Diagnostic Interview for Children
DISCO	Diagnostic Interview for Social and Communications Disorders
DISIDA	di-iso-propyl-imino-di-acetic acid (disofenin hepatobiliary scan)
DKA	diabetic ketoacidosis
DMO	dynamic movement orthosis
DMARDs	disease-modifying antirheumatic drugs
DMD	Duchenne muscular dystrophy
DMSA	di-mercapto-succinic-acid
DNA	deoxyribonucleic acid
DQ	developmental quotient

DS	Down syndrome
DSD	disorder of sexual development
dsDNA	double-stranded DNA
DSM-5	*Diagnostic and Statistical Manual of Mental Disorders*, 5th edition
DSS	Dejerine-Sottas syndrome
DTPA	Tc99m diethylene triamine penta-acetic acid
DW or DWS	Dandy-Walker syndrome
DXA	dual-energy X-ray absorptiometry
EACA	epsilon-aminocaproic acid
EBRT	external beam radiation therapy
EBV	Epstein-Barr virus
ECA	epilepsy childhood absence
ECG	electrocardiogram
ECMO	extracorporeal membrane oxygenation
EDIC	Epidemiology of Diabetes Interventions and Complications
EDMD	Emery-Dreifuss muscular dystrophy
EEG	electroencephalogram
EEN	exclusive enteral nutrition
EFD	eformoterol fumarate dihydrate
EGTCSA	epilepsy with generalised tonic-clonic seizures alone (aka EIG)
EHBA	extrahepatic biliary atresia
EHL	extended half-life
EIEE	early infantile epileptic encephalopathy
EIG	epilepsy, idiopathic generalised (aka EGTCSA)
EJA	epilepsy juvenile absence
EJM	epilepsy juvenile myoclonus
ELBW	extremely low birthweight
EMA	endomysial antibody
EM-AS	epilepsy with myoclonic atonic seizures (Doose syndrome)
EME	early myoclonic encephalopathy
EMG	electromyogram
ENFL	epilepsy nocturnal frontal lobe
ENT	ears, nose and throat
EPR	early-phase allergic response
EPS	electrophysiologic study
ER	endoplasmic reticulum *and/or* extended release
ERA	enthesitis-related arthritis
ERCP	endoscopic retrograde cholangiography
ERG	electroretinogram
ERPT	endorectal pull-through procedure
ESLD	end-stage liver disease
ESM	ethosuximide *and/or* ejection systolic murmur
ESR	erythrocyte sedimentation rate
ESRD	end-stage renal disease
ESRF	end-stage renal failure
FA1AT	faecal alpha-1-antitrypsin excretion test
FAS/FASD	fetal alcohol syndrome/fetal alcohol spectrum disorders
FBC	full blood count
FDA	Food and Drug Administration

FET	forced inspiratory time
FEV1	forced expiratory volume in one second
ffDNA	cell-free fetal DNA
FFEVF	familial focal epilepsy with variable foci
FFP	fresh frozen plasma
FHM	familial hemiplegic migraine
FISH	fluorescence in situ hybridisation
F-IX	factor 9
FLAIR	fluid attenuation inversion recovery sequences
FLE	frontal lobe epilepsy
fMMC	fetal myelomeningocele
fMRI	functional MRI
FP	fluticasone proprionate
FRDA	Friedreich ataxia
FS	febrile seizures
FS+	febrile seizures plus
FSGS	focal segmental glomerulosclerosis
FSH	facio-scapulo-humeral *and/or* follicle stimulating hormone
FVC	forced vital capacity
FVIIa	activated factor 7
FVIII	factor 8
FX	factor 10
G6PD	glucose-6-phosphate dehydrogenase
GABA	gamma-amino butyric acid
GABR	gamma-amino butyric acid receptor
GAD	glutamic acid decarboxylase
GADA	glutamic acid decarboxylase antibodies
GARS	Gilliam Autism Rating Scale
GBM	glomerular basement membrane
GBS	Guillain-Barre syndrome *and/or* group B streptococcus
GCDH	glutaryl-CoA dehydrogenase
G-CSF	granulocyte colony stimulating factor
GEFS+	generalised epilepsy with febrile seizures plus
GFR	glomerular filtration rate
GGT	gamma glutamyl transferase
GH	growth hormone
GI	glycaemic index
GIST	gastrointestinal stromal tumours
GIT	gastrointestinal tract
GLUT1-DS	glucose transporter 1 deficiency syndrome
GM-CSF	granulocyte-macrophage colony stimulating factor
GMFCS	gross motor functional classification system
Gn	gonadotrophin
GN	glomerulonephritis
GNAQ	guanine nucleotide-binding protein Q polypeptide
GnRH	gonadotrophin-releasing hormone (aka LHRH)
GOR	gastro-oesophageal reflux
GORD	gastro-oesophageal reflux disease
GSD	glycogen storage disease
GSTM1	glutathione-S-transferase

GTCS	generalised tonic clonic seizures
GTT	glucose tolerance test
GVHD	graft versus host disease
HACAs	human anti-chimeric antibodies
HAT	hepatic artery thrombosis
Hb	haemoglobin
HbA1C	haemoglobin A1C: glycosylated haemoglobin
Hb AS	haemoglobin AS (sickle cell trait)
HBB	haemoglobin subunit beta globin gene
HBeAg	hepatitis B e antigen
Hb C	haemoglobin C
Hb F	haemoglobin F (fetal)
Hb S	haemoglobin S (sickle cell)
Hb SC	haemoglobin SC (sickle cell/haemoglobin C disease)
HBsAg	hepatitis B surface antigen
Hb SS	homozygous sickle cell disease
HC	head circumference
HCC	hepatocellular carcinoma
hCG	human chorionic gonadotrophin
HCM	hypertrophic cardiomyopathy
HCV	hepatitis C
HD	haemodialysis *and/or* Huntington disease
HDL	high-density lipoprotein
HEADS	home, education/employment/eating/exercise, activities, drugs and alcohol, sexuality/sexual health/suicide/self-harm and depression/safety
HFA	hydrofluoroalkane
HFI	hereditary fructose intolerance
HGPRT	hypoxanthine guanine phosphoribosyl-transferase
HHT	hereditary haemorrhagic telangiectasia
HIDA	hepatobiliary iminodiacetic acid
HINE	Hammersmith infant neurological examination
HIV	human immunodeficiency virus
HKAFO	hip-knee-ankle-foot orthosis
HLA	human leucocyte antigen
HLHS	hypoplastic left heart syndrome
HMPOA	hexamethylpropylene-amine oxime
HNF	human nephron filter
HP	hypothalamic-pituitary
HPA	hypothalamic-pituitary-adrenal (axis)
HPE	holoprosencephaly
HPG	hypothalamic–pituitary–gonadal (axis)
HPOA	hypertrophic pulmonary osteoarthropathy
HPFH	hereditary persistence of Hb F
HPLC	high-performance liquid chromatography
HRCT	high-resolution CT
HRQOL	health-related quality of life
HS	hippocampal sclerosis
HSCT	haematopoietic stem cell transplantation
HSE	herpes simplex encephalitis

HSP	Henoch–Schönlein purpura
HSTCL	hepatosplenic T-cell lymphoma
HSV	herpes simplex virus
HTC	haemophilia treatment centre
HU	hydroxyurea
HUS	haemolytic uraemic syndrome
HVZ	herpes varicella-zoster
Hx	history
Hz	hertz
IA-2	tyrosine phosphatase
IAA	insulin autoantibodies
IBD	inflammatory bowel disease
IBW	ideal body weight
IC	intracranial
ICA	internal carotid artery
ICD	implantable cardioverter defibrillator
ICD-10	international classification of diseases
ICE-GTC	intractable childhood epilepsy with generalised tonic-clonic seizures
ICH	intracranial haemorrhage
ICP	intracranial pressure
ICS	inhaled corticosteroids
ICSI	intracytoplasmic sperm injection
ICU	intensive care unit
ID	intellectual disability
IDDM	insulin-dependent diabetes mellitus
IEM	inborn error of metabolism
IGF	insulin-like growth factor
IGFBP	insulin-like growth factor bonding protein
Ig	immunoglobulin
IHH	intermittent hypercarbic hypoxia *and/or* idiopathic hypogonadotrophic hypogonadism
IHH	idiopathic hypogonadotrophic hypogonadism
IIMs	idiopathic inflammatory myopathies
ILAE	International League Against Epilepsy
ILAR	International League Against Rheumatism
IM	intramuscular *and/or* infectious mononucleosis
IMP	inosine monophosphate
IMRT	intensity-modulated radiation therapy
INCS	intranasal corticosteroid
INR	international normalised ratio
INS	idiopathic nephrotic syndrome
IPTAS	isolated patients' travel and accommodation scheme
IQ	intelligence quotient
IRT	immunoreactive trypsin
IT-BLF	intrathecal baclofen
ITI	immune tolerance induction
ITT	immune tolerance therapy
IU	international units
IUGR	intrauterine growth retardation

IV	intravenous
IVH	intraventricular haemorrhage
IVIG	intravenous immunoglobulin
IVC	inferior vena cava
JA	juvenile arthritis
JAE	juvenile absence epilepsy
JBS	Johanson–Blizzard syndrome
JDM	juvenile dermatomyositis
JIA	juvenile idiopathic arthritis
JLNS	Jervell and Lange–Nielsen syndrome
JME	juvenile myoclonic epilepsy (Janz syndrome)
JMML	juvenile myelomonocytic leukaemia
JPsA	juvenile psoriatic arthritis
JVP	jugular venous pressure
KAFO	knee-ankle-foot orthosis
KCl	potassium chloride
KCN	potassium channel
KD	ketogenic diet
KF	Kayser-Fleischer
KSS	Kearns-Sayre syndrome
KTW	Klippel-Trénaunay-Weber syndrome
LABA	long-acting beta-2 adrenoreceptor agonist
LAM	lymphangioleiomyomatosis
LCM	lacosamide
LCR	locus control region
LDH	lactate dehydrogenase
LDL	low-density lipoprotein
LDLT	living-donor lobar transplantation
LDS	Loeys-Dietz syndrome
LEOPARD	lentigines, ECG, ocular, pulmonary (stenosis), abnormal (genitalia), retarded growth, deafness
LEV	levetiracetam
LFTs	liver function tests
LGL	Lown–Ganong–Levine syndrome
LGS	Lennox-Gastaut syndrome
LH	luteinising hormone
LHRH	luteinising hormone-releasing hormone (aka GnRH)
LJM	limited joint mobility
LKS	Landau–Kleffner syndrome
LMN	lower motor neurone
LNS	Lesch–Nyhan syndrome
LP	lumbar puncture
LPR	late-phase allergic response
LQTS	long QT syndrome
LRD	living related donor
LS	lower segment
LSD	lysosomal storage disorder
LTG	lamotrigine
LTM	leukotriene modifier
LTRAs	leukotriene receptor antagonists

LTx	liver transplantation
LV	left ventricle
LVEF	left ventricular ejection fraction
LVF	left ventricular failure
LVH	left ventricular hypertrophy
LVOTO	left ventricular outflow tract obstruction
LVS	levamisole
MACE	Malone Antegrade Continence Enema
MACS	manual ability classification system
MAE	epilepsy with myoclonic absences
MAG-3	mercapto-acetyl-triglycine (chelated to technetium-99m)
MAHA	microangiopathic haemolytic anaemia
MAIS	mycobacterium avium-intracellular-scrofulaceum
MAS	macrophage activation syndrome
MATCHES	MAIS, ALL, TB, CMV, HIV, EBV, Streptococcus
MCA	middle cerebral artery
McC-A	McCune–Albright
M-CHAT	Modified Checklist for Autism in Toddlers
MD	myotonic dystrophy
MDA	muscular dystrophy association
MDI	metered dose inhaler
MDLS	Miller-Dieker lissencephalopathy syndrome
MDS	myelodysplastic syndrome
MEI	myoclonic epilepsy in infancy
MEN2b	multiple endocrine neoplasia type 2b
MEP	maximum expiratory mouth pressure
MERRF	mitochondrial encephalopathy with red ragged fibres
MesPGN	mesangial proliferative glomerulonephritis
MG	myasthenia gravis
MHC	major histocompatibility complex
MI	meconium ileus
MIBG	radioactive iodine metaidobenzoguanidine
MIM	Mendelian inheritance in man
MIP	maximum inspiratory mouth pressure
MIS/AMH	müllerian inhibiting substance/anti-müllerian hormone
MLD	metachromatic leucodystrophy
MLDS	myeloid leukaemia of Down syndrome
MLPA	multiple ligation probe amplification
MMC	myelomeningocele
MMF	mycophenolate mofetil
MMR	measles-mumps-rubella
MOM	mometasone
MPC	model-predictive control (algorithm)
MPGN	membranoproliferative glomerulonephritis
MPH	methylphenidate *and/or* mid-parental height
MPNST	malignant peripheral nerve sheath tumours
MPS	mucopolysaccharidosis
MRA	magnetic resonance angiography
MRD	minimal residual disease
MRE	magnetic resonance enterography

MRI	magnetic resonance imaging
mRNA	messenger RNA
MRSA	methicillin-resistant staphylococcus aureus
MSG	monosodium glutamate
MSU	mid-stream urine
MTLE with HS	mesial temporal lobe epilepsy with hippocampal sclerosis
mTOR	mechanistic target of rapamycin
MTX	methotrexate
MVA	motor vehicle accident
MVP	mitral valve prolapsed
MW	molecular weight
Mx	management
NAC	National Asthma Council
nAChR	nicotinic acetyl choline receptor
NaCl	sodium chloride
NAI	non-accidental injury
NCSE	non-convulsive status epilepticus
NCSI	National Cancer Survivorship Initiative
NDSS	National Diabetes Syringe Scheme
NEC	necrotising enterocolitis
NEJM	New England Journal of Medicine
NF1	neurofibromatosis type 1
NF2	neurofibromatosis type 2
NFNS	neurofibromatosis Noonan syndrome
NGS	next generation sequencing
NH&MRC	National Health and Medical Research Council
NHF	National Haemophilia Foundation
NICU	neonatal intensive care unit
NIV	non-invasive ventilation
NPPV	non-invasive positive pressure ventilation
NREM	non-rapid eye movement
NS	Noonan syndrome *and/or* nephrotic syndrome
NSAID	non-steroidal anti-inflammatory drug
NTBC	2-(2-nitro-4-trifluoromethylbenzoyl)-1,3-cyclohexenedione
NTD	neural tube defect
OB	bronchiolitis obliterans
OCD	obsessive compulsive disorder
OCPill	oral contraceptive pill
OCS	oral corticosteroids
ODD	oppositional defiant disorder
OI	osteogenesis imperfecta
OMIM	online Mendelian inheritance in man
OPG	optic pathway glioma
OSA	obstructive sleep apnoea
OT	occupational therapist
OXC	oxcarbazepine
P2	pulmonary component of the second heart sound
P-A	posterior anterior
$paCO_2$	partial pressure carbon dioxide, arterial
PADP	program of aids to disabled people

PAH	pulmonary arterial hypertension
PAIS	partial androgen insensitivity
pANCAs	perinuclear antineutrophil cytoplasmic antibodies
PAPVD	partial anomalous pulmonary venous drainage
PAPVR	partial anomalous pulmonary venous return
PB	phenobarbitone
PBAC	Pharmaceutical Benefits Advisory Committee
PBID	paucity of bile interlobular ducts
PBM	peak bone mass
PBS	Pharmaceutical Benefits Scheme
PCC	Prothrombin complex concentrate
PCDAI	paediatric Crohn's disease activity index
PCF	peak cough flow
PCM	protein calorie malnutrition
PCO	polycystic ovary syndrome
PCR	polymerase chain reaction
PDA	patent ductus arteriosus
PDD-NOS	pervasive developmental disorder not otherwise specified
PDDST	Pervasive Developmental Disorders Screening Test
PDHD	pyruvate dehydrogenase deficiency
PDL	pulsed dye laser
PEDS	Parents' Evaluation of Developmental Status
PedsQL	Pediatric Quality of Life Inventory Generic Core Scales
PEEP	positive end expiratory pressure
PEF	peak expiratory flow
PEFR	peak expiratory flow rate
PEG	percutaneous endoscopic gastrostomy *and/or* poly ethylene glycol
PELD	Pediatric End-stage Liver Disease
PEP	positive expiratory pressure
PERT	pancreatic enzyme replacement therapy
PET	pre-emptive transplantation *and/or* positron emission tomography
PFE	pulmonary fat embolism
PFIC	progressive familial intrahepatic cholestasis disorders
PFTs	pulmonary function tests
PGD	preimplantation genetic diagnosis
PGE	primary generalised epilepsy
PGH	preimplantation genetic haplotyping
PHPT	pseudohypoparathyroidism
PHT	phenytoin *and/or* pulmonary hypertension
PI	protease inhibitor *and/or* pancreatic insufficiency
PID	proportional-integrative-derivative (algorithm)
PIH	pyridoxal isonicotinoyl hydrazone
PIP	peak inspiratory pressure
PK	pharmacokinetic
PKDTS	polycystic kidney disease, infantile, severe, with TSC
PKU	phenylketonuria
PKWS	Parkes-Weber syndrome
PLE	protein-losing enteropathy

PLMD	periodic limb movement disorder
PMA	postmenstrual age
pMDI	pressurised metered-dose inhaler
PME	progressive myoclonic epilepsies
PML	progressive multifocal leukoencephalopathy
PND	prenatal diagnosis
PNF	primary non-function
PPS	peripheral pulmonary arterial stenosis
PPV23	polysaccharide pneumococcal vaccine
PR	per rectum
PRA	plasma rennin activity
PS	pancreatic sufficiency *and/or* pulmonary (valve) stenosis
PSG	polysomnography
PT	prothrombin time *and/or* physiotherapist
PTC	percutaneous transhepatic cholangiography
PTH	parathyroid hormone
PTLD	posttransplant lymphoproliferative disorder/disease
PTSD	posttraumatic stress disorder
PUVA	psoralen plus ultraviolet light
PVH	periventricular haemorrhage
PVL	periventricular leukomalacia
PW	Prader–Willi
PWB	port wine birthmark
PWS	Prader–Willi syndrome *and/or* port wine stain
QEEG	quantitative EEG
QTc	corrected QT interval
RACP	Royal Australasian College of Physicians
RAS	renin angiotensin system
RAST	radioallergosorbent test
RBBB	right bundle branch block
RBC	red blood cell
RCDP	rhizomelic chondrodysplasia punctate
RCPCH	Royal College of Paediatrics and Child Health
RCT	randomised controlled trial
RDA	recommended daily allowance
R-DPSDQ	revised Denver pre-screening developmental questionnaire
REM	rapid eye movement
RF	radiofrequency *and/or* rheumatoid factor
rFIX	recombinant factor 9
fFVIII	recombinant factor 8
rhDNase 1	dornase alfa (recombinant human deoxyribonuclease 1)
rhGH	recombinant human growth hormone
r-HuEPO	recombinant human erythropoietin
RLD	restrictive lung disease
RLS	restless legs syndrome
RNA	ribonucleic acid
ROP	retinopathy of prematurity
RRT	renal replacement therapy
RSV	respiratory syncytial virus
RSV-Ig	RSV intravenous immune globulin

RTA	renal tubular acidosis
RTx	renal transplantation
RV	right ventricle
RVF	right ventricular failure
RVG	radionuclide ventriculography
RVH	right ventricular hypertrophy
RVOTO	right ventricular outflow tract obstruction
Rx	treatment
S1	first heart sound
S2	second heart sound
S3	third heart sound
S4	fourth heart sound
SABA	short-acting beta-2 adrenoreceptor agonist
SaO_2	oxygen saturation
SAP	serum alkaline phosphatase
SBBOG	small bowel bacterial overgrowth
SBDS	Shwachman–Bodian–Diamond syndrome
SBE	subacute bacterial endocarditis *and/or* small bowel enteroclysis
SBFT	small bowel follow through
SBS	short bowel syndrome
SBVCE	small bowel video-capsule endoscopy
SC	subcutaneous
SCA	sickle cell anaemia *and/or* spinocerebellar ataxia, AD
SCAIP	single-condition amplification internal primer sequencing
SCAR	spinocerebellar ataxia, AR
SCD	sickle cell disease *and/or* sudden cardiac death
SCFE	slipped capital femoral epiphysis
SCN	sodium channel
SCQ	social communication questionnaire
SCT	stem cell transplantation
SDB	sleep disordered breathing
SDR	selective dorsal rhizotomy
SDS	Shwachman–Diamond syndrome *and/or* standard deviation score
SE	status epilepticus
SEGA	subependymal giant cell astrocytoma (aka SGCT)
SEMLS	single-event multilevel surgery
SEN	subependymal nodules
SGA	small for gestational age
SGCT	subependymal giant cell astrocytoma (aka SEGA)
SGD	speech-generating devices
SHL	standard half-life
SI	sacroiliac
SIADH	syndrome of inappropriate antidiuretic hormone secretion
SIDS	sudden infant death syndrome
SLD	specific learning difficulties
SLE	systemic lupus erythematosus
SMA	spinal muscular atrophy
SMCP	submucosal cleft palate
SMEB	severe myoclonic epilepsy borderline

SMEI	severe myoclonic epilepsy in infancy (Dravet syndrome)
SMO	supramalleolar orthosis
SOD	septo-optic dysplasia *and/or* superoxide dismutase
SOJIA	systemic onset juvenile idiopathic arthritis
SPAX	spinocerebellar ataxia with prominent spasticity
SPECT	single-photon emission computed tomography
sPLA2	secretory phospho-lipase A2
SQUID	superconducting quantum interference device
SRY	sex-determining region on the Y chromosome
SSPE	subacute sclerosing panencephalitis
SSRI	selective serotonin reuptake inhibitor
ST	speech therapist
STAR	steroidogenic acute regulatory protein
STE	speckle tracking echocardiography
SUNDS	sudden unexpected nocturnal death syndrome
SVAS	supravalvular aortic stenosis
SVC	superior vena cava
SVT	supraventricular tachycardia
SWD	sphenoid wing dysplasia
SWS	Sturge-Weber syndrome
SX	salmeterol xinafoate
T1DM	type 1 diabetes mellitus
TAB	tiagabine
TAC	tacrolimus (aka TRL) *and/or* tolerisation advisory committee
TAM	transient abnormal myelopoiesis
TAND	TSC-associated neuropsychiatric disorder
TAPVD	total anomalous pulmonary venous drainage
TAR	thrombocytopenia absent radius syndrome
TB	tuberculosis
TBI	total body irradiation *and/or* traumatic brain injury
Tc-99m	technetium-99m
TCA	tricyclic antidepressant
TCD	transcranial Doppler
TDI	tissue Doppler imaging
TdP	torsades de pointes (twisting of points)
TED	thyroid eye disease
TEV	talipes equinovarus
TGA	transposition of the great arteries
TIBC	total iron-binding capacity
TIPSS	transjugular intrahepatic portosystemic stent shunt
TL	transient leukaemia
TLE	temporal lobe epilepsy
TMD	transient myeloproliferative disease
TMJ	temporomandibular joint
TMP-SMX	trimethoprim with sulfamethoxazole
TNF	tumour necrosis factor
TNF-α	tumour necrosis factor alpha
TOF	tetralogy of Fallot *and/or* tracheo-oesophageal fistula
TORCH	toxoplasmosis, other (syphilis), rubella, CMV, HSV/HVZ
TPM	topiramate

TPMT	thiopurine methyltransferase
TPN	total parenteral nutrition
TRF	teacher report form
TRJV	tricuspid regurgitant jet velocity
TRL	tacrolimus
TS	Turner syndrome *and/or* tuberous sclerosis
TSC	tuberous sclerosis complex
TSH	thyroid stimulating hormone
tTG	tissue transglutaminase
UAC	umbilical arterial catheter
UACR	urine albumin:creatinine ratio
UC	ulcerative colitis
UCB	umbilical cord blood
UCBT	umbilical cord blood transplantation
UMN	upper motor neurone
UMOD	uromodulin (gene)
UPPP	uvulopharyngopalatoplasty
URSO	ursodeoxycholic acid
URTI	upper respiratory tract infection
US	upper segment *and/or* United States of America
UTI	urinary tract infection
VA	ventriculoatrial
VACTERL	vertebral, anal, cardiac, tracheo-esophageal, renal, limb (anomalies)
VBT	vigabatrin (one of two widely used abbreviations; the other is VGB)
VCFS	velocardiofacial syndrome
VCR	vincristine
VER	visual evoked response
VF	ventricular fibrillation
VGB	vigabatrin (preferred abbreviation)
VLCFAs	very long chain fatty acids
VNS	vagal nerve stimulation
VNTR	variable number of tandem nucleotide repeats
VOC	vaso-occlusive crises
VOCA	voice output communication aids
VOE	vaso-occlusive pain events
VP	ventriculoperitoneal
VPA	valproate
VPI	velopharyngeal incompetence
VSD	ventricular septal defect
VT	ventricular tachycardia
VUR	vesicoureteric reflux
vWF	von Willebrand's factor
WAGR	Wilms, aniridia, genital (anomalies), retardation syndrome
WBSCR	Williams–Beuren syndrome critical region
WD	Wilson disease
WFH	World Federation of Hemophilia
WGA	whole gene amplification
WHO	World Health Organization

WHtR	waist-to-height ratio
WISC-R	Wechsler Intelligence Scale for Children—revised
WPPSI	Wechsler preschool and primary scale of intelligence
WPW	Wolff–Parkinson–White syndrome
WS	Williams syndrome
Wt	weight
XRT	radiotherapy
YSR	youth self-report
ZNS	zonisamide

Introduction

This book is designed primarily to assist candidates in passing clinical examinations in paediatrics, particularly at the postgraduate level. The first edition was found helpful in many countries with many different clinical examination scenarios, although it was specifically designed to tackle the clinical section of the FRACP Part 1 Examination in Paediatrics and the MRCP (now the MRCPCH) Part 2 Examination. Written examinations, which must be passed in most countries before any clinical examination can be sat, are not covered other than in the brief outline given below.

Basic training requirements

Most potential candidates should be familiar with these. Comprehensive information on training can be downloaded from the websites of the various learned colleges. For Australia, New Zealand, the United Kingdom and Canada, the relevant addresses are as follows:

- Fellowship in the Royal Australasian College of Physicians (FRACP): http://www.racp.edu.au
- Membership of the Royal College of Paediatrics and Child Health (MRCPCH): http://www.rcpch.ac.uk
- Fellowship of the Royal College of Physicians and Surgeons of Canada (FRCPSC): http://www.royalcollege.ca

The written examination

The written examination for the FRACP can be sat once a minimum of 24 months of basic training has been completed successfully. The College is changing to computer-based testing (CBT) for the divisional written examination from 2018, replacing the previous paper and pencil format.

The written examination comprises a medical sciences paper (70 questions, of which four are extended matching questions [EMQs], while 66 are one-correct answer multiple-choice questions), and a clinical applications paper (100 questions, of which eight are EMQs while 92 are one-correct multiple-choice questions). The pass mark is not set for the written examination until after the papers have been marked, each year.

The best preparation for any written examination involves doing as many past examination questions as possible, and extensive reading of major texts and journals. The most useful textbooks and journals are listed under Suggested reading at the end of the book. There are no set curricula specified for most paediatric examinations.

The college regularly releases previous examination papers. These are essential reading. There are also a number of papers that are composites of remembered questions that previous candidates have written down after their examination, which have been 'handed down' over the years. The main problem with 'remembered' papers is their inaccuracy. However, most candidates seem to find these helpful.

The RACP produces self-assessment questions for paediatricians, the Australian Self-Assessment Programme (ASAP), which are strongly recommended.

Generally, books of multiple-choice questions available in any medical bookshop are of much less value.

Remember, repeated practising of multiple-choice questions is the most valuable preparation.

The clinical examination

This book is aimed at assisting in preparing for clinical examinations. Chapter 1 details a general approach. It will be noted that certain cases are emphasised, not because they are more important than others but because they are good examples of the complicated material required for long and short cases.

The mini-clinical evaluation exercise (mini-CEX)

This is used by the RACP as a formative assessment tool to evaluate trainees in real-life medical settings, in their normal working environment, as part of the Physician Readiness for Expert Practice (PREP) Program. A variety of environments should be evaluated during the trainee's basic training, not just one favoured hospital department. Skills assessed include history taking, communication skills, physical examination and management strategies. A mini-CEX is not unlike a hybrid long case/short case, so becoming proficient at these will assist trainees in handling short and long cases. Trainees receive valuable feedback to assist their learning, although the mini-CEX does not contribute to decisions regarding eligibility for progression through the PREP programme. Trainees are rated in the following areas as listed on the mini-CEX evaluation sheet: medical interviewing skills; physical examination skills; professional qualities/communication; counselling skills; clinical judgment; and organisation/efficiency. The trainee is responsible for organising their own mini-CEX encounters. Each of these assessments should focus on a few specified competencies. Each case should take around 15–20 minutes, immediately followed by feedback from the assessor, with this feedback being the most useful component of the mini-CEX process. For more information, trainees should go to http://www.racp.edu.au or http://www.racp.org.nz

Achievement psychology: the psychology of passing

Chapter 4 discusses the psychological aspects of the preparation for, and performance in, the examination. This is a very important area that should not be overlooked.

Chapter 1

Approach to the Examination

Positive mindset

All paediatric clinical examinations test the following aspects:

1. Clinical skills—history taking, physical examination, interpretation of findings, construction of a diagnosis or differential diagnoses, method of investigation, overall management of the patient.
2. Attitudes.
3. Interpersonal relationships.

Candidates invited to postgraduate clinical examinations have usually satisfied their relevant learned college regarding their factual knowledge. Consequently, their factual knowledge should be at a standard appropriate for making management decisions in the case being examined.

Clinical skills are usually taught adequately to most candidates at the hospitals where they were trained. However, little if any attention is paid to developing proper attitudes and interpersonal relationship skills. Advertisers and sales representatives know the importance of personal contact. They realise that appearance, personality and speech are crucial in successful negotiations. The 'viva' is very similar in that candidates have to 'sell' themselves and their knowledge to the examiners. Successful candidates usually possess certain characteristics, namely:

1. A positive, confident response to personal confrontation. People with strong personalities have little trouble, but those who are easily embarrassed and shy away from confrontation between equals may do poorly. This response can be changed by the methods described in this book.
2. Ability to sort out relevant from irrelevant information. Those who 'think', ask questions, seek explanations and try to understand rather than learn by rote do well.
3. Familiarity with the method of examination.
4. Endurance. Candidates who are 'streetwise' and naturally confident tend to have little difficulty, whereas their less confident colleagues are left to learn the hard way and eventually succeed or fail.

Preparation for the 'viva' requires effective communication skills during physical confrontation. Attitudes, interpersonal skills and projection of a confident, professional consultant image can be learned and developed.

Techniques include:
- Mental rehearsal, visualisation, affirmations (see Chapter 4, Achievement psychology).
- Body language.
- Eye contact.
- Breath control.
- Dress sense.
- Speech training.
- Development of equanimity.
- Ability to summarise.
- Reasoning skills.
- Examiner assessment.

Body language

Non-verbal communication in the form of a person's gestures is a very accurate indicator of his or her attitudes, emotions, thoughts and desires.

In order to learn body language, set aside a couple of minutes a day to study and read other people's gestures. Examine your own body language. Copy the body language of people you admire and respect, such as a consultant who you feel would have no difficulty passing the clinical examination. The model you choose does not necessarily have to be a real person: he or she may be a composite of ideal body language.

There is an old saying: 'If you would be powerful, pretend to be powerful'. One way to adopt an attitude that helps you achieve any objective is to act 'as if' you were already there. If you change your posture, your breathing patterns, your muscle tension, your tone of voice, you instantly change the way you feel. For example, if you feel depressed, consciously stand up straight, throw your shoulders back, breathe deeply and look upward. See if you can feel depressed in that posture. You'll find yourself feeling alert, vital and confident.

An important component of body language is consistency. If you are giving what you think is a positive message, but your voice is weak, high-pitched and tentative and your gestures reveal poor self-confidence, you will be unconvincing and ineffective. Individuals who consistently succeed are those who can commit all of their resources, mental and physical, towards reaching a goal.

One way to develop consistency is to model yourself on individuals who are consistent. Copy the way they stand, sit and move, their key facial expressions and gestures, their tone of voice, their vocabulary, their breathing patterns and so on. You will begin to generate the same attitudes that they experience, and experience the same successful results. Effectiveness comes from delivering one unified message.

When you next attend a place where people meet and interact, study the individuals who have adopted the gestures and postures of the individuals with whom they are talking. This mimicry is how one individual tells another that he or she is in agreement with their thoughts and attitudes. You can use this unconscious mimicry to your advantage. One of the best ways of establishing effective personal communication is through mimicking the breathing patterns, posture, tone of voice, gestures, words and phrases of the person or people with whom you are interacting. Once you establish contact with someone, you create a bond and reach a stage where you begin to initiate change rather than just mimicking the other person, a stage where you have established so much mutual contact that when you change, the other person unconsciously follows you. If, when you try to lead someone, he or she does not follow, it simply means there is insufficient rapport. Mimic, strengthen the mutual contact and try again.

Eye contact

When answering questions or making a point, look the examiner straight in the eye. Powerful individuals have always been characterised by exceptional eyes. If you have difficulty maintaining eye contact, there are a few techniques you can use to develop a more effective gaze.

Work on not blinking. Practise unblinking eye contact, especially when under pressure. If you are intimidated and unable to look directly into the examiner's eyes, a little trick is to concentrate your gaze on a point midway between the examiner's eyes. Another helpful hint is to imagine a triangle on the examiner's forehead, with the apex at the highest point and the base of the triangle formed by an imaginary line between both eyes. Keep your gaze directed at this area. In the mirror, practise narrowing your lids a bit but do not squint. When you move your eyes from one point to another (as from one examiner to another), do it without blinking. When you look from one person to another without blinking, it is unnerving for anyone watching you. To further emphasise this powerful gaze, move your eyes first without blinking and then follow with your head movement just behind the eye movement. Slightly lowering your head forwards while maintaining the gaze also adds power to the eye movement.

Breath control

Often, especially in a 'viva' voce or an important interview, you find yourself struck by a sudden panic attack. Breath control can be particularly useful to regain composure, prevent fear, reduce stress or fatigue, and generate energy. It is a technique developed by the samurai to regain control during life and death struggles. Take a deep breath, then exhale slowly and imperceptibly. As you are exhaling, contract your abdominal muscles so that you feel as though you are tightening a corset. Relax the muscles at the end of exhalation. Do not expel all the air. Leave about 20% in the lungs. Then inhale gently. Your lips should be slightly parted, expelling your breath over your lower teeth with your tongue gently touching your hard palate. You may repeat breath control as often as required. Practise breath control until it is second nature and then use it whenever you are under any physical or mental stress.

Dress and grooming

You have to 'sell' yourself and your knowledge. Your appearance is your most important 'equipment' for the clinical examination. It must reflect the public expectations of the professional person. Look around at what is worn by successful individuals in the respected professions (such as your examiners). Ask yourself: 'Do I look like a mature, careful, conservative and respected junior consultant?'

Male candidates should avoid colourful suits, jackets and trousers, and unusual ties. Dark suits (greys, navy blue, pin-stripes, non-committal ties, red ties) are more suitable (this is termed 'power dressing' by image consultants). Female candidates should preferably avoid revealing or tight dresses as well as showy jewellery. Footwear should be clean and appropriate.

Long hair and beards should probably be avoided, but if you cannot bear to shave your beard, at least keep it neat and trimmed. It is safer to be clean-shaven and have tidy hair. Visit the hairdresser a couple of days before (and not on the day of) the clinical examination so that it does not appear as though you have had it done just for the examination.

If you have difficulties with perspiration when under pressure, use an unscented antiperspirant on the day of the examination. Apply the antiperspirant to your forehead, hairline and neck to prevent beads of sweat appearing during the 'viva' (one of the previous co-authors used this method successfully).

Speech training

Poor speech will definitely adversely affect your 'viva' performance and is surprisingly common. By poor speech we mean poor diction, inaudible voice and bad vocabulary. Record yourself speaking, using your mobile phone or a digital recorder, or have someone sit about 2 metres from you and listen to you speak. Then note:

1. Whether or not every word was heard clearly.
2. Whether or not what you said was understood.
3. Whether or not you used jargon, slang or abbreviations.

Addressing these three points will help you assess whether or not your speech is a problem. Take note of the pitch and rapidity of your speech. If you do speak too quickly, make a conscious effort to slow down by reading aloud at a pace that allows a listener to make a note of the content of your speech. Another useful exercise is to study the speech of newsreaders. Note that they speak clearly, concisely and slowly so that every word is understood. They also use very little jargon, slang or abbreviations. Try mimicking a newsreader's speaking style the next time you present a case.

Other methods of improving your speech are:

1. Enrolment with a professional teacher.
2. Using your mobile phone video camera to film your efforts and then playing back the result.

Equanimity

Sir William Osler suggested that physicians should possess equanimity: composure under pressure, and when faced with the adversities of life. This is particularly true during the clinical examination, where your long case may be an uncooperative, crying child, for example. Candidates may experience stress as a result of physical confrontation, inadequate knowledge, low self-confidence and poor physical health. Equanimity, although coming more easily to phlegmatic personalities, may be cultivated. Knowledge and experience create confidence, which in turn leads to calmness.

The above causes of stress can all be overcome by more study (to improve knowledge base), more practice, mental reprogramming and then actively seeking out stressful situations to increase experience. Adequate exercise, a well-balanced diet and enough sleep should go a long way towards maintaining physical health.

Ability to summarise

The ability to summarise, encapsulate the essence and emphasise the major issues without losing too much detail requires understanding and experience. However, it is a necessary skill for the physician, and therefore needs to be developed through practice. Remember: practice makes the impossible possible. Note that the limit of effective retention of verbal information is usually less than 15 seconds, so the better you can convey the essential details to the examiners in the 'viva', the greater the effect.

Reasoning skills

Reasoning skills involve the ability to analyse a problem rapidly, break it down into manageable parts and then formulate a solution. An adequate knowledge base, experience and rational thinking are needed.

To assist in developing these skills, make a habit of meticulously examining every detail of a child's clinical records. Analyse the data, learn to pick out any vital information that is missing and ignore irrelevant information. Deduce from available data what other information you need to justify your conclusions.

Assessment of examiner

An ancient Chinese general, Sun Tze, once stated, 'Know the enemy and know yourself, and you can fight a hundred battles with no danger of defeat'. Although examiners are not exactly the enemy, you still need to assess:

1. Whether or not the examiner is friendly or unhelpful.
2. The quality of communication between the examiner and yourself.
3. The strength of the examiner's personality compared to yours.

The clinical examination
Preparation

The road to success in any 'viva' usually entails doing a large number of long and short cases. You need to begin seeing cases at least several months before the clinical examination. Your service commitment should provide you with all the material you require for training and preparation. Treat each patient you see during the course of your daily work as a practice long or short case. Endeavour to do at least one (but preferably two or three) long case(s) per week. Try to expose yourself to as many different examiners as possible.

Preparation for the short case requires much practice, especially when more candidates fail their short cases than their long cases. If possible, visit other hospitals, especially if these have a reputation for teaching. Experience as a 'bulldog' (i.e. observing an actual examination and assisting the candidate) is also invaluable in gaining insight about the conduct of the examination and the expectations of the examiners. Taking turns as an examiner during practice sessions with your colleagues is worthwhile because it allows you to experience first-hand the annoying habits of candidates. Mental rehearsal of short cases (and long cases) will accelerate learning (see Chapter 4, Achievement psychology).

Most major teaching hospitals hold trial and mock examinations a few weeks before the actual 'viva'. These simulated examinations provide invaluable feedback about your progress.

Part of your preparation involves obtaining all the relevant information from the appropriate learned college about the requirements for paediatric training; this is invariably available in booklet form or is downloadable from the college's website. Familiarise yourself well with the contents and study the regulations. About 6 months before the examination, apply to the college for an application form. Fill in your application form a few months before the examination and ensure that the form and your examination fee reach the college before the closing date. Remember to apply for examination leave from your employer.

If possible, in the last few weeks before the 'viva', do some reconnaissance work and locate the examination venue as far as you can. Check it out in relation to where you will be staying, ascertain the suitable modes of transport, public transport timetables and the length of time it will take to travel to the venue at the times scheduled for the examinations. Remember to check your accommodation arrangements in advance.

In the week before the examination, check the clothing you intend to wear (make sure it fits!), check that you have the right equipment and remember the appointment with the hairdresser. In the few days before the examination, try to get some mental rest and leave study aside. Avoid any major changes in your daily routine and lifestyle.

A checklist (prepared in advance) of what you need to do on the day may be helpful. Make sure you arrive at least 30 minutes before the examination is due to start, so that you can recover from the trip, relax, go to the bathroom and so on. The longer the travelling distance, the more provision you need to make to cover delays during travel (one of the previous co-authors experienced car trouble on the day of the 'viva').

There are certain 'rules' that you need to obey at the 'viva'. Do not enter the examiner's room until asked. Do not sit down until invited. Do not slouch when seated but sit four-square and upright (it creates the impression that you mean what you say). Minimise nervous hand movements. If you tend to fidget, turn your hand movements into gestures. Bags should be placed under the chair (or given to the 'bulldog', or Examination Assistant) and removed when leaving. Do not stare, smile politely and always answer courteously. Remember to speak up and be as brief and factual as possible.

Avoid jargon, slang, clichés, abbreviations, brand names (of medications), meaningless expressions, and rising inflections at the end of sentences. Most importantly, do not antagonise or argue with the examiners. You will always lose! Some examples of antagonising behaviour include patronising answers, appearing to show little or no interest in the subject matter and a negative response to criticism.

If you decide to use beta-blockers during the examination, it would be wise to use the drug during at least one practice session, particularly if you have asthma. It would be inconvenient to have an asthma attack at the examination, as happened to a colleague who took a cardioselective beta-blocker. After 12 puffs or so of salbutamol, he passed.

Equipment

Candidates have to bring their own stationery and their own equipment to the examination. It would be wise to take the following with you:

1. Pens (more than one and make sure they work), pencils and blank paper/cards; proformas and templates are not permitted.
2. Watch, preferably with a sweeping second hand.
3. Your own stethoscope (and not electronically augmented, except with permission).
4. A handheld eye chart for testing visual acuity (with a piece of string attached to the chart, the length of which is the recommended distance from eye to chart; this allows you to quickly position the chart at the correct distance from eye).
5. A red-topped hat pin for visual field testing in the older child.
6. Standard handheld ophthalmoscope (not a pan-ophthalmoscope).
7. Pocket torch with new batteries and bulb.
8. Standard auroscope.
9. Tuning fork.
10. Tendon hammer.
11. Cotton wool (for fine sensation).
12. Single-use neurological examination pins (for testing sensation).
13. Pocket tape measure (for head circumference, and measuring sizes of liver, leg etc.).
14. Toys for developmental assessment: red woollen ball on a thread to test visual fields in infants; small container of hundreds and thousands (or equivalent) to test

hearing; raisins (pincer grip); coloured cubes for stacking; other equipment for developmental assessment.

15. Standard growth charts.

Candidates must not bring mobile phones, tablets or other data-storing or recording devices. Taking in unauthorised material can lead to disqualification from the examination. Any candidate found with a mobile phone or other recording device automatically fails.

Chapter 2

The Long Case

Most candidates have a small leather briefcase (or equivalent carrying bag) for their equipment. Be absolutely familiar with the equipment you have in your bag. Nothing looks worse than a candidate fumbling through his or her bag or, worse still, his or her pockets at the vital moment.

On the day of the examination, in Australia, there are two long cases, one in the morning cycle and one in the afternoon cycle, and the candidate is examined by two sets of examiners. For each long case, the candidate is given 60 minutes with the patient and parent(s); then 10 minutes organising the case, and finally 25 minutes with the examiners. The candidate must take a full history, perform a relevant physical examination and synthesise a management plan that is sensible and appropriate for the particular child. The examiners will not interrupt the presentation of the history and examination findings unless there is, exceptionally, a specific key point that requires clarification. The entire presentation should take between 10 and 12 minutes, generally 7–8 minutes presenting the history, 2–3 minutes presenting the physical examination then 1 minute for a summary, before launching into management. Practice is the key to success.

Practising long cases is extremely beneficial for improving your clinical skills, irrespective of the examination looming in the distance. Practice cases should be performed under examination conditions whenever possible. Most consultant paediatricians are quite willing to spare 20–30 minutes to listen to candidates presenting cases. Advanced trainees who have recently passed are also usually prepared to act as examiners for candidates.

Obtaining the history

The aim of the long case is chiefly to assess how you would manage the child, his/her problems and his/her family. The examiners want to know whether or not you can competently care for a patient in practice. The history in the majority of cases will provide you with the diagnoses.

You must allocate your time with care. Generally, 20 minutes should be spent on the history, 10–15 minutes on the physical examination and the remainder of the time on recording, reviewing and organising the information for presentation. This time spent on organisation is the most important.

Making notes is vital. Two commonly used methods are:
1. Using a small spiral-bound pad.
2. Using a small card system: numbering the cards, and using headings such as 'examination findings'.

Remember to keep to the essentials and to include the following:
- Identification of the child's details—age, date of birth, home address.
- Identification of the clinical problem(s).
- Specific inquiry of system involvement.
- Relevant past medical history: include birth history, immunisation history.
- Present treatment.
- Growth and development.
- Social history: always ask about parental relationships, number of children, family income, financial support, other siblings' reactions to the patient's illness, schooling.

Always introduce yourself to the child and parent(s). Always be courteous, diplomatic and tactful, use basic English and never order them about. Explain to the parent(s) that this is a very important examination.

The following questions have been found useful by many candidates:
1. What exactly is wrong with your child?
2. Is your child an inpatient at the moment?
3. What are the names of the doctors taking care of your child?
4. What tests have been done on your child? Have any new tests been done lately? How often do you come for review? How many times has your child been admitted?
5. What treatment is your child on? Have there been any recent changes in your child's treatment?
6. What is worrying you the most?
7. What is worrying the doctors the most?
8. What is worrying the child the most?
9. What complications of treatment are there?
10. What of the future? For the family? For the patient?
11. Is there anything that someone else has done or asked that I haven't done or asked?

Remember, do not accept the patient's history without questioning.

Make a list of all the important problems and then organise this list so that the most important or current issue is presented first, followed by the other problems in decreasing order of importance.

Physical examination

Remember to keep to essentials and look at the front, back and both sides. Ask the parent(s) what the examiners looked for when they examined the child. A detailed examination should be done of those regions related to the child's main complaint. Following the specific examination, other systems need to be assessed. Remember to assess growth parameters, vital signs including blood pressure, oral cavity and the skin.

Preparation to meet the examiners

After completing the history and examination, always ask yourself: 'Have I left anything out?' and 'Can this be anything else?'

Study your notes thoughtfully, underline or highlight positive findings and 'box' all relevant negative findings. This is the information you will present to the examiners.

Ask yourself whether the case is mainly a management or a diagnostic problem. If it is a diagnostic problem, remember that 'common things occur commonly'. If more than half of your findings support your first diagnosis, then it is most likely the correct one. For your alternative diagnoses, take the main positive findings and have three possible diagnoses for each. Make a summary of the possible diagnoses that occur three or more times.

Create an introduction that is clear, concise, arouses interest and summarises the main problems. It should last no longer than 30 seconds. Remember: first impressions are important, so spend time mentally rehearsing the delivery of your introduction. (See below for a long-case proforma.)

Mentally rehearse your order of presentation; present the most important issues first. Keep some issues in reserve so that when the examiners ask you about them, you will be able to provide immediate answers, rather than laying all your cards on the table immediately. Your conclusion should re-emphasise the main problems in order of decreasing importance. The entire presentation of the history should last no longer than 7–8 minutes.

Try to anticipate possible lines of questioning, and think up reasonable answers in advance. Common questions asked by examiners include:

- 'Tell me about your patient'. You should be able to give a clear, concise presentation lasting less than 10–12 minutes.
- 'What is your conclusion about this case?' You should respond by giving a most likely diagnosis and differential diagnoses. Avoid giving an over-comprehensive list of differential diagnoses.
- 'How would you manage this patient?' You should prepare an outline of management and be able to support it. You are probably going to be asked about relevant investigations. You should have reasons for doing each test and be able to discuss the test in detail. Write down any test results given and comment on their significance.

Assume that the examiners are there to help you. If an examiner continues to ask a question even though you do not immediately know the answer, he or she may be attempting to establish a very basic fact. Try to step back mentally for a moment; the answer is often forthcoming. Do not waffle. If you do not know the answer to a question, do not be afraid to admit it, but do so confidently. This allows the examiner to change the line of questioning and, hopefully, ask you a question that you *can* answer. Always be prepared to justify any statement you make in the 'viva'.

A long-case proforma

Although proformas cannot be taken into the examination, it is very useful to have a standard commencement to a long-case presentation that is second nature to you. It is suggested that you may use proformas in practice cases; the author used the proforma below successfully with each and every long case.

Opening statement

'I have just seen [name of child], a [age in months or years] old boy/girl with a [duration of time] history of [presenting complaint], who is currently in hospital for [reason for being in hospital that day]. [Name of child]'s problems include [list of each diagnosis in order of importance, or in the case of a multi-system disease, each aspect as it arose in chronological order]. I shall discuss the history of each problem in this order.'

Details and history

Next, the presenting complaint is set out in detail.

Then, for each problem listed in the opening statement, make four columns, with the headings *Dates (or age of child)*, *Past history*, *Current status*, *Recent changes*. The history is listed in chronological order under each heading. For example, if the problem was nephrotic syndrome it could be listed as in Table 2.1.

Remaining history

When you have completed the problem-listing sheets, remember to ask the parent supplying the history, 'What did the examiners ask you?' Then the rest of the history can be obtained. The prompts given in Table 2.2 may help.

Table 2.1

Details of problem list

DATES (OR AGE OF CHILD)	PAST HISTORY	CURRENT STATUS	RECENT CHANGES
12 months	Presented with generalised oedema		
16 months	Renal biopsy diagnosed MCGN, started cyclophosphamide		
24 months	Moved interstate and weaned off prednisolone		
2 years 3 months	Changed hospitals and management reintroduced steroids		
4 years	Prednisolone stopped		
4 years 3 months	Admitted with oedema		
Present		On alternate day prednisolone	Reintroduction of steroids after representation with oedema

Table 2.2

Remaining history details

BIRTH HISTORY

Date of birth _____/Birth weight _____/Hospital _____

Pregnancy: Drugs _____/Bleeding _____/Illnesses _____

Hyper/hypotension _____/Hospitalisations _____

Ultrasounds _____/Other tests _____

Polyhydramnios: _____/Fetal movements: _____

Planned? _____/Gestation _____/Delivery method _____

Apgar scores _____ at 1 minute _____ at 5 minutes

PERINATAL HISTORY

Respiratory distress _____/Oxygen requirement _____

Feeding: Breast _____/Bottle _____/Tube _____

Jaundice _____/Weight gain _____/Other problems _____

Discharge date/age _____/Discharge weight _____

Continued

Table 2.2 (continued)

FEEDING HISTORY

Currently _____/Breast/bottle: until _____/Solids: since _____

Past feeding history _____

MILESTONES

Good baby? _____/Hearing _____/Smiled _____

Compared to sibs _____/Sat _____/Sleeping behaviour _____/Crawled _____/

Feeding self _____/Walking _____

Toilet trained _____/Talking: Single words _____ Sentences _____

School compared to sibs _____/Vision _____

Current developmental abilities/problems:

Vision _____/Hearing _____/Gross motor _____

Fine motor _____/Language _____/Personal social _____

FAMILY HISTORY

Mother: Name _____ Age _____ Job _____ Health _____

Father: Name _____ Age _____ Job _____ Health _____

Note any consanguinity _____/Planning any more children? _____

Relevant family history _____/Other diseases in family _____

Previous marriages _____

Past pregnancies: Terminations _____/Miscarriages _____

Children who have died _____

Family interactions _____/Family supports _____

Family's understanding of disease: Mother/Father/Sibs _____

SOCIAL HISTORY (CAN BE THE MOST IMPORTANT)

Financial status _____/Private health insurance _____

Home _____/Car _____/Allowances _____

Family supports _____/Other supports _____

Societies _____/Magazines _____

How long in Australia? _____

SCHOOL HISTORY

School attended _____/Grade _____/Performance _____

Subjects _____/Sports _____/Friends _____

Ambitions _____/How much school has been missed? _____

Repeated any grades? _____

Table 2.2 (continued)
PARENTS
Change in social life _____/Parents' friends _____
Last holiday? _____/Respite care? _____
HOME
Any structural changes to cope with the illness? _____
TRANSPORT TO SCHOOL/DOCTOR
Need for special transport _____/Financial burden of transport _____
OTHER PAST HISTORY
Infections _____/Fractures _____
Operations _____/Hospitalisations _____
IMMUNISATION
Up to date? _____/Given on time? _____
Any missed? _____/Adverse reactions? _____
ALLERGIES
Presenting symptoms: Rash _____/Angio-oedema _____/
Anaphylaxis _____ Requirement for adrenaline? _____/MedicAlert bracelet _____
MOST SERIOUS PROBLEM
Mother's opinion _____/Father's opinion _____
Patient's opinion _____/Doctor's opinion _____
PARENTS' UNDERSTANDING OF DISEASE
_____
COMPLIANCE
_____
ALTERNATIVE MEDICINE
_____
SYSTEMS REVIEW
Cardiovascular/Respiratory/Ear, nose, throat/Eyes/Gastrointestinal tract/Central nervous system/Skin/Joints/Endocrine/Renal/Haematological

Continued

Table 2.2 (continued)		
HOME MANAGEMENT		
Medications Side effects Levels Note: List the above under headings: many long-case patients are on multiple drugs.		
OTHER MANAGEMENT		
Physiotherapy _____/Occupational therapy _____		
Speech therapy _____/Other therapy _____		
Daily routine _____		
Clinics attended _____		
Specialists seen regularly (what do they ask/do/examine?) _____		
Local doctor _____		
Paediatrician _____		

Examination

For the examination, it is always best to start with a general description of the patient, as if you were describing a photograph over the telephone. Again using the example of nephrotic syndrome, an opening line could be: 'On examination [name] was a 4-year-old Cushingoid boy, with moon face, a swollen abdomen and a swollen scrotum, with an intravenous line in the left forearm'.

Next, describe the parameters (head circumference, weight, height) and show the examiners the centile chart (which you have of course plotted at high speed). The vital signs (pulse, respiratory rate, blood pressure, temperature and, if relevant to the presentation, urinalysis) may then be given, and then the findings in the organ system most relevant to the child's current clinical problems. Still using the nephrotic syndrome example, this would be similar to the following: 'Examination of the renal system was as follows: periorbital oedema, ascites, tense scrotum, no effusions, Cushingoid features (buffalo hump, loss of supraclavicular fossa), but no striae, cataracts, not short, no acne, no bone pain, no bruising'.

During the examination of the child, ask the parent again, 'What did the examiners look at yesterday?' After the relevant system, examine the other systems too: cardiovascular, chest, abdomen, ear, nose and throat, central nervous system, and where appropriate, developmental assessment.

After the examination findings, present a summary, reiterating the important points. Following this you have the opportunity to discuss the management plan that you, the candidate, would initiate. There are several useful phrases that may help you start this discussion, such as:

- 'As regards management, my main concerns are …', *or*
- 'With respect to [problem], as the paediatrician looking after [patient], I would …', *or*
- 'In the line of investigations, I would …'

Remember to have a list of issues ready to discuss confidently.

The criteria used to assess performance in the long case have five headings (assessment domains): history, examination, synthesis and priorities, impact of illness on patient and family, and management plan. One of the examiners will have already taken the history and examined the patient 'cold', before the first candidate, and presented to their fellow examiners, without seeing any notes or prepared history, such that the circumstances are as close as possible to those the candidate will experience; the examiners know what sort of historian the parent may be, and will have determined the priority list of clinical problems for themselves.

The examiners then spend some 20 minutes reviewing the notes and a prepared long-case summary sheet, which outlines the diagnoses, problems and the examiners' key issues. Also, all examiners will have undergone a calibration session in the weeks before the examination, to ensure consistency and fairness.

Chapter 3

The Short Case

The short-case section of any postgraduate examination covers a number of systems (typically cardiovascular, respiratory, abdomen, neurological), and different countries' learned colleges vary in their approach. In Australia, the individual FRACP short case tends to have a lead-in that is fairly broad (e.g. 'Examine the gait') and a comprehensive examination is expected. Each short-case examination lasts 15 minutes.

On the day of the examination, in Australia, there are four short cases, two in the morning cycle and two in the afternoon cycle, and the candidate is examined by four sets of examiners. There is a 10-minute break between the two short cases in each cycle. For each short case, the candidate is given 15 minutes with the patient. The candidate is supplied with a written introduction on a card that is posted outside the door of the examination room, outlining a short history and indicating the system(s) to be examined, such as 'Ian is a 7-year-old boy who has had increasing trouble climbing stairs over the last 6 months. Please examine his gait'. The candidate has 2 minutes to read this introduction before meeting the patient. The same introduction is used for all candidates. The candidate should perform a relevant physical examination; the examiners are interested in the method of examination, and appropriate interpretation of signs elicited. Practice is the key to success.

In the United Kingdom, the individual MRCPCH short cases tend to have a lead-in that is more directed, so a more focused examination is in order: the examiner may say 'Listen to the heart', and that is what the candidate must do—not pick up the hands, take the pulse and look for clubbing, but get the stethoscope and listen. The short cases here are deliberately set out in the 'comprehensive' approach; it is easy to adapt the relevant portion of the examination to whichever lead-in the examiner gives. A short case tests the candidate's ability to examine a child with the ease and accuracy of a consultant paediatrician, rather than a paediatric registrar, although the examiners are judging the candidate at his or her expected level of training.

A short-case examination should be sufficiently comprehensive for the lead-in given, but directed. It should be confidently performed, quick enough to be within the confines of examination timing, and above all conducted kindly and with consideration for the patient and the parent.

The emphasis is as much on the method of physical examination as on the interpretation of the signs elicited. Remember that the examiners are judging you as a (future) peer. Thus a high standard is mandatory.

Proficiency in short cases, even more so than in long cases, is dependent upon months of practice, preferably on a daily basis, perfecting a coherent approach to every possible clinical problem likely to be presented.

Several examination problems, such as short stature or precocious puberty, require a great deal of clinical material to be covered in 15 minutes, so a well-prepared routine is essential. This book gives an outline of an approach to most of the commonly seen short-case topics.

For several of the short cases outlined, there is an accompanying diagram that visually supplements the content of the text. The author found it easier to remember a diagram than a long list written on a card.

The time allotted to the short-case section varies between countries. Irrespective of the time allocated, it is usual that at least four systems are assessed. Often, the examiners will instruct that you may either talk as you proceed, or examine in silence and summarise at the completion of the examination. Most candidates prefer the former method, as it allows the examiners to see, and hear, how you think, and should a questionable finding be noted, the examiners may guide you at that point.

It is crucial to read carefully the written introduction to the case, which is provided before the candidate meets the patient, to get into the correct frame of mind and plan the appropriate approach. The introduction gives clear instructions as to the approach required. Several points here need emphasising. The introduction has been carefully formulated by the examiners, to be concise and realistic and fairly neutral, without obvious directed diagnostic clues. Do what the introduction instructs. If the request is to perform an abdominal examination, do not start with the hands—start with the abdomen.

In any short case, it is always worthwhile spending at least 20–30 seconds standing back and getting an overall impression of the patient; otherwise, signs such as chest or limb asymmetry, or a recognisable pattern of dysmorphism, may well be overlooked.

It helps to visualise yourself as a consultant before you commence any short case. It may be useful to imagine you are a locum paediatrician, being asked for a second opinion on any child you see. One sign of being stuck in 'registrar mode' is prefacing every potential action with 'I'd like to'. Do not say 'I would now like to look at …'—just do it! You do not see one consultant asking another's permission to proceed during each step of an examination.

However, do not overstep the boundaries of confidence. Do not argue with the examiners under any circumstances. Very rarely you may be right, but you may fail and be thought arrogant. If you become angry with an uncooperative child, you may fail; if you inadvertently hurt a child, such as in a joint examination, you may well fail. If you do not follow the instructions of the provided introduction, you will fail; as one examiner was heard to say (in a mock exam, thankfully): 'Answer the bloody question!'

At the completion of your examination, you may mention further areas that you would examine next, should time permit, and then present a succinct summary of your findings with the most likely diagnosis, followed by a logically presented differential diagnosis. The differential diagnosis need not be exhaustive. In particular, it should never be a rote-learnt list for a certain type of case, but it should be relevant only to the particular child you have just examined.

Be careful that the first diseases you mention are not inappropriate suggestions. For example, an infant with jaundice and a Kasai scar on the abdomen should not be given a diagnosis of metabolic liver disease as the most likely possibility. So, beware of 'automatic list' responses.

Should you see a particularly confusing patient, and you are quite unable to work out their signs, do not bluff. It would be appropriate to admit that you find the signs confusing, but approach this methodically and logically. For example, if a child has a large array of heart murmurs, and the underlying diagnosis is completely unclear, it may be sensible to say, 'This child has complex congenital heart disease, but I am uncertain as to the exact anatomical diagnosis. However, taking each murmur individually …', and proceed to give a differential diagnosis for each murmur, mentioning that an electrocardiogram and a chest X-ray may clarify the diagnostic possibilities. You do not have to get the diagnosis absolutely correct to pass. Conversely, getting the diagnosis correct does not equal passing: if a child has an obvious aortic stenosis, missing neck auscultation for murmur radiation, and giving no thought to assessing the severity of the lesion, will not help you to pass.

Many candidates over the years have had acting lessons and training in elocution to improve their presentation. For many, overcoming mumbling is a major hurdle. A successful solution for some candidates has been to film their performance using their mobile phone or tablet video camera, and then replay this to see how they would appear to the examiners.

An important point in presentation is correct coinage. Do not use terms such as 'I think there perhaps might be a little bit of asymmetry of the chest'; either there is asymmetry, or there is not. Similarly, 'perhaps a tinge cyanosed' is not an appropriate description. You should try to eliminate words of uncertainty from your vocabulary.

As well as avoiding the 'I think perhaps' syndrome, you need to consciously tighten up your description of the patient's signs; for example, 'acyanotic' is far preferable to 'pink', and 'paucity of spontaneous lower limb movement' is preferable to the 'legs aren't moving quite as much as I'd expect them to'. Use the correct medical terminology every time; avoid all colloquialisms.

Do be aware that the examiners themselves have examined the children on the morning of the examination, without the aid of the child's notes and with a similar introduction to the one that the candidates receive. This means that they too have examined the child 'blind', and thus any conflicting or questionable findings can be noted so as to maximise the suitability of the case, and assess whether the lead-in is appropriate.

The most useful form of practice is to be critically assessed by a consultant, and optimally one who is an examiner. Being examined by an advanced trainee who has recently passed is also very beneficial. The most easily accessible form of practice is, of course, with your fellow candidates.

It makes sense to practise at a number of different hospitals and to be exposed to as many different examiners as possible, so as not to become accustomed to one particular pattern of criticism and questioning.

The criteria used to assess performance in the short case have five headings (assessment domains): approach to patient, examination technique, examination accuracy, interpretation of physical findings and discussion of investigations. One of the examiners will have already examined the patient 'cold', before the first candidate, without seeing any prepared notes, such that the circumstances are as close as possible to those the candidate will experience; the examiners know how easy (or otherwise) the child may be to examine, and whether any particular signs are difficult to elicit. The examiners then spend some time reviewing the notes, and a prepared short-case summary sheet, which lists the written introduction (stem), the diagnosis and the examiners' agreed signs. Remember, all examiners will have undergone a calibration session in the weeks before the examination, to ensure consistency and fairness.

Chapter 4

Achievement Psychology

Positive mindset

As a man thinketh in his heart, so is he.
PROVERBS 23:7

The essence of any successful candidate's mental attitude is positive thinking. If you expect success, you get success; but if you expect failure, you eventually get failure. Negativism is one of life's great cop-outs, because it allows you to accept life's little failures without embarrassment. If you expect to fail—and you have communicated this belief to those around you—you will not look that bad when you do fail. But if you expect and communicate success, then fail, you end up looking a fool.

It is risky to expect positive things to happen to you, but positive self-expectancy is the only sure way of being successful. 'What can be conceived and believed can be achieved'—but it takes more than saying 'I can' to pass exams or achieve any other goal.

One of the presuppositions of neurolinguistic programming is that *if one person can do something, anyone can learn to do it.* Therefore confidence, self-discipline, self-esteem, mental toughness, persuasion, concentration and decisiveness are all qualities and skills you can learn and develop, just as you have learned to tie your shoelaces, drive a car or ride a bicycle. You need to develop an effective strategy by using role models. Find someone who is achieving the success you want. Find out what that individual is doing. Do the same things and you will achieve the same results. The price you pay is to take consistent action and to do it repeatedly until you acquire the winning habits that will allow you to achieve those results. This chapter will provide you with strategies that will empower you to realise your goals.

Self-motivation

Great souls have wills, feeble ones have only wishes.
CHINESE PROVERB

Candidates who do not persist with their desire to succeed do so out of choice! They have chosen not to exercise self-discipline and persistence to work diligently towards their goal. You can choose to be a success or failure: 'Whether you think you can or think you can't, you're right'. Realise that nothing is final until you accept it as such. We all make mistakes, we all fall down and we have all at some time given up under adversity. However, to stay down once you've fallen is a matter of choice.

Commitment

If success has an entry fee, the cost is total commitment.
DENIS WAITLEY

There is no lasting success without absolute commitment. Achievers are willing to *do whatever it takes* to succeed. This commitment to 'paying the price' is the essential quality in the mindset of an achiever. Heed Goethe's advice:

Until one is committed, there is hesitancy, the chance to draw back, always ineffectiveness. Concerning all acts of initiative (and creation), there is one elementary truth the ignorance of which kills countless ideas and splendid plans: that the moment one definitely commits oneself, then Providence moves too. All sorts of things occur to help one that would never otherwise have occurred … Whatever you can do or dream you can, begin it now. Boldness has genius, power, and magic in it.

Remember the words of the Jedi Master Yoda in *Star Wars*: 'Try not. Do, or do not. There is no try'.

Why do you do the things you do?

If you cannot answer this question, you are just going through the motions, drifting. 'I guess I'm doing what I'm supposed to' becomes the theme of your life. This lack of total commitment may keep you from regressing, but it does not encourage peak performance. Successful candidates always have a *purpose* in mind for their actions. The quality of your life is directly related to your willingness to put your plans into action. Purpose creates motivation. If you want the power of purpose, you need to identify your mission and always act in a way that will further your efforts to reach it.

Create a priority purpose—a *mission* for yourself. Ask yourself:

1. Why do I do the things I do?
2. What is most important to me?
3. What am I willing to invest?
4. How much am I willing to endure?
5. What am I willing to give up?
6. How much responsibility am I willing to take?
7. Am I willing to begin where I am?
8. Am I willing to settle for anything less than my full potential?

Answering these questions will aid you in determining your mission. *Focus* on that mission in your thoughts and actions.

To further your efforts to fulfil your mission, ask yourself:

1. Do I understand the aims and requirements of the examination?
2. Do I have the determination to study seriously? Do I give top priority to study at the expense of time with family and friends?

3. Does my employment provide adequate experience? Do I use my employment to gain experience?
4. Have I discussed my plans with a supervisor or sympathetic consultant paediatrician? Do others feel I have the aptitude for paediatrics?
5. Can I accept constructive criticism from those who want to help me?

You must understand that in any endeavour, obstacles and conflict are inevitable. In your efforts to overcome these factors, at some stage you will experience the pain of present limitation. The only way to overcome the limitation is to *push through* the limitation towards your objective.

Goal-setting

If you fail to plan, plan to fail.

Once you have made up your mind to become a paediatrician, you must chart a course towards this ultimate goal. This means intelligent goal-setting. Goal-setting is not easy. To be effective it requires constant review and change.

Goal-setting involves *writing out the steps* it will take to accomplish your mission. It may take 5 months, it may take 10 years, but the mission must be broken down into smaller units so that you know what you are to achieve in each area every day, week and month.

Goal-setting will allow you to plan your time for study most effectively. Service commitments, domestic demands and social obligations are the main factors affecting study time. Organise your working time to your greatest advantage by sensibly reviewing your commitments. Ensure that realistic time periods are allotted. Decide an order of priority in their execution and then do it! A small amount of time used at the start of the day reviewing what tasks need to be done pays off in time saved for studying. Remember always to differentiate between *important* tasks and *urgent* tasks.

Here are some guidelines for setting goals:
- **Set specific goals.** Specific goals are much more productive than general goals that merely stress 'doing your best'.
- **State goals positively.** For example, set aside 2 hours every evening to study Nelson's textbook. Effective goals need a positive mental image of yourself achieving what you want or being what you want to become. You cannot picture a negative goal.
- **Set challenging goals.** Psychologist Edwin Locke found that 'the higher the level of intended achievement [that is, the higher the goal], the higher the level of performance'.
- **Set measurable goals.** Goals need to be measurable in terms of what is achieved and when it is achieved. A goal of 'increasing performance in the long case' is not measurable. Rather, a goal of 'completing 20 long cases within 3 months' is measurable.
- **Set realistic and achievable goals.** A goal must not be too difficult, otherwise you will not want to try. But it must not be too easy—there is no challenge. State what results can be realistically achieved, given your resources. For a medical student to say 'My goal is to be professor of paediatrics within 12 months' is unrealistic. 'My goal is to be professor of paediatrics in 20 years' is a more realistic goal, especially if the student sets down the intermediate goals.
- **Set tangible goals.** Some of your goals will be intangible. You can accomplish these intangible goals by achieving related tangible ones. The goals you set should always

be tangible. For example, if you lack self-confidence, the intangible goal of 'achieving greater confidence' is not measurable. How will you know when you have enough confidence? Setting specific, tangible goals fostering development of confidence will be effective (e.g. 'I speak up at grand rounds').

- **Make sure goals include behavioural changes.** You must set goals of becoming, of developing whatever characteristic you lack before you achieve your tangible goal. You cannot expect to become proficient in short cases if you continue to avoid doing them. You need to alter your behaviour.
- **Write out your goals in present tense.** Written goals ensure that you clearly describe what you want and that you commit yourself to its accomplishment. Written goals need to be in the positive present tense, so that your mind accepts them. Written goals force you to establish priorities, for often two very desirable goals will come into conflict. Prioritise your values to determine which is the most important.
- **Vividly imagine your goals.** Develop the habit of several times a day vividly imagining yourself achieving your goal.
- **Write down the benefits of reaching your goals.** Writing down the benefits of reaching your goals improves motivation and desire.
- **Write out a plan to reach your goal.**
- **Write out a list of obstacles that hinder you in reaching your goals.** Listing the obstacles that hinder goal achievement allows you to focus on what needs to be done: 'A problem stated is a problem half-solved.'
- **Set short-term and long-term goals.** Set time-priority goals: a 5-year plan, a 1-year plan, a daily 'to do' list. Every day, write down the six most important things that need to be done. Rank the six items with the hardest first down to the easiest last. Start on number 1. If interrupted, take care of the interruption and return to finishing number 1. Check off each item as it is completed and carry over into the following day those that were not accomplished. Every night, make out a new list for the next day.
- **Set goals to maintain a balanced life.** True happiness can be reached only by living a balanced life. To ensure a balanced life, set goals in the following areas: physical, mental/career, spiritual, financial, family and social.

The secret of success lies in establishing a *clearly defined goal*, writing it down and then hammering it into your subconscious mind with unrelenting practice—daily rehearsal with words, images and emotions as if you had already accomplished it.

Affirmation

Destiny is not a matter of chance, it is a matter of choice—it is not a thing to be waited for, it is a thing to be achieved.
W. BRYAN

An affirmation is a positive statement describing what you want to be, have or do. The constant repetition of positive thought day in and day out displaces stored negative thoughts in your subconscious mind. In the words of Benjamin Franklin, 'Little strokes fell great oaks'. Here are a few guidelines for constructing affirmations.

- **Use the first person, 'I'.**
- **State affirmations positively.** 'I will not be afraid when I perform in long cases' is not as effective as 'I enjoy the challenge and sense of achievement I feel when I perform in long cases'.

- **State affirmations in the present tense.** Even though you know it is not true yet, affirmations need to be worded in the present tense. Therefore state 'I am a paediatrician', rather than 'I will be a paediatrician' and see yourself already in possession of your goal.
- **State affirmations with emotion.** The more feeling you can generate when repeating the affirmations, the more effective they will be.
- **Write out affirmations.** Write out your affirmations, with copies on your mobile phone, tablet and also on 3 × 5 cm cards, and carry them with you (in your pocket, wallet, etc.) and place them in areas where you will see them (e.g. study desk, bathroom mirror, dressing table, dashboard). Repeat them throughout the day, especially first thing upon awaking and before going to sleep.

Self-talk

We can do anything we want to do if we stick to it long enough.
HELEN KELLER

Another application of affirmation is self-talk. You are constantly having an internal dialogue with yourself about events that are occurring in your internal and external environment. The self-talk has a very strong effect on emotions and behaviour. It usually happens subconsciously, but with practice you can learn to listen to it and control it. Most of the inner dialogue is negative; for example, 'I can't do it. I'm not good enough. I'll mess it up. It's too hard. There is no point going on. They'll think that I'm stupid and useless' and so on. Negative self-talk creates pressure.

Candidates in a pressure situation, such as being unable to answer a question in the long case, may react in the following ways:
- Magnify the obstacles and underestimate their own resources.
- Think irrationally and feel that the examiners dislike and are 'out to get' them.
- Visualise the outcome they fear or do not want to happen and not concentrate on what they want to achieve.
- Try too hard with 'do nots' and 'must nots'.
- Worry about criticism, rejection by others and embarrassment.

Self-defeating thoughts are difficult but not impossible to control. Some of the strategies used are given below:
- Repeating negative thoughts aloud as soon as they come to mind helps some individuals get rid of them.
- Thought-stopping. As soon as you are aware of negative thoughts, say 'STOP!', 'CANCEL!' and/or imagine a red light or the word 'STOP!', and then focus on something else, such as your breathing. Another technique is to wear an elastic band around the wrist, and to pull and flick it each time a self-defeating thought comes to mind.
- Being aware that everyone has negative thoughts, particularly in pressure situations, helps to lessen their impact.
- If you fight negative thoughts, you concentrate on them and make them worse. You need to replace them with positive thoughts.
- Encouraging negative thoughts to go through your mind and then allowing them to pass out may also get rid of them (e.g. saying to yourself 'Come on, I'm waiting for you').

- Asking yourself questions such as 'Why am I doing this?', 'What's my plan?', 'What do I have to do now?' and 'What's the worst thing that can happen?' may also reduce self-defeating thoughts.
- You can stop undesirable self-talk by taking a few slow deep breaths and thinking positive affirmations. For example, say to yourself 'Take a few deep breaths, relax and take control', 'You can do it!', 'Relax and flow', 'Slow down', 'I perform better under pressure'.
- As James Rohn states, 'Don't say "If I could, I would". Say, "If I can, I will"'.

Visualisation

Men's natures are alike; it is their habits that carry them far apart.
CONFUCIUS

Visualisation or mental rehearsal is the technique of picturing the results you would like to see happen, and using these images to focus all your energies on attaining your goals. Visualisation reinforces affirmations. Visualisation becomes several times more effective when three or more senses (sight, smell, touch, taste, hearing) are involved in the process. There are two aspects to visualisation. One is picturing a future desired result as being already in existence (e.g. picturing yourself seeing your name on the 'pass' list for an exam, being congratulated by your colleagues, friends and spouse and then savouring the emotions of joy and happiness you feel).

The other is mentally rehearsing a physical act, the actual process or performance (e.g. picturing yourself going through a perfect short case). There are slightly different guidelines for each form of visualisation.

Research has shown that the subconscious mind cannot differentiate between a real event and one that is vividly imagined. When you repeatedly imagine something with feeling, your subconscious mind accepts these images as reality, storing them for future use. When in a future situation similar to the one you have visualised, your subconscious mind with its stored information will go to work for you, helping you to live out the event as near to the one in your vivid mental rehearsal as possible. Capture the feelings of success. Clearly picture yourself in conclusion enjoying the rewards of your success.

An important requirement of practising mental rehearsal of an actual process is that the *mental images must involve movement*; that is, they should be mental images of actions rather than static postures. Recall the moment of your best performance or the best segment of a performance (e.g. long-case introduction). You must actually see yourself going through the *complete action*, and the *timing* of the images you create should be as close as you can make it to the duration of the actual event. The best test of a visualisation is that after mentally rehearsing the activity three or four times you should be able to run through it effortlessly.

At this stage, choose a single word that accurately describes or names the event or action you are rehearsing. You can use this 'trigger word' to elicit a replay of what you mentally rehearsed whenever you want to use it. For example, just before a cardiac short case, you could close your eyes momentarily, repeat your trigger word 'cardiac short case' and replay the rehearsed mental image to prime yourself.

Not only will proper mental rehearsal enhance your ability; it can also be superior to actual physical practice because the mental rehearsal will be letter perfect, whereas the actual performance is often filled with errors that can lead to bad habits or discouragement.

The perfect visualisation will eliminate any potential bad habits. You will later go through the performance physically *in the same perfect manner* as you have visualised.

Apply the technique as follows. Lie down as still as possible, let your eyelids close and relax completely by concentrating on your breathing. As you exhale, mentally repeat the word 'calm'. As you do, generate the feeling of calmness and imagine the 'calm' flowing through you. When you are deeply relaxed, mentally see, feel and experience yourself as dynamic, confident, competent and successful, an individual of superior ability. Don't just watch this mental movie; *become* this individual. Think the thoughts, feel the feelings and experience yourself as this peak performer *as if it is an already accomplished fact!*

Remain with your mental movie for 10–15 minutes, then focus your attention on your breathing. If you are doing this visualisation before sleep, mentally repeat the word 'drowsy' as you exhale and let the associated sensations deeply relax you. To return to full alertness, see yourself slowly climbing five steps. While climbing, suggest to yourself that at the top you'll feel relaxed, revitalised and alert. When you reach the top step, open your eyes, breathe in deeply and stretch. For maximum benefits, this technique should be practised *twice daily* (once in the morning upon awaking, and then just before going to sleep). It is best to *set aside a specific time* each day for practice.

It is crucial that you practise this reprogramming exercise *consistently*, because establishing a new conditioned, stimulus-response (thinking, feeling and acting differently) needs *continuous* reinforcement of the programming in your subconscious. Your subconscious mind becomes so familiar with *seeing and feeling* yourself being the 'successful you' that in time you'll find yourself actually behaving this way. This technique should be used each day and night until you've experienced a satisfactory change (usually takes between 21 and 90 days).

Mental toughness

Surrounded by a forest of enemy spears—enter deeply and learn to use your mind as a shield.
MORIHEI UESHIBA

Mental toughness is the ability to consistently perform at your best during the heat of competitive battle, despite adversity. It is the capacity to handle and thrive in stressful situations. Some tips for developing mental toughness are as follows:
- Learn everything you can about individuals who have overcome adversity and succeeded.
- You do not need to experience a setback to get ahead.
- Provide solution-oriented feedback when problem-solving.
- Expect the unexpected—stretch yourself beyond your comfort zone. Expect the best, but plan for the worst.
- Strengthen your abdomen. According to sports psychologist James Loehr, 'The foundation of mental toughness is grounded in the physical. You want to develop a tremendous capacity for absorbing physical stress'. Your abdomen determines your posture and breathing, and supports your lower back. To strengthen your abdomen, do 100 abdominal crunches daily.
- Practise interval training by contrasting periods of stress with rest and recovery. Aim to exercise your body for 30 minutes daily, using the interval training principle. For example, if you are a jogger, run fast and then slowly.

- Develop performer skills. Acting 'as if' you feel a certain way, such as confident, causes biochemical changes in your body. Physically relax, breathe and hold for about five heartbeats between each inspiration and expiration until your mind is calm. Recall a positive emotionally loaded memory and get fully associated with it, then magnify it many times and step into it. Repeat with a second positive memory, then see and feel yourself facing the impossible and succeeding. Open your eyes and perform your task. Remember: 'practice makes the impossible possible'.
- Practise winning rituals. Establish a consistent schedule of eating, exercising and studying. Highly ritualised routines will enhance your effectiveness when so much of your life is out of control.

Failure

What if you do all the right things and still fail? Remind yourself that you can never really fail if you refuse to accept 'failure'. Failure is a temporary setback and is never final until you accept it as such. Hemingway said that 'man can be defeated but not destroyed'. Defeat is not the end of the world. Every failure carries with it the seed of an equivalent or greater success.

The main reasons for failure are the following:
- Difficulty comprehending questions.
- Succumbing to the 'stress' of physical confrontation.
- Fatigue.
- Relying on luck rather than planned preparation. Remember that luck is where preparation meets opportunity.
- Inadequate teaching and training in paediatrics.
- Lack of aptitude for paediatrics.

Turn each defeat to your advantage by examining how and why you have been unsuccessful and determine that you will never be defeated in the same way again. You need to ask yourself honest questions about the following:

1. Your attitude and approach.
2. Whether or not your experience was adequate to allow you to deal with the examinations.
3. Whether or not you studied sufficiently, sought the necessary experience and avoided distractions during your training.
4. Whether or not your training is of the required standard.

If your training is inadequate, then what is your plan to overcome this? To formulate your plan, you need to answer the following questions:

1. Am I going to sit again?
2. How am I going to get the missing experience?
3. Do I require more intensive study?
4. Is this the correct career for me?
5. What are my motives for doing paediatrics?
6. Do I need to seek help from a trusted senior colleague or clinical psychologist?

In this way, failure becomes an opportunity for growth, 'a teacher', and by reframing it in positive and beneficial terms you become more resourceful. Instead of seeing your experiences as random events, use each and every one of them. Even the most boring or demeaning occurrence can serve you by allowing you to take control. Likewise, the most demanding or stressful event is also an opportunity to learn. As Nietzsche said, 'that which does not kill you only makes you stronger'.

Further reading

- Ariely, Dan. *Predictably Irrational, Revised and Expanded Edition: The Hidden Forces That Shape Our Decisions.*
- Bowden, Mark. *Tame the Primitive Brain: 28 Ways in 28 Days to Manage the Most Impulsive Behaviors at Work.*
- Bowden, Mark. *Winning Body Language: Control the Conversation, Command Attention, and Convey the Right Message without Saying a Word.*
- Brown, Dr Jeff, Fenske, Mark, Neporent, Liz. *The Winner's Brain: 8 Strategies Great Minds Use to Achieve Success.*
- Buzan, Tony. *The Ultimate Book of Mind Maps.*
- Cain, Susan. *Quiet: The Power of Introverts in a World That Can't Stop Talking.*
- Cialdini, Robert B. *Influence: Science and Practice.* 5th edition.
- Divine, Mark. *Unbeatable Mind: Forge Resiliency and Mental Toughness to Succeed at an Elite Level.*
- Dobelli, Rolf. *The Art of Thinking Clearly.*
- Everly Jr, George S, Strouse, Douglas A, McCormack, Dennis K. *Stronger: Develop the Resilience You Need to Succeed.*
- Gladwell, Malcolm. *David and Goliath: Underdogs, Misfits, and the Art of Battling Giants.*
- Gladwell, Malcolm. *Outliers: The Story of Success.*
- Goulston, Mark, Ullmen, John. *Real Influence: Persuade Without Pushing and Gain Without Giving In.*
- Greene, Robert. *The 48 Laws of Power.*
- Helgoe, Laurie. *Introvert Power: Why Your Inner Life Is Your Hidden Strength.*
- Holiday, Ryan. *The Obstacle is the Way: The Ancient Art of Turning Adversity to Advantage.*
- Kahneman, Daniel. *Thinking, Fast and Slow.*
- Kahnweiler, Jennifer. *Quiet Influence: The Introvert's Guide to Making a Difference.*
- Laney, Marti Olsen. *The Introvert Advantage: How to Thrive in an Extrovert World.*
- McGonigal, Kelly. *The Willpower Instinct: How Self-Control Works, Why It Matters, and What You Can Do to Get More of It.*
- McNab, Andy, Dutton, Kevin. *Sorted! The Good Psychopath's Guide to Bossing Your Life.*
- McNab, Andy, Dutton, Kevin. *The Good Psychopath's Guide to Success.*
- Morland, Polly. *The Society of Timid Souls: or, How to Be Brave.*
- Navarro, Joe, Karlins, Marvin. *What Every BODY is Saying: An Ex-FBI Agent's Guide to Speed-Reading People.*
- Shelleman, Joyce M. *The Introvert's Guide to Professional Success: How to Let Your Quiet Competence Be Your Career Advantage.*
- Siegel, Daniel J. *Mindsight: The New Science of Personal Transformation.*
- Spackman, Kerry. *Winner's Bible: Rewire your Brain for Permanent Change.*
- Taleb, Nassim Nicholas. *Antifragile: Things That Gain from Disorder.*
- Wiseman, Richard. *The Luck Factor: The Scientific Study of the Lucky Mind.*

Chapter 5

Behavioural and Developmental Paediatrics

LONG CASE: Anorexia nervosa (AN)

The eating disorders anorexia nervosa (AN) and bulimia nervosa (BN) are potentially lethal conditions, and two of the leading bio-psychosocial developmental disorders among adolescents, both female and male, described in many countries, not just wealthy countries with Western culture. The *Diagnostic and Statistical Manual of Mental Disorders* (5th ed.; DSM-5; American Psychiatric Association, 2013) revised significantly the diagnostic aspects of AN and BN as they were enumerated in the previous DSM-IV manual (1994), to cut down on the 'residual category diagnosis' of 'Eating Disorder Not Otherwise Specified', which essentially included 50% of eating disorders.

An excellent review of the changes and of current clinical guidelines by the Royal Australian and New Zealand College of Psychiatrists was published by the College in 2014, and can be accessed at www.ranzcp.org under 'Guidelines and resources for practice'. The section of the DSM-5 devoted to 'Feeding and Eating Disorders' now includes three eating disorders (AN, BN and binge eating disorder [BED]) and three feeding disorders (pica, rumination disorder [RD]), and avoidant/restrictive food intake disorder [ARFID]); BED and the latter three do not involve disturbed perception of body image.

Eating disorders are significantly more common in females than in males. Lifetime prevalences of eating disorders are: AN: 1% females, < 0.5% males; BN: 2% females, 0.5% males; BED: 3.5% females, 2% males.

AN involves an inability to maintain a body weight that is normal for the patient's age and height, or failure to gain weight when growing, with fear of gaining weight and disturbed perception of body weight and/or shape, and endocrine complications of nutrition such as amenorrhoea (this has been removed as a criterion in the DSM-5). There are two subtypes: the restrictive type alone, and the binge-purge subtype that includes bulimic behaviour or overexercising (note that vomiting per se does not make a diagnosis of BN, and in the context of low weight and vomiting, the diagnosis of AN takes precedence).

The aims of this long-case section are as follows:

- To give an overview of current management strategies employed in treating children and adolescents diagnosed as having AN by correctly interpreted criteria of ICD-10 (*Classification of mental and behavioural disorders: clinical descriptions and diagnostic guidelines*, World Health Organization [WHO], 1992; soon to be replaced with the ICD-11) or the DSM-5. This section predominantly follows DSM-5.
- To suggest a directed examination technique for detecting salient physical findings, and to guide the ordering of appropriate investigations that will enable accurate diagnosis of AN and its common complications.
- To give guidelines regarding need for hospitalisation and a review of the mechanisms of the irreversible, life-threatening complications of AN.

This long case deals exclusively with AN. The long case can be challenging, but offers a wide discussion base regarding management. As AN is the third most common chronic illness in adolescent girls in Australia, the United Kingdom and the United States, there are always long-term patients available in hospitals where examinations are held.

Background information

There is increasing evidence of a strong biological predisposition to AN. AN is a neuro-psychiatric disorder arising from a complex interaction of genes, biology and the environment. It is a chronic condition where the patient has distorted perceptions about food and body image that interfere with normal functioning and involve the establishment of a range of unhealthy behaviours. Illness denial is a common feature of AN with many patients denying or minimising the severity of their illness. Although, historically, many texts have described disturbed parent–child relationships as often underpinning the development of eating disorders, current research does not support abnormal parent interactions as aetiological.

There is no single aetiology for eating disorders but rather a combination of genetic predisposition and environmental risks. Twin and family studies suggest that AN heritability ranges between 50 and 83%. There is now good evidence that recurrent exposure to 'ideally thin' body images can lead to body dissatisfaction. The other significant risk factor for AN is rapid weight loss due to dieting. For many adolescents, overall self-esteem is linked directly to body esteem.

Risk factors creating susceptibility for the development of eating disorders include:

- Eating disorders, substance use disorder, affective disorders, in family members.
- Obsessional, perfectionist personalities with negative self-evaluation.
- Comorbid clinical problems such as depression, anxiety, obsessive-compulsive disorder (OCD), posttraumatic stress disorder (PTSD) and substance use disorders.

The development of a sudden desire to have a 'healthy' diet, to become a vegetarian or to lose weight by dieting can become extreme, with the development of disordered eating.

Dieting is a clear risk factor for onset of AN. The risk is greater the more extreme the dieting behaviours. However, because of the greater prevalence of moderate dieting, more cases of AN arise in moderate rather than extreme dieters.

Other risk factors include being involved in sports that place great emphasis on a particular body size and shape (e.g. ballet, gymnastics, athletics), or having type 1 diabetes mellitus (T1DM)—a chronic illness that causes a significant life stress, involves special attention to diet, is associated with increased risk of depression and anxiety (which themselves are risk factors for AN), and involves challenges and stresses in the parent–child relationship.

Trigger factors may include adolescence itself, with its concomitant developmental strivings, identity definition and need for independence, or traumatic life events such as the recent loss of a loved family member or animal, a move to a new school, starting high school, a move to a new home, family disruption (marital discord, domestic violence, divorce), a fight with a close friend, or being picked on or bullied at school. It can also be triggered by less extreme issues, such as comments by a sports coach about being overweight.

Perpetuating factors include, most importantly, the biological effects of being underweight and undernourished (from sustained caloric malnutrition and self-starvation), which include the classic psychological responses of food obsession, depressed mood, food-related rumination and aberrant food-related behaviours.

Inadvertent positive reinforcement can occur if the patient was initially overweight, and the initial weight loss was greeted with support for dieting efforts. Parents' accidental tacit agreement by complying with demands of the eating-disordered child (buying diet foods, allowing vigorous exercise schedules) can reinforce the evolving 'anorexic identity'.

AN is a misnomer. There is little evidence to suggest these patients could be *anorectic*; they have, traditionally, been viewed as having normal appetites. Recently, there have been investigations into whether there could be appetite hormone dysregulation (in the neuropeptide Y [NPY]-PYY appetite regulatory system); this is unresolved. AN patients can exert their control, by lack of recognition of their (initially) ordered physiology. *If a child or adolescent labelled as having AN does complain of anorexia,* and does not have body image distortion, then *that patient needs to be assessed for an organic problem* such as inflammatory bowel disease or occult malignancy (for the differential diagnosis of AN, see the short-case approach to weight loss in … 8, Gastroenterology).

History

Ideally, the history should be taken from the patient and the parent, but the logistics of an examination situation makes it prudent to take the history from one or the other predominantly; the history from the parent will (hopefully) not be as divorced from reality as that of the patient. The examiners need to know that the candidate appreciates the need to get the contrasting histories from both parties, in order to have a comprehensive overview of the dynamics of the patient and their family unit. The candidate must appreciate that the patient can reliably inform him/her about other aspects of his or her life, such as school, and peer relationships.

PRESENTING COMPLAINT

This should be the reason for presence at the examination. It may be a current admission: often a critical drop in weight, cardiovascular instability (e.g. bradycardia, hypotension), constant vomiting, safety concerns (e.g. self-harm or suicidality), hypothermia (seen in around one-third of patients) or serious electrolyte abnormalities (very uncommon in the absence of vomiting, even in the presence of very severe weight loss).

CURRENT STATUS

Behavioural symptoms: the A to F of AN

Summary: **A**ctivity (much), **B**ody image (abnormal), **C**ognitive (rigid thoughts), **D**rugs (laxatives), **E**ating (how, when), **F**ood (what).

1. **A**ctivity: exercise (compulsive, at unusual hours, solitary, not part of competitive sport, prolonged duration, long-distance running, sit-ups or stomach crunches a favourite), constant movement, standing rather than sitting. Ask 'How long and how much do you exercise each day?'

2. **B**ody image: negative comments (unhappy with thighs, abdomen, hips), frequent weighing of self, not happy with new lower weight, chooses baggy clothes to hide weight loss. Ask 'What do you think about your weight? Are you average, skinny or overweight? What would be a healthy weight for you?' Document how large the patient judges his or her body to be. Body checking: repeated weighing, pinching, measuring body parts, checking protrusion of particular bones, checking certain clothes fit, mirror gazing, comparison with others' bodies. Body avoidance: the opposite to body checking, avoiding the above, refusal to weigh, avoidance of mirrors. Minimising symptom severity. Shape concerns. Overvaluation of weight and shape in determining self-worth. Fear of weight gain. Disturbance in how their own body is experienced. Note that many young people choose not to share these concerns with a candidate because they are shameful emotions.

3. **C**ognitive aspects: rigid thought processes, impaired judgment, obsessive thoughts, rigid beliefs (e.g. cannot eat this food with that food; cannot eat after specified time, such as 6 p.m., as will not digest food), ritualised behaviour associated with purchase, preparation and consumption of food.

4. **D**rug aspects: use of laxatives, diet pills, diuretics, stimulants, thyroxine, cigarette smoking, diabetic (T1DM) patients withholding insulin. Ask: 'What [medicines] do you have?'

5. **E**ating behaviour: missing meals, eating very slowly (e.g. cutting food into very small pieces), hiding food, feeding her or his food to pets, feigning eating (e.g. pushing food around plate), avoiding social events involving eating, self-induced vomiting after meals, spitting, prolonged fasting (over 8 waking hours), strict rules about eating, little variety in foods (extreme vegan diets, avoidance of fat), secret eating, cooking for others but not eating themselves.

6. **F**ood intake: types of eating—restrictive (eating less), selective (limiting intake to a range of preferred foods), restrained (controlling type and amount of foods); refusal to eat foods perceived as fattening (e.g. meat, dairy products, fat, carbohydrates); high intake of water, diet drinks, vegetarian foods; claims 'allergy' to various foods; immediate guilt after eating (may induce vomiting, or exercise excessively).

Physical symptoms of AN

Summary: decreased vital signs, decreased energy, delayed puberty, delayed gastrointestinal function, dermatological features, dislike cold.

1. Current weight, height, age-appropriate body mass index (BMI) centile, % BMI calculated from matching centiles on growth charts or 50% centile BMI for age, rate of weight loss, fluctuations in weight, lowest weight, highest weight.

2. Amenorrhoea, oligomenorrhoea. Absence of at least three consecutive menstrual cycles. Ask: 'Are you having regular periods?', 'When was your last period?'

3. Pubertal delay: Tanner staging required.

4. Lethargy, weakness, fatigue. Ask: 'How are your energy levels now compared to when you were at a healthier weight?'

5. Constipation (including the use of laxatives). Ask: 'Have you had any laxatives for this?' 'How often?'

6. Hair and skin: hair loss, dry skin, purplish skin peripherally, oedema.

7. Circulation: poor peripheral circulation and peripherally cool, dizziness, lightheadedness, near-syncope, palpitations. Ask: 'Have you had any dizziness, fainting, shortness of breath, palpitations/feeling your heart going really fast, or any chest pain?'

8. Sensitivity to cold. Ask: 'Does cold weather bother you?' 'Do you feel the cold more easily than other people?'
9. Symptoms in postpubertal adolescents: reduced libido, reduced hair and beard growth, and reduced waking erections in adolescent males.

Complications of AN

1. Acute (and potentially fatal): medical instability—bradycardia, hypothermia, hypotension, severe hypokalaemia, hypophosphataemia (leading to arrhythmias), congestive cardiac failure, (and, very rarely, refeeding syndrome). A key issue is hypophosphataemia; need daily bloods to check for low phosphate and to check electrolytes).
2. Chronic: growth deceleration, pubertal arrest, bone loss (osteopenia or osteoporosis) or failure of normal bone accretion. Depression can be part of the biological effects on the brain from loss of weight, as well as part of the premorbid personality issues. Always ask about suicidal ideation; the two commonest causes of death from AN in adulthood are complications of malnutrition per se and suicide.

Current management of AN for inpatients

1. Multidisciplinary list of team: members (e.g. paediatrician or physician specialising in adolescents, psychiatrist, psychologist, dietician, occupational therapist, physiotherapist, social worker, nurse, teacher, art therapist, music therapist) together, with clarity about case management role; degree of engagement with patient (against wishes, perhaps) and parents; degree of success so far; whether the team addresses issues adequately in the opinion of patient/parents.
2. Approach to weight gain: eating meals and snacks provided; need for nasogastric tube, now or earlier in the admission; prescription of psychotropic medication during this admission.
3. Procedures of management program: usual measurements made (how patient is weighed—e.g. in underwear with gown; frequency of weighing), whether bladder scan is done (to subtract volume of urine from weight; note that this is inaccurate if patient drinks just prior to scan) or urine specific gravity checked (to detect water loading) unless salt loaded; whether there is a target weight known by patient; how height is checked; how often blood tests are performed; whether bone density is checked and how often; whether calcium supplements are given, whether the team has a target weight for the patient.

Comorbid psychiatric diagnoses

Ask about any psychiatric diagnoses made, especially mood disorders and anxiety disorders. AN is associated with very high rates of comorbid psychiatric illness, with 30–50% of children having major depression and around 50% having anxiety disorders, including OCD, so the candidate should ask about this in the history. Comorbidities may be treatable (e.g. depression). Ask about current or past psychotropic medication.

PAST HISTORY OF AN

Initial symptoms, investigations and management before diagnosis, diagnosis (when, where, how), subsequent investigations and management, progress of disease, hospitalisation details (frequency, duration, usual treatment), complications of disease, specialists and therapists involved (child psychiatrist, paediatrician, psychologist), approach to treatment (family-based treatment, individual psychotherapy), outpatient or other clinics attended, any recent change in symptoms or management.

SOCIAL HISTORY

Disease impact on patient

Growth, development, self-image, independence, requests for transfer to adult care, compliance with management program, schooling (attendance, performance, teacher awareness of disorder, peer interactions), employment prospects, effects on activities of daily living, comorbid pathology issues including depression.

Disease impact on parents

Marriage stability, depression, denial, guilt, fears for the future.

Disease impact on siblings

Sibling rivalry, hostility, support, similar disordered thoughts developing.

Social supports

Extended family, close friends, AN 'social network' (this is usually a negative support, disseminating pro-AN ideation websites), community nurses or social workers.

Coping

Who attends with patient, who supervises eating, confidence with management, parents' main concerns, degree of understanding of disorder, expectations for future, understanding of prognosis (by patient and parent).

Access

To local doctor, paediatrician, psychiatrist, psychologist, hospital.

FAMILY HISTORY

Other members with AN, whether other siblings are demonstrating similar disordered thoughts, other family members with any psychiatric diagnoses particularly depression or anxiety.

IMMUNISATION

Routine.

Examination for anorexia nervosa

The approach given in Table 5.1 assesses patients with AN for disease severity and current status. It omits the various negative findings that would be relevant in a patient in whom the diagnosis was only suspected, but not yet proven. For the differential diagnosis for AN, see the short case on weight loss in Chapter 8, Gastroenterology.

Investigations

Most centres treating AN patients have an initial work-up that involves, as a minimum, several blood tests: full blood count and film (to detect anaemia, neutropenia), urea and electrolytes (to check for hypokalaemia), magnesium, phosphorus, calcium, vitamin D, coeliac screen, liver function tests (especially transaminases, albumin, protein), thyroid function tests (low T_3, euthyroid sick syndrome) and an electrocardiogram (ECG) if there is evidence of bradycardia (to detect arrhythmias, Q-Tc abnormalities).

Other investigations that may be helpful in ongoing monitoring include: serum zinc, follicle-stimulating hormone (FSH), luteinising hormone (LH) and oestradiol (useful measures of malnutrition in postpubertal females); bone density studies (for osteopenia, osteoporosis); bone age; body composition.

Table 5.1
Examination for anorexia nervosa
1. Introduce self
2. General inspection
Parameters • Weight • Height
Percentiles • Weight age versus height age • Weight for height (quantitate)
Sick or well, cachectic, depressed affect, nasogastric tube
3. Demonstrate fat and protein stores
Subcutaneous fat: mid-arm, axillae, subscapular, suprailiac
Muscle bulk: biceps, triceps, quadriceps, glutei
4. Skin
Pallor, acrocyanosis
Yellowish hue (from hypercarotenaemia)
Petechiae—limited to superior vena cava (SVC) distribution (vomiting)
Dry, scaling
Dermatitis artefacta (e.g. cigarette-burns, other self-injury)
Excoriated acne
Hypertrichosis—lanugo-like, fine downy hair
Eczematous scaling around mouth, elbows, knees, genitals, anus (zinc deficiency)
5. Head and neck
Hair: loss of discrete areas (trichotillomania), thinning, brittle, pluckable
Eyes: conjunctival pallor (anaemias), cataract
Palate: scarring from self-induced vomiting
Teeth: erosion of enamel (purging)
Contour of lower face: prominent salivary glands (vomiting)
6. Upper limbs
Hands: Russell's sign (calluses, scars or erosions over dorsal surface of hands, especially metacarpophalangeal joints, with self-induced vomiting)
Nails: bitten, brittle
Pulse: bradycardia, irregular (atrial arrhythmia)
Blood pressure: hypotension—check for postural drop
7. Chest
Tachypnoea (metabolic acidosis)
Subcutaneous emphysema (with pneumomediastinum)

Table 5.1 (continued)
8. Abdomen
Scars (dermatitis artefacta), Tanner staging—pubertal delay Faecal loading
9. Lower limbs
Muscle bulk, pretibial oedema
10. Other
Bruising over spine and ischial tuberosity due to excessive exercise
Urinalysis: high specific gravity (dehydration)
Temperature chart: hypothermia

Monitoring of disease

ROUTINE CLINIC VISITS

Patients are seen weekly to monthly until they have recovered weight and are eating normally. Note target weight, weight, height (used to calculate BMI), menstrual history. Hormone levels are routinely assessed and electrolytes are checked if vomiting is suspected.

DOCUMENTATION OF DISEASE PROGRESSION

Progression is documented at intervals of 6 months to 1 year. The following may be done: bone density checked using DXA (**d**ual-energy **X**-ray **a**bsorptiometry) machine (at 12-monthly intervals; Medicare only reimburses annually); gonadotropin levels (low); FSH; LH; oestradiol (low).

Management

In this age of evidence-based medicine, AN remains a condition with significant morbidity (potential mortality), especially in adults with chronic disease, but in which until recently there has been little high-level evidence to support any particular form of intervention that could be said to approach a 'gold standard'.

Large randomised controlled trials (RCTs) of family-based treatments (FBTs), particularly Maudsley Family Therapy, demonstrate efficacy for adolescents less than 19 years old with a duration of illness of less than 3 years. Maudsley FBT is manualised, with 20 sessions over 12 months. Follow-up data over 5 years demonstrates the ongoing efficacy of this treatment. FBTs that focus on eating disorder behaviours and weight gain have demonstrated efficacy in adolescent AN management. FBTs have shown superiority over many forms of individual therapies.

Consensus opinion is that FBT should be first-line therapy for adolescents with AN aged under 19 and with an illness duration under 3 years. FBT does require families to commit fully to the treatment, so lack of compliance is considered a relative contraindication; however, there is a lack of evidence to suggest which patients may do better with individual therapy than FBT.

Current recommendations from FRANZCP include the following: treatment as an outpatient is preferable; treatment should be multidisciplinary, including FBTs for younger patients, and specialist-led manual-based psychological therapy; management needs to be culturally informed.

Hospitalisation

Most patients with AN manage to avoid admission to hospital. A number of parameters are used to assess the need for hospitalisation. Those who are admitted for stabilisation ideally should be admitted to a specialised child and adolescent eating disorders unit, as found in most tertiary paediatric referral centres.

Indications for admission to hospital can be divided into those requiring psychiatric admission and those needing medical admission; the RANZCP has produced a table of consideration for admission based on this distinction, for adults, plus a table for inpatient admission for children. Below is a mnemonic that includes the recommendations of the paediatric version.

INDICATIONS FOR ADMISSION: PAEDIATRIC AND ADOLESCENT

(Mnemonic: **POLICE WT**, police weight)

Physiological instability; **P**ostural hypotension (drop in systolic pressure of over 20 mmHg, from lying to standing)/**P**urpuric rash
Obvious (over 5%) dehydration/**O**xygen saturation < 85% (exceedingly rare)
Loss of weight: 1. to the point of significant cardiovascular compromise, *or* 2. < 75% expected body weight; *or* 3. rapid weight loss/**L**ow white cells (neutropenia)
Intractable vomiting
Cardiovascular compromise (hypotension [BP < 80/50], bradycardia [< 50 bpm], postural tachycardia [> 20/min.], slow capillary return, cyanosed extremities)
Electrolyte abnormalities: hypokalaemia < 2.5 mmol/L, hyponatraemia < 130 mmol/L, hypophosphataemia < 0.5 mmol/L/**E**CG changes: prolonged QTc interval > 450 msec (particularly with low potassium)

Worrying ideation (parasuicidal, depression, self-harming)/**W**eak muscles: squat test—'Get down/squat on your haunches and stand up without using your hands'—unable to get up without use of arms for leverage
Temperature low (hypothermia: < 35.5°C)

Different interest groups have different criteria for when to admit to hospital, whether to admit under medical or psychiatric teams, and whether to admit as a voluntary or involuntary patient, depending on the guidelines of the relevant Mental Health Act. In general, the admission will be 'medical' if the BMI is under 12 (this is extremely low) or there are significant medical complications, such as heart rate under 50 bpm. Admission to psychiatric units is more common for psychiatric symptoms such as self-harming or suicidal ideation. Admission practices differ significantly between paediatric and adult units. To illustrate this point, the following are adult versions based on current clinical practice guidelines for adults from the RANZCP, using the same mnemonic stem.

INDICATION FOR HOSPITAL ADMISSION: ADULT PSYCHIATRIC

Postural hypotension (drop in systolic pressure of > 10 mmHg, from lying to standing); **P**rotein (albumin) low

Over 1 kg weight loss per week/**O**ngoing weight loss despite community treatment

Liver enzymes mildly elevated

Inadequate caloric intake < 100 kcal/day/**I**ndex (BMI) < 14

Cardiovascular effects (hypotension [systolic BP < 90])/**C**old/blue extremities

Electrolyte (and other blood) abnormalities: hypokalaemia < 3.5 mmol/L, hyponatraemia < 130 mmol/L, glucose < 3.5 mmol/L, neutrophils < 1.5 × 10⁹/L

Worrying ideation (parasuicidal, depression, self-harming)

Temperature low (hypothermia: < 35.5°C)

INDICATIONS FOR HOSPITAL ADMISSION: ADULT MEDICAL

Postural hypotension (drop in systolic pressure of over 20 mmHg, from lying to standing)/**P**rotein low (albumin < 30 g/L)

Over 1 kg weight loss per week/**O**ngoing weight loss despite community treatment

Loss of weight to point of significant cardiovascular compromise/**L**iver enzymes markedly elevated (AST or ALT > 500 U/L)

Inadequate caloric intake < 100 kcal/day/**I**ndex (BMI) < 12

Cardiovascular compromise (hypotension [BP < 80 systolic], bradycardia [< 40 bpm, or > 120 bpm, or postural tachycardia > 20/min.], slow capillary return, cyanosed extremities)

Electrolyte (and other blood) abnormalities: hypokalaemia < 3.0 mmol/L, hyponatraemia < 125 mmol/L, hypoglycaemia < 2.5 mmol/L, hypomagnesaemia < 0.7 mmol/L, hypophosphataemia < 1.3 mmol/L, neutrophil count < 1.0 × 10⁹ /L/**e**CG changes: any arrhythmia, prolonged QTc interval (particularly with low potassium), non-specific ST or T wave changes/**e**GFR: rapidly dropping (25% drop in a week) or < 60 mL/min/1.73 m²

Worrying ideation (parasuicidal, depression, self-harming)

Temperature low (hypothermia: < 35.0°C)

Medical stabilisation can take weeks. It is important to avoid the refeeding syndrome, which can be very dangerous; the four main nutrients affected are phosphate, magnesium, potassium and thiamine; these can all drop to dangerous levels during refeeding.

Some units check phosphate, magnesium and potassium on a daily basis for the first week, and some give thiamine parenterally for the first 3 days, although this would only be for extreme cases.

BMI centiles can indicate likely return of endocrine function to normal: clinically, between the 14th and 39th BMI percentiles for age, and ultrasonically (ovarian follicle reappearance) between the 13th and 30th centile. There are accepted BMI centile charts for children, which can be used when determining weight goals, available from websites of the Centers for Disease Control and Prevention (CDC; also provides the Epi Info program to calculate age-related percentiles), and the World Health Organization (WHO; also provides the WHO AnthroPlus program to calculate age-related percentiles).

In the past, generally the plan has been to medically stabilise patients including normalising heart rate, temperature and blood pressure and achieving a minimum BMI of about 75% expected body weight (EBW) or BMI percentile (this is a better measure in adolescence; e.g. 17 kg/m^2 for a 12-year-old girl is > 25th centile BMI, compared to a 17-year-old, where it is < 5th centile) before the patient is ready for outpatient treatment; this is achieved by restoring 1–2 kg/week, until a minimum weight is achieved and the young person is eating orally.

Most inpatient programs for AN involve a multidisciplinary team, which may include paediatricians, dieticians, nurses, paediatric psychiatrists and psychologists, occupational therapists, physiotherapists, social workers, teachers and art/music therapists.

The parents must be engaged with the plan, which is not usually problematic. Engagement of the patient, however, can be difficult, as it not infrequently conflicts with the patient's agenda, which is to lose more weight. Most inpatient management plans deal directly with ongoing, perpetuating issues rather than delving into the aetiological reasons for the development of the disorder.

A helpful aspect of treatment is to 'externalise' the eating disorder, separating the thoughts attributable to the perpetuation of the disorder and its associated behaviours per se, and the thoughts of the patient. This then leads to there being two parts to the patient; one being the eating disorder/illness, and the other the person who is sick of AN, sick of doctors, and wants to be with friends and family. The goal is to make the latter part stronger than the former. It is critically important to involve the family in the treatment plan.

In hospital, regular eating of three meals and three snacks a day is encouraged to optimise physical health and gain weight. No medication has been found effective in overcoming AN, but psychotropic medications (atypical antipsychotics) can sometimes be required for inpatients who are particularly distressed by gaining weight. Educational needs have to be provided, and normalisation of interactions with the (non-AN) peer group are encouraged. The most difficult aspect is getting the patient to relinquish the eating-disordered lifestyle and achieve a normal non-AN (healthy) lifestyle.

The mainstay of FBT is to restore weight by using the family to take control over the young person's eating. The focus is not on exploring the aetiological factors that may or may not be responsible for the onset of the disorder. Once a healthy weight has been achieved, wider developmental and emotional concerns are able to be addressed.

Monitoring parameters

A target weight must be calculated for each patient, based on their height (measured with a stadiometer), their premorbid weight, their current weight (many units weigh patients in their underwear, wearing a gown, post-passing urine in the toilet and before eating/drinking, checking for hidden weights and performing an ultrasound of the bladder to subtract the volume of urine), their previous maximum weight and their minimum weight, and their Tanner staging. The target weight will need ongoing revision, until epiphyseal fusion. Some patients, when they become aware of their target weight, have the uncanny ability to produce that number when on the scales. Most units specify a target weight range.

Food and eating

Any appeal that food may have had has usually gone by the time a patient with AN commences eating; previous positive feedback from the smell and taste of food are almost eradicated by severe weight loss and food deprivation. Oral eating is encouraged.

Nasogastric feeding is only used for medically unstable patients. Most units offer three meals and three snacks a day and may safely refeed at 10 000 KJ/day. In the initial phase, the goal is to achieve a weight gain of at least 1 kg a week.

Measurement of electrolytes for refeeding syndrome should occur daily for the first week. The website http://rcpsych.ac.uk gives access to MARSIPAN (MAnagement of Really SIck Patients with Anorexia Nervosa) guidelines for refeeding.

The patients may well complain of fullness and bloating after eating; these feelings eventually resolve. A very rare complication of refeeding is the superior mesenteric artery syndrome, where the patient complains of chronic abdominal pain and feeling full after a meal, with subsequent vomiting, which can be due to compression of the superior mesenteric bundle and the third part of the duodenum (which is no longer protected by the fat pad around the bundle, the fat pad having disappeared).

Bone disease

Patients with AN have low bone density, increased bone fragility and increased risk of fractures, including stress fractures. Patients should have their bone density measured by DXA annually. DXA assesses the femoral neck, the lumbar spine and the forearms, and can also assess body composition—the body's proportion of bone mineral (calcium), lean body mass (muscle) and fat. Low bone density is caused by the combination of low weight, low hormonal levels such as oestrogen and inadequate nutrient intake, specifically calcium.

Prescription of the contraceptive pill has not been helpful in restoring bone. However, in 2011, a RCT showed treatment with physiological doses of oestrogen (given as patches) and progesterone improved bone density. Most units prefer patients to have between four and six serves of dairy a day (the recommendation for healthy adolescents is five serves a day). Resolution of AN may not lead to resolution of osteopenia.

Long-term effects on physical health

Long-term effects include some irreversible medical consequences, especially affecting the skeleton and teeth, the brain and the reproductive systems. Growth retardation, osteopenia and osteoporosis in the lumbar spine and proximal femur can occur within 12 months and can progress to produce fractures, kyphoscoliosis and chronic pain. Bone density is variably restored by weight gain.

Prognosis

In comparison to adults with established AN, adolescents with AN generally have a more optimistic course with about two-thirds making a complete recovery. Those with a shorter duration of illness at the time of accessing clinical services (e.g. less than 1 year) generally have a better outcome.

There is a distinct mortality rate in adults with long-standing AN, usually due to suicide or secondary to the metabolic, electrolyte or cardiac derangements of AN. The mortality rate of adolescents with AN who are receiving treatment is very low. Prolonged malnutrition can lead to osteopenia, osteoporosis, pubertal delay and growth failure.

LONG CASE: Attention deficit hyperactivity disorder (ADHD)

Introduction

A child with attention deficit hyperactivity disorder (ADHD) as the primary problem is an infrequent long-case subject, but many children with chronic conditions have ADHD symptomatology within their problem list. The criteria for ADHD have been modified by the publication of the DSM-5. ADHD is considered a dyad of symptoms involving: 1. inattention; and 2. hyperactivity and impulsivity. There are subtypes within the ADHD diagnosis: the inattentive subtype comprises 20–30%, the hyperactive-impulsive subtype comprises 15%, with the remaining 50–75% of patients having the combined subtype. ADHD is known as hyperkinetic disorder in countries which use the WHO's International Classification of Diseases diagnostic criteria (this includes all of Europe).

A genetic predisposition is well described, with twin studies demonstrating a mean heritability of around 75%. The investigational armamentarium for ADHD in any child with additional developmental delay, or autistic features, now includes as first-line treatment chromosomal microarray analysis (CMA), which can detect submicroscopic genomic deletions and duplications or copy-number variants (CNVs) smaller than 5 megabases (Mb). Whole exome sequencing (WES) can be used also.

Online Mendelian Inheritance in Man (OMIM) describes several conditions considered to cause susceptibility to ADHD (MIM#143465). Loci include: ADHD1 (MIM%608903; at 16p13), ADHD2 (MIM%608904; at 17p11), ADHD3 (MIM%608905; at 6q12), ADHD4 (MIM%608906; at 5p13), ADHD5 (MIM%612311; at 2q21.1), ADHD6 (MIM%612312; at 13q12.11), ADHD7 (MIM#613003; at 12q21.1, gene TPH2 [tryptophan hydroxylase 2; this is the rate-limiting enzyme in serotonin synthesis]), gene DRD4 (dopamine receptor D4) at 11p15.5, gene DRD5 at 4p16.1, gene SLC6A3 (which codes for dopamine transporter, DAT) at 5p15.33, gene SNAP25 (synaptosomal-associated protein, 25-KD) at 20p12.2 and gene HTR1B (serotonin 5-HT-1B receptor) at 6q14.1.

Summarising, this linkage analysis data suggests involvement of the following chromosomes: 2, 4, 5, 6, 8, 11, 12, 13, 16, 17 and 20. Association with ADHD has been described in mutations of genes which encode: the dopamine transporter (DAT), the enzyme tryptophan hydroxylase 2 (TPH2), dopamine receptors D4 and D5, the serotonin transporter gene, the synaptosomal-associated protein 25-KD and the serotonin 5-HT-1B receptor.

There is clear evidence that methylphenidate and dexamphetamine are highly effective for treating the symptoms of ADHD in the short term. Improvements in long-term academic or behavioural outcome have not been established, but previous concerns about cardiovascular side effects of stimulants have been re-analysed and modified. Stimulants are not recommended in preschoolers.

Globally, the prevalence of ADHD diagnoses is around 5% of children, and about 2.5% of adults. In the United States (US), ADHD is diagnosed in 8–11% of children aged 3 to 17 years; it may be more common in African American children and less common in Hispanic children. ADHD is more frequent in males, in a ratio of between 2:1 and 10:1 (the latter in outpatients seen in a clinic setting, more likely populated with disruptive boys). Girls are more likely to have the inattentive subtype and less comorbidities (oppositional defiant disorder, conduct disorder) but more likely to have co-existent anxiety and learning difficulties. ADHD is more likely to be diagnosed in children from families living in poverty, those with lower income and those of lower socioeconomic class, and this condition may be a factor that places them in poverty. Many studies, including the British Longitudinal Cohort study, show an increased incidence of housing, drug, employment and parenting issues in the ADHD population.

Independent of parental ADHD, exposure to cigarettes and alcohol in utero increases the risk of ADHD. Of all 'environmental' factors, those with the strongest evidence for an association with ADHD are low birthweight and maternal smoking. Children diagnosed with ADHD are likely to have social and academic impairments and low self-esteem. Having ADHD is associated with increased risk of academic failure, early school drop-out, delinquency, substance abuse, traffic accidents and criminal offences. Less than 10% of children diagnosed as having ADHD do not respond to stimulants or cannot tolerate them due to adverse side effects. Atomoxetine, a non-stimulant medication, is used widely, as are longer-lasting stimulant medications, but is generally considered to be less effective than the psychostimulants.

The aims of this long-case section, as well as of the subsequent short-case section, are as follows:

- To give a practical guide to the management of children diagnosed as having ADHD by the DSM-5 or hyperkinetic disorder by ICD-10. This section follows the DSM-5.
- To enable diagnosis of conditions that can be misinterpreted as ADHD.
- To enable the candidate to define not only that symptoms are present (to fulfil criteria) and to exclude relevant differential diagnoses, but also to define the developmental predicament—which areas of development are adversely affected by ADHD self-control problems.
- To provide clear guidelines regarding the use of stimulants, including dosage and timing recommendations, side effects, contraindications and appropriate follow-up.
- To enable the candidate to articulate a long-term management program based on routine regular visits to the paediatrician, developmental and mental health optimisation, and a plan to eventually get the child off medication (akin to epilepsy management).

The candidate needs to understand that ADHD involves neuropathology which can be lifelong. There needs to be a long-term management structure such as we would regard as routine for other chronic conditions such as diabetes or cystic fibrosis, and is a condition which can have a huge impact on family function, especially when there is associated oppositional defiant disorder (ODD) and executive function issues.

Background information

Few diagnostic labels have caused as much unhelpful and misguided media controversy and divergence of opinion as ADHD. Despite different rates of diagnosis in different countries, similar prevalence rates are reported across different cultures when standard diagnostic criteria are applied rigorously. Traditionally, ADHD is diagnosed very commonly in the US, where the American Academy of Child and Adolescent Psychiatry (AACAP) produced a Practice Parameter for ADHD management in 2007; this states:

Although scientists and clinicians debate the best way to diagnose and treat ADHD, there is no debate among competent and well-informed healthcare professionals that ADHD is a valid neurobiological condition that causes significant impairment in those whom it afflicts.

ADHD is diagnosed less frequently in Europe including the United Kingdom (UK). Diagnosis rates within Australia are somewhere in-between the US and European rates, although attitudes are rapidly changing with a decrease in use of the less helpful term 'hyperkinesis' (still used in many countries) and an increase in use of the term 'ADHD'.

There is still uncertainty as to whether ADHD represents the dysfunctional end of a continuum of normal temperamental characteristics or whether it represents a discrete qualitatively different biological or psychological condition.

The name for this behavioural syndrome has changed over the years, from labels that were unpopular with parents ('minimal brain damage') to 'minimal brain dysfunction', 'hyperkinetic child syndrome', 'minimal cerebral dysfunction', 'psycho-organic syndrome of childhood', to 'attention deficit disorder' (ADD) and finally 'attention deficit hyperactivity disorder' (ADHD), which has been the most widely accepted term in the US and Australasia, although as mentioned earlier throughout Europe it has been known as 'hyperkinetic syndrome'.

There is no single diagnostic test for ADHD. The DSM-5 sets out the criteria grouped under the following headings:

- Symptoms of inattention that are maladaptive and inconsistent with developmental level.
- Symptoms of hyperactivity and impulsivity that are maladaptive and inconsistent with developmental level.
- Age of onset criteria that specify that symptoms need to be present before age 12 years.
- Some impairment from the symptoms present in at least two settings (e.g. at school and at home).
- Clear evidence of clinically significant impairment in social or academic functioning.
- The symptoms must not occur exclusively during a psychotic disorder (such as schizophrenia) or be better explained by another mental disorder (such as bipolar disorder, personality disorder, anxiety, substance intoxication or withdrawal). The presentation is further specified as either **combined** (if both inattention and hyperactivity-impulsivity are met for the last 6 months), **predominantly inattentive** or **predominantly hyperactive-impulsive**. Other specifications noted include whether **in partial remission**, and current severity of impairment in social or occupational functioning (**mild**, **moderate** or **severe**).

The criteria set out in the DSM-5 should be fulfilled, at the very least, before a diagnosis of ADHD is entertained. In the age of evidence-based medicine, some cynics note that the criteria used in the DSM-5 are described using terminology that is not entirely succinct; the words 'often' and 'some' figure strongly in the criteria, although they are not concise quantitative or even qualitative terms, but the meaning they impart is integral in the determination as to whether the criteria are met. However, the requirement that six or more of nine symptoms of inattention and/or six or more of the nine symptoms of hyperactivity/impulsivity must be 'often' present defines a group of children of primary school age statistically who are more deviant than 90% of other children the same age. There is some valid statistical basis for these terms. As for the exclusion criteria, accurate and comprehensive appraisal of childhood psychiatric diagnoses is beyond the comfort zone and/or professional scope of most paediatricians.

It would be overly simplistic to equate the symptoms of ADHD with the disability or problems experienced by the child with ADHD, or to equate successful symptom control with successful treatment. A two-step approach can be followed. The first step is to confirm that the symptoms are present, to fulfil the criteria and to exclude differential diagnoses. The second step is to assess the child's development pattern and ask whether the symptoms are a problem. It only becomes a disorder if the symptoms lead to developmental delays, or problems in other areas such as learning, social development, self-esteem, mental health, fine motor abilities and organisational skills. The candidate needs to define the developmental predicament: which areas of development are impacted on by the self-control problems seen in ADHD.

Comorbidities are common and are discussed later. However, the nature of the comorbidity can very much affect the clinical presentation, and the impact of the condition on the child and family. It can also can mask and blur the underlying diagnosis of ADHD.

Parents and health workers can get 'hung up' on whether a child has ADD or ADHD. This differentiation is unimportant. The hyperactivity in a child's condition does not alter the principles behind treatment, and is often the least of the family's problems. The hyperactivity in ADHD refers more to restlessness and increased minor motor function rather than 'swinging from the trees'. The condition does not refer to 'naughty children'. Children who destroy your office are not demonstrating the hyperactivity to which the 'H' in ADHD refers.

ADHD may be regarded as a spectrum disorder. Children with ADHD have varying degrees of the different characteristics that make up the condition, which include inattention, impulsivity, overactivity, insatiability, disorganisation and social clumsiness.

One of the difficulties of diagnosis is that all children can have the characteristics comprising the diagnostic criteria to some degree. Most 3 year olds could comfortably meet all the criteria. The difficulty is in determining when these characteristics become pathological or at the severe end of normal development, and are causing impairment. These characteristics may lead to difficulties in learning, social interaction and behaviour. The home environment may accentuate the severity of subsequent symptoms and difficulties with which children and their families have to deal. Poor parenting skills are not the cause of true ADHD, but they may well exacerbate matters.

For the strict clinical diagnosis of ADHD, refer to the ICD-10 and DSM-5 criteria. Confusion in the diagnosis can result from difficulty in differentiating other disorders that can cause inattention and hyperactivity, and in identifying comorbid diagnoses. A comprehensive differential diagnosis is listed in the short-case section. It includes the normal, active preschool child, autism spectrum disorder, conduct disorder, ODD, reaction to social problems/environment (poor parenting skills, disruptive family dynamics), expressive language disorders, giftedness, hearing impairment and epilepsy syndromes (e.g. childhood absence epilepsy).

Comorbid diagnoses include the following:

- Specific learning difficulties (SLD).
- Conduct disorder (repetitive, persistent pattern of behaviour, where the basic rights of others or major age-appropriate societal norms or rules are violated; see the DSM-5).
- ODD, a pattern of negativistic, hostile, defiant behaviour (see the DSM-5).
- Anxiety, depression, OCD, tics.
- Poor fine motor and gross motor function.
- Expressive language delay.
- Autism spectrum disorders.

It has been hypothesised that there is a delay in maturation of inhibitory processes in the brain; this presents a useful working model of this condition. A loss of inhibition could explain decreased ability to concentrate, impulsive behaviour and motor hyperactivity. Children with ADHD have similar problems to children with frontal lobe deficits (problems with executive functions). A delay in functional cortical maturation of the frontal lobes has been hypothesised, with some support from some preliminary research studies of non-invasive functional MRI (fMRI) and quantitative EEG (QEEG), although these tests are not useful clinical tools at present.

The frequency of diagnosis varies between countries. In some states of the US, over 25% of boys are taking stimulant medication for ADHD. In Australia, it has been estimated to affect between 1 and 5% of the population. Difficulty arises in diagnosis because the condition is considered a delay in maturation of normal learning processes. Poor short-term memory, lack of concentration, impulsiveness and hyperactivity are all normal in a child at 3 years of age. By age 5–7, however, these characteristics are usually controlled. This is the reason why many kindergarten and primary school teachers describe these children as immature. Approximately 95% of children will be capable of controlling these characteristics by 5–7 years of age. Although parents, teachers and health professionals seem quite comfortable with the concept of a spectrum of developmental *motor* function (some normal children walk at 10 months, others at 18 months), any apparent delay within the spectrum of the (normal) development of *learning* engenders great concern. It should help to remember that the brain is continually growing, doubling in size in the first 12 months of life, with neuronal growth occurring throughout adolescence and adult life. Obviously, this growth and development will not occur at the same rate in all children.

Children with ADHD tend to have selective concentration. They can become obsessive in concentration if the situation or task interests them, such as a video game or television, but are unable to concentrate on a task of no specific interest.

These children have difficulty concentrating in a group situation. It is as if they are unable to filter information coming into the brain from sight, hearing and/or touch; they may be unable to differentiate, for example, between the teacher talking, the birds singing outside and little Johnny dropping his pencil in the classroom. All this sensory information appears to be presented to the brain at the same level of importance. In a mature learning system, the brain is able to sift and differentiate, excluding useless information and only processing what is important at the time. It is important not to be put off the diagnosis of ADHD because the child can concentrate on things interesting to him/her, but to assess whether or not, on the basis of the feedback available, the child is able to focus on the less interesting and whether this is problematic.

Parents will often describe their child with ADHD as bright, but lacking concentration and persistence in a task, and usually relatively underachieving. Children with ADHD tend to have poor organisational skills, be argumentative and impulsive, tend not to read body language well and make poor eye contact. Some will be said to display poor 'eye–hand coordination'; cynics also dislike, and question the usefulness of, this term, pointing out that most of the central nervous system is interposed between the eye and the hand. These children may have difficulty with reading and writing. If one considers the sensory–motor processing required for these two functions, it is not surprising. Most parents will report that these children respond well to a one-on-one learning situation.

The age at diagnosis often reflects the difficulty these children are having, and the likely difficulty the physician will experience in their management. They may present in the early years of schooling with poor behaviour, lack of concentration, fidgetiness and impulsiveness. These characteristics may be described by teachers as immature behaviour. For some children, this leads to poor school performance and loss of self-esteem, and worsening general behaviour. Other children's problems are not recognised until they reach secondary school, when poor organisational skills result in decreased work performance and subsequent loss of self-esteem. The workload is difficult because they have not obtained the basic building blocks/foundations in their education. In this situation, some children may present with depression or symptoms of chronic lethargy. Disruptive behaviour in the classroom may develop as an avoidance technique.

Developments in ADHD management

Recent evidence-based data has emerged that is challenging the way this condition has been managed previously. Important studies have been released, which have called into question several aspects of typical stimulant prescribing and use. There has been debate for years as to whether short-term effects of stimulants lead to any long-term benefits; so far there has been a paucity of well-designed studies to answer this issue. Some studies show academic improvement in the short term, but benefits gone by 3 years; some show no effect of stimulant use on academic outcomes, and some have found long-term academic gains, particularly in mathematics.

THE RAINE STUDY

Long-term outcomes associated with stimulant medication in treating children with ADHD have been evaluated in the Western Australian Pregnancy Birth Cohort (Raine) Study, which is a unique ongoing longitudinal study following 2868 children, with data collection since 1989, and with data at 1, 2, 3, 5, 8, 10, 14 and 17 years of age. Of the 1785 adolescents in the sample, 131 (7.3%) had received a diagnosis of ADHD. The demographics are as follows: 75.6% males (versus 48.95% male in non-ADHD), 22% lower-income families (versus 12.0% of non-ADHD diagnosed), 14.6% mothers under 20 years (versus 8.8% non-ADHD), 18% did not have the biological father living in same house at the time of birth (versus 9.4% of non-ADHD). Of the 131 with ADHD, 16% reported stimulant use at all three follow-up points (8, 10 and 14 years), 32.1% at two follow-up points, 29.8% at one follow-up point and 22.1% no use of stimulants at any follow-up point.

Outcome measures at 14 years of age included social, emotional, educational, physical and cardiovascular aspects. This study found that: there were no significant differences based on medication use for depression, self-perception and social functioning; there was no effect of stimulants on depressive symptoms; there was poorer self-perception in children diagnosed with ADHD (versus non-ADHD), with no effect from stimulant exposure on adolescent self-perception profile; and there was a lower level of social functioning within children diagnosed with ADHD, with no effect of stimulant exposure on the social functioning score.

Regarding academic performance, of the ADHD children 49.4% were performing 'below age level' according to their teacher, whereas 16.5% of non-ADHD were performing below age level, and school enjoyment levels were lower in ADHD children, which was not altered by stimulants. Regarding physical effects, there were no significant differences in average weight or height (at age 14) when comparing children consistently receiving medication to those never medicated.

Children who received stimulants consistently at all time points had significantly greater diastolic blood pressure than children who never had stimulants (10.79 mmHg greater); these children also had higher diastolic blood pressure than children who currently received stimulants but not previously (7.05 mmHg higher). On parent-rated measures, externalising behaviour and attentional problems did not change between the ages of 5 and 14, irrespective of whether or not medication was given.

Of course, the major limitation of this study is that children with ADHD were not randomised to stimulant medication treatment or non-treatment. Those treated with stimulants are likely to have more severe problems at onset than those not treated with stimulants. Comparing outcomes at adolescence is therefore highly questionable, and certainly not indicative that stimulant medication treatment has no positive impact on symptoms in the long term. Most clinicians consider that carefully fine-tuned management, involving not only medication where appropriate, but also other supports, has a beneficial effect. However, the transition between childhood and adulthood needs to be managed very carefully to achieve optimal long-term results. There is often a problem at this interface in service delivery.

It is highly unlikely that a long-term RCT of treatment versus no treatment will ever be conducted to answer this question.

The question of medication-induced cardiac effects

In 2017 this question has been answered. Healthy children without an underlying cardiac diagnosis do **not** have an increased risk of a serious cardiovascular event when taking stimulants, and do not require an ECG or an echocardiogram. However, children with a preexisting cardiac diagnosis, or symptoms that suggest a cardiac diagnosis in the child or the family, should be referred to a cardiologist before considering a trial of stimulants.

The American Heart Association (AHA) has noted that certain cardiac diagnoses are associated with an increased risk of ADHD, including hypoplastic left heart survivors (two-thirds have attention deficits), patients with 22q11 micro-deletion (35–55% have ADHD symptomatology) and patients with total anomalous pulmonary venous drainage (50% have ADHD symptomatology); in these children, there could be an increased risk of cardiovascular complications.

For any children with ADHD without a known cardiac diagnosis, before prescribing stimulants the AHA recommends taking a thorough cardiac history, including a comprehensive family history, and cardiovascular examination. The particular conditions to be uncovered are those that increase the risk of sudden cardiac death (SCD). SCD has three main groups of causes: cardiomyopathies, primary electrical disease and congenital heart disease (especially cyanotic or repaired). A more comprehensive list is as follows (mnemonic: **ABCD HELPs WPWMarfan**):

Arrhythmogenic right ventricular dysplasia
Brugada syndrome
Coronary artery anomalies
Dilated cardiomyopathy

Hypertrophic cardiomyopathy (HCM)
Ex-cardiac surgery (especially TGA, TOF, HLHS, AS, ASD, AV canal)
Long QT syndrome (LQTS)
Pulmonary hypertension/**P**rimary ventricular fibrillation or tachycardia

Wolff–**P**arkinson–**W**hite syndrome
Marfan's syndrome

The Royal Australasian College of Physicians (RACP) and the National Health and Medical Research Council (NHMRC) made available draft Australian ADHD Guidelines on 30 November 2009. These draft guidelines, however, were not endorsed by the NHMRC because of conflict of interest sanctions declared against one of the US-based researchers highly referenced in that document. Concerns about compromised research are serious in all areas of medicine, and particularly so in ADHD research. Subsequent to this, many critics have raised issues regarding the validity of much of the published ADHD material, with an emerging concern that research into ADHD interventions may be too unreliable to afford useful guidance.

Critics of ADHD research point out the following areas of concern: there is a population bias towards boys aged 6–12 years (although 50% of children diagnosed fall outside of that group); outcome measures lack consistency; follow-up on medication interventions are very brief (usually under a month); almost all studies have small sample sizes; many studies compare psychosocial interventions with pharmacological interventions (it is difficult to compare such different modalities of treatment).

In 2012 the NHMRC published 'Clinical practice points on the diagnosis, assessment and management of ADHD in children and adolescents'. This is very useful for candidates, and could be used as a major reference for the management of ADHD, as it is very comprehensive and well written. It is available at http://nhmrc.gov.au.

History
PRESENTING COMPLAINT
Reason for current admission/presentation for the examination.

CURRENT SYMPTOMS
1. *Inattention.* Failure to attend to details, careless mistakes in schoolwork, difficulty sustaining attention in tasks or play activities, not seeming to listen, not following through on instructions, failing to finish schoolwork, difficulty organising tasks, avoiding tasks requiring sustained mental effort, losing things necessary for tasks, easily distracted, forgetful in daily activities; note duration.
2. *Hyperactivity.* Fidgeting, squirming in seat, leaving seat when should be seated, running or climbing excessively, 'on the go', talking excessively.
3. *Impulsivity.* Blurting out answers before questions completed, difficulty awaiting turn, interrupting or intruding on others.
4. *Comorbid problems.*
   - Symptoms of *conduct disorder*: aggression to people or animals (e.g. bullying, using a weapon, cruelty to animals or people), destruction of property (e.g. lighting fires), deceitfulness, theft, violation of rules.
   - Symptoms of *oppositional defiant disorder*: negativistic, hostile, defiant behaviour—losing temper, arguing with or defying adults, deliberately annoying people, blaming others for mistakes, touchy or easily annoyed by others, angry, spiteful.
   - Learning disabilities: difficulties at school with writing, reading, spelling and arithmetic.
   - Minor motor problems: clumsiness, lack of ball-game skills.
   - Depression/anxiety/tics.

PAST HISTORY

Previous therapies tried, previous medication tried, past medical investigations (e.g. serum ferritin, psychometric testing, audiology, EEG).

Birth history

Pregnancy complications, gestational age, mode of delivery, Apgar score, resuscitation required, birthweight, need for oxygen, nursery care, neonatal period, any intracranial pathology (e.g. neonatal encephalopathy in term baby, intraventricular haemorrhage in premature infants, periventricular leukomalacia, hydrocephalus).

Developmental history

Age at which milestones achieved.

Family history

Any family history of ADHD or specific learning difficulties (SLD).

Current management

Usual medication at home, stimulants (e.g. dexamphetamine, methylphenidate) used currently or previously, other drugs (e.g. antidepressants, clonidine), dosage regimen, side effects noted (e.g. stimulants may cause decreased appetite, insomnia, rebound moodiness, irritability or hyperactivity), any therapies (e.g. occupational therapy), school issues (e.g. any school assistance, where the desk is positioned in the classroom—hopefully not next to a hyperactive twin, or at the back where the teacher cannot see the child), psychosocial interventions (e.g. behavioural therapies, educational tutoring), professionals seen (e.g. local doctor, psychologists, paediatricians, psychiatrists), activities to promote concentration and self-discipline (e.g. martial arts), alternative therapies tried (e.g. homeopathic preparations), educational internet resources.

SOCIAL HISTORY

Impact of condition on parents, siblings, friends, children in their class at school, family financial situation (e.g. private health insurance, cost of stimulant medications, visits to multiple professionals, government benefits received), social supports (e.g. social worker, extended family, respite care, ADHD parent groups).

Understanding of problems and prognosis

By parents, degree of education regarding ADHD, consideration of ongoing stimulant medication into adulthood, realistic career/occupational choices (e.g. not wise to try for air traffic controller).

Examination

See the short-case section in this chapter.

Teacher report

A report from the teacher, outlining the child's academic and social strengths and weaknesses, can be extremely useful in further assessment of the child's performance. Allowing the teacher to write a freehand report provides useful information, and gives the physician insight into the teacher's understanding of the child's problems. Teacher reports are necessary for clinical diagnosis, and are an extension of examination, rather than additional investigations.

Rating scales

These are also an extension of the examination. The most widely used scales in the US are the Conners rating scales, which include a parent questionnaire and a teacher questionnaire. Other scales include the DuPaul ADHD rating scales, the child behaviour checklist (CBCL), the teacher report form (TRF), the youth self-report (YSR) described by Achenbach and Edelbrock, and the Rowe behavioural rating inventory scale, described by Rowe and Rowe.

Diagnosis of ADHD

There is no single diagnostic test for ADHD. For the diagnosis to be made, documentation is required of specific impairing symptoms of the disorder in at least two settings, according to the criteria set out in the current ICD-10 and DSM-5 diagnostic manuals. These criteria act as a guide, as do the various ADHD rating scales (see above) for parents, teachers and the child. A thorough clinical history is essential. The history may enable the exclusion of differential diagnoses (especially social causes) and the inclusion of comorbid conditions. The examination can be very rewarding in excluding ADHD impersonators (see the short-case section in this chapter). Several evaluation tools can be used, but no test commonly employed by school-based psychologists (such as the Wechsler Intelligence Scales) can distinguish children with ADHD from normal children, with any reliability.

EDUCATIONAL AUDIOLOGY ASSESSMENT

An educational audiology assessment allows documentation of auditory processing, and may reveal difficulties with short-term auditory processing and hearing in association with competing background noise. A standard audiology assessment is of limited assistance.

EDUCATIONAL PSYCHOLOGY ASSESSMENT

Assessment by an educational psychologist is essential. This may well reveal that the child has a normal or high IQ. It will also help to identify children with specific learning difficulties and/or a low IQ; it will assess difficulties with concentration and spatial orientation, screen for ADHD characteristics and help to exclude conditions such as autism spectrum disorder. The Wechsler scale WISC-IV gives full IQ, verbal and performance IQ scores, and factors for freedom from distractibility plus speed of information processing.

DIAGNOSTIC INTERVIEWS

These are not recommended, but are mentioned for completeness. These semi-structured interviews are used particularly in a research setting. They include the Diagnostic Interview Schedule for Children (DISC-2C and DISC-2P), child and parent versions, the Diagnostic Interview for Children and Adolescents (DICA), and the Child Assessment Schedule (CAS). (Acronymophilia has been, and continues to be, rampant in scales and interviews concerned with ADHD.)

VIGILANCE TESTING

Again, note that these tests are not recommended. They aim to indicate an objective measurement for sustained attention. They include the Conners Continuous Performance Test (CCPT) and the Vigil Continuous Performance Test. The main problem is lack of standardisation or comparability.

EEG

It is not uncommon for children with ADHD and/or learning difficulties to have non-specific changes on EEG. Some clinics still perform quantitative EEGs, although these are not considered helpful by most clinicians. EEG will be useful to exclude *absence epilepsy* if this is suggested by the presentation.

OPHTHALMOLOGY EVALUATION

Standard eye examination is important to exclude visual deficits. In specific subgroups of children, further assessment of eye tracking and visual processing may be useful.

MISCELLANEOUS INVESTIGATIONS

Suspicion of other diagnoses should lead to the relevant investigations to exclude them (e.g. molecular genetic testing for fragile X syndrome, serum ferritin for iron deficiency, serum lead levels for lead toxicity, EEG [as above] for suspected absence epilepsy, overnight oxygen saturation or formal sleep studies for obstructive sleep apnoea impersonating as ADHD).

A number of functional neuro-imaging techniques have been used in evaluating ADHD, including positron emission tomography (PET), which measures glucose metabolism in areas of the brain concerned with attention processes; single-photon emission computed tomography (SPECT), which measures cerebral blood flow; functional magnetic resonance imaging (fMRI); and proton magnetic resonance spectroscopy (pMRS). There are differences in children with ADHD compared to control children in basal ganglia activation, frontal lobe activation and in cortico-striatal-thalamic connectivity. None of these, however, has established sensitivity or specificity, and none is recommended.

Management

Correct diagnosis is essential for appropriate management. It is important to establish that drug therapy is not the only option for treating this condition, although stimulant medication has been proved more effective than any form of behavioural therapy. Adolescent patients may gain sufficient understanding of their difficulties that they do not require drug treatment, but rather develop strategies to cope. There are children who will not respond to basic behavioural management/assisted teaching techniques without the use of medication.

A child with ADHD can have significant problems with communication, which may be exacerbated by the family's behaviour. Some households have the television turned on most of the day, and during dinner the children are asked to be quiet so that dad can listen to the news. Significant improvement in behaviour can be achieved simply by asking the family to turn the television off during dinner. Encouraging parents to learn how to communicate with, rather than talk at, their children, is important. While obvious to most physicians, this can be a startlingly new concept to many families. Adolescent patients in particular should not have a television in the bedroom. This will only lead to more reclusive behaviour and reinforce poor communication skills. One approach is to turn the television off after 6 p.m. and encourage the parents to help children with their homework, or alternatively play family games, which promote communication and learning to take one's turn. Simple techniques such as these can be effective in changing the child's behaviour. Most social skills and behaviour are learned at home, not at school.

SCHOOL STRATEGIES (EDUCATIONAL MANAGEMENT PRINCIPLES)

School difficulties are almost universal in children with ADHD. Specific problem areas may include mathematics, reading, writing or abstract thinking. Parents and teachers should be aware that these children may have difficulty with loud background noise. Short-term auditory processing is difficult, and the children need to be brought back on task. Instructions should be short, direct and repeated. Eye contact with the child is important when giving instructions. These children perform best in small classes.

Teachers who have a firm, fair, consistent teaching style will find that the student copes better. Some children with significant problems may need the assistance of an integration aide. Children with poor fine/gross motor coordination may need the assistance of occupational or physical therapy. Some children will have speech difficulties requiring speech therapy.

Tutoring on a one-to-one basis can help these children significantly. A good tutor can liaise with the teacher to document specific deficiencies in the child's knowledge base. It is important to ensure that, for each child, the proper foundation stones for their education are laid. This will enable them to go to the next step. As these children succeed, their self-esteem will improve markedly.

The areas of difficulty in the classroom can be divided into eight groups as follows, with three sample suggestions for each area:

1. *Inattention.* Maximise attention by: (a) seating the child at the front of class, near a good role model; (b) breaking longer assignments into smaller sections, so the child can see an endpoint to the work, and mastering material within his or her attention span; (c) pairing written instructions with oral instructions.
2. *Impulsiveness.* Counter this by: (a) complementing positive behaviour and increasing immediacy of rewards; (b) using time out for misbehaviour, avoiding lecturing or criticism; (c) supervising carefully at transition times.
3. *Motor activity.* Reduce overactivity by: (a) allowing the child to run errands that involve movement; (b) allowing the child to stand at times during schoolwork; (c) providing breaks between academic tasks.
4. *Socialisation.* Improve this by: (a) giving frequent praise to appropriate behaviour; (b) encouraging cooperative learning tasks with other children; (c) encouraging the child to take up an activity with supervised socialisation (e.g. sporting groups, scouts).
5. *Academic skills.* Overcome learning difficulties by: (a) organising remedial assistance for specific problem areas; (b) if mathematics is a problem, allowing a calculator, and providing additional time for maths; (c) if written language is weak, allowing non-written project submissions (using a tape recorder or a word processor).
6. *Mood.* Increase self-esteem by: (a) setting easily obtainable goals initially, then increasing the difficulty of tasks; (b) assisting the child to feel his or her contributions to the class are significant; (c) providing reassurance and encouragement.
7. *Compliance.* Increase compliance by: (a) seating the child near the teacher; (b) ignoring minor misbehaviour and reinforcing good behaviour; (c) recognising the positive behaviour of a child seated nearby.
8. *Organisational planning.* Help the child to follow instructions by: (a) checking homework assignments written down in a homework diary; (b) encouraging neatness but not criticising sloppiness; (c) encouraging the child to use notebooks with dividers and folders to organise schoolwork.

There are many internet-based resources available that help children with ADHD to improve their skills in mathematics, spelling, reading and abstract writing. Computerised learning techniques provide audiovisual reinforcement and allow the child to learn in a more efficient manner, and can be graded to the child's current ability.

Ideally, the above matters should be addressed before considering drug therapy. If the child is not responding to these techniques, then medication may be considered. While drugs are not a panacea in the management of a child's condition, if used appropriately they can be very helpful. Children require close supervision if medication is to be used; as the brain is continually developing, the response to medication may vary over time.

An understanding by the teacher of the true nature of ADHD, that it is an explanation, rather than an excuse, and that the use of medication is to make the child more available for learning, are all essential for effective school management.

MEDICATION

If drugs are used in a child with ADHD, the paediatrician (the candidate) managing the child needs to ensure that the drugs have treated the symptoms successfully. However, symptom treatment does not mean that the development will suddenly normalise. There is more to management than just knowing the drugs used and their side effects. The candidate should be able to delineate how the educational, social, behavioural and emotional problems are currently being managed to rehabilitate the child.

Stimulants

In concert with behavioural therapy, these are the mainstay of treatment for ADHD. Stimulants cause increased 'free brain levels' of noradrenaline and dopamine, by blocking their presynaptic neuronal reuptake and stimulating their release.

Controversy remains as to whether stimulants cause long-term growth suppression. A recent study (Multimodal Treatment Study of AD/HD [MTA]) showed at 3-year follow-up, in children with combined type ADHD, stimulant treatment was associated with 2 cm less height gain and 2.7 kg less weight gain. It is established that stimulant treatment does not result in substance abuse disorders during treatment, and their use most likely protects against developing substance abuse later in life. Stimulants may be short-acting (3–6 hours) or long acting (8–12 hours, which can be given once daily).

Short acting: dexamphetamine, methylphenidate (MPH)

The most widely used are dexamphetamine and methylphenidate (MPH). Dexmethylphenidate is the d-isomer of MPH and a newer preparation; it is more active than the l-isomer, has fewer side effects, requires half the standard MPH dose and lasts 4–6 hours. Dexamphetamine's mechanism of action involves increasing extracellular synaptic dopamine, inhibiting noradrenaline reuptake and exerting weak effects on the serotonin system. Its average duration of action is 5 hours and its half-life is 3–6 hours. MPH's mechanism is thought to involve selective binding of the presynaptic dopamine transporter (DAT) in striatal and prefrontal areas, with the effect of increasing extracellular dopamine levels, as does dexamphetamine. MPH also acts on the noradrenaline system by blocking the noradrenaline transporter; its average duration of action is around 3 hours and its half-life is 2–4 hours. The stimulant effect commences between 30 and 60 minutes after taking the dose.

Both medications have similar side-effect profiles, and in head-to-head trials neither appears to have an advantage over the other; each works in around 70% of children diagnosed with ADHD. In children with comorbid psychiatric disorders, stimulants may worsen the symptoms of the condition, especially in those with tic and mood disorders.

Dexamphetamine: dose range 0.2–1.0 mg/kg/day (usually 0.3–0.7 mg/kg/day; maximum 40 mg/day).

MPH: dose range 0.25–2.0 mg/kg/day (usually 0.3–0.7 mg/kg/day; maximum 60 mg/day).

The side-effect profiles for both drugs are similar: anorexia, weight loss (often 1–2 kg in the first 3 months), emotional lability, insomnia, social and emotional withdrawal, and occasional psychotic reaction. Most side effects are dose related. Both drugs have a good safety record.

In 2013, the US Food and Drug Administration (FDA) issued a warning that MPH products can rarely cause priapism, with painful erections lasting over 4 hours; the median age for this complication is 12.5 years (range 8–33 years). It is also a rare complication of dexamphetamine, and is also described with use of the non-stimulant drug atomoxetine (see overleaf), but has been under-recognised previously.

It is suggested that at first the dose is small (say, a morning dose of 5 mg), gradually increasing every 3–4 days to help reduce unwanted side effects. Generally, short-acting stimulant medication is best given two or three times a day. An afternoon dose at 3 p.m. often helps older children with their homework. Suggested dose times are with breakfast (7–8 a.m., to achieve therapeutic levels while in class during the morning), lunch (around 12 noon, to achieve therapeutic levels in class during the afternoon; often a smaller dose than at breakfast) and immediately after school (3–4 p.m., a smaller dose than at lunch, to avoid the phenomenon of rebound hyperactivity as that dose wears off; later or higher doses can lead to insomnia).

Long acting (8–12 hours): extended-release MPH tablets, long-acting MPH capsules, lisdexamfetamine dimesilate

These were developed because many children and adolescents do not like taking multiple daily doses of any drug; also, they dislike having attention drawn to them when they have to go to the school office for their medication. These can be given once daily.

MPH is available in Australasia as extended-release (ER) tablets or long-acting (LA) capsules. The ER tablets are available in strengths 18 mg, 36 mg and 54 mg, and last 12 hours. The LA capsules are available in strengths 20 mg, 30 mg and 40 mg, and last 8 hours. The MPH capsules contain 50% immediate-release and 50% sustained-release beads, allowing immediate release of MPH followed by a second delayed release of MPH. In the US, a transdermal patch form of MPH is available.

Lisdexamfetamine is a prodrug of dexamphetamine. It has a peak plasma concentration at 3.5 hours and lasts 12 hours. It is available in capsules of 30 mg, 50 mg or 70 mg.

Non-stimulants
Atomoxetine

This is a highly selective inhibitor of the presynaptic noradrenaline transporter, and is considered a first-line drug, as it is said to be as effective as the stimulants, although most clinicians in the field would not agree with this appraisal, and find it far less effective than stimulants.

Its efficacy is based on three double-blind, placebo-controlled studies. It can be used when parents are opposed to stimulant medication. It increases extracellular noradrenaline and dopamine levels in the prefrontal cortex. It is metabolised by cytochrome P450 2D6; drugs that inhibit this (such as selective serotonin reuptake inhibitors [SSRIs]) can increase levels and side effects of atomoxetine. Adverse effects include decrease in appetite, nausea, vomiting, fatigue, sedation, dizziness, mood swings and decreased growth velocity. The manufacturers have added a warning that atomoxetine can increase suicidality. It can also cause priapism, painful erections lasting over 4 hours, as can stimulants. Parents must be fully informed of all these potential side effects.

Clonidine (an alpha-2 noradrenergic agonist)

A second-line option, clonidine is not as effective as stimulants in ADHD, but can be useful if there is a comorbid tic disorder. It can cause loss of appetite, and sedation. Clonidine has been used for years, despite concerns about its efficacy and safety, to reduce impulsive behaviour, aggressive tendencies and oppositional-defiant symptoms. It has been used in combination with stimulants, as it allows a lower dosage of these medications to be used; there have been sporadic reports of death from this combination, however. One side effect of clonidine is drowsiness for 60–90 minutes, approximately 30 minutes after taking the tablet, which excludes its use as a morning dosage in children. The duration of behavioural effects is 3–6 hours (oral preparation). In the US, a patch form is available that can last 5 days. In patients in whom drowsiness is not a problem, it may be useful in a twice-daily dosage.

Nocturnal dosage of clonidine, with the side effect of drowsiness, counteracts the insomnia in patients that occurs with the stimulants dexamphetamine and methylphenidate, and can help in ADHD patients with primary sleep problems. Tics are not uncommon in children with ADHD, and it is now recognised that tics do not increase if these children receive stimulant medication; clonidine can be useful in the management of tics. Low doses are used in ADHD (1–3 µg/kg/dose). The Tourette's Syndrome Study Group reported a RCT that found that clonidine plus methylphenidate together lead to significant improvement in ADHD symptoms, tic severity and global functioning. The dosages of clonidine used in ADHD rarely affect blood pressure.

Parents must be told all the significant side effects of clonidine, including the cardiotoxicity of overdosage, and the uncommon but recognised complication of sudden discontinuation, which results in rebound hypertension. Other side effects include depression, dry mouth, hypotension (rare), confusion (with high doses) and local irritation with the transdermal form. Parents must be fully informed as to all the potential side effects of this alpha-2 noradrenergic agonist, including the several reports of death associated with the use of clonidine together with stimulants.

Other medications previously used: tricyclic antidepressants (TCAs; imipramine, desipramine), bupropion, venlafaxine

These are only mentioned here for completeness, as there are still occasional children encountered who are taking these. These drugs have been recommended as second-line options in the past, but now are rarely used as they are less effective and less safe than the stimulants, atomoxetine or clonidine.

TCAs had been used for decades. The mechanism of action of TCAs is to increase dopamine and noradrenaline levels in the brain. They may have potential benefits in children with ADHD and comorbid mood disorders, anxiety disorders and tic disorders, but they have **major potential cardiotoxicity**. Children who have not been coping well with ADHD can develop low self-esteem and depression. Rather than initiate antidepressant medication, it is preferable to address the specific problems of the child. If co-existing depression, sadness or anxiety are severe, then antidepressants may be warranted, and they may clarify thinking and improve concentration.

For ADHD without depression, antidepressants are rarely justified. As with clonidine, overdosages may be cardiotoxic (heart block and rhythm disturbances that, rarely, can be fatal). There have been reports of sudden, unexpected death in four children treated with desipramine. The author has encountered children admitted to paediatric intensive care units after an overdose of (inadvertent poisoning by) antidepressants, prescribed for 'ADHD' in children as young as 3 years of age, has been taken by the patient(s) themselves or by their friends or siblings, because no drug safety precautions were taken in the home. Antidepressants are much less popular with patients and parents than stimulants. Parents must be fully informed as to all the potential side effects of TCAs, including the cardiotoxicity.

Bupropion was another second-line option, an antidepressant that has indirect dopamine agonist and noradrenergic effects. It has been used for ADHD with comorbid depression. A significant side effect is **severe hypertension**; other side effects include insomnia, irritability and drug-induced seizures, particularly in adolescents with bulimia (in whom, thus, it is contraindicated). It is being used to help adult cocaine addicts who have ADHD and, in another formulation, is useful to help adult nicotine addicts stop smoking. It has been used in adolescents with ADHD and substance abuse who smoke, but has fallen out of favour because of its serious side effect profile.

Venlafaxine is a serotonin/noradrenaline reuptake inhibitor, another second-line drug, which has mainly been used to treat depression and anxiety disorders in adults. There has been interest in using it to treat adult ADHD with comorbid mood disorders. One study showed monotherapy with venlafaxine to be as efficacious as combined stimulant and antidepressant treatment. This study was in adults and cannot be generalised to children.

Melatonin

This hormone, produced by the pineal gland, is being used more frequently in recent years to enable children with ADHD to get to sleep. The common preparation available on prescription in Australasia has a dose of 2 mg, although doses from 0.5 mg to 5 mg have been used, with other preparations being available to buy over the internet. It has a far preferable, safer side-effect profile than other medications, such as clonidine, that have been used to initiate sleep in children with ADHD.

ALTERNATIVE TREATMENTS

The management of children diagnosed as having ADHD can be an emotional minefield. Parents at the end of their tether will try many and varied treatments, and any suggested 'cure' or quick fix will invariably lead some parents to try unorthodox treatments suggested by 'practitioners' of no fixed ability, representing a range of 'therapies'. Challenging this approach may damage the doctor–patient/parent relationship. While unusual 'therapies' can 'work' in children who do not really have ADHD, the fact remains that stimulants are the most effective treatment, but as long as there are desperate parents, there will be charlatans who will make money from treatments that have no scientific basis. Most alternative treatments are 'justified' by the suggestion that drug therapy will not be necessary; universally, their theoretical justification is inconsistent with current scientific knowledge. Included within the many non-traditional approaches are: optometric training, tinted lenses, megavitamins, patterning, kinaesthesiology, homeopathic substances to counter 'allergens', and sound therapy. Most of these therapies have not undergone controlled clinical trials, and their use is based on anecdotal testimony. The disadvantages to these approaches include high cost, wasting valuable time, delay in commencing recognised treatments, and damage to self-esteem caused by suggestions that the child's eyes, brain or ability to handle food are abnormal.

Diet has been suggested as a cause of ADHD. To date, many diets have been tried without success. The picture here is somewhat cloudy, as there are some children who appear to become hyperactive when exposed to certain food dyes or preservatives. This phenomenon is seen in normal children as well as in children with ADHD, but the behavioural changes are somewhat exacerbated in children with ADHD. Most parents are aware of changes in their child's behaviour when exposed to these foods (e.g. tomato sauce, chocolate and various types of 'junk food'). Rather than adopting specialist restrictive diets, the best approach is to keep a simple food diary to identify the particular culprit and then restrict this from the diet. Despite some mythology about sugar (quote from one parent, 'He can't have sugar, it sends him hypo! He had it once, he went mad for a week!'), sugar is never the culprit.

Prognosis

If ADHD can be considered a delay in the normal maturational processes of a developing brain—in particular, the frontal cortex and its connections—then there is an analogy with the maturational delay in nocturnal enuresis; as occurs in children with nocturnal enuresis, the problem may continue into adulthood. Many children either grow out of their ADHD (myelination in the frontal lobes is not completed until adolescence) or, as adults, learn to cope with the specific characteristics that cause them difficulty. As the condition is dynamic rather than static, children with this condition require regular review.

It is not appropriate to prescribe medication and see the child once or twice a year for renewal of the prescription. It is more appropriate to follow them on a minimum 3-monthly basis to assess both social and academic progress.

During adolescence, which is often a difficult time for any child, patients may require more frequent follow-up. It is not uncommon for the adolescent patient to require a decrease in stimulant dosage. Always ask about **HEADS**: **H**ome, **E**ducation and Employment, **A**lcohol and Activities, **D**rugs, **S**exuality and Suicide/depression. Assessment of drug effect/side effects/compliance is critical, along with assessment of sleep patterns, growth/eating habits and blood pressure if taking medication.

Children with ADHD and comorbid conduct disorder represent a poor prognostic group. It is not uncommon for these children to leave school at an early age. Children with poorly controlled conduct disorder have a high probability of being in trouble with the law by the age of 21 years (in reality, it is usually much earlier). Sometimes the best that can be achieved for these children is the teaching of life skills. They are often not candidates for stimulant medication, as it is usually abused with other drugs or sold for money. Principles for life skills include the teaching of budgeting, communication skills and organisational skills. If taught to budget, then these children are less likely to resort to unlawful means of obtaining money. Good communication skills may allow them to cope within the workforce and can increase the likelihood of establishing a stable relationship with a spouse.

Above all, candidates need to recognise the reality of the family and child dysfunction caused by ADHD and put this across in the long case, with an understanding of the harm it does, and the importance of using carefully fine-tuned medications together with the most appropriate other non-medical, evidence-based interventions to support the child and the family.

LONG CASE: Autism spectrum disorder (ASD)

Since the publication of the DSM-5, ASD is now considered a dyad of impairments, involving (a) defects in reciprocal social interaction; and (b) repetitive, restricted, stereotyped behaviours and interests. Speech delay per se is no longer a separate major diagnostic criterion. The previous individual domains of social and language impairment have been merged into the single domain of impaired social communication and social interactions. Within ASD, there is a range from mild eccentricities to severe developmental disabilities. Increased emphasis on earlier diagnosis of children with ASD stems from consensus that early intensive behavioural interventions are likely to be beneficial to children with ASD. Twin and family studies infer that most ASD arises from genetic factors, although more recent studies have reduced the heritability from 90% to 50% of variance.

The investigational armamentarium now includes, as first-line treatment, CMA, which can detect submicroscopic genomic deletions and duplications or CNVs smaller than 5 megabases (Mb). Increasingly, whole exome sequencing (WES) is used as well. If children with ASD, and no preexisting known genetic diagnosis, undergo both CMA and WES, a genetic cause is uncovered in around 16%.

The term 'ASD' replaces (and includes) the previous diagnoses of classic autism and its milder 'variants' such as Asperger's syndrome and pervasive developmental disorder—not otherwise specified (PDD-NOS). This section deals with the more severe end of the autism spectrum. The new diagnosis in DSM-5 for milder cases is social communication disorder.

There are a limited number of medications which can be useful in autism, although strictly their role is in the treatment of comorbid psychiatric disorders. These include: clonidine, an indirect noradrenergic blocker, methylphenidate (MPH, a noradrenaline-dopamine reuptake inhibitor), risperidone (a dopamine D2 receptor blocker), aripiprazole (a dopamine D2 receptor partial agonist), fluvoxamine and fluoxetine (both being SSRIs). In any child with a developmental disorder or abnormal brain there is a reduced rate of efficacy compared with a mainstream population and an increase in the rate of side effects. However, the secondary disability from the comorbid mental health problem and the lack of alternative psychological interventions makes their need for psychotropic medication greater.

Clonidine acts for 4 hours, and at 25 μg is valuable as a treatment for anxiety and overarousal, a second-line adjuvant treatment for ADHD and at higher doses it provides sleep initiation. It can be useful as needed for agitation and aggression, and on occasion it can be valuable to complete a consultation. It is water soluble and can be used flexibly to anticipate stressful situations (maximum of 350 μg in 24 hours). MPH can decrease hyperactivity, but less so than in neurotypical children, and at the expense of increased sensitivity to side effects which can include social withdrawal, increased anxiety and stereotypic behaviour or thinking and irritability and aggression. Risperidone can decrease irritability and improve restricted repetitive behaviours, but has no effect on social or communication difficulties; its use is limited by adverse effects (weight gain, drowsiness, prolactinaemia and tremor). Aripiprazole, which is used in the US, can lead to improvements in the Aberrant Behavior Checklist and in the Clinical Global Impression rating scale and improve irritability and aggression. Fluvoxamine may lead to decrease in repetitive thoughts/behaviours and improve language (remember flu**v**oxamine affects **v**oice/**v**erbal [i.e. language]. Fluoxetine can lead to a decrease in repetitive behaviours or OCD symptoms (remember flu**o**xetine affects **O**CD). The latter two SSRI drugs may have these positive effects at the expense of an increase in agitation, hostility and even suicidal ideation. The risk of behavioural activation is greater in those with developmental problems.

The aims of this long-case section are as follows:

- To give a practical guide to the management of children diagnosed as having ASD by correctly interpreted criteria of the DSM-5 or of the ICD-10 (to be replaced by the ICD-11, when it is released in 2018). This section follows the DSM-5 and discusses the classic severe end of the autism spectrum.
- To enable diagnosis of conditions that can be misinterpreted as autism (which can be a pitfall in the environment of increased diagnoses of 'ASD').
- To clarify which potential aetiological factors have some evidence, and which do not but receive adverse publicity, to counter much misinformation in the lay press.
- To give clear guidelines regarding therapies for which there is evidence of efficacy and therapies for which there is insufficient evidence to support their use. Autism is an area in which 'complementary' and 'alternative' medical therapies (CAM) are widely used. While parents appreciate their doctor's support for their use of their chosen CAM, it is also important to caution them against therapies that could have significant detrimental effects on their child's health (and on their finances). False unrealistic hope is also harmful, and deters families from seeking evidence-based treatments that promote development but which may be in short supply.

Background information

Autism is a very heterogeneous disorder. The prevalence of ASD is around 1 in 100; although some studies suggest up to 1 in 64. There is a male predominance. There seems to have been a rise in prevalence, partially due to changed criteria that include milder forms within the spectrum of autism, and partially due to increased recognition by both the public and professionals. There is no single diagnostic test for ASD. The DSM-5 sets out the diagnostic criteria for ASD grouped under five headings as follows:

1. Symptoms of impaired social communication/social interaction. These can include impaired non-verbal behaviours (e.g. eye-to-eye gaze), failure to develop peer relationships, lack of seeking to share (e.g. interests) and lack of emotional reciprocity.
2. Symptoms of restricted, repetitive behaviours and stereotyped behaviour patterns. These can include preoccupation with restricted patterns of interest, inflexible adherence to specific rituals, stereotyped repetitive motor mannerisms and persistent preoccupation with parts of objects.
3. Symptoms must have their onset in early childhood, although may not be noted until demands of social interaction exceed abilities or learned coping strategies are insufficient.
4. Symptoms lead to clinically significant impairments in important aspects of present functioning (such as occupational or social).
5. Disturbance is not better accounted for by intellectual disability or global developmental delay.

For ASD associated with a known genetic diagnosis, say, Rett syndrome, the terminology used is: 'ASD associated with Rett syndrome'. The severity should be specified by the level of support required (e.g. requiring very substantial support for whichever criterion).

Intellectual abilities should be specified next (e.g. with/without intellectual impairment). Next, language abilities are recorded (e.g. with/without language impairment).

Finally, if catatonia is present, it is noted separately as it can be associated with a range of conditions. Additional diagnoses should be mentioned next, whether neurodevelopmental, psychiatric or behavioural (e.g. enuresis, encopresis, ADHD and other disruptive behaviour disorders, anxiety, OCD, disruptive mood dysregulation disorder [DMDD] including mood lability, Tourette's syndrome, depression).

The criteria set out in DSM-5 should be fulfilled before a diagnosis of autism is entertained.

There are a number of 'red flags', or developmental warning signs, of possible ASD that can be identified and divided into four age groups: infants, preschool age, school age and adolescents.

Infant warning signs:
- At 6–9 months, poor eye contact, absent facial expression, decreased social smiling, delayed babbling.
- At 9–12 months, less turning to name, not following a point when adult indicates and points to an object, tuning into environmental sounds more than human voice, infrequent babbling.
- At 12–15 months, absence of any words, lack of pointing, lack of showing objects of interest to others, failure to follow simple verbal command with a gesture, failure to wave bye-bye.
- At 15–18 months, lack of imitation, lack of engagement with other people, loss of previously acquired words, decreased variety of play, limited symbolic play.

Preschool-age warning signs:
- No pointing, no pretending, no perception (of others).
- No taking turns, no taking interest (in others), no taking part (in games).
- No speech, no sharing (pleasure), no starting games, no social play.
- Unable to communicate non-verbally, unusual mannerisms, unusual reactions to sensory stimuli.

School-age warning signs:
- Cannot follow games, cannot follow trends (classroom 'norms'; overly critical of teachers), cannot follow social cues (in relation to adults, too intense or no relationship at all), cannot follow social 'norms' (overwhelmed by social situations).
- Cannot cope with altered environments (unstructured situations such as school camps), or large/open environments (not sure how to organise self in unstructured space, hugging perimeter of sports fields), or a totally new environment (cannot cope with change).

Adolescence warning signs:
- Difficulty making/keeping friends in peer group (gets on more easily with adults or younger children), difficulty 'getting' jokes (taking things literally, does not 'get' sarcasm or metaphor), difficulty adapting style of communication (can be too formal or, conversely, too familiar).
- Rigid thinking (lacking imagination), rigid behaviour (ritualistic, repetitive).
- Unaware of personal space invasion, unaware of peer group 'norms'.
- Talking 'at' rather than with, talking with unmodulated (flat) and repetitive speech pattern, talking about very limited range of topics of own interest only.

Aetiology

Autism can be an intricate component of an increasingly large number of recognised genetic disorders. Fragile X syndrome, tuberous sclerosis, Angelman syndrome and

Down syndrome can cause children to have symptomatology that fulfils the criteria of DSM-5. Over 25% of autistic children have a recognisable aetiological disorder. Twin studies demonstrate a significant genetic component. Monozygotic twins have 50–90% concordance for ASD. Dizygotic twins and siblings have a 10% concordance for ASD and 30% for other developmental issues, including personal/social issues as well as speech and language delays. Some refer to autism in association with genetic conditions as 'syndromic autism/ASD' or 'autism/ASD plus'. The following list includes many of the genetic diagnoses that can have ASD as a component.

TACT FREE MANNERS (references lack of emotional reciprocity in ASD):

Tuberous sclerosis complex (TSC)
Angelman syndrome
CHARGE/**C**FC (cardiofaciocutaneous)/**C**ATCH-22 (22q11.2 deletion)/
    Channelopathies/**C**iliopathies (e.g. Joubert)/**C**ohen/**C**ornelia de lang/**C**ostello/
    Cowden/**C**NTNAP2 (at 7q35)
Trisomy 21/**T**imothy

Fragile X syndrome
Rett syndrome
Epilepsies: named: channelopathies, creatine deficiency, pyridoxine deficiency
Epilepsies: initialled: SYN1; SSADH (succinic semialdehyde dehydrogenase)
    deficiency; *CNTNAP2* (think: 'can't nap 2'; association of insomnia with autism);
    UBE*3A* duplication or triplication

Mitochondrial cytopathies/**M**etabolic disorders/**M**yotonic dystrophy
Autism spectrum disorders (OMIM) numbers: AUTS1, AUTS3–AUTS18; X-linked:
    AUTSX1–AUTSX6
NF1 (neurofibromatosis type 1)/**N**RXN1 (neurexin1) deletion
Noonan
Epilepsies: numbered: **1**q21.1 del, **7**q11.23 dup, **15**q11.1q13.3 del and dup,
    16p11.2 del, **17**q12 del, **18**q12.1, **22**q11.2 (CATCH-22)
Rubinstein–Taybi/**R**enpenning
SHANK3 mutations (Phelan-McDermid, 22q13.3 del)/**S**impson–Golabi–Behmel
    (both overgrowth syndromes)/**S**mith–Lemli–Opitz (SLOS)/**S**mith–Magenis
    (SMS)/**S**torage diseases (e.g. lysosomal storage diseases [LSDs])

Theories attempting to explain autistic thought processes include: 'executive dysfunction' (inability to plan, inability to inhibit socially inappropriate responses, inability to flexibly shift attention), 'weak central coherence' (inability to integrate pieces of information into a meaningful whole) and 'lack of theory of mind' (lack of the ability to attribute feelings and belief systems to others and appreciate they are different to one's own).

The brain regions known to be hypoactive in ASD in tasks where cognition and social perception are used include the following (mnemonic: **FAST Pre-med**):

Fusiform gyrus
Amygdala
Superior temporal sulcus
Temporoparietal junction

Prefrontal cortex
medial aspect

Misinformation about autism is common in the lay press. An article in a well-respected journal in 1998 proposed an association between autism and the measles, mumps and rubella (MMR) vaccine; it subsequently was shown to be incorrect—was debunked and then withdrawn. It is now clear that *there is **no** causative association between autism and the administration of the MMR vaccine.* There have been many other spurious claims regarding causation of autism which, like the MMR belief, seemed to endure well after they have been debunked effectively in medical and scientific literature. Hypotheses on aetiology lead to hypotheses on treatment. Claims for various treatment modalities have had similar levels of credibility, but persist (see below). As autism is without cure, and parents will explore any avenue that might help their child, it is not surprising that many parents of children with autism have tried many unproven therapies and may not follow rational advice.

History

PRESENTING COMPLAINT

Reason for current admission/presentation for the examination. This is often related to a co-existent diagnosis, in syndromic ASD (e.g. any of the conditions in the above list).

CURRENT SYMPTOMS

1. *Impaired social interaction.* Impaired non-verbal behaviours (level of eye contact, cuddling family members, hugging, facial expressions, body posture, gestures used), any friends of similar age, any attempts at sharing of interests, enjoyment, achievements, show-and-tell at preschool, showing toys to friends and family, bringing or pointing out objects of interest, any demonstration of empathy, social or emotional.
2. *Behaviour patterns.* Preferring own company, tendency to be a loner, 'in his own world', wandering aimlessly, preoccupation with specific areas of interest (e.g. able to talk only about *Star Wars*). Depends not on the presence of special interests, but on the level of handicap from the time spent with and intrusion on routines and family members. For the less able, may involve primary sensory stimulation; for example, fascination with noises, lights, patterns, textures, tastes and movements of objects or part objects. The underlying deficit is a lack of reciprocity in social interaction, communication and imagination.
3. *Most problematic behaviours.* Those at present (e.g. rituals, anxiety, aggression, self-injury) and the impact of these on family, educational facility (e.g. special school), therapists and carers.
4. *Comorbid developmental diagnoses*:
   - Intellectual disability (ID)/regression (in 34–55%; see the short case on ASD in this chapter).
   - Specific learning disabilities: difficulties at school, writing, reading, spelling, arithmetic.
   - Language disorders/impaired communication: current level of spoken language, ability to converse with another, quality of language, any unusual patterns of speech quality and content, including echolalia, repetition, pronoun reversal and semantic pragmatic language disorder.
   - ADHD symptomatology (in 28–44%; see the long case on ADHD in this chapter).

- Tic disorders (in 14–38%; see the short case on involuntary movements in Chapter 13).
- Motor problems (hypotonia, motor delay, clumsiness, lack of ball-game skills, deficits in gait, balance, coordination, movement preparation, planning).
- Severe deprivation can lead to an ASD-like presentation leading to debate as to whether these are ASD cases or a look alike.
- Attachment disorders.

5. Comorbid general medical problems:
   - Features of genetic syndromes (in 5%; see above list).
   - Co-existent epilepsy (in 8–30%; see the long case on seizures and epileptic syndromes).
   - Macrocephaly: followed up in OPD for enlarged head circumference (in 17–20%).
   - Symptoms of sleep disorders (in 50–80%; see the long case on obstructive sleep apnoea [OSA]).
   - Gastrointestinal problems (in 9–70%; constipation, [related] food selectivity).
   - Symptoms of immune dysregulation (in < 38%; allergies, autoimmune disorders). Important to consider causes of silent pain in those who are non-verbal (e.g. constipation, gastro-oesophageal reflux, helicobacter infection, dental and sinus pain/infection).

6. *Comorbid psychiatric diagnoses.* Ask if diagnosed with any of the following:
   - Anxiety (in 42–56%; especially social anxiety, more in higher functioning).
   - Depression (in 12–70%; less in children, more as ageing, more in higher functioning).
   - OCD (in 7–24%).
   - ODD (in 16–28%): negativistic, hostile, defiant behaviour, losing temper, arguing with/defying adults, deliberately annoying people, blaming others for mistakes, touchy, easily annoyed by others, angry, spiteful.
   - Psychotic disorders (rare in children, mainly adults [in 12–17%], especially recurrent hallucinations; ASD-like behaviour can precede schizophrenia). However, with a lack of theory of mind or an intellectual disability, a child may lack capacity for describing subjective mental phenomena and can be mistaken for pseudohallucinations, pretend friends and stereotypic rumination or repetition of imaginary ideas.
   - Substance abuse (in < 16%); substances used to relieve anxiety.
   - Eating disorders (in 4–5%; can be a misdiagnosis; both can have rigid thinking, self-focus, attention to details).

7. *Comorbid behavioural disorders.* Ask if diagnosed with any of the following:
   - Aggressive behaviour (up to 68%; particularly aimed at caregivers; may be related to frustration of communication problems, sensory overload, routine disruption).
   - Self-injury (up to 50%; may be related to frustration with communication problems, sensory overload, routine disruption).
   - Pica (in 36%; more likely with co-existent intellectual impairment).
   - Suicidal ideation/attempt (in 11–14%; more risk with depression, teasing, bullying).

8. *Comorbid personality disorders (PDs).* Ask if diagnosed with any of the following:
   - Obsessive-compulsive PD (in 19–32%).
   - Avoidant PD (in 13–25%); may be related to social experiences being unsatisfactory.
   - Schizoid PD (in 21–26%).
   - Schizotypal PD (in 2–13%).
   - Paranoid PD (0–19%; may be related to misunderstanding others' intentions).
   - Borderline PD (in 0–9%; attributing hostile intentions wrongly; affect dysregulation).

- Personality disorders such as OCPD, schizoid PD and schizotypal are recognised long-term outcomes of ASD in adulthood.

PAST HISTORY

Any illnesses predating first features of autism (e.g. meningitis, encephalitis, other intracranial pathology, head injury). Details of past history of co-existent diagnoses (e.g. tuberous sclerosis complex). Symptoms leading to the diagnosis may include symptoms referrable to the following:

- *Lack of social interaction.* For example, not smiling socially, very 'independent', treating others as object rather than person, lacking or only superficial interest in other children, lack of or restricted eye contact, seeming to be in 'own world', seeming to 'tune out', lack of cuddling, no development of expected social skills.
- *Behavioural issues.* For example, temper tantrums, uncooperative, overactive, lining things up, obsessions with certain things (such as water, wheels, mechanical devices), odd motor movements, not playing with toys, unusual attachments to objects, refusal to wear anything but favourite outfit (e.g. dressing exclusively as Batman every day for many months), preoccupations, unusual sensory reactions, toe walking.
- *Language delay.* For example, not responding to name, no babbling, no pointing or waving by 12 months, no sharing of interest in objects, no single words by 16 months, appearing deaf, no spontaneous (non-echolalic) phrases/word combinations by 24 months, loss of words, language.
- Previous therapies tried, previous medication tried, past medical investigations (e.g. serum ferritin, chromosomal analysis, psychometric testing, audiology, EEG).

BIRTH HISTORY

Pregnancy complications, gestational age, mode of delivery, Apgar score, resuscitation required, birthweight, need for oxygen, nursery care, neonatal period, any intracranial pathology (e.g. neonatal encephalopathy in term baby, intraventricular haemorrhage in premature infant, periventricular leukomalacia, hydrocephalus).

DEVELOPMENTAL HISTORY

Age at which all major milestones achieved, especially speech and language acquisition, and personal–social interaction (25% of children with autism demonstrate regression in language and socialisation skills before 18 months of age).

FAMILY HISTORY

Any family history of ASD (recurrence is 10–20% in subsequent siblings). The genetic risk for a second child with non-syndromic ASD is over 5%.

IMMUNISATION

Is immunisation up to date? Do parents have any concerns regarding possible aetiological link? Timing of immunisation and noting of first symptoms (there will, of course, be temporal coincidence as the timing of some immunisations may well coincide within a few months of the noting of symptoms).

CURRENT MANAGEMENT

Psychoeducation and parent training such as Stepping Stones Triple P have good evidence of benefit. Some of their effect is due to better developmental attunement and preventing/improving secondary attachment disorders. Usual routine at home, any medications used (e.g. SSRIs, stimulants used [e.g. dexamphetamine, methylphenidate] currently or previously, other drugs for ADHD-like symptoms (e.g. antidepressants, clonidine), dosage regimen, side effects noted (e.g. stimulants may cause decreased appetite, insomnia, rebound moodiness, irritability or hyperactivity), any therapies (e.g. occupational therapy). School issues (e.g. which sort of school, any school assistance, where the desk is positioned in the classroom), psychosocial interventions (e.g. behavioural therapies [in particular Applied Behavioural Analysis has good levels of evidence of benefit], educational tutoring).

Professionals seen (e.g. local doctor, psychologists, paediatricians, psychiatrists), activities to promote concentration and self-control (e.g. relaxation or exercise), alternative therapies tried (e.g. homeopathic preparations), educational websites. Speech therapy and developmental treatments such as TEACCH have evidence of improvement.

SOCIAL HISTORY

Impact of condition on parents, siblings, friends, children in same class at school, family financial situation (e.g. private health insurance, cost of stimulant medications, visits to multiple professionals, government benefits received), social supports (social worker, extended family, respite care, autism associations).

UNDERSTANDING OF PROBLEMS AND PROGNOSIS

By parents, degree of education regarding autism, realistic long-term plans for care/career/occupational choices.

Examination

See the short-case section. Most children with autism have entirely normal physical appearance, other than macrocephaly in around 25%. A recognisable aetiological disorder/genetic mutation is associated in around 15–25% cases with ASD (tuberous sclerosis, fragile X syndrome, various less well-known mutations found on CMA or WES testing). Others may have minor abnormalities of uncertain significance, such as on EEG or brain scan.

Diagnosis of autism

There is no pathognomonic sign, no definitive biological marker and no diagnostic laboratory test for autism. To make the diagnosis, specific impairing symptoms of the disorder must be documented according to the criteria set out in the current DSM-5 or ICD-10 diagnostic manuals. Multidisciplinary teams are involved in the diagnosis of autism in Australia, the UK and the US. They comprise a range of professionals that usually include a doctor (paediatrician or psychiatrist), psychologist, speech therapist, occupational therapist and social worker. A thorough neurological and general medical examination must be performed (as per the short-case approach).

Several evaluation tools can be used. Autism may be suspected by routine developmental surveillance (see the next page). The next step involves a number of autism-specific screening tests (see the next page). The traditional tool for developmental screening, the Denver-II (DDST-II, formerly the Denver Developmental Screening Test—Revised), is regarded as being insensitive and lacking in specificity. Similarly, the Revised Denver Pre-Screening Developmental Questionnaire (R-DPSDQ) is not recommended for primary-care developmental surveillance.

There is a wide differential diagnosis for the ASDs. In children with neurogenetic disorders, autistic behaviour can be a prominent aspect of their medical condition. The most common of these disorders are fragile X syndrome (affected gene FMR1), which comprises less than 5% of autism, and tuberous sclerosis complex (affected genes TSC1 and TSC2, encoding hamartin and tuberin, respectively), which comprises less than 3% autism (but 8–14% of autism with epilepsy). Neurofibromatosis type 1 (NF1) also can cause autistic features. See long and short cases on TSC and NF1.

As set out in the mnemonic, dysmorphic syndromes associated with autism are many and varied. Several deletion syndromes (16p11 [gene PRKCB1], 22q13 [gene SHANK 3], 2q37 [genes KIF1A, GBX2]) and duplication syndromes (15q duplication and 16p duplication) have specific associations with autism.

Chromosomal abnormalities have been described in 15–25% of patients with ASD. The prevalence of intellectual impairment with autism is around 50–75%.

Karyotyping cannot detect submicroscopic genomic deletions and duplications or CNVs smaller than 5 megabases. Because of the strong genetic component to ASDs, routine testing has been extended to chromosomal microarray analysis (CMA), and whole exome sequencing (WES). Over 9% of females with ASD and over 7% of males with ASD have abnormalities on CMA, and a similar number have abnormalities on WES.

Several inborn errors of metabolism can cause autistic features, notably phenylketonuria, creatine deficiency syndromes, adenylosuccinate lyase deficiency, metabolic purine disorders and mitochondrial disorders. Metabolic diseases lead to accumulation of toxic metabolites, reduction of myelin, loss of neurons, and altered dopaminergic and serotoninergic neurotransmissions.

The differential diagnoses are listed in the short-case section.

SCREENING TESTS AND DIAGNOSTIC INSTRUMENTS
Routine developmental surveillance

- Ages and Stages Questionnaire, second edition (ASQ).
- BRIGANCE Screens.
- Child Development Inventories (CDI).
- Parents' Evaluation of Developmental Status (PEDS).
- Pervasive Developmental Disorder Screening Test II (PDDST-II, a parent-completed survey of the early features of ASD).

Autism-specific screening tests—younger children

- Infant Toddler Checklist (ITC; administer at 6–24 months).
- Early Screening of Autistic Traits (ESAT; administer at 14 months).
- Checklist for Autism in Toddlers (CHAT; administer at 18 months).
- Modified Checklist for Autism in Toddlers (M-CHAT; administer at 16–30 months).
- Quantitative Checklist for Autism in Toddlers (Q-CHAT; administer at 18–24 months).

Autism-specific screening tests—older children and adolescents

- Autism Spectrum Screening Questionnaire (ASSQ, administer at 7–16 years).
- Autism-Spectrum Quotient (AQ), child/adolescent: administer at 4–11 years/ 10–16 years.
- Social Communication Questionnaire (SCQ; administer at age 4 years or over).
- Social Responsiveness Scale (1st or 2nd edition, SRS, SRS-2, administer > 2.5 years).
- Childhood Autism Screening Test (CAST; administer at 4–11 years).

Diagnostic structured parental interviews

- Autism Diagnostic Interview—Revised (ADI-R).
- Diagnostic Interview for Social and Communications Disorders (DISCO), which takes a developmental framework, and can be administered at any age.

- Developmental, dimensional, and diagnostic interview (3Di); administer > age 2 years.

Diagnostic observational instruments

- Childhood Autism Rating Scale (1st/2nd edition, CARS, CARS-2; administer > 2 years).
- Autism Diagnostic Observation Schedule (1st/2nd edition, ADOS, ADOS-2; age > 1 year).

INVESTIGATIONS

Blood tests

1. High-resolution chromosomal analysis (karyotype).
2. DNA test for fragile X syndrome (3–25% of fragile X syndrome children have ASD). Molecular testing shows a trinucleotide repeat (CGG repeats) expansion and methylation pattern in the FMR1 gene.
3. Specific genetic testing for:
   - Rett syndrome (RTT, mainly caused by MECP2 mutation; gene map locus Xq28, Xp22; DNA sequencing/deletion screening) in girls; see the long case on RTT.
   - Angelman syndrome (AS, mainly due to deletion of maternally inherited 15q11–q13); analyse parent-specific DNA methylation imprints in the 15q11.2-q13 region (will diagnose 80%), plus UBE3A sequence analysis (will diagnose an additional 11%).
   - Smith–Magenis syndrome (due to deletion of a portion of 17p11.2), if clinically indicated.
   - 15q duplications, and 16p duplications or deletions (detected by CMA).
   - Neurocutaneous syndromes, tuberous sclerosis (TS), NF1 and HI can be diagnosed by clinical criteria or molecular genetic testing.
   - Any dysmorphic features present suggests chromosomal rearrangements even if the karyotype is normal; CMA or WES would be appropriate in this circumstance.
4. Serum lead levels for lead toxicity (especially if there is a history of pica, or living in an old house with lead-containing paint).
5. Serum amino acids to detect phenylketonuria (PKU).
6. Serum 7-dehydrocholesterol to detect Smith-Lemli-Opitz, if this is suspected.

Urine test

Metabolic screen (if initiated by the presence of suggestive clinical findings, such as cyclic vomiting, lethargy, early seizures, dysmorphic or coarse features, intellectual impairment).

Neurophysiological testing

1. Audiology is required to exclude impaired hearing as a contributing cause of speech delay.
2. EEG is not a routine requirement, but if a seizure has occurred, it may be indicated.

Ophthalmological assessment

Formal assessment by a paediatric ophthalmologist is appropriate to exclude any unrecognised visual impairment that could contribute to restriction of eye contact.

Other

Often, many more tests than the above are ordered. There is inadequate evidence to support the following (which may well be requested by parents): routine EEG, routine neuroimaging, coeliac disease serology, allergy testing, immunological studies, hair analysis, testing for micronutrients such as vitamins and trace elements, heavy metal screen, thyroid function tests, non-selective screening for mitochondrial disorders, intestinal permeability studies, stool analysis, urinary peptide levels—the list can go on and on. Many obscure investigations may be sent to the Great Plains Laboratory in Kansas; what to do with the results, if some are abnormal, remains unclear.

Educational psychology assessment

Assessment by an educational psychologist may be useful. This may reveal that the child has a normal or high IQ. It can help identify children with specific learning difficulties and/or a low IQ. The Wechsler scale WISC-III gives full-scale IQ, verbal and performance IQ scores.

Teacher's report

A report from the special school teacher, aide or regular school teacher outlining the child's academic and social strengths and weaknesses can be extremely useful in further assessment of the child's performance. Allowing the teacher to write a freehand report gives useful information, and gives the physician insight into the teacher's understanding of the child's problems.

Management

Prognosis depends on intellect and the establishment of functional communication by the age of 5 years.

Management can be divided into seven groups of headings, with the mnemonic **SPECIAL**:

School-based special education (for children over 3 years)
Pharmacotherapeutic intervention
Education of, and support for, parents
Community supports
Intervention
Alternative treatments
Learning/**L**inks: useful websites

SCHOOL-BASED SPECIAL EDUCATION

For most children with autism, education authorities assess the particular level of additional teaching/support required to optimise their education. Many public schools have special education development units that cater for children with autism.

Pharmacotherapeutic intervention

In autism, an effective medical treatment has yet to be found for the core problems involving language and social cognition, although the atypical antipsychotic agent risperidone does show some promising effects in improving social relatedness, and managing interfering, stereotyped and repetitive behaviours. Its use should be limited to associated behavioural and psychiatric problems of aggression, self-injury, hyperactivity, anxiety or stereotypes.

Irrespective of which drug is used, informed consent should be obtained regarding potential benefits and potential adverse side effects. Safe storage of medication in the home is essential. Careful and regular review must be carried out to monitor response, and carers, schoolteachers and general practitioners must be kept apprised of any change in, or new addition to, the therapeutic armamentarium.

Four main groups of behaviours may show a positive response to medication, as follows.

1. ADHD-like behaviours

Here, the same medications may be tried as are used in ADHD:

- The stimulants dexamphetamine and methylphenidate have poorer response rates and greater side effects in those with intellectual disability and autism. Side-effect profiles are similar, with anorexia, weight loss (often 1–2 kg in the first 3 months), emotional lability, tics, insomnia, social and emotional withdrawal, and occasional psychotic reaction. Most side effects are dose-related.

  Both drugs have a good safety record. Neither is recommended in patients with marked anxiety, motor tics or a family history of Tourette syndrome (for a discussion, see the long case on ADHD in this chapter).

- Atomoxetine and amitriptyline have a noradrenergic pathway effect and are often better for impulsiveness and aggression. These drugs have a different side-effect profile to that of stimulants.

- The antihypertensive clonidine, to reduce impulsive behaviour, aggressive tendencies, oppositional-defiant symptoms, anxiety and sleep initiation difficulties. Low doses are used in autism, as in ADHD (1–3 μg/kg/dose), and rarely affect blood pressure. Parents must be told all the significant side effects of clonidine, including the cardiotoxicity of overdosage, and the uncommon but recognised complication of sudden discontinuation, which results in rebound hypertension (again, for a discussion, see the long case on ADHD in this chapter).

  It can be helpful to consider stimulants as first-line treatment for ADHD, clonidine, atomoxetine and amitriptyline as second line, and mood stabilisers and major tranquillisers as third line.

2. Ritualistic/compulsive behaviours

- SSRIs, such as fluoxetine, sertraline, fluvoxamine and paroxetine, have been used in treating repetitive behaviours and aggression. Abnormalities of serotonin function have been noted in patients with ASD, and there is dysregulation of serotonin in OCD. Although these drugs are selective, they can still cause serotonin syndrome, from an excess of serotonin. Symptoms may include aggression, agitation, autonomic dysfunction, tremor, sweating, chills, restlessness, confusion, impaired coordination, fever, hyperreflexia, myoclonus, coma and, very rarely, death. The most common side effect is behavioural activation. SSRIs are safer than tricyclic antidepressants as regards cardiac side effects; tricyclics can cause prolongation of corrected QT interval, which can lead to fatal arrhythmias, but SSRIs have lower cardiotoxicity. SSRIs may cause behavioural activation (which can lead to an increase in impulsive self-harm) or a switch to hypomania.

  Atomoxetine is often used as a second-line ADHD medication in ASD, but is also prone to side effects. Amitriptyline can be a valuable treatment for ADHD in ASD, where anxiety is such a common concomitant. Amitriptyline requires an ECG to check the QT interval and a warning of a danger in overdosage.

- Risperidone (see point 4 on the next page).

3. Sleep disturbances

The types of problems noted in autism include dyssomnias (problems with initiating sleep, maintaining sleep, excessive sleepiness) and parasomnias (problems with arousal, partial arousal, sleep stage transitions) and disoriented awakening. One medication that has proved useful is melatonin.

4. Difficult behaviours (e.g. aggression, self-injury, temper tantrums)

- If aggression is related to impulsivity, then stimulants may be useful.
- If aggression is related to anxiety or stereotypic rigidity, then SSRIs or mood stabilisers (e.g. carbamazepine, sodium valproate) may be useful.
- If aggression is intractable, then the newer atypical antipsychotic drugs (e.g. risperidone) may be useful. Risperidone blocks postsynaptic dopamine and serotonin receptors. Side effects may include increased appetite, mild fatigue (usually short-lived), tremors and, upon discontinuing this drug after long-term use (over 6 months), mild, reversible withdrawal dyskinesias. Children receiving risperidone may show improvements in disruptive behaviours (including aggression, self-abuse, temper tantrums), plus improvements in degree of irritability, social withdrawal, hyperactivity and inappropriate speech.

Education of, and support for, parents

In Australia, there are autism associations in each state and territory. In the US, there are national and regional parent support organisations such as the Autism Society of America. Similar parent support organisations exist in most countries; they can be a good source of information and very beneficial to families. Parents must be warned about misinformation, particularly from internet sources, regarding aetiology (e.g. the alleged association with MMR) and management (e.g. alleged miracle cures). Parents should be provided with reliable and relevant information, specifying useful websites such as those listed overleaf.

Community supports

The amount of community support the family of an autistic child requires depends on the family's situation (e.g. there may be close relatives nearby, friends, neighbours, church groups), as well as the supports and therapies available at the local educational facility. There are many agencies serving children with autism; government-run education departments may offer specified amounts of aide time (several hours) per week. In Australia, the parents of all children with a diagnosis of autism (but not ASD) are eligible to receive a carer's allowance. Also, families can obtain allied health therapies through the Medicare Enhanced Primary Care program.

Intervention

There is adequate evidence to support the short- and medium-term benefits of early intervention. Intervention should begin as early as possible. Early interventions may take place in the child's home, in preschools with support, in special playgroups and in childcare facilities, and are individualised. The time required is around 15–25 hours of specific therapy per week: the National Initiative for Autism Plan in the UK recommends that 15 hours a week should be available to all; some have suggested that 40 hours is required, but this adds financial constraints without definite benefit. Early intervention may include behaviour management strategies, early developmental education, communication therapy, speech therapy, occupational therapy, physiotherapy, structured social play and much parent training. Once the child is old enough to enter the school system, it is essential to find the best educational facility available for that child's intellectual ability, language, communication and socialisation skills, and safety (many parents wish to avoid schools on main or busy roads, or near bodies of water).

Alternative treatments

The management of children with autism can be an emotional minefield. Parents at the end of their tether will try many and varied treatments, and any suggested 'cure' will invariably lead some parents to try unorthodox treatments. Challenging this approach may damage the doctor–patient/parent relationship. As long as there are desperate parents, there will be people who make money from treatments with no scientific basis. Included within the many non-traditional approaches are the examples listed below. The disadvantages to these approaches may include cost, wasting valuable time, delay in trying recognised treatments and potential public health issues (e.g. refusing to get a child immunised for fear of autism). Subjecting an already distressed child to further encumbrance may make the situation worse.

Diet has been suggested as a cause of autism. To date, many diets have been tried (e.g. gluten-casein free) without success. As many children with autism have restricted diets as a result of their self-imposed eating routines, their parents appreciate sensible guidelines on healthy eating. This advice should be the same as for any child, including avoiding caffeinated drinks and excessive fruit juice, and encouraging the intake of adequate water, fibre and fresh foods.

Some alternative treatments for autism are tolerated and have few safety concerns; these include the following (although none have sufficient evidence to support them):
- *Omega-3 fatty acids.*
- *Secretin.* This lacks evidence from RCTs and requires injections.
- *Vitamin B$_6$ with magnesium.* Vitamin deficiencies were found in disturbed children in one study in 1979. B$_6$ is a coenzyme in several metabolic processes, including neurotransmitter synthesis. Early studies in the 1980s suggested a positive behavioural response; there are methodological flaws in all studies.
- *Gluten-casein-free diet.* The hypothesis is that gluten (and casein) are absorbed through a 'leaky gut' and form exorphins, thus mimicking opioids that affect the brain; constant exposure leads to less endogenous opioid released during social interaction. Studies show no association between autism and coeliac disease or gluten challenge and behaviour. A gluten-casein-free diet can further isolate already socially handicapped patients and families.

Other alternative treatments include agents with significant safety concerns and no evidenced benefits:
- *Chelation with dimercaptosuccinic acid (DMSA).* This is an oral preparation for lead poisoning. The hypothesis is that exposure to heavy metal accumulation from vaccines or the environment may be causing autism. No RCTs exist investigating chelation and autism.
- *Hyperbaric oxygen therapy.*
- *Intravenous immunoglobulin.*
- *Antifungal agents.*

Useful websites

The following may be useful both for candidates and for parents of children with autism:
- Autism Society (US), www.autism-society.org
- First signs, www.firstsigns.org
- Developmental and Behavioral Pediatrics, American Academy of Pediatrics, www.dbpeds.org
- Australian Advisory Board on Autism Spectrum Disorders, www.autismaus.com.au
- Autism, Department of Health, New York State, www.health.ny.gov/community/infants_children/early_intervention/autism/
- The National Autistic Society (UK), www.autism.org.uk

LONG CASE: Rett syndrome

Children with Rett syndrome (RTT, OMIM #312750) may be involved in long- or short-case examinations. The following is an approach to long-case management, including an approach to directed physical examination that could be utilised as a short-case approach, and a mnemonic, based on the most common genetic cause, which covers most aspects of RTT.

Background information

Rett syndrome (OMIM #312750) is an X-linked dominant neurodevelopmental disorder (NDD), most commonly due to mutations in the gene on the X chromosome, which codes for methyl-CpG-binding protein-2 (MeCP2, OMIM *300005), a chromosomal protein which binds to methylated DNA, and is involved in transcriptional repression, via interacting with a co-repressor, SIN3A (another transcriptional regulatory protein), and activating histone deacetylase (which removes acetyl groups allowing histones to tightly wrap DNA, which affects DNA expression). More recently, it has been found that MeCP2 can bind unmethylated promoter regions and act as an activator of their associated genes. Expression of the MECP2 gene is widespread throughout the central nervous system, particularly in the brainstem and thalamus. RTT is the first disorder in humans proved to be due to mutations in proteins that control gene expression via effects on DNA. Loss of MeCP2 protein's function causes dysregulated expression of genes with which it typically associates. Chromatin structure is altered in RTT. Astrocyte function is not normal in RTT.

Most cases of RTT are caused by mutations in MECP2, but not all mutations in MECP2 cause RTT. RTT is sporadic in 99% of cases, and due to, almost always, paternally derived de novo, MECP2 mutations. The three main types of MECP2 mutations are missense, nonsense and frameshift mutations, but exonic or even whole gene deletions are seen. There are over 300 known pathogenic mutations of the MECP2 gene, and of these, there are nine which account for almost 80% (for completion, these are: p.Arg106Trp, p.Arg133Cys, p.Arg168*, p.Arg2558, p.Arg2708, p.Arg2948, p.Ag306Cys, p.Trp158Met and C-terminal truncations). There is little consistent genotypic–phenotypic correlation. Some mutations seem associated with mild features of RTT (p.Arg133Cys, p.Arg294* and C-terminal truncating mutations), whereas other are associated with more severe disease (p.Arg2708 and p.Arg255* genotypes). Other genes can cause RTT: mutations in FOXG1 at 14q12 (OMIM #164874) cause a congenital (Rolando) variant of RTT, and mutations in CDKL5 at Xp22.13 (OMIM #300203) cause an early seizure (Hanefeld) variant of RTT, although more recently it has been recognised that CDKL5 mutations cause a distinct disorder.

RTT was described in the DSM-IV under the heading of pervasive developmental disorders (PDDs), but has been removed in the DSM-5, so as not to be considered a specific form of ASD. Occurring almost solely in females, RTT shares some features of ASD behaviours, but only for a limited time during development (Stage II, overleaf).

Development typically slows, or stops, between 6 and 30 months (particularly between 6 and 18 months), and then regresses, with loss of previously acquired skills, including speech, the evolution of stereotypic movements of the extremities, particularly the hands, and evolution of gait abnormalities, accompanied by intellectual impairment and the development of epilepsy. It is a progressive disorder. Prior to the discovery of the MECP2 gene as the cause of RTT, RTT was described as having four stages; while of limited value, these at least allow some prediction of issues likely to arise throughout the affected child's life.

Diagnostic criteria

The criteria for diagnosing RTT were revised in 2010. There are two requirements for diagnosis of classic RTT: regression followed by stabilisation, and meeting **all** the main four criteria (below), with no exclusionary aspects:

1. Loss of **speech**
2. Loss of *purposeful* **hand** movements
3. Abnormal, dyspraxic **gait**, and
4. Development of *stereotypic* **hand** movements (just remember *speech, hand, gait, hand*, or *two hands gait speech*).

There are two exclusionary criteria for typical RTT: first, significantly abnormal psychomotor development in the first 6 months, and second, cerebral injury due to trauma, neurometabolic disease or significant infection that leads to neurological impairment.

There are also 11 supportive criteria that are not required for the diagnosis of typical RTT, are commonly found and upon which diagnosis of *atypical RTT* can be *based*. These can be organised into the mnemonic **BASED**:

Breathing abnormalities (awake)/**B**ruxism
Abnormal muscle tone
Screaming (and laughing) spells/**S**coliosis/**S**mall cold hands and feet/**S**leep pattern disturbed
Eye pointing
Deceleration of growth of head, then height and weight/**D**ecreased pain response/**D**isturbed peripheral vasomotor function

For atypical RTT, the requirements for diagnosis are regression followed by stabilisation, two of the main four criteria and 5 of the 11 supportive criteria.

Stages (mnemonic: DRUM)

Stage I: **D**elay or arrest in development/early onset stagnation; onset: 6–18 months; duration weeks to months; developmental delay, postural delay, includes bottom-shuffling, gross motor delay, decreased eye contact, decreased play, less cuddly, less facial expression, deceleration of head growth, and the start of hand wringing. Some of these infant RTT girls suddenly seem to need less attention from their mothers; others can be less interactive but more irritable and cry frequently. Postural developmental progress continues, but at a slower rate than previously. Sitting unsupported may be achieved, and bottom-shuffling used to get around, but a significant proportion of these infants never achieve walking. Language development also progresses, albeit slower, with some single words, and babbling.

Stage II: **R**egression in development/rapid deterioration/destructive phase; onset: 1–4 years of age, onset tempo: rapid to gradual. The duration of this stage can last several weeks to a year. Stage II is marked by loss of two abilities—1. acquired purposeful hand skills; and 2. language/communication (fine motor, babbling, active play)—and the evolution of two new aspects—1. stereotypical hand movements; and 2. gait abnormalities (walking unsteady, ataxic) (mnemonic: Stage 2: age 2, lose 2, gain 2).

During this stage, cognitive impairments become apparent, breathing abnormalities become apparent, including episodes of hyperventilation and apnoea, eye contact is preserved but diminished, autistic-like symptoms are noted (loss of social interaction, loss of communication). Reaching for toys is replaced with pulling at hair, or other hand stereotypies (mainly midline) including clapping, clasping behind back, grasping, holding hands at sides, unusual posturing of wrists, releasing, tapping, touching, twisting fingers, washing and wringing occur, and initiating of motor movements can be difficult.

Some important points:

- *Loss of speech* occurs at a median of *2 years*.
- *Majority (90%)* of RTT patients *learn to sit* (range 6–39 months; 10% never learn to sit).
- *Majority (55%)* of RTT patients *learn to walk*; (median: 19 months; 45% never learn to walk).
- *Loss of language* or hand function is *unlikely after age 4* years of age.

Stage III: **U**napparent slow deterioration/pseudostationary/post-regression/static period/improved behaviour + hand use + communication period; onset 2– 10 years (preschool to school years); duration years to decades; retained ambulation, some restoration of communication, regression of motor abilities, which is very slow. During this stage particular problems include epilepsy and apraxia (unable to execute learned movements despite understanding and preparedness to do so), and worsening control of motor abilities, with poor coordination of gait. However, some areas improve, there is less irritability, less crying, less ASD-like behaviours, more interest in surroundings. Several aspects can improve/increase, including alertness, attention span and communication skills. It is at this stage that intense eye communication becomes noted, with intense staring utilised to express wishes, which can develop into a quite sophisticated 'eye-pointing' language to make up for their loss of spoken language. It is also during this stage that lower limb deformity evolves, with the feet adopting a fixed supinated flexed position, caused largely by continual dystonic posturing.

Stage IV: **M**otor deterioration (late); onset when ambulation stops (teenage years); duration decades; wheelchair-dependent; wasting.

Each child with RTT follows their own unique trajectory, or colloquially, their own drumbeat. Accordingly, the mnemonic DRUMBEATS combines asking about the usual stages (mnemonic: DRUM), plus directed questioning about particular features relevant to many RTT children, including their functional severity, current management and prognosis (mnemonic: BEATS). The long-case presentation should address the major problems as the parent sees them, and as the various caregivers (e.g. doctors) see them; the interpretation may be quite different.

It is advisable to cover areas that were of interest to the examiners when they took the history and examined the child. Ask yourself: 'What did the examiners ask about? What areas did they examine?'

Variant forms of RTT
CONGENITAL VARIANT (ROLANDO VARIANT)

Unlike classic RTT, development is very abnormal from birth, with marked delay in both cognitive and motor domains, and these infants do not learn to walk; their head circumference decelerates, and development regresses, much earlier than classic RTT, with microcephaly occurring before 4 months and developmental regression by 5 months. These children do not get the Rett eye gaze. They do get the breathing abnormalities and autonomic peripheral vasomotor features. There are some unusual movement findings specific for the Rolando variant: stereotypies of the tongue, and jerky limb movements. (mnemonic for stereotypies: Roll lingual for Rolando). Unusual tongue movements affect oropharyngeal transfer patterns and swallowing in classic RTT but only the Rolando variant has specific lingual stereotypies. The gene mutation here is usually in FOXG1 (F for Foetal, i.e. Congenital).

PRESERVED SPEECH VARIANT (ZAPPELLA VARIANT)

The name of the preserved speech variant (Zappella variant) is reminiscent of 'a cappella', which is singing without accompaniment. This variant has less severe clinical features. Regression still occurs between 1 and 3 years, but is followed by a longer duration plateau, with much less epilepsy, much less hand skill loss, less significant scoliosis and/or kyphosis, much less autonomic dysfunction, and normal growth parameters. But the feature that gives this variant its name is the regaining of language post-regression, the average age of recovery being 5 years; these children attain single words or phrases and have less cognitive impairment than occurs in classic RTT, although autistic behaviours are common. The gene mutation here is usually in MECP2, as in classic RTT.

Differential diagnoses

Any child with RTT may see a number of doctors before the diagnosis becomes clear. Particularly in the earlier stages, there can be a very broad array of differential diagnoses put forward. Candidates should be familiar with conditions which can be confused with RTT. The mnemonic **PLACED** lists several disorders which can be considered when the diagnosis of RTT is still too unclear to place:

Pitt-Hopkins syndrome (PTHS): mutation in gene TCF4 on chromosome 18; developmental delay, intermittent hyperventilation and apnoea, but distinctive facial features including wide mouth)
Lennox-Gastaut syndrome (LGS)/**L**eucodystrophies
Autism spectrum disorder (ASD)/**A**ngelman (15q11-13 maternal deletion) syndrome/**A**taxias (spinocerebellar ataxia [multiple types], spastic ataxia)
Cerebral palsy (CP)
Encephalitis
Deletion (micro-deletion) syndromes, affecting chromosomes 12 to 22/**D**eafness/**D**isturbed vision

In children with suspected RTT, where there are no RTT-related pathogenic mutations of MECP2, FOXG1 or CDKL5, then investigations for the above differential diagnosis list may be performed if clinically appropriate, but if they are all unremarkable, then the diagnosis of RTT can still be made if the clinical criteria for RTT are fulfilled.

Epilepsy

This affects 80–90% of RTT patients. Seizures are very rare under 2 years, but increase in frequency with age until 30 years when the proportion affected is 86%, and above that age there is no increase. Seizures affect around one-third of RTT children under 5, 60% of RTT children under 10 and three-quarters of RTT children under 15. All forms of epileptic seizures have been described in RTT; most common are complex partial, tonic-clonic, tonic, myoclonic; absences and clonic seizures less so; convulsions especially occur in Stages II or III, CDKL5 mutation features early onset seizures. EEG is abnormal in all patients with RTT, and changes through time, following the clinical staging. There are no RCTs evaluating anti-epileptic drugs (AEDs) in this group. A large retrospective study suggested the most effective AEDs of first choice to be lamotrigine (LTG), especially for RTT patients developing epilepsy later, and sodium valproate (VPA) and carbamazepine (CBZ) for those patients developing seizures at an earlier age.

Intractable epilepsy can occur in up to 50% of patients with RTT. Some brainstem-derived episodes can include eye blinking, twitching of the face, or hypocapnoeic attacks with hypocalcaemic tetany and cyanosis. Parental perception of the occurrence of seizures has been shown to be at variance with EEG evidence of these events actually being seizures; parents can interpret RTT behaviours, such as 'vacant episodes' where activities are suddenly paused or frozen, being misconstrued as absences (but without EEG change correlations), or constant hand wringing misinterpreted as epileptiform automatisms (but without EEG change correlation). Similarly, in some RTT children there are seizures not recognised as such by parents, and occult fits during sleep. The most concerning aspect of seizures in these patients is that status epilepticus and aspiration are well recognised causes of mortality.

Motor disturbances

The key terms are extrapyramidal dysfunction, hand stereotypies, gait ataxia and apraxia.

EXTRAPYRAMIDAL MOTOR FINDINGS

These can be a **PROBLEM**: **P**roximal myoclonus, **R**igidity, **O**culogyric crises, **B**ruxism, **B**radykinesia, **L**ack of expression (hypomimia), **E**xcessive drooling and **M**uscle dystonia.

HAND STEREOTYPIES

These are mainly midline, many and varied; these can be virtually continuous during wakefulness, and include (in alphabetical order, with duplicated first letters in bold): **c**lapping and **c**lasping, finger kneading, grasping, holding hands at sides, mouthing, opposition of hands, posturing of wrists, **p**atting and **p**ill-rolling, **r**ubbing and **r**eleasing, **t**apping, **t**wisting and **t**ouching, **w**ashing and **w**ringing. Each RTT patient has their own repetitive manoeuvres, repeated over and over again. These movements tend to become more simplified as the child progresses through to Stage IV.

GAIT ATAXIA AND APRAXIA

The gait in RTT is classically described as being ataxic or apraxic. There are also some quite specific forms of walking: dynamic equinus gait and two distinct modes of ground contact during walking: *plantigrade* gait (during stance phase, the heel is in direct contact with the ground), and *digitigrade* gait (during stance phase, the first or fifth metatarsal is in direct contact with the ground [not the heel]). The *plantigrade* gait can also involve significant lateral trunk movement and a wide base. The *digitigrade* gait can also involve favouring one lower limb during walking, preferring to put it forward at every step.

Musculoskeletal system
SCOLIOSIS

Scoliosis occurs in over 50% of RTT patients, and typically is noted between 8 and 11 years. It is more likely to progress rapidly if there is hypotonia, or extrapyramidal asymmetrical dystonia, and particularly for non-ambulatory patients. There are two recognised forms:
1. a double curve, where the upper curve is longer, and usually *dextroconvex* (convex to the right), and the lower curve is shorter, and *sinistroconvex* (convex to the left); and
2. a single C curve. The single curve tends to worsen more rapidly. Kyphosis can also occur, particularly high deformities, and mainly in ambulant girls.

BONE DENSITY AND FRACTURES

Bone density is decreased in RTT, irrespective of whether patient is ambulatory. RTT patients have four times the risk of fractures of the general population.

HYPOPLASTIC COLD HANDS AND FEET

These are thought to be due to autonomic dysfunction. The feet become discoloured, with red- and blue-hued areas, and abiotrophic changes. The toes become clenched, and progress through to the feet becoming fixed in equinus, equinovarus or equinovalgus position, caused by continual dystonic posturing, extrapyramidal or pyramidal syndromes, and shortening of the Achilles tendon.

Sleep and nocturnal behaviours

The majority of RTT children have some form of sleep disturbance; these include lack of regular sleep times, long duration sleeps or waking periods, increased daytime sleeps, decreased night-time sleeps, and nocturnal awakenings with screaming or with crying and screaming.

Preschool children with RTT often wake up laughing during the night; these episodes are loud, can last hours and can be disturbing to the family.

Autonomic dysfunction

This affects particularly the gastrointestinal, cardiovascular and respiratory systems, and accounts for several of the classic RTT findings, including hyperventilation episodes, hypoventilation, breath-holding episodes, apnoea, Valsalva manoeuvres, air swallowing and consequent abdominal distension. The abnormality is due to dysfunction of the cardiorespiratory centre in the brainstem, involves the serotonergic system, and unusual integration within the 'wakefulness drive' areas of the hypothalamus and the limbic cortex. Autonomic dysfunction also manifests as episodes of agitation, panic-like episodes, sleep disturbances, fluctuating mood and episodes of pupillary dilation, which can last for many hours.

Gastrointestinal manifestations

FEEDING ISSUES (NUTRITION, FEEDING IMPAIRMENT)

Difficulties with food, including chewing difficulties, choking episodes and swallowing problems, involve dysfunctional oropharynx (includes ineffective chewing, with residual liquid or food left at the pyriform sinuses and small amounts of liquids and solids entering the larynx during swallowing) and upper gastrointestinal tract (GIT) (includes oesophageal dysmotility), relating to autonomic nervous dysfunction.

GASTRO-OESOPHAGEAL REFLUX DISEASE (GORD)

GORD is common in RTT, and may manifest as vomiting, regurgitation, rumination or respiratory symptoms including aspiration. It can be due to increased oesophageal motility. Complications may include aspiration pneumonia, oesophagitis and weight loss. Conservative approaches are preferred initially, with small frequent feeds, upright posturing and pharmacological agents, avoiding surgical treatment unless GORD cannot be controlled with medications. Fundoplication carries with it risk of gastric perforation in patients with significant aerophagia.

CONSTIPATION

Constipation is almost universal in RTT. This can be due to decreased gut motility. Constipation occurs more often in cases with decreased mobility or with scoliosis.

Management includes adequate fluid intake, physical exercise/activity and regular toileting, but tends to avoid paraffin-based laxatives because of the risk of aspiration and the complication of chemical pneumonitis.

AEROPHAGIA AND ABDOMINAL BLOATING

Air swallowing can lead to massive abdominal bloating and distension, which can be complicated by abdominal pain, or even perforation of the stomach or bowel. For this reason, fundoplication increases risk of gastric perforation, as on the previous page.

GROWTH (SUBOPTIMAL WEIGHT GAIN) AND NUTRITIONAL ASSESSMENT

Children with RTT have deceleration in head growth noted first, then there may be deceleration in other growth parameters. However, microcephaly is no longer an absolute requirement for the clinical diagnosis.

Cardiac abnormalities

Prolonged QTc (> 0.45) occurs with increased incidence in RTT. For this reason, prokinetic agents such as domperidone, cisapride and erythromycin should be avoided. Around a half to three-quarters of patients with RTT have autonomic nervous system abnormalities, including increased sympathetic tone. The incidence of sudden unexpected death is much higher in RTT girls than that seen in the general population; this is presumed to be largely because of electrical instability of the heart, related to the autonomic dysfunction. There is a wide range of cardiac conditions, other than prolonged QTc, reported in RTT including arrhythmias, atrioventricular dissociation, sinoatrial block, sinus bradycardia and ventricular tachycardia. There are several differences between echocardiography findings in RTT and those in matched controls, measurements which demonstrate cardiac dysfunction in RTT.

Breathing dysfunction

Disordered breathing when awake occurs in around three-quarters of RTT patients, usually with periods of hyperventilation (and hypocapnia) alternating with periods of hypoventilation and apnoea (up to 120 seconds) leading to cyanosis; between episodes breathing is normal, although a quarter have their usual respiratory rate at almost double that expected for girls of their age. Hyperventilation happens more when these children are excited, whereas apnoea occurs when children seem quiet and smile. This abnormal breathing does not cause seizures despite the hypoxaemia. Valsalva breathing can occur, and can lead to bloated abdomen due to swallowing air. The pathophysiology relates to faulty control measures for exhalation of carbon dioxide.

Breathing during sleep is typically normal in patients with RTT, but some RTT girls have been described with central apnoea at night, which requires treatment with continuous positive airway pressure (CPAP) or bilevel positive airways pressure (BiPAP). It is also noted that in RTT children requiring sedation for lumbar puncture, there is a greater risk of prolonged apnoea than in other children.

Screaming episodes

Teenage and older patients with RTT can have attacks of what sounds to be violent screaming, which are initially interpreted as being due to pain. Some have been severe enough to warrant consideration of an acute abdomen, but time reveals there to be no somatic cause. These are a more disturbing stereotypic symptom. It has been suggested that RTT girls are at increased risk of gallbladder/gallstone disease.

Decreased sensitivity to pain

Girls with RTT often have poor pain discrimination, and this can seem like a delay in pain perception as much as decrease in nociception. The altered pain perception can present quite differently as reflex sympathetic dystrophy. Some girls with RTT have been reported to put their hand into a flame and laugh in response, after a few seconds' delay.

History

Ask about the following.

PRESENTING COMPLAINT

Reason for current admission.

EVOLUTION OF SYMPTOMS (STAGES)/CURRENT SYMPTOMS/FUNCTION (DRUMBEATS)

1. **D**elayed development (Stage I): milestones (e.g. age when first smiled, sat, spoke, crawled, stood, walked)
2. **R**egression of development (Stage II): loss of acquired skills (e.g. language, hand use), loss of interest in toys, loss of social interaction
3. **U**napparent slow deterioration (Stage III): return of any abilities
4. **M**otor deterioration (late) (Stage IV): loss of ambulation, use of wheelchair, requirements for interventions (e.g. gastrostomy)
5. **B**reathing irregularities (almost always awake; rarely asleep; nocturnal central apnoea (rare): CPAP, BiPAP)/**B**ruxism/**B**lue hands and feet
6. **E**ye contact (decrease during regressive stage)/**E**ye pointing, or 'Rett's gaze' (developing during Stage III)/**E**pilepsy/**E**xpression (facial) and interpretation of others' expressions
7. **A**utism spectrum disorder—like symptomatology/**A**taxia/**A**praxia/**A**pnoeic episodes
8. **T**one abnormalities: hypotonic (early), spasticity, rigidity (later)
9. **S**pinal deformities: **S**coliosis (double curve or single C curve), kyphosis/**S**tereotypies (mainly midline, hand stereotypies) including clapping, clasping behind back, grasping, held at sides, releasing, tapping, touching, washing, wringing/**S**leep phenomena (including screaming, laughing, occasionally central apnoea)

Other aspects:

10. Activities of daily living (ADLs; bathing, cleaning teeth, combing hair, dressing, writing and other hand usage, toileting, menses).
11. Behaviour (hyperactivity), affect (depression).
12. Cognitive abilities (daycare, preschool, school progress).
13. Growth (head circumference, height, weight; often deceleration of growth in first 2 years).
14. Speech, and communication problems (use of: communication boards, computers, eye gaze technology).
15. Vision (usually normal acuity) and hearing (usually normal).

BIRTH HISTORY

Any notable findings at birth. Birth parameters are important to know to track deceleration of growth. Birth history typically unremarkable; usually born at term after unremarkable pregnancy and delivery.

DEVELOPMENTAL HISTORY

Age at which milestones achieved (including quality of attainment: e.g. bottom-shuffling, bunny-hopping, gross motor development, early hand preference in fine motor development).

Any family history of RTT.

MANAGEMENT

Recent management in hospital, usual treatment at home, daily routine, frequency of therapies, (e.g. physiotherapy, occupational therapy, speech therapy), usual doctors seen (e.g. local doctor, local paediatrician, subspecialists such as orthopaedic surgeon, neurologist), compliance with treatment, alternative therapies tried (e.g. acupressure, patterning).

SOCIAL HISTORY

Impact on parents and siblings, disruption to family routine, family financial considerations (e.g. private health insurance, visits to multiple specialists, cost of hospitalisations, surgical procedures, aids, home modifications, drugs, benefits received such as Child Disability Assistance Payment), social supports (social worker, extended family, respite care, involvement of Cerebral Palsy Alliance, self-help groups), legal proceedings surrounding perinatal care.

UNDERSTANDING OF PROBLEMS AND PROGNOSIS

Parents' and siblings' understanding; degree of education regarding RTT; question of resuscitation.

Examination

See the separate short case on Rett syndrome in this chapter. The procedure outlined there can be used for a long- or short-case examination. When presented in the long case, the examination of the child with RTT should convey to the examiners an overall picture of the patient (e.g. 'an intellectually disabled microcephalic girl with dystonic posturing, a broad-based ataxic gait, intense eye gaze, periods of hyperventilation, constantly wringing her hands, and not making any vocalisations') as the initial introduction.

IMPORTANT SIGNS IN EXAMINATION OF THE CHILD WITH RTT

A mnemonic that may be useful lists many features of RTT is **RETTS MECP2 BASED**:

Regression: fine motor (loss purposeful hand movement); cognition; communication/**R**ecovery (partial) post-regression, then slow worsening

Epilepsy: in 90%; many seizure types, except absence; infantile spasms (severe) in separate cause from MECP2 gene: CDKL5 gene mutation

To and fro rocking and retropulsion/**T**witching/**T**rembling/**T**urning head

Twisting hands plus squeezing, wringing, clapping/**T**one: rigidity

Speech lost/**S**lowing (early) head growth/**S**tagnation of development/**S**low deterioration after partial recovery phase/**S**tereotypic movements (licking, grabbing)/**S**creaming/**S**tages; four described

Methyl-CpG binding protein 2 encoded by MECP2, on Xq28; mutations in 95–97% RTT/**M**alnutrition; nutrition supplements with gastrostomy/**M**yoclonic jerks

Eating: impaired (problems: chewing; swallowing; choking; regurgitation)

Cardiac: increased QTc, **C**oding regions MECP2 gene: 3; multiple mutations (e.g. truncations/missense proteins)/**C**-shaped scoliosis worsen rapidly

Parameters (growth): decreased head, then weight, then height percentiles/**P**ubertal changes in height and weight diminished/**P**erforation of stomach or bowel (from aerophagia, especially with fundoplication)

(over) 250 known MECP mutations can cause RTT

Bradykinesia/**B**reathing disorder: *awake*: hyperventilation; hypoventilation; apnoea/**B**road-based gait/**B**ruxism/**B**one density decreased/**B**ack: scoliosis +/– kyphosis

Autonomic dysfunction (peripheral vasomotor anomalies; cold feet)/**A**spiration/ **A**bsence-like stopping (non-epileptic): staring, breath-holding, pupil dilation/ **A**praxic/**A**taxic gait/**A**bsent walking (later)/**A**berrant response to pain (delayed and diminished)/**A**erophagia (swallowing air)

Sporadic mutations cause RTT/**S**ympathetic tone increased/**S**leep architecture abnormal (waking disruptive, crying, laughing, screaming; shortened duration night)/ **S**coliosis

Expression (facial) diminished (masking of facial expression = hypomimia)/ **E**xtrapyramidal motor dysfunction: hands, gait/**E**yes: oculogyric crises

Drooling/**D**ystonic and **D**yskinetic tongue movements/**D**ysfunctional oropharynx/**D**ysmotile upper GIT/**D**ystonia/**D**eceleration of head growth +/–, weight +/– and height/**D**ouble-curved scoliosis thoracic + lumbar common

Management

MEDICATIONS

There are several medications that have been shown to be effective in numerous areas of RTT.

SEIZURES

1. Anti-epileptic drugs (AEDs) which have been found useful include: carbamazepine, clobazam, lamotrigine, levetiracetam, phenobarbitone, sulthiame, topiramate, valproate and vigabatrin.
2. Ketogenic diet can be beneficial in treating recalcitrant seizures.
3. Vagus nerve stimulation can be beneficial in treating recalcitrant seizures also.

DYSTONIC SPASMS AND RIGIDITY

1. Treatments have included: baclofen, benzhexol (trihexyphenidyl), carbidopa-levodopa, clonazepam, diazepam, gabapentin and tizanidine (central alpha 2 adrenergic agonist).
2. Botulinum toxin (which also can be used for extreme cases of bruxism).
3. Other treatments include swimming, warm baths and massage.

DROOLING

1. Glycopyrrolate.
2. Atropine eye drops given orally.
3. Botulinum toxin given orally.

RESPIRATORY DYSFUNCTION

1. Insulin-like growth factor 1 (mecasermin), given subcutaneously (twice daily for 4 weeks, daily for 20 weeks) has been described as decreasing apnoea episodes.
2. Naltrexone has been used for central apnoea.
3. Theophylline has been used for shallow breathing.

SLEEP DISORDERS

1. Melatonin decreases latency of onset of sleep (orally once daily at bedtime).
2. Additional agents tried with success in RTT include chloral hydrate, clonidine, cyproheptadine, diphenhydramine, lorazepam, mirtazapine (noradrenergic and specific serotonergic antidepressant), trazodone (tetracyclic antidepressant) and

zaleplon (a pyrazolopyrimidine hypnotic agent, which acts on the same receptors as benzodiazepines).

CARDIAC DYSFUNCTION

Avoidance of several medications which can lengthen the QT interval; for example; antibiotics (erythromycin), antipsychotics (thioridazine), antidepressants (imipramine), antiarrhythmics (sotalol, amiodarone), anaesthetic agents (thiopentone, succinylcholine). To treat prolonged QT interval, beta blockers may be useful, or for more severe cases, cardiac pacing may be needed.

AGITATION

Low dose risperidone, buspirone, clorazepate, naltrexone, quetiapine and SSRIs have been used to treat agitation.

GASTROINTESTINAL ASPECTS

1. Urso can be used in RTT patients with gallstones.
2. Anti-reflux medications are used for GORD.
3. Laxatives are often needed, but avoiding paraffin oil preparations.

MUSCULOSKELETAL ASPECTS

1. Bisphosphonates such as alendronate, or pamidronate have been used for osteoporosis.
2. Vitamin D, calcium and phosphorus preparations have been used if there is demonstrated biochemical or nutritional deficiency; RTT is known to be associated with decreased serum 25-hydroxyvitamin D levels, although the levels are not low enough to cause fractures. The increased risk of fractures in RTT is typically unrelated to serum 25-hydroxyvitamin D levels.

REPRODUCTIVE ASPECTS

As girls with RTT go through normal sexual development, they can become pregnant, so birth control and menstrual hygiene issues become important.

NEWER MEDICATIONS

In 2015 the FDA in the US granted Orphan Status to a new medication: trofinetide. Trofinetide is a synthetic analogue of a peptide based on IGF-1. In animal models, it has many beneficial effects including decreasing neuro-inflammation, improving microglial function and correcting synaptic dysfunction.

SURGERY

There are many operative procedures that can benefit RTT patients.

Surgical interventions for gastrointestinal/feeding problems

1. Gastrostomy tube is useful for RTT patients with poor growth, very slow feeding or a significant risk of aspiration.
2. Gastrojejunostomy or PEG-J tube may be preferred with severe GORD.
3. Fundoplication may be considered for very severe reflux, while being cognisant that RTT patients with aerophagia are at increased risk of gastric perforation if they have a fundoplication.
4. Cholecystectomy can be indicated for cholecystitis biliary dyskinesia, and cholelithiasis.
5. Surgery for drooling: tympanic plexus neurectomy, partial removal of salivary glands, redirection of salivary ducts.

Surgical interventions for scoliosis

1. Posterior spinal fusion and unit rod instrumentation can decrease curvature from around 70 degrees to under 30 degrees. Some studies show a high complication rate (including respiratory, gastrointestinal and infective complications).
2. Computer-assisted posterior segmental pedicle screw fixation from T1 to L3 has been successful without complications in a case report.

THERAPIES

1. Conventional effective therapies: physiotherapy, occupational therapy, speech therapy; these are aimed at maintaining or improving walking, balance, hand function and communication, and preventing deformities.
2. Other effective therapies: music therapy, massage therapy, horseback riding (hippotherapy), hydrotherapy.

EYE GAZE AND EYE TRACKING TECHNOLOGY

Eye gaze control is another form of communication available to patients with RTT, giving them access to computers for educational or fun activities. Children with RTT use eye gaze to select things to show what they want or need. Video-based eye tracker systems are being used in RTT, as the computer essentially can determine what the person is looking at. An example is the Tobii PCEye, a device that can be used with most personal computers, which converts movement of the eyes to a cursor, allowing eye control of the computer.

PROGNOSIS

Life expectancy is currently over 50 years for RTT. The causes of death are usually lower respiratory tract infection, respiratory failure, aspiration or asphyxiation (and possibly sudden cardiac arrhythmias). One-quarter of RTT girls die unexpectedly, suddenly; some of these deaths are attributed to cardiac disease, some to seizure activity and some due to respiratory complications.

Useful websites

- RettBASE, http://mecp2.chw.edu.au
- EuroRETT, www.erare.eu/financed-projects/eurorett
- InterRett, https://interrett.ichr.uwa.edu.au
- Genetica Medica, www.biobank.unisi.it/Elencorett.asp
- MeCP2.org.uk, www.mecp2.org.uk
- Rett Syndrome Database Network, www.rettdatabasenetwork.org
- Rettsyndrome.org, www.rettsyndrome.org

SHORT CASES

SHORT CASE: Suspected ADHD

The lead-in here could be: 'This child does not seem to concentrate at school', or 'This boy has trouble paying attention' or 'The parents are worried he has ADHD. Could you assess please?'

Given that so many conditions can present with inattention and hyperactivity, a fairly comprehensive mnemonic may help.

ACCURATE DIAGNOSIS HIGHLY DESIRABLE contains the vast majority of diagnoses or problems that must be excluded, or taken into consideration, before ADHD is diagnosed.

Autism spectrum disorder (ASD)/**A**norexia nervosa (AN, overactive to lose weight)
Cerebral palsy (CP)/**C**erebrovascular accident (CVA)/**C**erebral tumour (frontal lobe)
Conduct disorder/**C**ongenital heart disease (22q11, cyanotic, TAPVD, HLHS)
Urea cycle disorders
Reaction to social set-up (new partner/blended family)/**R**eactive attachment disorder
Acquired brain injury (ABI, especially frontal lobe damage, e.g. post-MVA), **A**buse/
    Attachment/**A**djustment/**A**nxiety disorders/**A** duplicate of a hyperactive dad
Teratogens in utero (cocaine, heroin, methadone)/**T**ourette syndrome/**T**wins ('hype'
    each other when *together*)/**T**uberous sclerosis complex (TSC)
Expressive language disorder/**E**ncephalitis/meningitis sequelae

Deafness/**D**rugs (illicit)/**D**isrupted family (divorce)/**D**isruptive mood dysregulation
Intellectual impairment/**I**mpaired: vision, hearing, speech, language, reading
Alcohol: fetal alcohol spectrum disorder (FASD)/**A**lcoholic parents
Global developmental delay (later termed intellectual impairment; various causes)
Neurocutaneous syndromes (e.g. NF1)/**N**ICU graduate (ex-premmie, < 1500 g)
Obstructive sleep apnoea (OSA)/**O**ppositional defiant disorder (ODD)
Small for gestational age (SGA)/**S**moking in pregnancy/**S**chizophrenia
Iron deficiency/**I**nborn errors of metabolism (e.g. phenylketonuria, PKU)
Syndromes: fragile X, Down, Williams, XXY, XYY, Sturge-Weber (SWS), Sotos

Hydrocephalus/**H**ead injury/**H**aemorrhage (IVH/ICH in ex-premmie)
Intrauterine disorders: infections (TORCH)/teratogens (cocaine, heroin)
Graves' hyperthyroidism/**G**overnment benefits: faking ADHD to obtain (parent
    instructs child to trash paediatrician's office to prove he needs stimulants)
Hypothyroidism ('dreamy' inattention)/**H**ypoxic insult (drowning, strangulation)
Lead intoxication/**L**eukaemia survivor (cerebral irradiation)
Young/inexperienced parents (unrealistic beliefs; e.g. 12 month old referred!)

Depression/**D**rug acquisition (faking ADHD to get dexamphetamine, to make 'ice')
Epilepsy: childhood absence epilepsy (CAE, 'petit mal') or 'temporal lobe absences'
Sickness in family member (reaction to)/**S**ubstance use disorder/**S**tereotypies
Iatrogenic (phenobarbitone/beta-2-sympathomimetics/antihistamines/thyroxine)
Reaction to trauma (posttraumatic stress disorder)/**R**eaction to food/food additives
Attention seeking/**A**cting out/**A**bsent dad: 'Acute **D**ad **D**eficiency'
Bright but bored (i.e. gifted and curious)/**B**ipolar disorder
Learning disorder (specific, SLD)/**L**anguage disorders/**L**ack of stable family
Environmental stressors at school or home (doing poorly in class; chaotic house)

Remember that ADHD has no single diagnostic test; the diagnosis is based on criteria, many of which can apply to a multitude of conditions, both normal and abnormal (see the long case on ADHD in this chapter). All the DSM-IV criteria can be met by a normal 3 year old; hence, the reluctance of many paediatricians to diagnose ADHD in children under 6 years.

Just as 'all that wheezes is not asthma', so to 'all that is inattentive and/or hyperactive is not ADHD'. Furthering that analogy, if all wheezing were treated simply with bronchodilators, then diagnoses such as inhaled foreign body would be missed and the treatment would not work. Similarly, if all inattentiveness, impulsiveness or hyperactivity were treated simply with stimulants, diagnoses such as obstructive sleep apnoea, iron deficiency and lead intoxication would be missed and the stimulants would not work.

These conditions can mimic ADHD or can coexist with ADHD. Most have been encountered by the author. Several causes listed may seem far-fetched (e.g. faking ADHD just to get government benefits, or to get dexamphetamine to sell); these will be relevant in the real world, rather than in the examination format, but are noted for completeness.

In practice, the really important and more common issues are teasing out the effects of the environment, such as parental separation, absent dad, abuse in different ways, medical issues including sleep apnoea, having a learning difficulty, specific or otherwise, or being gifted and in the wrong environment at school.

Examination

The examination is to detect (exclude) any of the above diagnoses. It comprises a combined neurological, developmental and dysmorphic assessment, plus growth percentiles, vision and hearing.

GROWTH PARAMETERS

Head circumference (increased with hydrocephalus, decreased with ABI), weight (decreased with AN, thyrotoxicosis, SGA syndromes), height (decreased: SGA, increased: XYY). In adolescents, note Tanner staging (delayed in AN).

UPPER LIMBS

Nails (koilonychia), palmar creases (iron deficiency), pulse (slow in hypothyroid, anorexia; fast in hyperthyroidism, or with sympathomimetic side effects), blood pressure (low in anorexia, or secondary to clonidine treatment; high in some cases of neurofibromatosis, and with stimulant side effects; important baseline measurement before commencing on stimulant medication). Check for tremor (hyperthyroidism). Note any involuntary movements (e.g. tics, from comorbid primary tic disorder) or abnormal posturing (CP).

DYSMORPHOLOGY EXAMINATION

(Dysmorphology examination is of the head and neck at this stage; the remainder of dysmorphic assessment is performed when proceeding through neurological examination.) There are many dysmorphic syndromes with countless dysmorphic features; note any dysmorphic aspects and refer to synthesising a diagnosis using websites or reference books on recognition of patterns of malformation. Significant features associated with fragile X (prominent ears, elongated face)/Williams syndrome (elfin face, large mouth, up-turned nose)/FASD (short palpebral fissures, smooth to absent philtrum).

HEAD

Look for shunt (hydrocephalus), scars (surgery for trauma/tumours), bony defects (encephalocele).

EYES

Vision, visual fields, external ocular movements, conjunctival pallor (iron deficiency).

EARS

Note any hearing aids, check eardrums, check hearing (irrespective of result, comment on need for formal audiology).

SPEECH

Evaluate quality, content (impression of whether age-appropriate) as examination proceeds, and mention this later.

MOUTH

Check for angular cheilosis or pale tongue (iron deficiency), and size of tonsils (OSA).

NECK

Check for goitre.

SKIN

Look for neurocutaneous lesions: café-au-lait macules (NF1), hypopigmented macules (TSC), vascular malformation in trigeminal distribution (SWS).

NEUROLOGICAL EXAMINATION

Look for any evidence of brain injury or other cerebral pathology. Examination is best commenced with the gait, followed by the motor system. During the neurological examination, certain so-called 'soft' signs (minor motor anomalies, such as asymmetry; e.g. positive Fog test) may be noted. These are not infrequent in children diagnosed as having ADHD or learning disorders, but are in no way diagnostic of any condition and should not be thought to influence in any way the diagnosis of ADHD. Soft signs resolve with developmental maturation and are common in young children; they tend to persist in clumsy children who are developmentally immature. Many children diagnosed as having ADHD have associated motor problems, including developmental coordination disorder (DCD) (clumsiness).

Note the importance of observing the child out of the corner of your eye while you are talking to the parents; observe how he plays, does he switch off, is there any evidence of absence epilepsy, how does he relate to his parents, what are his verbal communication and expression like?

DEVELOPMENTAL ASSESSMENT

Gross motor, personal–social, fine motor adaptive, language. Check spoken language (chat about an area of interest for that child). A specimen of handwriting could be very useful, as poor legibility may indicate poor fine motor organisation. Regarding gross motor assessment, most normal children can hop by 5 years, skip by 6 and (by report from parent) ride a bike without training wheels by 7.

Also, a tennis ball is very useful to test a child of an appropriate age. A child can usually throw a ball to the examiner's (your) hand by age 4, catch a tennis ball bounced to his or her hands by $5\frac{1}{2}$ years, catch a ball in the air with the hands (when thrown to the child's hands) by 6 years, move to a ball to catch it by $7\frac{1}{2}$ and catch a ball in a container by $8\frac{1}{2}$.

Mention to the examiners that there are standardised tests that may be useful, both to identify ADHD and to note comorbid pathology. Irrespective of what the tests show, you, the candidate, are trying to make a clinical diagnosis, determining whether or not a child meets DSM-5 criteria—that is, is excessively inattentive, hyperactive, impulsive or inattentive at home and school; is this significant; and is there a better differential diagnosis for this. You are then assessing for the comorbidities.

The tests include behaviour rating scales, psychometric profiles (e.g. Wechsler scales), reading test booklets, drawing tests such as the draw-a-person test (which gives an indication of general intelligence and also of any graphomotor disability) and the kinetic family drawing test (a drawing of the child's family with each person doing something, which can reveal underlying psychopathology).

SIDE EFFECTS OF TREATMENT

If the child has already been labelled as having ADHD, and is on medication such as dexamphetamine, methylphenidate or clonidine, then evidence of any side effects of these drugs should be sought as included above (check the blood pressure and pulse rate). See the long case on ADHD in this chapter for a discussion of management. Note that when discussing medications with parents, put side effects into perspective, explain what you are trying to achieve with the medications (i.e. not just about medication), but that educational and other strategies are always important.

Careful fine tuning and small adjustments in medication doses can be very important. But the emphasis should be on how important other strategies are (see the long case in this chapter). The candidate needs to be able to discuss the range of medications, short and long acting, and how to adjust the dose and minimise side effects.

SHORT CASE: Suspected ASD

The approach given here can be used for a short-case approach to a child suspected of having autism or autism spectrum disorder (ASD), or to guide the examination of a child with autism who presents as a long case.

The differential diagnosis for autism/autistic spectrum disorder is broad. The mnemonic used here is **DIFFERENT CHILD**:

Deafness (hearing loss alone, or combined with visual impairment [can cause poor eye contact, stereotypic head nodding, hand/finger flapping])/**D**isordered mood (bipolar or unipolar mood disorders)/**D**own syndrome
Intellectual impairment (any cause)
Fragile X syndrome
Fetal (intrauterine) TORCH infections/**F**etal alcohol syndrome (FAS)
Expressive language disorder
Rett syndrome (females almost exclusively)
Elective mutism
Neurodegenerative conditions/**N**eurocutaneous conditions (other than tuberous sclerosis, which has the strongest association, ASD also has been associated with neurofibromatosis type 1 [NF1] and hypomelanosis of Ito)/**N**eglect (or abuse)
Tuberous sclerosis complex (TSC)

Cerebral palsy/**C**erebral tumour/**C**hildhood schizophrenia/**C**hromosomal syndromes (Smith-Lemli-Opitz, Smith–Magenis, Cohen, Joubert, Timothy, 15q and 16p duplication)
Hyperactivity with attention deficit disorder/'**H**appy puppet' (Angelman) syndrome
Inborn errors of metabolism (presenting with encephalopathy) (PKU)
Landau–Kleffner syndrome (acquired epileptic aphasia)/**L**ead intoxication
Disintegrative disorder

Examination

A suggested order for the examination is as follows.

1. INTRODUCE SELF TO PARENT AND PATIENT

Note the child's degree of eye contact (ASD children classically avoid eye contact), gain an impression of hearing ability, note quality of speech. Decreased vocalisation occurs in severe ASD, hearing impairment and Rett syndrome. In girls, look for any unusual pattern of respiration, such as periods of hyperventilation or breath-holding and midline hand wringing (Rett). Observe how the child interacts with the surroundings. Note any compulsive replacement of any objects moved by the child to their exact original positions (ASD).

2. QUALITY OF MOVEMENT AND POSTURE

In females, note any Rett features (e.g. tortuous wringing of hands, flapping, pill-rolling, rocking body movements, jerky truncal ataxia). Note any features suggesting cerebral palsy (e.g. hemiplegic posturing, choreoathetoid movements).

3. GROWTH PARAMETERS

Head circumference (decreased with intrauterine TORCH infections; deceleration on progressive percentiles in Rett syndrome; markedly enlarged in Bannayan–Riley–Ruvalcaba).

4. DYSMORPHOLOGY EXAMINATION

(Dysmorphology examination is of the head and neck at this stage; the remainder of dysmorphic assessment is performed when proceeding through neurological examination.) Note any features associated with fragile X (prominent ears, elongated face). There are many dysmorphic syndromes with countless dysmorphic features; note any dysmorphic aspects and refer to synthesising a diagnosis using reference books or websites on recognition of patterns of malformation.

5. EYES

Vision, visual fields, external ocular movements (particularly important in children who are not demonstrating any eye contact), fundi: retinopathy (TORCH), grey flat retinal lesions (TS).

6. EARS

Look for hearing aids, check eardrums, check hearing (irrespective of result, comment on need for formal audiology).

7. SPEECH

Evaluate quality and content (impression of whether age-appropriate). Return to this later.

8. SKIN

Hypopigmented macules (TS), café-au-lait spots (NF1).

9. FULL NEUROLOGICAL EXAMINATION

Look for any evidence of brain injury or other cerebral pathology. Examination is best commenced with gait, followed by the motor system. This must include inspection of the back, looking for scoliosis (Rett, cerebral palsy, fragile X). During the neurological examination, certain so-called 'soft' signs (minor motor anomalies, such as asymmetry; e.g. positive Fog test) may be noted. These are not infrequent in children diagnosed with co-existent learning disorders, but are in no way diagnostic of any condition and should not be thought to influence in any way the diagnosis of autism. Soft signs resolve with developmental maturation, and are common in young children. They tend to persist in clumsy children who are developmentally immature. Many children diagnosed with co-existent behavioural disorders have associated motor problems, including DCD (clumsiness).

10. DEVELOPMENTAL ASSESSMENT

Gross motor, personal–social, fine motor adaptive. Be aware that the Denver-II lacks specificity (see the long case in this chapter). Check spoken language (chat about an area of interest for that child, such as trains, wheels). The draw-a-person test is a good clinical measure of IQ/conceptual development. Reading age can be clinically estimated by testing the length of word the child can read. In autism, reading recognition is frequently better than comprehension. A specimen of handwriting can be useful, as poor legibility may indicate poor fine motor organisation.

Regarding gross motor assessment, most normal children can hop by 5 years, skip by 6 and (by report from parent) ride a bike without training wheels by 7. Also, a tennis ball is very useful to test a child of an appropriate age. A child can usually throw a ball to the examiner's (your) hand by age 4, catch a tennis ball bounced to his or her hands by $5\frac{1}{2}$ years, catch a ball in the air with the hands (when thrown to the child's hands) by 6, move to a ball to catch it by $7\frac{1}{2}$, and catch a ball in a container by $8\frac{1}{2}$.

Mention to the examiners that there are various levels of assessment for autism. These can be listed under the headings of routine developmental surveillance, autism-specific screening tests, diagnostic parental interviews and diagnostic observation instruments (see the long case in this chapter for more detail).

The diagnostic criteria as noted in the DSM-5 should be mentioned to demonstrate the candidate's knowledge (see the long case in this chapter).

11. SIDE EFFECTS OF TREATMENT

If the child has already been diagnosed with autism, and is on medication such as dexamphetamine or risperidone, then evidence of any side effects of these drugs should be sought (check the blood pressure, note any tics). See the long case in this chapter for a discussion of management.

12. INVESTIGATIONS

After the candidate has completed the physical examination, the examiners may ask which investigations might be appropriate. This depends on the individual child, as there may be features (e.g. dysmorphism) that will direct this. See the long case on ASD in this chapter for a list of investigations that may be found useful when contemplating autism as a diagnosis.

SHORT CASE: Rett syndrome (RTT)

The approach given here can be used for a short-case approach to a child known to have RTT or for a child suspected of having RTT, or to guide the examination of a child with RTT who presents as a long case.

The 'stem' may involve any of a large number of introductions that may be given; for example, 'not walking', 'not developing as well as her siblings', 'has unusual movements', 'has unusual repetitive hand movements', or more directed introductions such as 'This girl has Rett syndrome; please assess her for complications of this condition', or 'This girl has developmental regression; please assess her for an underlying cause'.

In each case, the initial 1 to 2 minutes spent standing back and inspecting should identify RTT as the most likely problem and direct the examination accordingly.

There are two mnemonics that may be useful.

The first is a fairly comprehensive list of many features of RTT: **RETTS MECP2 BASED**.

The second is a simple guide to remembering the order the examination can take, based on an alliterative mnemonic: **G**rowth, **G**ait, **G**aze, **G**asping (irregular breathing patterns), **G**rasping (hand stereotypies), **G**rinding (teeth), **G**elastic episodes (laughter, unprovoked).

Important signs in examination of the child with RTT: **RETTS MECP2 BASED**.

Regression: fine motor (loss of purposeful hand movement); cognition; communication/**R**ecovery (partial) post-regression, then slow worsening

Epilepsy: in 90%; many seizure types, except absence; infantile spasms (severe) in separate cause from MECP2 gene: CDKL gene mutation

To and fro rocking and retropulsion/**T**witching/**T**rembling/**T**urning head

Twisting hands plus squeezing, wringing, clapping/**T**one: rigidity

Speech lost/**S**lowing (early) head growth/**S**tagnation of development/**S**low deterioration after partial recovery/**S**tereotypic movements (licking, grabbing)/**S**creaming/**S**tages: 4

Methyl-*C*p*G* binding *p*rotein 2 encoded by MECP2, on Xq28; mutations in 95–97% RTT/**M**alnutrition; nutrition supplements with gastrostomy/**M**yoclonic jerks

Eating: impaired (problems: chewing; swallowing; choking; regurgitation)

Cardiac: increased QTc; sudden death in 0.3%/**C**oding regions MECP2 gene: 3; multiple mutations (e.g. truncations/missense proteins)/**C**-shaped scoliosis worsen rapidly/**C**ataracts (traumatic; self-injurious, from repetitive tapping with agitation)

Parameters (growth): decreased head, then weight, then height percentiles/**P**ubertal changes in height and weight diminished/**P**erforation of stomach or bowel (from aerophagia, especially with fundoplication)

250 known MECP mutations can cause RTT

Bradykinesia/**B**reathing disorder: *awake*: hyperventilation; hypoventilation; apnoea/**B**road-based gait/**B**ruxism/**B**one density decreased/**B**ack: scoliosis +/– kyphosis

Autonomic dysfunction (peripheral vasomotor anomalies; cold feet)/**A**spiration/**A**bsence-like stopping (non-epileptic): staring, breath-holding, pupil dilation/**A**praxic/**A**taxic gait/**A**bsent walking (later)/**A**berrant response to pain (delayed and diminished)/**A**erophagia (swallowing air)

Sporadic mutations cause RTT/**S**ympathetic tone increased/**S**leep architecture abnormal (waking disruptive, crying, laughing, screaming; shortened duration night)/**S**coliosis

Expression (facial) diminished (masking of facial expression = hypomimia)/**E**xtrapyramidal motor dysfunction: hands, gait/**E**yes: oculogyric crises

Drooling/**D**ystonic and **D**yskinetic tongue movements/**D**ysfunctional oropharynx/**D**ysmotile upper GIT/**D**ystonia/**D**eceleration of head growth +/– weight +/– height/**D**ouble-curved scoliosis thoracic + lumbar common

Examination

A suggested order is as follows: General observations, Gait, Growth, Grinding, Gaze, Gelastic, Gasping, Grasping, Gas.

1. INTRODUCE SELF TO PARENT AND PATIENT (GENERAL OBSERVATIONS)

Note the following:

- Any dysmorphic features (there should not be any in classic RTT).
- Parameters: head circumference (often obvious microcephaly), weight (often failing to thrive), height (usually decreased), progressive percentile charts.
- Vital signs: respiratory rate (hyperventilation, apnoea); heart rate (can be bradycardic); medical equipment (Kangaroo pump, tubing for PEG, walking aides, wheelchair).
- Posture (dystonia, scoliosis, kyphosis).
- Movement: 1. involuntary (e.g. dystonic spasms; seizures); 2. voluntary (e.g. hand stereotypies; clapping and clasping, patting and pill-rolling, tapping and twisting; ataxic/apraxic gait pattern with wide base; jerking of limbs; bradykinesia; rocking to and fro; retropulsion).
- Behaviour (e.g. lack of interaction with environment, crying, laughing, screaming).
- Eye signs (e.g. relative lack of eye contact [very early], Rett gaze [later]).
- Bulbar signs (e.g. drooling).

In particular, note the child's degree of eye contact (RTT children classically may avoid eye contact during their 'ASD' phase, later developing intense eye communication including eye pointing, or 'Rett gaze'), gain an impression of hearing ability, note quality of speech. Decreased vocalisation occurs in Rett syndrome.

Look for any unusual pattern of respiration, such as periods of hyperventilation or breath- holding; note any panting, hypersalivation, spitting and midline hand wringing.

Observe how the child interacts with the surroundings. Some children may be agitated due to unrestrained sympathetic activity. If presented with a box of toys, magnetic shapes or building blocks, there is a distinct lack of interest in playing with them.

2. QUALITY OF MOVEMENT AND POSTURE (GAIT)

Note any of the following features: tortuous wringing of hands, flapping, pill-rolling, rocking body movements, 'jerky' truncal ataxia.

3. GROWTH PARAMETERS, NUTRITIONAL ASSESSMENT AND TANNER STAGING (GROWTH)

Check head circumference (deceleration on progressive percentiles), plus height and weight. Perform a nutritional assessment (see the short case on nutritional assessment in Chapter 8, Gastroenterology). Note any aids for nutritional support (e.g. gastrostomy).

4. DYSMORPHOLOGY EXAMINATION (HEAD AND NECK) (GRINDING)

This is to exclude certain differential diagnoses. Girls with RTT usually have no dysmorphic features, but this is worth checking in any child suspected of having symptoms where RTT is one of several possible diagnoses. Look at the teeth (if cooperation allows) for any dental damage or wear from bruxism, or decay targeting back teeth from acid reflux with GORD.

5. EYES (GAZE)

As part of developmental assessment, check visual acuity, visual fields, external ocular movements (particularly important in children who are not demonstrating any eye contact; in adolescents, there can be 'eye pointing'). Check the retinal reflex for traumatic self-injuriously induced cataracts from tapping on the eyes. Also check for strabismus.

6. EARS AND HEARING

As part of developmental assessment, check hearing, look for hearing aids, check eardrums (if cooperation allows). Irrespective of result, comment on need for formal audiology, if there is minimal vocalisation.

7. SPEECH (GELASTIC)

Evaluate quality and content of any speech (for any age-appropriate aspects).

8. CARDIORESPIRATORY SYSTEM (GASPING, GELASTIC)

Watch the breathing pattern, noting any hyperventilation, possibly alternating with hypoventilation/apnoea. Take the pulse or auscultate heart to look for bradycardia. Note any unprovoked laughter.

9. FULL NEUROLOGICAL EXAMINATION (GAIT, GAZE, GRASPING)

Examination is best commenced with gait, followed by checking lower limbs, then upper limbs, then motor cranial nerves. This must include inspection of the back, looking for scoliosis. Any scoliosis should be fully assessed as per the specific short-case approach on scoliosis.

10. DEVELOPMENTAL ASSESSMENT (GAIT, GAZE, GRASPING)

In a younger child (under 2 years of age), a developmental assessment can precede a neurological examination, much as a gait examination commences a neurological examination in an older child. A recommended order to proceed is starting with the infant on her parent's lap for checking vision and hearing, then fine motor, personal–social and language, as set out in the short case on developmental assessment. Be aware that the Denver-II lacks specificity. Check spoken language.

The draw-a-person test is a good clinical measure of IQ/conceptual development. Reading age can be clinically estimated by testing the length of word the child can read. A specimen of handwriting can be useful, as poor legibility may indicate poor fine motor organisation. Regarding gross motor assessment, most normal children can hop by 5 years, skip by 6 and (by report from parent) ride a bike without training wheels by 7. Also, a tennis ball is very useful to test a child of an appropriate age.

A typical child can usually throw a ball to the examiner's (your) hand by age 4, catch a tennis ball bounced to his/her hands by $5\frac{1}{2}$ years, catch a ball in the air with the hands (when thrown to the child's hands) by 6 years, move to a ball to catch it by $7\frac{1}{2}$ and catch a ball in a container by $8\frac{1}{2}$.

Mention to the examiners that there are various levels of assessment for components of Rett syndrome. These can be listed under the headings of routine developmental surveillance, autism-specific screening tests, diagnostic parental interviews and diagnostic observation instruments.

The diagnostic criteria should be mentioned to demonstrate the candidate's knowledge.

11. ABDOMINAL EXAMINATION (GAS; SWALLOWED AIR)

In up to 50% of RTT patients, there can be significant air swallowing to the degree that there is distension (bloating) of the abdomen, so extreme that it can mimic the appearance of pregnancy, and it can be complicated by perforation of the stomach or the intestine. Also some RTT patients can have significant constipation, such that there may be palpable faeces on abdominal examination.

12. SIDE EFFECTS OF TREATMENT

If the child has already been diagnosed with RTT, and is on medication such as dexamphetamine or risperidone, then evidence of any side effects of these drugs should be sought (check the blood pressure, note any tics).

13. INVESTIGATIONS

After the candidate has completed the physical examination, the examiners may ask which investigations might be appropriate. Blood testing for DNA analysis for MECP2 mutations should be tested first, in a girl with typical signs of RTT. In girls with clinical presentations consistent with atypical RTT, if the congenital form is considered DNA analysis for FOXG1 mutations should be sought; in the early seizure variant, CDKL5 mutations should be sought.

For children with similarities to RTT, but where there is insufficient evidence to place a diagnosis of RTT, then a useful differential diagnosis is given by the mnemonic **UNPLACED** (see the long case on RTT in this chapter) and one could list the investigations for any conditions in this differential list that may be relevant.

Neuromuscular assessment

The request to perform a neuromuscular assessment does not mean that the problem is neuromuscular disease. A common error is to assume that there is neuromuscular pathology, even when the patient has an obvious problem such as hemiplegia or spastic paraparesis. The candidate should first form an opinion as to whether the problem is neuromuscular. Having determined that it is, another common problem in differential diagnosis is to fail to think of major levels of lesion (anterior horn cell, peripheral nerve, neuromuscular junction and muscle fibre).

There are several possible introductions; for example, 'This boy has increasing difficulty climbing stairs' or 'This girl has been having trouble with increasing tiredness and weakness'.

Essentially, a neuromuscular assessment is a modified neurological examination. Specific manoeuvres are included that aim at eliciting relevant signs of various neuromuscular disorders. The procedure outlined below describes several of these.

Start with general observations. Enquire whether the child can stand for you. Then, focus your attention systematically on the following:

1. Posture (e.g. as in Duchenne's muscular dystrophy [DMD]; see the long case in Chapter 13, Neurology).
2. The face: for myopathic facies, ptosis, presence of nasogastric tube or oxygen catheter, tongue fasciculations (spinal muscular atrophy [SMA]).
3. The neck: for tracheostomy tube, or scars from a previous tracheostomy, goitre (hyperthyroidism can cause myopathy), muscle bulk (for facioscapulohumeral dystrophy), contractures (Emery-Dreifuss muscular dystrophy [EDMD]). Weakness of neck flexors is a good pointer to DMD.
4. Upper limbs: for horizontal axillary skin folds (DMD), proximal muscle wasting (most myopathies), distal muscle wasting (myotonic dystrophy [DM], neuropathies), fasciculations (SMA), scars (tendon releases or transfers), contractures.
5. The back: for scoliosis, kyphosis, lordosis.
6. Lower limbs: for proximal or distal wasting, fasciculations, scars (tendon releases or transfers), contractures, foot deformity such as pes cavus.

Remember to glance at the parents for any evidence of myopathic facies, peroneal atrophy or pes cavus.

After this, ask whether the child can walk for you. Have the child go through a full gait examination (i.e. walking normally, walking on toes, walking on heels, walking heel to toe, running, hopping, jumping, using stairs, stepping up onto a chair or stool, squatting and rising, lying on floor and rising, performing push-ups). This may give very valuable clues to help differentiate between neuropathy and myopathy.

Next, ask the child to hold up both arms above the head, to test for proximal upper limb weakness. Have the child make a fist and then quickly open the hand (easier to assess than a handshake) and finally percuss the thenar eminence (these manoeuvres involving the hands are to detect myotonic dystrophy). If positive, go on to tap the deltoid muscle with a tendon hammer, for myotonia, and ask the mother to make a fist and then open her hand quickly and percuss over her thenar eminence as well.

Next, ask the child to look upwards at the roof (unless there is already ptosis) for a full 30 seconds (screening for myasthenia gravis).

Following these screening tests, perform a standard neurological examination of the lower limbs and upper limbs (including palpating for hypertrophied lateral popliteal, ulnar and greater auricular nerves), followed by the motor cranial nerves. By this stage, the type of problem should be apparent and will allow guidance as to what else should be examined.

If a myopathic process is most likely, then at the completion of the neurological examination, it may be wise to examine the cardiorespiratory system next (cardiac muscle can be involved in DMD, Pompe's disease [in infants]; conduction defects can occur in DM, EDMD and mitochondrial cytopathies), and then the abdomen (for storage diseases).

Chapter 6

Cardiology

LONG CASE: Cardiac disease

This chapter deals with problems that are likely to be discussion areas in the long-case section. Cardiac long-case patients may have complex cyanotic heart disease, or heart disease and other medical problems either causally related, as in Noonan syndrome or congenital rubella, or as a complication of their heart disease or its treatment (e.g. hemiparesis with cyanotic heart disease).

Background information
IMPORTANT CARDIAC CONDITIONS
Cyanotic congenital heart defects (CCHDs)

There are eight lesions worth knowing in detail, as outlined below: 6 **T**s, 1 **P** and 1 **H**. Most can be diagnosed with a combination of clinical acumen, chest X-ray (CXR) and ECG interpretation.

1. **T**ransposition of the great arteries (TGA): the aorta and pulmonary arteries have swapped places, the aorta arising from the right ventricle anterior to, above and to the right of the pulmonary artery (Fig. 6.1). Isolated TGA has no murmur, may be loud S2 due to anterior aortic valve closure (Fig. 6.2). CXR: 'egg on string' heart, narrow pedicle, normal or increased pulmonary vasculature (Fig. 6.3); ECG may be normal. Most common cause of CCHD presenting in neonates. Initially requires a balloon atrial septostomy (BAS). Corrected by the arterial switch operation (Fig. 6.4).

2. **T**etralogy of Fallot (ToF): (a) right-ventricular outflow tract obstruction (RVOTO; subvalvular [infundibular] and/or valvular and/or supravalvular); (b) right-ventricular hypertrophy (RVH); (c) ventricular septal defect (VSD); (d) overriding (of the interventricular septum) aorta, which is dextropositioned (see Fig. 6.5). Systolic murmur over pulmonic area, due to RVOTO (not VSD); may be RV prominence/ heave on palpation, a left sternal edge thrill and an aortic click. Continuous murmurs can occur with collaterals (Fig. 6.6). CXR: 'boot' shape, concave left upper heart border, pulmonary oligaemia (Fig. 6.7). ECG: may be normal, or T wave positive in V1, or may be RVH with tall R waves in V4R and V1, and S wave in V5, V6.

2. **T**etralogy of Fallot (continued)

Commonest cause of CCHD after first year of life; historically, untreated ToF mortality rate was 50% by 6 years. (See Fig. 6.8.)

Infants (especially around 2–6 months) may have 'Fallot's attacks' or 'tet spells' (increased right-to-left shunting, infant becomes blue, tachypnoeic, may lose consciousness; may *squat* to alleviate [compensatory mechanism]); remember '*only Fallot's squat*'; these attacks are due to infundibular spasm. During these hypercyanotic episodes, murmurs may disappear. Management of ToF may include: prostaglandin E1 (PGE1) (neonate, duct-dependent); beta blockers (to treat 'spells'; to decrease both heart rate and systemic vascular resistance [SVR]); spells may need knee-chest positioning, oxygen, morphine, fluid bolus, phenylephrine; primary surgical repair around 6–24 months. (See Fig. 6.9.)

3. **T**ricuspid atresia (TA): absent tricuspid valve, no communication between right atrium and right ventricle, survival depends upon right-atrial blood being able to reach the lungs, which requires patency of foramen ovale, (initially) patent ductus arteriosus (PDA) and presence of an atrial septal defect (ASD), and, most importantly, a ventricular septal defect (VSD). There is often accompanying pulmonary stenosis. Systolic murmur (VSD) and single second heart sound. CXR: pulmonary oligaemia (unless large VSD); ECG: left-axis deviation (LAD); cyanosis plus LAD means TA usually. (See Figs 6.10 and 6.11.)

Treatment: first, a shunt between the aorta or a branch of it, and a pulmonary artery branch; second, a bidirectional cavo-pulmonary shunt (BCPS) where the superior vena cava (SVC) is connected to the right pulmonary artery (RPA); then third, at around 2 years, the definitive Fontan procedure, which diverts all the blood from the venae cavae (both SVC and IVC) directly to the pulmonary arteries, achieved by channelling the IVC blood into the pulmonary arteries (the SVC already diverted by BCPC), thus bypassing the right ventricle (and the left atrium). (See Figs 6.12 and 6.13.)

4. **T**ricuspid 'ectopia': (**E**bstein's anomaly; claiming mnemonic privilege); two of the tricuspid valve leaflets (septal and posterior) have **e**ctopic attachments to the **e**ndocardium, below the annulus fibrosus, whereas the anterior leaflet arises normally; valve is narrowed, conical and incompetent, and functionally the heart above it acts as atrium, effectively providing downward displacement of the valve within the right ventricle; often patent foramen ovale (PFO) or ASD. Small volume pulse, S1 may be loud (thickened valve leaflets), systolic murmur (of TI, tricuspid incompetence), scratchy diastolic murmur at left sternal edge (of tricuspid flow/stenosis). CXR: may be massive cardiomegaly in neonate; in lesser cases, may be just prominent right atrium. ECG: pathognomonic; P waves in lead 2 peaked, tall, higher than QRS complexes. Other findings may include a prolonged PR interval, right bundle branch block (RBBB) and pre-excitation such as Wolff–Parkinson–White (WPW) syndrome. Repair depends on severity; palliation early with Norwood staged repair, closure of ASD later, then tricuspid valve replacement. (See Figs 6.14, 6.15 and 6.16.)

5. **T**runcus arteriosus: persistence of primitive truncus arteriosus which fails to divide into aorta and pulmonary artery, leaving a single, common arterial trunk with both great arteries having a single origin; blood from each ventricle passes through a VSD into the truncus; truncus valve has 2 to 6 cusps, and is typically incompetent. Presents with cyanosis and heart failure. Bounding pulses (Corrigan's sign, collapsing or 'water-hammer' pulse). Active praecordium, systolic ejection click, single S2, systolic murmur with thrill, diastolic murmur of truncus valve incompetence, may be mitral flow murmur. CXR: enlarged heart, pulmonary plethora, congestive cardiac failure. ECG: LVH, RVH, BVH (biventricular hypertrophy); can be changes of ischaemia.

   Complete repair usually around 4–8 weeks and includes aortic reconstruction, separating the pulmonary artery from the truncus, inserting a pulmonary conduit between the right ventricle and the pulmonary artery, and closing the VSD with a patch. (See Figs 6.17 and 6.18.)

6. **T**otal anomalous pulmonary venous *drainage* (TAPVD) (or *connection* or *return*): all four pulmonary veins (hence 'total') do not drain directly to the right atrium. They drain to anomalous sites, which may be: *supracardiac* (to left innominate vein or SVC), *cardiac* (to right atrium or coronary sinus) or *infracardiac* (to portal vein, ductus venosus, IVC, or hepatic vein); the supracardiac and cardiac forms are mainly 'non-obstructive' (no obstruction to pulmonary venous flow), with a large volume flow of arterial blood into the right atrium; infracardiac forms are associated with pulmonary venous obstruction, have less blood to right atrium, and are more cyanosed than those with non-obstructive pulmonary venous drainage. Often have other cardiac anomalies. Physiology determined by amount of shunting to left heart, and mixing of blood through PFO, PDA or ASD. (See Fig. 6.19.)

   Obstructed TAPVD (infracardiac, or occasionally with drainage to left innominate vein) presents with: cyanosis and tachypnoea, cough; loud S2, may be no murmur, crackles over lung fields; CXR: pulmonary oedema; ECG: normal or RVH.

   Non-obstructed TAPVD (supracardiac or cardiac) presents with respiratory symptoms and lack of weight gain; tachycardia, right-ventricular heave, loud S1, clearly split S2 with loud P2, can be gallop rhythm, ejection systolic RVOT murmur due to high pulmonary flow, may be diastolic murmur due to high tricuspid flow. CXR: right-atrial and ventricular enlargement ('snowman', 'figure of 8' or 'cottage loaf' appearance with TAPVD to innominate vein), and pulmonary plethora. ECG: right-axis deviation (RAD), RAH (right-atrial hypertrophy), RVH. Treatment may involve PGE1, BAS, initially, then surgical repair, connecting the main pulmonary venous trunk to the left atrium, division/disconnection of the anomalous pulmonary veins, and closure of the ASD; can be complicated by residual pulmonary hypertension. (See Fig. 6.20.)

7. **P**ulmonary atresia (PA): there are two main presentations. (a) *PA-VSD* (PA with VSD), presents similarly to ToF (indeed is a form of ToF), but presents earlier, and with no spells; all RV blood enters aorta via VSD; very active praecordium, continuous murmurs may be heard, posteriorly and anteriorly, due to flow through collateral vessels to the lungs. CXR: similar to ToF, but less pulmonary blood flow, and longer left heart border. ECG similar to ToF, with RAD, RAH, RVH. Survival depends on ductal patency or collateral vessels; initial PGE1; most need initial shunt from aorta to pulmonary artery branch; complete repair is carried out after 12 months, involving insertion of a conduit from RV to pulmonary artery, and closure of VSD.

7. **P**ulmonary atresia (continued)
There are two subgroups within PA-VSD: those with a PDA (*PA-VSD + PDA*), and those with multiple aortopulmonary collateral arteries (*PA-VSD + MAPCAs*; surgery here may involve connecting multiple collateral vessels). (b) *PA-IVS* (PA with intact ventricular septum): blood cannot leave right ventricle, blood from right atrium goes through PFO or ASD to left heart; cyanosed at birth, tachypnoea, heart failure; may be systolic murmur due to flow through PDA or through tricuspid regurgitation. CXR: prominent RA, pulmonary oligaemia. ECG: peaked P waves from RAH, normal axis, V1 and V2 low RV activity. Survival depends on ductal patency; initial PGE1; most need shunt from aorta to pulmonary artery branch. (See Figs 6.21, 6.22 and 6.23.)

8. **H**ypoplastic left heart syndrome. The most severe cardiac malformation; the entire left side of heart underdeveloped, may be atretic aortic valve, rudimentary LV (left ventricle); commonest cause of heart failure first 2–3 days of life; appear normal at birth, develop cyanosis, tachypnoea, pulmonary oedema and right-sided heart failure with hepatomegaly; as duct closes, peripheral pulses diminish, pallor and shock supervene; loud single S2, may be no murmurs. CXR: enlarged heart, pulmonary plethora/pulmonary oedema. ECG: RAD, RVH, minimal left-ventricular activity. Treatment with surgery (Norwood procedure) or heart transplantation. Norwood is a three-stage procedure. First procedure is connecting origin of pulmonary artery to aorta, so RV can become main ventricular pump for the systemic circulation; atrial septum removed; shunt placed between right subclavian artery and right pulmonary artery (or conduit between RV and pulmonary artery). Second procedure is BCPS at around 3 months, blood from SVC being channelled to pulmonary arteries. Third procedure is the Fontan operation (see earlier), at 3 or 4 years; the Fontan anatomy includes the IVC attached to a conduit, this conduit and the SVC attached to the pulmonary artery; and there is usually a fenestration permitting blood flow between right atrium and conduit. Heart transplantation is a definitive treatment but obviously limited by availability. (See Figs 6.24 and 6.25.)

One line summaries regarding cyanotic congenital heart diseases cover the main clinical feature, CXR and ECG, with 'classic features' in bold italics (6 **T**s, 1 **P** and 1 **H**):

TGA: Listen: loud S2, no murmur. ***CXR: egg on string***. ECG: may be normal

ToF: RV heave; ***murmurs: RVOT, collaterals. CXR: boot***. ECG varies: T +ve V1, RVH

Tricuspid atresia: single S2, VSD murmur. *CXR: pulmonary oligaemia*. ***ECG: LAD***

Tricuspid ectopia (Ebstein): TI murmur. ***CXR: cardiomegaly. ECG: P waves > QRS***

Truncus: ***truncal valve regurgitant murmur***. *CXR: pulmonary plethora*. ECG: LVH, RVH

TAPVD: loud S1, split S2, flow murmurs (RVOT, tricuspid). ***CXR: snowman***; ECG: RAD

PA: (a) **PA-VSD**, continuous murmurs: CXR, ECG like ToF; variants **+ *PDA*, + *MAPCAs***. (vii) (b) **PA-IVS**, murmurs: PDA, TI. CXR: big RA, pulmonary oligaemia ECG: peaked P

HLHS: loud single S2. CXR: cardiomegaly, pulmonary plethora. ECG: RAD, RVH

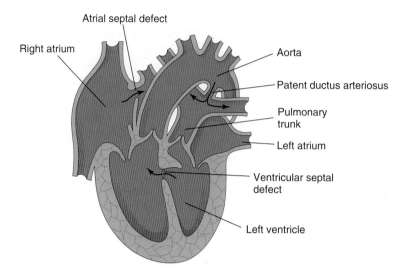

Figure 6.1 Drawing of a heart illustrating transposition of TGA. The ventricular and atrial septal defects allow mixing of the arterial and venous blood. TGA is the most common single cause of cyanotic heart disease in neonates. This birth defect is often associated with other cardiac defects as shown (i.e. ventricular septal defect and atrial septal defect).

Source: Moore, Keith, Persaud, T.V.N. & Torchia, M. (2015). *The Developing Human: Clinically Oriented Embryology* (10th ed.). Philadelphia: Saunders.

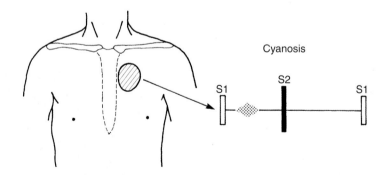

Figure 6.2 Cardiac findings of transposition of the great arteries. Heart murmur is usually absent, and the S2 is single in the majority of patients.

Source: Park, M.K. (2014). *Park's Pediatric Cardiology for Practitioners* (6th ed.). Philadelphia: Elsevier. Figure 14.1.

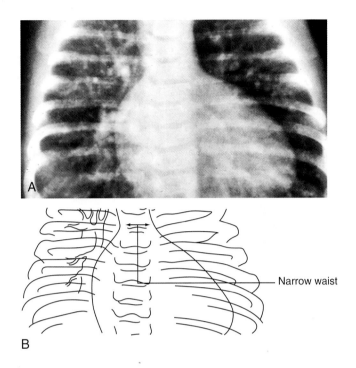

Figure 6.3 **Transposition of the great arteries. Note the 'egg on a string' heart shadow, which results from the position of the main pulmonary artery posterior and slightly to the left of the aorta, contributing to the narrow waist (the 'string').**

Source: Zitelli, B.J., McIntire, S.C. & Nowalk, A.J. (2012). *Atlas of Pediatric Physical Diagnosis* (6th ed.). Philadelphia: Elsevier. Figures 5.21A and B.

TRANSPOSITION OF THE GREAT ARTERIES

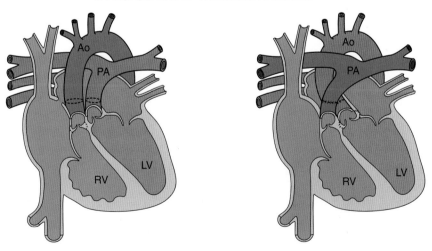

Arterial switch
(Jatene procedure)

Figure 6.4 **Arterial switch (Jatene) procedure for transposition of the great arteries. Ao = aorta; LV = left ventricle; PA = pulmonary artery; RV = right ventricle.**

Source: Zitelli, B.J., McIntire, S.C. & Nowalk, A.J. (2012). *Atlas of Pediatric Physical Diagnosis* (6th ed.). Philadelphia: Elsevier. Figure 5.67.

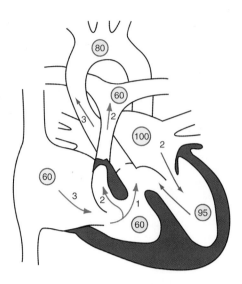

Figure 6.5 Physiology of the tetralogy of Fallot. Circled numbers represent oxygen saturation values. The numbers next to the arrows represent volumes of blood flow (in L/min/m²). Atrial (mixed venous) oxygen saturation is decreased because of the systemic hypoxemia. A volume of 3 L/min/m² of desaturated blood enters the right atrium and traverses the tricuspid valve. Two litres flow through the right-ventricular outflow tract into the lungs, whereas 1 L shunts right to left through the VSD into the ascending aorta. Thus, pulmonary blood flow is two-thirds normal (Qp:Qs of 0.7:1). Blood returning to the left atrium is fully saturated. Only 2 L of blood flows across the mitral valve. Oxygen saturation in the left ventricle may be slightly decreased because of right-to-left shunting across the VSD. Two litres of saturated left-ventricular blood mixing with 1 L of desaturated right-ventricular blood is ejected into the ascending aorta. Aortic saturation is decreased, and cardiac output is normal.

Source: Behrman, R.E., Kliegman, R.M. & Jenson, H.B. (2015). *Nelson Textbook of Paediatrics* (20th ed.). London: Saunders. Figure 423.1.

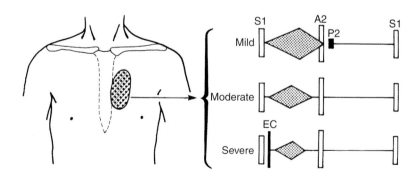

Figure 6.6 Cardiac findings in cyanotic ToF. A long ejection systolic murmur at the upper and mid-left sternal border and a loud, single S2 are characteristic auscultatory findings of ToF. EC = ejection click.

Source: Park, M.K. (2014). *Park's Pediatric Cardiology for Practitioners* (6th ed.). Philadelphia: Elsevier. Figure 14.18.

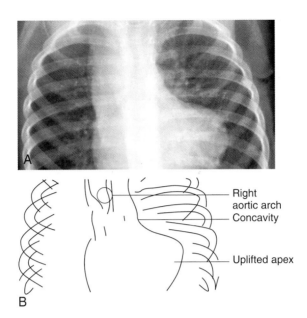

Figure 6.7 **ToF with pulmonic stenosis produces a 'boot-shaped' heart, which results from right-ventricular hypertrophy, upward tilt of the apex, and the concavity at the left upper heart border caused by a small right-ventricular infundibulum and main pulmonary artery. Note also the right aortic arch.**

Source: Zitelli, B.J., McIntire, S.C. & Nowalk, A.J. (2012). *Atlas of Pediatric Physical Diagnosis* (6th ed.). Philadelphia: Elsevier. Figures 5.22A and B.

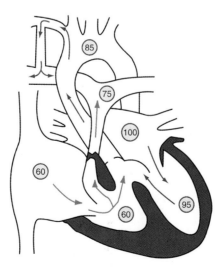

Figure 6.8 **Blalock–Taussig shunt in the patient with ToF. Circled numbers represent oxygen saturation values. The intracardiac shunting pattern is as described for Fig. 6.5. Blood shunting left to right across the shunt from the right subclavian artery to the right pulmonary artery increases total pulmonary blood flow and results in a higher oxygen saturation than would exist without the shunt (Fig. 6.5).**

Source: Behrman, R.E., Kliegman, R.M. & Jenson, H.B. (2015). *Nelson Textbook of Paediatrics* (20th ed.). London: Saunders. Figure 423.5.

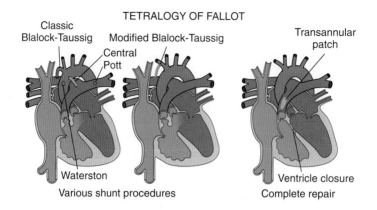

Figure 6.9 Palliative shunt procedures and definitive operative procedure for ToF.

Source: Zitelli, B.J., McIntire, S.C. & Nowalk, A.J. (2012). *Atlas of Pediatric Physical Diagnosis* (6th ed.). Philadelphia: Elsevier. Figure 5.62.

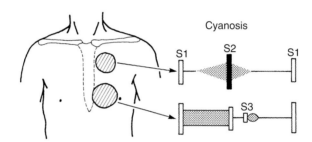

Figure 6.10 Cardiac findings of tricuspid atresia associated with PDA and VSD. 'Superior' QRS axis on the electrocardiogram and cyanosis are characteristic of the defect.

Source: Park, M.K. (2014). *Park's Pediatric Cardiology for Practitioners* (6th ed.). Philadelphia: Elsevier. Figure 14.35.

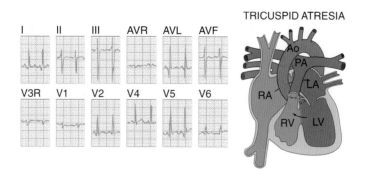

Figure 6.11 Electrocardiogram of a child with tricuspid atresia. Note the left-axis deviation, left-atrial enlargement and left-ventricular hypertrophy. Ao = aorta; LA = left atrium; LV = left ventricle; PA = pulmonary artery; RA = right atrium; RV = right ventricle.

Source: Zitelli, B.J., McIntire, S.C. & Nowalk, A.J. (2012). *Atlas of Pediatric Physical Diagnosis* (6th ed.). Philadelphia: Elsevier. Figure 5.36.

TRICUSPID ATRESIA

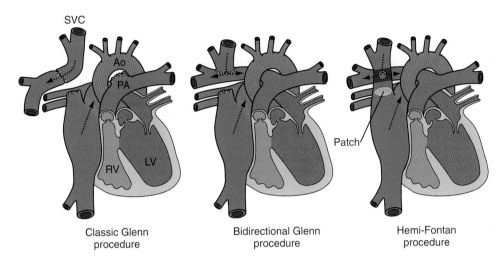

Classic Glenn
procedure

Bidirectional Glenn
procedure

Hemi-Fontan
procedure

Figure 6.12 Various initial palliative procedures for a functionally single ventricle, such as tricuspid atresia.

Source: Zitelli, B.J., McIntire, S.C. & Nowalk, A.J. (2012). *Atlas of Pediatric Physical Diagnosis* (6th ed.). Philadelphia: Elsevier. Figure 5.64.

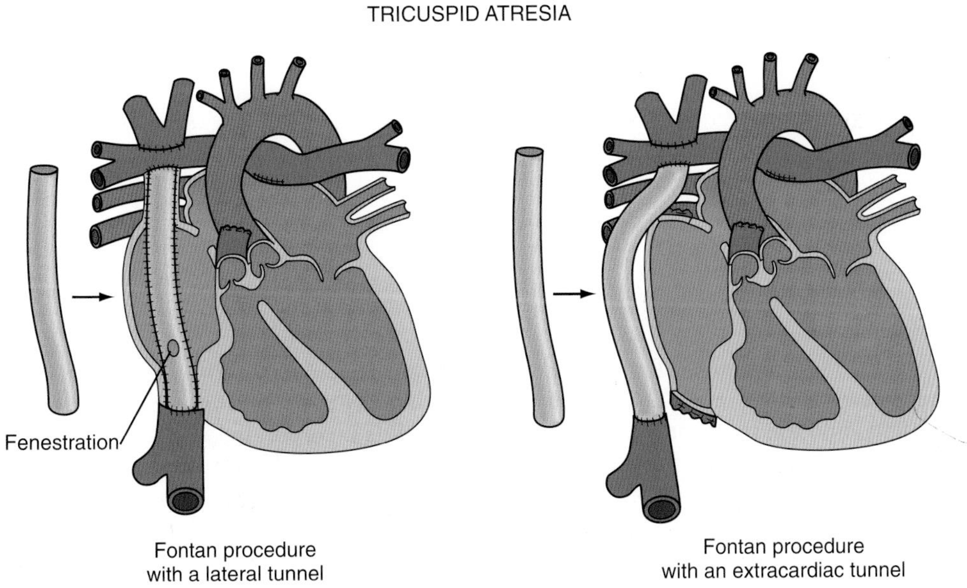

TRICUSPID ATRESIA

Fenestration

Fontan procedure
with a lateral tunnel

Fontan procedure
with an extracardiac tunnel

Figure 6.13 Completion of palliation for a functionally single ventricle, such as tricuspid atresia.

Source: Zitelli, B.J., McIntire, S.C. & Nowalk, A.J. (2012). *Atlas of Pediatric Physical Diagnosis* (6th ed.). Philadelphia: Elsevier. Figure 5.65.

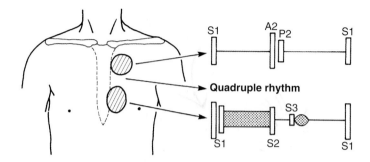

Figure 6.14 Cardiac findings of Ebstein's anomaly. Quadruple rhythm and a soft, regurgitant systolic murmur (of tricuspid regurgitation) are characteristic of the defect.

Source: Park, M.K. (2014). *Park's Pediatric Cardiology for Practitioners* (6th ed.). Philadelphia: Elsevier. Figure 14.52.

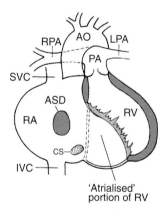

Figure 6.15 Diagram of Ebstein's anomaly of the tricuspid valve. There is an apicalward displacement of the tricuspid valve, usually the septal and posterior leaflets, into the right ventricle (RV). Part of the RV is incorporated into the right atrium (RA) ('atrialised' portion of the RV). Regurgitation of the tricuspid valve results in RA enlargement. An ASD is usually present. Ao = aorta; CS = coronary sinus; IVC = inferior vena cava; LPA = left pulmonary artery; PA = pulmonary artery; RPA = right pulmonary artery; SVC = superior vena cava.

Source: Park, M.K. (2014). *Park's Pediatric Cardiology for Practitioners* (6th ed.). Philadelphia: Elsevier. Figure 14.51.

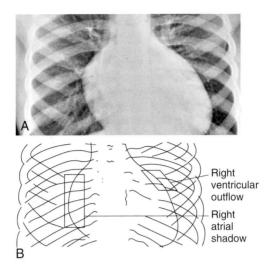

Figure 6.16 **Ebstein anomaly of the tricuspid valve. Note the radiographic appearance of a 'box-shaped' heart, enlarged right atrium and prominent right-ventricular outflow tract.**

Source: Zitelli, B.J., McIntire, S.C. & Nowalk, A.J. (2012). *Atlas of Pediatric Physical Diagnosis* (6th ed.). Philadelphia: Elsevier. Figure 5.25.

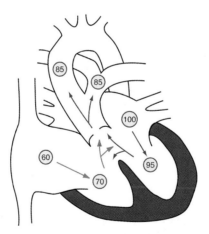

Figure 6.17 **Physiology of truncus arteriosus. Circled numbers represent oxygen saturation values. Right-atrial (mixed venous) oxygen saturation is decreased secondary to systemic hypoxemia. Desaturated blood enters the right atrium, flows through the tricuspid valve into the right ventricle and is ejected into the truncus. Saturated blood returning from the left atrium enters the left ventricle and is also ejected into the truncus. The common aortopulmonary trunk gives rise to the ascending aorta and to the main or branch pulmonary arteries. Oxygen saturation in the aorta and pulmonary arteries is usually the same (definition of a total mixing lesion). As pulmonary vascular resistance decreases over the first few weeks of life, pulmonary blood flow increases dramatically and mild cyanosis and congestive heart failure result.**

Source: Behrman, R.E., Kliegman, R.M. & Jenson, H.B. (2015). *Nelson Textbook of Paediatrics* (20th ed.). London: Saunders. Figure 424.6.

TRUNCUS ARTERIOSUS

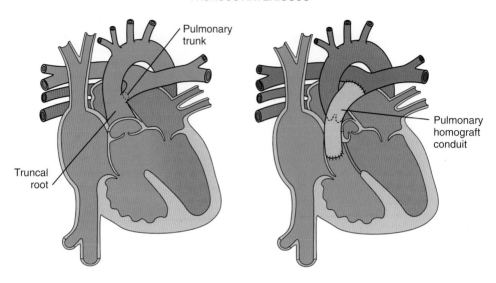

Rastelli procedure

Figure 6.18 Creation of a right ventricle-to-pulmonary conduit and closure of a ventricular septal defect for truncus arteriosus (Rastelli procedure).

Source: Zitelli, B.J., McIntire, S.C. & Nowalk, A.J. (2012). *Atlas of Pediatric Physical Diagnosis* (6th ed.). Philadelphia: Elsevier. Figure 5.68.

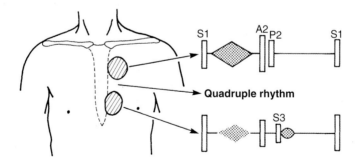

Figure 6.19 Cardiac findings of total anomalous pulmonary venous return without obstruction to pulmonary venous return.

Source: Park, M.K. (2014). *Park's Pediatric Cardiology for Practitioners* (6th ed.). Philadelphia: Elsevier. Figure 14.31.

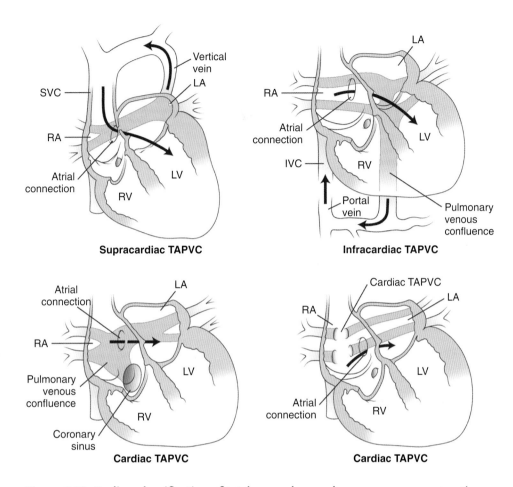

Figure 6.20 **Darling classification of total anomalous pulmonary venous connection (TAPVC). With supracardiac TAPVC, pulmonary venous connection is to a vertical vein, draining to the left brachiocephalic vein and superior vena cava (SVC). With infracardiac TAPVC, the pulmonary veins connect to a systemic venous vessel below the diaphragm (the portal vein in this diagram). With cardiac TAPVC, the pulmonary veins connect either to the coronary sinus or directly to the right atrium (RA). The direction of systemic blood flow (dark arrows) is shown. Note that blood must flow through an atrial connection to reach the left side of the heart. IVC, Inferior vena cava; LA, left atrium; LV, left ventricle; RV, right ventricle. (From Wilson A. Total anomalous pulmonary venous connection, E-Medicine, March 28, 2006.)**

Source: Coley, B.D. (2014). *Caffey's Pediatric Diagnostic Imaging*, 2-Volume Set (12th ed.). Philadelphia: Saunders. Figure e72.7.

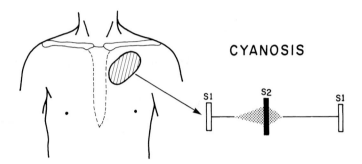

Figure 6.21 **Cardiac findings of pulmonary atresia. These are non-specific for the defect and may be found in tetralogy of Fallot with pulmonary atresia as well.**

Source: Park, M.K. (2008). *Park's Pediatric Cardiology for Practitioners* (5th ed.). Philadelphia: Elsevier. Figure 14.45.

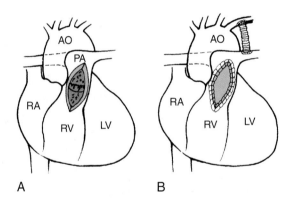

Figure 6.22 **Initial surgery for tripartite or bipartite type of pulmonary atresia. A. A longitudinal incision is made across the pulmonary annulus. The pulmonary valve is incised and the right-ventricular outflow tract is carefully widened. B. A piece of pericardium is used for the transannular patch. A left-sided Gore-Tex shunt is made between the left subclavian artery and the left pulmonary artery (PA). AO = aorta; LV = left ventricle; RA = right atrium; RV = right ventricle.**

Source: Park, M.K. (2014). *Park's Pediatric Cardiology for Practitioners* (6th ed.). Philadelphia: Elsevier. Figure 14.45.

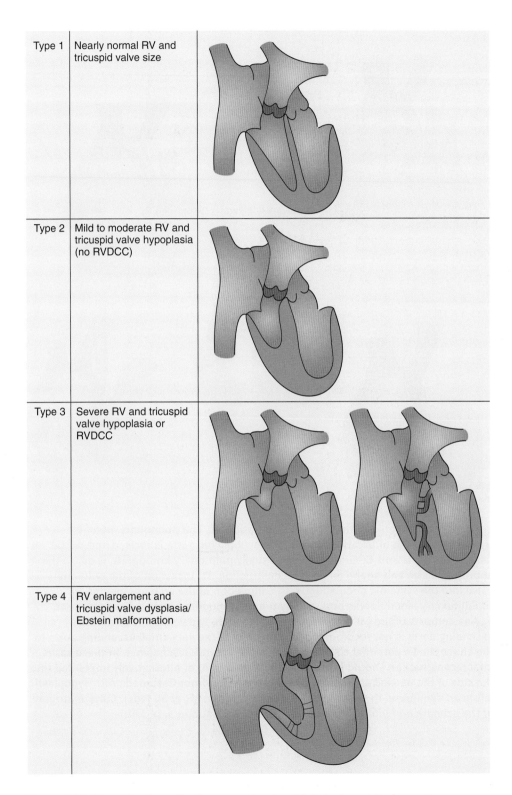

Type 1	Nearly normal RV and tricuspid valve size
Type 2	Mild to moderate RV and tricuspid valve hypoplasia (no RVDCC)
Type 3	Severe RV and tricuspid valve hypoplasia or RVDCC
Type 4	RV enlargement and tricuspid valve dysplasia/ Ebstein malformation

Figure 6.23 Classification of pulmonary atresia with intact ventricular septum.

Source: Crawford, M.H., DiMarco, J.P. & Paulus, W.J. (2010). *Cardiology* (3rd ed.). Philadelphia: Mosby. Table 116.1.

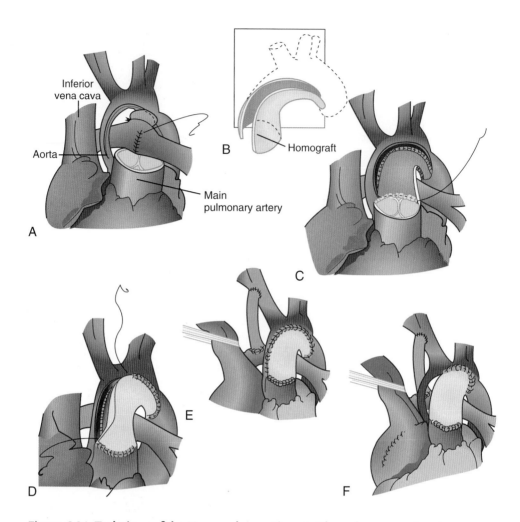

Figure 6.24 Technique of the Norwood operation. A. The pulmonary artery is transected and the bifurcation closed. The hypoplastic aorta is incised and ductal tissue excised. **B and C.** Graft material, usually pulmonary homograft, is cut to the appropriate size and shape for arch reconstruction. **D.** Inclusion of the pulmonary valve into the systemic circulation, with completion of the arch augmentation. **E.** Pulmonary blood flow is provided by the right modified Blalock-Taussig shunt. **F.** Anastomosis of the pulmonary artery to the arch; bypassing the diminutive ascending aorta is not recommended. Proximity of the very small ascending aorta to the shunt allows potential coronary steal and myocardial ischaemia. In these cases, arch reconstruction should proceed as illustrated in A, or alternatively implanted into the side of the neoaorta. (Reprinted with permission from Castañeda AR: Hypoplastic left heart syndrome. In Castañeda AR, Jonas R, Mayer JE, et al. (eds). *Cardiac surgery of the neonate and infant*, Philadelphia, 1994, WB Saunders, p. 371.)

Source: Sellke, F.W., Del Nido, P.J. & Swanson, S.J. (2016). *Sabiston and Spencer Surgery of the Chest* (9th ed.). Philadelphia: Elsevier. Figure 128.2.

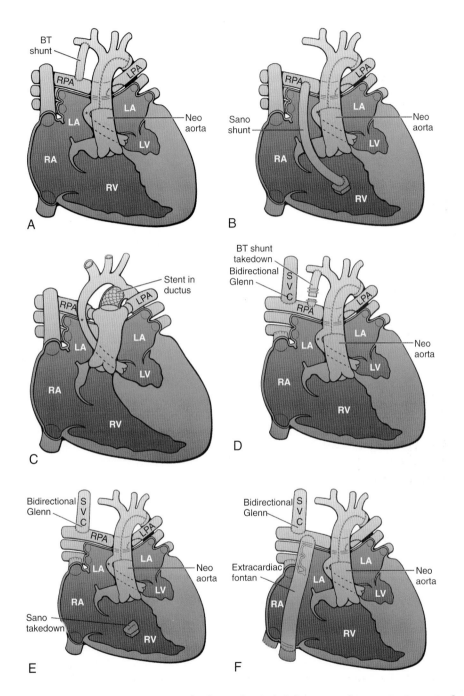

Figure 6.25 **Staged reconstruction for hypoplastic left heart syndrome. A. Stage I of the Norwood reconstruction using a modified Blalock-Taussig (BT) shunt. B. Stage I of the Norwood reconstruction using the Sano modification. C. Hybrid procedure. D. Stage II of the Norwood reconstruction. E. Stage II of the Norwood reconstruction using the Sano modification. F. Fontan procedure. * = Native ascending aorta; LA = left atrium; LPA = left pulmonary artery; LV = left ventricle; RA = right atrium; RPA = right pulmonary artery; RV = right ventricle; SVC = superior vena cava.**

Source: Coley, B.D. (2014). *Caffey's Pediatric Diagnostic Imaging*, 2-Volume Set (12th ed.). Philadelphia: Saunders. Figure 75.4.

Aortic disease: bicuspid aortic valve, aneurysmal aortic dilatation

Bicuspid (or bicommissural) aortic valve (BAV) is a condition in which the aortic valve is anatomically or functionally bileaflet in structure. The commonest form has a trileaflet valve with fusion of predominantly one commissure, most commonly between the right and left coronary cusps, rendering the valve functionally bicuspid. Less common is a structurally bileaflet valve without evidence of a third commissure. Both forms are generically/collectively termed 'bicuspid aortic valve'. It affects approximately 1% of the general population, making it the most common congenital heart condition, with a male predominance.

BAV is associated with increased risk throughout life (from infancy to adulthood) of aneurysmal dilatation of the ascending aorta, with possibility of dissection of the thoracic aorta in adult life. Specific situations can increase risk of dissection in young adults such as high-intensity weightlifting. Isolated aortic aneurysm can occur in the absence of BAV as a random or familial abnormality. Aortic disease with its familial associations is more common than any of the syndromes involving cardiac disease. It is now mandatory to screen all first-degree relatives of patients with BAV. There is a significant (perhaps 10%) incidence of often unrecognised aortopathy in relatives, with up to 37% of families with more than one member having BAV pathology. BAV is an autosomal dominant trait with reduced penetrance.

The aortopathy associated with BAV demands lifelong surveillance. It is rare for a patient with BAV to retain normal valve function lifelong. Most patients have aortic stenosis, regurgitation or mixed function of varying degree. Over 50% of patients will develop ascending aortic dilatation, often detected in infancy or childhood. The risk of aortic aneurysm does not appear dependent on the basic nature of the aortic valve, with no apparent difference between the fundamentally tricuspid or bileaflet valve.

The hallmark of BAV is an ejection click at the apex with murmurs of stenosis or regurgitation along the left lower sternal edge radiating to the base.

Incidence of aortic stenosis (AS) in BAV is around 25–33% (aortic valve stenosis; see Fig. 6.26). Treatment for severe advanced AS is aortic valve replacement.

Incidence of isolated aortic regurgitation (AR) in BAV is around 1.5–10%, with most patients having mixed lesions. BAV is the most common cause of AR (Fig. 6.27). AR is often mild and not clinically apparent, but mild AS is easily detected clinically. The AR is then detected on echo in association with AS. In BAV, 3–6% patients have surgery for AR alone. Treatment of AR comprises valve replacement (Fig. 6.28) or repair. Endocarditis is increased in BAV patients, with an incidence of 2–3%. In children, BAV is second only to ToF in incidence of infective endocarditis. However, antibiotic prophylaxis is no longer recommended for BAV.

Dissection of the aorta is more common in those with BAV than in those with a tricuspid aortic valve. Prophylactic replacement or repair of the aortic root is generally recommended when the diameter of the aortic root or ascending aorta is above 5 cm to 5.5 cm; if aortic valve replacement is required for severe AS or AR, the ascending aorta is also replaced if the diameter is at or above 4.5 cm. (see Fig. 6.29.) After aortic valve replacement, patients with BAV still remain at risk of long-term aortic complications including aneurysm and dissection, and require close surveillance with global imaging modalities such as MRI or CT in addition to echocardiography.

BAV with AS, AR and aortic aneurysm (AA) have important implications in pregnancy, in regard to severity of lesions, how the pregnancy may be conducted, natural delivery or caesarean section, and surveillance of AA during pregnancy. Pregnancy is associated with increased cardiac output, increased left-ventricular stroke volume (which increases until 25 weeks' gestation), as well as increased blood volume (reaching 150% of pre-pregnancy

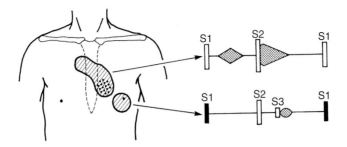

Figure 6.26 Cardiac findings of aortic regurgitation. The S1 is abnormally soft (black bar). The predominant murmur is a high-pitched, diastolic decrescendo murmur at the third left intercostal space.

Source: Park, M.K. (2014). *Park's Pediatric Cardiology for Practitioners* (6th ed.). Philadelphia: Elsevier. Figure 21.4.

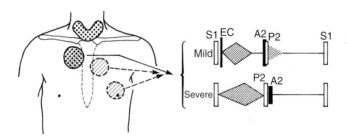

Figure 6.27 Cardiac findings of aortic valve stenosis. Abnormal sounds are indicated in black. Systolic thrill may be present in areas with dots. EC = ejection click.

Source: Park, M.K. (2014). *Park's Pediatric Cardiology for Practitioners* (6th ed.). Philadelphia: Elsevier. Figure 13.6.

AORTIC VALVE DISEASE

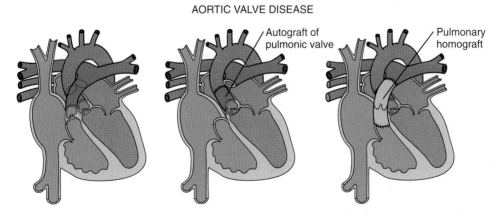

Figure 6.28 Replacing the diseased aortic valve with the native pulmonary valve (Ross procedure).

Source: Zitelli, B.J., McIntire, S.C. & Nowalk, A.J. (2012). *Atlas of Pediatric Physical Diagnosis* (6th ed.). Philadelphia: Elsevier. Figure 5.69.

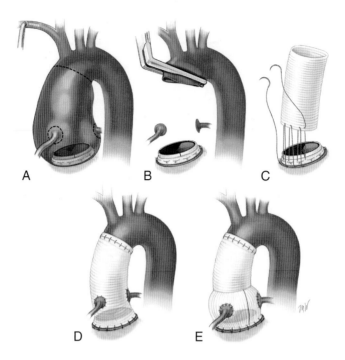

Figure 6.29 Completion Bentall procedure. A. Aortic root aneurysm with normally functioning mechanical aortic valve prosthesis. **B.** With the aneurysm resected, and with normal valve function confirmed, the root is mobilised and 'buttons' are fashioned containing the coronary ostia. **C.** A graft is sutured to the valve cuff with three 2-0 polypropylene sutures, including the valve sewing cuff and the aortic remnant with each pass of the suture. **D.** With the graft secured in position, the coronary buttons and distal anastomosis are constructed. **E.** Completion Bentall procedure using a Valsalva graft.

Source: Malekan, R., Spielvogel, D., Saunders, P.C., Lansman, S.L. & Griepp, R.B. (2011). The completion Bentall procedure. Annals of Thoracic Surgery, 92, 362–363. © 2011 by The Society of Thoracic Surgeons.

volume by 32 weeks) and increased oxygen consumption. Cardiac output further increases by 50% in labour, and each contraction forces 300–500 mL of blood back into the circulation. These all increase the stress on the aorta.

All aortopathies are associated with increased risk of dissection and/or rupture in pregnancy, perinatally and postnatally. The relevant aortopathies, in addition to BAV, include: Marfan syndrome (MFS), Ehlers–Danlos syndrome (EDS, vascular subtype [IV]), Loeys–Dietz syndrome (LDS), coarctation of the aorta, and Turner syndrome (TS, particularly after assisted reproductive technologies [ART], although 2–5% of TS patients may become pregnant naturally, especially with a mosaic karyotype; in TS an indexed aortic diameter > 25 mm/m^2 is considered dilated and at risk of dissection). Surveillance echocardiography is very important during pregnancy. Repair before pregnancy is recommended for: uncorrected coarctation; MFS if the aortic root diameter is > 4.7 cm (the risk of dissection is 10% in MFS during pregnancy if the aortic root diameter is > 4.0 cm).

Elective caesarean delivery is recommended for unrepaired coarctation, LDS (as this is associated with increased dissection risk even with normal pre-pregnancy aortic root diameter) and MFS if the aortic root diameter is > 4.5 cm. If the aortic root diameter in MFS is < 4.5 cm, then epidural anaesthesia and assisted delivery have been recommended, although coexistent dural ectasia in MFS can lead to spinal anaesthesia being less effective.

In women with congenital aortic stenosis, there is a complication rate in 10% of pregnancies, and repair before pregnancy is preferable; severe AS is associated with late complications including heart failure, arrhythmias, need for cardiac intervention, and cardiac death. Should women with severe AS become symptomatic during pregnancy, balloon aortic valvuloplasty during the second trimester may afford adequate palliation if the valve is sufficiently compliant.

BAV is associated with several congenital heart disorders, including VSD, PDA, coarctation of the aorta, supravalvular aortic stenosis and subvalvular aortic stenosis. BAV is also associated with several syndromes mentioned on the previous page, including Turner syndrome, and connective tissue disorders such as MFS.

Exercise restriction/limitation in adolescents with AS and AA is an important area. Athletes with AS need yearly assessment to ascertain whether engagement in sports should continue. Those with mild AS and normal exercise testing can engage in all sports. Those with moderate AS can engage in low to moderate dynamic competitive sports if exercise testing is satisfactory. Those with severe AS, whether asymptomatic or symptomatic, should not engage in competitive sports. Athletes with AR also need yearly assessment to ascertain safety in sports involvement. Those with mild to moderate AR, if they have normal exercise testing, can participate in all competitive sports; those with severe AR and symptoms should not engage in any competitive sports.

Acute aortic dissection or rupture can occur in BAV and in other aortopathies, in the context of increased BP causing aortic stress during physical exertion. Low-intensity non-competitive exercise with low likelihood of significant bodily contact, is generally acceptable as a baseline.

Athletes with BAV and normal-sized aortic root and ascending aorta may engage in competitive athletics. Athletes with BAV and mild aortic dilation should have yearly echocardiograms and MRA, and may engage in low to moderate static and dynamic sports with low likelihood of significant bodily contact, and should avoid intense weight training. Athletes with BAV and moderate aortic dilatation may engage in low-intensity competitive sports with low chance of bodily contact; with BAV and severe aortic dilatation, competitive sports that involve chance of bodily collision should be avoided; with BAV and marked aortic dilatation, all competitive sports should be avoided.

Athletes with MFS, vascular Ehlers-Danlos syndrome or Loeys–Dietz syndrome should not engage in any competitive sports that involve bodily collision. Athletes with MFS may engage in low to moderate static to low-dynamic sports if they do not have aortic root dilatation, significant mitral regurgitation, significant left-ventricular dysfunction or a positive family history of aortic dissection at an aortic diameter < 50 mm.

History

PRESENTING COMPLAINT

Reason for current admission.

DIAGNOSIS

When made (birth, days, weeks or months); where; symptoms at diagnosis (e.g. cyanosis, tachypnoea, poor feeding, failure to thrive, recurrent infection); how (initial investigations: CXR, electrocardiography, echocardiography, angiography).

INITIAL TREATMENT

1. Surgical (e.g. palliative, such as balloon septostomy or shunting procedures, or corrective, such as patent ductus ligation).
2. Pharmacological (e.g. diuretics, angiotensin-converting enzyme [ACE] inhibitors) and side effects thereof.

PAST HISTORY

1. Aetiology (e.g. rheumatic fever, pregnancy complicated by maternal rubella, smoking, alcoholism, or drugs such as lithium, warfarin or phenytoin).
2. Indications for, and number of, previous hospital admissions.
3. Pattern and timing of change in condition (e.g. when cyanosis or heart failure developed, when and how it was controlled).
4. Episodes of infective endocarditis.
5. Other complications of disease (e.g. cerebral thrombosis or cerebral abscess with cyanotic heart disease).

TREATMENT

1. Past surgery, complications thereof, plans for further operative procedures.
2. Past interventional catheter procedures.
3. Past ablation therapy, pacemaker or defibrillator placement.
4. Medications, past and present, the side effects of these, monitoring levels (e.g. digoxin), treatment plans for future.
5. Exercise restrictions (may be inappropriately applied by parents).
6. Recommendations for antibiotic prophylaxis for dental procedures; maintenance of dental hygiene.
7. Compliance with treatment.
8. Any need for identification bracelet.
9. Instructions for air travel and high altitude.
10. Any recent investigations monitoring treatment (e.g. Holter monitoring; oxygen saturation).
11. Any recent changes in treatment regimen, and indications for these.

CURRENT STATE OF HEALTH

Note any of the following:

- Symptoms of cardiac failure, such as fatigue and shortness of breath (in comparison with peers), cough, sweating, poor feeding, recurrent chest infections.
- Cyanosis, squatting with 'Fallot turns'.
- Episodes suggestive of arrhythmias, such as syncope, alteration of consciousness, dizziness, shortness of breath, palpitations in older children (what was the rate; i.e. faster than when usually playing or excited), or a 'funny feeling' in the chest, sweating, nausea, vomiting or the parents being unable to count the rapid pulse rate, suggesting a tachyarrhythmia.
- Chest pain (e.g. myocardial ischaemia versus musculoskeletal, pleural or pericardial causes) or headache (e.g. polycythaemia in cyanotic heart disease, severe hypertension, cerebral abscess).
- Recent change in condition. Note the temporal relationship between associated symptoms with any tachycardia or palpitation: they should coincide—functional chest pain can be followed by a reflex sinus tachycardia.

OTHER ASSOCIATED PROBLEMS

These may either be related to the main diagnosis (e.g. Down, Marfan) or be more general problems (e.g. poor growth, developmental delay, especially involving gross motor abilities, exercise limitations and psychological effects).

SOCIAL HISTORY

1. Disease impact on child; for example, growth, development, schooling (academic performance, sports restrictions, teachers' attitudes, peers' attitudes, teasing, amount of school missed and whether schooling is appropriate).
2. Disease impact on parents; for example, financial situation, financial burden of disease so far, government allowances being received, marriage stability, restrictions on social life, plans for further children, genetic counselling, or at least an awareness of the risks of recurrence, and availability of fetal echocardiography.
3. Disease impact on siblings; for example, sibling rivalry, effect of family financial burden.
4. Social supports; for example, social worker, contact with other families of children with similar problems, break from managing child.
5. Coping: contingency plans (e.g. plan if child develops severe febrile illness); parents' degree of understanding regarding cause, prognosis, exercise restriction, and antibiotic prophylaxis for operations and dental procedures.
6. Access to local doctor, paediatrician, cardiac outpatients clinic (where, how often), other clinics attended.

FAMILY HISTORY

Any early cardiovascular death (e.g. hypertrophic cardiomyopathy [HCM]), unexplained death (e.g. long QT syndrome [LQTS]) or arrhythmias (e.g. Wolff–Parkinson–White [WPW] syndrome); any known cardiovascular diagnoses (e.g. cardiomyopathies); any known syndromes (e.g. Marfan).

IMMUNISATIONS

Any unnecessary delays, local doctor attitudes, parents' understanding of importance.

Examination

The physical examination of the cardiac long case includes a full cardiological appraisal (see the short-case section of this chapter), plus assessment of associated problems, either aetiologically associated (e.g. findings of syndromal diagnoses such as Down syndrome) or complicating the course of the disease (e.g. hemiplegia).

Management issues

The following covers most areas of management that may be relevant in the long-case context, but use of this section should be tailored to the case you are discussing.

1. GENERAL DEVELOPMENT, GROWTH AND NUTRITION

Most children with congenital heart disease develop normally, but children seen in the examination context often have cyanotic heart disease, congestive heart failure or underlying syndromal diagnoses, all of which may be associated with some degree of developmental delay.

Children with cyanotic heart disease or chronic congestive cardiac failure may have delay in their motor milestones. Other children can have prolonged periods of hospitalisation or overprotective family or schooling environments, which can adversely affect social development. Parents should be counselled regarding development. In an otherwise normal child, the degree of delay associated with heart disease is not severe, and provision of a stimulating environment and encouragement of normal schooling should be discussed.

Chronic left-to-right shunts sufficient to cause cardiomegaly often cause growth retardation. This may be an indication for surgical correction even in the absence of other indications such as pulmonary hypertension. Marked hypoxia may be associated with growth retardation, but the hypoxia has to be severe to do so. Most patients who have Eisenmenger's syndrome with cyanotic heart disease and pulmonary hypertension do not have increased energy requirements or inadequate caloric intake, and do not have growth retardation. It takes profound hypoxia to cause growth retardation.

Nutrition is an important issue in general development. Issues to discuss regarding feeding include role of solids, undesirability of fluid restriction, requirements for additional caloric intake, dangers of iron deficiency in cyanosed patients and, perhaps most importantly, support for the mother regarding the above. There is some evidence that more intensive nutritional treatment and early corrective surgery may optimise outcomes in some children with correctable lesions that have previously been associated with poor growth.

2. PROPHYLAXIS AGAINST SUBACUTE BACTERIAL ENDOCARDITIS (SBE) RISK
Dental procedures and dental care

Antibiotic prophylaxis with dental procedures is recommended only for cardiac conditions with the highest risk of endocarditis: prosthetic material (valve [especially—the highest risk], other device [first 6 months after placement], patch, material); cyanotic congenital heart disease (unrepaired; includes palliative shunts and conduits); previous endocarditis; and cardiac transplantation recipient with cardiac valvular disease.

Tetralogy of Fallot has the highest risk of developing SBE of known cardiac conditions, and almost 10% of patients with CHD and endocarditis will have aortic insufficiency. Tooth brushing has been shown to yield positive blood cultures in 23%, compared to 33% for tooth extraction with SBE prophylaxis, and 60% for tooth extraction without SBE prophylaxis; hence tooth brushing represents the greatest risk of SBE, given the frequency of tooth brushing. A high level of dental hygiene should be maintained, and problems such as carious teeth and periodontal disease should be dealt with promptly, with appropriate antibiotic cover.

Endocarditis has a bimodal peak in age, the largest groups being patients under 12 months, and over 16 years. In a study reviewing a national database, between 2000 and 2003, most children diagnosed with endocarditis (900 out of 1558) had no preexisting heart disease, but had various medical conditions that predisposed them to increased risk of SBE.

Four risk groups have emerged: 1. patients with multiple interventions, including chronic line placements; 2. immune compromised patients (e.g. primary immune deficiencies [such as 22q11.2 deletion syndrome, 22q11.2DS], sickle cell anaemia, secondary immune deficiencies [immunomodulator therapies]); 3. unrepaired cyanotic heart disease and those with prosthetic materials; and 4. older patients with CHD.

Prophylaxis is usually given as amoxycillin, 1 hour before the procedure, orally, or when anaesthesia is needed, parenterally. The usual oral dose is 3 g for a child over 10 years, and 1.5 g if under 10 years of age. If the patient is allergic to penicillin, then a cephalosporin can be used.

For patients with prosthetic heart valves, who have the highest risk of acquiring endocarditis from any procedure; some units add an aminoglycoside to the usual cover for other valve disease. All children with congenital heart disease who require prophylaxis should be given a letter or card to show any dentist or doctor, explaining the need for antibiotic prophylaxis for any dental or similar procedure (e.g. tonsillectomy), including the recommended doses.

Genitourinary and gastroenterological surgery

As enterococci are the usual problem, the recommended treatment should adequately cover these organisms; thus parenteral gentamicin and ampicillin is an appropriate choice.

Non-cardiac surgery

Generally, it is sensible to consult with the child's cardiologist before any surgical procedure, as the concerns are not only those of bacteraemia, but of acid–base and electrolyte balance and oxygenation. The patient groups of most concern are those with severe congestive cardiac failure, pulmonary hypertension, severe cyanosis or severe outflow tract obstruction. Other children who need careful monitoring are those with conduction disturbances and those with significant arrhythmias. Polycythaemic cyanotic patients must have adequate hydration and intravascular volume maintained, to avoid risks of thrombosis, hypoxia and acidosis.

During any procedure, monitoring of blood pressure, oxygenation (with provision of supplemental oxygen if necessary, although avoid unnecessary oxygen in patients with failure due to left-to-right shunts), arterial pH and electrolyte balance are of paramount importance. Preoperatively, checking of electrolyte levels is mandatory. Digoxin need be stopped only for bypass operations. Diathermy is contraindicated in patients with pacemakers.

3. INFECTION

Common infections

Viral upper respiratory tract infections can cause significant problems in children with cardiac failure or cyanosis (e.g. respiratory syncytial virus) because of the effect of hypoxia on pulmonary vascular resistance (especially in Down syndrome).

Gastroenteritis can lead to dehydration and result in thromboses in polycythaemic patients; care must be taken to avoid dehydration. Gastroenteritis can also lead to hypokalaemia in patients taking diuretics, or cause toxicity in patients taking digoxin.

Any febrile illness may precipitate cardiac decompensation via the increase in the body metabolic needs. Appropriate cultures should always be taken; if subacute bacterial endocarditis is suspected antibiotics are contraindicated until multiple blood cultures have been taken, unless the child is very sick.

Cerebral abscess

Children over 2 years of age with cyanotic congenital heart disease have an increased incidence of brain abscess, the severity of which relates to the degree of hypoxia. They may present with fever, headache, seizures or focal neurological signs.

Immunisation

There is no contraindication to immunisation, with the exception of associated immune defects (e.g. asplenia, 22q11.2DS). Children with heart disease are particularly at risk if not immunised.

4. SOCIAL ISSUES

Impact of disease

The young child may be pampered and overprotected. During adolescence, issues such as anxiety regarding contraception, sexual performance and peer approval become important.

Parents tend to overprotect and pamper the child and give the other siblings less attention. Parents should be given adequate education regarding the nature of the defect; they should appreciate the need for antibiotic prophylaxis for dental and other surgical procedures and understand the rationale for treatment (e.g. with digoxin) and be supplied with clear guidelines as to age-appropriate activities and any exercise restrictions (see later). Common problem areas can be anticipated and dealt with before they become a concern.

Siblings receiving less parental attention than expected in a normal family is a commonly encountered problem.

Schooling

The teachers and school nurse need sufficient education regarding the disease to help them understand the most likely type of future employment (e.g. sedentary) for that patient, the symptoms that warrant referral for a medical opinion, and in the case of athletics, whether restrictions apply (see below).

Recommendations regarding sports participation and exercise

Parents and school teachers often ask about exercise. It is a difficult area, and parents' questions must be answered on an individual patient basis. Many units let children set their own levels rather than try to enforce restrictions, but may suggest avoidance of strenuous or competitive sport (and anaerobic exercise) if there is severe pulmonary hypertension, or more than mild aortic stenosis, subaortic stenosis or hypertrophic cardiomyopathy (HCM).

Patients with haemodynamically insignificant heart lesions with left-to-right shunts such as ASD, VSD and PDA may engage in all sports. However, patients with haemodynamically significant ASD, VSD or PDA who have pulmonary hypertension (> 25 mmHg) have decreased capacity for exercise and when exercising can develop chest pain, arrhythmias, syncope and even sudden cardiac death (SCD).

Patients with right-to-left shunts develop increased cyanosis when they exercise, and they are at high risk of SCD.

Patients with pulmonary stenosis (PS) that is mild, with normal function, or those treated with surgery or balloon valvoplasty with PS pressure below 40 mmHg, may engage in all sports. PS that is moderate or severe, restricts patients to low-intensity sports, as does pulmonary incompetence (PI).

Patients with mild AS (mean < 25 mmHg, or peak < 40 mmHg) may engage in all sports; those with moderate AS (mean 25–40 mmHg, or peak 40–70 mmHg) may engage in low-intensity sports; those with severe AS (mean > 40 mmHg, or peak > 70 mmHg) should be restricted from all competitive sports. Patients with untreated coarctation of the aorta without any significant aortic dilatation may engage in all sports. Patients post-repair (surgical or stent) of coarctation should avoid sports with bodily collisions, and any high-intensity static exercise.

In patients with unrepaired cyanotic heart disease, if clinically stable and asymptomatic, low-intensity sports may be considered, after a full evaluation. In postoperative ToF, patients with no significant RVOTO, ventricular dysfunction or arrhythmias may be able to engage in moderate- to high-level sports, but only after completing exercise testing without any concerning exercise-induced symptoms or signs.

In postoperative ToF with severe RVOTO or recurrent arrhythmias, patients should avoid engaging in any competitive sport. In post-arterial switch procedure for TGA, if there are no cardiac symptoms, normal ventricular function and no tachyarrhythmias, then patients may engage in all competitive sports.

In post-Fontan procedure, after exercise testing, if there is no symptomatic heart failure, low-intensity exercise may be permissible. Patients with mild to moderate Ebstein's anomaly may engage in all sports, but patients with severe Ebstein's anomaly should be restricted to low-intensity sports only.

Adolescence

The problems of non-compliance, peer group acceptance, non-participation in sporting activities, decisions regarding future career possibilities, delayed puberty and anxiety related to sexual performance are commonly encountered. Other issues include contraception, pregnancy, genetic counselling (see later), eligibility for life insurance and obtaining a driving licence (if suffering recurrent syncope).

Some teenagers have never had their heart disease explained to them, as it has been discussed only between doctors and parents in the past; this area should be considered.

Pregnancy

Pregnancy is contraindicated in the setting of Eisenmenger's syndrome (pulmonary hypertension with right-to-left shunting), or severe pulmonary hypertension (from any cause), because of a high risk of maternal and fetal morbidity and mortality. Relative contraindications to pregnancy include severe congestive cardiac failure and severe cyanosis, with oxygen saturation below 80%. Several other problems (e.g. aortopathies including BAV, MFS and LSD [see Aortic Disease section], severe aortic valve disease, cardiomyopathy, hypertension) also carry an increased risk to both mother and fetus.

Teratogenic drugs (e.g. warfarin) should be ceased for the pregnancy. Fetal echocardiography can be performed to detect congenital heart disease and, at birth, prophylaxis against endocarditis is given. Breastmilk from mothers who are taking warfarin, propranolol or quinidine can produce toxic effects in the baby; digoxin, however, is safe in this respect.

Genetic counselling

Most parents will ask about the risk of recurrence. The answer depends on whether the heart disease is the only problem, or whether it is part of a syndromal diagnosis, such as Marfan or Noonan syndrome. Most cardiac defects have a multifactorial inheritance, with a recurrence risk of between 1% and 4% if one sibling has the condition, and between 2% and 4% if one parent has the condition; the percentage may be higher in some conditions, such as truncus arteriosus. A notable exception is HCM, which has an autosomal dominant mode of inheritance. Those with syndromal diagnoses will have the recurrence risk of that syndrome. The parents should be advised about fetal echocardiography (available from around 18 weeks' gestation).

Travel

All these children should carry information (such as on their [parents'] mobile phone, a USB or hard copy as a letter) explaining the nature of their heart lesion, their usual medications, and the name of their doctor or usual treatment centre, and have access to a hospital if they have a disease prone to sudden deterioration (e.g. Fallot spells). An identification bracelet should also be worn.

Those with pacemakers in particular should carry written details regarding their unit and its program. Patients with severe congestive cardiac failure, severe cyanosis or pulmonary hypertension must avoid high altitudes (e.g. above 1500 m) and require supplemental oxygen to be available during commercial air travel. Hot climates can be a problem in children with polycythaemia, and adequate hydration must be maintained. The child's exercise tolerance must be considered when planning the trip itinerary.

5. SPECIFIC PROBLEMS
Drugs
The more common medications prescribed for congenital heart disease include diuretics, ACE inhibitors (e.g. captopril) and antiarrhythmics. Most candidates will be fairly familiar with these agents. The candidate should be familiar with vasodilators. ACE inhibitors, such as captopril, are often used in the treatment of cardiac failure, as they reduce afterload, mainly, and preload. Important side effects of captopril include hypotension, renal impairment and hyperkalaemia.

The issues to consider include whether the dose is appropriate, noting any adverse side effects, and whether regular monitoring of levels, and of electrolytes, has been performed. In children with prosthetic valves receiving warfarin therapy, the prothrombin ratio should be checked regularly. Drug interactions can pose problems; these should be considered when changing drugs or adding any new drug to the treatment regimen.

Contraception
Patients need to be aware of the theoretical risk of thrombosis potentiated by oestrogens, and therefore a low-oestrogen formulation of contraceptive pill is preferred; alternatives include Depo Provera, Implanon or low-dose minipill, *plus* one other method (e.g. barrier methods). The combined oral contraceptive pill is not contraindicated, but should be used with caution in girls with prosthetic heart valves, cyanotic heart disease or pulmonary hypertension. Intrauterine devices are potentially a source of bacteraemia, causing endocarditis. The risks of pregnancy for each patient must be assessed and suitable counselling given.

Specific syndromes: cardiac involvement
Marfan syndrome (MFS)
MFS (OMIM#154700) is an autosomal-dominant condition caused by defective *fibrillin*, a protein important to the integrity of connective tissue (Fig. 6.30). The relevant gene (*FBN1*) has been mapped to chromosome 15q21.1.

The cardiac features are the most important and life-threatening aspects of MFS manifesting in childhood in 25% of those affected. The cardiac involvement is progressive in around one-third of these children.

Features include the major diagnostic criterion of dilatation of the ascending aorta with or without aortic regurgitation, and involving at least the sinuses of Valsalva or dissection of the ascending aorta. Minor diagnostic criteria for MFS include mitral valve prolapse with or without mitral valve regurgitation, dilatation of the main pulmonary artery in the absence of another anatomic cause (before age 40), calcification of the mitral annulus (before age 40), and dilatation or dissection of the descending thoracic or abdominal aorta (before age 50).

Parental education regarding the importance of avoiding strenuous exercise and competitive or contact sports is important, and should begin before preschool, placing less emphasis on the importance of sporting activities. Non-strenuous activities should be encouraged (e.g. walking, fishing, golf). The symptoms of aortic dissection must be discussed, including chest pain and syncope.

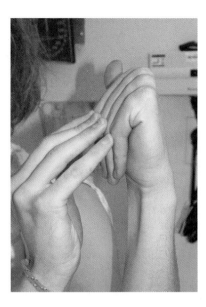

Figure 6.30 Marfan syndrome—joint hypermobility.

Source: Jones, K. (2005). *Smith's Recognizable Patterns of Human Malformation* (6th ed.). Philadelphia: Elsevier Saunders, p. 550.

The following lists are mnemonics which include most of the features of MFS. The first list is based on the letter **D**. The second list is based on the acronym **MARFANS**. After these two lists, the scoring system is described:

Dilatation or **d**issection of *aorta* at level of sinuses of Valsalva

Displacement of *lens* (ectopia lentis); directed upward; cataract formation

Dural ectasia (lumbosacral)

Dolichostenomelia: disproportionately long extremities; decreased upper to lower segment ratio (US:LS < 0.85 for older children/adults) or arm span to height ratio > 1.05; other diagnostic skeletal features include the following

Deformation of spine (scoliosis > 20°, or spondylolisthesis)

Deformation of sternum (pectus: excavatum or carinatum, requiring surgery)

Deep acetabulum with accelerated erosion (protrusio acetabulum)

Decreased elbow extension (< 170°) (in contradistinction to hypermobility of other joints)

Digit-related eponymous signs: 1. the thumb (Steinberg) sign, this being an extension of the whole distal phalanx of the thumb beyond the ulnar border of the hand when apposed across the palm (Fig. 6.31); and 2. the wrist (Walker–Murdoch) sign, this being overlapping of the distal phalanx of the thumb with the distal phalanx of the little finger when encircling the opposite wrist (Fig. 6.32)

Downward (medial) rotation of medial malleolus causing pes planus; four of these skeletal features are considered one major criterion

Distinctive facial features (**d**olichocephaly, **d**own-slanting palpebral fissures, **d**eeply set eyes [enophthalmos], **d**ecreased malar prominence [malar hypoplasia], **d**iminished jaw [retrognathia])

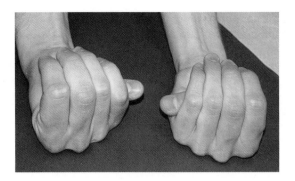

Figure 6.31 Steinberg thumb sign.

Source: Jones, K. (2005). *Smith's Recognizable Patterns of Human Malformation* (6th ed.). Philadelphia: Elsevier Saunders. Figure 2B.

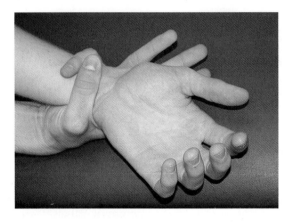

Figure 6.32 Walker–Murdoch wrist sign.

Source: Jones, K. (2005). *Smith's Recognizable Patterns of Human Malformation* (6th ed.). Philadelphia: Elsevier Saunders. Figure 2C.

The acronym **MARFANS** also can be used as an (alternative) aide-mémoire:

Mitral prolapse ± **M**itral regurgitation

Ascending aorta dilatation (involving sinuses of Valsalva)/dissection/**A**rched palate (high arched, with tooth crowding)/**A**cetabuli (protrusio acetabuli)

Regurgitation of aorta/mitral valve/**R**etinal detachment/**R**educed US:LS ratio

Fibrillin defective/**F**acial gestalt (dolichocephaly, down-slanting palpebral fissures, deeply set eyes [enophthalmos], decreased malar prominence [malar hypoplasia], diminished jaw [retrognathia])/**F**lat cheek bones/**F**lat cornea/**F**lexible joints (joint hypermobility)

Apical blebs (on CXR)/**A**ir leaks (spontaneous pneumothorax)/**A**rachnodactyly

Near-sightedness (myopia)/**N**eurological involvement related to dural ectasia; stretching of dural sac in the lumbosacral region/**N**erve entrapment: CSF leak from dural sac (causing postural hypotension and headache)

Scoliosis/**S**ternal deformation/**S**keletal dolichostenomelia/**S**acral dural ectasia

In teenage years, important issues include consideration of beta blockers to slow the progress of aortic dilatation, and counselling to teenage girls about the risks of pregnancy, as rupture of the aorta can occur during pregnancy or at delivery.

Medical therapy for MFS syndrome with angiotensin II receptor blockers (ARBs) has been shown to decrease the risk of aortic root dilatation, after a specific metabolic defect of the aortic wall was discovered that improved with ARBs.

The revised diagnostic criteria for MFS (Loeys et al. 2010) utilise family history, plus personal history, plus examination findings, plus echocardiography (or other cardiac imaging) and slit lamp findings.

There are two findings with major significance: aortic root enlargement and ectopia lentis. Features other than these are weighted and grouped to obtain a 'systemic score' as per the National Marfan Foundation Website.

A composite score adds the values attributed to discerning signs; a value of three is given to positive wrist *and* thumb signs; a value of two is given for pectus carinatum, hindfoot deformity, pneumothorax, dural ectasia or protrusio acetabulae; and a value of one is given to wrist *or* thumb sign, pectus excavatum *or* chest asymmetry, plain flat foot (pes planus), reduced upper segment/lower segment *and* increased arm span/height ratios, scoliosis or thoracolumbar kyphosis, reduced elbow extension, 3 of 5 facial features, skin striae, myopia and mitral valve prolapse.

If *no family history* of MFS, diagnosis can be made in a proband if there is aortic root enlargement and one of: ectopia lentis, a pathogenic *FBN1* variant, or a systemic score of 7 or more; or, if there is ectopia lentis and an *FBN1* pathogenic variant previously associated with aortic enlargement.

If *there is a family history* of MFS, diagnosis can be made with a reduced number of physical findings; the diagnosis in a first-degree relative of the proband can be established if there is ectopia lentis, a systemic score of at least 7 and aortic root enlargement.

The molecular genetic testing done for MFS is sequence analysis of *FBN1* (*FBN1* is the only gene where pathogenic mutations cause classic MFS). Either of the following confirm the diagnosis of MFS: pathogenic variant proven to segregate with MFS in families; or, de novo pathogenic variants (with paternity proven, and absence of MFS in parents), if there is 1 of 5 specified forms of variant. There may be a requirement to exclude similar conditions if there is a lack of discriminating features; these conditions are vascular Ehlers-Danlos syndrome, Loeys–Dietz syndrome and Shprintzen-Goldberg syndrome. If any of these are possible, then collagen biochemical testing and molecular genetic testing of *TGFBR1, TGFBR2, SMAD3, TGFB2, COL3A1* should be performed.

Management of MFS

Recommended surveillance includes, at a minimum, annual echocardiography and also annual ophthalmological examination. The ascending aorta must be monitored carefully; once the aortic root diameter is increasing at a rate of more than 1 cm a year, or there is progressive, or severe, aortic regurgitation, then aortic root surgery should be performed.

In adults, once the aortic root diameter reaches 4.5 cm, then echocardiography should be performed more often than annually. If the rate of aortic dilation exceeds 0.5 cm/year in an adult, and there is significant aortic regurgitation, then the entire aorta should be evaluated by intermittent MRA or CT scans. The most common surgical repair in MFS in children is not that of the aorta, but repair of the mitral valve if there is progressive and severe mitral valve regurgitation with ventricular dysfunction. If dental work is needed, SBE prophylaxis is required for those with aortic or mitral valve regurgitation.

Parental education regarding the importance of avoiding strenuous exercise and competitive or contact sports is important, and should begin before preschool, placing less emphasis on the importance of sporting activities. Non-strenuous activities should be encouraged (e.g. walking, fishing, golf). The symptoms of aortic dissection must be discussed, including chest pain and syncope.

In teenage years, important issues include consideration of beta blockers to slow the progress of aortic dilatation, and counselling to teenage girls about the risks of pregnancy, as dissection and/or rupture of the aorta can occur during pregnancy, at delivery or in the postpartum period. The increased risk is believed to be related to the increased aortic wall stress caused by the hyperdynamic circulation of pregnancy; also, hormonal changes are thought to accelerate pathological change in the aortic wall. Pre-conceptual aortic dilatation predicts increased likelihood of aortic dissection.

Medical therapy for MFS syndrome with ARBs has been shown to decrease the risk of aortic root dilatation, after a specific metabolic defect of the aortic wall was discovered that improved with ARBs.

There are several activities and agents that must be avoided in MFS: drugs or other agents that stimulate the cardiovascular system, such as caffeine and decongestants; drugs or other agents that cause vasoconstriction such as sumatriptan and other triptans; and laser eye surgery.

Other treatments needed may include: surgery to correct scoliosis and pectus deformities (the latter is for cosmetic reasons only); eyeglasses for most eye problems, although ectopia lentis may require removal of a dislocated lens and implanting of an artificial lens (ideally once growth is complete); orthotics for pes planus; positive pressure ventilation should be avoided if possible in those with predisposition to pneumothoraxes.

Noonan syndrome (NS)

NS (OMIM#163950) is an autosomal-dominant condition, associated with several genes, mutations of which alter proteins involved in signalling through RAS, so NS is a RASopathy. Related RASopathies are cardiofaciocutaneous syndrome, Costello syndrome, NS with multiple lentigines, and NS-like syndrome with loose anagen hair. In 50% of cases, the associated gene locus is at 12q24.1, with mutations in *PTPN11*, the gene encoding the non-receptor type protein, tyrosine phosphatase SHP-2.

The other genes include *SOS1* (10–13% cases), *RAF1* (5%), *RIT1* (5%), *KRAS* (< 5%), *BRAF* (< 2%), *MAP2K1* (< 2%). Almost all patients with NS have some cardiac defect, particularly a dysplastic (and often stenotic) pulmonary valve, which is more common with a PTPN11 mutation, or hypertrophic cardiomyopathy (HCM), which affects around 20–30% of NS children, but is less common with a PTPN11 mutation. The ECG frequently shows left-axis deviation and a dominant S wave over the praecordial leads, even in NS patients with no known cardiac disease; the cause for this is not known. Phenotypic features of NS include dysmorphic facial features, short stature, webbed neck and skeletal anomalies (see Fig. 6.33 and the short case on dysmorphism).

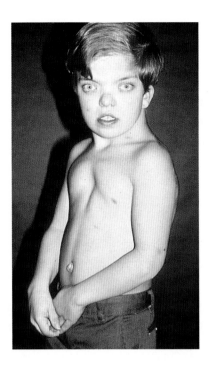

Figure 6.33 Noonan syndrome. Note the widely spaced eyes, low-set ears, webbing of the neck, shield chest, pectus and increased carrying angle of the arms.

Source: Zitelli, B.J., McIntire, S.C. & Nowalk, A.J. (2012). *Atlas of Pediatric Physical Diagnosis* (6th ed.). Philadelphia: Elsevier. Figure 5.9.

The acronym **NOONANS** can be used as an aide-mémoire of the various features:

Neurodevelopmental problems: 25% learning disability, 10-15% special education, < 30% mild intellectual impairment, 72% articulation problems, nonverbal abilities better than verbal, specific learning problems/**N**euromuscular: hypotonia (floppy strong); joint hyperextensibility/**N**eurosurgical: Arnold–Chiari type I

Obstructive heart lesions: RVOT (pulmonary valve); left-ventricular outflow tract (LVOT) (HCM)/**O**ther: ASD, VSD, ToF, coarctation of aorta, branch pulmonary artery stenosis

Ocular anomalies in up to 95%: strabismus, refractive errors, amblyopia, nystagmus; hypertelorism, epicanthic folds, droopy eyelids, vivid blue or blue - green irises

Neoplasia risk: juvenile myelomonocytic leukaemia (JMML); myeloproliferative disorders; Noonan-like/multiple giant-cell lesion syndrome (granulomas and joint and bone anomalies); hepatosplenomegaly (related to subclinical myelodysplasia)

Abnormal coagulation (33% have one or more defects)/**A**bnormal lymphatics: lymphoedema (hands/feet/scrotum/vulva), lymphangiectasia (lung, gut or testis)

Neck webbing, with low-set posteriorly rotated ears/**N**ipples widely set/**N**ephrological anomalies: duplex collecting systems, renal hypoplasia

Sternal deformity (superior carinatum, inferior excavatum)/**S**hort stature (GH responsive)/**S**econdary sexual characteristics: delayed puberty, cryptorchidism in males/**S**kin: pigmented naevi (25%), café-au-lait patches (10%), lentigines (3%)

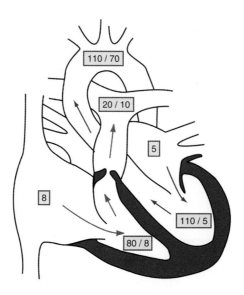

Figure 6.34 **Physiology of valvular pulmonary stenosis. Boxed numbers represent pressure in mmHg. Because of the absence of right-to-left or left-to-right shunting, blood flow through all cardiac chambers is normal at 3 L/min/m². The pulmonary-to-systemic blood flow ratio (Qp:Qs) is 1:1. Right-atrial pressure is increased slightly as a result of decreased right-ventricular compliance. The right ventricle is hypertrophied, and systolic and diastolic pressure is increased. The pressure gradient across the thickened pulmonary valve is 60 mmHg. The main pulmonary artery pressure is slightly low, and poststenotic dilatation is present. Left heart pressure is normal. Unless right-to-left shunting is occurring through a foramen ovale, the patient's systemic oxygen saturation will be normal.**

Source: Behrman, R.E., Kliegman, R.M. & Jenson, H.B. (2015). *Nelson Textbook of Paediatrics* (20th ed.). London: Saunders. Figure 420.1.

NS patients with dysplastic pulmonary valves can have rapid progression of pulmonary valvular obstruction and may require review more frequently than for non-NS pulmonary valve lesions. Also, NS-associated valve obstruction is more likely to require surgical intervention. (See Fig. 6.34.)

Balloon valvoplasty is usually unsuccessful in abolishing the obstruction, and simple valvotomy may be inadequate. Often complete excision of the valve, resection of the right-ventricular outflow muscle and occasionally an outflow tract patch may be needed.

ASDs (Fig. 6.35) and pulmonary artery branch stenoses may coexist with valvular pulmonary stenosis. Other infrequent findings with NS include VSDs (Fig. 6.36) and ToF.

HCM in NS does not have a clearly defined natural history. HCM can become progressive in infancy, or may not develop or be recognised until late in childhood. Symptomatic HCM in NS can lead to sudden cardiac death, even in infancy. Treatment is as for non-syndromic HCM, including cardiac transplantation. See the section on familial HCM later in this case.

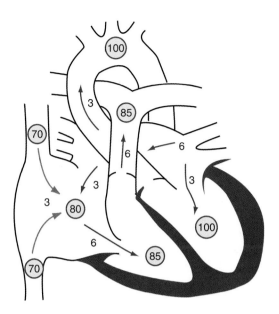

Figure 6.35 **Physiology of atrial septal defect (ASD). Circled numbers represent oxygen saturation values. The numbers next to the arrows represent volumes of blood flow (in L/min/m²). This illustration shows a hypothetical patient with a pulmonary-to-systemic blood flow ratio (Qp:Qs) of 2:1. Desaturated blood enters the right atrium from the vena cavae at a volume of 3 L/min/m² and mixes with an additional 3 L of fully saturated blood shunting left to right across the ASD; the result is an increase in oxygen saturation in the right atrium. Six litres of blood flows through the tricuspid valve and causes a mid-diastolic flow rumble. Oxygen saturation may be slightly higher in the right ventricle because of incomplete mixing at the atrial level. The full 6 L flows across the right-ventricular outflow tract and causes a systolic ejection flow murmur. Six litres returns to the left atrium, with 3 L shunting left to right across the defect and 3 L crossing the mitral valve to be ejected by the left ventricle into the ascending aorta (normal cardiac output).**

Source: Behrman, R.E., Kliegman, R.M. & Jenson, H.B. (2015). *Nelson Textbook of Paediatrics* (20th ed.). London: Saunders. Figure 419.1.

The diagnosis can be established with an NS multigene panel, by serial single-gene testing (starting with *PTPN11* then being guided by phenotype, such as *RIT1* if HCM present), or by genomic testing, such as whole-exome sequencing or whole-genome sequencing.

NS can be mimicked by other conditions with NS-syndrome-like facies, which can be related at a genetic level in many cases:

• *NS with multiple lentigines (NSML)* is a RASopathy, which closely resembles NS. Lentigines are freckle-like small hyperpigmented skin lesions, which appear on the face trunk and limbs, numbering in the thousands, by 5 years of age. HCM

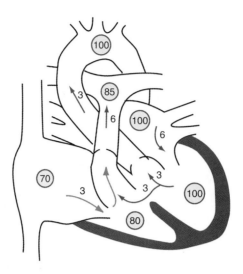

Figure 6.36 Physiology of a large ventricular septal defect (VSD). Circled numbers represent oxygen saturation values. The numbers next to the arrows represent volumes of blood flow (in L/min/m²). This illustration shows a hypothetical patient with a pulmonary-to-systemic blood flow ratio (Qp:Qs) of 2:1. Desaturated blood enters the right atrium from the vena cava at a volume of 3 L/min/m² and flows across the tricuspid valve. An additional 3 L of blood shunts left to right across the VSD, the result being an increase in oxygen saturation in the right ventricle. Six litres of blood is ejected into the lungs. Pulmonary arterial saturation may be further increased because of incomplete mixing at right-ventricular level. Six litres returns to the left atrium, crosses the mitral valve and causes a mid-diastolic flow rumble. Three litres of this volume shunts left to right across the VSD and 3 L is ejected into the ascending aorta (normal cardiac output).

Source: Behrman, R.E., Kliegman, R.M. & Jenson, H.B. (2015). *Nelson Textbook of Paediatrics* (20th ed.). London: Saunders. Figure 419.5.

occurs in 80% of cases, the most of any RASopathy, but it usually has a fairly benign prognosis. Sensorineural deafness is commoner in this (occurring in 20%) than in NS (occurs in 5%). It was previously known by a mnemonic, **LEOPARD** syndrome (**L**entigines, **E**CG abnormalities [axis deviations, unilateral or bilateral hypertrophy, conduction abnormalities], **O**cular hypertelorism, **P**ulmonary stenosis, **A**bnormalities of genitalia, **R**etardation of growth and **D**eafness). Two genes associated: *PTPN11* and *RAF1*; testing these finds mutations in 93% of affected people.

- *Cardio-facial-cutaneous 1 (CFC1) syndrome* (OMIM#115150) is a RASopathy. Cardiac lesions occur in 75% of cases, most commonly pulmonary valve stenosis, and hypertrophic cardiomyopathy (HCM) occurs in 40%; also, ASDs occur). The facial aspects include marked macrocephaly, and dolichocephaly, with prominent forehead, bitemporal narrowing, coarsening of features, hypertelorism, squint, nystagmus and absent eyelashes/eyebrows. The cutaneous findings (ectodermal dysplasia) include hyperkeratosis, haemangiomata and ichthyosis. CFC has similar lymphatic findings to NS. Other differentiating features include neurological aspects (cognitive impairment, hypotonia) and gastrointestinal problems (food aversion, failure to thrive, severe constipation). Four genes are associated with CFC1: *BRAF* (75%), *MAPK1 + MAPK2* (20–25%) and *KRAS*.

- *Costello syndrome* (OMIM#218040) is another RASopathy, gene map locus 11p15.5. Gene: the *HRAS* proto-oncogene; phenotypic overlap with NS and CFC. Features: short stature, pulmonary stenosis, HCM (in two-thirds, hence more frequently than in NS; a quarter of patients will need a septal myotomy), coarse features, hypertelorism, epicanthic folds, intellectual development variable; distinctive features include papillomata, splayed fingers with ulnar deviation, and increased risk of neuroblastoma or rhabdomyosarcoma. Mnemonic: **COSTELlo**: **C**ardiac (PS, HCM), **O**cular (epicanthic folds, hypertelorism), **S**hort stature, **T**umours (papillomata, neuroblastoma, rhabdomyosarcoma), **E**ducational difficulties, **L**imb involvement (splayed fingers, ulnar deviation).
- *NS-like disorder with loose anagen hair* (*NSLH*, OMIM#607721), another RASopathy, includes ectodermal findings of darkly pigmented skin, eczema or ichthyosis, and loose anagen hair. It is caused by heterozygous mutation to *SHOC2*.
- *NS-like disorder with or without juvenile myelomonocytic leukaemia (JMML)* (*NSLL*, OMIM#613563) is another RASopathy, and is due to a heterozygous mutation in the *CBL* gene. This causes more neurodevelopmental features (hypotonia, developmental delay, language delay) and less cardiac features than NS (aortic stenosis, mitral regurgitation), plus (variable) short stature and undescended testes.

Non-RASopathies

Non-RASopathies, which resemble NS include:

- *Neurofibromatosis–Noonan syndrome* (*NFNS*, OMIM#601321); allelic with NF1 and Watson syndrome (see below); gene map locus 17q11.2; caused by mutations in the neurofibromin gene, *NF1*; the clinical overlap between NFNS and NS is explained by the respective gene products, neurofibromin and SHP2, exerting their modulatory effects via a common pathway.
- *Watson syndrome (WTSN*, OMIM#193520); allelic with NFNS and NF1 (see above); gene map locus 17q11.2; caused by mutations in the neurofibromin gene, *NF1*. Features: short stature, pulmonary valve stenosis, pigmented skin lesions (café-au-lait spots), intellectual development variable. Phenotype overlaps with NF1 as well as NS.

Management of NS

There are a number of guidelines available, by various consortiums. The treatment of the various complications of NS are standard and the same as those in the general population with the same conditions. There are recommendations for investigations and ongoing follow-up and monitoring:

- Growth should be monitored and parameters plotted on NS growth charts.
- Imaging should include X-ray of spine and rib cage, echocardiography (annually until 3 years, then at 5 and 10, looking for HCM), renal ultrasound, brain and cervical spine MRI if neurological symptoms present. An ECG should be done, plus audiology.
- Bloods can be taken for coagulation screen, including full blood count, film, PT and aPPT, as 50–89% patients have bleeding or abnormal coagulation on laboratory testing.
- Assessments by cardiologist, endocrinologist (to test GH axis if decreased height growth velocity; pre-pubertal NS children with GH deficiency respond to hGH at the same rate as girls with Turner syndrome, but not as well as idiopathic GH deficiency patients), ophthalmologist, and developmental paediatrician.

22q11.2 deletion syndrome (22q11.2DS): conotruncal defects

This includes these syndromes: DiGeorge (DGS), velocardiofacial (VCFS), Shprintzen, conotruncal anomaly face (CTAF), Caylor cardiofacial, and autosomal-dominant Opitz G/BBB.

Deletion of chromosome 22 is the most common chromosome deletion, affecting 1 in 4000 live births. The deletion most commonly spans three megabases of DNA and contains almost 30 genes. A wide variety of cardiac defects are described in patients with microdeletions in band 11 of the long arm of chromosome 22 (22q11 deletions). The acronym **CATCH-22** (**C**ardiac defects, **A**bnormal facies, **T**hymic hypoplasia and T-cell deficiency, **C**left palate, **H**ypoparathyroidism and **H**ypocalcaemia) can be useful.

Other findings include renal anomalies, developmental delay and late-onset psychiatric problems. These children may be born with duct-dependent complex cyanotic heart disease. Around one-third of children with non-syndromal conotruncal cardiac defects have 22q11.2 deletions as well. Deletions of 22q11.2 have also been identified in children with various forms of familial, and sporadic, congenital heart disease.

Similar phenotypic characteristics may occur in association with microdeletions on chromosomes 5, 10 and 17, as well as 22. The 22q11.2DS-associated cardiac defects include **T**runcus arteriosus, **T**etralogy of Fallot and **T**ricuspid atresia with d-malposition of the aorta (3 **T**s); **A**ortic arch interruption, **A**trial septal defect and **A**berrant right subclavian artery (3 **A**s); and **P**ulmonary atresia and ventricular septal defect, **P**ulmonary valve absence and **P**atent ductus arteriosus (3 **P**s).

Deletions of 22q11.2 can also be seen in isolated heart disease (e.g. found in 30% of interrupted aortic arch, 20% of truncus arteriosus and 8% of ToF).

The acronym **CATCH-22** can expand to **CATCHING-22** to include more features:

Cardiac: 74%; Conotruncal; 3 Ts, 3 As, 3 Ps (3 TAPs; see above); causes > 90% of all deaths/**C**orneal: posterior embryotoxon (PE; 69%), and other ophthalmological findings: tortuous retinal vessels (58%), strabismus (13%)

Abnormal face: long face, malar flatness, hypertelorism, hooded eyelids, ptosis, ear anomalies (overfolded helices, cupped, microtic, protuberant ears, preauricular pits), prominent nasal root, bulbous nasal tip, nasal dimple, asymmetric crying face/**A**utoimmune: Graves, vitiligo, juvenile idiopathic arthritis (JIA), coeliac disease

Thymic hypoplasia, T-cell deficiency; 77% have *immunodeficiency*

Cleft palate, palatal anomalies: velopharyngeal incompetence (VPI), submucosal cleft palate (SMCP), bifid uvula, cleft lip; palatal problem in 69%/**C**raniosynostosis, other skeletal anomalies: Cervical spine anomalies (50%)/**C**roup-like: laryngotrachealoesophageal anomalies: vascular ring, laryngeal web

Hypoparathyroidism/**H**ypocalcaemia/**H**earing loss (conductive/sensorineural)

Intellectual: learning problems (nonverbal), 70–90%; mean full scale intelligence quotient (IQ) 75–80; neuropsychological: ADHD, autism; schizophrenia, bipolar, anxiety, depression/**I**mpaired swallowing/feeding: dysmotile pharyngoesophageal area, derived from 3rd and 4th pharyngeal pouches; nasopharyngeal reflux, abnormal cricopharyngeal closure

Neurologic: unprovoked fits, neural tube defects, cerebellar atrophy, tethered cord/**N**ephrologic: dysplastic kidneys, horseshoe kidney, duplicated kidney (37% in all)/**N**eoplastic: 'blastomas': neuroblastoma, nephroblastoma (Wilms), hepatoblastoma, renal cell carcinoma

Growth hormone deficiency/**G**enitals: hypospadias, cryptorchidism, absent uterus/ **G**astrointestinal: atresias (oesophageal, jejunal, anal), malrotation, Hirschsprung/ *GP1BB* mutation can cause coexistent Bernard–Soulier syndrome (BSS) with thrombocytopaenia and giant platelets; risk of bleeding significant

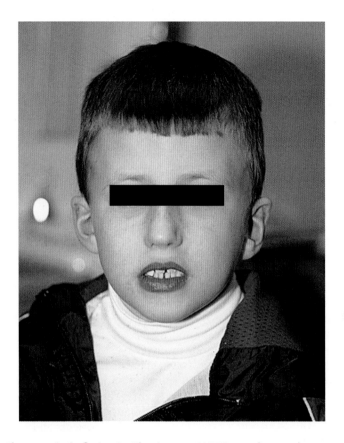

Figure 6.37 Characteristic facies in Shprintzen (VCFS) syndrome.

Source: Hay, B.N. (2007). Deletion 22q11: spectrum of associated disorders. *Seminars in Pediatric Neurology*, *14*(3), 136–139. Figure 1. Copyright © 2007 Elsevier Inc.

Dysmorphic facial features include a myopathic facial appearance, unusually shaped ears, a long nose with a broad bridge, a small mouth, micrognathia, short upward slanting palpebral fissures, and a cleft or high palate (may be accompanied by hypernasal speech). (See Fig. 6.37.)

With any patients with these anomalies, genetic assessment and counselling is warranted, with chromosomes and fluorescence in situ hybridisation (FISH) for the 22q11.2 microdeletion. The parents should be tested for 22q11.2 deletion, and must be educated as to the associated problems (e.g. problems with the palate, immunodeficiency, learni ng difficulties, developmental delay), the likelihood of further syndromal traits developing and the risk of transmitting the deletion to their offspring (50%).

More details on selected aspects discussed, presented in the **CATCHING-22** order:

Cardiac findings. Conotruncal anomalies of the outflow tract are the most frequent; the most individual common conditions within 22q11.2DS are, in order, ToF, then interrupted aortic arch (IAA), VSD and TA. There is a small but significant group who have aortic root dilatation, but how this evolves is still being investigated. **C**orneal findings of PE (which is seen on slit lamp as a thin greyish white arcuate ridge on the inner surface of the cornea) is the most common ophthalmologic finding; others include strabismus, amblyopia, cataracts and colobomas.

Abnormal facies. The facial features are very variable, and there may be no discernible abnormalities in some. **A**utoimmune conditions can include JIA (especially polyarticular; 20–100 × general population rate) and idiopathic thrombocytopaenic purpura (ITP; 200 × general population rate).

T-cell immunodeficiency. This is due to impaired T-cell production and occurs in two-thirds of patients. Recurrent infection also may be due to aspiration pneumonia, related to palatal dysfunction, or gastro-oesophageal reflux, plus dysphagia can lead to a degree of malnutrition. Up to one-third of older children have recurrent sinusitis or otitis media.

Cleft palate. Palatal anomalies occur in 69% of 22q11.2 DS patients. The most common is velopharyngeal incompetence (VPI) which may be due to structural (due to short palate), or functional (due to hypotonia) problems, or both; submucous cleft palate is more common than overt cleft palate or cleft lip. **C**ervical spine abnormalities include: posterior fusion C2–C3, hypoplastic C1; dysmorphic C2, instability on flexion/extension X-rays; increased motion at two or more vertebral levels; episodes of spinal cord compression, albeit rare, have occurred. Other skeletal findings include butterfly vertebrae, hemivertebrae, scoliosis (15% patients), hypoplastic scapulae, extra ribs or absent ribs, polydactyly and syndactyly.

Hypocalcaemia. This occurs in 17–60% of 22q11.2DS patients and is usually most severe as a neonate, normalising with increasing age, although it can recur with intercurrent illness, puberty or pregnancy.

Intellectual issues. Younger children with 22q11.2DS often have developmental delay; they are often nonverbal until 2 or 3; preschoolers assessed with WPPSI-R had a mean full scale IQ of 78; 40% had significant language delay. Around 20% of younger 22q11.2DS children fulfil criteria for autism spectrum disorder. In school-aged children, 30% are in the range of intellectual disability. Older children have better verbal IQ scores than performance IQ scores; they tend to have nonverbal learning disorder; they are better at rote verbal learning. **I**mpaired feeding occurs in 30–40% of children, sometimes necessitating nasogastric tube feeding or placing a gastrostomy tube. This predominantly is due to dysmotility of phases of swallowing (oro-pharyngeal and crico-oesophageal) rather than palate or heart issues.

Neurological issues. Most 22q11.2DS infants have hypotonia. Microcephaly occurs in 18–50% of cases. Around 7% have unprovoked seizures. Functional MRI scan have shown decreased volume of posterior brain, especially white matter loss in the left posterior occipital and parietal regions, which correlates with problems experienced with mathematics, visuospatial abilities and executive functioning. **N**ephrology. Renal or other genitourinary system abnormalities occur in 31–45%, including horseshoe kidney, renal tubular acidosis, hydronephrosis, hypospadias, inguinal herniae and undescended testes. **N**eoplastic conditions. These include three 'blastomas'; the absence of *COMT* which normally permits detoxification of environmental carcinogens, and is normally within the area deleted in 22q11.2DS, is thought to be the cause.

Growth charts. These have now been developed for 22q11.2DS. Around 41% cases are below the 5th centile for height. A number have GH deficiency, and respond to human growth hormone (hGH) treatment.

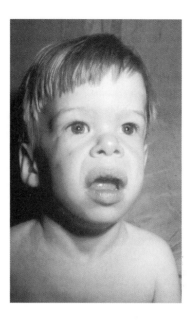

Figure 6.38 Williams syndrome. Note the depressed nasal bridge, epicanthal folds, periorbital fullness, anteverted nares, long philtrum and prominent lips with large mouth.

Source: Jones, K. (2005). *Smith's Recognizable Patterns of Human Malformation* (6th ed.). Philadelphia: Elsevier Saunders. Figure 1A.

Investigations of 22q11.2DS may include:

- Imaging: heart (CXR, which will also find thoracic vertebral anomalies, echocardiogram, chest MRI if vascular ring suspected); cervical spine (X-ray including six views; flexion, extension, AP, lateral, open mouth, skull base); kidneys (ultrasound).
- Bloods: Ca^{2+}, PTH, TSH, T4, T3, full blood count plus film, (if low lymphocytes, then T-cell and B-cell subsets), immunologic testing (flow cytometry, immunoglobulins, T-cell function).
- Assessments: cardiology, ophthalmology, audiology, speech and language pathology.

Williams syndrome (WS)

WS is due to a deletion of a region of chromosome 7, termed the Williams–Beuren Syndrome Critical Region; it comprises 1.5–1.8 million base pairs and has 26–28 genes (Fig. 6.38). This area is predisposed to misalignment, during meiosis, of 'duplicons', which are low-copy-repeat blocks of homologous groups of genes and pseudogenes flanking the WBSCR. Hemizygosity for the elastin gene (*ELN* deletion) leads to the elastin arteriopathies supravalvular aortic stenosis (SVAS), peripheral pulmonary arterial stenosis (PPS) and other vascular stenoses. Hemizygosity for the gene *LIM-kinase 1* leads to impaired visuospatial construction cognition.

WS is a polyendocrine disorder that can involve all endocrine organs, and it is also a neurodevelopmental disorder. Children with this condition are friendly, outgoing and gregarious, are easily noticed and approach strangers readily. It is inherited as autosomal dominant. Cardiovascular conditions seen in WS include: SVAS, PPS, mitral valve prolapse, ventricular and ASDs, renal artery stenosis with hypertension, and hypoplastic aorta.

The mnemonic **WILLIAMS HYPERCALCAEMIA** lists the main features of WS:

Williams–Beuren Syndrome Critical Region (WBSCR); chromosome locus 7q11.2
Intelligence quotient (IQ) average 50–60/**I**mpaired vision: reduced stereopsis
Low tone (hypotonia)/**L**ow pitched or hoarse voice, vocal cord paralysis
Lax joints (joint hypermobility)/**L**oquacious, over-friendly, excessively empathic
Impaired feeding; tactile sensory defensiveness (difficulty with food textures); vomiting
ADHD symptomatology/**A**nxiety (somatisation can lead to abdominal pain)
Mitral valve prolapse (MVP)
Supravalvular aortic stenosis (SVAS)/**S**coliosis, kyphosis/**S**ternum: excavatum

HYpercalcaemia, **HY**percalciuria, **HY**pertension
Peripheral pulmonary arterial stenosis (PPW)/**P**uberty early (but not precocious)
Elastin arteriopathy (SVAS, PPS, aortic insufficiency, stenosis of mesenteric arteries)/**E**ndocrine: hypothyroidism; IDDM in adults/**E**lfin face (see below under A)
Renal anomalies (nephrocalcinosis, pelvic kidney)
Chronic otitis media (50%)/**C**haracteristic personality: over-friendly, people-orientated, empathic
Audiological: high-frequency sensorineural hearing loss, hyperacusis (in 90%)
Linear growth failure; postnatal growth rate 75% of normal/**L**oquacious personality
Cognitive: good verbal short-term memory, language; poor visuospatial construction
Appearance: broad brow, bitemporal narrowness, medial eyebrow flare, short palpebral fissures, epicanthic folds, blue stellate iris, short nose, full nasal tip, full cheeks, malar hypoplasia, long philtrum, full lips, wide mouth, small jaw, prominent earlobes
Eyes: hypotelorism, strabismus (50%), amblyopia, refractive errors (hyperopia in 50%)
Malocclusion, microdontia, enamel hypoplasia, widely spaced teeth, missing teeth
Intestinal problems: constipation, diverticulosis, coeliac disease
Abdominal pain: reflux oesophagitis; cholelithiasis; diverticulitis; ischaemic bowel

Management of WS
There are a number of guidelines available. The treatment of most of the various complications of WS are standard and the same as those in the general population with the same conditions:
- Growth should be monitored and parameters plotted on WS growth charts.
- Investigations may include: imaging (echocardiogram, ultrasound of kidneys and bladder); bloods for urea and electrolytes, Ca^{2+}, TSH, T4 and T3; and assessments by an audiologist and ophthalmologist.
- Surgical correction may be required for SVAS (in around 20–30% of cases), mitral valve incompetence or renal artery stenosis. Hypertension has been treated medically by calcium channel blockers. Hypercalcaemia management may involve diet to keep Ca^{2+} intake below 100% of recommended daily allowance; refractory hypercalcaemia may require oral corticosteroids, and symptomatic hypercalcaemia in infancy may be treated with intravenous pamidronate. Development of nephrocalcinosis or hypercalciuria would warrant involving a paediatric nephrologist.
- Hyperacusis can be treated with ear protection. ADHD and anxiety may require pharmacologic treatment (see the long case on ADHD in Chapter 5, Behavioural and developmental paediatrics).

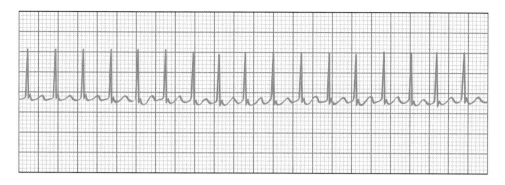

Figure 6.39 Supraventricular tachycardia. Note the normal QRS complex tachycardia at a rate of 214 beats/minute without visible P waves.

Source: Zitelli, B.J., McIntire, S.C. & Nowalk, A.J. (2012). *Atlas of Pediatric Physical Diagnosis* (6th ed.). Philadelphia: Elsevier. Figure 5.44.

Supraventricular tachycardia (SVT)

The commonest sustained tachyarrhythmia in children, SVT is caused mainly by an additional electrical connection between the atria and ventricle (accessory atrioventricular connection [AAVC]) in those under 12; in teenagers, atrioventricular node re-entry tachycardia (AVNRT; has the functional equivalent of an extra connection within the AVN) may be a cause. Those with AAVCs often have 'orthodromic' tachycardia, with antegrade conduction down the atrioventricular (AV) node and retrograde conduction up the AAVC (the right way down the right path, the wrong way up the wrong path). Some patients have an AAVC that conducts in an antegrade fashion as well (giving 'antidromic' tachycardia, with retrograde conduction either up the AV node or the AAVC). (See Fig. 6.39.)

Re-entry, the mechanism underlying these forms of SVT, requires two electrophysiologically distinct pathways around an insulated core, such as the AV valve annulus. Most cases of re-entrant SVT are sporadic.

Accessory connections include: 1. the concealed accessory connection, where the connection is not seen on ECG in normal sinus rhythm, and it conducts in a retrograde fashion from ventricle to atrium, a unidirectional retrograde accessory pathway; and 2. permanent junctional reciprocating tachycardia, where the accessory connection acts like a concealed connection, but the transmission through the connection is slow, such that during SVT the rate may be quite slow (130–150 beats/min) compared to other forms of SVT. Other additional pathways are named Wolff–Parkinson–White (WPW), Lown–Ganong–Levine (LGL) and Mahaim, as follows:

- *Wolff–Parkinson–White (WPW)* syndrome is a combination of pre-excitation on surface ECG and episodic SVT, whether orthodromic or antidromic. In WPW, the ECG shows a short PR interval, a delta wave (initial slurring of the QRS complex) and a wide QRS complex. During episodes of tachycardia the ECG develops either a narrow QRS tachycardia with a retrograde P wave after the QRS (orthodromic SVT) or a wide QRS (antidromic SVT). Children with WPW can develop atrial flutter, and also have a small risk of sudden cardiac death (SCD) from extremely fast atrial tachycardias (e.g. atrial flutter or atrial fibrillation being conducted down the AAVC, producing ventricular tachycardia [VT] or ventricular fibrillation [VF]). (See Fig. 6.40.)

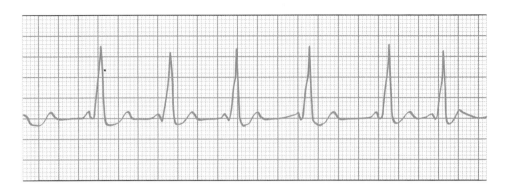

Figure 6.40 Wolff–Parkinson–White syndrome. Note the characteristic findings of a short P–R interval, slurred upstroke of QRS (delta wave), and prolongation of the QRS interval.

Source: Zitelli, B.J., McIntire, S.C. & Nowalk, A.J. (2012). *Atlas of Pediatric Physical Diagnosis* (6th ed.). Philadelphia: Elsevier. Figure 5.45.

- *Lown–Ganong–Levine (LGL)* syndrome is another form of pre-excitation and episodic SVT, where the ECG shows a short PR interval and normal QRS complex; in LGL, the upper AV node is bypassed by James fibres that connect the atrium and the bundle of His, producing a short PR, but the ventricles are depolarised normally.
- *Mahaim-type* pre-excitation and episodic SVT is a third form, which has a long QRS with a delta wave, but a normal PR interval; here, the bundle of His is bypassed by Mahaim fibres, which connect the AV node and one of the ventricles.

Treatment modalities for acute SVT include vagal manoeuvres (e.g. Valsalva, blowing up balloons with nose occluded, blowing into the end of a syringe [trying to move/blow the plunger outward], application of icepack to face, doing a 'headstand', carotid body massage), IV adenosine (the preferred IV drug, given rapidly and can be increased incrementally) or IV propranolol, digoxin, procainamide or amiodarone. Adenosine is the treatment of choice in the haemodynamically unstable child; if unsuccessful, or there is difficult venous access, synchronised cardioversion (0.5–1.0 joule per kg) can be used. Verapamil is best avoided; IV verapamil is contraindicated in infants, in whom it can be lethal because it can produce AV block.

SVT in infants spontaneously resolves in the majority, and medical management is the first choice in the first year; also, transcatheter ablation has increased risk, and is avoided at this age. Beyond infancy, for long-term treatment, radio-frequency (RF) catheter ablation has a success rate, of around 90–95%.

RF ablation comprises delivery of a high-frequency (500 kHz), low-energy electric current to the relevant cardiac area by an intracardiac catheter. This raises the temperature and burns the arrhythmia substrate. Risks of RF catheter ablation include inadvertent AV block and cardiac perforation; these are both very rare, the overall complication rate for RF ablation being below 4%. The other form of ablation is cryoablation, which does not cause unintentional heart block, but this enhanced safety has to be balanced against a potentially higher recurrence rate.

Long-term pharmacological treatments are aimed at modifying the conduction properties of the AVN, and usually involve beta blockers, digoxin or calcium channel blockers (however, digoxin and calcium channel blockers are contraindicated in those with WPW, as they can precipitate arrhythmias by enhancing AAVC conduction). For cases that are more difficult to control, other useful agents include the more potent antiarrhythmics, such as the sodium channel blocker flecainide (but this is avoided in structural or ischaemic heart disease), the combined beta blocker and potassium channel blocker, sotalol (but this can lead to QT prolongation and proarrhythmia), procainamide and amiodarone. In the absence of cardiomyopathy or structural heart disease, the prognosis for SVT is very good. WPW does have a small but real risk of SCD, the main risk indicator being symptoms (such as syncope or palpitations) in adults; 55% of asymptomatic children and adolescents become symptomatic by the age of 40, and symptomatic patients have an overall lifetime risk of 3–4% of SCD. All children with WPW should be referred to a paediatric electrophysiologist.

Long QT syndrome (LQTS)

Children with arrhythmias (e.g. sick sinus syndrome, severe bradycardia, complete AV block), congestive cardiac failure, myocarditis or anthracycline cardiotoxicity, or those on certain medications (e.g. several antiarrhythmics [especially quinidine], some antibiotics, diuretics [by causing acute/chronic hypokalaemia], promotility agents, [cisapride]) have an increased risk of developing LQTS, and subsequent 'torsades de pointes' (TdP, twisting of points) ventricular tachycardia, which can present with **S**udden death, **S**yncope or **S**eizures (the 3 **S**s). Recent molecular breakthroughs are unravelling the congenital forms of LQTS.

A scoring system has been established to make a clinical diagnosis of LQTS. Points are attributed for ECG, clinical history and family history findings. A QTc of 480 ms or above scores 3 points; QTc 460–479 ms scores 2, QTc 450–459 ms (males only) scores 1 and QTc of 480 ms or over, during the fourth minute of recovery after an exercise stress test, scores 1 also. Other ECG findings score as follows: *torsades de pointes* (2), T wave alternans (1), notched T wave in three leads (1), low heart rate for age (0.5). Clinical history of syncope with stress scores 2, without stress scores 1. Family member with definite LQTS scores 1, and unexplained sudden cardiac death under the age of 30 in immediate family scores 0.5. A total score is then given; 3.5 or above gives a high likelihood of LQTS. Diagnosis is made if there is the risk score of 3.5 or above, if there is a QTc above 500 in repeated ECGs (in the absence of a secondary cause for prolongation of QTc) or if there is identification of a pathogenic mutation in one of the (at least) 15 genes in which mutation is known to cause LQTS.

Molecular testing may be by a multigene panel which includes all known LQTS genes, or by single gene testing based on the phenotype (T wave pattern, and syncope triggers). Around two-thirds of cases are due to pathogenic mutations of *KCNQ1, KCNH2, or SCN5A* (see below). These correspond to LQTS types 1, 2 and 3 respectively. The remaining dozen types are rare.

LQTS is usually inherited as an autosomal dominant cardiac electrophysiological disorder, characterised by LQTS and T wave abnormalities on ECG, and by TdP; TdP is usually self-terminating and causes syncope particularly with exercise or emotional stress, with no warning—sometimes at rest, or in sleep. TdP can degenerate to VF and causes sudden death, or aborted cardiac arrest if defibrillated successfully. Molecular genetic testing has identified the genes associated with LQTS that code for potassium or sodium channels: *KCNQ1* (chromosome 11p15.5; type 1, 30–35% of LQTS), *KCNH2* (chromosome 7q35–q36; type 2, 25–30% LQTS), *SCN5A* (chromosome 3p21; type 3, 5–10% of LQTS); the remaining genes coding for K+ or Na+ channels, occur in < 1%: *KCNE1 (type 5), KCNE2 (type 6), KCNJ2 (type 7), KCNJ5 (type 13), SCN4B (type 10)*. Other genes occurring in < 1% LQTS: *ANK2 (type 4), CACNAIC (type 8), CAV3 (type 9), AKAP9 (type 11), SNTTA1 (type 12), CALM1 (type 14), CALM2 (type 15)*.

Three clinical phenotypes are recognised: LQT1, due to mutations in *KCNQ1* causing IKs potassium channel dysfunction, and cardiac events triggered by exercise and emotion; LQT2 is due to mutations in *KNH2* causing IKr potassium channel dysfunction, and cardiac events triggered by exercise, emotion and sleep; and LQT3 is due to mutations in SCN5A, the cardiac sodium channel gene, causing INa channel dysfunction, and cardiac events triggered by sleep. Syncope is most common in LQTS1 (63%), followed then by LQTS2 (46%), and then LQTS3 (18%). In patients between 0 and 18 years of age, the cumulative mortality rates are 2% for LQTS1, 3% for LQTS2 and 7% for LQTS3. Management for the LQT1 and LQT2 phenotypes is beta blocker or pacemaker if beta blocker produces symptomatic bradycardia; recurrence of events while receiving beta blockers is usually the result of inadequate dosing; for the LQT3 phenotype, implantable cardioverter–defibrillator (ICD); ICD may also be required for the LQT1 and LQT2 if resistant to beta blockers or there is a past history of cardiac arrest. Automatic external defibrillators should be readily available at home, school and work. It is very important these patients avoid drugs that increase QT: see www.azcert.org for an updated list (this stands for Arizona Centre for Education and Research on Therapeutics).

LQTS also can occur with phenotypes that include extracardiac features.

Jervell and Lange–Nielsen syndrome (JLNS) is an autosomal recessive condition is characterised by congenital profound bilateral sensorineural hearing loss and LQTS, with the corrected QT interval being greater than 500 ms (markedly prolonged, at 557 ± 65 ms). It is caused by an abnormality in a potassium channel, which is found in two places in the body; the stria vascularis of the cochlea, and the heart. It classically presents as a deaf child having syncopal episodes when stressed or frightened, or when exercising. The diagnosis requires the presence of two disease-causing mutations of the genes *KCNQ1* or *KCNE1*, the only two genes known to be associated with JLNS. *KCNQ1* and *KCNE1* encode the alpha and beta subunit proteins (KvLQT1/minK) for the slow potassium current IKs of the cochlea and the heart. Mutations are found in *KCNQ1* or *KCNE1* in 94% of patients with JLNS; 90% of these are attributable to *KCNQ1* and 10% to *KCNE1*. Mutations can be found in all coding exons. Around one-third are compound heterozygotes.

In JLNS, abnormal cardiac depolarisation and repolarisation can lead to prolonged QT interval and tachyarrhythmias, including VT, TdP and VF, which can cause syncope or sudden death: 50% of patients will have cardiac events before 3 years of age, triggered by emotions and exercise. Corrected QT prolongation in JLNS is associated with increased risk of sudden infant death syndrome (SIDS), and if untreated, more than half of the children with JLNS will die prior to 15 years of age. Up to 95% of people with JLNS have a cardiac event before adulthood.

Although the sex ratio among patients with JLNS is equal, females have lower risk of SCD. Heterozygotes have normal hearing; in some heterozygotes, there is no QT prolongation; in others, there can be QT prolongation with fainting and risk of SCD, which is RWS as above. Only the genes *KCNQ1* and *KCNE1* are involved in both RWS and JLNS.

Andersen–Tawil syndrome (LQTS type 7) is characterised by episodic flaccid muscle paralysis, and facial dysmorphic features, due to mutations in *KCNJ2*.

Timothy syndrome (LQTS type 8) is associated with syndactyly, dysmorphic facial features and neurological disorders; average age of death from VT 2.5 years; calcium channel gene *CACA1C*; the recommended treatment is ICD).

Acquired causes for LQTS include electrolyte abnormalities (hypokalaemia, hypocalcaemia and hypomagnesaemia), malnutrition, myocardial disease (cardiomyopathy, myocarditis) and drugs, including some vasodilators, tricyclic antidepressants, antihistamines and phenothiazines; the full list is at www.azcert.org, as mentioned earlier.

More than 50 mutations in four cardiac ion (sodium or potassium) channels on the myocyte have been delineated; medications implicated in causing LQTS affect these same channels. Symptomatic LQTS can be triggered by physical activity (e.g. swimming), intense or sudden emotions, or awakening, all of which cause adrenergic arousal. Syncopal events can be precipitated by competitive sports, amusement park rides, scary movies and jumping into cold water.

Any child (with cardiac disease in particular) who is due to commence any of the drugs known to trigger LQTS must have an ECG to measure the corrected QT interval (Bazett formula: QT (corrected) = QT/square root of the R–R interval; QT is measured from the start of the Q to the end of the T), which should be less than or equal to 0.46. If it is greater than this, avoid all drugs known to precipitate LQTS.

Not all LQTS can be detected on a standard resting ECG; exercise ECG will unmask the 5% of those with the LQTS gene who have absent QT prolongation at rest.

As untreated LQTS has a mortality rate of around 50%, appropriate therapy should be commenced quickly once the diagnosis is made. Treatment options include, for the hearing impairment, cochlear implantation (CI), which does not interfere with bipolar pacemakers, but precautions still need be made during anaesthesia for this procedure because of the increased risk of arrhythmia.

For the cardiac problem, the traditional first-line treatment has been beta blockers, which do reduce mortality, but unlike the situation with LQTS1, cardiac events in JLNS still can occur frequently despite beta blockade; the mortality rate for beta blockade treatment alone is 35% over 5 years, and 86% of patients will have a cardiac event.

Implantable cardioverter–defibrillators (ICDs) are advisable in those with a history of cardiac arrest, or high risk: corrected QT interval > 550 ms, syncope before 5 years old and male gender older than age 20 years with KCNQ1 mutation. Left cervicothoracic sympathetic ganglionectomy (also called left cardiac sympathetic denervation, LCSD) has been successful in some patients.

Sodium channel blockers can be useful in treating LQTS3, who have a QTc interval > 500 ms, as they can shorten the QTc interval by 40 ms.

Family members of those with JLNS should be trained in cardiopulmonary resuscitation (CPR), there should be availability of automated external defibrillators in the home, the school and, for older adolescents, the workplace; local emergency/ambulance services should be made aware of high-risk patients such as those with JLNS, and all patients should have a MedicAlert bracelet explaining their diagnosis.

LQTS should be sought/excluded in any child with breath-holding attacks, seizures precipitated by emotion or exertion, all initial afebrile seizures, unexplained syncope and congenital deafness.

Brugada syndrome

Described in 1992, this is an inherited cardiac disease causing ventricular tachyarrhythmias in patients with structurally normal hearts, presenting with syncope or cardiac arrest, and a strong family history of syncope or sudden death. It is inherited as autosomal dominant. There are 11 types of Brugada syndrome listed in OMIM. For Brugada syndrome 1, the gene known to be associated is *SCN5A*, located at 3p22.2, which encodes the sodium channel protein type 5 subunit alpha in cardiac myocytes; there are over 160 known mutations in *SCN5A*. Mutations in *SCN5A* are found in 20–25% of patients with Brugada syndrome. It has a characteristic ECG pattern: right bundle branch block (RBBB) and ST elevation in V1 to V3; some patients with normal resting ECGs can have the classic changes induced by giving ajmaline, an antiarrhythmic medication. Implantable cardioverter–defibrillators (ICDs) can be placed in patients with a history of syncope or cardiac arrest, to prevent life-threatening arrhythmias; this is the only therapy known to be effective in these patients. Isoproterenol infusion can be used for electrical storms. Quinidine also has been used to prevent symptoms and resolve ECG features.

Brugada syndrome 2 is due to a mutation in the *GPD1L* gene; Brugada syndromes 3 and 4, phenotypes of which include a shortened QT on ECG, are caused by the mutations *CACNA1C* and *CACNB2*, respectively; Brugada syndrome 5 is caused by mutation in *SCN1B*; Brugada syndrome 6 is caused by mutation of the *KCNE3* gene; Brugada syndrome 7 is due to mutation in the *SCN3B* gene; and Brugada 8 is caused by mutation in the *HCN4* gene.

Drugs to avoid include Class 1C antiarrhythmic drugs (including flecainide and propafenone) and Class 1A drugs (including procainamide and disopyramide). Drugs that unmask the Brugada ECG include tricyclic antidepressant drugs, alpha-adrenergic agonists, beta-adrenergic antagonists, first-generation antihistaminics (dimenhydrinate), anaesthetics and anti-psychotic drugs with sodium-blocking effects. Cocaine toxicity, vagotonic agents and being febrile, also unmask the Brugada ECG.

Brugada syndrome has three different ECG patterns. The diagnosis can be confirmed by finding: 1. Type 1 ECG (elevation of J point [junction between QRS complex and ST segment] at least 2 mm with a negative T wave and an ST segment that is of 'coved' type and gradually descending) in more than one right precordial lead (V1–V3), with or without administration of a sodium channel blocker (flecainide, pilsicainide, ajmaline or procainamide); and 2. at least one of documented VF, self-terminating polymorphic VT, a family history of SCD, 'coved-type' ECGs in family members, electrophysiological inducibility, syncope or nocturnal agonal respiration; and/or (c) a mutation of any of the following: *SCN5A, SCN1B, SCN2B, SCN3B, GPD1L, CACNA1C, CACNB2, CACNA2D1, KCND3, KCNE3, KCNEIL (KCNE5), KCNJ8, HCN4, RANGRF, SLMSAP or TRPM4.*

Brugada syndrome should be considered with the following: Type 2 ECG (elevation of J point at least 2 mm, with a positive or biphasic T wave; the ST segment has a 'saddle back' pattern and is elevated at least 1 mm) in more than one right precordial lead, with conversion to Type 1 ECG following challenge with a sodium channel blocker; and Type 3 ECG (elevation of J point at least 2 mm, with a positive T wave; the ST segment has 'saddle back' configuration and is elevated < 1 mm) in more than one lead, with conversion to Type 1 ECG following challenge with a sodium channel blocker.

The parameter used for clinical decision-making is inducibility during electrophysiological study (EPS), which is highly predictive of subsequent events.

Brugada syndrome has a high risk of ventricular arrhythmias and sudden death. Males with easily induced arrhythmias and spontaneously abnormal ECGs have a 45% chance of an arrhythmic event at any time during life. Brugada syndrome usually manifests during adulthood, the mean age of sudden death being 40 years. It can present as SIDS, or as sudden unexpected nocturnal death syndrome (SUNDS). Most patients who have Brugada syndrome diagnosed have inherited it from a parent; the proportion caused by *de novo* mutations is around 1% only; the family history may still be negative because of failure to recognise the condition.

Myocardial disease
Dilated cardiomyopathy (DCM)—familial dilated cardiomyopathy (FDC) and idiopathic dilated cardiomyopathy (IDC)

The most common form of cardiomyopathy, DCM, is characterised by left-ventricular enlargement, systolic dysfunction and reduced myocardial contraction force. It can present with Dysrhythmia, Congestive failure and Mural thrombus, leading to thromboembolic disease. The term 'DCM' can have a generic meaning (describing two features: left-ventricular enlargement and systolic dysfunction), and can be familial dilated cardiomyopathy (FDC), idiopathic dilated cardiomyopathy (IDC), which may in fact be familial in 20–50% of cases, or it may be secondary to therapeutic toxins (anthracyclines), radiation, inflammatory conditions, myocarditis, long-standing severe hypertension or thyroid disease. DCM (FDC) has been researched at the molecular level, identifying over 30 genes which account for 40–50% of autosomal dominant FDC, the commonest ones encoding the structural proteins of cardiac muscle: lamin-A/C, gene *LMNA* (7–8%); myosin 7, gene *MYH7* (5–8%); sodium channel protein type 5 subunit alpha, gene *SCN5A* (2–4%), at least two genes for X-linked DCM, these genes encoding the proteins—dystrophin, gene *DMD*, and tafazzin, gene *TAZ*, and one gene for autosomal recessive inheritance DCM, encoding troponin I, cardiac muscle, gene *TNNI3*. Other genes are involved in metabolic causes, such as deficiencies of enzymes needed for myocardial fatty acid oxidation. First-degree relative screening should include the medical history, physical examination, an echocardiogram and ECG.

Symptomatic DCM indicates late disease. Symptoms may be those of congestive cardiac failure (CCF) (oedema, orthopnoea, paroxysmal dyspnoea), palpitations, chest pain, or exercise intolerance or syncope; signs include hypotension, weak peripheral pulses and hepatomegaly, with investigations showing cardiomegaly (CXR), arrhythmias (ECG), dilatation of the left ventricle and left atrium (echocardiography).

Treatment options include controlling CCF with antifailure therapy, including beta blockers (especially carvedilol) and ACE inhibitors, controlling arrhythmias with antiarrhythmics, consideration of pacemakers and implantable cardiac defibrillators, minimising the risk of thromboembolism with anticoagulants and antiplatelet drugs and, for those more refractive to treatment, a ventricular assist device or transplantation. Cardiac transplantation is still the definitive treatment for DCM refractory to medical, or device, therapy. Training in cardiopulmonary resuscitation is advisable for family members and caregivers.

Familial hypertrophic cardiomyopathy (FHCM): also called hypertrophic obstructive cardiomyopathy (HOCM) and idiopathic hypertrophic subaortic stenosis (IHSS)

Inherited most often as an autosomal dominant trait, HCM penetrance is incomplete in early childhood, increasing with age. Over 1500 mutations have been identified in the 16 genes that account for HCM, which encode various sarcomeric proteins, including, most commonly: myosin heavy chain, cardiac muscle beta isoform, gene *MYH7* (40%); myosin-binding protein C cardiac-type, gene *MYBPC3* (40%); troponin T, cardiac muscle, gene *TNNT2* (5%); troponin I, cardiac muscle, gene *TNNI3* (5%).

Particular mutations determine prognostic factors, including risk of early death. HCM is occasionally transmitted as a mitochondrial disorder (i.e. maternally inherited).

Symptoms include failure to thrive, CCF, cyanosis, shortness of breath on exertion, dyspnoea, fatigue with exercise, chest pain, presyncope, syncope and palpitations. Signs include prominent left-ventricular apical impulse or lift, systolic murmur (increased by exercise, standing, straining; decreased by squatting), extra heart sounds (S3 and S4) and mid-diastolic rumble (mitral flow murmur with severe mitral regurgitation, with systolic anterior motion of the mitral valve).

LVOT or intracavity obstruction may need provocative manoeuvres to detect their presence, such as the Valsalva manoeuvre, standing from squatting, and exercise. Investigations show cardiomegaly (CXR), right- and left-ventricular hypertrophy (RVH and LVH) in infants, LVH and abnormal Q waves in older children, LQTS in infants or older children, or arrhythmias (ECG), asymmetric septal hypertrophy, and concentric and apical hypertrophy (echocardiography or cardiac MRI).

Other tests may include gated technetium-99m labelled blood pool scan (assess ejection fraction), thallium perfusion scan (regional perfusion abnormalities) and positron emission tomography (regional metabolic abnormalities).

In children under the age of 4, there is a differential diagnosis of: 1. inborn errors of metabolism (the main one being glycogen storage disease II [Pompe disease], which presents in the first few months of life); 2. malformation syndromes (the main one being NS; see earlier in this case); and 3. neuromuscular disorders (the main one being Friedreich ataxia, FRDA, with slow-onset ataxia between 10 and 15 years, and diagnosed on molecular genetic testing of FXH). Other (rarer) secondary causes of HCM include Beckwith-Wiedemann syndrome, and mitochondrial diseases.

Treatment includes beta blockers (e.g. propranolol, atenolol) or calcium channel blockers (e.g. verapamil, nifedipine) for those who are symptomatic (*note:* verapamil excluded in infants under 12 months, or in those with major conduction disturbances), and consideration of the same treatment for asymptomatic children with a worrying family history. Disopyramide may be used if the other drugs are unsuccessful. Children with lethal, refractory arrhythmias may be treated with amiodarone.

If there is a high risk of cardiac arrest, or the patient is a survivor of cardiac arrest, then an implantable cardioverter–defibrillator (ICD) is recommended. Endocarditis prophylaxis is important. Resistant atrial fibrillation may warrant anticoagulation.

Active sports participation is exceedingly unwise. *It is important to avoid the following*: competitive endurance training, heavy weight training, sprinting, dehydration, hypovolaemia, and medication that increases afterload (ACE inhibitors, ARBs) and other direct vasodilators.

Surgery is an option for failed medical therapy, to ease subaortic obstruction; the Morrow operation (myotomy/myectomy) can relieve symptoms and prolong life. Cardiac transplantation is a further option for high-risk patients. Around 5–10% of HCM progress to end-stage disease; without transplant, annual mortality is 11%.

Congestive cardiac failure (CCF)

CCF, irrespective of the cause, involves some form of cardiac injury that activates compensatory and deleterious pathways, which can cause chronic progressive deterioration that ultimately can hasten the demise of the patient. CCF is the most common cause for children with heart disease being prescribed medication, and accounts for at least half of paediatric referrals for heart transplantation. Around 40% of paediatric patients with cardiomyopathy develop heart failure to the degree that will be fatal without a transplant, and around 20% of children with structural heart disease will develop CCF. Symptoms may be feeding difficulties due to dyspnoea, getting tired easily and failure to thrive; signs may include mild to severe intercostal and subcostal recession, grunting, tachycardia, gallop rhythm (S3, S4) and hepatomegaly.

Principles/aspects of managing CCF can be listed as follows (mnemonic **ASPECTS**):

Afterload reduction: ACEIs, ARBs, brain natriuretic peptide (BNP), milrinone, nitrates
Sympathetic inhibition: beta blockers, BNP, digoxin
Preload reduction: BNP, diuretics
Enhanced contractility (inotropy): digoxin
Cardiac remodelling prevention: mineralocorticoid inhibitors (spironolactone)
Timely surgical repair of structural congenital heart disease
Systemic disease recognition and treatment (of pathology underlying CCF)

ACE inhibitors (e.g. captopril) are very useful in lowering afterload and have been shown to decrease mortality in adults (but must be avoided in HCM, as per earlier); they are usually started in hospital due to the risk of initial dose hypotension and the worsening of any unrecognised renovascular pathology. Diuretics (e.g. combined low-dose loop and thiazide diuretics) give rapid symptomatic relief; diuretics reduce preload, which prevents high cardiac filling pressures (which could lead to pulmonary oedema). Mineralocorticoid inhibitors (e.g. spironolactone) can help prevention of maladaptive cardiac remodelling and interstitial fibrosis. Digoxin is still widely used; it acts as an inotrope, but its use remains controversial and in adults it does not increase survival in CCF—indeed, there are no studies demonstrating its efficacy. Beta blockers (e.g. metoprolol, carvedilol) also are used increasingly in carefully graduated doses. Growth hormone has been used in a small number of patients (e.g. pre-transplant) and has been associated with improved indices on echocardiography, increased exercise capacity and decreased myocardial oxygen consumption.

Nesiritide, which is a recombinant form of BNP, causes both diuresis and vasodilation, decreases both preload and afterload, inhibits the sympathetic nervous system, promotes cardiac myocyte survival and inhibits cardiac fibroblast activation; it shows promise as a third-line therapy, but studies in the paediatric age group are lacking at this stage.

There are surgical forms of circulatory support other than transplantation. External left-ventricular support devices and second-generation implantable devices have been developed, which provide prolonged mechanical unloading and can be used in myocarditis.

These surgical support methods can act as a 'bridge' to transplantation, or a 'bridge' for biding time until the myocardium recovers in cases of myocarditis with acute cardiogenic shock. Advances in the technology of axial flow impeller pumps are producing smaller devices (e.g. the Jarvik 2000 impeller pump, smaller than a finger, but capable of a flow of 3 L/min). Another procedure for end-stage disease is partial left ventriculectomy and mitral valve replacement/repair (the Batista operation). This has been successful in children with DCM. The ultimate therapy for CCF refractory to medical treatment is cardiac transplantation.

Cardiac transplantation

Transplantation is now a well-established procedure for infants and children with severe congenital heart disease with ventricular failure (accounting for around two-thirds of cases) or end-stage cardiomyopathies (around one-third of cases), and survival rates continue to improve: 90% at 1 month, 85% at 1 year, 68–75% at 5 years, 58–65% at 10 years and 40% at 20 years. In the older population of children (beyond infancy), cardiomyopathies account for most transplantations: 55% of those aged 1–10 years, and 64% of those in adolescents. For transplantation to be considered, generally the life expectancy is below 1 or 2 years, and/or quality of life is very poor. Prognosis is worse for those under 1 year of age and those with assistive devices.

Survivors of childhood cancer with cardiomyopathy due to anthracyclines represent a growing number of potential recipients, as do babies requiring primary transplantation for hypoplastic left heart syndrome. A small percentage are retransplantations (around 3–5% of all paediatric transplants).

Indications for heart transplantation can be divided into two broad groups: life-saving indications and life-enhancing indications:

- *Life-saving*: (**CC**, **UU**, **RR**): **C**CF with symptomatic ventricular dysfunction secondary to myocardial disease or palliated CHD; **C**omplex CHD with failed surgical correction; **U**nresectable tumours; **U**nresectable ventricular diverticula; **R**hythm disturbances: life-threatening (arrhythmias), resistant to therapy; **R**etransplantation (graft vasculopathy, ventricular dysfunction).

- *Life-enhancing*: (**CC**, **FF**, **II**): **C**CF associated with pulmonary hypertension; **C**ardiomyopathy—restrictive, with poor survival overall; **F**ontan circulation with protein-losing enteropathy resistant to medical therapy; **F**ontan failing with decreased exercise tolerance, and declining quality of life; **I**noperable AV valve or aortic regurgitation; **I**noperable CHD with severe oxygen desaturation.

Transplant surgery may involve the biatrial technique, where there is anastomosis of donor and recipient aortas, pulmonary arteries and atrial cuffs; this can be associated with conduction disturbances, and a pacemaker is needed in 4–15% of patients; also, this can cause higher thromboembolism rate, poorer atrial synchrony and AV valve regurgitation (due to atrial anatomy being altered). The other transplant technique is the bicaval approach, where the right atrium remains intact as the donor and recipient superior vena cava (SVC) and inferior vena cava (IVC) are anastomosed; this is associated with fewer of the above complications.

The major problem is finding suitable donors. The donor pool for infants under 12 months can include ABO-incompatible (ABO-I) transplants, as these have been shown to have equal long-term survival compared to ABO-compatible transplantations. Administration of blood products during and following ABO-I transplants must be done very carefully, to ensure there are no isohaemagglutinins against the donor or the recipient.

For combined heart–lung transplantation (which is only indicated for severe pulmonary parenchymal or vascular disease with poor left-ventricular function, single ventricle anatomy, or a lesion requiring exceedingly complicated repair with excessive ischaemic time) the usual requirements are ABO and CMV compatibility plus donor–recipient chest size compatibility within 10%. The main immunosuppressive drugs used include the antiproliferatives (azathioprine [AZA], sirolimus or mycophenolate mofetil [MMF], which increasingly is replacing AZA in many centres), the calcineurin inhibitors (cyclosporin [CSA] or tacrolimus [TRL]) and steroids. Most centres have a triple immunosuppression protocol involving one agent from each group.

Allograft rejection occurs to a moderate or severe degree in most children, with the risk of rejection being highest in the first 6 months, and remains the most common cause of mortality in the first 3 years posttransplant. Risk factors for rejection are older age at transplant, CMV, gender mismatch or a previous episode of rejection. Rejection can be asymptomatic, but severe acute rejection can cause tiredness, poor appetite, nausea, poor feeding, abdominal pain, weight gain or fever.

Haemodynamically significant rejection is associated with an increased mortality rate. However, there is no blood test proven to screen accurately for rejection; in most centres, endomyocardial biopsy is the diagnostic gold standard. Infections remain a significant cause of morbidity.

Early infections (up to a month after transplant) are usually bacterial or fungal; intermediate (2–6 months after transplant) infections are often viral (e.g. Epstein-Barr virus [EBV], cytomegalovirus [CMV]); and late infections include viruses (EBV, varicella) and fungi (e.g. *Aspergillus* genus).

The commonest long-term side effects are related to immunosuppression:

- *Coronary artery disease* in up to 75% examined by intravascular ultrasound 5 years after transplant. Symptoms can include presyncope, syncope, exercise intolerance and chest pain (rare due to denervation of the transplanted heart). This form of chronic rejection is an accelerated graft vasculopathy that presents at a median of 6 years. To assess risk, coronary angiography can be done 1–2 yearly and, if positive, infers severe disease. Other imaging studies can be used: myocardial perfusion scanning, dobutamine stress echocardiography and MRI studies. Several agents are being investigated for prevention of vasculopathy, including calcium antagonists,

ACEIs, vitamin E, statins, aspirin, MMF and rapamycin. Coronary artery disease may lead to need for retransplantation.

- *Hypertension* in up to 60% at 5 years; more in those on steroids and CSA; less with CSA alone; least with TRL alone. Aggressive treatment is required, usually with an ACE inhibitor or the calcium blocker diltiazem. For those with relevant congenital heart pathology, evaluation for residual pathology (e.g. residual coarctation) is required; check renal function yearly; nuclear scans may be needed to calculate the glomerular filtration rate (GFR).
- *Neoplasia* in 20%, most commonly lymphoproliferative diseases, at 6 months to 6 years after transplantation.
- *Abnormal renal function* in up to 25% at 5 years. With longer survival, a small number of patients are developing end-stage renal disease (ESRD) and then have a renal transplant; increased use of MMF and sirolimus (no renal toxicity) may allow decreased use of CSA and TRL and thus less nephrotoxicity.
- *Osteoporosis* probably occurs in 100%: steroids and calcineurin inhibitors decrease bone formation and increase bone destruction; steroids decrease calcium absorption. Supplemental calcium and vitamin D are recommended; protocols have been developed that include biphosphates, calcitonin and hormone replacement, although paediatric data is scant. Yearly bone density (DXA) scanning is useful.

Other long-term issues include psychological issues (up to a third of children have behavioural problems at 5 years posttransplant—neurocognitive and neuropsychiatric support are important), non-compliance in adolescents and altered lifestyle requirements (need to get routine exercise 3–4 times a week, for at least 30 minutes, stop smoking, and maintain a heart-healthy diet, avoiding saturated fats and cholesterol).

Contraindications to transplantation are becoming fewer over the years. Currently (2016) the only contraindications are: 1. severe irreversible end organ damage or multi-system organ failure; 2. severe irreversible pulmonary hypertension; 3. active infection; 4. anatomical features that technically preclude transplant, such as severe hypoplasia of branch pulmonary arteries (as distal branch arteries are from the recipient and cannot be corrected with transplantation) and severe pulmonary vein stenosis or atresia (as the recipient veins are connected to the donor left atrium); 5. a severe or progressive non-cardiac condition with limited survival (mitochondrial disorders, untreatable metabolic disorders, Duchenne muscular dystrophy, cancer); and 6. psychological issues—non-compliance, smoking, drug abuse and psychiatric conditions.

There are some fetal indications for listing on the transplant waiting list. These include: hypoplastic left heart syndrome, where transplantation is primary therapy; intractable arrhythmias; unresectable cardiac tumours; cardiomyopathies with poor ventricular function; right-atrial isomerism syndromes; and single ventricle anatomy, with risk factors for surgical palliation (severe atrioventricular valve regurgitation, decreased function).

Candidates are listed from 35 weeks' gestation and weight over 2.5 kg; if a donor heart becomes available, then patients are delivered by caesarean section, followed by immediate transplantation.

Telemedicine

Advances in telecommunications technology, with the widespread introduction of integrated services digital network (ISDN) lines, allows transmission of echocardiogram images from peripheral to tertiary centres, with a paediatric cardiologist interpreting the transmitted images and guiding the performance of the scan to ensure that the best possible views are obtained. This approach has been used successfully in many countries. The defects that must be correctly diagnosed early include those causing cyanosis, obstructive lesions of the left and right heart, and total anomalous pulmonary venous drainage (TAPVD), the latter providing the greatest diagnostic difficulty. The other two lesions that can be difficult to diagnose are coarctation of the aorta (obtaining good aortic arch views can be challenging) and PDA (and, if present, ascertaining how much it contributes clinically).

Cardiac imaging

Positron emission tomography (PET) scanning is being used to assess the cross-sectional functioning of the myocardium after significant cardiac insults related to coronary artery problems, such as in Kawasaki disease, corrective surgery for congenital heart disease (coronary occlusion can complicate the arterial switch procedure for transposition of the great arteries) and coronary arteriopathy seen in cardiac transplantation (here, there may be few clues; chest pain does not occur as the heart is denervated). Cardiac PET studies can assess regional substrate metabolism, chemical recognition (of receptors and enzymes) and regional blood flow. It can accurately differentiate between areas that can be reperfused (so-called 'stunned' areas) and infarcted areas from irreversible ischaemia.

SHORT CASE

SHORT CASE: The cardiovascular system

As one of the most common examination cases, a cardiac case is expected to be performed extremely well. A slick, complete examination, followed by a logical, relevant differential diagnosis and sensible interpretation of CXRs and electrocardiograms (ECGs) are all minimum requirements.

Introduce yourself. Stand back and give a brief general description of the child. Note the child's colour (blue or pink), work of breathing (any respiratory distress), any dysmorphic features (Down, Williams, 22q11 [DiGeorge], Turner, Noonan syndromes) and general growth parameters (failure to thrive, short stature [above syndromes], or tall stature [Marfan]). Then the child's chest needs to be exposed appropriately. Positioning older children standing directly in front of the candidate allows thorough inspection for chest asymmetry, including walking around the child, checking carefully for scars; school-aged children may be positioned lying at 45°, younger children may be on their mother's lap.

During general inspection of chest and body build, one should consider connective tissue disorders including Marfan (MFS) and Loeys–Dietz (LDS) syndromes, as these cases are seen in examinations. Looking for additional or peripheral clues to these diagnoses can be left until the cardiac signs have been elicited (see the next page).

Look for any scars. *Median sternotomy scars* may indicate any complex cardiac surgery, pulmonary artery (PA) banding, or bypass surgery. Do not miss the scar of a Blalock-Taussig (BT) shunt (posterolateral thoracotomy) on either side, which may be associated with an absent radial pulse on that side (with classical BT shunt; 'newer' BT shunts may have pulse present).

Look carefully for scars over the back, in the infrascapular regions: in addition to BT shunts, *left thoracotomy scars* may indicate previous repair of coarctation of the aorta, ligation of a patent ductus arteriosus (PDA), or PA banding (or non-heart-related reasons for thoracotomy).

Right thoracotomy scars may indicate BT shunt, PA banding (or non-heart-related reasons for thoracotomy, repair of tracheo-oesophageal fistula in VACTERL association, repair of congenital diaphragmatic hernia [10% have associated heart defects]). Other causes for scars include pacemaker insertion and intercostal drain tubes.

Pick up the child's hands, check the fingernails for clubbing, peripheral cyanosis and capillary return, and check the toenails. Feel the radial pulse, noting the rate, amplitude and character; the upper limb can be lifted straight up to detect hyperdynamic pulsation (Watson's water-hammer sign in aortic incompetence [AI]). Note the respiratory rate at this stage (tachypnoea from pulmonary oedema in left-ventricular failure). Feel both radial pulses and femoral pulses: absent left radial pulse may be found with repaired coarctation and in BT shunt; absent or decreased femoral pulses, with normal or increased brachial pulses, suggest coarctation (brachiofemoral delay is found only in adults with coarctation.). Inspection of the femoral region may reveal catheter scars. If you cannot feel pulses, it is safe to say pulses are 'difficult to feel'. (See Fig. 6.41.)

Although it is rare to see a patient with coarctation of the aorta in the exam, the author scored a child with corrected coarctation, plus additional complex heart disease, and a BT shunt; the signs included chest wall asymmetry with left chest wall prominence, no radial or brachial pulse on the left, no radial pulse on the right with linear scar over radial artery, normal brachial pulse on right, decreased femoral pulsations with overlying scars bilaterally, and five distinct murmurs. Asking for the BP next led to the examiners challenging this candidate to measure it.

Therefore, next ask for (or offer to measure) the BP in both upper limbs. Usually, the examiners will give the values, but at other times you may be given a sphygmomanometer to measure it yourself. Check the jugular venous pressure (JVP) in older children, by sitting them at 45° in the standard manner.

Look at the tongue and state whether the patient is cyanosed; if uncertain, comment on the need to look again in natural daylight (if the room is artificially lit), or use a torch, or compare to the parent. Babies and infants may need dummies removed to visualise their tongues. Avoid saying 'pink' or 'blue': say 'not cyanosed' or 'cyanosed'. So far, the examination should have taken less than a minute.

Now, turn your attention to the chest. If not already done, check for scars and asymmetry carefully. If clinically suggestive, consider connective tissue disorders as mentioned above. At this point, lie the child down on the examination bed. Look for the apex beat and then palpate for it. Describe the location (make a show of counting down the intercostal spaces) and the quality of the impulse. Beware of dextrocardia (as in Kartagener syndrome) if the apex appears elusive. After the apex, feel the parasternal border and substernal region for heaves, and the suprasternal and supraclavicular regions for thrills, and feel over the pulmonary area for palpable closure of the pulmonary valve (i.e. 'palpable S2').

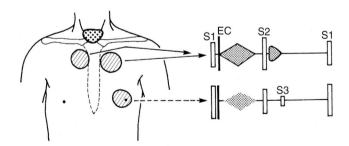

Figure 6.41 Cardiac findings of coarctation of the aorta. A systolic thrill may be present in the suprasternal notch (area shown by dots). EC = ejection click.

Source: Park, M.K. (2014). *Park's Pediatric Cardiology for Practitioners* (6th ed.). Philadelphia: Elsevier. Figure 13.16.

By the time auscultation is performed, a short list of possibilities should have been formulated, based on previous findings, by considering the following points as you proceed:

1. Cyanotic or acyanotic.
2. Heart failure or not heart failure.
3. Peripheral findings (pulses, blood pressure, JVP).
4. Praecordial findings.
5. Syndromic conditions.

The key to successful auscultation is to listen carefully to each segment of the cardiac cycle while mentally blocking out the rest. A limited number of cycles should be sufficient for each segment: first heart sound, systole, second heart sound, diastole in order. This is performed at each relevant site. Auscultation should commence at the apex, with the diaphragm of the stethoscope initially and then the bell (for diastolic murmurs). Listen at the apex (mitral area), work across to, and up, the parasternal border; listen over the tricuspid area (lower left sternal edge [LSE], the fourth left intercostal space, also where VSDs are heard best) and listen over pulmonary (upper LSE, the second left intercostal space) and aortic (upper right sternal edge [RSE], the second right intercostal) areas. Listen to each component of the cardiac cycle carefully. Note the intensities of S1 and S2 and whether S2 splits normally on inspiration. In adults, the closure of the aortic and pulmonary components of S2 are separated by 40 msec during inspiration. A split S2 excludes diagnoses such as isolated outflow tracts (Fontan circulation, pulmonary atresia) or pulmonary hypertension.

A fixed split occurs with ASD, due to prolongation of right-ventricular systole (see Fig. 6.42 for ASD findings). Listen for added sounds, in particular any ejection click, noting the point of maximal intensity, or any opening snap (mitral stenosis; rare) and then systolic and diastolic murmurs.

Note radiation of any murmurs to axillae or carotids. Mitral murmurs radiate to axillae, left-ventricular outflow tract (LVOT) murmurs such as classically radiate up the carotids, but in younger children especially other murmurs can be heard in the neck. Next, sit the child up and listen to any murmur's variation with this change in position. Listen with the child in full expiration for the subtle early diastolic murmur of AI.

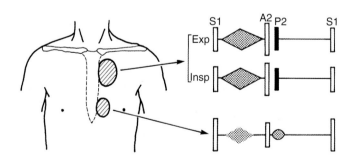

Figure 6.42 Cardiac findings of ASD. Throughout this book, heart murmurs with solid borders are the primary murmurs, and those without solid borders are transmitted murmurs or those occurring occasionally. Abnormalities in heart sounds are shown in black. Exp = expiration; Insp = inspiration.

Source: Park, M.K. (2014). *Park's Pediatric Cardiology for Practitioners* (6th ed.). Philadelphia: Elsevier. Figure 12.2.

When describing your findings, do not say 'heart sounds dual', as this merely confirms the patient is alive, but does not advance one's standing with the examiner, nor one's diagnostic precision. In the manner described above, one can then accurately describe the findings in each area. Describe each heart sound, then added sounds, then murmurs, then point of maximal intensity, then grade of the murmur. Added sounds such as clicks are of particular diagnostic importance but will only be appreciated by the careful method described. The aortic click is *best* heard at the *apex* and may be the *only* finding with a bicuspid aortic valve which does not produce flow disturbance. The click from PS is best heard along the left sternal border and pulmonary area.

Listen to the back for radiation of any murmurs and for any pulmonary adventitious sounds (inspiratory crackles with left-ventricular failure; variable findings with coexistent chest infection in Kartagener's primary ciliary dyskinesia [PCD] syndrome).

Lie the child down again and examine the abdomen for hepatomegaly (CCF), and pulsatile liver (tricuspid incompetence [TI]). Then feel for ankle oedema (right-ventricular failure).

Generally, it is not worth spending time looking for signs of more obscure diseases in the exam, although they are listed in most books on clinical examination.

If you suspect a connective tissue diagnosis such as MFS, or LDS, when relevant (*after* eliciting cardiac signs), spare a thought to examine quickly for arachnodactyly, hyperflexibility, pes planus and obvious chest wall deformity, such as pectus excavatum or carinatum. Does the patient wear glasses? A top candidate will score points if, with such a patient, one notes the presence of gastrostomy button (gastroenterological abnormalities are a part of LDS spectrum, not MFS) and when examining the oropharynx, one checks the uvula. Even experienced clinicians have been embarrassed after years of following patients with the diagnosis of MFS, to have a registrar make the diagnosis of LDS by noting facial dysmorphism (hypertelorism) or bifid elongated uvula. (Note that a bifid uvula, however, can be a normal variant in isolation.) Although enshrined in medical undergraduate folklore, the high-arched palate is both subjective, unreliable and not regarded as a useful sign by clinicians in the field.

The following are further down the list of priorities as they are exceptionally rare in the exam: only after the main signs have been elucidated should the candidate have time to even consider looking for signs of SBE (looking for dental caries, splinter haemorrhages, splenomegaly, Roth spots, blood in urine, elevated temperature), rarer conditions like Pompe disease (splenomegaly), or scleral icterus (due to mechanical valve haemolysis, or CCF affecting the liver).

Give a succinct differential diagnosis based on your clinical findings; only after this should you request the CXR and ECG.

You do not have to give a specific diagnosis immediately; this is fraught with danger. If, for example, you hear an ejection systolic murmur over the aortic area, and you are sure that a patient has valvular AS, you should say so. But if there is any uncertainty, it is prudent to give as a diagnosis 'LVOT obstruction' (LVOTO) and then proceed to delineate which of the various causes of LVOTO (supravalvular, valvular or subvalvular) is most likely and why. Supravalvular LVOTO has a thrill, valvular LVOTO has a click and a thrill, and subvalvular LVOTO has neither.

If you hear an ejection systolic murmur in the region of the pulmonary valve, the possibilities include a pulmonary flow murmur, an ASD (which is technically also a pulmonary flow murmur) or a right-ventricular outflow tract obstructive (RVOTO) lesion. It is prudent to describe it initially as a RVOT murmur, and then delineate at which level it could be, if there are clues as to an obstructive lesion (supravalvular, valvular or subvalvular). (For pulmonary stenosis types see Fig. 6.43.)

If you hear a systolic ejection click, then you can be confident this is at the valvular level. If there is a thrill at the upper left sternal border, or in the suprasternal notch, then the lesion could be at a valvular level or above, the click differentiating the two. (See Fig. 6.44 for pulmonary stenosis findings.)

The most commonly heard diastolic murmurs, in the exam format, are those of AI and pulmonary incompetence (PI). PI may be heard (accompanying a PS murmur) in patients with a median sternotomy scar, from repaired tetralogy of Fallot (ToF); other signs of repaired ToF include single S2, and there may be additional scars of previous shunts.

Continuous murmurs may be encountered, due to PDA, where the patient will be pink, have no clubbing and no scars, or due to collateral vessels in patients with pulmonary atresia with VSD due to significant aortopulmonary collateral arteries, where the patient may be cyanosed, may have clubbing and a median sternotomy scar.

If a child is cyanosed and has a confusing array of murmurs, you do not have to give an anatomically correct diagnosis. It is better to start in general terms, such as: 'This child has complex cyanotic congenital heart disease'.

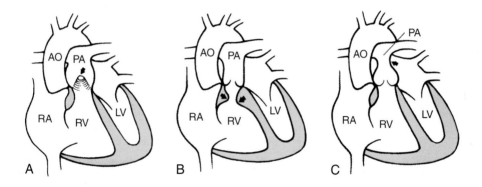

Figure 6.43 **Anatomic types of pulmonary stenoses (PSs). A.** Valvular stenosis. **B.** Infundibular stenosis. **C.** Supravalvular PS (or stenosis of the main pulmonary artery [PA]). Abnormalities are indicated by arrows. AO = aorta; LV = left ventricle; RA = right atrium; RV = right ventricle.

Source: Park, M.K. (2014). *Park's Pediatric Cardiology for Practitioners* (6th ed.). Philadelphia: Elsevier. Figure 13.1.

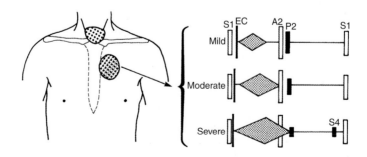

Figure 6.44 **Cardiac findings of pulmonary valve stenosis. Abnormal sounds are shown in black. Dots represent areas with systolic thrill. EC = ejection click.**

Source: Park, M.K. (2014). *Park's Pediatric Cardiology for Practitioners* (6th ed.). Philadelphia: Elsevier. Figure 13.2.

If you have a reasonable idea of the likely anatomical diagnosis, say so, but if not, it is sensible to take each murmur in turn and give a brief differential diagnosis of each (provided that these are relevant to a child with cyanotic congenital heart disease). When the CXR and ECG have been examined, the precise diagnosis may become apparent.

Additional manoeuvres may be needed to clarify suspected diagnoses. The Valsalva manoeuvre is useful in identifying hypertrophic obstructive cardiomyopathy (HOCM), as it increases the intensity of the murmur (via increased intrathoracic pressure, decreased venous return and hence decreased intracardiac volume and more severe LVOTO), and in mitral valve prolapse, where the murmur is also increased and the systolic click is heard earlier. Innocent systolic outflow tract murmurs decrease in intensity in response to the Valsalva manoeuvre.

Exercising the child is especially useful in bringing out a tricuspid diastolic murmur in an ASD (see Fig. 6.35); this is most easily achieved by having the child do several sit-ups. In patients with VSDs and ASDs, the appearance of a mid-diastolic murmur suggests a pulmonary blood flow at least twice that of the systemic circulation, and in patients with mitral or tricuspid incompetence, such a murmur suggests at least a moderate degree of regurgitation. (See Fig. 6.45 for sites of various murmurs.)

With any findings strongly suggestive of a specific diagnosis, make a point of going beyond simple diagnosis of the said lesion, and be aware of clinical signs indicating the severity of that lesion. For example, with a ventricular septal defect, assess the size of the shunt, as outlined earlier; with pulmonary stenosis, assess the severity by the timing of the peak of the murmur, the associated presence or absence of a click, movement of S2 with respiration, and clinical signs of right-ventricular hypertrophy.

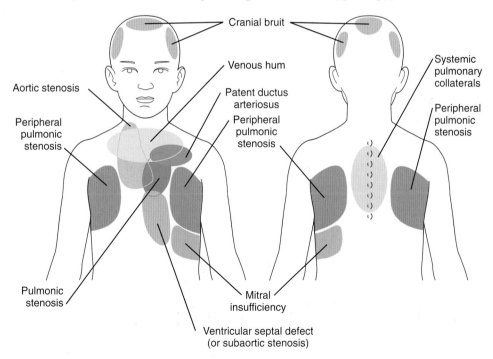

Figure 6.45 Sites where murmurs resulting from various cardiovascular lesions are best heard.

Source: Zitelli, B.J., McIntire, S.C. & Nowalk, A.J. (2012). *Atlas of Pediatric Physical Diagnosis* (6th ed.). Philadelphia: Elsevier. Figure 5.5.

With an infant or fractious toddler, the approach is different, and the order may need to be completely rearranged. Distant observation is very important, noting size, colour, respiratory rate and perfusion. It is appropriate to tell the examiners that you are going to start with auscultation while the baby is quiet; if the baby does become restless, a breast or bottle may be a life saver. With a very uncooperative child, the key is to do what you can, while you can, without becoming angry or overtly frustrated. Your approach to this is just as important as your differential diagnosis or ECG interpretation.

One final point concerns correct coinage in cardiac cases. Do not use abbreviations when presenting your findings or in your discussion: do not say 'VSD', but say 'ventricular septal defect'; do not say 'ECG', but say 'electrocardiogram'.

Fig. 6.46 shows the major points just outlined.

A more comprehensive listing of possible findings on cardiovascular examination is given in Table 6.1 (see also Figs 6.47 and 6.45).

Table 6.1
Additional information: possible findings on cardiovascular examination
GENERAL OBSERVATIONS
Height • Short (Down, Williams, Noonan, Turner; heart disease causing failure to thrive, e.g. large atrioventricular canal) • Tall (Marfan; check arm span if you suspect this)
Weight: failure to thrive (congenital rubella, severe heart disease, cyanosis or congestive cardiac failure)
Head circumference: small (congenital rubella)
Dysmorphic syndromes: Down, Williams, 22q11 (DiGeorge), Turner, Noonan, Marfan
Scars • Median sternotomy (all open-heart corrections) • Lateral thoracotomy (e.g. coarctation repair, pulmonary artery banding, ligation of PDA or vascular ring, pulmonary artery reconstruction, shunts) • Groin (cardiac catheters)
Chest asymmetry • Left chest prominence (chronic right-ventricular hypertrophy) • Right chest prominence (dextrocardia with chronic ventricular hypertrophy)
Respiratory rate: tachypnoea with left-ventricular hypertrophy
UPPER LIMBS
Nails: check both hands and both feet • Clubbing (cyanotic heart disease, suppurative lung disease; e.g. Kartagener): note any differential clubbing (e.g. clubbed toes, normal fingers in Eisenmenger's syndrome with patent ductus)
Pulses • Rate, amplitude, character (lift arm to detect hyperdynamic pulsation of AI) and rhythm • Radial (both sides, for radioradial delay) • Brachial and femoral together (for brachiofemoral delay in older adolescents) • Femorals (both sides): reduction of one femoral only is not due to coarctation, but to local trauma (cardiac catheter)
BLOOD PRESSURE
Both upper limbs
All four limbs if any suggestion of coarctation
Jugular venous pressure (sit child at 45°): elevated in right-ventricular failure

1. Introduce self

2. General inspection
Position patient: lying down
Well or unwell
Growth parameters
Dysmorphic syndromes
Scars
Chest asymmetry
Respiratory rate

3. Upper limbs
Nails
Clubbing
Pulses
Blood pressure

4. Head and neck
Jugular venous pressure
Eyes:
    Conjunctival pallor (anaemia)
    Scleral icterus (fragmentation
    Haemolysis with artificial valves)
Lips: cyanosis
Tongue: cyanosis
Teeth: caries

5. Chest
Inspect
Scars
Symmetry
Apical pulsation
Palpate:
    Apex position (beware dextro-
    cardia) (count down the ribs)
    Heaves (parasternal, substernal,
    apical)
    Thrills (substernal, supraclavicular)
    Palpable pulmonary valve closure
    (pulmonary hypertension)

    Auscultate (use diaphragm initially,
    then bell)
        Areas: apex, parasternal border,
        pulmonary, aortic areas; roll to
        the left to accentuate mitral murmurs
        Heart sounds (intensity, splitting)
        Added sounds
        Murmurs (systolic, diastolic or
        continuous, site of maximal intensity,
        character, grade)
        Radiation of murmurs: axilla (mitral),
        neck (aortic), back (pulmonary,
        coarctation)
        Variation of murmurs: sitting, inspiration,
        expiration

Manoeuvres (if appropriate):
Valsalva, exercise
    Lung fields: Adventitious sounds
    (LVF, infection with Kartagener's)
After this, palpate back for Sacral
oedema (RVF)
Collaterals (if coarctation suspected;
also check deep in axillae)

6. Abdomen
    Liver (palpate edge and measure
    span by percussion)
    Enlarged (RVF)
    Pulsatile (tricuspid incompetence)
Spleen:
    Enlarged (SBE)

7. Lower limbs
Inspection:
    Clubbing (if not already done)
    Splinter haemorrhages (if not done)
Palpation:
    Ankle oedema (RVF)

8. Other
Urinalysis: blood (SBE)
Temperature chart (SBE)
Fundoscopy for Roth spots if SBE seems
likely

9. Investigations
After presenting a differential diagnosis,
    request CXR/ECG

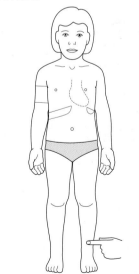

RVF = right ventricular failure; SBE = subacute bacterial endocarditis.

Figure 6.46 **The cardiovascular system.**

Source: Park, M.K. (2014). *Park's Pediatric Cardiology for Practitioners* (6th ed.). Philadelphia: Elsevier.
Figure 3.20.

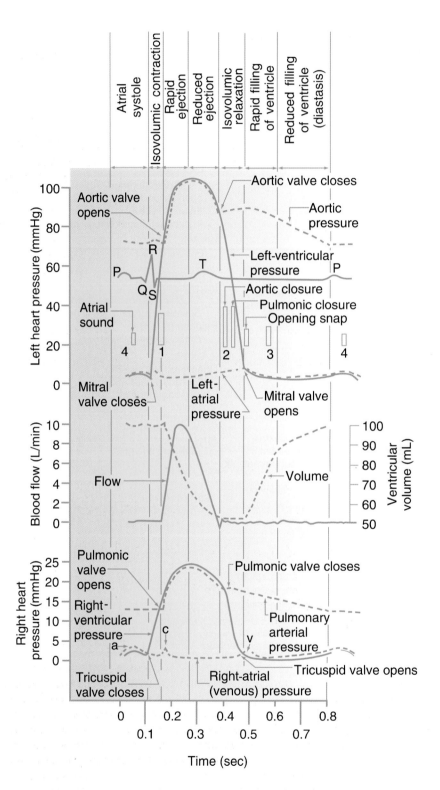

Figure 6.47 Idealised diagram of the temporal events of a cardiac cycle.

Source: Behrman, R.E., Kliegman, R.M. & Jenson, H.B. (2015). *Nelson Textbook of Paediatrics* (20th ed.). London: Saunders. Figure 415.3.

Chest X-ray (CXR) and electrocardiography (ECG)

At the completion of the cardiac short case, it is customary to request the accompanying CXR and ECG.

CXR

When describing a CXR, first note the name and date, and then which side is marked right (the position of the gastric air bubble on the left can help unless there is complete situs inversus) to avoid the embarrassment of missing dextrocardia twice (once clinically and then again on the CXR). Then comment on the centring and penetration of the film, and the degree of inspiration. The cardiac diameter should be measured and compared to chest width at the level of the right hemidiaphragm (cardiothoracic ratio); normally this ratio is less than 50% (but up to 55–60% in neonates). (See Fig. 6.48.)

Next, the cardiac contour can be assessed, particularly for the size of the pulmonary artery and the position of the aortic arch. Then, the lung fields should be evaluated, with particular emphasis on pulmonary vascularity (see below). Finally, the bony structures are assessed, especially for rib notching in older children with possible long-standing coarctation.

In cyanosed children, check whether pulmonary vascularity is increased or decreased. Note, however, that most of these conditions (such as the 'increased pulmonary vascularity' list overleaf) will not be seen in the exam context, as they pertain only to the early neonatal period and will all be subject to early repair. Some of the decreased vascularity list may be seen in the exam context, such as pulmonary atresia with multiple aortopulmonary collaterals (MAPCs), although this is uncommon.

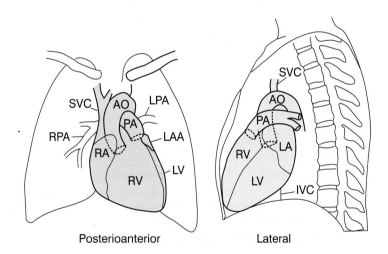

Figure 6.48 Posteroanterior and lateral projections of normal cardiac silhouette. Note that in the lateral projection, the right ventricle (RV) is contiguous with the lower third of the sternum and that the left ventricle (LV) normally crosses the posterior margin of the inferior vena cava (IVC) above the diaphragm. AO = aorta; LA = left atrium; LAA = left atrial appendage; LPA = left pulmonary artery; PA = pulmonary artery; RA = right atrium; RPA = right pulmonary artery; SVC = superior vena cava.

Source: Park, M.K. (2014). *Park's Pediatric Cardiology for Practitioners* (6th ed.). Philadelphia: Elsevier. Figure 4.2.

Increased pulmonary vascularity (pulmonary plethora) occurs in the following:
1. Truncus arteriosus.
2. Total anomalous pulmonary venous drainage (TAPVD).
3. Transposition of the great arteries (TGA; in neonate).

Decreased pulmonary vascularity (pulmonary oligaemia) occurs in the following:
1. Pulmonary atresia with intact ventricular septum (Fig. 6.49).
2. Tricuspid atresia (Fig. 6.50).
3. Ebstein's anomaly (Fig. 6.51).
4. Tetralogy of Fallot: 25% of these have a right-sided aortic arch.
5. Critical pulmonary stenosis associated with a right-to-left shunt (in neonate) (Fig. 6.52).

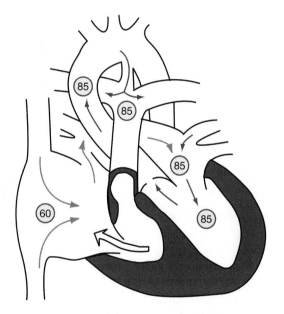

Figure 6.49 Physiology of pulmonary atresia with an intact ventricular septum.
Circled numbers represent oxygen saturation values. Right-atrial (mixed venous)
oxygen saturation is decreased secondary to systemic hypoxemia. A small amount
of the blood entering the right atrium may cross the tricuspid valve, which is often
stenotic as well. The right-ventricular cavity is hypertrophied and may be hypoplastic.
No outlet from the right ventricle exists because of the atretic pulmonary valve;
thus, any blood entering the right ventricle returns to the right atrium via tricuspid
regurgitation. Most of the desaturated blood shunts right to left via the foramen
ovale into the left atrium, where it mixes with fully saturated blood returning from the
lungs. The only source of pulmonary blood flow is via the PDA. Aortic and pulmonary
arterial oxygen saturation will be identical (definition of a total mixing lesion).

Source: Behrman, R.E., Kliegman, R.M. & Jenson, H.B. (2015). *Nelson Textbook of Paediatrics* (20th ed.).
London: Saunders. Figure 423.6.

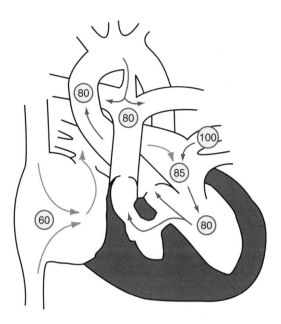

Figure 6.50 Physiology of tricuspid atresia with normally related great vessels. Circled numbers represent oxygen saturation values. Right-atrial (mixed venous) oxygen saturation is decreased secondary to systemic hypoxemia. The tricuspid valve is non-patent, and the right ventricle may manifest varying degrees of hypoplasia. The only outlet from the right atrium involves shunting right to left across an ASD or patent foramen ovale to the left atrium. There, desaturated blood mixes with saturated pulmonary venous return. Blood enters the left ventricle and is ejected either through the aorta or via a VSD into the right ventricle. In this example, some pulmonary blood flow is derived from the right ventricle, the rest from a PDA. In patients with tricuspid atresia, the PDA may close or the VSD may grow smaller and result in a marked decrease in systemic oxygen saturation.

Source: Behrman, R.E., Kliegman, R.M. & Jenson, H.B. (2015). *Nelson Textbook of Paediatrics* (20th ed.). London: Saunders. Figure 423.7.

ECG

As with the CXR mentioned earlier, when describing a ECG, first check it belongs to this patient, note the name and date, and then the recording speed (routine speed is 25 mm/sec; so 1 mm equals 0.04 seconds, 5 mm equals 0.20 seconds [one large division between heavier lines], 30 mm equals 1.20 seconds and 300 large divisions equal 1 minute) and the scale (1 millivolt causes a deflection of 10 mm, but the amplitude is read as millimetres; the calibration should be checked as some machines automatically change the sensitivity to a half or a quarter if deflections are too large to be recorded; values need be doubled or quadrupled accordingly). (See Figs 6.53 and 6.54.)

Determine the ventricular rate (roughly—do not waste time), the rhythm and then the axis.

The ventricular rate can be determined by dividing 300 by the number of large divisions (large squares) between two R waves, so if there are three large squares between consecutive R waves, the rate would be 300/3 = 100/minute; this is easier at slower heat rates; alternatively count RR cycles over 6 large squares and multiply by 50; this is easier with faster rates.

This is also the time to look at the shape of the complexes for any typical ventricular conduction disturbances, such as right bundle branch block (RBBB). RBBB may be seen

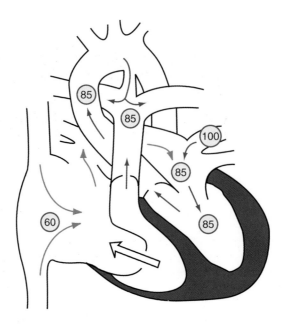

Figure 6.51 Physiology of the Ebstein anomaly of the tricuspid valve. Circled numbers represent oxygen saturation values. Inferior displacement of the tricuspid valve leaflets into the right ventricle has resulted in a thin-walled, low-pressure 'atrialised' segment of right ventricle. The tricuspid valve is grossly insufficient (clear arrow). Right-atrial blood flow is shunted right to left across an ASD or patent foramen ovale into the left atrium. Some blood may cross the right-ventricular outflow tract and enter the pulmonary artery; however, in severe cases, the right ventricle may generate insufficient force to open the pulmonary valve, and 'functional pulmonary atresia' results. In the left atrium, desaturated blood mixes with saturated pulmonary venous return. Blood enters the left ventricle and is ejected via the aorta. In this example, some pulmonary blood flow is derived from the right ventricle, the rest from a PDA. Severe cyanosis will develop in neonates with a severe Ebstein anomaly when the PDA closes.

Source: Behrman, R.E., Kliegman, R.M. & Jenson, H.B. (2015). *Nelson Textbook of Paediatrics* (20th ed.). London: Saunders. Figure 423.10.

in postoperative cases where there has been a right ventriculotomy, during repair of a VSD, or ToF; there is an 'M' pattern in V1 with a tall secondary R wave (rsR pattern), and 'W' pattern in V6 with a slurred S wave (qRS pattern). Right ventriculotomy interferes with the subendocardial Purkinje fibre network of the right ventricle, which causes RBBB without actually damaging the main right bundle branch.

RBBB also occurs in ASD; here the mechanism is right-ventricular volume overload, with ventricular activation (and QRS duration) lengthened, due to a structurally longer pathway, as the RV volume can be several times the normal volume in ASD. (See Figs 6.55 and 6.56.)

The rhythm is checked next. Arrhythmias are very unlikely to be encountered in exams (apart from normal 'sinus arrhythmia' with breathing, heart rate increasing during inspiration).

The frontal QRS axis can be calculated most simply by using lead 1 and lead aVF voltages as vectors on a graph. By plotting lead 1 on the x-axis (lead 1 looks at the heart at

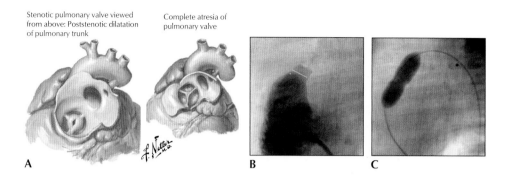

Stenotic pulmonary valve viewed from above: Poststenotic dilatation of pulmonary trunk

Complete atresia of pulmonary valve

A   B   C

Figure 6.52 Pulmonary valvular stenosis and atresia. A. The anatomic features of congenital pulmonary stenosis and atresia are illustrated. B. A lateral-view right ventricular angiogram in a neonate with critical pulmonary valve stenosis shows the doming valve with an annulus diameter of 5.9 mm and a tiny poststenotic jet. C. A lateral view of an 8-mm-diameter balloon dilation catheter fully inflated across the annulus. The balloon has been passed over a guide wire that had been placed across the ductus to the descending aorta.

Source: Frantz, E.G. (2016). Catheter-based treatment of congenital heart disease. *Thoracic Key*, 12 June. Figure 52.2. Retrieved from: http://thoracickey.com/catheter-based-treatment-of-congenital-heart-disease/

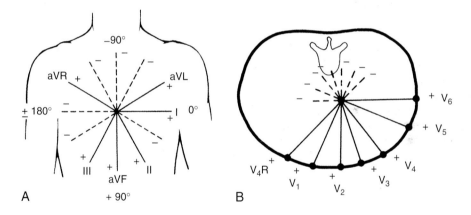

A   B

Figure 6.53 Hexaxial reference system.

Source: Park, M.K. (2014). *Park's Pediatric Cardiology for Practitioners* (6th ed.). Philadelphia: Elsevier. Figure 3.1.

0°), and 'minus' lead aVF on the y-axis (lead aVF looks at the heart at +90°), the frontal axis can be estimated to be in one of four quadrants. The net vector in each lead must be calculated by positive deflection (R wave, measured in small squares) minus negative deflection (Q plus S waves, measured in small squares). For lead 1, the vector is marked along the x-axis, and for lead aVF, the vector is marked down the y-axis towards aVF. The resultant net vector/frontal axis is the angle formed by the vector. (See Fig. 6.57.)

Next, systematically look at the P waves, (checking there is a P wave before each QRS); the PR interval, then the QRS complexes, the ST interval and finally the T waves. Several patterns give important clues to the diagnosis. The age of the child must always be taken into consideration.

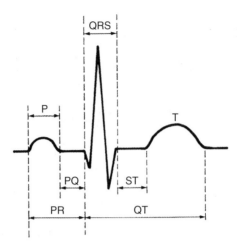

Figure 6.54 Diagram illustrating important intervals (or durations) and segments of an electrocardiographic cycle.

Source: Park, M.K. (2014). *Park's Pediatric Cardiology for Practitioners* (6th ed.). Philadelphia: Elsevier. Figure 3.13.

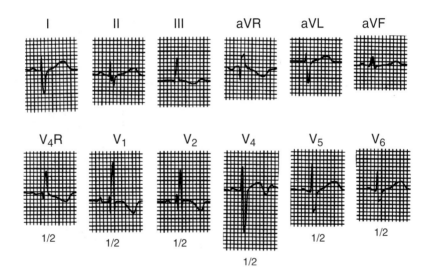

Figure 6.55 Tracing from a 7-year-old girl with large secundum atrial septal defect.

Source: Park, M.K. & Guntheroth, W.G. (2006). *How to Read Pediatric ECGs* (4th ed.). Philadelphia: Mosby. Figure 6.6.

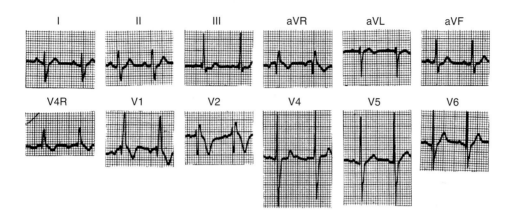

Figure 6.56 Tracing from a 6-year-old boy who had corrective surgery for ToF that involved right ventriculotomy for repair of a ventricular septal defect and resection of infundibular narrowing.

Source: Park, M.K. (2014). *Park's Pediatric Cardiology for Practitioners* (6th ed.). Philadelphia: Elsevier. Figure 3.11.

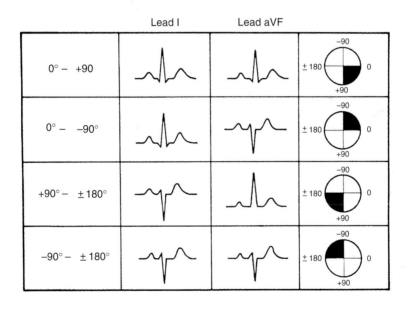

Figure 6.57 Locating quadrants of mean QRS axis from leads I and aVF.

Source: Park, M.K. (2014). *Park's Pediatric Cardiology for Practitioners* (6th ed.). Philadelphia: Elsevier. Figure 3.11.

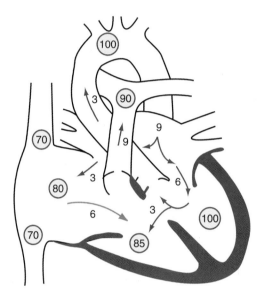

Figure 6.58 **Physiology of atrioventricular septal defect (AVSD). Circled numbers represent oxygen saturation values. The numbers next to the arrows represent volumes of blood flow (in L/min/m²). This illustration shows a hypothetical patient with a pulmonary-to-systemic blood flow ratio (Qp:Qs) of 3 : 1. Desaturated blood enters the right atrium from the vena cavae at a volume of 3 L/min/m² and mixes with 3 L of fully saturated blood shunting left to right across the ASD; the result is an increase in oxygen saturation in the right atrium. Six litres of blood flows through the right side of the common AV valve, joined by an additional 3 L of saturated blood shunting left to right at the ventricular level, further increasing oxygen saturation in the right ventricle. The full 9 L flows across the right-ventricular outflow tract into the lungs. Nine litres returns to the left atrium, with 3 L shunting left to right across the defect and 6 L crossing the left side of the common AV valve and causing a mid-diastolic flow rumble. Three litres of this volume shunts left to right across the VSD, and 3 L is ejected into the ascending aorta (normal cardiac output).**

Source: Behrman, R.E., Kliegman, R.M. & Jenson, H.B. (2015). *Nelson Textbook of Paediatrics* (20th ed.). London: Saunders. Figure 419.2.

The following lists outline several important points regarding age-related changes and clues to certain diagnoses.

Frontal plane QRS axis—normal values vary with age:
1. Birth: +60° to +180°.
2. 1 year: 0° to +110°.
3. 10 years: −15° to +110°.

Right-axis deviation (RAD) (i.e. an axis at +90° to +180°, after infancy)—often is associated with right-ventricular hypertrophy.

Left-axis deviation (LAD) (i.e. an axis at −90° to 0°) has numerous causes, including atrioventricular (AV) canal (Fig. 6.58), tricuspid atresia and conduction anomalies.

Definitions of ventricular hypertrophy

Right-ventricular hypertrophy
1. R greater than S in V1 after 1 year.
2. Upright T wave over right praecordial leads after 1 week of age.
3. sV6 greater than 15 mm at 1 week.
4. sV6 greater than 10 mm at 6 months.
5. sV6 greater than 5 mm at 1 year.

Left-ventricular hypertrophy
1. sV1 + rV6 greater than 30 mm to 1 year.
2. sV1 + rV6 greater than 40 mm after 1 year.

Causes of atrial hypertrophy

Right-atrial hypertrophy (RAH) is seen in the following:
1. Tricuspid atresia.
2. Complex congenital heart disease.
3. Hypoplastic right heart.
4. Ebstein's anomaly.
5. Pulmonary atresia.

Left-atrial hypertrophy (LAH) is seen in the following:
1. Mitral valve disease.
2. Cardiomyopathy.
3. Large PDA or large VSD (any large left-to-right shunt).

QRS and Q wave abnormalities

Prolonged QRS is seen in the following:
1. Bundle branch block (especially postoperatively).
2. Ventricular hypertrophy.
3. Others: digoxin therapy; hyperkalaemia; hypothyroidism.

Q waves occur in the following circumstances. They are normal in leads II, III, aVF, V5 and V6, and abnormal in other leads. Think of:
1. Hypertrophic cardiomyopathy.
2. Congenitally corrected transposition.
3. Anomalous left coronary artery.

Particularly large Q waves occur in:
1. Septal hypertrophy.
2. Infarction.

Specific diagnosis by ECG

Although a pathophysiological approach is, of course, preferable to a mnemonic or list in cardiology, ECGs do lend themselves to the latter. Table 6.2 is one such list, but rather than rote-learning this, the candidate should endeavour to understand the pathophysiology and always consider the ECG in the context of the clinical findings.

Table 6.2	
Electrocardiographic findings and associated pathologies	
IF THE FINDING IS	**THINK OF**
Prolonged P–R interval	Endocardial cushion defect
	Ebstein's anomaly
	Acute rheumatic fever
	Congenital block (maternal SLE)
Partial RBBB	
with LAD	Ostium primum ASD
with RAD	Ostium secundum ASD
with RAH, delta waves	Ebstein's anomaly
Complete RBBB	Post-ventriculotomy
LAD	Endocardial cushion defect
	Tricuspid atresia
	Hypertrophic cardiomyopathy
	Inlet VSD
RAH	Ebstein's anomaly
without RVH	Tricuspid atresia (LAD)
	Pulmonary atresia with intact septum
with axis over 90°	Truncus arteriosus
	Tetralogy with large VSD
Deep Q waves	Hypertrophic cardiomyopathy
	Transposition of great arteries
	Anomalous left coronary artery

ASD = atrial septal defect; LAD = left-axis deviation; RAD = right-axis deviation; RAH = right-atrial hypertrophy; RVH = right-ventricular hypertrophy; VSD = ventricular septal defect.

Reference

Loeys, B.L. et al. (2010). Revised Ghent criteria for the diagnosis of Marfan syndrome (MFS) and related conditions, *Journal of Medical Genetics*, 47, 476–485.

Chapter 7

Endocrinology

LONG CASE: Congenital adrenal hyperplasia (CAH)

Background information

Congenital adrenal hyperplasia (CAH) refers to a number of inherited defects in adrenal steroidogenesis, which cause impaired synthesis of cortisol from cholesterol in the adrenal cortex. The most common of these, accounting for around 90% of cases of CAH, is 21-hydroxylase deficiency (21-OHD), which is caused by a range of mutations in one gene—the CYP21A2 gene on chromosome 6p21.33, which codes for 21-hydroxylase (P450C21). The end result is a lack of cortisol (and usually aldosterone) synthesis by the adrenal cortex. This leads to increased adrenocortical stimulation by hypothalamic corticotrophin-releasing hormone (CRH) and pituitary adrenocorticotropic hormone (ACTH), which induces adrenal glandular hyperplasia—hence the term 'CAH'. CAH is inherited in an autosomal recessive manner. This long case deals with the common form of CAH due to 21-OHD, the preferred term for which, under current nomenclature, is 21-OHD CAH (OMIM#201910).

21-OHD CAH can present in two forms: classic (previously called early onset) and non-classic (previously called late onset or attenuated). The 21-OHD CAH heterozygote carrier rate has been estimated at around 1.5% for classic CAH and at around 10% for non-classic 21-OH CAH. The incidence of the classic form of 21-OH CAH is 1 in 15 000 live births overall, but there are varying prevalences in different populations: 1 in 300 in Yupik Eskimos of Alaska, 1 in 5000 in Saudi Arabia, 1 in 21 000 in Japan and 1 in 23 000 in New Zealand. The prevalence of the non-classic form of 21-OH CAH is 1 in 100 in the general heterogeneous New York City population, highest in Ashkenazi Jews (1 in 27).

The majority (up to three-quarters) of patients with 21-OH CAH have the classic salt-losing form and can develop adrenal insufficiency in the early weeks of life, presenting with hyponatraemia, hyperkalaemia, hypoglycaemia and shock (see below), which can be lethal. This is due to a lack of adequate aldosterone production to maintain normal sodium balance. A further result of the excess adrenal stimulation in 21-OHD CAH is synthesis of adrenal sex hormone precursors and their by-products. This variably leads to androgenisation of females in utero, or to virilisation of either sex later in childhood.

Females with classic 21-OHD CAH are born with ambiguous genitalia. The degree of virilisation of the external genitalia is scored by the Prader scale (see the short case on ambiguous genitalia in this chapter). Males with classic salt-wasting 21-OHD CAH may appear normal at birth (although affected male neonates can have increased genital pigmentation and penile size), but then deteriorate with adrenal insufficiency after 1–4 weeks. In these babies, adrenal aldosterone production is insufficient for the distal tubules to reabsorb sodium, leading to salt loss as well as deficiency of cortisol and an excess of androgens. Symptoms can include poor feeding, failure to thrive, vomiting, loss of weight, dehydration, hypotension, hyponatraemia, hypoglycaemia and hyperkalaemic metabolic acidosis, leading to adrenal crisis with vascular collapse and a significant mortality rate. Some degree of aldosterone deficiency occurs in all forms of 21-OHD CAH. Also, some component of hypotension and hypoglycaemia can be attributed to suboptimal adrenaline synthesis in the adrenal medulla, as cortisol usually stimulates phenylethanolamine N-methyl-transferase, which is the final enzyme in the adrenaline biosynthesis pathway.

Females with non-classic 21-OHD CAH may present with clitoromegaly, early development of pubic hair, hirsutism, acne, increased growth rate, advanced bone age and gynaecological problems such as oligomenorrhoea, abnormal menses or infertility. Males with non-classic 21-OHD CAH may develop early penile growth, pubic hair, increased growth rate and increased musculature.

Deficiency of cytochrome P450 enzyme 21-hydroxylase (CYP21A2) causes 90% of 21-OHD CAH cases. Ten types of mutation in CYP21A2 account for more than 90% of affected cases, although well over 100 have been described, including point mutations, small deletions, small insertions and complex rearrangements of the gene. 21-OHD CAH demonstrates a heterogeneous phenotype, with concordance between phenotype and genotype. The Human Gene Mutation Database, Cardiff (http://www.hgmd.org) lists all known mutations.

Macro-deletions, comprising a quarter of 21-OHD CAH cases, always cause a severe salt-wasting form. Patients with classic salt-wasting 21-OHD CAH possess two mutant alleles that obliterate 21-OH activity (CYP21 deletion).

Patients with non-classic 21-OHD CAH with simple virilisation tend to have one severe mutant allele and one moderate mutant allele. The latter can include the point mutation Ile172Asn in exon 4, which permits about 2% of normal enzyme activity.

The majority of cases with non-classic 21-OHD CAH have two mildly compromised alleles; many are associated with a valine-to-leucine missense mutation at amino acid position 281 (termed 'Val281Leu') in exon 7, which permits around 50% of normal enzyme activity. Genotyping of CYP21 can be useful in establishing the requirement for glucocorticoid and mineralocorticoid replacement. In over 95% of cases, phenotype correlates with genotype. Many children with CAH are compound heterozygotes. These children tend to present with clinical features more in keeping with the less deleterious allele.

Diagnosis

21-OHD CAH can be diagnosed at different ages, as follows.

HIGH-RISK PREGNANCIES: PRENATAL DIAGNOSIS OF 21-OHD CAH

Only performed in mothers with a previously affected child with 21-OHD CAH, prenatal diagnosis of 21-OHD CAH is possible through molecular genetic studies of chorionic cells or annulus fibrosus (AF) cells. After pre-pregnancy genetic counselling, molecular genetic testing is undertaken on the proband, and on both parents, to ascertain the mutation in the CYP21A2 gene, and document that both parents are carriers.

When pregnancy is confirmed, before 9 weeks' gestation and before any prenatal testing, in some countries the pregnant mother is prescribed daily dexamethasone, to suppress fetal adrenal androgen secretion to prevent virilisation of an affected female (this is not done in Australia; here the use of antenatal steroids is controversial and would only be considered in a research study; it is difficult to justify the maternal side effects and also treating 7 out of 8 infants unnecessarily). Chorionic villus sampling (CVS), in those countries that use antenatal steroids, can then be performed at 9–12 weeks, to determine the sex of the child; if the karyotype is male, the dexamethasone is stopped. CVS is preferable to amniocentesis, as the latter is performed at 15–18 weeks, and management decisions depend on prenatal testing; the earlier the better.

If the fetus is female, and the proband has two CYP21A2 disease-causing mutations, then molecular testing of fetal DNA is undertaken to identify whether the fetus has inherited both disease-carrying alleles. If the fetus is female and unaffected, dexamethasone is stopped. If the fetus is female and is found by DNA analysis to have classic 21-OHD CAH, dexamethasone is continued to term. Prenatal treatment is solely to prevent virilisation of the genitalia in affected females. It has no effect on any later requirement for hormone replacement therapy. There are no significant side effects of dexamethasone treatment; there is no increased risk of congenital anomalies, and no effect on birth weight, length or head circumference.

LOW-RISK PREGNANCIES: PRENATAL DIAGNOSIS OF 21-OHD CAH

Genital ambiguity is occasionally detected on prenatal ultrasound. If this occurs, then a fetal karyotype and tertiary ultrasound examination for müllerian structures should be performed; if the karyotype is a normal female 46,XX, with a normal-appearing uterus, then classic 21-OHD CAH is a diagnostic consideration. It is useful to know to optimise the medical management once the child is born.

PREIMPLANTATION GENETIC DIAGNOSIS (PGD) OF 21-OHD CAH

This may be offered to families in which the disease-causing mutations have been identified.

NEONATAL DIAGNOSIS OF 21-OHD CAH

This may follow neonatal screening. Screening occurs in all 50 states in the United States, and in many other countries, including New Zealand. It does not occur in Australia yet, but it is being advocated for strongly in recent years, and that advocacy is continuing. The sample is taken (ideally) between days 2 and 3 of life, 17-OHP levels are analysed and those above cut-off levels have diagnostic testing: false negatives are very rare, but have occurred in infants treated with dexamethasone for the management of unrelated problems; false positives can occur in premature, small-for-gestational-age (SGA), very unwell infants, or if the sample is taken too soon (in the first 24 hours, 17-OHP can be elevated in all infants). In classic 21-OHD CAH, 17-OHP serum levels are markedly elevated. Levels of 17-OHP are normally high in the first two days after birth, and then fall in healthy babies by day 2–3, but levels rise in those affected by 21-OHD CAH. In affected infant girls, serum testosterone may be elevated, and in infants of either sex androstenedione is elevated.

NEONATAL PRESENTATION OF 21-OHD CAH AT 1–4 WEEKS

Neonates with 21-OHD may present with ambiguous genitalia (affected girls) or adrenal crisis (especially affected boys) between 1 and 4 weeks. Diagnosis of patients with symptoms of classic CAH is by elevated serum 17-OHP (and in those with ambiguous genitalia, ultrasound of the abdomen and genital tract: for more details, see the short case on ambiguous genitalia in this chapter).

NON-CLASSIC FORMS OF 21-OHD CAH

Patients presenting with the non-classic forms of 21-OHD CAH usually manifest with androgen excess (late onset). If the basal 17-OHP level is unconvincing, further investigation using the ACTH stimulation test can be considered. The level of serum 17-OHP should show a significant rise 60 minutes (to a peak > 30 nmol/L) after an intravenous bolus of ACTH. The cortisol is also measured: the 17-OHP:cortisol ratio will be elevated. Urine steroid profiling can assist with differentiating different types of CAH; if a baby is suspected to have CAH, a urine should if possible be collected before any steroid is given.

CAH DUE TO 11-BETA-HYDROXYLASE DEFICIENCY

Patients with CAH due to 11-beta-hydroxylase deficiency (11-OHD CAH) may present in a similar way to 21-OHD CAH, with virilisation of the affected female fetus. These patients, however, can also present with hypertension, due to accumulation of salt-retaining aldosterone precursors. Paradoxically, some infants with 11-OHD CAH are transiently salt losers and become hypertensive at a later stage. They also have mildly elevated 17-OHP levels and can easily be misdiagnosed as 21-OHD clinically unless molecular genetic testing is performed. 11-OHD represents around 8% of CAH cases, and is seen more frequently in children of Iranian, Jewish or Moroccan descent.

OTHER FORMS OF CAH

There are five forms of CAH. Patients with other forms of CAH (< 2% of CAH patients) may present at various ages. Impaired enzyme function at each step of adrenal steroidogenesis leads to a unique set of excess precursors and reduced products. 17-OHD CAH is due to mutation in the gene CYP17A1 on chromosome 10q24.3, which codes for 17-hydroxylase (P450C17). CAH caused by deficiency of 3-beta-hydroxysteroid dehydrogenase (3Beta-HSD) is due to mutation in the gene HSD3B2, on chromosome 1p12. HSD3B2 encodes 3-hydroxyacyl-CoA dehydrogenase type II, a mitochondrial protein that catalyses a number of steroids, fatty acids and alcohols. CAH caused by deficiency of steroidogenic acute regulatory protein (STAR) is due to mutation in the STAR gene; the protein encoded by the STAR gene allows the transfer of cholesterol across the mitochondrial membrane, after which it is converted into pregnenolone. For further discussion, see the short case on ambiguous genitalia in this chapter.

MECHANISM OF VIRILISATION

Dihydrotestosterone (DHT) is the most potent of androgens at virilising the external genitalia. DHT is normally synthesised from testosterone by 5-alpha-reductase, which is situated in the genital tissues' skin. High levels of steroidogenic precursors are converted to testosterone and DHT. Steroidogenic tissue also can convert precursors (progesterone, 17-OH progesterone), to DHT by an alternate pathway which bypasses testosterone.

GOLD STANDARD OF DIAGNOSIS

The ACTH stimulation test (also called the Cosyntropin, Synacthen or Tetracosactide stimulation test) using a dose of 0.125–0.25 mg of ACTH can allow measurement of a full panel of adrenal hormones, and can differentiate 21-OH CAH from other enzyme deficiencies.

History

PRESENTING COMPLAINT

Reason for current admission.

INITIAL DIAGNOSIS

1. Initial symptoms:
   - *Neonate*: ambiguous genitalia, adrenal insufficiency, vomiting, seizures (from hyponatraemia or hypoglycaemia); near-death episodes resembling SIDS have been reported.
   - *Older child*: symptoms associated with virilisation, recurrent sinus or pulmonary infections (from poor response to stress of infection).
   - *Adolescent*: syncope or near-syncope, hypotension (21-OHD); hypertension (11-OHD); tempo of onset (developing over days, weeks or months before diagnosis).
2. Immediate pre-diagnosis symptoms:
   - Symptoms of *adrenocortical failure*: for example, lethargy, disorientation (cortisol lack), salt craving (aldosterone lack), weakness, anorexia, vomiting, weight loss (lack of cortisol and aldosterone), hypoglycaemia.
   - Symptoms associated with *virilisation*: for example, girls—clitoromegaly, other genital virilisation, increased pigmentation of genital skin, pubic hair, increased height, abnormal menses, hirsutism, acne, oligomenorrhoea; boys—increased penile growth, increased pigmentation of genital skin, pubic hair, increased height, increased muscle growth, bone age advancement.
3. Where, when and how the diagnosis was made, length of hospital stay, education given, any treatment of the mother with steroids while the fetus was in utero, treatment in hospital, treatment at discharge.

PROGRESS OF THE DISEASE

1. Details of subsequent hospitalisations (frequency, indications, usual length of stay, usual outcome).
2. Complications of the disease; for example, the need for corrective genital surgery, episodes of adrenal crisis, abnormal growth and development, psychosexual developmental aspects (e.g. girls with male-type play, physical aggression, low interest in babies or maternal nurturing behaviours; increased incidence of same-sex relationships), inadequately treated hyperandrogenism, hypoglycaemic reactions.
3. Complications of treatment; for example, overtreatment with steroids causing deceleration of linear growth, too much fludrocortisone causing hypertension, degree of control (number of episodes of adrenal crisis), inadequate steroid treatment leading to bone age advancement and potential compromise of final height.
4. Monitoring of the disease: how often seen in clinic, the usual investigations performed, how often seen by local doctor.
5. Changes in management; for example, the usual increases in steroid dosage on sick days. Is there an emergency steroid injection to administer, and does the family know the dose, have they been educated, is there a written emergency plan, are they linked in with the state ambulance service (candidates should know if the patient lives a long way from medical care [isolated]) versus close to hospital? Is there a glucometer (if prone to hypoglycaemia), is there a 'hypo' plan (which could include glucagon)?
6. At what age was the patient administering his or her own steroids?
7. Compliance; for example, previous refusal to take steroids in teenage males.

CURRENT STATUS

1. General health: lethargic or energetic.
2. Current medications: type (e.g. hydrocortisone, fludrocortisone, salt supplement), regimen (how much, when, given by whom, modifications with intercurrent illness), salt craving (not enough fludrocortisone), hypertension (too much fludrocortisone), compliance with treatment.
3. Adrenal insufficiency: how often, what symptoms (e.g. vomiting, lethargy, crying, convulsions, near-syncope, syncope, loss of consciousness), usual precipitants, anticipatory strategies for prevention, response.
4. Hypoglycaemia: any episodes, any suggestion of this (e.g. sweating, pallor, tremulousness, hunger, headache, odd behaviour, lethargy, crying, bad temper, lack of coordination, dizziness, vomiting, convulsions, loss of consciousness).
5. Symptoms attributable to virilisation: acne, increased linear growth, amenorrhoea.
6. Other problems; for example, compliance problems, adolescent self-image, gender identity issues (gender identity in females with CAH is usually female; females with virilising CAH can have more 'masculine' interests), urinary issues; can review surgical correction (e.g. vagina/urinary issues in adolescence).

SOCIAL HISTORY

1. Impact on child: self-image, reaction of school friends, effects (e.g. virilisation), coping with taking steroids, amount of school missed.
2. Impact on siblings: sibling rivalry, risk of CAH.
3. Impact on parents: family finances, employment, concern regarding future complications, genetic counselling.
4. Social supports: parents' groups, access to social worker, government benefits obtained.
5. Coping: who attends the clinic with the patient, the level of education of the child and parents, contingency plans for intercurrent illnesses or severe adrenal crisis causing loss of consciousness, access to local doctor, paediatrician, hospital.

FAMILY HISTORY

Record details of other affected members.

IMMUNISATION

List all routine immunisations. Fluvax is recommended by many clinics.

Examination

For a neonate, see the short case on ambiguous genitalia and for an older child the short cases on precocious puberty and on virilisation in the postnatal period (in this chapter). The main areas to focus on are sequential growth parameters and pubertal development (Tanner staging), pigmentation and blood pressure.

Management

All patients with CAH, regardless of type, require treatment with glucocorticoids. These replace cortisol (which is deficient) and provide negative feedback, suppressing ACTH secretion. This then prevents continued adrenal stimulation, inhibiting excess androgen production (as 17-OHP is not available as a substrate for excess androgen production; this prevents virilisation). Patients with the salt-losing form (for practical purposes, all those with a raised plasma renin activity [PRA]) also require mineralocorticoid replacement to normalise the sodium balance associated with aldosterone deficiency. Girls with moderate to severe clitoral enlargement and all those with fused labia are offered corrective surgery. The timing of this, and the place of surgery for mild degrees of clitoromegaly, is now a very controversial area, as previous surgical approaches are considered to have led to some loss of clitoral sensation. Some centres have moved to late surgery, where the young person can be involved in the decision, discuss the pros and cons, the surgeons may suggest advantages of early surgery are compliant tissues and small distances. The overall principles of treatment are given below.

CONTROL OF STEROID REQUIREMENTS
Glucocorticoids

The usual preparation used in growing children is oral hydrocortisone (this is the preferred hormone, because cortisone is only active after conversion to hydrocortisone in the liver). It is given at a dosage of 10–20 mg/m^2 per 24 hours, in three divided doses, as hydrocortisone has a short half-life of 90–120 minutes. The usual doses are: for infants, 2–4 mg three times a day; and for children, 4–8 mg three times a day. The morning dose is given as early as possible, to blunt the early morning corticotrophin release. The dose can be adjusted according to symptoms, signs, weight and height velocity, and tests (serum 17-OHP and PRA). Because of concerns about the side effect profile and growth suppression when using longer-acting steroids (such as dexamethasone or prednisolone), these agents are used only in patients who have completed their linear growth.

Mineralocorticoids

These are required for patients with disturbed electrolyte regulation (salt losers) and elevated PRA. The usual preparation used is fludrocortisone acetate (also called 9-alpha-fluorocortisol; fluorination at the 9-alpha position enhances all biological actions of corticosteroids), given at a dosage of 0.05–0.3 mg daily. The dose can be adjusted according to blood pressure and PRA.

Additional salt supplementation (6 mmol/kg per day sodium chloride) may be required. This is necessary in almost all cases occurring in the first 3 months of life and may need to be given throughout the first year in very hot climates.

Non-salt-losing CAH

Non-salt-losing CAH, especially in boys, may lead to a bone age more than 5 years in advance of their chronological age when these patients are first diagnosed. Starting glucocorticoid therapy can slow growth and bone maturation towards normal rates. There is a high risk that treatment of such children with hydrocortisone would precipitate the onset of true puberty. Before treatment with hydrocortisone, the elevated androgens exert a 'maturing' effect on the hypothalamus, but gonadotropin secretion is suppressed by the androgens. When the androgen levels are suddenly suppressed by the hydrocortisone treatment, gonadotropins are released from the pituitary gland. This form of precocious puberty must then be managed with a long-acting luteinising hormone-releasing hormone (LHRH, also known as GnRH) analogue, in combination with hydrocortisone and fludrocortisone.

Most non-salt-losers excrete excessive salt in the urine, even though they are asymptomatic or nearly so. If they have high PRA levels, they should be treated with fludrocortisone.

Other potential approaches to treatment

The combination of an antiandrogen (blocking androgen effects) and an aromatase inhibitor (blocks conversion of androgen to oestrogen) may require a lower dose of hydrocortisone. Adrenalectomy has been advocated to eliminate the problem of inadequate adrenal androgen suppression.

Prevention of acute complications

Adrenal crises can be averted by anticipatory strategies. All patients with CAH need extra steroid cover for stress: this includes any acute medical condition (such as gastroenteritis, or other viral illnesses), any surgical procedure requiring an anaesthetic and any significant orthopaedic injury (such as a major fracture). Treatment may include hydrocortisone 25–100 mg parenterally (IM or IV), repeated 4–6 hourly until recovery from the acute aspect of the illness: triple the usual dose for 2 days, then double the usual dose for 3 days. All patients should have an emergency identification bracelet, such as MedicAlert.

Optimum growth and development

Timely diagnosis of CAH may prevent precocious puberty leading to short stature. Adequate education of patient and parents is essential to ensure compliance with recommended treatment. It should be explained to parents that the doses of hydrocortisone and fludrocortisone must be adjusted to be optimised for each child, and that optimised doses allow normal growth, normal response to stress and illness, and normal pubertal development. Parents must be made aware of the dangers of too little or too much hydrocortisone and fludrocortisone: too little hydrocortisone leads to ongoing pituitary stimulation and ongoing overproduction of androgens, while too little fludrocortisone leads to salt craving and low blood sodium; too much hydrocortisone leads to slowed growth; and too much fludrocortisone leads to high blood pressure. They need to know that the normal hydrocortisone dose should be tripled at the start of any illness and that if the child needs surgery for any reason, they must inform both the anaesthetist and the surgeon that extra hydrocortisone is needed to cover that stressful procedure.

Psychological support

The treating paediatrician should ensure adequate access to appropriate social supports. In females who were born with ambiguous genitalia, who have had surgical procedures for virilised external genitalia as a neonate or who have virilisation, issues regarding sexuality may need to be discussed. Surgery should be avoided between the ages of 2 and 12 years as far as possible. Girls should not be subjected to repeated genital examinations. Clinical photography is only justified when the parents and patient (if she is old enough) consent to it in order to have a visual record of the anatomy before surgery. Usually, the photograph would be taken when the patient was undergoing a procedure under general anaesthetic.

The following basic principles are important:

1. Minimise the number of days off school.
2. Involve the child in management of his or her CAH as appropriate to age and ability.
3. In times of 'adolescent rebellion', support and encourage; never resort to threats.
4. Identify and treat negative family responses to CAH, including overindulgence, over-anxiousness, neglect and disinterest, resentment and overcontrolling parents.
5. When the initial diagnosis is made, be aware of depression in patients, siblings and parents, and counsel accordingly. It is important that the parents and child have a full understanding of the pathophysiology of CAH, and all elements of the psychosexual aspects that can arise should be openly discussed with the parents, and when it is age-appropriate, with the child. There should be no secretive aspects to

the family's handling of this diagnosis, as this could be damaging. There is significant value in sexual counselling for many of these patients and their families.

For the purposes of the long case, the usual problem is that of a non-compliant adolescent. Unfortunately, it is in adolescence—the least receptive time of the patient's life—that it is crucial to avoid serious complications. For a teenager, immediate peer acceptance, which may involve nights out at parties or hotels, far outweighs the long-term benefits of adequate steroid replacement. Most teenagers with CAH require additional emotional support, which may be achieved through attendance at discussion groups or talking one-on-one with a clinical psychologist.

Problems affecting adolescents can be foreseen and discussed with the parents before they occur. Generally, parents should be encouraged to emphasise the positive aspects of adequate control, to explain the need for increased steroid dosage during illness, and to be supportive and avoid chastisement during rebellious episodes. By 18 years of age, most adolescents will be more responsible in caring for their CAH.

Social supports

All families of children with CAH should have access to an experienced social worker. The disease represents a significant financial burden for many families, and the social worker can make them aware of the various government benefits to which they may be entitled. Contact with CAH groups will allow access to many helpful people and ideas. Social workers also offer psychological support and are able to screen the family from the outset for social risk factors.

Routine follow-up

Children with CAH should be seen every 3–4 months. On each occasion, the child's growth (height and weight percentiles), Tanner staging, blood pressure and evidence of any complications should be documented, and then managed accordingly. Investigations should include serum 17-OHP, PRA and electrolytes. Hydrocortisone dosing can be optimised by testing 17-OHP dried blood spot profiles. Bone age should be checked annually.

Types of corticosteroids

The examiners will expect you to be familiar with the various types of steroids and their equivalents. Table 7.1 is a brief guide; refer to the latest *MIMS*, *British National Formulary* or equivalent publication for the names of the various preparations available.

21-OHD CAH prenatal diagnosis and intervention

This area may be mentioned in the long-case discussion. Prenatal treatment of CAH attributable to 21-OHD by administration of corticosteroids (dexamethasone) to the mother is most commonly performed in females with a previously affected child. This is a very controversial area. Informed consent must be obtained from the parents before prenatal treatment is contemplated. There are possible maternal adverse effects with CAH, the genital outcome is variable and there may be long-term effects on children, which are presently unknown. Masculinisation of the external genitalia begins at 6–7 weeks' gestation; if treatment before this suppresses the fetal pituitary–adrenal axis, it could prevent ambiguous genitalia. Of reported cases where prenatal treatment has occurred, it was successful in three-quarters of them (one-third normal genitalia, two-thirds mildly virilised) and unsuccessful in a quarter.

Maternal complications from dexamethasone have included features of Cushing's syndrome, marked weight gain, irritability, mood swings, diabetes, hypertension and

Table 7.1		
Corticosteroids: glucocorticoid and mineralocorticoid activities		
STEROID	RELATIVE GLUCOCORTICOID ACTIVITY	RELATIVE MINERALOCORTICOID ACTIVITY
Hydrocortisone (cortisol)	1	1
Cortisone acetate (11-deoxycortisol)	0.8	0.8
Prednisone	4	0.8
Prednisolone	4	0.8
Methylprednisolone (6-alpha-methylprednisolone)	5	0.5
Fludrocortisone (9-alpha-fluorocortisol)	10	125
Betamethasone (9-alpha-fluoro-16-beta-methylprednisolone)	25	0
Dexamethasone (9-alpha-fluoro-16-alpha-methylprednisolone)	25	0

significant striae with permanent scarring. These adverse effects occurred in about one-third of women treated until delivery; of these women, one-third would not undergo such treatment again in a future pregnancy. The diagnostic tests (DNA for *CYP21A2* from chorionic villous cells) are obtained at 8–9 weeks' gestation. This means that treatment has to be commenced (at 5 weeks) before it is known what sex the fetus is (at 9 weeks) and whether the fetus has CAH. If the fetus is a male or an unaffected female, maternal treatment can be ceased. This means that eight mothers and babies will have to be treated to prevent the disease in one baby, as only one in eight will be an affected female.

Mothers who have previously had some medical conditions themselves—such as psychiatric diagnoses, hypertension or diabetes—should not be treated. If mothers do opt for treatment, the usual dose is 20–25 μg/kg per day in three divided doses, started no later than the ninth week of gestation. Maternal monitoring must continue throughout pregnancy, including serum oestriol to determine adequacy of fetal adrenal suppression and fasting blood sugar monthly.

Management of acute adrenocortical insufficiency (adrenal crisis)

Candidates can explore thoroughly their understanding and practical application of the underlying pathophysiology of CAH through discussion of a hypothetical presentation of the long-case patient with 21-OHD CAH in adrenal crisis.

Adrenal crisis is most commonly seen with an intercurrent illness. Precipitating stresses include febrile illnesses, vomiting and diarrhoea, surgery or anaesthesia. Symptoms are attributable to cortisol deficiency (lethargy, disorientation), aldosterone deficiency (acute dehydration and collapse, salt craving, diarrhoea) or a deficiency of both (nausea, vomiting, weight loss, muscular weakness).

Signs include shock, dehydration, muscular weakness, hypotension and decreased pulse pressure (dehydration, decreased vasomotor tone). Examination should include a finger-prick blood glucose level. Hypoglycaemia occurs from decreased gluconeogenesis.

Investigations should include diagnostic pre-treatment blood chemistry—decreased serum sodium and chloride, increased serum K, raised blood urea, low blood glucose, and acidosis on blood gas. An ECG may demonstrate low-voltage, wide PR interval, peaked T waves from hyperkalaemia due to lack of aldosterone. PRA is elevated in mineralocorticoid deficiency and ACTH is elevated. Electrolyte abnormalities take a few days to develop and may not be present in an acute crisis.

IMMEDIATE MANAGEMENT

1. Assess and secure the airway, breathing and circulation (the ABCs).
2. Insert an IV cannula; take blood as per the previous page.
3. Restore the circulating volume with an infusion of normal saline (isotonic, 0.9%) with added glucose to make up to 5% glucose. Start with a 20 mL/kg bolus. Correct hypoglycaemia. Aim to replace fluid and electrolytes over the next 24–48 hours.
4. Give bolus hydrocortisone IV (or IM if IV access is difficult):
   - Dose under 2 years: 25–50 mg.
   - Dose 2–5 years: 50–100 mg.
   - Dose over 5 years: 100 mg.
   - Another option is 100 mg/m^2/dose as initial dose, and then 25 mg/m^2.
   - Repeat hydrocortisone dose 6-hourly. Although both cortisol and aldosterone are low, only cortisol is needed during acute treatment. Avoid corticosteroids with negligible mineralocorticoid activity (e.g. dexamethasone) during resuscitation. (Remember that *dex*amethasone only affects *dex*trose, it is not appropriate in an adrenal crisis; whereas *hydro*cortisone is called this because it affects *water* balance via its effects on sodium absorption—that is, it has a *mineralocorticoid* effect— so it is the drug of choice in adrenal crisis, as it has both glucocorticoid and mineralocorticoid effects.)
5. Hyperkalaemia may need further correction with salbutamol, insulin, glucose and calcium.
6. Treat precipitating stress: sepsis, trauma.

LONG CASE: Type 1 diabetes mellitus (T1DM)

There have been many recent advances in the knowledge, understanding and management of T1DM (also called insulin-dependent diabetes mellitus, IDDM). Insulin pumps are core therapy worldwide; in 2014, in diabetic children over 6 years old, these were used by 47% of patients in the United States, 41% in Germany, 40% in Austria, and 14% in England; in Australia the number was around 12% in 2014. Augmented closed-loop systems have been developed, with continuous glucose monitoring (CGM; interstitial fluid glucose concentration is measured every 5 minutes using a fine glucose-sensing subcutaneous cannula) allowing fully automated blood glucose control, decreasing rates of hypoglycaemia. In development are two devices to be released by 2020.

The Medtronic 640G insulin pump device is a hybrid closed-loop system, which allows background insulin delivery but still requires patient/parent input for calibration and to administer mealtime boluses and correction boluses; it comprises an insulin pump, a fourth-generation CGM system and a control algorithm. A pivotal study of the Medtronic 640G showed a significant improvement (decrease) in the amount of time patients had plasma glucose levels (commonly termed 'blood sugar levels' or BSLs) either too high (> 10 mmol/L) or too low (< 4 mmol/L), and no patient developed diabetic ketoacidosis (DKA).

The Beta Bionics iLet device, also called the 'bionic pancreas', can dispense both insulin and glucagon. It can be used as a single chamber device (dispensing just insulin or glucagon) or a dual-chamber bihormonal device. A key study of a closed-loop glucagon-only system showed a 75% reduction in duration of hypoglycaemia plus a reduction in nocturnal hypoglycaemia by 91%. The Beta Bionics company is developing a more stable glucagon analogue for use in the iLet.

Important aspects of any hybrid closed-loop/artificial pancreas system include the control algorithm and supervisory modules. There are two main types of algorithm used: the proportional-integrative-derivative (PID) control, which is essentially reactive to current BSLs; and the model-predictive control (MPC), which is proactive, predicting future BSLs in response to insulin and meals and activity. Supervisory modules add to the safety of control algorithms by stopping insulin delivery when BSLs are too low. A combination of PID and MPC algorithms is used to run devices using both insulin and glucagon.

Cell-based therapies are being pursued, and various types of stem cells investigated (embryonic, fetal stem and adult derived). Pancreatic islet cell allo-transplantation uses islet cells derived from the pancreas of an adult cadaver, purified, processed and transferred by injecting a small volume (several millilitres) of purified tissue into the patient. There are two approaches, the first of which is into the portal vein by a percutaneous trans-hepatic approach. A newer approach is to spread a collection of cells across the omentum, which is then folded over and held in place by a gel comprising plasma and thrombin; this latter approach is to minimise any inflammatory reaction, plus it still drains directly to the liver. Both approaches require ongoing immunosuppression. In Australia, islet isolation and transplantation are performed at St Vincent's Hospital in Melbourne, Westmead Hospital in Sydney and the Royal Adelaide Hospital, with around 44% of patients free of needing insulin at 3 years post-procedure.

Pancreatic transplantation is another approach, which can be done in conjunction with kidney transplantation, as the immunosuppression covers both; in Australia this procedure is performed at the Westmead National Pancreas Transplant Unit in Sydney and the Monash Medical Centre in Melbourne, with pancreatic graft survival around 60% at 5 years.

The incidence of T1DM continues to rise worldwide at 3–5% per year, presenting at a younger age. In Australia, the incidence of T1DM has doubled in the last 20 years, raising the question of a possible pathogenic role for epigenetic or environmental factors. Best practice guidelines have been produced to guide transition of young people with T1DM from paediatric to adult care. There have been further advances in understanding the interplay between genetic susceptibility and environmental factors in the pathogenesis of T1DM. The Environmental Determinants of Islet Autoimmunity (ENDIA) study is an Australian study following 1400 infants with first-degree relatives with T1DM from second trimester of pregnancy into childhood to examine prospectively the relationship between prenatal and postnatal environmental factors and the development of islet autoimmunity and T1DM (see www.endia.org.au).

Children and adolescents with diabetes represent a large and readily available group of patients who frequently are suitable as long cases. They may have problems related to inadequate control of their disease, compliance with treatment (especially adolescents), prevention of complications, difficult-to-manage behavioural problems, associated coexistent diseases such as autoimmune thyroid disease or coeliac disease, or other underlying chronic illnesses such as cystic fibrosis or β-thalassaemia major.

Background information

T1DM affects 1 in 1000 children (and 1 in 400 by adolescence), with a male-to-female ratio of 1.5 : 1 (in European populations). Type 1A diabetes mellitus refers to autoimmune destruction of islet cells; type 1B diabetes mellitus refers to non-autoimmune destruction of islet cells. This discussion uses the term 'T1DM' to refer to type 1A only. The incidence of T1DM increases with age, starting around 1 year, peaking around 8 years; children comprise 50% of those with new-onset T1DM.

The main genetic factor determining susceptibility to T1DM lies within the major histocompatibility complex (termed 'IDDM1'). There is an association with certain HLA haplotypes: more than 90% of children under 7 years with T1DM have HLA-DR3 DQB1*0201 and/or HLA-DR4 DQB1*0302 (class II antigens located on the short arm of chromosome 6, at 6p21). For children who carry both of these highest-risk HLA haplotypes (DR4/DR3), the risk of being diagnosed with T1DM by 15 years is 1 in 20. T1DM is most prevalent in European populations (especially in Scandinavia), less prevalent in African populations, less prevalent again in Hispanic populations and least prevalent in Asian populations (lowest in Japan and China). In African Americans, the haplotype with greatest association with developing T1DM is DRB1*0701-DQA1*0301-DQB1*0201, whereas there is a haplotype which protects against developing T1DM: DRB*0701-DQA1*0201-DQB1*0201.

Non-HLA genes, recognised as contributing to family aggregation of T1DM, include INS (the insulin gene, coding for pre-proinsulin) situated on chromosome 11p5.5. INS is next to a variable number of tandem nucleotide repeats (VNTR) polymorphism. Different sizes of the VNTR are associated with a risk of T1DM, the long form of VNTR being associated with protection from T1DM.

A meta-analysis of data combined from most of the genome-wide studies of linkage to T1DM has been carried out by the Type 1 Diabetes Genetics Consortium; this shows that most of the genetic risk for T1DM is conferred by the class II genes encoding HLA-DR and HLA-DQ, as well as one or more additional genes within the HLA region. Another gene associated with an increased risk of T1DM is the protein tyrosine phosphatase, non-receptor type 22 (lymphoid) gene (PTPN22); a single nucleotide polymorphism in this gene is associated with increased risk of T1DM, rheumatoid arthritis, systemic lupus erythematosus (SLE), vitiligo, Graves' disease, but a decreased risk of Crohn disease.

At least 50 inherited susceptibility loci for T1DM are known. Almost every chromosome has at least one locus identified. Apart from the genes in the HLA region, the majority of these loci affect T-cell function, including antigen-driven T-cell activation and cytokine signalling, proliferation or maturation.

Sibling studies previously had shown that approximately two-thirds of the susceptibility to developing T1DM is linked to the HLA system. Compared to the proband, identical twins have a 40–50% chance of developing diabetes, HLA identical siblings have a 15–20% risk, HLA haploidentical siblings a 5–8% risk and non-identical siblings only a 1–2% risk. Regarding parents, if a mother has T1DM, the risk of her child developing T1DM is around 2–3%; if a father has T1DM, the risk of his child developing T1DM is around 5–6%, and this occurs about 1–2 years earlier than if the mother is the proband; if both parents have T1DM, the risk of developing T1DM is 30%; and if the parents developed the disease earlier than 11 years of age, this increases the risk further.

The role of viral agents in the aetiology has been discussed for years. Children with congenital rubella have a far greater incidence than the general population: this is the only environmental trigger conclusively associated with T1DM.

T1DM is associated with other autoimmune-type diseases, such as coeliac disease (occurs in 6% of T1DM), Hashimoto's thyroiditis (occurs in 3% of T1DM), Graves' disease, Addison's disease, primary ovarian failure, vitiligo and ulcerative colitis. T1DM is considered a T-cell-mediated disease; islet tissue from patients with recent-onset T1DM shows insulitis, with an infiltrate made up of CD4 and CD8 T-lymphocytes and macrophages.

The development of T1DM in relatives of T1DM patients can be predicted by detecting islet-related antibodies; detection of two or more autoantibodies (GAD65 [glutamic acid decarboxylase 65] antibodies, IA-2 [insulinoma-associated protein-2] antibodies, ICA [islet cell cytoplasmic autoantibodies], IAA [insulin autoantibodies] or ZnT8 [zinc transporter 8] antibodies) has a positive predictive value of more than 90%.

Immunotherapy studies show promise in prolonging the honeymoon period. The most effective intervention so far is anti-CD3; stem cell autologous transplants from cord blood stored at birth is also effective. The TrialNet Natural History Study of the Development of T1DM studies first-degree relatives of people with T1DM with positive T1DM-related autoantibodies, affording them the opportunity to be part of intervention studies to prevent progress to T1DM.

Prevention of complications of T1DM

The Diabetes Control and Complications Trial (DCCT) involved 1441 volunteers with T1DM, ages 13–39, who had had T1DM for at least 1 but less than 15 years, and no, or minimal, diabetic eye disease. It compared intensive control of blood glucose (keeping HbA1c [glycosylated haemoglobin] as close to 6% as possible) versus standard control of blood glucose. Patients were studied for an average of 6.5 years. The DCCT study showed that intensive blood glucose control (HbA1c 7.1% versus HbA1c 9.1%) decreases the risk of eye disease (retinopathy) by 76%, kidney disease by 50% and nerve disease (neuropathy) by 60%. The trial ended, and was reported, in 1993, but 90% of patients were followed up and a second study, the Epidemiology of Diabetes Interventions and Complications (EDIC) study reporting in 2005, assessed both microvascular (eye, kidney and nerve) and macrovascular disease, including incidence and predictors of various forms of cardiovascular disease (including myocardial infarction, cerebrovascular accidents and requirement for cardiac surgery). The EDIC study showed that intensive blood glucose control decreases the risk of any cardiovascular disease event by 42%, and non-fatal myocardial infarction, cerebrovascular accident or death from any cardiovascular cause by 57%. The EDIC study showed that the benefits noted for the microvascular complications involving the eyes, kidneys and nerves during the DCCT study persisted after that study was completed. This longer-lasting benefit from tight glucose control has been termed 'metabolic memory'. A HbA1c of 7% is associated with a three-fold risk of cardiovascular disease (CVD), compared to controls; a HbA1c of > 10% is associated with a ten-fold risk of CVD.

Screening for microvascular complications should be performed from 12 years of age, annually (fundoscopy for retinopathy, clinical examination for neuropathy, urine albumin:creatinine ratio [UACR] for nephropathy). If albuminuria is confirmed (UACR elevated in 2 of 3 monthly samples), an angiotensin-converting enzyme (ACE) inhibitor may be prescribed. Also, a 24-hour BP recording should be performed; it may show a loss of night dip in BP as the first sign of pathology. Cardiovascular risk factors also should be considered: smoking (by the parents) should be discussed at any age, and hypertension and lipid profiles should be pursued in those 12 years or older; if lipids are elevated, the family should be checked for hyperlipidaemia.

Diagnosis

Type 1 diabetes can be diagnosed in children as follows:
- Patients with the 'classic' symptoms of T1DM, namely the triad of polydipsia, polyuria and weight loss despite polyphagia, are diagnosed by having a random BSL > 11.8 mmol/L. In practice, the diagnosis is usually clear cut.

- Asymptomatic patients require two criteria: a fasting BSL > 7.0 mmol/L, plus a 2-hour postprandial BSL > 11 mmol/L. Alternatively, a formal oral glucose tolerance test (GTT) demonstrating a sustained elevation in BSL > 11 mmol/L at 2 hours is required, as well as a similarly elevated intervening value taken between the time the glucose load (which is 1.75 g/kg, up to 75 g) is given and the 2-hour value. Again, this is fairly theoretical, as doubtful cases requiring a GTT for diagnosis are very rare.
- DKA comprises around 30–40% of presentations; in these patients there is a small but significant risk of death from several complications, including cerebral oedema (see section later this chapter), especially in younger patients (under 2 years). These children may be late presentations and there is a significant occurrence of posttraumatic stress disorder (PTSD) associated with the admission, linking with fears in the future. Initial education should discuss targets for BSLs (including overnight) and should include discussions addressing fear of death from nighttime hypoglycaemia.

History

PRESENTING COMPLAINT

Reason for current admission.

INITIAL DIAGNOSIS

1. Initial symptoms: for example, early symptoms preceding the classic triad, lack of weight gain, nocturia, behaviour change, altered school performance, changed vision (blurring), tempo of onset (developing over days, weeks or months pre-diagnosis).
2. Immediate pre-diagnosis symptoms: polydipsia, polyuria, weight loss despite polyphagia.
3. Symptoms associated with ketoacidosis: for example, vomiting, abdominal pain, clouding of consciousness.
4. Where, when and how the diagnosis was made, length of hospital stay, education given, treatment in hospital, treatment at discharge.
5. Length of honeymoon period. Hypoglycaemic episodes, hypoglycaemia un/awareness, fears, time off school, conflicts over food, routines, pump/injections.

PROGRESS OF THE DISEASE

1. Details of subsequent hospitalisations (frequency, indications, usual length of stay, usual outcome).
2. Complications of the disease: for example, eye problems with cataracts, retinopathy, joint problems with limited joint mobility (LJM), severe hypoglycaemic reactions.
3. Complications of treatment (e.g. fat atrophy or hypertrophy, insulin allergic reactions); degree of control (number of episodes of ketoacidosis, frequency of hypoglycaemic symptoms).
4. Monitoring of the disease: how often seen in clinic, usual investigations performed, how often seen by local doctor.
5. Changes in management: for example, increase in insulin administration from daily to twice daily with additional short/ultra-short-acting or basal bolus regimen, use of insulin pump, altered dosages due to occult nocturnal hypoglycaemia, changeover from human insulin to analogues, use of CGM.
6. At what age did the patient begin to administer his or her own insulin?

CURRENT STATUS

1. General health: lethargic or energetic.
2. Insulin type, dose, regimen (which sort, how much, when, given by whom, where, rotation of sites; modifications with raised BSL, sporting activities, intercurrent illness or dining out), compliance with treatment.
3. Diet or dose adjusted for normal eating; whether portions/exchanges used, glycaemic index, recommended foods, diet actually taken, alcohol intake (adolescents), involvement of dietician, any restrictions (adhered to or not), timing of meals, suspension of choices, ability to count carbohydrates, snack sizes, missed boluses.
4. Hypoglycaemia: how often, what symptoms (e.g. sweating, pallor, tremulousness, hunger, headache, odd behaviour, lethargy, crying, bad temper, lack of coordination, dizziness, vomiting, convulsions, loss of consciousness, early morning headaches after nocturnal 'hypo', restless sleep); usual precipitants; anticipatory strategies for prevention of 'hypos'; response to 'hypos' such as taking fast-acting sugars (e.g. glass of orange juice with added sugar, glass of lemonade, jelly beans) followed by a small protein and complex carbohydrate snack (e.g. bread, biscuits); ever any need for intramuscular glucagon? (*Note*: if no 'hypos' have occurred, BSL may have been too high.) Any evidence of 'hypoglycaemia unawareness'?
5. Control: hypoglycaemia (see above); hyperglycaemia (e.g. any nocturia, polyuria, blurred vision, weight loss, excessive weight gain, disturbance of menstrual periods in postpubertal girls); BSL readings (usual levels, when performed, how often, by whom, response to high level); usual HbAlc levels; urine testing (how often, what indications); amount of school missed in the last few months, vaginal thrush, other infections such as pilonidal sinus, infected ingrown toenail.
6. Other problems: for example, adolescent self-image, compliance issues.

SOCIAL HISTORY

1. Impact on child: self-image, reaction of school friends, coping with giving insulin, dietary restrictions, exercise, amount of school missed.
2. Impact on siblings: sibling rivalry, risk of diabetes.
3. Impact on parents: family finances, employment, concern regarding future complications, genetic counselling.
4. Social supports: Diabetes Association, access to social worker, government benefits obtained; if insulin pump, is this supplied by private health insurance or subsidised by the Australian Government's Insulin Pump Program.
5. Coping: who attends the clinic with the patient, level of education of the child and parents, contingency plans for intercurrent illnesses or severe hypoglycaemia causing loss of consciousness, access to local doctor/paediatrician/hospital.
6. Peer pressures, risk-taking behaviours.

FAMILY HISTORY

Other affected members, other autoimmune diseases (e.g. thyroid disease).

IMMUNISATION

Influenza vaccine (recommended).

ASSOCIATED DISEASES

Autoimmune (e.g. thyroid disease), underlying chronic illness (e.g. cystic fibrosis, congenital rubella).

Examination

See the short case on diabetes in this chapter.

Management

This involves the use of insulin, diet and regular exercise, with the following aims:

1. Control of BSL: maintaining close to normoglycaemia.
2. Prevention of acute complications; for example, hypoglycaemia, ketoacidosis.
3. Ensuring optimum growth and development.
4. Maintaining a normal lifestyle.
5. Adequate education of the patient and parents.
6. Early detection and treatment of associated disease (e.g. Hashimoto's thyroiditis).
7. Provision of psychological support and counsel.
8. Ensuring adequate access to appropriate social supports.
9. Reducing long-term complications by maintaining good metabolic control.
10. Regular screening for complications and early intervention when they appear (ACE inhibitors for hypertension or proteinuria, etc.).
11. No readmissions with T1DM.

AGE-SPECIFIC ASPECTS OF CONTROL

The expectations at different ages vary. There are three groups:

1. Infants to preschoolers: the main goal is to avoid hypoglycaemia and preserve cognitive function (in line with the findings of the DCCT). The acceptable range for BSLs at this age is between 6 and 15 mmol/L, and the HbA1c between 8.0 and 9.5 gm%.
2. School-age to puberty: again, avoidance of hypoglycaemia is a top priority. Acceptable ranges are BSL 4–10 mmol/L, HbA1c 8.0 gm%.
3. Adolescence: acceptable ranges are BSL 4–8 mmol/L, HbA1c as low as possible. It may be that postpubertal control is more important than prepubertal; this is unclear.

INSULIN THERAPY

Average dosage requirements are as follows:

1. 'Honeymoon' period: 0.5 units/kg/day (or less).
2. Preadolescent: 1.0 unit/kg/day.
3. Adolescent: 1.0–2.0 units/kg/day (increase with pubertal growth spurt and reduce later when growth has finished).

The 'honeymoon' period, which tends to commence about 2 weeks after diagnosis, occurs in about two-thirds of newly diagnosed patients (especially older boys); the nadir of insulin requirements is at an average of 13 weeks' post-diagnosis.

Traditionally, regular insulin was given 30 minutes before a meal. The ultra-short-acting insulin analogues (insulin lispro, insulin aspart, insulin glulisine) can be given with, or just after, the commencement of a meal. It has become apparent since the development of insulin lispro that the short-acting insulins may also be effective if given *with* the meal.

Candidates should be familiar with the various insulin regimens. These include:

1. Daily (longer-acting only, or mixed short and longer).
2. Twice daily (see below).
3. Twice daily with additional short or ultra-short.
4. Basal bolus (three pre-meal short or ultra-short, plus longer in evening; only used in motivated adolescents).

5. Premixed (biphasic) insulin (only used for non-compliance, or inability to mix insulin).
6. Insulin pumps.

Traditionally, the most common regimen, worldwide, has been a twice-daily dosage based on the 'two-thirds/one-third' rule. This is also termed a 'split/mixed regimen', and is based around intermediate-acting insulin.

The total daily insulin dosage is divided up as follows:
- *Two-thirds* is given in the *morning* (before breakfast).
- *One-third* is given in the *evening* (before dinner).

And for each time it is given:
- *Two-thirds* is given as *longer-acting* (intermediate) insulin.
- *One-third* is given as *short-acting* insulin.

This may give insufficient control (which may well be the case in the complicated long-case patient). Most newly diagnosed diabetics are started on the twice-daily regimen, although some very young patients may require only intermediate- or long-acting insulin.

The second most common regimen is the 'basal bolus' regimen, where the basal insulin provides background/baseline, or fasting, insulin needs, while the bolus covers eating and drinking (food and drink needs), and correction for any significant hyperglycaemia.

The basal insulin is provided by long-acting insulin analogues (insulin detemir, insulin glargine, [insulin degludec in Europe]) given once or twice daily, or in the case of insulin pumps, rapid-acting insulin given at a basal rate.

TYPES OF INSULIN/INSULIN ANALOGUE

The examiners will expect you to be familiar with the various types of human insulin, the types of insulin analogues and their durations of action. The following is a brief guide, noting the action after subcutaneous (SC) injection; refer to the latest *MIMS* or equivalent publication for the names of the various preparations available. There are five groups, based on onset and duration.

Rapid-acting (or ultra-short-acting) insulin analogues (insulin lispro, insulin aspart, insulin glulisine)

These are the standard insulins to be used in pumps. Ultra-short-acting analogues can be very useful in toddlers, as it can be given after food. They may improve management compliance with adolescents, and can reduce nocturnal hypoglycaemia. They can be given as an additional dose during illness or when eating extra food. Disadvantages can include the rapid fall in blood sugar, which is especially a problem in toddlers. They do not suit all patients. The action of rapid-acting (or ultra-short-acting) insulins is:
1. Onset at 5–15 minutes.
2. Peak effect at 30–120 minutes.
3. Total duration of 3.5–6 hours.

Insulin analogues can replicate the prandial aspects of insulin replacement more accurately than human insulins. Appropriate use of insulin analogues allows more flexibility in timing of meals, snacks and exercise. Also, the occurrence of hypoglycaemia is less common with analogues.

Short-acting (clear) insulins (neutral/regular/soluble insulin)

These are the standard human insulins. Their action is:
1. Onset at 30–60 minutes.
2. Peak effect at 2–5 hours.
3. Total duration of 6–8 hours.

Intermediate-acting insulins (isophane insulin)

The action of isophane insulins after SC injection is:
1. Onset at 1–2 hours.
2. Peak effect at 4–12 hours.
3. Total duration of 16–24 hours.

Long-acting insulins (basal insulins)

There are three long-acting human insulin analogues: insulin glargine (IGlar), insulin detemir (IDet) and insulin degludec (IDeg). Their action is:
1. Onset at 30–60 minutes (IGlar, IDet), and 30–90 minutes (IDeg).
2. For IGlar, there is little peak effect: this is a 'peakless basal insulin'; IGlar's half-life is around 12 hours; for IDet, the time to maximal effect is between 3 and 14 hours; for IDeg there is no peak, the half-life is 25 hours, and it reaches a steady state in just 3 days.
3. Total duration of 16–24 hours for IGlar and IDet; 24–42 hours for IDeg. Detemir has a shorter time profile than glargine, and may require twice-daily injections. Degludec has been used in Europe, and shows similar glucose control to glargine, but with less hypoglycaemic episodes.

Biphasic insulins

These are premixed preparations of short-acting insulin (comprising 25–30%, depending on the preparation) and intermediate-acting insulin (making up 70–75%).

Action after SC injection is:
1. Onset at 30 minutes.
2. Peak effect at 1–12 hours.
3. Total duration of 16–24 hours.

MODIFYING INSULIN DOSAGES; SELF-TITRATION BOLUS INSULIN

Self-titration calculations for teenagers and adults utilise the carbohydrate ratio (CHR) and insulin sensitivity factor (ISF); the CHR is the number of grams of carbohydrate (CHO) covered by 1 unit of insulin, and the ISF is the drop in BSL (measured in mmol/L) effected by 1 unit of insulin. The prandial insulin dose (just to cover the CHO) should be the CHO load (in grams) divided by the CHR (CHO/CHR); for example, if the CHR was 10, and the meal had 40 g of CHO, then the prandial dose would be $40/10 = 4$ units. The correctional insulin dose (to correct the current BSL to the target BSL) will be [difference between current BSL and target BSL] divided by the ISF; for example, if the current BSL was 14, and the target was 5, and the ISF was 3, then the correctional dose would be $[14 - 5]/3 = 3$ units of insulin. The total dose in this example would be prandial (4 units) plus correctional (3 units) = total 7 units of short-acting insulin.

THE GLYCAEMIC INDEX (GI)

This measures how rapidly a foodstuff can raise the blood sugar. Glucose is the fastest carbohydrate available, except for maltose. Glucose is given a value of 100; other carbohydrates are rated compared to glucose. Faster-acting carbohydrates have higher numbers, and are useful to alleviate hypoglycaemia and to cover brief periods of exercise. Slower-acting carbohydrates are useful to prevent nocturnal hypoglycaemia, and for prolonged periods of exercise.

OTHER POINTS ABOUT INSULIN

1. Insulin given intramuscularly has a higher peak and shorter duration than when given subcutaneously.
2. Insulin absorption rate varies with the site of the injection: it is most consistent when injected into the abdominal wall, followed by the upper limbs and then the lower limbs.
3. Insulin should not be injected into an area that is going to be exercised, so if playing tennis, inject into the abdomen, but if doing sit-ups, inject into the thigh.
4. Lipohypertrophy can occur when the same site is used repeatedly for injection. The injection into this lipohypertrophied area slows the absorption of insulin dramatically and so the insulin appears not to work. This can be avoided by ensuring rotation of injection sites.

SPECIFIC PROBLEM AREAS

Intercurrent illness

Insulin must be given irrespective of illness, and adequate carbohydrate intake must be kept up so that, in the absence of recurrent vomiting, an input of 10 g of carbohydrate every hour is a fair guide, in conjunction with regular BSL measurements (2-hourly). If the BSL is > 15 mmol/L, then checking for ketones in blood or urine, avoidance of carbohydrates, maintenance of low-calorie fluids and a stat dose of 20% of the usual daily insulin dose are appropriate. Some units recommend giving an extra 10–20% of total daily requirements as short-acting insulin regularly, every 2 to 4 hours. If there is recurrent vomiting or ketone levels are high, the BSL should be checked hourly, and admission to hospital may be appropriate. Patients should have a 'sick day' plan.

Hypoglycaemic episodes

The best treatment for hypoglycaemia is prevention, which is essentially anticipation of likely provoking circumstances, such as prolonged exercise (remember that low BSL readings can occur many hours after exercise).

Symptoms of a hypoglycaemic episode (e.g. tremor, hunger, sweating, pallor, confusion, headache) without access to a glucometer, or a BSL reading < 3.5 mmol/L, should be treated immediately. Fast-acting sugars should be given (e.g. half a glass of lemonade, four jelly beans, or two sugar cubes: each of these approximates half a portion) if consciousness is not impaired.

All family members should be instructed in intramuscular glucagon administration, in case loss of consciousness occurs. Generally, it takes 10 minutes or so before the child starts to feel better, so a delay of this duration should not prompt further amounts of fast-acting sugar to be given, which would result in hyperglycaemia.

If a meal is due within 30 minutes of such an episode, it should be given early. If not, then additional food should be given as a complex carbohydrate (e.g. a slice of bread or a banana).

Occult nocturnal hypoglycaemia can occur in association with early morning high blood sugar readings; this is believed to be due to the effect of insulin wearing off. Isophane insulins may peak around 1 a.m., thus a very low BSL can occur at this time, but by 6 or 7 hours later the BSL may be elevated. Nocturnal BSLs must be checked before attributing high early morning readings to insufficient evening insulin dosages. The importance of this is to recognise that the insulin dose should be decreased in the evening and not increased inappropriately by trying to 'chase' the hyperglycaemia.

All children with T1DM should have an identification bracelet stating that they have T1DM, the name of their usual doctor and the hospital they attend. If found unconscious, which usually will be due to a 'hypo', this will allow glucose to be administered. Hypoglycaemia-induced convulsions are common. Parents are advised to position the child appropriately, call an ambulance and administer IM glucagon. After any 'hypo', the patient and parents should ask why this particular episode happened. The family should have an emergency plan for hypoglycaemia.

In Australia in the last decade, the incidence of severe hypoglycaemia in children with T1DM has dropped from 17.3 to 5.8 per 100 patient-years.

ALTERNATIVE MODES OF INSULIN DELIVERY
Insulin pumps

An insulin pump is a small computerised device, which is programmed to supply a basal infusion of insulin, subcutaneously, with increases given at meal times. Pumps have become increasingly sophisticated, and increasingly adopted as a preferred mode of therapy among motivated individuals. They work particularly well in motivated families who are very comfortable with technology. Pumps cost $10 000, though private health funds do cover them. Blood glucose testing is required six times per day. The pump has to be programmed by the user/parent, based on those measurements, while considering food intake and exercise patterns. When used optimally, compared to standard therapy, the use of pumps is associated with better blood glucose control, lower HbA1c levels and improved body mass index (BMI), and reduction in the risk of long-term complications. Insulin delivery more accurately simulates the way a pancreas would deliver insulin, and pumps allow more flexibility with mealtimes, sleeping patterns and ease of adjustments when unwell, and are even associated with improved school performance. Potential disadvantages include not liking the thought of being attached to a piece of machinery/technology constantly, more blood testing, superficial skin infection (or even abscesses) at the infusion site, other site problems (lipohypertrophy, skin reactions to tape, air in lines, kinks in lines) and weight gain (too easy to bolus for unhealthy snacks).

A notable disadvantage of pumps is an increased risk of diabetic ketoacidosis (DKA); this can occur because only ultra-short-acting insulin is administered via pumps, so if the insulin runs out overnight, within a few hours the blood glucose may be rising very rapidly. For this reason, there should always be insulin and pens available at any time, so that the patient can revert to these should the need arise.

Pumps can be removed for short periods (up to 2 hours) to have a shower, go swimming or play sport. A pump is only as good as its operator.

Paediatric diabetes units have much experience in assessing whether a given patient/family is suitable for pump therapy. Most diabetic units have well-organised pathways to obtaining insulin pump management. Initially, there is a period of education, with provision of pump information, relevant web sites, usually pump information evenings, pump group education, meetings with various members of the team (the diabetic educator, dietician and the industry representative of the pump chosen) and trial periods of wearing the pump and loading it with saline. Once the decision is made to start on a pump, then usually a 2-day admission to hospital is appropriate and/or an intensive outpatient program over a few days to receive much technical training about the pump and cover the practicalities, such as the technique for insertion of the catheter, re-siting the catheter every 3 days and troubleshooting the more common pump problems. There should be 24-hour phone contact for a diabetic educator and paediatric endocrinologist or paediatrician, on call 24 hours a day, who can be contacted through the relevant hospital. There is very frequent telephone follow-up for the first few weeks/months, and there are pump clinics in the tertiary hospitals.

The aim of pump therapy is optimal blood glucose control. The National Institute for Health and Care Excellence (NICE) in the UK has set the recommended HbA1c level as < 6.5% (48 mmol/mol) for all children. To achieve these aims, targets must be set; the day can be divided into four segments: fasting (greater than 8 hours since last meal taken); pre-meal (just prior to main meals); postprandial (less than 3 hours after a meal is eaten); and bedtime (immediately prior to going to bed). For each of these time segments, there is a target BSL range. Generally, when fasting and pre-meals and snacks, the target BSL should be 4–7 mmol/L, when postprandial 5–10 mmol/L.

BSL testing should be performed before meals and snacks, 2 hours after each meal or snack, at midnight, at 3 a.m., and additionally 1 and 2 hours after any correction is made, 2 hours after a re-site or set exchange, and any other time where there is any concern. The reason for the midnight and 3 a.m. tests is the decrease in BSL that often seems to occur at those times in many patients.

Basal, or background, insulin rates, are organised to reflect requirements for different time periods during the day; most patients have 4–5 different rates during the day, with modified rates for sick days, or periods of exercise/sport. The basal insulin determines the fasting and pre-meal BSLs. Bolus doses are given for meals and snacks. The insulin-to-carbohydrate ratio, which is programmed into the pump, is used to work out the bolus of insulin given with meals, and determines postprandial BSLs. Pumps can work out the dose of insulin based on the BSL and the amount of carbohydrate to be eaten (which needs to be estimated by the patient), the numbers being entered by the patient. If the BSL is too high or low at the time, then an adjustment in bolus dose (correction bolus) can be given.

Patients should keep a written diabetes diary and not rely on the pump, as pumps can lose data. The patient/parent needs to take the responsibility for maintaining a 'back-up' written record of BSLs, food intake, the amount of insulin given and special circumstances (sport, sick days).

When just getting started with pump therapy, it is unwise to increase the total insulin by more than 10% in any one given 24-hour period; however, if hypoglycaemia should occur, it is acceptable to reduce the dosage by more than just 10%. Modifications in the longer term require ascertaining which of several bolus rates need to be adjusted initially; this must be worked through systematically, testing the basal rate first, then testing the correction bolus, then testing the meal bolus—this area is too complicated to discuss briefly here. It is worthwhile candidates spending time with their hospital's diabetic educators to work through such problems. An excellent resource has been produced by Diabetes Australia: a booklet entitled *I'm Considering an Insulin Pump; Information for People with Type 1 Diabetes* can be accessed at www.diabetesvic.org.au. Insulin pens are standard, as they allow insulin to be given easily and discreetly, particularly when dining out or at other social outings.

DIET

Normalisation of diet is important. The usual caloric requirements are 1000 kilocalories plus 100 kilocalories per year of life: 50% of this should comprise carbohydrate, approximately 35% protein and 15% fat. Generally, the child can be given what he or she normally eats, with some degree of modification and adjustment of insulin dosage.

The diet is planned using GI principles. There are few absolute restrictions. High carbohydrate, high fibre and low fat are preferable. The concept of 'portions' or 'exchanges' is less important than the use of the GI. The former terms describe set amounts of carbohydrate. One 'portion' contains 15 g of carbohydrate, which is equivalent to

60 kilocalories. (This is not universal; in some diabetic clinics, the size of a portion is 10 g of carbohydrate.)

The diabetes diet is planned with the help of a dietician, with the daily requirements usually divided into three main meals and three snacks. Some units use the concept of a 'traffic light' division of foods, namely foods that can be eaten relatively freely ('go', or green light, foods such as meat, fish, black coffee and clear soups), some that can be eaten in moderation ('caution', or amber light, foods such as bread, milk, cereals and pasta), and finally those that should be avoided in excess ('stop', or red light, or 'sometimes', foods such as chocolate, raw sugar, soft drinks and cakes).

EXERCISE

Exercise promotes glucose entry into cells and increases the number of insulin receptors. The positive effects of exercise include increased cardiovascular fitness and increased utilisation of glucose at the same insulin dosage. Exercise also allows certain normally 'red light' foods to be consumed, such as chocolate bars or lollies, due to the increased caloric needs.

The only difficulties are the additional considerations about diet and insulin (which are dealt with easily), and that certain groups of patients should avoid strenuous exercise, namely those with BSL readings > 20 mmol/L, with ketones present, significant retinopathy and hypertension.

During acute exercise, if the BSL readings remain within the normal range or fall, this suggests fairly good control. If the BSL levels remain above normal but the patient feels unwell, this suggests poor control. It is much easier to manipulate food intake than to modify the insulin dose; it may be necessary, during strenuous exercise, to have fast-acting carbohydrates frequently.

MONITORING AND CONTROL

Home BSL monitoring

The glucometer is used at least twice daily (if using a pump, five or six times daily) to record the BSL, stored on the glucometer or in a log book. It is useful for decisions regarding altering dosages of insulin, in particular longer-acting insulin. The goals are:
- Fasting (waking) BSL 4.0–7.0 mmol/L.
- Preprandial BSL 4.0–7.0 mmol/L.
- Postprandial BSL 5.0–10.0 mmol/L.
- At 3.00 a.m. BSL 5.0–8.0 mmol/L.
- When driving a car (16 years old and older), BSL at least 5.0 mmol/L.
- When starting exercise, BSL 5.0–14.0 mmol/L; if BSL is over 14.0, intense exercise can exaggerate hyperglycaemia.

Continuous glucose monitors are commercially available devices to monitor glucose continuously, usually used in conjunction with pump therapy. They can identify high and low BSLs and provide alarms for low BSLs.

GLYCOSYLATED HAEMOGLOBIN (HBA1c)

This is a useful indicator of metabolic control over the preceding 6 weeks to 3 months. Recently it has been recommended to describe HbA1c in units of mmol/mol, rather than as a percentage. NICE (UK) recommend < 6.5%, for all children.

There is a good correlation between HbA1c levels and average BSL readings. HbA1c levels, as percentages, mmol/mol and BSL correlates are:
- HbA1c: 5% = 31.1 mmol/mol → BSL: 5.4 mmol/L.
- HbA1c: 6% = 42.1 mmol/mol → BSL: 7.0 mmol/L.

- HbA1c: 7% = 53.0 mmol/mol → BSL: 8.5 mmol/L.
- HbA1c: 8% = 63.9 mmol/mol → BSL: 10.1 mmol/L.
- HbA1c: 9% = 74.9 mmol/mol → BSL: 11.7 mmol/L.
- HbA1c: 10% = 85.8 mmol/mol → BSL: 13.3 mmol/L.
- HbA1c: 11% = 96.7 mmol/mol → BSL: 14.9 mmol/L.
- HbA1c: 12% = 107.7 mmol/mol → BSL: 16.5 mmol/L.

HbA1c levels vary with ethnicity; African Americans have higher HbA1c levels than non-Hispanic whites, and higher fructosamine levels.

If the patient also has anaemia or a haemoglobinopathy, this can alter the accuracy of some HbA1c assay methods. 'Interfering' haematological diagnoses are listed at www.ngsp.org/interfer.asp.

'Interfering' treatments include blood transfusion and erythropoietin therapy. Haemolysis also interferes with some HbA1c assays. The HbA1c test should not be used for patients with Hb SS, Hb CC or Hb SC. HbA1c levels in haemoglobinopathy patients can be falsely high, overestimating actual BSL levels over the last 3 months. HbA1c levels can be falsely low with heavy bleeding or anaemia. HbA1c levels can be falsely high with low iron, kidney failure or liver failure.

GLYCOSYLATED ALBUMIN (FRUCTOSAMINE)

Like HbAlc, this gives an indication of recent glycaemic control, but over the preceding 2–4 weeks. This can be used when the HbA1c cannot, such as in patients with haemoglobinopathies.

KETONES

Blood ketones and/or urine ketones are important tests. Blood testing is easier, quicker and more recent, but costs more. It is important to check that the dipsticks are not out of date and spoiled (3 months after opening the pack). Ketones should be checked when the BSL is > 15 mmol/L.

ROUTINE FOLLOW-UP

Children with T1DM should be seen every 3 months. On each occasion, the child's growth (height, weight, percentiles, maturation), blood pressure and evidence of any complications should be documented (for the method of examination, see the short case in this chapter) and then managed accordingly. Proteinuria is checked for with dipstick testing, and if positive, a UACR is performed. Fixed proteinuria suggests significant nephropathy. Microalbuminuria above 20 μg in 24 hours is predictive of development of chronic renal failure within 10 years. (*Note*: 1–2% of normal children have microalbuminuria.)

The other important clinical point is regular eye examination by an ophthalmologist, annually from 12 years, to look for diabetic retinopathy or juvenile cataracts. In remote locations, retinal photographs can be taken and then checked by a paediatric ophthalmologist.

Routine investigations and screening should include the following:
1. Screening for *coeliac disease* (occurs in 3–5% of T1DM): IgA tTG (tissue transglutaminase) antibodies (sensitivity 95%, specificity 90%); IgA EmA (endomysial) antibodies (sensitivity 90%, specificity approaches 100%); in children under 2, antigliadin IgG antibodies (children under 2 have a limited ability to produce IgA antibodies); if IgA deficient, IgG antigliadin antibodies; if screening is positive, small bowel biopsy. Performed at diagnosis, and then yearly.

2. Screening for *thyroid disease*: thyroid function tests (TFTs), including TSH (3% of patients with T1DM develop Hashimoto's thyroiditis, and a third of these develop hypothyroidism); if TSH is abnormal, antithyroid antibodies should be tested. Performed at diagnosis, and then yearly.

3. Screening for *lipid disorders*, annually once the patient is over the age of 12 years (ideally after overnight fasting): total cholesterol, low-density lipoprotein (LDL) cholesterol, high-density lipoprotein (HDL) cholesterol, triglycerides.

4. If 12 years of age or more: check for *retinopathy* and for *cataracts*, annually.

5. If 12 years of age or more: check for *microalbuminuria*, and monitor for *hypertension*, annually. The initial screen is the albumin:creatinine ratio (ACR; normal range 3–30 mg/mmol).

6. If 12 years of age or more, or if poor control (HbA1c > 9%): check for *neuropathy* and examine the feet. This should include testing vibration sensation by tuning fork, testing sensation to light touch and testing ankle reflexes. Also look for any ulcers, infection, or Charcot arthropathy (although very unlikely).

EACH OUTPATIENT VISIT

Remember rarer complications and associations which can be overlooked easily, if not specifically assessing for these: Addison disease, necrobiosis lipoidica and juvenile cataracts.

Check for all the findings sought in the short-case approach, at every appointment, and it is unlikely anything important will be missed. Smoking prevention should be mentioned at every appointment. Smoking worsens macrovascular and microvascular complications. Smoking is associated with worse metabolic control in adolescents. Adolescents should also be reminded about drugs, alcohol, post-end-of-school celebrations, sexual health and contraception, in particular that pregnancy in adolescent girls can be associated with more significant and more frequent complications to both mother and baby, than in older women with T1DM. Also remind families about the importance of immunisation (such as annual immunisation against influenza in children over 6 years) and the importance of dental checks.

COMPLICATIONS

Complications are generally divided into microvascular, macrovascular and 'other'. Despite the advances in insulin treatment, over 50% of patients with childhood-onset T1DM will still develop complications such as incipient nephropathy and background retinopathy within 12 years of T1DM. If the glycaemic control in the first 5 years is suboptimal, this shortens the time lapse before complications occur. All children with T1DM should avoid any contact with cigarette smoke because smoking—either active or passive (second-hand smoke)—worsens vasculopathy.

MICROVASCULAR COMPLICATIONS

Risk factors for the development of microvascular complications include long duration of T1DM, poor control of BSL, family history of complications of T1DM, and associated medical problems, such as hypertension.

Retinopathy

This occurs to some degree in 90% or more of patients within 15 years of the onset of their T1DM. The most common lesions seen are 'background' lesions, which include microaneurysms, retinal haemorrhages (named according to appearance: dot, blot and flame), hard exudates, cottonwool spots (retinal nerve fibre infarcts) and venous calibre changes (loops, beading). Background retinopathy can be seen in up to one-quarter of adolescent patients. More advanced lesions of 'proliferative' retinopathy occur in 40% of T1DM patients after 20 years of disease, but are uncommon in adolescence. These changes include signs of neovascularisation, fibrous proliferation and haemorrhage into the vitreous (which can cause sudden visual loss or retinal detachment secondary to fibrosis and traction) and can lead to glaucoma (obstruction to aqueous humour from vascular overgrowth).

Severe loss of vision occurs within 5 years in 50% of those with untreated proliferative retinopathy. The other form of retinopathy, maculopathy, causes central visual loss, mainly due to oedema and hard exudate formation at the macula. Retinopathy is documented with colour or red-free retinal photography and the severity assessed with fluorescein angiography. The treatment for early background retinopathy is maintenance of near normoglycaemia, there being some evidence that the institution of improved glucose control can actually reverse some of the changes. The treatment used for both proliferative retinopathy and maculopathy is laser photocoagulation: panretinal for the former and focal for the latter. Photocoagulation can reduce the rate of visual loss by half.

Nephropathy

Patients may eventually develop end-stage renal failure (ESRF), although this is rare in childhood; around 2.2% of T1DM patients get ESRF 20 years after diagnosis, and 7.8% T1DM patients get ESRF 30 years after diagnosis. Diabetic nephropathy is associated with an increased risk of cardiovascular disease. A microvasculopathy affecting the glomeruli (diffuse or nodular glomerulosclerosis) is the cause of the depressed glomerular filtration rate (GFR). The first sign of this process is microalbuminuria of over 20 μg/minute. Intermittent microalbuminuria or 'borderline' levels (7.6–20 μg/minute) increase the chance of nephropathy. Once proteinuria is persistent and easily detected, there has already been a reduction in the GFR, which is an ominous sign. There is a 95% occurrence of retinopathy in newly uraemic diabetics, on the basis of the same pathological process, microangiopathy, afflicting both the glomerulus and the retina. This association has been called the 'renal–retinal syndrome'. A clinical point worth remembering is that eye status should be reviewed when any patient develops evidence of renal impairment, such as proteinuria.

Nephropathy is accelerated by hypertension, and control of the blood pressure will decrease the amount of proteinuria and slow the rate of fall in the GFR. ACE inhibitors delay progression to/of nephropathy. The renal function can be monitored by plotting 1 divided by serum creatinine versus time.

Once ESRF occurs, the treatment options include renal transplantation (or combined renal–pancreatic transplantation), peritoneal dialysis, haemodialysis or haemofiltration.

Neuropathy

There are several forms of neuropathy:
1. Symmetric distal neuropathy, which predominantly affects sensory neurons, causing paraesthesia or pain, but can also involve the motor system.
2. Autonomic neuropathy, which can lead to postural hypotension, arrhythmias (due to denervation hypersensitivity to catecholamines), gastroparesis and impaired response to hypoglycaemia, and may be associated with painless myocardial infarction.
3. Carpal tunnel syndrome, due to the neuropathy affecting the median nerve (often the ulnar nerve is involved as well).
4. Mononeuropathy, which particularly affects cranial nerves.

All of these are infrequent in the paediatric age range. However, nerve conduction studies demonstrating subclinical peripheral nervous system involvement and evidence of sensory neuropathy are not uncommon in adolescent diabetics. The underlying pathology is thought to be a combination of polyol pathway abnormality (conversion of glucose to sorbitol, then sorbitol accumulation in peripheral sensory nerves) and microangiopathy affecting the vasa vasorum, leading to axonal loss and segmental demyelination. Mononeuropathy of cranial nerves and motor neuropathy are due to vasa vasorum angiopathy.

MACROVASCULAR COMPLICATIONS

In 2016, risk factors for cardiovascular disease (CVD) were assessed in the long-term follow-up (averaging 27 years) of the DCCT T1DM cohort. Evaluating major atherosclerotic cardiovascular events (MACEs, meaning myocardial infarction or stroke, whether fatal or non-fatal) and 'any'-CVD (meaning MACEs plus angina, revascularisation, congestive cardiac failure), it was found that age and HbA1c were strongly related to any-CVD and MACEs, more so than other conventional factors such as high blood pressure, high lipids or not taking ACE inhibitors. *For each HbA1c percentage point increase, there was an increased risk for any-CVD of 31%, and for MACE of 42%.* Only age was a more important risk factor for CVD than HbA1c. In other words, it is now proven that the risk of CVD in T1DM is related closely to the HbA1c level.

Coronary atherosclerosis

Coronary artery disease is common in T1DM patients, the prevalence increasing with the duration of the disease. The extent of involvement of coronary vessels also tends to be greater (triple vessel disease more common), and it is more common in women. Clinical disease is rare in the childhood and adolescent population.

Peripheral vascular disease

Atherosclerosis is accelerated in T1DM. Peripheral vascular disease, like coronary arterial disease, is rare in the paediatric population, so that problems such as digit ischaemia are unlikely to be encountered.

OTHER COMPLICATIONS
Limited joint mobility (LJM)

Thought to be due to glycosylation of periarticular tissues, LJM occurs in approximately 40% of children with T1DM. It is a painless condition that does not cause any significant disability in its early form. It affects the hands (metacarpophalangeal, proximal and distal interphalangeal joints, initially of the fifth, then the more medial fingers), wrists, elbows, spine (cervical and/or thoracolumbar) or other large joints. There seems to be a correlation between LJM and retinopathy, with an increased risk of microvascular disease developing in patients with LJM.

Requirement for psychological support

For the purposes of the long case, the usual problem is that of a non-compliant adolescent. Adolescence encompasses many developmental tasks: becoming more independent from parents; getting an education and a job; coming to terms with sexuality (sexual self-concept); and fitting in with peers and being different ('man', 'dude', 'bro'). Teenagers can find themselves in single-parent families or moving between parents, in low-income situations, caring for siblings or parents, or feeling cramped. On top of this, dealing with the cognitive changes includes the ability to think in an abstract manner about their future, appreciate the consequences of their behaviour (in older adolescents), and formulate hypotheses and apply logical tests. Unfortunately, it is most important to avoid serious complications in adolescence, at exactly the least receptive time of the patient's life.

For a teenager, immediate peer acceptance, which may involve nights out at parties or hotels, far outweighs the long-term benefits of near normoglycaemia. Parents' fears at this time are of their teenagers taking risks (be they smoking, drinking, sexual risks or staying out late), and they feel out of control and worried. Parents become concerned about their teenager not managing themselves well, become frustrated, threaten about complications, and anxiety and confusion follow. Parent traps include being over-involved (parent, 'I nag.' versus teenager, 'Back off, mum!') or under-involved (parent, 'I give up—you do it!' versus teenager, 'Diabetes—who cares?'), whereas the favoured approach is guiding and expressing understanding while applying limits, where, hopefully the teenager will think, 'Diabetes is not that hard. I can do this'.

There are three important principles in parenting adolescents with a chronic illness: first, staying involved, which is paramount; second, expressing understanding while applying limits; and, third, working as a team. Teenagers want to be understood, but want to be different from their parents. Parents have to learn to accept some things with which they do not agree; one can accept something without agreeing with it (e.g. not wanting to take insulin at school), accept that it is annoying ('Yeah, it sucks. You must hate this—you must wish you could forget about it.') but, without agreeing to comply with the teenager's request, recognise that the issue must be solved ('How about we figure out a way to sort this out?').

Parents should make it as easy as possible to live with them, recognising that they, the parents, and their teens both will get frustrated but will continually agree that the necessary management aspects for diabetes must be attended to.

There are similar principles for the paediatrician managing adolescents: staying involved and expressing understanding while applying limits. Hence effecting 'good care' involves: staying involved; engaging the teenager by regular contact; semi-structured conversation; a friendly environment, non-judgmental and strictly confidential; explanation of the importance of optimal management, which is evidence-based (so the teenager can check the evidence themselves if they wish); a focus on positives, looking for resilience factors and returning control to the patient. Clinics for adolescents with diabetes are based on these principles. At each follow-up visit, the usual adolescent issues can be brought up (**HEADS**: **H**ome, **E**ducation, **E**mployment, **E**xercise, **E**ating, **A**ctivities, **A**lcohol, **D**rugs, **S**moking, **S**exuality, **S**uicide/depression/psychiatric issues, **S**ocial/psychological issues, **S**afety concerns).

Achievement of independence is the ultimate goal.

The things that doctors find difficult are the adolescent's poor glycaemic control (typically no glucose monitoring, omitting insulin, variable diet and activity), the variable attendance at follow-up, missing appointments, risk-taking behaviour and the low priority given to health. The doctors focus on weight, what the patient is eating, routines regarding insulin administration and BSL checks. The things that adolescent patients find difficult are having a chronic illness, and the repetitive ongoing nature of diabetic management. The adolescents focus on what their peers are eating, flexibility and spontaneity in socialising, and not being different.

In chronic illness in adolescence, non-adherence is usually due to comorbidities. Identified barriers to achieving and maintaining metabolic control include intrapersonal barriers such as: mental health issues in teens (e.g. weight and shape concerns, low mood, anxiety, substance abuse, oppositional behaviour); fear of hypoglycaemia; and learning and attention issues. There is never a problem with knowledge of diabetes *per se*. Interpersonal barriers include inadequate or ineffectual parental support, difficulties in the family system, single-parent families and financial stress. An effective intervention in recurrent DKA is that a responsible adult is the one who gives the insulin.

Families need access to supports: counsellors, psychologists, peer group support and diabetes camps. All of these help the patient and the parents cope with T1DM.

Eating disorders

Adolescent females with T1DM are more than twice as likely to develop an eating disorder than typical adolescents without T1DM. Around 10% of adolescent diabetic girls fulfil the DSM-5 criteria for an eating disorder; this has serious adverse metabolic consequences including worse microvascular disease, occurring sooner and progressing faster than in age-matched diabetic girls without an eating disorder.

COMORBID DISORDERS

Autoimmune thyroid disease occurs eventually in 3% of children with T1DM. The risk in the first 10 years after diagnosis is indicated by the presence or absence of thyroid autoantibodies when T1DM is first diagnosed. Hypothyroidism occurs more commonly than hyperthyroidism, and particularly occurs in adolescent females around puberty. For this reason, symptoms of thyroid dysfunction should be sought, any goitre noted and serum thyroid function tests be performed 12 monthly.

Addison disease can present with recurrent hypoglycaemia or with insulin requirements decreasing. The usual screening test is an 0800-hour serum cortisol, plus serum sodium and serum potassium.

Coeliac disease occurs in 4–9% of children with T1DM, although it is asymptomatic in two-thirds of these patients. It can present with frequent hypoglycaemia or poor metabolic control. The usual screening blood tests comprise anti-tissue transglutaminase antibody (anti-tTG), IgA class and Ig A levels. If the patient is IgA deficient, the alternative test is anti-tTG, IgG class.

Social supports

All families of patients with T1DM should have access to an experienced social worker. T1DM represents a significant financial burden for many families and the social worker can make them aware of the various government benefits to which they may be entitled.

These benefits may include Child Disability Allowance (CDA), the Child Disability Assistance Payment (CDAP), the Isolated Patients Travel and Accommodation Assistance Scheme (IPTAAS) if the patient lives more than 200 km from the hospital, and the Program of Appliances for Disabled People (PADP) which consists of scripts for needles, syringes and glucometer if the patient has a Health Care Card. Diabetes Australia provides access to many helpful people and ideas, including attendance at diabetic camps and the use of the National Diabetes Services Scheme (NDSS).

TRANSITION FROM PAEDIATRIC TO ADULT CARE

A well-structured transition program is important. It has been recognised that around one-third of patients with T1DM have, in the past, been lost to specialist follow-up during their (planned) transfer from paediatric to adult care. To address this, in Queensland, the Lady Cilento Children's Hospital and Queensland Health together have developed a comprehensive set of Best Practice Guidelines for health professionals. It provides clearly set out steps to guide the process, at key ages (12–13, 15, 16–17, 18+). It aims to actively involve young people in the transition process, allowing flexibility of timing, assigning a transition case worker, the choice of an adult diabetic care provider, and significant preparation and coordination. The family should have a concept, or plan, for transition.

PRE-DIABETES SCREENING AND INTERVENTION

Screening

Islet cell antibodies may be detected in (future) patients (first-degree relatives) with beta cell autoimmunity months or years before T1DM declares itself clinically. Islet cell antibodies include antibodies against insulin (insulin autoantibodies, IAA), plus non–beta-cell-specific proteins such as glutamic acid decarboxylase (GAD) and tyrosine phosphatase (IA-2).

Prevention

Many agents have been trialled to prevent T1DM; none has succeeded as yet. There continues to be an enormous amount of research in this area, which is beyond the scope of this book. There is a wealth of information about screening and prevention of T1DM available on the internet. A good starting point is https://clinicaltrials.gov.

ACUTE MANAGEMENT OF DIABETIC KETOACIDOSIS (DKA)

This is an area where the candidate's discussion of a hypothetical presentation of the long-case patient with DKA can explore thoroughly his or her understanding and practical application of the underlying pathophysiology of DKA.

The principles of treatment can be divided into five main areas, the 'diabetic pentathlon':
1. Water and sodium replacement.
2. Potassium replacement.
3. Correction of acid–base imbalance.
4. Insulin administration.
5. Prevention of treatment complications.

The first four areas should be well known to candidates and are not discussed here in detail. The fifth area, which can generate the most questions, will now be discussed briefly.

SOME COMPLICATIONS

Cerebral oedema (CO)

Subclinical cerebral oedema occurs frequently in children with DKA. Many children fall asleep during treatment, but failure to rouse easily or onset of headache should raise suspicion of CO (or hypoglycaemia, so checking BSL is mandatory). This typically occurs 2–24 hours after starting treatment, especially around 4–12 hours; two-thirds of cases occur within 7 hours of treatment. It has been described up to 48 hours after starting treatment, and it has been described before any treatment has started. Once it is clinically apparent, mortality rates reported have ranged from 25–64%.

CO is the most common cause of death in children presenting with DKA. Clinical CO occurs in 0.2–1.0% of children with DKA. Survivors of CO have a significant risk of residual neurological damage.

Other causes of depressed level of consciousness include: acidosis; hypoglycaemia; any rapid change in osmolality, serum sodium, serum glucose or pH; hyponatraemia; hypernatraemia; hyperosmolality; hypoxia; hypothermia; hypovolaemia; and neuroglycopenia. A cerebral CT scan should be considered if depressed level of consciousness does not respond to volume/colloid, or if it occurs during treatment.

There are three groups of criteria, described by Muir et al. (2004) to delineate CO:
1. *Diagnostic criteria* are four: (a) **P**ain response abnormal: verbal or motor; (b) **P**osture decorticate or decerebrate; (c) **C**ranial nerve palsy (especially III, IV, VI); (d) **C**heyne Stokes or other abnormal respiratory pattern (mnemonic 2 **P**s, 2 **C**s).

2. *Major criteria* are three: (a) **C**onsciousness level altered; (b) **C**ardiac deceleration (drop by > 20 beats per minute); (c) **C**ontinence lost (age-inappropriate incontinence) (mnemonic 3 **C**s).

3. *Minor criteria* are five: (mnemonic **HALVED**): (a) **H**eadache; (b) **A**ge young (< 5); (c) **L**ethargy: (d) **V**omiting/**E**mesis; (e) **D**iastolic pressure high (> 90 mmHg).

If a child has 1 diagnostic criterion, 2 major criteria, or 1 major and 2 minor criteria, then this gives 92% sensitivity, and 96% specificity for identifying CO soon enough to intervene.

Risk factors for CO are 10: (mnemonic: 10 **F**s): **F**ive years or under (especially under 2 years); **F**ast insulin (insulin given as bolus); **F**ast fluids/**F**looding with fluids (giving IV fluids [especially dangerous if hypotonic] too rapidly); **F**ailure to correct serum sodium (hyponatraemia developing with treatment, or failing to rise); **F**irst serum sodium high (especially > 160 mmol/L); **F**irst presentation of T1DM with DKA; **F**irst hour insulin (insulin given within first hour of treatment); **F**irst arterial PCO_2: low; **F**irst serum urea: high; **F**looding with bicarbonate (excessive administration).

Warning features are headache, deterioration in consciousness, irritability, with later (ominous) signs of hypertension, bradycardia and dilated pupils. On occasion, there may be a presentation of polyuria, secondary to diabetes insipidus, which can be misdiagnosed as osmotic diuresis.

Prevention strategies include slow correction of fluid and glucose abnormalities, and nursing children with the head elevated. Active treatment includes: 20% mannitol, 0.5–1.0 g/kg IV statim, repeated every 15 minutes; hypertonic (3%) saline 5–0 mL/kg IV, given over 30 minutes (as alternative to mannitol, or if mannitol unsuccessful); decreasing rate of fluid administration (to two-thirds maintenance); and intubation and hyperventilation (but keeping PCO_2 above 25 mmHg to avoid neurological sequelae).

Hypoglycaemia (BSL < 3.9 mmol/L)

This can present as an altered consciousness state, thus being confused with CO. Treatment is with a bolus of 10% glucose (2 mL/kg), plus a decrease in the insulin infusion rate.

Hypokalaemia (serum K^+ < 3.5 mmol/L; moderate hypokalaemia < 3.0; severe < 2.5)

This is a potential cause of cardiac arrhythmia and death. ECG changes are seen when serum K^+ < 2.7; these include: P wave: higher amplitude and wider; PR interval: longer; T wave: flattened and inverted; ST segment: depressed; U waves: prominent, more so than T waves; when U wave exceeds the T wave in amplitude, T and U waves fuse giving an *apparently* long QT interval (which is actually a long QU interval).

LONG CASE: Hypopituitarism

Children with hypopituitarism may be encountered in long-case settings. Hypopituitarism can present at any age, depending on the underlying aetiology, and it is often this aetiology which leads to the child being in the hospital at an opportune time for clinical examinations. Causes which typically present as a neonate include genetic disorders (e.g. PROP1-related combined pituitary hormone deficiency [CPHD], holoprosencephaly), CNS structural lesions which are mainly sporadic (e.g. septo-optic dysplasia [SOD]), and neonatal encephalopathy. Causes which present later, at any age, include tumour (e.g. craniopharyngioma), treatment for tumours (e.g. cranial radiotherapy) or trauma (e.g. acquired brain injury after motor vehicle accident). These can be recalled as the mnemonic **CRASH**:

Craniopharyngioma (and other intracranial tumours in hypothalamic/pituitary region)/**C**HARGE syndrome/**C**ombined pituitary hormone deficiency (CPHD)

Radiotherapy (cranial irradiation for CNS or non-CNS tumours, late effects of oncology treatment)

Acquired brain injury, including neonatal encephalopathy (can term **A**sphyxia purely for recall)

Septo-optic dysplasia (most common CNS structural cause)

Holoprosencephaly (failure of prosencephalon to divide adequately into two hemispheres)/**H**istiocytosis (Langerhans cell histiocytosis [LCH])

Craniopharyngioma

Craniopharyngioma arises from the craniopharyngeal cleft, which develops from the fusion of two primordial structures, Rathke's pouch and the infundibulum, in the fourth week of gestation. It is a benign tumour, situated in the suprasellar area. It is **C**alcified and **C**ystic, **S**low growing and **S**quamous **E**pithelial, and **E**xtra-axial (outside of brain) (2 **C**s, 2**S**s and 2 **E**s). The craniopharyngioma spectrum includes the predominantly childhood-prevalent adamantinomatous type (likely from embryologic remnants), and the mainly adult-prevalent squamous papillary type (from metaplastic foci, from mature anterior pituitary cells).

There can be 1 or 2 years between onset of first symptoms and diagnosis; the tumour usually has to be around 3 cm before symptoms occur. It is rarely diagnosed before 2 years of age; it tends to present between 5 and 14 years of age.

The exact site and direction of spread determine the symptomatology, due to the mass effect of the suprasellar tumour on adjacent structures (hypothalamus, pituitary gland, visual tracts, cerebrospinal fluid [CSF] pathways, frontal lobe, temporal lobe). Pre-chiasmal spread can lead to visual symptoms and signs. Retro-chiasmal spread can lead to raised intracranial pressure (ICP) either via direct mass effect or via obstruction of the third ventricle causing hydrocephalus. Intrasellar spread leads to endocrine symptoms and headache.

The tumour most likely to involve the pituitary, craniopharyngioma typically presents with headache (in 60–80%), which is mainly in the early morning, accompanied by projectile vomiting from raised ICP, although when a retrospective history is taken, the order of clinical problems appearing is: 1. the various endocrine hypofunctions (such as growth disturbance); 2. headache; and 3. visual symptoms. Children tend to be unaware of visual loss, but at presentation, 20–60% of children have visual field cuts (bitemporal hemianopia, unilateral temporal hemianopia [starting with superior field cut]), loss in acuity, diplopia or blurring of vision. Children are usually unaware of bitemporal field losses and may compensate with head turning. Within the endocrine symptoms (which may be overlooked), the usual order of appearance is those related to growth (GH, LH, FSH) first, followed by thyroid hypofunction next, followed by adrenal hypofunction, followed by diabetes insipidus if the posterior lobe of the pituitary is involved. The endocrine symptoms most likely to lead to presentation are growth failure, and polyuria and polydipsia from diabetes insipidus (DI). Other presenting symptoms include trouble waking, loss of balance, difficulty walking, change in energy level, sleepiness, hearing loss and change in personality.

Treatment comprises surgery (almost always), which has three functions: 1. establishing the diagnosis; 2. relieving problems due to mass effects; and 3. removing as much tumour as possible. Pre-operative assessment may involve elucidating and treating endocrine dysfunction, controlling raised ICP and oedema around tumour, shunting hydrocephalus and draining larger cystic areas.

Approach is determined by tumour site. Intrasellar tumours may be resected by transsphenoidal surgery, and suprasellar tumours by extended transsphenoidal surgery;

others may be approached by pterional craniotomy (pterion being where four bones join: squamous temporal, sphenoid, parietal and frontal).

Radiation therapy (RT) is used for residual disease or recurrence. RT techniques can include stereotactic radiotherapy (SRT) and stereotactic radiosurgery (SRS) using patient-specific coordinates, where radiation is aimed at the tumour only (fractionated in SRT, covering a large volume of tissue, or in the case of SRS, using a single fraction of radiation targeting smaller tumours), intracavity radiation (radioactive material placed inside tumour), intensity-modulated radiation therapy (IMRT) (a three-dimensional radiation therapy aiming protons or photons at the tumour) and external beam radiation therapy (EBRT) which utilises protons to deliver high radiation dosage to the target tumour volume. Using fractionated treatment, radiation doses above 55 Gy usually are effective in treating local recurrences, and doses less than 61 Gy largely avoid RT-induced endocrine, vascular and neurological complications. Recurrent tumour may also require chemotherapy (such as intracavitary chemotherapy) and biologic therapy (intracavitary).

Clearly post-treatment hormone profiles will be quite different to pre-treatment; many patients who are ACTH sufficient at diagnosis become ACTH deficient postoperatively. Indeed, post-treatment most children have panhypopituitarism (adrenal insufficiency, hypothyroidism, hypogonadism, growth hormone deficiency), some have hypothalamic dysfunction (DI, abnormal temperature regulation, obesity [with type 2 diabetes] and sleep disruption), and there are many potential neurological problems (intellectual impairment, behavioural problems, worsening of previous visual impairments), as well as vascular anomalies post-RT (aneurysms, moya, cavernoma), and transient ischaemic episodes or completed strokes post-multimodal therapy, and finally secondary tumours post-RT (e.g. meningioma).

A few important points:
1. All patients with craniopharyngioma, at presentation, should be considered ACTH deficient until proved otherwise.
2. All patients with craniopharyngioma require careful assessment of their fluid balance and checking of their serum electrolytes, before and after starting glucocorticoids, and before and after treatment/surgical removal of the tumour. In patients with both central adrenal insufficiency and DI, before treatment, the DI may be masked by the adrenal insufficiency; so, once glucocorticoid treatment commences, DI is unmasked.
3. Glucocorticoid replacement must occur *before* thyroid hormone replacement; otherwise adrenal crisis can be precipitated, so the mantra for craniopharyngioma (or other forms of hypopituitarism) is:
Steroids replaced first, then replace all the others, watch out for DI.

CHARGE syndrome

This is autosomal dominant, and comprises **C**olobomatous malformation of the eye (retinal coloboma the most common), **H**eart anomalies (e.g. tetralogy of Fallot), **A**tresiae of the choanae (bony and/or membranous), **R**etardation both cognitive and somatic growth, **G**enital anomalies and/or hypoplasia (males), **E**ar anomalies and/or deafness (OMIM#214800). Almost two-thirds of these patients have a mutation in the chromodomain helicase DNA binding protein-7 (CHD7) gene. CHD7 is an ATP-dependent remodelled of chromatin, and it binds to methylated histones. Hypopituitarism occurs as part of CHARGE syndrome, particularly as hypogonadotrophic hypogonadism (HH), GH deficiency and ACTH deficiency. There have been reported cases of the same genetic mutation in CHD7 causing both CHARGE and structural anomalies of the pituitary gland.

Combined pituitary hormone deficiency (CPHD)

A genetic diagnosis is still not known for most cases in clinical practice, although this will increase with modern genetic techniques. At the time of writing (2017), there were mutations recognised in at least eight known genes. Some of these are listed below with their location and hormones affected:

- *CPHD1* (OMIM#613038); gene: *POU1F1*; location 3p11.2; hormones decreased are GH, prolactin (PRL), and TSH only.
- *CPHD2* (OMIM#262600); gene: *PROP1*; location 5q35.3; sequential hormone loss occurs: GH, then gonadotrophin, TSH and finally ACTH.
- *CPHD3* (OMIM#221750); gene: *LHX3* (OMIM*600577); location 9q34.3; hormones affected: GH, LH/FSH, TSH and PRL.
- *CPHD4* (OMIM#262700); gene: *LHX4* (OMIM*602146); location 1q25.2; hormones affected: GH, LH/FSH, TSH and PRL.
- *CPHD5* (OMIM#182230); gene: *HESX1* (OMIM*601802); location 3p14.3; hormones affected: GH, LH/FSH, TSH, ACTH and antidiuretic hormone (ADH); mutation of this gene can cause septo-optic dysplasia (SOD) (see below).
- *CPHD6* (OMIM#613986): gene: *OTX2* (OMIM*600037); location 14q22.3; hormones affected: GH, ACTH, TSH, LH/FSH.
- Gene: *PITX2* (OMIM*601542); location 4q25; hormones affected: GH, PRL.
- Gene: *SIX6* (OMIM*606326); location 14q23.1; hormones affected: GH.
- *Culler-Jones syndrome* (CJS) (OMIM#615849); gene: *GLI2* (OMIM*165230); location 2q14.2; hormones affected: GH, GnRH, TSH; includes polydactyly; mutation of the GLI2 gene can cause holoprosencephaly.

Of all the CPHDs, the most common mutation is of the PROP1 gene which comprises 12–55% of known cases. The genes involved make transcription factors which act to control other genes and are essential to the process of pituitary development and cell type differentiation.

Isolated pituitary hormone deficiencies

IGHD1A (isolated growth hormone deficiency type 1A) (OMIM#262400); gene: *GH1*; (OMIM*139250); location 17q23.3; hormone affected: GH.

IGHD1B (isolated growth hormone deficiency type 1B) (OMIM#612781); gene: *GHRHR* (growth hormone-releasing factor receptor) (OMIM*139191); location 7p14.3; hormone affected: GH.

Isolated GH deficiency often presents later in childhood.

Kallmann syndrome (OMIM#308700); gene: *KAL1*; (OMIM*300836) location Xp22.31; hormones affected: LH/FSH. This syndrome includes anosmia or hyposmia. The protein product of KAL1, anosmin, is important in the embryonal migration of GnRH-synthesising neurons, and of olfactory neurons, to the hypothalamus. Anosmia, and hyposmia, occur depending on whether there is absence, or hypoplasia, of the olfactory bulbs, respectively.

nIHH (normosmic idiopathic hypogonadotropic hypogonadism) (OMIM#308700, same as Kallmann syndrome, but with normal sense of smell); gene: KAL1 (OMIM#300836); location: Xp22.31; hormones affected LH/FSH.

Hypogonadotropic hypogonadism 12 (OMIM#614841) with or without anosmia (OMIM#614841); gene: *GNRH1* (gonadotropin-releasing hormone 1) (OMIM*152760); location 8p21.2; hormones affected: LH/FSH.

Adrenal hypoplasia congenital + hypogonadotropic hypogonadism (OMIM#300200); gene: *NR0B1* (DAX1) (OMIM*300473); hormone affected: LH/FSH.

IAD (Isolated ACTH deficiency) (OMIM#201400); gene: *TBX19* (OMIM*604614); location 1q24.2; hormone affected: ACTH.

Hypothyroidism, congenital nongoitrous (OMIM#275100); gene: TSHB/TSH-Beta (OMIM*188540); location 1p13.2; hormone affected: TSH.

Thyrotropin-releasing hormone resistance, generalised; gene: TRHR (thyrotropin-releasing hormone receptor) (OMIM+188545); location 8q23.1; hormone affected: TSH.

Radiotherapy

Prophylactic or therapeutic radiation frequently lead to abnormalities in the hypothalamic–pituitary (HP) axis. However, radiation does not affect the posterior pituitary, only the anterior pituitary. Radiation at a dose of 18 Gy can cause GH deficiency. Doses of 30–50 Gy can cause GH deficiency in 50–100% within 3 to 5 years; this same dose can cause TSH and ACTH deficiency in 3–6% of patients. Effects on gonadotropin secretion are interesting: doses less than 30 Gy can cause precocious puberty, but doses above 30 Gy can cause gonadotropin deficiency and delayed puberty. Higher doses of radiation (above 60 Gy) can cause ACTH and TSH and LH/FSH deficiency in 30–60% in 10 years. Anterior pituitary hormone deficiencies induced by radiation are irreversible and progressive.

Acquired (traumatic) brain injury

Traumatic brain injury (TBI) is now well recognised as a major cause of pituitary dysfunction. The prevalence of anterior pituitary dysfunction overall is around a quarter of adults with TBI (range in adults 15–68%); it certainly occurs in children also, although the frequency is unclear. The adult literature gives the deficiencies of each axis as: somatotrophin, 12%; gonadotrophin, 12%; corticotrophin, 8%; and thyrotropin, 5%.

With time, there is an overall tendency to improvement, although the progress is unpredictable; some patients develop new pituitary deficiencies, and can evolve from having a single deficiency to multiple pituitary hormone deficiencies, months to years after injury.

Septo-optic dysplasia (SOD) (OMIM#1822390) is a heterogeneous disorder, clinically, with two or more of a classic triad of: 1. hypoplasia of the optic nerves; 2. hypoplasia of the pituitary gland (with variable levels of hypopituitarism); and 3. midline brain anomalies (absence of septum pellucidum, agenesis of corpus callosum). There can be associated anomalies such as cerebellar hypoplasia and schizencephaly. Neurological abnormalities, found in around 80% of patients, vary from focal involvement to global developmental delay/intellectual impairment. Wandering nystagmus can be the presenting feature, with optic nerve involvement, typically bilateral (in around 90%).

The spectrum of visual involvement can include unilateral optic nerve hypoplasia, mild to moderate visual impairment, microphthalmia, anophthalmia or blindness. Endocrine deficiencies can develop over time; these include isolated GH deficiency, TSH and ACTH deficiency, gonadotrophin-releasing hormone deficiency, gonadotrophin deficiency (with pubertal delay in adolescence), DI and multiple pituitary hormone deficiencies that can be caused by the gene HESX1 (OMIM*601802), which is then termed 'combined pituitary hormone deficiency', 5 (CPHD5), as mentioned earlier.

Mainly sporadic, SOD occasionally has a genetic cause, in about 1%, such as: mutations in aforementioned HESX1 (the Rathke pouch homeobox), LHX4, SOX2 and SOX3. There is no available treatment for the visual impairment of SOD. Endocrine replacement commences with hydrocortisone, before other hormones, so as not to precipitate adrenal crisis.

There are a number of other recognised associated features found in SOD including: obesity, obstructive sleep apnoea, autistic spectrum disorder and temperature instability. MRI may show hypoplasia of optic nerves (bilateral or unilateral), and optic chiasm, absent septum pellucidum, anomalies of corpus callosum and anomalies of the hypothalamic–pituitary region (e.g. may be hypoplasia of the anterior pituitary, absent infundibulum, ectopic posterior pituitary).

Holoprosencephaly (HPE)

There are multiple types of holoprosencephaly noted in OMIM (e.g. HPE1 [OMIM%236100], HPE2 [OMIM#157170] and many more). These all result from failure of prosencephalon to divide adequately into two halves, which usually happens at 3–4 weeks' gestation. It is the most common forebrain malformation. Aetiology can be genetic as mentioned (there is a multiplicity of genes associated; see OMIM, www.omim.org) or environmental (from maternal diabetes, drug, alcohol or maternal treatment with retinoic acid), or a combination of the two.

There are three classic subtypes in this continuum of incomplete separation, with loss of midline structures of the face and the brain, and a merging of the third ventricle and lateral ventricles:

1. *Alobar HPE*, where the thalami are fused, and there is one ventricle, with facial anomalies such as cyclopia.
2. *Semilobar HPE*, where there is more separation than alobar, but still fusion anteriorly, included fused thalami, and absence of olfactory tracts and corpus callosum.
3. *Lobar HPE*, the final and least affected of the three, has fusion of the cingulate gyrus and the thalami, with absent/hypoplastic olfactory tracts and absent/hypoplastic corpus callosum.

Two other less severe subtypes are: the middle interhemispheric fusion variant (MIHV) type (where posterior frontal and parietal lobes; and basal ganglia and thalami, fail to part), and there is a septo-pre-optic type (where non-separation only occurs in septal and pre-optic areas).

For many of the known genetic causes of HPE, molecular testing is available: 25–50% of HPE have a chromosomal anomaly (numeric or structural); 18–25% of patients with monogenic HPE have a syndrome; and 10% of patients with HPE have an abnormality in the biosynthesis of cholesterol.

There are many other structural CNS associations (abnormal midline structures, Dandy-Walker syndrome, caudal dysgenesis, anomalies of neuronal migration) and a continuum of craniofacial anomalies (in around 80%).

The mnemonic **HPE FUSED** includes selected features of HPE:

Hypotonia/**H**ypothalamic dysfunction/**H**ead size: microcephaly common, macrocephaly uncommon (**H**ydrocephalus)
Pituitary deficiency: posterior or anterior pituitary hormones; central DI/**P**neumonia (aspiration)
Epilepsy (often hard to control)

Feeding difficulties (multiple causes, including poor tone, poor suck)
Uncoordinated oral-sensory function
Spina bifida can accompany/**S**leep disturbances
Eating slow/**E**sophageal reflux
Developmental delay

While children with the more severe forms (e.g. alobar) usually die before their first birthday, over half the children with semilobar or lobar HPE survive beyond 12 months, and these survivors generally have normal vision and hearing, and can smile.

History

PRESENTING COMPLAINT

Reason for current admission.

CURRENT SYMPTOMS

1. Cognitive abilities, or present developmental status (e.g. intellectual impairment), schooling details (related to underlying diagnosis, complications of hypopituitarism per se [hypothyroidism, hypoglycaemia]; similar for 2, 3 and 4 below).
2. Learning issues at school (e.g. visual–spatial–perceptual skills, reading disability, executive functioning skills, any neuropsychometric testing by guidance officer), any help needed, attitudes of class teacher, fellow students.
3. Behavioural issues (e.g. ADHD, ASD [especially in SOD] symptomatology and any relevant medications such as stimulants), professionals involved in management (psychologist, psychiatrist, paediatrician, therapists).
4. Speech, hearing, communication problems, professionals involved.
5. Vision (e.g. decreased visual acuity, bitemporal visual field cuts [pituitary tumour], strabismus known optic nerve hypoplasia [SOD], progress with MRI results, frequency of ophthalmic/MRI evaluations).
6. Neurological symptoms seizures (SOD, HPE, previous hypoglycaemia).
7. Growth and puberty (e.g. short stature, delayed puberty).
8. Symptoms referrable to ACTH deficiency: weight loss, postural dizziness, weakness, fatigue, anorexia, nausea, myalgia, arthralgia; symptoms of hypoglycaemia, hyponatraemia and anaemia.
9. Symptoms referrable to TSH deficiency: weight gain, cold intolerance, depression, fatigue, constipation, menstrual disorders, myalgias.
10. Symptoms referrable to LH/FSH deficiency: fatigue, decreased cognition, altered mood, menstrual disorders.
11. Symptoms referrable to GH deficiency: short stature, decreased energy.
12. Symptoms referrable to ADH deficiency: polyuria, polydipsia, nocturia.
13. Symptoms referrable to craniopharyngioma: headache, trouble waking, loss of balance, difficulty walking, change in energy level, sleepiness, hearing loss, change in personality, current known tumours, current treatment regimen.
14. Symptoms referrable to radiotherapy and underlying diagnosis leading to radiation therapy.
15. Symptoms referrable to SOD: temperature instability, hearing impairment (sensorineural), anosmia, developmental milestones delayed, ASD behaviours, seizures, sleep disturbances, increased appetite.
16. Symptoms referrable to HPE: developmental milestones delayed, cognitive impairment, seizures, hydrocephalus, shunt, involuntary movements, unusual posturing (dystonia), requirement for surgery for craniofacial defects, hydrocephalus, feeding (gastrostomy).

BIRTH HISTORY

1. Maternal past history of miscarriages or infertility.
2. Pregnancy: hyperemesis, hypertensive disease of pregnancy, teratogenic medications, placental problems, clinical evidence of (or exposure to) infection (e.g. TORCH),

quality of fetal movements, gestational age. Prenatal ultrasonic identification of malformations of HPE (often obvious) or SOD (usually subtle).

3. Delivery: presentation (e.g. breech, face), instrumental delivery, Apgar score, resuscitation required, birth weight, need for oxygen, nursery care, recognition of dysmorphic features of HPE (microcephaly, microphthalmia, hypotelorism, cleft lip, palate) or SOD (nystagmus).

4. Neonatal period: hypothermia, hypoglycaemia, hyperbilirubinaemia (phototherapy or exchange transfusion), lethargy, respiratory distress, metabolic acidosis, hypotonia, feeding difficulties, seizures, hypoglycaemia, hyponatraemia, hyperbilirubinaemia (phototherapy or exchange transfusion), complications of prematurity (intraventricular haemorrhage [IVH], periventricular leukomalacia [PVL], hydrocephalus, retinopathy of prematurity [ROP]). Neonatal examination: tremors, irritability, abnormal Moro reflex, hypotonia, midline CNS defects, microgenitalia, hypoplastic scrotal sac, bilateral undescended testes. Whether diagnosis made as neonate, any treatment given as a neonate (IV dextrose, hydrocortisone, thyroxine).

PAST HISTORY

1. Initial diagnosis: what age informed diagnosis of hypopituitarism/underlying cause (e.g. SOD, CPHD, holoprosencephaly, craniopharyngioma).
2. Time period between being informed of hypopituitarism diagnosis and development of symptoms.
3. What investigations undertaken to confirm diagnosis.
4. Evolution of seizures, evolution/regression of development.
5. Number of hospitalisations and indications for these.
6. Development of complications (e.g. learning issues at school, ADHD and/or ASD symptomatology) and their management.
7. Previous medications tried.
8. Immunisations, allergies.

CURRENT MANAGEMENT

Present treatment in hospital, usual treatment at home (for underlying conditions such as TBI, SOD, HPE) including physiotherapy, occupational therapy, speech therapy, exercise, medications taken, future treatment plans, usual follow-up (by whom, where, how often), unproven (not really 'alternative') therapies tried (e.g. naturopathy).

SOCIAL HISTORY

1. Impact on child (e.g. delays or regression in development, difficulties at school, limitations on lifestyle, body image, self-esteem, peer reactions).
2. Impact on family (e.g. parental coping, difficulties between mother and father, effect on siblings, financial considerations, transport, hospitalisations, private health insurance).
3. Benefits received.
4. Social supports (e.g. social worker), early intervention services for children with disabilities (e.g. via the Australian Government's Department of Social Services at https://dss.gov.au, Better Start at www.betterstart.net.au).

FAMILY HISTORY

Any family members with hypopituitarism or underlying genetic causes (e.g. CPHD, CHARGE, SOD, HPE).

UNDERSTANDING OF DISEASE

By the child, by the family (e.g. parents, siblings, grandparents) and by teachers. Ask about the degree of previous education about hypopituitarism (e.g. in hospital, by local paediatrician), and contingency plans (adrenal crisis; status epilepticus).

At the completion of the history, think about what particular problems this family is experiencing at the moment, from the viewpoints of the child, the parents and the attending physicians. These three perspectives may be quite different.

Examination

The order for the examination can be remembered by the mnemonic **GREEN**:

GRowth (parameters, measurements)
Eye (acuity, fields)
Endocrine (Tanner stage, BP, pulse)
Neurological (gait, reflexes, disease-specific signs for underlying aetiology signs [e.g. SOD association, signs of raised ICP])

See the separate short case on hypopituitarism in this chapter.

Management

The candidate should be familiar with emergent issues which arise, not infrequently, in patients with hypopituitarism. Patients with panhypopituitarism (with posterior pituitary involvement) will have DI with potential hypernatraemic dehydration complicating management. The initial diagnosis may need to be followed by fluid resuscitation in acutely hypotensive infants, and immediate treatment of hypoglycaemia with intravenous dextrose and then glucocorticoid. This scenario can arise in neonates presenting, variously, with decreased oral intake, generalised irritability, hypothermia, hypotension, hypoventilation, hypoglycaemia, hyperbilirubinaemia or microgenitalia.

Around a fifth of neonates with hypopituitarism present with hypoglycaemia, which can manifest with a vast array of symptoms; hypoglycaemia can cause almost any symptom one can think of in a neonate, except for fever and colour change; therefore, the first symptom of hypopituitarism could be jitteriness, tremors, seizures, poor suck, poor feeding, refusal to feed, hypotonia, lethargy, tachypnoea, high-pitched cry, exaggerated reflexes or temperature instability.

The physical examination of the male neonate with hypopituitarism may only demonstrate micropenis (defined as measurement of less than 2.5 standard deviations below the mean in a full-term male [mean is 3.5 cm], which means less than 2–2.5 cm), and otherwise be normal. Another clue to hypopituitarism would be delayed separation of the umbilical cord, which can happen in hypothyroidism, either primary or secondary.

Glucocorticoid hormone replacement therapy

Glucocorticoids should always be given before (the next hormone) thyroxine. The reason is that thyroxine can increase the rate of metabolism of the glucocorticoid, which thus increases the risk of adrenal crisis, the most immediate life-threatening aspect of hypopituitarism.

Deficiency of adrenocorticotropic hormone (ACTH; also called corticotrophin) may be termed *central* adrenal insufficiency (CAI). Glucocorticoid replacement is essential in CAI, but mineralocorticoid replacement is not needed. ACTH is the major regulator of glucocorticoid production and secretion, whereas mineralocorticoid regulation is affected not solely by ACTH, but also by the renin–angiotensin system, plus by direct stimulation determined by serum electrolyte concentrations.

Mineralocorticoid secretion is maintained in CAI, so there are no features of mineralocorticoid deficiency (such as hypovolaemia, or hyperkalaemia or salt craving), and no increased skin pigmentation.

Hyponatraemia in CAI may occur, however, not involving any mineralocorticoid effect but due to inappropriate ADH secretion, caused by glucocorticoid deficiency or due to central hypothyroidism.

The candidate should be conversant with the following child recommendations for CAI:

1. *Acute (central) adrenal crisis*: for this scenario, a child will require intravenous fluids consisting of normal (0.9%) saline, with added glucose (between 5% and 10% dextrose, depending on the age of the patient [10% dextrose for neonates; between 5% and 10% dextrose for age up to 6 months, then 5% should be sufficient after 6 months, but this is a guide only; monitoring the plasma glucose will guide this more immediately]).

   In addition to fluid resuscitation, the child will need hydrocortisone, in 'stress' dosages. The initial dosage should be hydrocortisone 100 mg/m^2 IV (or IM) and then 100 mg/m^2/day in 3 or 4 divided doses. An easy-to-remember approximation to this is: in infants, 25 mg hydrocortisone; for school-aged children, 50 mg hydrocortisone; for adolescents, 100–150 mg hydrocortisone IV (or IM); these doses can be repeated each 6–8 hours and adjusted as needed. When the IV line is first placed, blood should be taken to check serum glucose and electrolytes, plus to check cortisol and ACTH, but never wait for these results before initiating treatment with fluids and steroids.

2. *Chronic adrenocortical deficiency*: for this scenario, a child will need maintenance therapy, which generally means oral hydrocortisone 8–15 mg/m^2/day in 3 or 4 divided doses, or equivalent dose of cortisone acetate (remember hydrocortisone 4 mg = cortisone 5 mg) plus a plan to increase the therapy in certain circumstances, which can be termed 'stress' therapy.

Physiological stresses include surgery, physical trauma, haemorrhage or any illness. It is very important that the child's parents are well versed in all the potentially 'stressful' circumstances that can occur. All children with hypopituitarism must have medical identification bracelets or tags or cards (or tattoos in some adolescents).

Children receiving medications which induce cytochrome P450 hepatic enzyme inducers need to take increased dosages of their usual glucocorticoid medication; this includes children receiving phenobarbitone, phenytoin, topiramate or rifampicin, each of which increases steroid clearance. Another reason to increase the usual dosage in older teenagers is mentioned for completion: pregnancy; here the dosage should be increased by at least 50%, in the third trimester.

Recommendations include *tripling or quadrupling the child's usual dose* for intercurrent febrile illnesses, minor surgery or minor trauma. This dosage would generally correlate to hydrocortisone 50–62.5 mg/m^2/day in 3 or 4 divided doses. An easy-to-remember approximation to this is 1 mg/kg hydrocortisone repeated every 6–8 hours and adjusted as needed.

For more significant surgery, for vomiting or diarrhoea, or for significant febrile illness requiring hospitalisation, the hydrocortisone should be given parenterally, which usually means IV.

IM hydrocortisone may be given in a number of scenarios, including at a general practice, where there may not be the set-up for intravenous cannulation, while awaiting an ambulance to transport the child to a paediatric facility.

All patients with hypopituitarism require regular follow-up of their growth, blood pressure and serum electrolytes in particular, looking for evidence of over- or under-replacement.

There is a very rare complication of preexisting pituitary pathology which has been reported occasionally in paediatric patients: pituitary apoplexy. This is caused by a sudden event, either haemorrhage or infarction, affecting the pituitary gland, usually within a preexisting but undiagnosed pituitary adenoma. A CT scan can identify quickly haemorrhage and necrotic tissue; treatment involves intravenous glucocorticoid, and may require transsphenoidal decompression in some patients. It is mentioned for completion.

Thyroid hormone replacement therapy

Thyroid hormone replacement should always follow confirmation of normal adrenal function, or adequate treatment of CAI, as mentioned earlier. The thyroxine tablet (levothyroxine) comes as 50 µg, so the dosage is rounded to the nearest that can be achieved by quartering a tablet. The recommended dose is 100 mg/m^2/day, given once daily. This approximates to: age 1–6 months: 7–12 µg/kg daily; age 6–12 months: 6–8 µg/kg daily; age 1–5 years; 4–6 µg/kg daily; age 5–10 years: 3–5 µg/kg daily; 10–20 years: 2–3 µg/kg daily.

Growth hormone (GH) replacement therapy

The mean commencement age for GH replacement in Australia is around 5 years. GH therapy may need to start in the neonatal period or infancy, especially if there is ongoing hypoglycaemia. GH deficient patients usually respond to doses in the range of 4.5–6 mg/m^2/week, delivered in divided daily doses. It is recognised that patients respond more effectively to GH in their first year of treatment, than in subsequent years. The dose is titrated upwards to an optimal maintenance dose. Each time the child is reviewed in clinic the height, weight and body surface area (BSA) should be recorded, and a bone age is useful.

Antidiuretic hormone (ADH) replacement therapy

Without antidiuretic hormone (ADH), the distal tubules and collecting ducts of the kidney cannot reabsorb water or concentrate urine, acting more like a sieve and permitting non-homeostatic loss of water. The result is massive volumes of water lost in the urine; urinary osmolality is very low (50–100 mOsm) and specific gravity of urine is < 1.005. Urinary sodium and potassium concentrations are low (sodium < 20 mEq/L, potassium < 10 mEq/L).

The standard treatment of choice for central DI is desmopressin (DDAVP), which is a synthetic drug, an analogue of ADH. Desmopressin can be given intranasally, orally, subcutaneously (SC) or IV; doses are not equivalent. Oral dosing is usually preferred for convenience and better stability of absorption compared to nasal. The dosing varies with the chosen mode of administration. The medication dose is started low and built up gradually, to control the symptoms of polyuria and polydipsia.

Water intake must be closely monitored. Fluid balance is vitally important in these children. They should not drink beyond their thirst being satisfied, because increased fluid intake can lead to hyponatraemia, which can be life-threatening.

The medical management of central DI is very complicated and beyond the scope of this book. Some general points are given below that are worth knowing if one encounters a child in the long-case scenario:

- For *nasal* DDAVP, starting dose is 1–5 µg/day given via nasal route, in 1 or 2 divided doses; the usual maintenance dose is *2–40 µg/day*.
- For *oral* DDAVP, starting dose is 50–100 µg/day, orally, in 1 to 2 divided doses; the usual maintenance dose is *200–1200 µg/day*.
- For *parenteral* DDAVP, starting dose is 0.1–0.5 µg/dose IV or IM; the usual maintenance dose is *0.2–4 µg/day IV or IM*. Parenteral doses are usually given

in postoperative or acutely very unwell patients. Urine specific gravity and urine osmolarity being kept at normal values is the goal.

The daily dose is specific to that which the individual patient requires to control diuresis.

In some infants, low-solute feeds with thiazide diuretics can be used instead of DDAVP. The paradoxical effect that thiazides have on DI has been recognised for over 50 years, but the mechanism remains unclear. Current theories support the effect being secondary to an increase in renal sodium excretion. Thiazide diuretics are known to act on the distal convoluted tubule (DCT) by inhibiting the NaCl co-transporter.

Gonadotropin hormone replacement therapy

The earliest gonadotropin replacement is needed in the male infant who has a micropenis, meaning below 2–2.5 cm length. These babies require testosterone. A typical preparation would be testosterone enanthate 25 mg IM three times every 4 weeks. Usually the penis will increase in length by at least 0.9 cm after the first dose; if it has not then the dose should be repeated.

Induction of puberty is the next time gonadotropin replacement becomes important. Induction of puberty usually commences at 11 years in girls and 12 years in boys. There are many different protocols and guidelines regarding each.

Induction of puberty in girls

The first aspect of induction is achieving adequate oestrogenisation by gradually increasing doses of oestrogen over 12–24 months, followed by introduction of cyclic progesterone (either medroxyprogesterone, at 5–10 mg/day, or norethisterone at 0.7–1.0 mg/day, added every 12–14 days), which may be when uterine breakthrough bleeding occurs, to induce menstruation. The initial medications used include conjugated oestrogens (0.15 mg daily or 0.30 mg alternate daily), ethinyl oestradiol (0.05–0.10 µg/kg/day) or 17-beta-oestradiol orally (5 µg/kg/day) or transdermal patches (0.85 µg/kg/day). The dose is generally increased every 6 months, over the next 2–3 years, until adult dose is reached or adequate adult breast size is reached.

Induction of puberty in boys

Testosterone undecanoate (Andriol, orally) is commonly used in the early stages of induction, often switching to injectable preparations or skin gels in the later stages. Long-acting injectable preparations are available for adult maintenance therapy (Reandron, testosterone undecanoate).

There is not a standard protocol for this. Some approaches commence at age 12, by gradually increasing doses of testosterone. Other preparations can include testosterone enanthate or testosterone cypionate, at a dose of 15–50 mg IM per month. The dose is kept low to ensure optimal growth. The dose is gradually increased every 6 to 12 months, over the following 3–5 years, until adult dosage is reached.

SHORT CASES

SHORT CASE: Disorders of sexual development (DSD) (ambiguous genitalia)

This is an uncommon, but exceedingly important, case. The inability to determine the sex of a newborn immediately at birth is one of the most difficult clinical problems. Some causes are life-threatening (CAH). A comprehensive approach is essential and, after the diagnosis is made, issues of sex of rearing give candidates much scope for fielding interesting questions. To understand this area, some background embryology is worth reviewing, as are pathways of steroid hormone synthesis. The latter are discussed in the long case on CAH (in this chapter); the former is outlined below. This problem is also termed 'intersex' by some.

There are five groups of babies:

1. 46,XX DSD: genetic females with ambiguous or male phenotype.
2. 46,XY DSD: genetic males with ambiguous or female phenotype.
3. Ovotesticular DSD: usually 46,XX, genitalia usually ambiguous, gonads contain both ovarian and testicular components.
4. Sex chromosome aneuploidy DSD: for example, 45,X/46,XY mosaicism, with one streak gonad and one dysgenetic testis (also known as mixed gonadal dysgenesis).
5. Other: dysmorphic syndromes, cloacal anomalies, bladder exstrophy etc.

The most common scenario of these is female with ambiguous genitalia due to CAH.

There are two groups of babies that can be mistakenly labelled as having 'ambiguous genitalia'. The first group are premature female infants with an unusual genital appearance; these apparent genital abnormalities are transient. The second group have perineal anatomy that is abnormal, but that is not due to any endocrine problem. They have anatomical anomalies that are not within the range of normal sexual differentiation, such as significant defects in caudal embryogenesis, which can be associated with complete aplasia of the genital tubercle such that neither a penis nor a clitoris are present. These babies do not have an intersex condition; they have anomalies of the perineum unaffected by hormones. Often, these are ano-genital malformations, not just genital ones. They are mentioned here for completeness.

There is a scoring system for the degree of masculinisation of the external genitalia described by Prader, numerically graded from 0 to 5. Prader 0 refers to normal female anatomy. Prader 5 refers to normal male anatomy. The numbers in between describe the transition from the embryological default outcome of female towards masculinity imposed by exposure to androgens. Prader 1 refers to an enlarged phallus, Prader 2 an enlarged phallus with visibly separate openings of urethra and vagina, Prader 3 refers to an enlarged phallus with a single urogenital sinus opening and Prader 4 an enlarged phallus with hypospadias.

Until 7 weeks' gestation, the internal genital tracts are bipotential in both XX and XY embryos. In both, the genital ducts are the wolffian (mesonephric) duct and the müllerian (paramesonephric) duct. In a normal male, the wolffian duct transforms into the epididymis, vas deferens and seminal vesicles. In a normal female, the müllerian duct transforms into the uterus, fallopian tubes and upper portion of the vagina.

If the SRY (sex-determining region on the Y chromosome) gene is present (as in a normal male), the indifferent (or ambisexual) gonad will develop into a testis. By 8 weeks' gestation, the Sertoli cells in the testis produce müllerian-inhibiting substance/anti-müllerian hormone (MIS/AMH), while the fetal Leydig cells produce testosterone and INSL3, a peptide hormone involved in the regulation of testicular descent. The müllerian duct regresses between 8 and 12 weeks, due to MIS/AMH. Concurrently between 8 and 12 weeks' gestation, androgens transform the genital primordium into normal male external genitalia. Testosterone is converted by 5-alpha-reductase into dihydrotestosterone (DHT). DHT causes the genital tubercle to develop into the penis, with the male urethra opening at the tip, the outer labioscrotal folds to fuse into the midline scrotal raphe, forming the scrotum, and the urogenital sinus to differentiate into the bladder and the prostatic urethra. From 12 weeks until full term, enlargement of the phallus to normal penile size occurs. All external virilisation is due to androgens.

If the SRY gene is absent (as in a normal female), the bipotential gonad will develop into an ovary. Lack of testosterone and MIS/AMH leads to regression of the wolffian duct and preservation of the müllerian ducts. In the absence of androgens, the genital tubercle and the urethral plate form the clitoris and short female urethra, the labioscrotal folds remain unfused to become labia majora, and the vaginal plate, part of the posterior wall of the urogenital sinus, canalises, so forming the lower vagina.

Sexual differentiation of the brain occurs between 15 and 25 weeks' gestation.

Examination for ambiguous genitalia

1. General examination:
   - Skin: hyperpigmentation (CAH); may be subtle; best seen in genitalia and areolae.
   - Syndromal diagnosis: head, heart, hands (e.g. Beckwith; see the short-case approach to the dysmorphic child in Chapter 9, Genetics and dysmorphology).
   - Hydration: assess for dehydration secondary to vomiting (CAH).
   - Blood pressure: elevated in CAH due to 11-beta-hydroxylase deficiency or 17-alpha-hydroxylase deficiency.
2. Abdomen/pelvis/genitalia:
   - Inspect for Prader grading of virilisation of external genitalia:
     - Prader 0: Normal female.
     - Prader 1: Enlargement of phallus (looks more like clitoris; abnormal exposure to androgens beyond 8 weeks' gestation).
     - Prader 2: Enlargement of phallus, vagina and urethra openings separate.
     - Prader 3: Enlargement of phallus, urogenital sinus (single opening).
     - Prader 4: Enlarged phallus with hypospadias.
     - Prader 5: Normal male.
   - Inspect the scrotum:
     - Fused, absent gonads (must exclude XX with CAH).
     - Bifid, bilateral gonads present (undervirilised XY; true hermaphrodite with bilateral ovotestes rarely).
     - Bifid, maldeveloped, bilateral gonads placed high (undervirilised XY, true hermaphrodite with ovotestes rarely, or XY gonadal dysgenesis [dysplastic testes]).
   - Examine the midline cleft/urogenital sinus:
     - Gently open cleft/sinus; confirm impression of Prader stage. Skin tags with purplish tinge imply hymen present.
   - Palpation for gonads:
     - Gonads palpable bilaterally, can be brought to base of scrotum (almost certainly testes and almost certainly male; bilateral ovotestes in true hermaphrodite rare).
     - Gonads palpable bilaterally but placed high (undervirilised XY, true hermaphrodite with ovotestes rarely, or XY gonadal dysgenesis [dysplastic testes]).

- Gonads palpable bilaterally but asymmetrical position/descent (true hermaphrodite with a testis on one side and an ovotestis on the other, or mixed gonadal dysgenesis with a testis on one side and a streak ovary with a hernia on the other).
- Single gonad palpable (almost certainly testis; other may be ovary, streak gonad [mixed gonadal dysgenesis] or ovotestis [true hermaphrodite]).
- Gonads impalpable bilaterally (cannot predict gonadal status).
- Rectal examination should be mentioned; the little finger can palpate the cervix and confirm a uterus.

At the completion of physical assessment, give a differential diagnosis, followed by a list of investigations appropriate for that patient. A suggested list for each follows.

Differential diagnosis

VIRILISED FEMALE

1. Congenital adrenal hyperplasia (CAH)—deficiency of:
   - **21-alpha-hydroxylase** (converts progesterone → **deo**xycortisone [DOC]; 17OH progesterone → 11 deoxycortisol); affected gene is CYP21A2; OMIM#201910; this is called 21-OHD CAH.
   - **11-beta-hydroxylase** (11 deoxycortisol → cortisol; 11 deoxycorticosterone → corticosterone); affected gene is CYP11B1; this also is called 11-OHD CAH.
   - **3-beta-hydroxysteroid-dehydrogenase** (pregnenolone → progesterone; 17OH pregnenolone → 17OH progesterone; **dehydroepia**ndrosterone [DHEA] → androstenedione; androstenediol → testosterone); affected gene is HSD3B2; this also is called HSDB3 deficiency.
2. Androgen exposure in utero (maternal androgens):
   - Progesterone.
   - Medroxyprogesterone.
   - 19 nortestosterones.

TESTICULAR FAILURE (UNDERVIRILISED MALES)

1. Deficiency of:
   - *Steroid acute regulatory protein (STAR)* (cholesterol → pregnenolone), causing lipoid congenital adrenal hyperplasia (LCAH); affected gene is STAR.
   - *3-beta-hydroxysteroid-dehydrogenase* (pregnenolone → progesterone; 17OH pregnenolone → 17OH progesterone; DHEA → androstenedione; androstenediol → testosterone); affected gene is HSD3B2; this is also called HSDB3 deficiency.
   - *17-alpha-hydroxylase* (pregnenolone → 17OH pregnenolone; progesterone → 17OH progesterone); affected gene is CYP17A1; this also is called 17-OHD CAH.
   - *17,20 lyase* (17OH pregnenolone → DHEA; 17OH progesterone → androstenedione); affected gene is CYP17A, same as above.
   - *17-beta-hydroxysteroid-dehydrogenase 17-HSD/17 ketosteroid reductase* (DHEA → androstenediol; androstenedione → testosterone); affected gene is HSD17B3.
   - *5-alpha-reductase* (testosterone → dihydrotestosterone, DHT); affected gene is SRD5A2.
2. Anatomic:
   - 46 XY pure gonadal dysgenesis (usually appear female).
   - 46 XY mosaic (45 X/46 XY) or isochromosome.
3. Partial androgen insensitivity (PAIS).

IMPORTANT POINTS

1. Males with STAR deficiency (OMIM#201710, also called LCAH), 3-beta-hydroxysteroid dehydrogenase deficiency (OMIM#201810, also called HSDB) or 17-hydroxylase deficiency (OMIM#202110, also called 17-OH CAH) have ambiguous or female genitalia, due to inadequate exposure to testosterone during the first trimester of fetal life.

2. Children with 11-beta-hydroxylase (gene CYP11B1) deficiency (11-OHD CAH, OMIM#202010) or 17-alpha-hydroxylase (gene CYP17A1) deficiency (17-OHD CAH, OMIM#202110) have hypertension, due to excessive production of deoxycorticosteroid, a mineralocorticoid.

3. Females with 17-alpha-hydroxylase deficiency are rarely diagnosed early, presenting with delayed puberty or hypertension.

Investigations

BLOOD TESTS

Chromosomes for karyotype, urea and electrolytes, 17OH progesterone, cortisol, ACTH, PRA, testosterone, DHT, DHEA, androstenedione.

PROVOCATION TESTS

HCG stimulation for testosterone or DHT synthesis. Also used to assess ratio of androstenedione to testosterone (elevated in 17-HSD). ACTH stimulation for differentiating types of CAH.

IMAGING

Pelvic ultrasound.

SPECIALISED TESTS

Androgen binding studies; androgen receptor gene mutation analysis.

SHORT CASE: Type 1 diabetes mellitus (T1DM)

The introduction for this case usually requests examination for complications of diabetes or for assessment of quality of control. The candidate needs to be aware not only of the complications, but also of their time course and relation to glucose control.

It may be another chronic disease process that is causing the diabetes, such as cystic fibrosis or β-thalassaemia major. This is worth keeping in the back of your mind when initially assessing growth and Tanner staging in particular. Thus, it is relevant to scan for thalassaemic facies and hyperpigmentation, or clubbing and cough, although usually the patient will only have type 1 diabetes. Other associations may be readily apparent, such as Friedreich ataxia (FRDA), Wolfram syndrome (features of which are known by the mnemonic **DIDMOAD: D**iabetes **I**nsipidus, **D**iabetes **M**ellitus, **O**ptic **A**trophy, **D**eafness) or Cushing's syndrome.

Examination

Begin by introducing yourself. Have the child adequately undressed to allow a complete examination: this usually means fully undressed down to underwear in younger children, but not necessarily in older children. Assess weight and height parameters, and percentile charts. Poor growth can be due to inadequate insulin dosage or poor compliance, associated impaired thyroid function or coexistent chronic disease. Assess pubertal status, hydration and whether the child looks sick or well. Look for any intravenous lines and read the labels on any intravenous fluid being administered.

Pick up the child's hands. Look for any cutaneous infection or trophic changes, and carefully inspect the fingertips for prick marks indicating regular blood glucose testing. Assess for LJM by asking the child to hold his or her hands in the 'prayer' position, and looking for lack of apposition of palmar aspects of the fingers (when positive, this is called the cathedral sign). If there is evidence of LJM, go on to extend the distal and proximal interphalangeal joints (normally extend to 180°), the metacarpophalangeal joints (normally extend to 60°), the wrist (normally extends to 70°) and the elbow (at least 180°). Note the colour of the palmar creases; they may be pigmented due to coexistent Addison disease, or underlying thalassaemia major with haemosiderosis.

Next, take, or request, the blood pressure (hypertension with nephropathy, postural hypotension with autonomic neuropathy or dehydration in ketoacidosis, hypotension with Addison disease).

Examine the eyes. Look carefully for squint, cataract and contact lenses (or nearby glasses). Check the visual acuity in each eye, and then the eye movements (for neuropathy). Check the pupillary reactions and the red reflex, and assess the retinae for diabetic retinopathy, of which there are three groups:

1. Background lesions include microaneurysms, retinal haemorrhages, hard exudates, cottonwool spots (small retinal infarcts) and venous beading.
2. Proliferative lesions include new vessel networks (arising from peripheral vessels or from vessels overlying the optic disc), vitreous haemorrhage and retinal detachment.
3. Maculopathy, which is rare, includes oedema and hard exudate deposition. Also look for optic atrophy (DIDMOAD).

Examine the mouth for ketotic breath and oral candidiasis, and to assess hydration. Then inspect for goitre, palpate the thyroid gland, assess movement with swallowing and auscultate if there is thyroid enlargement (associated autoimmune thyroid disease). Next, in girls, assess breast development (for delayed puberty; Tanner staging pictures on growth charts can be useful).

The abdomen is then inspected for injection sites, fat atrophy or hypertrophy, any distension (associated coeliac disease), pubertal status and insulin pump. Palpate the liver for hepatomegaly (from glycogen if 'overinsulinised' or fat if 'underinsulinised') and, in boys, note the size of the testes (for pubertal delay). Mention looking for perineal candidiasis in girls, but this does not need to be performed.

The legs are then assessed for injection sites on the thigh, and any associated fat atrophy or hypertrophy, and the lower legs for necrobiosis lipoidica diabeticorum. Look at, and between, the toes, for trophic changes or candidiasis. Finally, check for peripheral neuropathy: check the reflexes at the knee and ankle, and then examine for light touch, vibration and position sense.

Request urinalysis for glucose, ketones, protein or blood, and also the temperature chart for any infection that may have precipitated the presentation.

At this stage, the examiners may ask if there is anything further that you wish to do. Here, you can request a hearing test (DIDMOAD) and examine the ears, nose, throat and chest for any underlying infection. Finish by giving a succinct summary of the relevant findings and an overall assessment of disease control. You may then express interest in seeing the child's medication chart for insulin dosages, and the daily recordings of blood glucose levels before the current admission. Ask for the HbA1c, insulin dose regime, recent investigations such as TFTs, coeliac screening, lipid profile, urine microalbumin analysis. Ask for 24-hour BP profile. If unsure of diagnosis, ask for islet cell autoantibodies and MODY gene analysis.

Figure 7.1 summarises the examination for diabetes.

1. Introduce self

2. Position patient
Initial inspection standing, then lying,
   adequately undressed

3. General inspection
Parameters
Weight
Height
Percentiles
Well or unwell
Hydration
Intravenous lines
Tanner staging

4. Hands
Fingertip pricks
Trophic changes
Cutaneous infections
Limitation of joint mobility
Pigmented palmar creases (Addison)

5. Blood pressure
Hypertension (nephropathy)
Hypotension (Addison)
Postural hypotension (autonomic
   neuropathy, dehydration)

6. Eyes
Inspection
Squint
Cataract
Contact lenses
Visual acuity
Eye movements
Pupillary reactions
Red reflex (cataracts)
Fundi
Retinopathy
Optic atrophy (DIDMOAD)

7. Mouth
Hydration
Ketotic breath
Oral candidiasis

8. Thyroid
Inspect
Swallowing
Palpate
Auscultation

9. Abdomen
Injection sites
Fat atrophy, hypertrophy
Distension (coeliac disease)
Hepatomegaly

Tanner staging
Perineal candidiasis

10. Lower limbs
Injection sites
Fat atrophy, hypertrophy
Trophic changes
Candidiasis
Necrobiosis lipoidica
Reflexes
Sensation
Light touch
Vibration

11. Urinalysis
Glucose
Ketones
Protein
Blood

12. Other
Hearing (DIDMOAD)
ENT and chest (infection precipitating
   presentation)
Request insulin dosages and
   glucometer readings

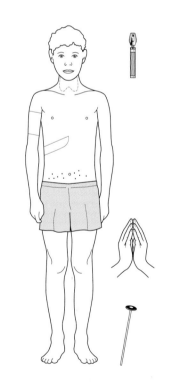

Figure 7.1 **Diabetes**

SHORT CASE: Short stature

This particular case covers more clinical ground than most and requires a very structured routine. The one outlined here proved successful both in practice cases and in the examination. It comprises four parts:

1. Observation.
2. Measurements.
3. Manoeuvres.
4. Systematic relevant examination.

Observation

First, listen carefully to the patient's age in the introduction. Then stand back and look for any evidence of an obvious diagnosis (e.g. Turner or Noonan syndromes), any dysmorphism and any disproportion (skeletal dysplasias, rickets), and visually assess the pubertal status. The pubertal status is particularly important.

Whether puberty is delayed, normal or precocious will determine the differential diagnoses to be considered as the examination progresses: for example, delayed puberty is consistent with constitutional delayed puberty, pituitary disorders and chronic diseases; normal puberty is consistent with familial short stature; and advanced pubertal staging is consistent with various causes of precocious puberty (see the short case on precocious puberty in this chapter). Comment on your findings.

Measurements

Explain what you are doing as you proceed. Ask for the height and offer to measure the patient yourself: stand the child against a wall, position the head and heels appropriately, and record the height. The lower segment (LS) is the distance from the pubic symphysis to the ground. The upper segment (US) is calculated by subtracting the LS from the total height. Work out the US:LS ratio: normal values are 1.7 at birth, 1.3 at 3 years, 1.0 at 8 years and 0.9 at 18 years.

INTERPRETATION OF THE US:LS RATIO AND ARM SPAN

- If the US:LS ratio is increased, it suggests short lower limbs (skeletal dysplasias, hypothyroidism).
- If the US:LS ratio is decreased, it suggests a short trunk (scoliosis, spondylodysplasia, osteogenesis imperfecta [OI]) or short neck (Klippel–Feil sequence).
- Next, measure the child's arm span, and compare this to the total height. The normal arm span minus height values: −3 cm from birth to 7 years, 0 cm from 8–12 years, +1 cm (girls) and +4 cm (boys) at 14 years.
- A short arm span can occur with skeletal dysplasias, and an apparently long arm span with a short neck, trunk or legs.
- If the span is less than the height with a high US:LS, this may indicate short limbs and a normal trunk, or normal limbs and a long trunk.
- If the span is greater than the height with a low US:LS, this indicates a short trunk and normal limbs.
- If the span is less than the height with a low or normal US:LS ratio, this indicates short trunk and limbs.

Measure the head circumference and request the weight. Request percentile charts and progressive measurements (if not given), and calculate the height velocity (be aware of the normal range and nature of percentile charts). Request the birth parameters (for intrauterine and chromosomal causes, such as being SGA) and the parents' heights and onsets of puberty (for family history of constitutional delayed puberty).

By now, you may well have a good indication of the type of short stature with which you are dealing.

After all these parameters have been evaluated, either: 1. proceed with the manoeuvres below, particularly if the child is very short, or has obvious skeletal anomalies or a clearly disproportionate short stature; or 2. commence a systematic head-to-toe examination, and slot in the manoeuvres along the way, should they appear relevant. The order adopted is unimportant; it is the demonstration of a comprehensive approach that is required.

The mid-parental height (MPH) may be calculated: for girls, MPH = mother's height plus (father's height − 13 cm)/2, ± 6 cm; for boys, MPH = father's height plus (mother's height + 13 cm)/2, ± 7.5 cm.

Manoeuvres
INSPECT FROM FRONT

A set of manoeuvres can be performed that very rapidly screens for a number of syndromes that may be relevant in assessing short children. With each manoeuvre, stand opposite the child and demonstrate, so that he or she will mirror your movements.

Screen for asymmetry: have the child put the palms together with the arms out straight, and stand with legs together. Asymmetry occurs in Russell–Silver syndrome. Focus on the upper limbs first, then evaluate the lower limbs.

Screen for carrying angle: have the child hold the arms by their side, with palms forwards. This angle can be increased in Turner or Noonan syndromes. Also, restriction of elbow extension may be detected (e.g. hypochondroplasia).

Screen for short limbs: have the child touch the tips of the thumbs to the tips of the shoulders. If the thumbs overshoot, there is proximal-segment (rhizomelic) limb shortening. If the thumbs do not reach the shoulders, there might be either middle-segment (mesomelic) or distal-segment (acromelic) limb shortening, or alternatively the limbs may be bent (camptomelic). Thus, this manoeuvre should detect proximal-segment shortening (e.g. achondroplasia), middle-segment shortening (e.g. Langer mesomelic dysplasia) or distal-segment shortening (e.g. acromesomelic dysplasia).

Screen the hands: have the child hold the palms up. Look for simian crease (Down syndrome) and clinodactyly (Russell–Silver syndrome). Note the structure of the fingers (e.g. short with hypochondroplasia), their number and any syndactyly (e.g. Apert syndrome). Turn the hands over (palms down), note the structure of the hand (e.g. trident deformity in achondroplasia) and check the nails (e.g. hyperconvex in Turner).

Ask the child to make a fist and look for a shortened fourth metacarpal (pseudohypoparathyroidism).

INSPECT FROM THE SIDE

The child should be standing with the arms by his or her side. Note whether there is a prominent forehead (e.g. achondroplasia), flat occiput (Down), proptosis (e.g. syndromes with craniosynostosis), micrognathia (e.g. Pierre Robin sequence) or prognathism (e.g. achondroplasia). Note how far the upper limbs reach; if the limbs are short, the fingers may only reach the proximal thigh; if the trunk is short, the fingers may reach the knees. Note the shape of the back, for lordosis (e.g. achondroplasia), thoracolumbar kyphosis (e.g. achondroplasia) or crouched posture (e.g. diastrophic dysplasia).

INSPECT FROM THE BACK

Examine for scoliosis (and any kyphosis, which should have been noted already). Have the child bend forwards and touch the toes to determine whether any scoliosis is structural. Scoliosis can occur in dozens of syndromes, including many skeletal dysplasias, several trisomies and a number of popular examination syndromes (e.g. Noonan). Do explain what you are doing as you proceed, so that the examiners will be aware of the significance of the manoeuvres.

Examination

The formal physical examination flows well if commenced at the hands, working up to the head, and then downwards: essentially a 'head-to-toe' pattern. Table 7.3 ('Additional information') at the end of this section outlines the findings sought at each point.

At the completion of the comprehensive physical examination, request results of urinalysis (e.g. type 1 diabetes mellitus [T1DM], chronic kidney disease [CKD]) and stool analysis (malabsorption from cystic fibrosis [CF], coeliac disease, inflammatory bowel disease [IBD]). Finally, summarise your findings succinctly and give a brief differential diagnosis, placing the most likely diagnosis first (see Fig. 7.2).

Investigations

At this stage, you may be asked what investigations you would perform. Depending on the findings, of course, the answers vary. Generally, a bone age is most useful and, in girls, a chromosomal analysis is always warranted to exclude Turner syndrome.

Other investigations often ordered include thyroid function tests (hypothyroidism), electrolytes, urea and creatinine (CKD), tissue transglutaminase antibodies (coeliac disease) and GH provocation testing (clonidine, arginine or glucagon), the latter only being performed after other preliminary testing is done (see Table 7.2), and poor height velocity is demonstrated. Low IGF-1 and IGFBP-3 levels are useful in predicting GH deficiency, or GH resistance, although normal levels do not exclude GH deficiency (see Table 7.2).

Table 7.2 lists some relatively simple investigations that may be useful in the child with short stature. More common diagnoses in examination settings include constitutional delay in growth and puberty (maturational delay) and Russell–Silver syndrome.

Aetiologies

The mnemonic **IS NICE** lists various headings/causes for aetiologies of short stature:

Idiopathic (constitutional delay in growth and puberty [maturational delay]; familial short stature)/**I**ntrauterine (SGA, TORCH, fetal alcohol syndrome [FAS])

Skeletal causes (dysplasias, OI)/**S**pinal defects (scoliosis, kyphosis)/**S**yndromes (Russell–Silver, Kallmann)/**S**epto-optic dysplasia (SOD)

Nutritional (e.g. malabsorption)/**N**urturing (4deprivation)

Iatrogenic (steroids, radiation)

Chronic diseases (CKD, congenital heart disease, CF, IBD)/**C**hromosomal (Turner, Down)/**C**raniopharyngioma (or other central tumour)

Endocrine (e.g. GH deficiency, GH insensitivity, hypopituitarism, hypothyroidism, Cushing's syndrome, T1DM, pseudohypoparathyroidism)

Two other lists worth remembering enumerate the conditions that cause short stature and obesity. They are not comprehensive, but they are simple to recall. There are five endocrine causes and five syndromal causes.

Endocrine:
1. Hypothyroidism.
2. Hypopituitarism.
3. GH deficiency.
4. Cushing's syndrome.
5. Pseudohypoparathyroidism.

Syndromal:
1. Prader–Willi (P–W).
2. Bardet–Biedl (B–B).
3. Alström.
4. Down.
5. Fröhlich.

1. Introduce self

2. General inspection
Position patient: standing, undressed
    adequately to allow examination
    without embarrassment (underwear
    in young children)
Diagnostic facies
Disproportionate stature
Tanner staging
Nutritional status
Skeletal anomalies
Colour
Tachypnoea
Skin

3. Measurements and manoeuvres
See Figure 7.3

4. Upper limbs
Structure
Fingertips
Nails
Palms
Pulse
Joints
Blood pressure

5. Head and neck
Head
Hair
Eyes (full examination)
Nose
Mouth and chin
Ears
Hairline
Neck (thyroid)

6. Chest
Tanner staging
Chest deformity
Praecordium
Lung fields

7. Abdomen
Full abdominal examination

8. Genitalia
Tanner staging
Anomalies

9. Gait, back and lower limbs
Inspect lower limbs
Gait (full examination)
Back
Lower limbs neurologically

10. Other
Urinalysis
Stool analysis

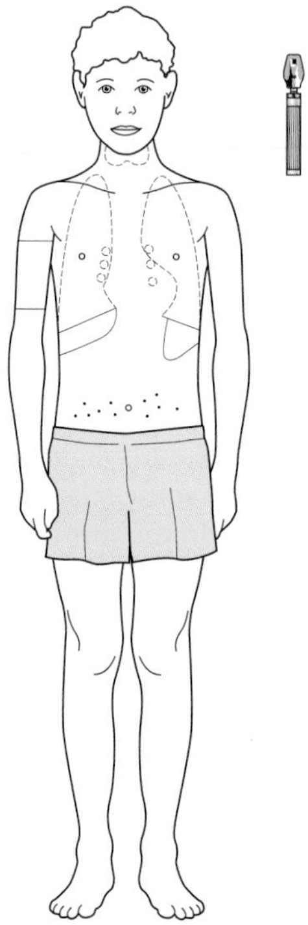

Figure 7.2 **Short stature: examination and observation**

Alternative introduction to short stature—endocrine

Occasionally, the lead-in for short stature has been: 'This child is short. Please examine the endocrine system'. For those who have learned a comprehensive approach such as that previously outlined, this can cause some concern. This should not be the case, as all that is required is some abbreviation of the previous system, with elimination of the irrelevant parts.

A. MEASUREMENTS

Height
Lower segment (LS)
Calculate upper segment
 (US) by subtracting LS from
 height
Calculate US:LS ratio

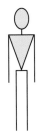

B. MEASUREMENTS

Arm span
Head circumference
Request weight
Assess percentile charts
Calculate height velocity
Request birth parameters
Request parents' percentiles
 and ages of puberty

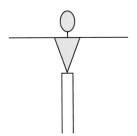

C. HANDS AND FEET
TOGETHER

To detect:
Asymmetry (Russell–Silver)
Approximation of shoulders
 (absent clavicles in
 cleidocranial dysostosis)

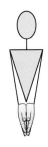

D. ARMS OUT STRAIGHT

To detect:
Cubitus valgus (Turner, Noonan)
 over 15° in girls;
 over 10° in boys

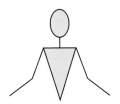

E. THUMBS ON SHOULDERS

To detect:
Proximal segment shortening
 (e.g. achondroplasia,
 hypochondroplasia)
Middle segment shortening
 (e.g. Len–Weill
 dyschondrostenosis,
 Langer mesomelic
 dysplasia)
Distal segment shortening
 (e.g. acromesomelic
 dysplasia)

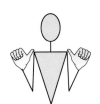

F. PALMS UP

To detect:
Simian crease (Down, Seckel)
Clinodactyly (Russell–Silver,
 Down, Seckel)

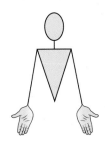

G. MAKE A FIST

To detect:
Short fourth metacarpal
 (pseudohypoparathyroidism,
 Turner, fetal alcohol)

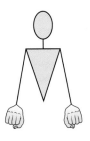

H. BACK

To detect:
Short neck (Klippel–Feil,
 Noonan)
Neck webbing (Turner, Noonan)
Low hairline (Turner, Noonan,
 Klippel–Feil)

I. BEND OVER AND
TOUCH TOES

To detect:
Scoliosis (e.g. Noonan,
 Klippel–Feil, Prader–Willi)

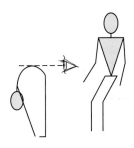

J. SIT UP

To commence systematic
 physical examination

Figure 7.3 Short stature: measurements and manoeuvres

Table 7.2

Some useful investigations in the child with short stature

INVESTIGATION	INDICATIONS/RELEVANCE
BLOOD	
Full blood examination and film	Chronic disease, anaemia
Erythrocyte sedimentation rate	Inflammatory bowel disease
Electrolytes, urea, creatinine	Chronic kidney disease
Fasting blood glucose	Diabetes
Calcium, phosphate, SAP	Rickets, hypophosphatasia
Liver function tests	CLD, nutritional deficiency
Tissue transglutaminase antibodies	Coeliac disease
Pancreatic isoamylase	Shwachman syndrome
Thyroid function tests, TSH	Hypothyroidism
Karyotype	Syndromes, e.g. Turner, Down
Somatomedin C (also called insulin-like growth factor, IGF1)	GH deficiency, coeliac, Crohn, malnutrition, hypothyroidism, T1DM (poorly controlled)
Insulin-like growth factor binding protein 3 (IGFBP-3)	GH deficiency
GH stimulation tests (arginine, clonidine, glucagon, GHRH)	GH deficiency
LH, FSH, prolactin, oestradiol, testosterone	Hypogonadism
Dexamethasone suppression test (combined high and low dose)	Cushing's syndrome
SWEAT	
Sweat conductivity	Cystic fibrosis
IMAGING	
Bone age	Maturational delay, precocious puberty, hypothyroidism, hypopituitarism
Skeletal survey	Skeletal dysplasias
Skull X-ray	Craniopharyngioma
MRI of brain	Intracranial tumour

CLD = chronic liver disease; FSH = follicle-stimulating hormone; GH = growth hormone; GHRH = growth hormone releasing hormone; LH = luteinising hormone; SAP = serum alkaline phosphatase; TSH = thyroid-stimulating hormone.

Remember that assessment for Turner syndrome is part of an endocrine assessment, as is evaluation for Kallmann syndrome, septo-optic dysplasia, craniopharyngioma or other central tumour (i.e. do not forget to test the visual acuity and visual fields, examine the optic fundi and perform a gait examination) and rickets. See Table 7.3 for additional information.

Table 7.3

Additional information: a more comprehensive listing of possible physical findings in children with short stature

GENERAL INSPECTION

Diagnostic facies
- Dysmorphic syndromes (Russell–Silver, Turner, Noonan, FAS)
- Endocrine disorders (GH deficiency, Cushing, hypothyroidism)
- Other (e.g. thalassaemia)

Disproportionate stature
- Skeletal dysplasias (achondroplasia)
- Metabolic bone disease (rickets)
- Connective tissue disorders (osteogenesis imperfecta [OI])

Tanner staging
- Advanced (precocious puberty)
- Delayed (constitutional delayed puberty [CDP]; chronic illness [CKD, CHD]; endocrine disorders [hypopituitarism, hypothyroidism])

Nutritional status
- Obese (endocrine causes, syndromal causes)
- Poor (malabsorption, undernutrition, chronic diseases)

Skeletal anomalies
- Asymmetry (Russell–Silver)
- Pectus excavatum (Noonan)
- Scoliosis (Noonan, Klippel–Feil)

Colour
- Pallor (thalassaemia, nutritional deficiency, CKD)
- Sallow (CKD)
- Jaundice (CLD)
- Cyanosis (CHD, CF)
- Pigmented (thalassaemia)

Tachypnoea
- Cardiac (CCF with large VSD)
- Respiratory (CF)

Irritability (coeliac disease)

Skin
- Various rashes related to nutritional deficiencies
- Erythema nodosum (IBD)
- Café-au-lait spots (NF1, Fanconi anaemia, Russell–Silver)

UPPER LIMBS

Structure
- Clinodactyly fifth finger (Russell–Silver, Shwachman, Seckel)
- Short fourth metacarpal (pseudohypoparathyroidism, Turner, FAS)
- Trident hand (achondroplasia)
- Polydactyly (Bardet–Biedl)

Fingertips: BSL testing (T1DM)

Continued

Table 7.3 (continued)

Nails
- Clubbing (CHD, CF, CLD)
- Brown lines (CKD)
- Leuconychia (CLD)
- Short (cartilage hair hypoplasia)
- Hyperconvex (Turner)
- Hypoplastic (FAS)

Fingers: swollen joints (JIA)

Palms
- Simian creases (Down)
- Crease pallor (anaemia from nutritional deficiency, CKD)
- Pigmented creases (thalassaemia, long-standing CAH)
- Erythema (CLD)

Wrists
- Swollen (JIA)
- Splaying (rickets)
- Deviation (JIA)
- A-V fistula (CKD)

Pulse
- Bradycardia (untreated hypothyroidism)
- Radiofemoral delay (coarctation of aorta with Turner, NF1)

Forearms: muscle bulk (malnutrition)

Blood pressure: elevated (CRF, Cushing, CAH, NF1, Turner with coarctation)

HEAD

Size
- Small (TORCH, syndromes)
- Large (intracranial tumour, toxoplasmosis)

Shape
- Triangular (Russell–Silver)
- Frontal bossing (rickets, thalassaemia)

Consistency: craniotabes (rickets)

Fontanelle
- Large (Russell–Silver, rickets, hypothyroidism)
- Bulging (intracranial tumour with raised ICP)

Hair
- Dry (hypothyroidism)
- Greasy (precocious puberty)

EYES

Inspection
- Photophobia (cystinosis)
- Hypertelorism (Noonan, William)
- Epicanthal folds (Noonan, William, Turner, Down)
- Ptosis (Noonan, pseudohypoparathyroidism)
- Squint (William, Prader–Willi, septo-optic dysplasia [SOD])
- Nystagmus (SOD)

Conjunctivae: pallor (CKD, malnutrition, thalassaemia)

Table 7.3 (continued)

Sclerae
- Icterus (CLD)
- Blue (OI)

Cornea: cloudy (rubella)

Visual fields: field defect (intracranial tumour, e.g. craniopharyngioma)

Eye movements
- Upward gaze palsy (pineal tumour)
- Lateral rectus palsy (intracranial tumour with raised ICP)

Cataracts (rubella, Cushing, treated thalassaemia, T1DM)

Fundi

Papilloedema (intracranial tumour with raised ICP)
- Optic nerve hypoplasia (SOD)
- Chorioretinitis (TORCH)
- Diabetic retinopathy (T1DM)
- Pigmentary retinopathy (abetalipoproteinaemia)

NOSE

Midface hypoplasia (FAS)

Midline dimple (hypopituitarism)

Nasal polyps (CF)

Anosmia (Kallmann)

MOUTH AND CHIN

Central cyanosis (CHD, CF)

Midline defects associated with hypopituitarism
- Cleft lip (repaired)
- Cleft palate (repaired)
- Single central incisor

Delayed dentition (hypothyroidism)

Glossitis (nutritional deficiency)

Facial hair or acne (precocity, Cushing)

Micrognathia (Russell–Silver, Turner, Seckel)

EARS

Low set (Turner, Seckel, Noonan)

Posteriorly rotated (Russell–Silver)

HAIRLINE

Low (Turner, Noonan)

NECK

Pterygium colli (Turner, Noonan)

Short (Klippel–Feil)

Scoliosis (Klippel–Feil)

Goitre (hypothyroidism)

Continued

Table 7.3 (continued)
CHEST
Inspection • Tanner staging in girls (for precocity or delay) • Wide-spaced nipples (Turner) • Hyperinflation (CF) • Sternal deformity (Noonan) • Rib rosary (rickets)
Palpation • Praecordium (CHD) • Ribs for rosary (rickets)
Percuss chest: hyperresonance (CF)
Auscultation • Lung fields (CF, CCF) • Praecordium (CHD)
ABDOMEN
Inspection • Distension • Weak muscles (coeliac, nutritional deficiency) • Ascites (CKD, CLD, nutritional deficiency) • Hepatosplenomegaly (thalassaemia)
Tanner-staging pubic hair (for precocity or delay)
Operative scars (Kasai, liver transplant, renal transplant)
Access devices (e.g. Tenckhoff catheter for CKD, access ports in CF)
Striae (Cushing)
Injection sites (insulin in T1DM, desferrioxamine in thalassaemia)
Palpation • Abdominal tenderness (Crohn) • Hepatomegaly (e.g. nutritional deficiency, T1DM, CF, Shwachman) • Splenomegaly (e.g. thalassaemia, storage diseases, CF, CLD) • Hepatosplenomegaly (e.g. thalassaemia, storage diseases) • Enlarged kidneys (e.g. polycystic kidneys or hydronephrosis with CKD) • Transplanted kidney (CKD)
Percussion: ascites (CKD, CLD)
Auscultation: renal artery stenosis (NF1)
Posterior aspect • Buttock wasting (malnutrition) • Perianal fistulae (Crohn)
GENITALIA
Tanner-stage genitalia • Measure penis length • Measure testes parameters; estimate testes volume • Advanced stage (causes of long-standing precocity, e.g. CAH) • Delayed stage (e.g. CKD, thalassaemia, hypopituitarism)
Penile anomalies • Micropenis (hypopituitarism) • Hypospadias (Noonan)
Testicular anomalies: cryptorchidism (Noonan)

Table 7.3 (continued)

GAIT, BACK AND LOWER LIMBS

Inspection of lower limbs
- Lower limb bowing (rickets)
- Proximal, middle or distal shortening (bony dysplasias)
- Joint swelling (JIA)
- Injection marks on thighs (T1DM)
- Erythema nodosum (IBD)
- Necrobiosis lipoidica (T1DM)
- Pyoderma gangrenosum (IBD)
- Oedema of dorsa of feet (Turner)
- Clubbing of toes (CF, CHD)

PALPATION: ANKLE OEDEMA (CCF WITH CHD, CLD)

Gait—standard examination screening for:
- Long-tract signs (IC tumour)
- Peripheral neuropathy (nutritional deficiency, CKD)
- Proximal weakness (Cushing)

BACK

- Scoliosis
- Kyphosis
- Focal spinal shortening (irradiation for malignancy)
- Midline scar (spina bifida)
- Spinal tenderness (Cushing, rickets)

LOWER LIMBS NEUROLOGICALLY

- Long tract signs (IC tumour)
- Neuropathy (CKD, nutritional deficiency)
- Delayed ankle jerk relaxation (hypothyroidism)

OTHER

Urinalysis
- pH (RTA)
- Specific gravity (CKD)
- Blood (CKD)
- Protein (CKD)
- Glucose (T1DM, Cushing)

Stool analysis
- Blood (IBD)
- Pus (IBD)
- Fat globules (CF)
- Fat crystals (coeliac)
- Glucose (T1DM, Cushing)

Stool analysis
- Blood (IBD)
- Pus (IBD)
- Fat globules (CF)
- Fat crystals (coeliac)

BSL = blood sugar level; CAH = congenital adrenal hyperplasia; CCF = congestive cardiac failure; CF = cystic fibrosis; CHD = congenital heart disease; CKD = chronic kidney disease; CLD = chronic liver disease; FAS = fetal alcohol syndrome; IBD = inflammatory bowel disease; ICP = intracranial pressure; JIA = juvenile idiopathic arthritis; LS = lower segment; NF = neurofibromatosis; OI = osteogenesis imperfecta; RTA = renal tubular acidosis; SCA = sickle cell anaemia; T1DM = type 1 diabetes mellitus; TORCH = intrauterine infections with toxoplasmosis, other (e.g. HIV, syphilis), rubella, cytomegalovirus, herpes (both simplex and varicella); US = upper segment; VSD = ventricular septal defect.

SHORT CASE: Tall stature

This is not a common case, but it can appear in the examination setting. The routine outlined is quite comprehensive. Like the short stature case, it comprises four parts:

1. Observation.
2. Measurements.
3. Manoeuvres.
4. Systematic relevant examination.

Observation

Start by noting the child's age in the introduction. This is important for appropriate assessment of the Tanner staging and intellect, which are essential in this case. Introduce yourself to the child and parent. Ask the child which grade he or she is in at school, and note whether the response seems age-appropriate (impairment of intellect can occur with Beckwith-Wiedemann [B-W] or Sotos syndrome, or with homocystinuria).

Now stand back and inspect for any evidence of a Marfanoid body habitus (e.g. Marfan syndrome; multiple endocrine neoplasia type 2b [MEN 2b]; homocystinuria) or a eunuchoid habitus (e.g. Klinefelter or Kallmann syndromes), and visually assess the Tanner staging. Note whether the child is wearing glasses (e.g. myopia in Marfan syndrome or homocystinuria). Note any skeletal anomalies such as asymmetry (e.g. in neurofibromatosis type 1 [NF type 1], B-W, Proteus or McCune–Albright syndrome), pectus carinatum or excavatum (e.g. in Marfan syndrome or homocystinuria) or scoliosis (e.g. Marfan syndrome, homocystinuria, NF type 1, Proteus syndrome, Sotos syndrome), and observe any unusual posturing (e.g. hemiplegia in homocystinuria, complicated by a cerebrovascular accident due to thrombotic tendency). Comment on your findings.

Look at the skin for areas of hyperpigmentation, such as café-au-lait spots (in NF type 1, Proteus syndrome, McCune–Albright syndrome [McC–A]) or larger areas (e.g. in the sacral area in McC–A syndrome, and the epidermal naevi in Proteus syndrome), as well as subcutaneous tumours (numerous types can occur in Proteus syndrome, such as lipomata, haemangiomata and lymphangiomata). Also note whether the child has acne (various causes of precocity).

Measurements

Next, measure the patient yourself. Stand the patient against a wall, position the head and heels appropriately and record the height. Measure the LS—that is, the distance from the pubic symphysis to the ground—then calculate the US, which is the height minus the LS. Work out the US:LS ratio. Normal values at various ages are listed in Table 7.4.

If the US:LS ratio is decreased, it suggests that the lower limbs are disproportionately long (e.g. Marfanoid body habitus, eunuchoid body habitus). If the US:LS is normal, this is more in keeping with diagnoses such as familial tall stature or pituitary gigantism.

Table 7.4	
Normal upper segment to lower segment ratios	
AGE	RATIO
Birth	1.7
3 years	1.3
8 years or more	1.0

Table 7.5	
Normal arm span minus height values	
AGE	VALUE
Birth to 7 years	−3 cm
8–12 years	0
14 years	+1 cm in girls

Next, measure the arm span and compare this to the total height. The normal arm span minus height values at various ages are given in Table 7.5. A long arm span occurs in Marfanoid or eunuchoid patients, or patients with other diagnoses complicated by a shortened trunk, caused by scoliosis (e.g. Sotos) or kyphosis (e.g. pituitary gigantism). If the arm span to height ratio is > 1.05, then this indicates long limbs (e.g. Marfan syndrome or eunuchoid body habitus).

Next, measure the head circumference and request the weight.

Request percentile charts, progressive measurements (if not given) and calculate the height velocity (be aware of the normal range and nature of percentile charts for this measurement). Request the birth parameters (B-W and Sotos can have large birth weights) and the parents' heights, percentiles and onsets of puberty (ask about age of menarche for women and age when men started shaving).

Manoeuvres

Next, a series of manoeuvres can be performed to screen for a number of possible causes of tall stature. With each manoeuvre, stand opposite the child and demonstrate, so that he or she will mirror your movements. First, ask the child to put the palms together with the arms straight, and stand with the legs together. This is to screen for asymmetry (as can occur in B-W syndrome, McC–A syndrome and in NF type 1) and also allows inspection for genu valgum (homocystinuria), genu recurvatum (Marfan syndrome) and pes planus (Marfan syndrome).

Next, ask the child to bend forwards and touch the toes; this is to check for scoliosis (can occur in Marfan syndrome, homocystinuria, MEN 2b or Sotos syndrome) or kyphosis (can occur in conjunction with scoliosis in the above diseases, as well as in pituitary gigantism/acromegaly); if the child can do this with ease, then ask him or her to put their palms flat on the floor, while reaching down/bending forwards, without any bending of the knees. This is one of the tests for hypermobility (Marfan) comprising the 'Beighton score'—the other tests include: 1. apposing thumb to forearm with wrist flexed; 2. passive hyperextension of the fifth finger over 90 degrees (Gorling's sign); and 3. hyperextension of knees greater than or equal to 10 degrees (genu recurvatum). In Marfan syndrome, the fifth component of the Beighton score (more than 10 degrees' hyperextension of the elbows) is not useful, as Marfan syndrome is paradoxically associated with decreased elbow extension (to < 170 degrees). If these tests show less mobility than normal, then homocystinuria is more likely. Next, test for arachnodactyly (Marfan), using two digit-related eponymous signs: 1. the thumb (Steinberg) sign—this is an extension of the whole distal phalanx of the thumb beyond the ulnar border of the hand when apposed across the palm; and 2. the wrist (Walker–Murdoch) sign—this is overlapping of the distal phalanx of the thumb with the distal phalanx of the little finger when encircling the opposite wrist. If both these tests are normal, then Marfan syndrome is a less likely diagnosis.

Table 7.6
Manoeuvres to assess for tall stature
HANDS AND FEET TOGETHER
To detect: • Hemihypertrophy (Beckwith, McCune–Albright, Proteus) • Unilateral growth arrest (homocystinuria with cerebrovascular accident) • Genu valgum (homocystinuria) • Genu recurvatum (Marfan) • Pes planus (Marfan)
BEND OVER AND TOUCH TOES
To detect: • Scoliosis (Marfan, homocystinuria, Proteus, Sotos, NF1) • Kyphosis (with scoliosis, as above, pituitary gigantism)
PALMS TO FLOOR/THUMB TO FOREARM/HYPEREXTENSION FIFTH FINGER/HYPEREXTENDED KNEES (BEIGHTON SCORE FOR HYPERMOBILITY)
To detect: • Hypermobility (Marfan) • Limitation of extension (homocystinuria)
ARACHNODACTYLY TESTS: STEINBERG (THUMB PAST ULNAR BORDER)/WALKER–MURDOCH (WRIST)
To detect Marfan syndrome
TREMOR
To detect hyperthyroidism

Finally, ask the child to hold the arms out straight in front with the fingers spread apart and check for tremor associated with hyperthyroidism.

For a list of manoeuvres, see Table 7.6.

Remember, as you proceed, to explain to the examiners what you are doing and why, so that the significance of each manoeuvre will be appreciated. The formal physical examination proceeds from the hands, working up to the head and then downwards; that is, head to toe, as outlined in Figure 7.3. A comprehensive listing of possible findings is given in Table 7.7 at the end of this section.

If the patient appears to be quite clearly Marfanoid, the examination outlined can be substantially abbreviated and can concentrate on the skeleton, eyes and heart. At the completion of your physical examination, summarise your findings succinctly and give a brief differential diagnosis.

Investigations

At this stage, you may be asked what investigations would clarify the diagnosis. This, of course, depends on the findings and may include: a slit-lamp ophthalmological assessment if Marfan syndrome or homocystinuria are possibilities; urine homocystine and blood homocystine and methionine levels if homocystinuria is likely; an electrocardiogram, chest X-ray and echocardiogram if Marfan syndrome seems likely; plasma somatomedin C concentration and a cerebral CT or MRI scan if a pituitary cause needs to be excluded; and skeletal X-rays if McC–A syndrome is likely (multiple areas of bony fibrous dysplasia) or to confirm and document the degree of scoliosis or kyphosis in patients likely to have Marfan syndrome or homocystinuria (Fig. 7.4).

Table 7.7

Additional information: details of possible findings in the child with tall stature

INTRODUCTION

Impression of mental state: intellectual impairment (homocystinuria, Sotos, Beckwith-Wiedemann [B-W], Klinefelter)

GENERAL INSPECTION

Body habitus
- Marfanoid (dolichostenomelia: Marfan, homocystinuria, MEN 2b)
- Eunuchoid (Kallman, Klinefelter)

Tanner staging
- Delayed (Kallmann, Klinefelter)
- Advanced (precocious puberty, virilisation, e.g. adrenal tumour, CAH)

Skeletal anomalies
- Asymmetry (Beckwith, NF1, McCune–Albright [McC–A], Proteus)
- Pectus excavatum (Marfan, homocystinuria, MEN 2b)
- Scoliosis (Marfan, Sotos, homocystinuria, MEN 2b, NF1)

Posture
- Hemiplegic (homocystinuria)

Skin
- Café-au-lait spots (NF1, McC–A, Proteus)
- Subcutaneous tumours, e.g. lipomata, haemangiomata (Proteus)
- Hyperpigmented areas (McC–A, Proteus)
- Acne (virilisation syndromes)

UPPER LIMBS

Arachnodactyly (Marfan, MEN 2b)

Large hands (Sotos, Proteus, pituitary gigantism)

Nails: thyroid acropathy (hyperthyroidism)

Palms
- Warm, sweaty (hyperthyroidism)
- Pigmented creases (CAH)

Pulse: collapsing (aortic incompetence in Marfan, hyperthyroidism)

Blood pressure
- Elevated (NF1, CAH, pituitary gigantism, MEN type 2b with phaeochromocytoma)
- Pulse pressure elevated (aortic incompetence with Marfan, hyperthyroidism)

Axillae: assess pubertal staging for precocity or delay, apocrine secretion, hair, odour

HEAD

Size
- Large (Sotos, NF1)
- Small (B-W)

Shape
- Frontal bossing (Sotos)
- Prominent occiput (B-W)

Hair
- Receding frontal hairline (Sotos)
- Dry, light, sparse (homocystinuria)
- Greasy (CAH)

Continued

Table 7.7 (continued)
Face • Asymmetry (B-W, Proteus, NF1, McC–A) • Fair complexion (homocystinuria) • Malar flush (homocystinuria) • Café-au-lait spots (NF1, McC–A) • Naevus flammeus (B-W)
Eyes Inspect: • Wearing glasses (myopia with Marfan, homocystinuria) • Blue irides (homocystinuria) • Prominent (B-W, hyperthyroidism) • Exophthalmos (hyperthyroidism) • Hypertelorism (Sotos) • Downslanting (Sotos) • Conjunctival neuromata (MEN 2b) • Bluish sclerae (Marfan) • Lens displacement (up in Marfan, down in homocystinuria)
Visual acuity • Myopia (Marfan, homocystinuria)
Visual fields • Bitemporal hemianopia (pituitary tumour) • Homonymous hemianopia (cerebral thrombosis with homocystinuria)
External ocular movements • Ophthalmoplegia (hyperthyroidism) • Sixth cranial nerve palsy (intracranial tumour)
Cataracts (homocystinuria)
Fundoscopy • Retinal detachment (Marfan, homocystinuria)
Glaucoma (Marfan, homocystinuria)
NOSE
Anosmia (Kallmann)
MOUTH AND CHIN
Lips: prominent (neuromata in MEN 2b)
Tongue • Big (B-W, pituitary gigantism) • Nodular (MEN 2b)
Teeth • Crowding (homocystinuria) • Separation (pituitary gigantism)
Palate • High, narrow (Marfan, Sotos, homocystinuria) • Cleft (Marfan)
Chin • Acne (sexual precocity) • Hair (pubertal staging) • Prognathism (Sotos, B-W, McC–A)

Table 7.7 (continued)

EARS

Linear fissures in lobules (B-W)

Punched-out depressions in posterior pinnae (B-W)

Large (Proteus, Marfan)

NECK

Examine for goitre (hyperthyroidism)

CHEST

Tanner-stage breasts in girls, hair in boys

Deformity: pectus carinatum or excavatum (Marfan, homocystinuria)

Praecordium: full assessment for Marfan cardiac complications, e.g. aortic regurgitation, mitral valve prolapse

ABDOMEN AND GENITALIA

Inspect:
- Café-au-lait spots (NF1, McC–A, Proteus)
- Herniae (Marfan, homocystinuria, B-W)
- Umbilical scar (repair of exomphalos with B-W)
- Tanner staging of pubic hair

Palpate
- Hepatomegaly (homocystinuria, B-W)
- Enlarged kidneys (Wilms' tumour in B-W)
- Adrenal mass (tumour; isolated or associated with B-W)
- Tanner staging of genitalia

LOWER LIMBS

Asymmetry (hemihypertrophy with B-W, NF1, Proteus; growth arrest with CVA in homocystinuria)

Large feet (Sotos, Proteus, pituitary gigantism)

Gait
- Shuffling gait; like Chaplin's Little Tramp (homocystinuria)
- Hemiplegic gait (homocystinuria with CVA)

CAH = congenital adrenal hyperplasia; CVA = cerebrovascular accident: MEN = multiple endocrine neoplasia; NF1 = neurofibromatosis type 1.

1. Introduce self

2. General inspection
Position patient: standing, adequately
   undressed to allow examination
   without embarrassment
Body habitus
Tanner staging
Glasses
Skeletal anomalies
Posture
Skin

3. Measurements
Measure:
- Height
- Lower segment (LS)
- US:LS ratio
- Arm span
- Head circumference

Request weight
Assess percentile charts
Calculate height velocity
Request:
- Birth parameters
- Parents' percentiles and ages of
  puberty

4. Manoeuvres
(See Table 7.7 for findings sought)
Standing with arms and legs together
Touching toes
Tests tor hyperextensibility
Tests for arachnodactyly
Arms and hands outstretched

5. Upper limbs
Hands
Pulse
Blood pressure
Axillae

6. Head and neck
Head (size, shape)
Hair
Face
Eyes (full examination)
Nose
Mouth
Chin
Ears
Neck

7. Chest
Tanner staging
Deformity
Praecordium

8. Abdomen and genitalia
Inspect (e.g. herniae)
Palpate (organomegaly)
Tanner stage genitalia

9. Lower limbs
Inspect
Gait

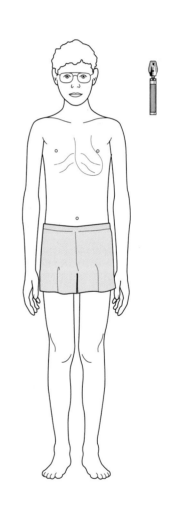

Figure 7.4 **Tall stature**

SHORT CASE: Obesity

There are a number of introductions to the examination of the obese child, and a number of parameters that are specifically useful in evaluating these children in the examination context. A widely used measure of total body fatness is the BMI, which is the weight in kilograms divided by the height in metres squared; there are BMI-for-age percentile charts that can be requested in the short-case format, if the candidate is familiar with them (see Fig. 7.5). A widely used measure of fat distribution is the waist circumference (measured at the narrowest or midpoint between the lower costal margin and the iliac crest), which correlates with abdominal fat and with cardiovascular risk factors; there are nationally derived waist-circumference-for-age percentile charts. The third useful measure is the waist-to-height ratio (WtHR); the aim is to keep the waist to less than half the height. The lead-in may include looking for an underlying cause, assessing the complications of obesity per se or, possibly, assessing a child for complications of corticosteroid therapy. In the latter case, the child may not be obese, but the structure of the physical examination is similar.

It is useful, also, to be aware of two medical 'laws' that are pertinent in terms of orthopaedic complications: 1. the Hueter–Volkmann law, that excess load across a growth plate retards growth, and reduced load across a growth plate accelerates growth; and 2. Wolff's law, that the structure of a bone adapts and remodels in response to the loads applied to it. These come into play with slipped capital femoral epiphysis (SCFE) and with Blount's disease.

Observation

The first step is to introduce yourself to the child. Note any obvious sleepiness in the response to your questions, which may indicate Pickwickian syndrome (gross obesity, somnolence, hypoventilation with episodes of periodic breathing and cyanosis mainly during sleep, secondary polycythaemia and right-ventricular failure). Note whether the child's reaction seems age-appropriate—intellectual impairment with Prader–Willi (P–W), Bardet–Biedl (B–B), Fröhlich or Down syndrome, untreated hypothyroidism, pseudohypoparathyroidism or some storage diseases.

Next, stand back and inspect for evidence of any dysmorphism (P–W, B–B) or obvious diagnosis (e.g. Cushing's syndrome), note the distribution of the obesity (truncal in Cushing's syndrome, and how fat tends to obliterate the supraclavicular fossae, which are preserved in other cases). In girls, note any signs of androgen excess, such as hirsutism or acne (polycystic ovary syndrome [PCOS]). Note any goitre. Note any hyperpigmentation (acanthosis nigricans, in PCOS, reflects hyperinsulinism; characterised by thickened velvety areas of hyperpigmentation in intertriginous areas such as the axillae, groin, antecubital and popliteal fossae, umbilicus and base of neck). Note any unusual posture/gait affecting the pelvis or lower limbs; look for SCFE, bowing of the tibia (Blount's disease, or tibia vara), or knock knees (genu valgum).

Note the parameters and request the percentile charts. If the child is short, a pathological cause is more likely. There are five well-known endocrine causes of a short obese child: Cushing's syndrome, hypopituitarism, hypothyroidism, growth hormone deficiency and pseudohypoparathyroidism (PHPT). If the child is tall, it is more likely to be simple obesity, but it can be pathological; for example, Klinefelter syndrome.

Take particular note of the size of the hands (small in P–W syndrome), any glasses (B–B) or hearing aid (Alström syndrome) and the Tanner staging (may appear advanced in simple obesity or in Cushing's syndrome, and delayed in hypothyroidism and the syndromal diagnoses).

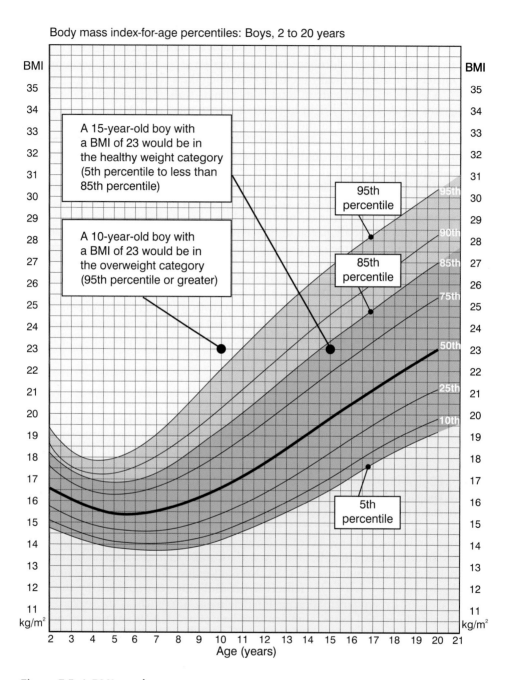

Body mass index-for-age percentiles: Boys, 2 to 20 years

A 15-year-old boy with a BMI of 23 would be in the healthy weight category (5th percentile to less than 85th percentile)

A 10-year-old boy with a BMI of 23 would be in the overweight category (95th percentile or greater)

95th percentile

85th percentile

5th percentile

Figure 7.5 A BMI graph

Redrawn from Nathan Bradford, Primary Care: Clinics Office Practice, Volume 36, Issue 2 (2009), p. 322, Figure 3. The BMI number has different meanings by age. An example of a 10-year-old boy and a 15-year-old boy who both have a BMI-for-age of 23. For a 10 year old, this BMI is obese but for the 15 year old, this is normal weight. The children of different ages are plotted on the same growth chart to illustrate a point. Normally the measurement for only one child is plotted on a growth chart. (From Centers for Disease Control and Prevention. Healthy Weight. Available at: http://www.cdc.gov/healthyweight/assessing/bmi/childrens _bmi/about_childrens_bmi.html.)

1. Introduce self

2. General inspection
Position patient: standing, adequately undressed to allow examination without embarrassment (underwear in younger children)
Dysmorphic features (PW, B–B)
Cushingoid features
Growth parameters
- Weight
- Height
- Head circumference
- Percentiles
Distribution of obesity
Skin
Tanner staging
Respiratory rate

3. Hands
Small (PW)
Short fourth metacarpal (PHPT)
Polydactyly (B–B)
Scars from removal of additional digit (B–B)
Temperature
- Cool (hypothyroidism)
- Warm (CO_2 retention in Pickwickian)
Pulse
Slow (hypothyroidism)
Bounding (CO_2 retention)
Hypotonic (PW)
Flap (CO_2 retention)

4. Blood pressure
Hypertension (Cushing's, or complication of obesity)

5. Head and neck
Head
Hair
Face
Eyes (acuity, fields, lens, retina)
Nose
Mouth and chin
Neck
Throat (tonsillar hypertrophy)

6. Back
'Buffalo hump', i.e. interscapular fat pad (Cushing's)
Kyphosis (Cushing's)
Scoliosis (with spina bifida, or osteoporosis with Cushing's)

Midline scar (repaired myelomeningocele)
Spinal tenderness (osteoporosis with Cushing's)

7. Abdomen
Striae
Hepatomegaly (RVF)
Adrenal mass
Genitalia

8. Lower limbs and manoeuvres
Inspect
Measure
Palpate
Manoeuvres (see text)
Hip examination
Ankle jerks

9. Cardiorespiratory
Full praecordial examination for evidence of cor pulmonale:
- Right-ventricular hypertrophy
- Loud second heart sound

10. Urinalysis
Glucose (PW, Alström's, Cushing's)

11. Hearing
Impaired (Alström's, Kallmann's)

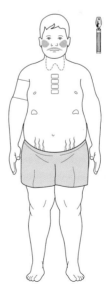

Figure 7.6 **Obesity**

Examination

After this initial assessment, a systematic physical examination can be performed, looking for most of the more common causes and complications. Depending on the 'lead-in' from the examiners, certain elements of this examination outline may need to be omitted.

The approach given here starts with the hands, followed by checking the blood pressure and then examining the head and neck. When examining the back, ask the child to touch the toes and check for scoliosis or kyphosis; next, ask the child to lie down and examine the abdomen, in particular the genitalia.

Following this, inspect and palpate the lower limbs. Then a series of manoeuvres can be performed to detect orthopaedic complications of obesity, such as SCFE, and certain features of Cushing's syndrome, such as proximal myopathy. The child is then returned to the bed for further assessment of the hip joints and lower limbs. Finally, the cardiorespiratory system is examined, having been deferred until now as the findings sought are complications rather than causes. Always request the urinalysis and do not forget to test the hearing if there is suspicion clinically of Alström or Kallmann syndrome. If the 'lead-in' is specifically for complications, then this is essentially a cardiorespiratory and lower limb examination, and the order will be somewhat different from the one outlined here. The various findings sought are enumerated in Table 7.8. A summary of the suggested approach is given in Figure 7.5.

Table 7.8
Additional information: details of possible findings on obesity examination
INTRODUCTION
Impression of mental state • Intellectual impairment (PW, B–B, Down, Fröhlich; hypothyroidism, PHPT, some storage disorders) • Sleepy (Pickwickian)
GENERAL INSPECTION
Growth parameters Height • Short (endocrine or syndromal causes) • Tall (simple obesity, Klinefelter)
Head circumference: enlarged (intracranial tumour, hydrocephalus with spina bifida)
Percentile charts
Calculate height velocity
Request • Birth parameters • Parents' percentiles
Distribution of obesity: central (Cushing)
Skin • Bruising (Cushing) • Poor wound healing (Cushing) • Café-au-lait spots (McCune–Albright syndrome)
Truncal striae
Tanner staging • Pseudoprecocity (Cushing) • Hypogonadism (syndromes: PW, B–B, Kallmann, Fröhlich) • Gynaecomastia (Klinefelter)

Table 7.8 (continued)

Respiratory rate
- Hypoventilation (Pickwickian syndrome)

HEAD

Shape: prominent forehead and bitemporal narrowing (PW)

Size: large (brain tumour, hydrocephalus with spina bifida)

Hair
- Dry, pluckable (hypothyroidism)
- Oily (Cushing)

Face
- Cherubic (round, immature face of GH deficiency)
- Moonface (Cushing)
- Plethora (Cushing, or secondary polycythaemia if Pickwickian)
- Telangiectasia (Cushing)
- Coarse features (hypothyroidism)
- Down syndrome facies

Eyes
- Eyebrows: loss of outer third (hypothyroidism)
- Almond-shaped eyes (PW)
- Squint (PW)
- Epicanthic folds (Down syndrome)
- Down-slanting (Down syndrome)
- Visual acuity: impaired (B–B, Fröhlich, Alström)
- Visual fields: bitemporal hemianopia (pituitary tumour)
- Cataract (posterior subcapsular in Cushing)
- Retinae

Retinitis pigmentosa (B–B, Alström)

Papilloedema (pituitary tumour, benign intracranial hypertension in Cushing)

Hypertensive retinopathy (Cushing)

Nose
- Anosmia (Kallmann)
- Midline dimple (hypopituitarism)

Mouth and chin
- Triangular upper lip (PW)
- Central cyanosis (Pickwickian)
- Midline defects associated with hypopituitarism or Kallmann

Cleft lip (repaired)

Cleft palate (repaired)

Single central incisor
- Delayed dentition (hypothyroidism)
- Oral candidiasis (Cushing)
- Tonsillar size (upper airway obstruction associated with hypoxia and hypercapnia in Pickwickian)
- Micrognathia (PW)
- Facial hair or acne (Cushing)

Continued

Table 7.8 (continued)
NECK
Goitre (hypothyroidism)
Obliteration of supraclavicular hollow, i.e. supraclavicular fat pads (Cushing)
Elevated JVP (RVF in Pickwickian)
ABDOMEN
Striae (Cushing)
Hepatomegaly (RVF with Pickwickian syndrome)
Adrenal mass (Cushing syndrome due to adrenal tumour)
Genitalia • Advanced development of hair or phallus (Cushing, hypothyroidism) • Delayed development (hypothyroidism; can advance or delay) • Hypogonadism (PW, B–B, Fröhlich, Kallmann, Klinefelter)
LOWER LIMBS
Inspection • Small feet (PW) • Skin: striae, bruises, poor wound healing (can all occur in Cushing syndrome) • Limb shortening (with SCFE or avascular necrosis of femoral head) • External rotation at hip (SCFE) • Genu valgus or varus (complications)
Measure: limb lengths (for shortening, as above)
Palpate: ankle oedema (RVF in Pickwickian)
MANOEUVRES
Stand child with legs together and re-inspect for: • Leg shortening (if not measured) • External rotation • Genu valgus or varus
Hold arms up against resistance (proximal myopathy in Cushing)
Squat (proximal myopathy); can 'race' child with repeated squats; normal child should win
Walk, looking for limp with: • Avascular necrosis femoral head (Cushing) • SCFE (complication of obesity)
Trendelenberg's test: positive with avascular necrosis of femoral head or SCFE
Lay patient down again for completion of lower limb examination
LOWER LIMBS COMPLETION
Hip examination: limitation of internal rotation or abduction (SCFE)
Ankle jerks: delayed relaxation (hypothyroidism)

B–B = Bardet–Biedl syndrome; GH = growth hormone; JVP = jugular venous pressure; PHPT = pseudohypoparathyroidism; PW = Prader–Willi syndrome; RVF = right ventricular failure; SCFE = slipped capital femoral epiphysis.

SHORT CASE: Normal puberty

Pubertal development in girls usually commences between the ages of 9 and 13 years, and in boys between 10 and 14 years. During puberty, there is development of the reproductive system and accompanying development of secondary sexual characteristics, as well as an increase in body size, a change in body composition, and acceleration in skeletal growth and muscle mass. It takes between 1.5 and 5.5 years (average 3.5 years) to go through puberty. Most of the changes are sex-specific, although some are common to females and males. The sequence of events tends to be relatively more consistent than the age at which they occur. Rating systems have been devised to indicate the stage that a child's pubertal development has reached.

Several terms are invariably used in discussing pubertal development, and these may be confused. Some definitions are as follows:

- *Adrenarche*: maturational increase in adrenal androgen (17-ketosteroid) production as normally occurs at puberty.
- *Pubarche*: pubic hair development as normally occurs at puberty.
- *Thelarche*: breast development as normally occurs at puberty.
- *Gonadarche*: development of pulsatile GnRH and gonadotropin activity resulting in enlarging gonads.
- *Menarche*: first menstrual period.

In the female, the first sign is breast development, then pubic hair development, although occasionally this order is reversed. Development of the uterus and the vagina parallels that of the breasts. The height spurt peaks at approximately breast Stage 4 and pubic hair Stage 3, at about 1–2 years before menarche, which is quite a late occurrence in the sequence. After menarche, girls tend to grow a further 6 cm, irrespective of age at menarche.

In the male, the first sign of puberty is enlargement of the testes and scrotum, with development of reddening and thickening of the scrotal skin; this is followed by pubarche and later growth of the penis and increase in growth velocity. The height spurt reaches its peak at approximately pubic hair Stage 4, which is usually about 2 years after the beginning of pubic hair growth. This is also the time at which axillary hair appears. Deepening, or 'breaking', of the voice tends to be a late occurrence, and can take place very gradually, so it is not, of itself, a reliable index of pubertal development.

Staging

The Tanner staging system is used in Australia. Stages (abbreviated) are as follows.

BREAST DEVELOPMENT

Stage 1: Preadolescent.
Stage 2: Breast bud.
Stage 3: Breast and areolae enlarged and elevated, but no separation of their contours.
Stage 4: Areola and papilla form a mound above the contour of the breast.
Stage 5: Mature.

PUBIC HAIR STAGES (FOR FEMALES AND MALES)

Stage 1: Preadolescent.
Stage 2: Long, fair, straight hair; sparse, mainly along labia or at base of penis.
Stage 3: Darker, coarser, curlier, sparse.
Stage 4: Adult-type hair; smaller area covered than in adult.
Stage 5: Adult; spread to medial surface of thighs.

Stage 1: Preadolescent.
Stage 2: Enlargement of scrotum, with reddening and thickening of scrotal skin.
Stage 3: Enlargement of penis; further growth of scrotum.
Stage 4: Further growth of penis and scrotum; darker scrotal skin.
Stage 5: Adult.

SHORT CASE: Precocious puberty

Sexual development is described as precocious if the onset is before 8 years in girls, and before 9 years in boys. True or central precocious puberty occurs when the hypothalamic control mechanism for puberty (the GnRH pulse generator) is prematurely turned on, leading to early gonadal maturation; this is gonadotrophin dependent.

Pseudoprecocious puberty, also called incomplete or peripheral precocity (in contrast), is not due to premature activation of the hypothalamic control system; this is gonadotrophin independent. However, to complicate the picture further, long-standing pseudoprecocious puberty can lead to premature activation of the central GnRH-generating mechanism, and thence to true precocious puberty. The puberty hormones prime the hypothalamic–pituitary–gonadal (HPG) axis, and release the tonic prepubertal inhibition of GnRH pulsatility.

True precocious puberty is far more common in girls than in boys. In girls, it is usually idiopathic, whereas in boys, the diagnosis is more often a central nervous system disorder; for example, an intracranial tumour or malformation.

The short-case approach covers a large amount of clinical ground, and requires a very structured routine to enable its completion in the examination's time constraints. The approach given is comprehensive and covers most relevant findings for girls and boys.

Examination

The examination essentially focuses on accurate staging of puberty and assessment of growth parameters, followed by evaluation of the central nervous system, the adrenal glands and the gonads. The other signs sought provide further evidence of suspected diagnoses, such as café-au-lait spots and scoliosis in neurofibromatosis type 1 (NF1).

Commence by introducing yourself to the patient and the parent; note the quality of the child's voice replying, particularly in boys, for deepening of the voice. Next, ask the child to undress as fully as possible without causing her or him undue embarrassment; underwear can be left on for this initial inspection. Visually scan the child and assess the Tanner staging, noting the androgen effects in boys and the oestrogen effects in the girls. Next, assess the growth parameters, commencing with the height. Precocious puberty per se can cause tall stature early in its course. Tall stature can also occur in underlying causes such as McCune–Albright (McC–A) syndrome (which can cause central or peripheral precocity), or NF1 (causes central precocity). Short stature can result from long-standing precocious puberty, but is also a feature of Russell–Silver syndrome and can occur in NF1 (not a misprint: NF1 can cause tall or short stature, just as it can cause large or small head circumference), two causes of true precocious puberty. Short stature may also occur in Cushing's syndrome (causes premature pubarche) and in severe hypothyroidism, which causes precocity by an unknown mechanism.

Weight is also important, as obesity can be a feature of hypothyroidism (true precocity) or Cushing's syndrome (premature pubarche). The head circumference may be increased (e.g. in hydrocephalus or intracranial tumours) or decreased, such as in previous severe head injury or in cerebral palsy. Other parameters of importance include arm span and US:LS ratio. The arm span is normally less than the height before the age of 8 years. If it is greater than the height before this age, it implies that the growth spurt has already occurred.

The US:LS ratio for the child's age may be increased in hypothyroidism, or decreased in children with NF1 who have scoliosis.

Next, inspect the skin for any evidence of hyperpigmentation, which can occur in CAH, or café-au-lait (CAL) spots, which can occur in NF1, McC–A syndrome or Russell–Silver syndrome (the CAL spots in McC–A syndrome tend to be bigger and more irregular than those in NF1). Also look for evidence of carotenaemia, which can occur in hypothyroidism, or increased sebaceous gland activity, which occurs with increased androgen secretion. Note any obvious dysmorphic or diagnostic features, such as Russell–Silver syndrome, Cushing's syndrome, McC–A syndrome or NF1.

The remainder of the examination commences at the upper limbs, initially checking for any asymmetry and then starting with the hands, working up to the head and neck, with particular emphasis on the eyes. Continue with the chest in girls, and to a lesser extent boys (e.g. pubertal gynaecomastia), and the abdomen, with accurate staging of the genitalia in boys. It is important to estimate the volume of the testes, as this is the best indicator of the maturational age. Prepubertal testes are usually less than 3 mL in volume, and the easiest way of measuring the volume is with an orchidometer. A rough approximation is that a prepubertal testis is the size of a small grape.

The penile length can be easily measured by using a cottonwool-tipped swab stick: the penis is measured up against the swab stick, with the cottonwool end on the abdominal wall, and the stick is broken at the point where the tip of the glans reaches, so the stick can then be measured accurately on a ruler.

This is followed by examination of the gait, back and lower limbs. The relevant findings sought are set out in Figure 7.6.

Investigations

At the completion of your examination, give a succinct summary and differential diagnosis, followed by a brief list of investigations you feel are appropriate. These investigations depend on the sex of the child and the particular findings in that child, but may include the following (see also Fig. 7.7).

BLOOD TESTS

1. Baseline LH, FSH; morning gonadal steroids: testosterone, oestradiol.
2. GnRH stimulation test (LH and FSH responses).
3. DHEAS (dehydroepiandrosterone sulfate), which may be extremely high in adrenal tumours.
4. hCG (can be produced by various tumours).
5. Thyroid function tests, including TSH level.

IMAGING

1. X-ray of left wrist and hand for bone age (the most important investigation). A normal bone age suggests, depending on the clinical picture, premature adrenarche, premature thelarche or ingestion of exogenous sex steroids. An accelerated bone age is more in keeping with central precocity (various causes), adrenal or ovarian pathology (such as tumour) or McC–A syndrome.
2. A skeletal survey for suspected McC–A syndrome (polyostotic fibrous dysplasia).
3. Ultrasound studies of the pelvis, testes and adrenal glands.
4. Brain MRI (for various intracranial pathologies, such as hypothalamic hamartoma, pinealoma, hydrocephalus, third ventricular cysts).

Additional information

Details of possible findings on precocious puberty examination are given in Table 7.9.

1. Introduce self
Quality of voice
- Deep (androgenised)
- Mature female (oestrogenised)
- Higher-pitched child's voice (normal for age)

2. General inspection
Position patient: standing, adequately undressed to allow examination without embarrassment
Visually assess Tanner staging
Boys (androgen effects)
- Male body habitus
- Muscle development
- Hair: facial, axillary
- Axillary odour
- Pubic hair (stage this)
- Increased size of genitalia (stage these formally later)
Girls (oestrogen effects)
- Female body habitus
- Fat distribution
- Breasts (stage these)
- Pubic hair (stage this)
Skin
- Syndromal diagnosis

3. Measurements
Height
- Short (e.g. Russell–Silver, NF1, hypothyroidism, Cushing's, long-standing precocity)
- Tall (e.g. recent onset precocity, NF1, McCune–Albright)
Lower segment
US:LS ratio (for age)
- Increased (hypothyroidism)
- Decreased (scoliosis, e.g. with NF1)
Arm span: greater than height before
- 8 years infers growth spurt has already occurred
Weight
- Increased (e.g. Cushing's, hypothyroidism)
Head circumference
- Increased (e.g. hydrocephalus, IC tumour)
- Decreased (previous severe head injury)
Assess percentile charts
Calculate height velocity
- Increased (true precocity)
Request parents' percentiles and ages of puberty

4. Upper limb
Symmetry
Fingers
Palms
Pulse
Blood pressure
Axillae

5. Head and neck
Head (size, scars, shunts)
Hair
Face
Eyes (full examination)
Mouth and chin
Neck

6. Chest
Breasts
Tanner staging in girls
Galactorrhoea (hypothyroidism, pituitary tumour, hypothalamic tumour)

7. Abdomen and genitalia
Liver
- Enlarged (hepatoblastoma producing hCG, in boys)
- Bruit (hepatoblastoma)
Adrenal glands
- Mass (tumour)
Ovaries
- Mass (tumour; mention rectal examination for completeness)

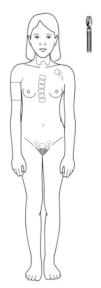

Continued

Figure 7.7 **Precocious puberty**

Uterus
- Size (stage of development; mention rectal examination for completeness)

Pubic hair
- Tanner staging

External genitalia (boys)
- Tanner staging
- Penis length (measure with swab stick)
- Testicular volume (estimate or request orchidometer, 3 mL or less is prepubertal)
- Scrotal rugosity

8. Gait, back and lower limbs
Full gait examination to screen for long tract signs (IC tumour, hydrocephalus, head injury)
Back: scoliosis (NF1)
Full lower limb examination to detect:
- Long-tract signs
- Delayed ankle jerk relaxation (hypothyroidism)

Figure 7.7, continued

Table 7.9
Additional information: details of possible findings on examination of precocious puberty
GENERAL INSPECTION
Skin • Hyperpigmentation (CAH) • 'Coast of Maine' café-au-lait spots (McCune–Albright [McC–A]) • 'Coast of California' café-au-lait spots (NF1) • Carotenaemia (hypothyroidism) • Dry, cool (hypothyroidism) • Sebaceous gland activity
Syndromal diagnosis (Russell–Silver, McC–A, NF1)
HEAD
Size • Large (hydrocephalus, NF1, IC tumours) • Small (head trauma, cerebral palsy) • Scars (cranial surgery) • Shunts (hydrocephalus)
Hair • Dry (hypothyroidism) • Greasy (CAH)
Face • Moonface (Cushing's) • Coarse (hypothyroidism) • Asymmetry (Russell–Silver, McC–A)
EYES
Inspect • Prominent (hyperthyroidism with McC–A) • Squint (sixth cranial nerve palsy with IC tumour) • Lisch nodules (NF1)
Visual fields • Bitemporal hemianopia (pituitary tumour) • Other field cuts such as homonymous hemianopia (IC tumour)

Continued

Table 7.9 (continued)
External ocular movements • Sixth cranial nerve palsy (IC tumour) • Loss of upward gaze (pineal tumour) • Ophthalmoplegia (hyperthyroidism with McC–A)
Pupils • Argyll Robertson pupils (pineal tumour)
Cataracts (Cushing's)
Fundoscopy • Papilloedema (IC tumour)
NOSE
• Comedones (androgens)
MOUTH AND CHIN
• Facial hair (androgens) • Acne (androgens) • Brown pigmentation (Peutz–Jeghers associated with granulosa cell tumours in girls)
NECK
• Goitre (hypothyroidism, hyperthyroidism with McC–A)
UPPER LIMB
Hands together in front • Asymmetry (McC–A, NF1, Russell–Silver)
Fingers • Clinodactyly (Russell–Silver)
Palms • Pigmented creases (CAH) • Cool, dry (hypothyroidism) • Warm, sweaty periphery (hyperthyroidism with McC–A)
Pulse • Slow (hypothyroidism) • Collapsing (hyperthyroidism with McC–A)
Blood pressure • Elevated (e.g. CAH, Cushing's, NF1)
Axillae • Hair, odour, apocrine secretion (androgens) • Freckling (NF1)

SHORT CASE: Delayed puberty

Sexual development is described as delayed if the onset of puberty has not occurred by two standard deviations from the mean; namely, 13 years in girls and 14 years in boys. Delay in puberty occurs in any condition where the bone age is delayed; bone age correlates with developmental and pubertal stage, and puberty normally occurs when the bone age is pubertal, irrespective of the chronological age.

Important causes of delayed puberty can be divided into three groups:

1. Constitutional delayed puberty (and growth) (CDP).
2. Gonadotrophin (Gn) deficiency (hypogonadotropic hypogonadism).
3. Primary gonadal failure (hypergonadotrophic hypogonadism).

CDP is the cause in up to two-thirds of boys, and one-third of girls, with pubertal delay. Boys with CDP are generally short (under the 3rd to 10th centiles), with normal prepubertal penile length (6–7 cm stretched), normal prepubertal testes size (under 2.5 cm length, under 4 mL in volume, measured using the Prader orchidometer); bone age typically delayed by more than 2 years; and there tends to be a positive family history. In CDP, puberty occurs at a bone age of 12 in girls (which usually occurs at a chronological age of 16), and a bone age of 14 in boys (chronological age of 18).

Functional Gn deficiency causing delayed puberty can occur with any cause of severe and chronic undernutrition; hormones such as leptin, which are synthesised in fat, are involved in regulation of Gn secretion. Such conditions, which retard bone growth, include causes of chronic malnutrition (e.g. anorexia nervosa [AN], cystic fibrosis [CF], Crohn's disease, coeliac disease); many chronic illnesses, especially those associated with poor appetite (e.g. thalassaemia, sickle cell anaemia [SCA], chronic kidney disease [CKD], cyanotic congenital heart disease [CHD], juvenile idiopathic arthritis [JIA], and other severe connective tissue diseases); and several endocrine conditions (e.g. hypothyroidism, GH deficiency, hypopituitarism).

In boys, Gn deficiency can be isolated, as in idiopathic hypogonadotrophic hypogonadism (IHH). IHH is usually caused by mutations in one of three genes: first, the KAL1 gene on the X chromosome, which encodes the neural cell adhesion molecule anosmin-1, and is a cause of X-linked recessive Kallmann syndrome, which includes hypo- or anosmia, and may also involve midfacial clefting, synkinesia (mirror movements—ask to raise one arm, raises both), cerebellar dysfunction and deafness; second, the FGFR1 (KAL2) gene, which can cause autosomal-dominant IHH, anosmic/hyposmic or normosmic, with similar associated neurological findings to X-linked Kallmann syndrome; and third, GNRHR, with normosmia. Also, Gn deficiency may be one of multiple pituitary hormone deficiencies (congenital hypopituitarism; craniopharyngioma).

In girls, the causes of Gn deficiency are very similar, except that the more common functional causes include AN, excessive exercise with decreased body fat (especially in three types of exercise: competitive swimming, ballet dancing and gymnastics) and emotional stress (neglect/abuse); and those girls who have Kallmann syndrome have a non-X-linked form.

Causes of primary gonadal failure in boys (hypergonadotrophic hypogonadism) include: Klinefelter syndrome (47, XXY karyotype; there may be small testes for the degree of androgenisation production; penile enlargement occurs at the usual age, with an increase in pubic hair, but the testes volume remains < 6 mL, length < 3 cm; often tall, and have learning problems); cryptorchidism; post-surgery for cryptorchidism; previous testicular torsion; and post-radiation to testes for malignancy.

Causes of primary gonadal failure in girls (hypergonadotrophic hypogonadism) include: Turner's syndrome (see the long case in Chapter 9; these girls have pubic hair because adrenal androgen production is not affected, but oestrogen is low or absent due to gonadal dysgenesis); autoimmune damage to ovaries (especially if associated autoimmune conditions such as type 1 diabetes or multiple autoimmune endocrinopathy syndrome [the latter can include hypothyroidism, hypoparathyroidism and Addison's disease]); or total body irradiation or chemotherapy for malignancy.

Unlike precocious puberty, pubertal delay is far more common in boys. Remember that CDP can occur in boys (more commonly) or girls; hypogonadism in boys may be hypogonadotropic (e.g. Kallmann) or hypergonadotrophic (e.g. Klinefelter); and, similarly, hypogonadism in girls may be hypogonadotropic (e.g. AN) or hypergonadotrophic (e.g. Turner). It should be remembered that pubic and axillary hair development and axillary odour are caused by increases in adrenal androgen secretion, which are independent of the hypothalamic–pituitary–gonadal (HPG) axis, so pubertal delay may well be present despite pubic hair growth having started if there is no breast development in girls or any penile or testicular growth in boys.

This short-case approach covers as much clinical material as precocious puberty and requires as structured a routine. It covers relevant findings in boys and girls.

Examination

The examination focuses on accurate staging of puberty and assessment of growth parameters, followed by evaluation for any underlying cause, evidence of chronic disease, syndromal features (e.g. Turner's, Noonan) or certain endocrine disorders (e.g. hypopituitarism). This is a case where it is very important to stand back and look at the child's general appearance, especially for dysmorphic features (Turner's, Noonan), growth parameters (boys with CDP usually very short), nutritional status (AN) and any abdominal distension (coeliac). In addition to CDP, think about conditions affecting nutrition, the pituitary gland or the gonads.

Begin by introducing yourself to the patient and parent, and note the quality of the child's voice replying, particularly in boys, for lack of deepening (but comment to the examiners that the voice 'breaking' is a late sign and is quite variable, not a reliable indicator of pubertal status). Next, ask the child to undress as fully as possible without causing undue embarrassment; underwear should be left on for this initial inspection. Visually scan the child and assess the Tanner staging, noting the lack of androgen effects in boys or oestrogen effects in girls.

Next, quickly note any obvious dysmorphic features suggesting a diagnosis such as Turner's, Noonan, P–W or B–B syndrome, or diagnostic facial features (e.g. thalassaemia). Note the nutritional status, as nutritional deficiency may occur in Crohn's disease, cystic fibrosis and anorexia nervosa, and excessive adipose tissue can occur with several endocrine disorders (e.g. hypopituitarism, hypothyroidism) or in syndromes (e.g. P–W, Fröhlich). Pallor may indicate a chronic anaemia (e.g. CKD, SCA or thalassaemia).

Measure (or request) the height. If the child is particularly short or tall, then the US:LS ratio and arm span are worth doing, but in a child of normal stature these additional measurements are not needed, unless there is the impression of disproportion. The LS is the distance from the pubic symphysis to the ground. The US is calculated by subtracting the LS from the total height. Measure the head circumference. Request the weight and the percentile charts, calculate the height velocity and interpret this appropriately. Finally, ask for the parents' percentiles and ages of puberty. The height and height velocity are especially important, as can be appreciated from the large number of causes of short stature listed in Table 7.3. If there is an impression of an eunuchoid body habitus, then measuring the US:LS ratio and the arm span helps to evaluate this. If the US:LS ratio is decreased in a boy, it suggests that the lower limbs are disproportionately long (eunuchoid body habitus can occur in Kallmann or Klinefelter syndromes). Also, a long arm span occurs in eunuchoid patients; if the arm span to height ratio is > 1.05, then this indicates long limbs. If the US:LS ratio is increased, it suggests short lower limbs (e.g. hypothyroidism).

The weight is also important in detecting diagnoses such as AN and chronic diseases in thin children, and endocrine and syndromal problems in obese children. Head circumference, if increased, may indicate an intracranial tumour. Always request the percentile charts and do not forget to calculate the height velocity. Finally, requesting the parents' ages of puberty may make a diagnosis of CDP apparent. If Kallmann syndrome is suspected in a boy, then questioning about the sense of smell is useful (ask the parent whether the child notices smells at home, or ask the child if there are smells he likes or ones he does not).

The remainder of the examination begins with the hands and proceeds up to the head and neck, with a strong emphasis on the assessment of any midline defects, visual field loss and particularly examining the optic fundi for optic atrophy (craniopharyngioma), and then moves on to the chest (check for galactorrhoea from prolactinoma), the abdomen and finally accurate staging of the genitalia in boys. The volume of the testes should be estimated, as this is the best indicator of the maturational stage. Prepubertal testes are usually less than 3 mL in volume, and less than 2 cm in length. An orchidometer can be requested if you are familiar with its use. Another measurement that may be used is the testicular volume index, which is the average length multiplied by the width of both testes. Prepubertally, it is usually between 1.0 and 1.4 cm^2.

Finally, request the urinalysis.

The procedure is outlined in Figure 7.8. A detailed listing of possible findings is given in Table 7.10.

Investigations

At the completion of the physical examination, the examiners may ask which investigations you would perform. These of course depend on the physical findings, but the following list covers some of the more useful investigations. The most important test is the bone age. Note, as mentioned earlier, that the various causes of hypogonadism are often divided into two groups, based on the serum gonadotropin levels: patients with primary hypogonadism (primary hypofunction of testis or ovary) have high gonadotropin levels, and are said to have hypergonadotrophic hypogonadism, while those with gonadal hypofunction secondary to lack of pituitary gonadotropic hormones (on the basis of hypothalamic or pituitary disease) have hypogonadotropic hypogonadism. Be aware that there are no tests that reliably distinguish CDP from Gn deficiency.

BLOOD TESTS

1. Baseline LH, FSH (LH and FSH are elevated in primary gonadal failure, but low in other conditions); prolactin; total testosterone in boys, oestradiol in girls.
2. GnRH stimulation test (LH and FSH responses).
3. Provocative testing for growth hormone release (arginine, clonidine or glucagon).
4. TRF stimulation testing (prolactin and TSH responses).
5. Thyroid function tests.
6. Karyotype (especially for Turner syndrome and androgen insensitivity in girls, Klinefelter syndrome in boys).
7. Full blood count and film (for chronic anaemias).
8. Electrolytes, urea and creatinine (for occult CKD).
9. ESR (for Crohn's disease).
10. Coeliac disease screen (including anti-tissue transglutaminase, IgA).

1. Introduce self
Quality of voice
- High-pitched (prepubertal)

2. General inspection
Position patient: standing, undressed
(consider leaving underwear on to
avoid embarrassing the child)
Visually assess Tanner staging
Boys (lack of androgen effects)
- Male body habitus
- Muscle development
- Facial or axillary hair
- Body odour
- Pubic hair (stage this)
- Size of genitalia (stage these
formally later)
Girls (lack of oestrogen effects)
- Female body habitus
- Fat distribution
- Breasts (stage these)
- Pubic hair (stage this)
Dysmorphic features
Body habitus
Nutritional status
Pallor

3. Measurements
Height
- Lower segment
- US:LS ratio
Arm span
Weight
Head circumference
Percentiles
Calculate height velocity
Request parents' percentiles and ages
of puberty

4. Upper limbs
Hands
Fingertips
Nails
Palms
Pulse
Forearms
Blood pressure
Axillae

5. Head and neck
Head
Hair
Eyes (full examination)
Nose

Mouth and chin
Ears
Hairline
Neck

6. Chest
Breasts
Sternal deformity
Lung fields
Praecordium

7. Abdomen
Inspection
Palpation
- Hepatomegaly
- Splenomegaly

8. Genitalia
Tanner stage genitalia
- Measure penis length
- Measure testes parameters;
estimate testes volume
Penile anomalies
- Micropenis (Kallmann's,
hypopituitarism)
- Hypospadias (Noonan's)
Testes anomalies
- Cryptorchidism (Klinefelter's,
Kallmann's, Noonan's)

9. Gait and lower limbs
Inspection
Gait
Lower limbs
neurologically

10. Other
Urinalysis
Low specific gravity
(CRF, diabetes
insipidus with
septo-optic
dysplasia)
Glucose (IDDM)

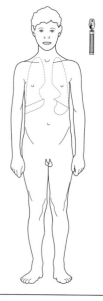

Figure 7.8 **Delayed puberty**

Table 7.10

Additional information: details of possible findings on delayed puberty examination

GENERAL INSPECTION

Dysmorphic features (various syndromes—Turner, Noonan, P–W, B–B)

Body habitus: eunuchoid (Kallmann, Klinefelter)

Diagnostic facies (e.g. Turner, Noonan, thalassaemia)

Nutritional status
- Poor (anorexia nervosa, Crohn's disease, coeliac disease)
- Excess adiposity (hypothyroidism, P–W, B–B, Fröhlich, hypopituitarism)

Pallor (thalassaemia, SCA, CKD)

Abdominal distension (coeliac)

MEASUREMENTS

Short stature
- Constitutional delay
- Chronic malnutrition (undernutrition, CF, Crohn)
- Chronic illness (thalassaemia, SCA, CRF, cyanotic CHD, JIA)
- Endocrine disorders (hypothyroidism, GH deficiency, hypopituitarism, severe T1DM)
- Syndromes (Turner, Noonan, P–W, B–B, Fröhlich, Kallmann)

Normal stature (excludes most of the above)
- Primary gonadal failure (dysplastic [Klinefelter]; absent [congenital anorchia, or removal due to gonadal tumour]; dysfunction [androgen insensitivity, or rarer forms of congenital adrenal hyperplasia])
- Anorexia nervosa
- T1DM

Tall stature
- Kallmann (can cause tall or short stature)
- Klinefelter

US:LS ratio
- Increased (hypothyroidism)
- Decreased (Klinefelter, Kallmann)

Arm span
- Over 4 cm more than height (eunuchoid habitus, e.g. Kallmann)

Weight
- Decreased (chronic illnesses, malnutrition; see above)
- Increased (endocrine disorders, syndromes; see above)

Head circumference
- Increased (intracranial tumour)

Height velocity
- Decreased (chronic illnesses, chronic malnutrition, endocrine disorders)
- Normal (constitutional delay, primary gonadal failure)

UPPER LIMBS

Hands
- Small (P–W)
- Polydactyly (B–B)

Fingertips: BSL testing (T1DM, thalassaemia, CF)

Continued

Table 7.10 (continued)

Nails
- Clubbing (CHD, CF, Crohn)
- Brown lines (CKD)
- Hyperconvex (Turner)

Palms
- Crease pallor (chronic anaemias, CKD)
- Crease pigmentation (thalassaemia)

Pulse
- Bradycardia (untreated hypothyroidism)
- Absent femorals (Turner with coarctation)

Forearms: muscle bulk (malnutrition)

Blood pressure: elevated (CKD, Turner with coarctation)

Axillae: lack of apocrine secretion, hair or odour (confirm delay)

HEAD

Midline scar (repaired frontal encephalocoele)

HAIR

Dry (hypothyroidism)

EYES

Inspection
- Hypertelorism (Noonan)
- Epicanthal folds (Noonan, Turner)
- Ptosis (Noonan)
- Squint (septo-optic dysplasia, P–W)
- Nystagmus (septo-optic dysplasia)

Conjunctival pallor (thalassaemia, CKD, malnutrition)

Visual acuity: diminished (pituitary tumour, T1DM, B–B)

Visual fields: bitemporal hemianopia (craniopharyngioma, pituitary tumour)

External ocular movements: sixth cranial nerve palsy (intracranial tumour)

Cataracts (T1DM)

Fundi
- Papilloedema (raised ICP, craniopharyngioma)
- Optic nerve hypoplasia (septo-optic dysplasia)
- Optic atrophy (raised ICP, craniopharyngioma)
- Diabetic retinopathy
- Retinitis pigmentosa (B–B)

NOSE

Anosmia (Kallmann)

Midline dimple (hypopituitarism)

Nasal polyps (CF)

MOUTH AND CHIN

Central cyanosis (CHD)

Midline defects associated with hypopituitarism
- Cleft lip (repair)
- Cleft palate (repair)
- Single central incisor

Table 7.10 (continued)
Delayed dentition (hypothyroidism)
Glossitis (malnutrition)
EARS
Low set (Turner, Noonan)
HAIRLINE
Low (Turner, Noonan)
NECK
Pterygium colli (Turner, Noonan)
Goitre (hypothyroidism)
CHEST
Breasts • Tanner staging in girls • Gynaecomastia (Klinefelter) • Galactorrhoea (breast discharge) (prolactinoma) • Well-developed but with no pubic or axillary hair (androgen insensitivity) • Wide-spaced nipples (Turner, Noonan)
Sternal deformity (Noonan)
Hyperinflation (CF)
Percuss for hyperresonance (CF)
Auscultate: chest (CF); praecordium (CHD)
ABDOMEN
Inspection • Tanner staging of pubic hair • Injection sites (T1DM, thalassaemia) • Scars (CF-meconium ileus; CKD-peritoneal dialysis, renal transplant; Crohn's disease surgery) • Venous access port (CF) • Perianal disease (Crohn)
Palpation • Hepatomegaly (thalassaemia, CF, T1DM, malnutrition, chronic active hepatitis) • Splenomegaly (thalassaemia, CF with portal hypertension)
GAIT AND LOWER LIMBS
Inspection • Injection marks on thighs (T1DM) • Erythema nodosum (IBD) • Necrobiosis lipoidica (T1DM) • Oedema of dorsa of feet (Turner) • Clubbing of toes (CF, CHD)
Gait, screening for • Long-tract signs (IC tumour) • Peripheral neuropathy (CRF, nutritional deficiency)
Lower limbs neurologically • Long-tract signs (IC tumour) • Neuropathy (CKD, nutritional deficiency) • Delayed ankle jerk relaxation (hypothyroidism)

B–B = Bardet–Biedl syndrome; CF = cystic fibrosis; CHD = congenital heart disease; CKD = chronic kidney disease; CLD = chronic liver disease; IBD = inflammatory bowel disease; ICP = intracranial pressure; T1DM = type 1 (insulindependent) diabetes mellitus; P–W = Prader–Willi syndrome; SCA = sickle cell anaemia.

IMAGING

1. X-ray of left wrist and hand for bone age (the most important investigation; in CDP bone age is typically delayed by over 2 years; this can allow prediction of adult height).
2. Brain MRI (for intracranial pathologies, such as craniopharyngioma). The later the puberty, the more reason there is to consider this.
3. Pelvic ultrasound (if suspect imperforate hymen or vaginal agenesis).

SHORT CASE: Disorders of sexual development (DSD) (virilisation in post-neonatal period)

This is an uncommon case. The presentation/lead-in can be of, usually, adolescent girls with hirsutism, with hair in the 'beard' distribution, over the chest or back, or early or excessive growth of axillary and pubic hair (with a masculine distribution), acne, the evolution of a masculine body habitus, decreasing breast size, clitoromegaly or, in the case of polycystic ovary syndrome (PCOS), obesity and acanthosis nigricans. Occasionally, a younger girl may present with increased growth and body odour as the key presenting symptoms. The short-case lead-in will direct the candidate accordingly. The introduction could be 'early pubic hair development' (before any other signs of puberty), and then the approach would need to differentiate between premature pubarche, precocious puberty and virilisation.

If the lead-in gives more information, such as associated oligomenorrhoea, this effectively eliminates simple premature pubarche as a possibility, and makes polycystic ovary syndrome and 21-OHD CAH more likely.

PCOS comprises androgen excess in association with hirsutism, secondary amenorrhoea, obesity, infertility, hyperinsulinism and bilaterally enlarged polycystic ovaries. PCOS is a diagnosis that requires excluding all other possible causes of androgen excess. There are three separate guidelines with slightly different criteria to diagnose PCOS: the 1990 National Institutes of Health Criteria, the 2003 Rotterdam Consensus Criteria and the 2006 Androgen Excess Society Criteria; these criteria can include hyperandrogenism, oligo- or amenorrhoea, and polycystic ovaries on ultrasound. A mnemonic for PCOS, which includes most of the features of virilisation per se (plus common features of PCOS asterisked), is **HYPERANDROGENISM**:

Hirsutism (excessive growth in androgen-dependent sites; differentiate from hypertrichosis, which is excessive vellus or non-androgen responsive hair)
Y (chromosome, i.e. male) body habitus; remodelling of limb–shoulder girdle
Pubic hair towards umbilicus (male escutcheon)
Enlarged larynx (and elevated lipids: dyslipidaemia)
Reduced ovulation
Acanthosis (velvety hyperpigmentation: neck, axilla, under breasts, genitals)
Nigricans (*)
Deepening of the voice (vocal cord coarsening)
Reduced breast size
Obesity (*) in around 55% of patients with PCOS (and OSA increased [*])
Genital enlargement (clitoromegaly) (in sexually mature females, > 35 mm^2)
Enlarged striated muscle mass (masculine musculature)
Non-insulin-dependent diabetes mellitus (type 2 diabetes mellitus) (*)
Insulin level elevated; insulin resistance (*)
Skin; seborrhea, acne
Menstrual disturbance (oligo- or amenorrhoea)/**M**etabolic syndrome (*)

Pubertal development is termed 'isosexual' when the secondary sexual characteristics are appropriate for the sex of the child, but 'heterosexual' when secondary sexual characteristics of the opposite sex manifest themselves, the latter being the case in virilisation.

Hirsutism can be graded by the Ferriman–Gallwey score, assessing 11 androgen-sensitive areas (the upper lip, chin, chest, upper back, upper arm, forearm, upper abdomen, lower abdomen, lower back, thigh and leg), with the grade for each area ranging from 0 (no terminal hair) to 4 (overtly virile); more than 8 is considered hirsutism; the axilla and pubic areas are not included, as terminal hair grows here at normal androgen levels.

Only three forms of CAH can present with virilisation, these being deficiencies of:

- **21-alpha-hydroxylase** (converts progesterone → **d**e**oxyc**ortisone [DOC]; 17OH progesterone → 11 deoxycortisol).
- **11-beta-hydroxylase** (11 deoxycortisol → cortisol; 11 deoxycorticosterone → corticosterone).
- **3-beta-hydroxysteroid-dehydrogenase** (pregnenolone → progesterone; 17OH pregnenolone → 17OH progesterone; **d**e**h**ydro**epi**androsterone [DHEA] → androstenedione; androstenediol → testosterone).

Girls with non-classic 21-OHD CAH may present with clitoromegaly, early development of pubic hair, hirsutism, acne, increased growth rate, and gynaecological problems such as oligomenorrhoea, abnormal menses or infertility. Girls with CAH due to 11-beta-hydroxylase deficiency (11-OHD CAH) may present in a similar way to 21-OHD CAH, as above; these patients, however, can also present with hypertension due to accumulation of salt-retaining aldosterone precursors. Extremely rare is deficiency of 3-beta-hydroxysteroid dehydrogenase (HSD3B CAH), which also can present in a similar way to 21-OHD.

Cushing's syndrome (of endogenous origin: pituitary tumour secreting ACTH, adrenal tumour secreting cortisol, and androgens, ectopic tumour secreting ACTH) can present with pubic hair as its first sign, and can also cause hypertension. Virilising tumours of the adrenal glands or the ovaries must be excluded, and although it is unusual to palpate these, this should be attempted; discussion as to appropriate imaging can occur after the physical examination. To understand this area, it is worth reviewing pathways of steroid hormone synthesis. The latter are discussed in the long case on CAH (at the start of this chapter).

A differential diagnosis of the causes of premature and/or excessive development of pubic hair in girls (not just virilising conditions) follows (mnemonic **PREMATOUR**):

Pituitary causes: true precocious puberty (see the short case on precocious puberty); gonadotrope neoplasia or hyperplasia/**P**olycystic ovary syndrome (PCOS)

Remote (ectopic) causes: chorionic-gonadotropin secreting tumours: hepatoblastoma; pineal dysgerminoma; retroperitoneal tumours

Exogenous: anabolic steroids; corticosteroids (Cushing's syndrome)

Metabolic: congenital adrenal hyperplasia: three forms: 21-OHD, 11-OHD, HSD3B

Adrenal causes: premature adrenarche, CAH (above), tumour (below), Cushing's syndrome

Tumour, virilising: adrenal—adrenocortical carcinoma, adenoma; ovary— arrhenoblastoma (usually benign); pineal—dysgerminoma; pituitary— gonadotrophin-releasing tumours

Ovarian causes: virilising tumour (arrhenoblastoma); PCOS

Unexplained (and unimportant pathology-wise): premature pubarche

Reductase (5-alpha-reductase) deficiency in an undervirilised XY child (can suddenly virilise at puberty, from previously phenotypically normal female)

The examination focuses on accurate staging of puberty, thorough evaluation of androgen effects and oestrogen effects, and assessment of growth parameters, followed by evaluation of the blood pressure, the adrenal glands, the gonads and the central nervous system. The other signs sought provide further evidence of suspected diagnoses, such as acanthosis nigricans in PCOS, or buffalo hump in Cushing's syndrome.

Commence by introducing yourself to the patient and the parent; note the quality of the child's voice replying, for deepening of the voice. Next, ask the child to undress as fully as possible without causing her undue embarrassment; underwear can be left on for this initial inspection. Visually scan the child and assess the Tanner staging, noting the androgen effects and the oestrogen effects. Next, assess the growth parameters, commencing with the height. Hyperandrogenism per se can cause tall stature early in its course. Short stature can result from long-standing hyperandrogenism. Short stature may also occur in Cushing's syndrome. Weight is also important, as obesity can be a feature of PCOS or Cushing's syndrome. The head circumference may be increased (e.g. intracranial [IC] tumours).

Next, inspect the skin for any evidence of hyperpigmentation, two forms of which may be found in hyperandrogenism. CAH can cause hyperpigmentation over extensor surfaces of joints, and areolae. PCOS can be associated with acanthosis nigricans, which is velvety, verrucous, hyperpigmented skin on the neck, axillae, under the breasts or on the vulva; it is usually a sign of insulin resistance in PCOS. Look for evidence of increased sebaceous gland activity (androgens) or abdominal striae (Cushing's syndrome). Note any obvious dysmorphic or diagnostic features, such as Beckwith-Wiedemann syndrome (associated with adrenocortical carcinoma or hepatoblastoma), or Cushing's syndrome.

Next, measure the blood pressure. This is very important, as it is elevated in 11 OHD CAH, but not the other forms of CAH; blood pressure also can be elevated in adrenocortical carcinoma, adenoma, Cushing's syndrome and in some patients with PCOS.

Next, check for any asymmetry (Beckwith-Wiedemann syndrome), then check the eyes (external ocular movements, fields and fundi) for any evidence of an intracranial tumour.

Examine the abdomen carefully for adrenal masses or ovarian masses, and mention that a rectal examination could be used to clinically evaluate the ovaries, but this is theoretical, and in reality ultrasound or MRI would be used to evaluate ovarian size. Mention the importance of inspecting the external genitalia to detect virilisation, in particular, clitoromegaly; in the interests of patient modesty, the examiners may indicate whether this is present without insisting on direct inspection.

Finally, examine the gait and lower limbs for any evidence of long-tract involvement (IC tumour) or proximal weakness (Cushing's syndrome). The relevant findings sought are set out in Table 7.11 (see also Fig. 7.9).

Table 7.11
Virilisation
1. INTRODUCE SELF
Quality of voice • Deep (androgenised) (androgen-induced enlargement of larynx) • Mature female (oestrogenised) • Higher-pitched child's voice (normal for age)
2. GENERAL INSPECTION
Position patient: standing, adequately undressed to allow examination without embarrassment
Visually assess Tanner staging
Oestrogen effects • Female body habitus • Fat distribution (decreased with hyperandrogenism; increased with PCOS) • Breasts (stage these) (decreased breast size with hyperandrogenism; no palpable breast tissue in premature pubarche from premature adrenarche [differential diagnosis])
Androgen effects • Masculine body habitus • Muscle development • Hirsutism: hair: facial, axillary, chest, back, perianal (differentiate from hypertrichosis) • Axillary odour • Pubic hair (stage this; look for male-type escutcheon, spreading up the linea alba) • Increased size of genitalia; clitoromegaly (offer to stage formally later)
Syndromal diagnosis (Beckwith-Wiedemann [associated adrenal tumours]; Cushing's)
Hemihypertrophy (Beckwith-Wiedemann; see short case on dysmorphology)
Skin • Acne (androgens) (head, neck and upper back distribution) • Hyperpigmentation: CAH (ACTH-induced: extensor surfaces of joints; and areolae) • Hyperpigmentation: acanthosis nigricans (PCOS) (velvety, verrucous, hyperpigmented skin on neck, axillae, under breasts, on vulva; usually sign of insulin resistance in PCOS) • Sebaceous gland activity (androgens) • Striae—abdominal (Cushing's) • Bruising (Cushing's)
Head and neck: appearance
Hair: greasy (androgens)
Face: moonface (Cushing's); squint (sixth cranial nerve palsy with IC tumour); nose:
comedones (androgens); mouth and chin: facial hair (androgens); acne (androgens)
Buffalo hump (Cushing's)
MedicAlert bracelet (CAH; risk of Addisonian crisis; alert to treat with hydrocortisone)
3. MEASUREMENTS
Height • Short (Cushing's, long-standing hyperandrogenism) • Tall (recent-onset hyperandrogenism)
Weight • Increased (Cushing's, PCOS)

Continued

Table 7.11 (continued)
Assess percentile charts
Calculate height velocity (acceleration of linear growth with androgens) • Increased (recent-onset hyperandrogenism)
4. BLOOD PRESSURE
Elevated in 11 OHD CAH, Cushing's, PCOS, adrenal tumours
5. HEAD AND NECK
Visual fields • Bitemporal hemianopia (pituitary tumour) • Other field cuts such as homonymous hemianopia (IC tumour)
External ocular movements • Sixth cranial nerve palsy (IC tumour) • Loss of upward gaze (pineal tumour: dysgerminoma)
Ophthalmoscope: cataracts (Cushing's)
Fundoscopy: papilloedema (IC tumour)
6. ABDOMEN AND GENITALIA
Liver • Enlarged (hepatoblastoma producing hCG) • Bruit (hepatoblastoma)
Adrenal glands • Mass (tumour)
Ovaries • Mass (tumour; mention rectal examination for completeness) (arrhenoblastoma)
Pubic hair • Tanner staging
External genitalia • Clitoromegaly (does not occur in premature pubarche, due to premature adrenarche)
7. GAIT, BACK AND LOWER LIMBS
Full gait examination to screen for signs of proximal weakness (Cushing's) or long-tract signs (IC tumour)

11-OHD CAH = congenital adrenal hyperplasia due to 11-beta-hydroxylase deficiency; IC = intracranial; PCOS = polycystic ovary syndrome

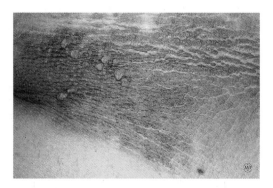

Figure 7.9 Acanthosis nigricans

Pigmentary Disorders. Medical Clinics of North America, Volume 93, Issue 6 (November 2009) Copyright © 2009 W. B. Saunders Company, p. 1235, Figure 8. Acanthosis nigricans. Areas of creases are usually involved and have a 'velvety' texture. (Reproduced with permission from the American Academy of Dermatology, Copyright © 2009. All rights reserved.)

Investigations

PROVOCATION TESTS AND OTHER BLOOD TESTS

If the patient is pubertal, then the most useful initial test is an LHRH test (also called gonadotrophin-releasing hormone [GnRH] test), as this assesses the pituitary response in any disorders of puberty or gonadal function. GnRH stimulates LH and FSH release from the pituitary gland, which in turn stimulate sex steroid release from the ovaries; testosterone and oestradiol are measured.

If there are no signs of puberty but obvious virilisation, then blood should be taken in the morning for: testosterone (to confirm hyperandrogenism—if very high, an adrenal or ovarian tumour is more likely); DHEAS (dehydroepiandrosterone sulfate; adrenal tumour marker); androstenedione; SHBG (sex hormone-binding globulin); and 17-hydroxyprogesterone (17-OHP) and PRA (CAH).

If the 17-OHP is elevated, then a short ACTH (Synacthen) stimulation test can be performed. This tests the stimulated cortisol response of the adrenal cortex, and in CAH can be useful in detecting milder or rare enzyme blocks by evaluating ratios of adrenal steroids to their precursors; for example, the ratio of 17-OHP to cortisol.

If the adrenal androgens are very high, then a dexamethasone suppression test (e.g. combined low and high dose) can be organised; this can determine whether an adrenal tumour is likely, and can be used to diagnose Cushing's syndrome.

Chromosomes for karyotype is appropriate if 5-alpha-reductase deficiency is suspected; steroid 5-alpha-reductase 2 catalyses the conversion of testosterone to dihydrotestosterone (DHT), so the DHT level will be very low. Mutations in the gene *SRD5A2* cause 5-alpha-reductase deficiency; a handful of laboratories around the world can directly test for these mutations.

IMAGING

MRI of the pituitary, adrenal glands and/or ovaries may be appropriate.

SHORT CASE: Thyroid disorders

These are not uncommon cases, but there are a number of possible introductions that may be used, including examining the neck, the thyroid (specified) or the eyes, or examining for causes of irritability, nervousness or even cold intolerance. Probably the most common introduction is to examine the neck. The approach outlined below is for children beyond infancy; in infants, the approaches for congenital hypothyroidism or hyperthyroidism are somewhat different and are discussed at the end of this section.

Most cases will have an autoimmune thyroid disease, such as Graves' disease or Hashimoto's thyroiditis. These may be associated with other autoimmune diseases, such as insulin-dependent diabetes mellitus (IDDM), Addison's disease and less commonly hypoparathyroidism, pernicious anaemia, vitiligo and hypogonadism.

Graves' disease comprises three components, namely a hyperfunctioning goitre, an ophthalmopathy and a dermopathy. The ophthalmopathy comprises exophthalmos (due to infiltration of orbital contents, excluding the eyeball, by inflammatory cells) and the findings of sympathetic overactivity, which are found in hyperthyroidism irrespective of cause. The dermopathy usually occurs over the dorsal aspect of feet or legs, and is termed 'pretibial myxoedema'.

Hashimoto's disease, or autoimmune thyroiditis, includes chronic lymphocytic thyroiditis and primary myxoedema. Most patients with this diagnosis are initially euthyroid but eventually become hypothyroid. A small percentage are initially hyperthyroid, and may have ophthalmopathy: this is called 'hashitoxicosis'.

The approach outlined assesses for the presence of autoimmune thyroid disorders, as well as associated autoimmune diseases. It also assesses for other underlying diagnoses, causing hyperfunction (e.g. toxic adenoma) or hypofunction (e.g. endemic cretinism, fetal iodine deficiency or haemosiderosis from thalassaemia).

Examination

Begin by introducing yourself to the child and the parent. Note any hoarseness in the child's voice when he or she replies (hypothyroidism in older children), and ask the child which school he or she attends and which grade, for an impression of mentation (slow in hypothyroidism, restless in hyperthyroidism).

Next, stand back and inspect the child for any obvious signs associated with hyperthyroidism (such as exophthalmos, tremor) or hypothyroidism (such as short stature, thyroidectomy scar, yellow skin discolouration due to carotenaemia, facial myxoedema). Note the height and weight parameters, and request the percentile charts. Hyperthyroidism is associated with tall stature and decreased weight, while hypothyroidism is associated with short stature and increased weight.

If the child is short, or hypothyroidism seems likely, then the US:LS ratio should be measured to see if it is increased. Now, ask the child to sit on a chair for examination of the neck. Inspect the neck from all angles, noting any redness overlying the thyroid region (thyroiditis) and any obvious swelling. Note the size, shape and symmetry of any swelling, and confirm that it is the thyroid gland by obtaining a glass of water and having the child swallow a small amount. Do not be tempted to rush in and palpate before careful inspection during swallowing. The thyroid is best palpated from behind in the first instance, with the child's chin lowered and the head slightly inclined towards whichever side is being examined, to relax the overlying sternomastoid muscle.

The palpation of the thyroid gland itself should be along similar lines to that of any lump (after first checking with the child that it is not exquisitely tender). Note the site, size, shape, symmetry (symmetrical enlargement is the rule in thyrotoxicosis), surface (smooth in thyrotoxicosis, irregular in multinodular goitre), consistency and mobility (any degree of fixation to surrounding structures suggests malignancy). Tenderness is present in subacute thyroiditis (de Quervain's; very rare in children) or acute suppurative thyroiditis. Thyrotoxicosis may be accompanied by a thrill, due to the increased vascularity of the gland, which can be felt by lightly laying your hand over the lateral lobes; this needs to be differentiated from transmitted carotid pulsation. Also note that if the carotid pulsation cannot be felt on one side, this may be due to malignancy surrounding the artery. Check for involvement of draining lymph nodes (in malignant thyroid tumours) and distortion of normal anatomy (such as a retrosternal goitre displacing the trachea).

Next, check for retrosternal extension of thyroid enlargement by percussing across the upper portion of the manubrium sterni (e.g. from right to left) to assess for any retrosternal dullness. Next, auscultate for any bruits (a systolic bruit can accompany a thrill in thyrotoxicosis).

Finally, assess for any direct effects on other neighbouring structures, by quickly checking the child's eyes (for Horner's syndrome due to involvement of the cervical sympathetic chain in malignant thyroid disease) and the voice (for hoarseness due to malignant involvement of the recurrent laryngeal nerve).

Then check for Pemberton's sign of thoracic inlet obstruction (due to retrosternal thyroid enlargement), by asking the child to raise both arms fully and checking a few seconds later for facial plethora and distended jugular veins, and note any evidence of inspiratory stridor. Ask the child to take a big breath in, through an open mouth, to check more formally for stridor.

Only when the thyroid gland itself has been fully evaluated should the examination proceed to look for signs of hyperfunction or hypofunction; a suggested format is as follows.

The examination flows well if you start at the neck and then move to the head (in particular, the eyes). Make a point of thoroughly inspecting the eyes from all angles, especially from above, over the child's forehead. Next, examine the upper limbs (these aspects can be checked with the child sitting on a chair), followed by a series of manoeuvres and then the lower limb examination, the praecordium and the lung fields (looking for complications such as congestive cardiac failure) and then the abdomen. Finally, request the temperature chart, urinalysis and, depending on the findings so far, check the child's development and/or hearing, and/or test for signs of hypoparathyroidism (essential if a thyroidectomy scar is present).

It can be difficult to assess a child who is being treated for either problem, as many expected signs, such as a slow pulse, are not present and this may fluster the inexperienced candidate. Should this happen to you, try to remain calm and simply perform a comprehensive examination, looking for all the signs mentioned, until it becomes apparent whether hypofunction or hyperfunction is the problem, and then proceed with a more directed assessment. For a summary of the examination, see Fig. 7.10.

1. Introduce self
Mentation

2. General inspection
Position patient: standing for initial
   inspection, then sitting
Obvious signs of:
 • Hyperthyroidism
 • Hypothyroidism
Parameters
 • Height
 • US/LS (if short or suspect
   hypothyroidism)
 • Weight
 • Percentile charts
 • Height velocity
Skin

3. Neck – thyroid gland
Examine with patient sitting
Inspection for goitre
Swallowing
Palpation (from behind)
Percussion (for retrosternal extension)
Auscultate for bruit (+)
Assess direct local effects
Check for Horner's syndrome and for
   hoarse voice (if possibility of
   malignancy)
Pemberton's sign (for retrosternal
   extension)

4. Head
Hair
Face
Eyes (full examination)
Mouth

5. Upper limbs
Hands
Fingertips
Nails
Palms
Pulse
Manoeuvres for hyperthyroidism
 • Hands out
 • Take pulse with arm elevated
 • Proximal strength
Blood pressure

6. Lower limbs
Inspection
Manoeuvres
Power
Reflexes
Sensation

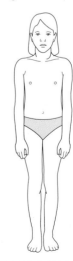

Figure 7.10 **Thyroid disorders**

Investigations

At the completion of your examination, the investigations worth mentioning are as follows.

HYPERTHYROIDISM

Blood tests

1. Thyroid function tests, including TSH level.
2. Thyroid autoantibodies found in Graves' disease, including the following:
   - Thyroid-stimulating immunoglobulin.
   - TSH-binding inhibiting immunoglobulin.
   - Exophthalmogenic immunoglobulin.
   - Dermopathy-associated immunoglobulin.
3. Other autoantibodies found in associated diseases:
   - Pancreatic islet cell antibody.
   - Adrenal cell antibody.

Imaging

Radionuclide scanning.

HYPOTHYROIDISM

Blood tests

1. Thyroid function tests, including TSH.
2. Thyroid autoantibodies found in Hashimoto's disease, including the following:
   - Antithyroglobulin antibody.
   - Antimicrosomal antibody.
3. Other autoantibodies found in associated diseases:
   - Pancreatic islet cell antibody.
   - Adrenal cell antibody.

Imaging

1. Bone age.
2. Radionuclide scan.
3. Cranial MRI if a pituitary lesion is suspected.

SHORT CASE: Thyroid disorders in infants

The most common scenario is a baby with hypothyroidism, although a neonate with hyperthyroidism may occasionally be encountered. Transient neonatal thyrotoxicosis is usually due to transfer of thyroid autoantibodies across the placenta. In these cases, the examination can proceed in the same order as that outlined for the older child, but with much more emphasis on assessing lack of weight gain, and also watching the baby feed. These children are usually tremulous, irritable and do not gain weight; sweating and tachycardia are prominent. The nappy of such a baby should be checked, as diarrhoea is the rule. After assessing the baby with hyperthyroidism, remember to ask to examine the mother for manifestations of Graves' disease.

Congenital hypothyroidism is not uncommon, although screening has afforded most infants prompt diagnosis and treatment. The examination of the infant with suspected hypothyroidism commences with general inspection, after taking particular note of the age of the baby.

Inspection may reveal jaundice, somnolence, respiratory difficulties (noisy respirations, apnoeic episodes due to large tongue), delayed separation of the umbilical cord, umbilical hernia, protuberant abdomen, peripheral cyanosis, oedematous extremities and genitalia. The growth parameters are usually normal at this early stage.

Next, inspect the head and neck. Note the facial features: the hairline may reach a long way down on the forehead; the eyes may seem far apart; the eyelids swollen; palpebral fissures narrowed; the nose broad with a depressed nasal bridge; the mouth open and the tongue large. The neck may appear short and thick, with an increase in adipose tissue (above the clavicles and between the neck and the shoulders). In an older infant, there is a delay in the development of the teeth. Now, palpate the hair, which may be coarse and brittle.

Feel the head; the scalp may be thickened and the fontanelles wide open. Look at the conjunctivae for pallor. Look in the mouth with a spatula for a lingual thyroid. Next, with the infant lying prone on the mother's lap, look for goitre; this is best palpated with the baby in this position. Following this, examine the heart and the abdomen, in the standard fashion, looking for evidence of cardiomegaly, constipation and oedema of the external genitalia.

Perform a gross motor developmental assessment to evaluate for delay and hypotonia. Finally, request the temperature chart (for hypothermia) and ask to watch the child feed; there may be disinterest in feeding, poor effort and choking episodes. Remember to ask to examine the mother for hyperthyroidism in neonates with a goitre (transplacental delivery of antithyroid medication).

The most useful investigations are thyroid function tests, including TSH level, and a thyroid scan, to differentiate between dyshormonogenesis and ectopic or absent thyroid tissue.

Table 7.12 gives detailed possible findings on examination of a child with a thyroid disorder.

Table 7.12
Additional information: details of possible findings on examination of a child with a thyroid disorder
1. INTRODUCE SELF
Quality of voice: hoarse (−)
Mentation • Impaired (−) • Irritable (+)
2. GENERAL INSPECTION
Obvious signs associated with: • Hyperthyroidism (e.g. exophthalmos, tremor, sweating, nervousness) • Hypothyroidism (e.g. short stature, coarse facies, thyroidectomy scar) • Associated autoimmune diseases (e.g. Addison, vitiligo) • Causes of hypofunction (thalassaemia)
Tanner staging • Precocity (−) • Delay (−)

Continued

Table 7.12 (continued)
Skin • Yellow tinge (−) • Vitiligo (autoimmune association) • Hyperpigmentation (Addison, thalassaemia) • Pretibial myxoedema (Graves)
Hair • Dry (−) • Alopecia (autoimmune association)
Face • Flushed, sweaty, anxious (+) • Coarse, bloated, yellow (−) • Rodentoid features (thalassaemia) • Hyperpigmented (Addison)
Eyes
Inspection (from above and from side) • Exophthalmos (Graves) • Thyroid stare (+) • Lid lag (+) • Lid retraction (+) • Strabismus (fetal iodine deficiency, exophthalmic ophthalmoplegia) • Nystagmus (fetal iodine deficiency)
Conjunctivae • Pallor (hypothyroidism per se or secondary to thalassaemia; associated pernicious anaemia) • Oedema, inflammation (in exophthalmos)
Cornea (ulceration in exophthalmos)
Visual fields: bitemporal hemianopia (pituitary tumour causing hypothyroidism)
Extraocular movements: muscle paresis in exophthalmos (in order) • Inferior oblique (first affected) • Adductors (muscles of convergence: medial, superior, inferior recti) • Lateral rectus • Test for lid lag (+)
Lens: cataracts (associated T1DM)
Retina • Optic atrophy (with exophthalmos) • Diabetic retinopathy (associated T1DM)
Mouth
Pigmented buccal mucosa, gums (Addison)
Lingual thyroid (−)
Poor dentition (−)
3. UPPER LIMBS
Hands • Dry, cool, puffy (−) • Peripheral cyanosis (−) • Peripheral neuropathy (−) • Tremulous, warm, sweaty (+)

Table 7.12 (continued)

Fingertips: prick marks from BSL testing (T1DM)

Nails
- Onycholysis (+)
- Thyroid acropathy (+)

Palms
- Erythema (+)
- Crease pallor (−, pernicious anaemia)
- Crease pigmentation (Addison, thalassaemia)

Pulse
- Slow (−)
- Rapid (+)
- Ectopic beats (+)
- Atrial fibrillation (+)
- Collapsing pulse (+)

Manoeuvres for hyperthyroidism
- Hands out in front (tremor)
- Take pulse with arm elevated (collapsing pulse)
- Test proximal muscle strength (proximal myopathy)
- Reflexes (brisk)

Blood pressure
- Decreased (Addison)
- Wide pulse pressure (+)

4. LOWER LIMBS

Inspection (standing)
- Onycholysis (+)
- Acropathy (+)
- Pseudohypertrophy (−)
- Pretibial myxoedema (Graves)
- Injection sites on thighs (T1DM)

Manoeuvres
- For hyperthyroidism: squat and stand (proximal myopathy)
- For hypothyroidism: gait (normal and heel–toe)
- High stepping (peripheral neuropathy)
- Ataxia (endemic cretinism)
- Spasticity (endemic cretinism)

Kneel on chair to test ankle jerks (delayed relaxation)

Neurological examination (on bed)

Power
- Proximal myopathy (+)
- Generally decreased (−)

Reflexes
- Brisk (+, endemic cretinism)
- Slow relaxation (−)

Sensation: diminished (demyelinating neuropathy in hypothyroidism)

BSL = blood sugar level; T1DM = insulin dependent diabetes mellitus.
If a finding is related to hyperthyroidism, it is marked with a plus sign (+), and if to hypothyroidism, with a minus sign (−).

SHORT CASE: Hypopituitarism

The lead-in for this case could include introductions which mention short stature, delayed puberty, or neonatal presentation with severe hypoglycaemia, jaundice and microgenitalia, or delayed separation of cord. Other introductions could make mention of craniopharyngioma, cranial irradiation, septo-optic dysplasia or acquired brain injury. Assessment specifically for signs of hypopituitarism could be requested.

If the patient is a girl aged over 13, or a boy over 15, then assess carefully for Tanner staging. Remember, sexual development is described as delayed if the onset of puberty has not occurred by two standard deviations from the mean, namely, 13 years in girls and 15 years in boys. Delay in puberty occurs in any condition where the bone age is delayed, which includes hypothyroidism, growth hormone deficiency and panhypopituitarism. This short-case approach covers a large amount of clinical material and requires a structured routine.

The simplest way to recall the key areas to check is the acronym **GREEN**.

GRowth (parameters, measurements)
Eye (acuity, fields)
Endocrine (Tanner stage, BP, pulse)
Neurological (gait, reflexes, disease-specific signs for underlying aetiology signs [e.g. SOD association, signs of raised ICP])

Examination procedure

The examination focuses on accurate staging of puberty and assessment of growth parameters, and evaluation for underlying causes and clinical effects of hypopituitarism.

Begin by introducing yourself to the patient and parent, and note the quality of the child's voice replying, particularly in boys, for lack of deepening (voice 'breaking' is a late sign, variable, not a reliable indicator of pubertal status). Next, ask the child to undress as fully as possible without causing undue embarrassment; underwear should be left on for this initial inspection. Visually scan the child and assess the Tanner staging, to note whether any lack of androgen effects in boys or oestrogen effects in girls.

Next, quickly note any obvious facial dysmorphic features (e.g. cleft lip, hypotelorism), suggesting a diagnosis such as holoprosencephaly, or other diagnostic features (e.g. nystagmus, or wearing glasses, suggesting visual problem, perhaps SOD, CHARGE). Note the nutritional status, as nutritional deficiency may occur in: children with acquired traumatic brain injury: children with tumours treated with radiotherapy, or hypothalamic tumours or craniopharyngioma causing diencephalic syndrome; or central adrenal insufficiency (CAI). Excessive adipose tissue can occur with hypopituitarism, or hypothyroidism. Also note the body habitus (e.g. eunuchoid habitus: i.e. arm span significantly greater than height, and lower segment greater than upper segment length) suggestive of hypogonadotrophic hypogonadism (HH).

The measurements of height, lower segment, US:LS ratio and arm span should then be carried out (or requested of the examiners), followed by the head circumference. Request the weight and the percentile charts, calculate the height velocity and interpret this appropriately. If the lead-in mentioned pubertal delay, ask for the parents' percentiles and ages of puberty. The height and height velocity are especially important.

Measuring the US:LS ratio and the arm span helps to evaluate whether there is any eunuchoid body habitus, which can occur in HH, and also detects a short lower segment, such as classically occurs in hypothyroidism.

The weight is important in detecting diagnoses such as tumours, HPE or acquired brain injury, in thin children, and endocrine problems such as hypopituitarism or hypothyroidism in obese children. Head circumference, if increased, may indicate an intracranial tumour, whereas microcephaly could be due to neonatal encephalopathy, or HPE. Always request the percentile charts and do not forget to calculate the height velocity.

The remainder of the examination begins with the hands, checking the blood pressure, and proceeds up to the head and neck, with particular emphasis on assessment of any midline defects or visual field loss, and then to the chest to check for heart defects, and then abdomen and accurate staging of the genitalia in boys.

The volume of the testes should be estimated, as this is the best indicator of the maturational stage. Prepubertal testes are usually less than 3 mL in volume, and less than 2 cm in length. An orchidometer can be requested if you are familiar with its use. Another measurement that may be used is the testicular volume index, which is the average length multiplied by the width of both testes. Prepubertally, it is usually between 1.0 and 1.4 cm^2.

Next, CNS signs are sought by a gait examination followed by checking the lower limb tone, power and reflexes, which may demonstrate upper motor neuron signs with diagnoses associated with raised intracranial pressure, hydrocephalus, brain tumours or pyramidal tract dysfunction secondary to previous insults of TBI or neonatal encephalopathy.

Finally, request the urinalysis. A specific gravity of 1.005 or less suggests diabetes insipidus (DI). Candidates can request urine osmolality, which should be below 200 mOsm/kg in DI.

A fairly detailed listing of possible findings is given in Table 7.13.

Table 7.13
Details of possible findings on hypopituitarism examination
GENERAL INSPECTION
Dysmorphic features (CHARGE, HPE)
Body habitus: eunuchoid (HH)
Diagnostic facies (e.g. HPE, CHARGE)
Nutritional status • Poor (e.g. neonatal encephalopathy, HPE) • Excess adiposity (hypothyroidism, hypopituitarism)
MEASUREMENTS
Height • Short stature: hypothyroidism, GH deficiency, hypopituitarism) • Normal stature (unusual): adequately treated hypopituitarism • Tall stature: chiasmal tumour, HH
US:LS ratio • Increased (hypothyroidism) • Decreased (HH)
Arm span: over 4 cm more than height for older adolescent (eunuchoid habitus, e.g. HH)

Continued

Table 7.13 (continued)
Weight • Decreased (malnutrition from TBI, HPE, tumours, diencephalic syndrome) • Increased (hypothyroidism, hypopituitarism, GH deficiency)
Head circumference • Increased (intracranial tumour, hydrocephalus) • Decreased (neonatal encephalopathy, acquired brain injury, HPE)
Height velocity • Decreased (hypopituitarism, hypothyroidism, GH deficiency, chronic malnutrition) • Normal (treated hypopituitarism, hypothyroidism, GH deficiency)
UPPER LIMBS
Fingertips: BSL testing (hypoglycaemia with CAI, unwell)
Pulse: bradycardia (untreated central hypothyroidism); tachycardia (undertreated DI, ACTH deficiency, CAI)
Forearms: muscle bulk (malnutrition with HPE, tumours)
Blood pressure: low (CAI, undertreated DI)
Axillae: lack of apocrine secretion, hair or odour (can support pubertal delay)
HEAD
Scalp: scar (resected brain tumour, ventriculo-peritoneal shunt [VP shunt])
Hair: dry (hypothyroidism)
EYES
Inspection • Hypotelorism (HPE) • Squint (septo-optic dysplasia [SOD], HPE, CHARGE) • Nystagmus (SOD)
Coloboma (CHARGE)
Visual acuity: diminished (SOD, pituitary tumour, HPE, CHARGE)
Visual fields: bitemporal hemianopia (craniopharyngioma/other pituitary tumour)
External ocular movements: sixth cranial nerve palsy (intracranial tumour)
Fundi • Papilloedema (raised ICP, craniopharyngioma) • Optic nerve hypoplasia (SOD) • Optic atrophy (SOD, raised ICP, craniopharyngioma)
NOSE
Anosmia (HH, SOD)
Midline dimple (HPE)
MOUTH AND CHIN
Central cyanosis (e.g. Tetralogy of Fallot, from CHARGE)
Midline defects associated with HPE or SOD • Cleft lip (repair) • Cleft palate (repair) (use a torch) • Single central incisor
Delayed dentition (central hypothyroidism)

Table 7.13 (continued)
EARS
Dysmorphic (CHARGE); hearing aid (CHARGE, SOD)
CHEST
Breasts: Tanner staging in girls
Auscultate: praecordium (CHD from CHARGE)
ABDOMEN
Inspection • Tanner staging of pubic hair • Scars (VP shunt)
GAIT AND LOWER LIMBS
Upper motor neurone signs (intracranial tumour, HPE, TBI, neonatal encephalopathy)
Delayed ankle jerk relaxation (undertreated central hypothyroidism)

Investigations

At the completion of the physical examination, the examiners may ask which investigations you would perform. These of course depend on the physical findings, but the following list covers some of the more useful investigations.

Note that those with gonadal hypofunction secondary to lack of pituitary gonadotropic hormones (on the basis of hypothalamic or pituitary disease) will have HH.

Hormone studies are best performed in pairs, with pituitary-stimulating hormones and their corresponding target organ hormones. Provocative/stimulation testing for each of these may be needed.

BLOOD TESTS

1. ACTH stimulation test (e.g. Synacthen stimulation test); morning (e.g. 9 a.m. at private labs) baseline bloods for cortisol and ACTH; Synacthen is then administered IV (or IM) (dose 10 µg/kg in children under 25 kg), blood is taken at 30 minutes for cortisol and then at 60 minutes for cortisol (to diagnose central ACTH deficiency).
2. Provocative testing for growth hormone release (with exercise, insulin induced hypoglycaemia, arginine infusion or levodopa).
3. TRF stimulation test: preparation: no caffeine for 24 hours before test; procedure: blood pressure is checked first, baseline bloods are taken for TFTs (thyroxine T4 and T3), prolactin and TSH; TRF is given over 2 minutes intravenously (IV) (as has caused arrest if given more rapidly), dose 5 µg/kg (up to 200 µg at 40 kg) blood is collected at 20 and 60 minutes, post-TRF, for TSH and prolactin assays).
4. Baseline LH, FSH, testosterone, oestradiol.
5. Gonadotropin-releasing hormone (GnRH) stimulation test (LH and FSH responses).
6. Serum electrolytes, glucose, urea and creatinine (CAI, DI).
7. Simultaneous plasma and urinary osmolality (for DI).
8. Plasma ADH (to diagnose DI; central DI has low ADH when plasma osmolality is elevated).
9. Water deprivation test (rarely needed) (to diagnose DI).

10. Vasopressin stimulation test (to diagnose central DI).
11. Gene testing:
    - PIT-1 (pituitary-specific transcription factor [OMIM*173110], responsible for pituitary growth and hormone expression, also called POU1F1; mutation can lead to CPHD1 [OMIM#613038], which causes decreased production of GH, prolactin [PRL] and TSH).
    - PROP-1 (Prophet of Pit-1; [OMIM*601538]; mutation can lead to CPHD2 [OMIM#262600]).
    - Neurophysin II (arginine vasopressin [AVP]) [OMIM*192340]; mutation can lead to neurohypophyseal DI [OMIM#125700]).

These three gene tests are readily available for children with congenital hypopituitarism.

IMAGING

1. X-ray of left wrist and hand for bone age (a very useful investigation).
2. MRI (for intracranial pathologies, such as craniopharyngioma, SOD, HPE).

Reference

Muir, A., Quisling, R., Yang, M., et al. (2004). Cerebral edema in childhood diabetic ketoacidosis; natural history, radiographic findings and early identification. *Diabetes Care*, 27, 1541–1546.

Chapter 8

Gastroenterology

LONG CASE: Inflammatory bowel disease (IBD)

The incidence of inflammatory bowel disease (IBD) in children has doubled, worldwide, in the last decade. Australia has the highest incidence of IBD in the world. Although the pathogenesis remains incompletely understood, there seem to be three components: genetic predisposition, environmental priming (related to commensal microbes) and then some triggering effect. Genome-wide association studies have found over 99 non-overlapping genetic risk loci, with 28 shared between Crohn's disease (CD) and ulcerative colitis (UC). There is an increasingly large number of genes associated with CD and UC, including genes which affect the function of the intestinal epithelial barrier and some which affect host defences. This increased understanding of genetic susceptibility suggests CD and UC may represent a mechanistic continuum of disease.

Research continues into identifying genotypic and phenotypic aspects which could allow prediction of a primary non-response to biologic agents. With the recent shift in the IBD management paradigm, mucosal healing is now used as an end point rather than a clinical indicator of remission, recognising that endoscopic lesions and symptoms may not correlate. Exclusive enteral nutrition (EEN) emerged as the ideal induction therapy for children with CD, although its uptake in adult practice has been limited.

A risk stratification has evolved, with those at higher risk of severe CD—predictors of more aggressive disease including younger age of onset, extensive small bowel disease, deep colonic ulcers, perianal disease and early need for corticosteroids—receiving more aggressive therapy, with earlier use of immunomodulators and biological agents; this is termed 'top-down' therapy (as opposed to the traditional approach of escalating, or 'step-up' therapy).

Long-term, poorly controlled CD or UC is associated with an increased risk for malignancy. There is now more awareness of the need for screening for immunisation status, and catch-up immunisation at diagnosis, prior to commencing any immunosuppressant regimens. Recommended vaccinations include: influenza, pneumococcal polysaccharide, hepatitis B and human papillomavirus. Immunisation against varicella-zoster virus (VZV) is recommended if VZV serology is negative, and if the child is not yet receiving immunosuppressants.

Patients with CD and UC are often used as long case subjects. With the incidence of CD and UC rising, there will be more patients seen in the examination format. Both diseases are commonly complicated by extraintestinal manifestations (EIMs), including arthralgia, erythema nodosum, uveitis and primary sclerosing cholangitis (PSC); CD is more associated with sacroiliitis, ankylosing spondylitis and peripheral arthritis, and UC is more associated with PSC, which can appear independent of activity of colitis. Either may present with these EIMs years before IBD is diagnosed. Both may require surgical intervention at some stage in their course. All candidates should be familiar with the differentiating features between the two. Candidates should know the medications used to *induce* remission: mnemonic in CD is **BEEN SAS** (**B**iologics, **EEN**, **S**teroids, **A**ntibiotics, **S**urgery); in UC it is **BASS** (**B**iologics, **A**minosalicylates, **S**teroids, **S**urgery); and those used to *maintain* remission is **BIAS** (**B**iologics, **I**mmunomodulators, **A**minosalicylates, **S**upplementary enteral nutrition in CD, **S**urgery in UC) in each condition. Steroids and antibiotics have *no* place in maintaining remission. Most agents used to treat acute attacks in UC can be used to maintain remission (except, obviously, for steroids).

History
PRESENTING COMPLAINT
Reason for current admission.

GASTROINTESTINAL SYMPTOMS
Interval/current: weight loss, growth, abdominal pain (site, interference with sleep, precipitation by eating), anorexia, nausea, vomiting, odynophagia or dysphagia (oesophageal CD), diarrhoea, urgency, tenesmus, incontinence, nocturnal defaecation, rectal bleeding, fistulae (CD, usually enterocutaneous), perirectal disease (CD).

EXTRAINTESTINAL SYMPTOMS
Interval/current: rashes (e.g. erythema nodosum [more in CD], pyoderma gangrenosum [more in UC]), itch (PSC), mouth involvement (e.g. aphthous ulcers), liver involvement (e.g. PSC, chronic active hepatitis), joint disease (e.g. arthralgias, spondyloarthropathies), visual problems (e.g. uveitis), vascular complications (e.g. vasculitis), renal tract involvement (e.g. nephrolithiasis), hypertension, myocarditis, pericarditis, fever, pubertal delay, neurological problems (e.g. peripheral neuropathy), haematological disease (e.g. anaemia), musculoskeletal weakness (e.g. vasculitic myositis, steroid-induced myopathy), pancreatitis, extraintestinal neoplasia (e.g. lymphoma), amyloidosis, thromboembolic disease (e.g. cerebral, retinal).

PAST HISTORY
Initial presentation, symptoms, when, where and how diagnosed, response to treatment, subsequent course, doctors involved, clinics attended, previous hospitalisations, past surgery, previous complications of disease and treatment, coexistent congenital immunodeficiencies (e.g. common variable immunodeficiency, neutrophil disorders), previous misdiagnoses (e.g. avoidance of food, thinness and pubertal delay as in anorexia nervosa, joint disease as in juvenile arthritis, severe perirectal disease as in child sexual abuse). Drug side effects are common and should be identified.

OTHER RELEVANT MEDICAL HISTORY
Immunisations (are they up to date, any missed due to treatment); past operations (e.g. appendicectomy); cigarette smoke exposure (exacerbates CD, but protects against UC).

TREATMENT

Drugs, nutritional therapy (enteral and parenteral, used either to induce a remission or to re-nourish a malnourished patient), surgical, alternative medicine, side effects of treatment (e.g. steroids, immunosuppressants), past courses of antibiotics (*Clostridium difficile* colitis).

SOCIAL HISTORY

1. Impact on child

Problems of chronic disease: energy levels, behavioural problems, chronic hospitalisation, altered self-image, school absence, depression, feeling of missing out due to disease exacerbations and energy levels, initial denial of interference with life, frustration, anger about physical symptoms (pain, diarrhoea, faecal incontinence), altered appearance, unpleasant and demanding treatments, lack of independence, lack of control of choices of activities (school, leisure, employment, sport), isolation.

Steroid effects, short stature, delayed sexual development (adverse effects on socialisation, self-esteem), effect on overall quality of life, perception of long-term effects on peer group recognition, whether and when desired transition to adult care, refusing counselling (not 'cool').

2. Impact on family

Financial burden of multiple hospitalisations, surgical procedures, parents' worries (how disease will affect future, problems at school, medication side effects, guilt), conflicts with parents (concerning eating habits and compliance with medication), siblings' worries (being kept ignorant of disease and treatment, jealousy of attention and overprotection of patient).

3. Social supports

Social worker, parent support groups, psychologist (IBD has one of the highest effects on mental health of chronic diseases in children), online 'chat groups' for teenagers, camps for adolescents with IBD.

FAMILY HISTORY

Inflammatory bowel disease, ankylosing spondylitis, rheumatoid arthritis, other autoimmune disorders.

Examination

The examination is essentially a modified gastrointestinal system short case, incorporating a nutritional assessment plus added elements to look for EIMs. This examination should thus include assessing the skin, joints, eyes and mouth. Perianal inspection must not be forgotten; it is particularly important in CD. Skin findings may include erythema nodosum, pyoderma gangrenosum, jaundice, and scratching from pruritus (PSC). The joints can be rapidly screened, including tests for sacroiliitis (spring pelvis) or spondylitis (bend over, touch toes, estimate degree of forward flexion); see Chapter 16's short case on joints.

The neurological consequences of relevant deficiencies (vitamins B_1, B_6, B_{12}, E) can be sought, by an abbreviated gait examination (walk, tandem [heel toe], on toes, on heels, Romberg, squat) plus lower and upper limb reflexes.

The salient findings sought on physical examination are listed in Figure 8.1.

Investigations

Investigations to clarify the diagnosis and those to assess disease activity are undertaken concurrently, so they are listed together here. In 10–15% of cases, it is not possible

1. General inspection
Weight
Height
Percentiles
Tanner staging
Nutritional status (muscle bulk,
    subcutaneous fat, peripheral
    oedema)
Pallor
Jaundice
Cushingoid appearance
Abdominal scars and stoma
Joint swelling (especially lower limbs)
Skin rashes (erythema multiforme,
    erythema nodosum, pyoderma
    gangrenosum)

2. Upper limbs
Clubbing (especially CD)
Palmar crease pallor (anaemia from
    dietary deficiency, iron loss in gut,
    folate malabsorption, vitamin B_{12}
    malabsorption, chronic disease, or
    side effects of salazopyrine)
Arthritis (wrists, elbows)
Palpable epiphyseal enlargement
    (vitamin D deficiency)

3. Head and neck
Cushingoid facies
Conjunctival pallor (anaemia)
Conjunctivitis
Scleral icterus (sclerosing cholangitis,
    chronic active hepatitis)
Iritis
Corneal xerosis or clouding (vitamin A
    deficiency)
Cataracts (if on steroids)
Aphthous stomatitis

4. Abdomen
Scars
Stoma
Striae (if on steroids)
Tenderness
Mass (matted loops or abscess)
Hepatomegaly (sclerosing cholangitis,
    chronic active hepatitis)
Ascites (protein deficiency, protein-
    losing enteropathy in CD)
Enlarged kidneys (hydronephrosis in CD
    from ureteral compression by
    inflammatory mass or fibrosis)

Fistulae (CD)
Gluteal wasting
Perianal disease (anal fissures, fistulae,
    abscesses, anal tags)
Rectal examination (blood, pus on
    glove)

5. Lower limbs
Joint swelling (knees, ankles)
Tibial bowing (vitamin D deficiency)
Erythema nodosum, pyoderma
    gangrenosum
Toe clubbing

6. Stool and urine
Stool
  • Inspection for blood, pus
  • Analysis for white cells reducing
    substances
Urinalysis
  • Urinary tract infection (recurrent in
    CD with enterovesicular fistulae)
Calculi: oxalate (CD), urate (UC)

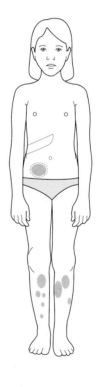

CD = Crohn's disease; UC = ulcerative colitis.

Figure 8.1 **Inflammatory bowel disease**

to differentiate CD from UC; these patients have 'indeterminate' colitis (an interim diagnosis).

STOOL

Mainly to differentiate other causes of symptoms:

1. Faecal multiplex polymerase chain reaction (PCR) to detect enteric bacteria and enteric protozoans including: *Campylobacter* species (sp.), *Shigella* sp., *Salmonella* sp., *Aeromonas* sp., *Yersinia enterocolitica*, *Giardia* sp., *Blastocystis* sp., *Entamoeba histolytica*, *Dientamoeba* sp., *Cryptosporidium* sp.; most laboratories prefer this method over the older methods of microscopy for cysts, ova, parasites, and culture and sensitivity (MCS) for bacteria. Faeces MCS still has a place in detecting pathogens not identified by particular laboratories' multiplex PCR panels, such as enteropathogenic *Escherichia coli*, and in providing a profile of any bacterial pathogen's susceptibility to antimicrobial agents.
2. Clostridium difficile toxin.
3. Alpha-1-antitrypsin level (screen for protein loss from bowel).
4. Neutrophil-derived proteins:
   a. Calprotectin: 95% sensitivity, 91% specificity for diagnosis of IBD.
   b. Lactoferrin: 80% sensitivity, 82% specificity for diagnosis of IBD.
   c. S100 calcium binding protein A12: 97% sensitivity, 97% specificity.

These stool markers provide useful measures of mucosal inflammation, improving as patients go into remission.

BLOOD

1. Full blood count (leucocytosis found in two-thirds of CD; anaemia plus high ESR has 96% specificity in diagnosing IBD in a referred patient population with suspected IBD).
2. CRP (elevated in 70–100% of CD and 50–60% of UC; also useful to prognosticate disease course)/ESR (elevated in 80–90% IBD patients).
3. Liver function tests (liver dysfunction as part of IBD; low albumin, total protein from protein-losing enteropathy).
4. Vitamins: folate (serum and red cell), vitamin B_{12} (ileal disease), vitamins A, D, E and prothrombin time for vitamin K (fat malabsorption).
5. Minerals: calcium, magnesium, phosphate, iron, ferritin, zinc, copper, selenium.
6. Electrolytes, urea and creatinine (associated renal disease).
7. Thiopurine methyl transferase (TPMT) (potential future treatment with a thiopurine); some patients are slow metabolisers, with increased risk of toxicity.
8. Serology for *Yersinia* species (*enteropathica* and *pseudotuberculosis*) to exclude this as a diagnosis. *Yersinia* colitis can present with erythema nodosum and arthralgia, as can CD.
9. Serology for varicella (if no clear history of vaccination; may need catch-up vaccines).
10. Serology for coeliac disease (1.4% of IBD patients have concurrent coeliac disease).
11. Immunological testing for tuberculosis (TB), such as the 'QuantiFERON-TB Gold' assay. Abdominal TB can mimic Crohn's disease.

The following investigations, the *serological biomarkers*, have limited clinical applications, but are included for completeness. Each has insufficient sensitivity and/or specificity to establish the diagnosis of IBD, or to distinguish clearly between CD and UC; p-ANCA and Anti-*Saccharomyces cerevisiae* antibodies (ASCAs) are the most frequently tested.

12. Perinuclear antineutrophil cytoplasmic antibodies (pANCAs) to neutrophil proteins, with an atypical staining pattern, may be elevated in UC (in 40–80%) or CD (in 5–25%); for diagnosing UC, sensitivity 55%, specificity 89%. May be helpful.
13. ASCAs are present in 50–60% of patients with CD, 20% of healthy first-degree relatives of those with CD, 10–15% of patients with UC and 0–5% of controls. The combination of ASCA and ANCA may be helpful to differentiate UC from CD.

Only in the setting of known IBD could serological profiles help distinguish CD from UC. The combination of *positive ASCA* and *negative p-ANCA* is specific for *CD*, while the opposite, *negative ASCA* and *positive atypical p-ANCA*, is specific for *UC*.

IMAGING

Magnetic resonance imaging (MRI) and *ultrasound* (US) have become the primary imaging investigations. The goals of imaging include making the diagnosis of IBD, then determining which type, its extent, how it is progressing (whether it is penetrating, stricturing or inflammatory) and whether there are complications.

The two main issues are the technical difficulties of obtaining an excellent view of the small bowel, and the amount of radiation needed for some of the investigations, to obtain these views.

Magnetic resonance enterography (MRE) involves no radiation, it is reproducible with less inter-observer and intra-observer bias than ultrasound, it has superior soft tissue contrast and can differentiate acute active disease from chronic disease, plus it can assess for extraintestinal complications. It is particularly useful in defining small bowel disease.

Some studies have shown a reclassification rate of over 10% when patients are assessed by MR; either indeterminate IBD reclassified as CD, or UC reclassified as CD.

MRE and *MR enteroclysis* both have a sensitivity of 88% for detecting IBD. MR enterography has a specificity of 92–100% for detection of small bowel IBD. Gadolinium-enhanced MRI has improved intestinal image resolution: CD shows transmural enhancement of the colon, and bowel wall thickening of the terminal ileum or proximal small bowel; UC shows mucosal enhancement and submucosal sparing extending proximally from the rectum. The technique is cheaper than endoscopy, but still requires bowel cleansing. MR provides detailed images of perianal fistulae and is the dominant imaging technique for assessing perianal disease in CD. MRE is preferable to CTE because of lack of radiation, and because of superior images that can distinguish active inflammation from fibrosis.

US of abdomen and pelvis identifies inflammation by increased bowel wall diameter and altered pattern of mural stratification, and Doppler studies can detect increased blood flow. US may be useful in delineating intra-abdominal masses (e.g. solid lesions or bowel loops), including abdominal or pelvic abscesses. US for the initial diagnosis of IBD has a sensitivity of 75–94%, with a specificity of 67–100%, can identify bowel wall thickening, and differentiate fibrosis from oedema.

Contrast-enhanced ultrasound (using the new microbubble contrast agent that lasts a few minutes in the bloodstream) can evaluate the bowel wall and assess disease activity with a sensitivity of 93% and a specificity of 93%.

Imaging modalities involving radiation are used rarely now, in favour of MRI and US. Some of the following imaging techniques are still used, but less frequently:

- *Bone age.* Assessment of growth delay in CD; left wrist X-ray.
- *Bone densitometry (DXA; dual energy X-ray absorptiometry).* Baseline; measures bone mineral density (BMD); used to detect osteopenia at diagnosis and after steroid treatment.

- *Plain abdominal X-ray*, erect and supine. May see evidence of incomplete bowel obstruction with distended bowel loops and air/fluid levels in CD.
- *Chest X-ray.* Used to help detect TB, a cause of chronic bowel inflammation. Its utility depends on the endemicity of TB.
- *CT scanning.* Multiplanar imaging can visualise overlapping bowel loops, and complications such as fistulae or abscesses. *Traditional CT* uses a contrast agent such as barium or iodine, which highlights intraluminal filling defects such as masses. *CT enterography* (CTE) uses neutral (low-density) oral contrast and intravenous contrast to accentuate the distinction between the enhancing small bowel wall and the low-attenuation gut lumen, to visualise the bowel wall and mucosa. *CT enteroclysis* comprises placement of a nasojejunal tube, and infusing a contrast agent into the proximal small bowel. CTE and CT enteroclysis may detect segmental mural enhancement, and wall thickening, consistent with active inflammation; reactive mesenteric adenopathy also may be found, supporting the diagnosis of active inflammation. For any CT study, the benefits must be weighed against the cumulative deleterious effects of ionising radiation, especially in younger children.
- *Positron emission tomography* (PET) scanning. This can identify areas of active inflammation, in UC. PET uses [F18] fluoro-2-deoxy-D-glucose to spot areas of increased metabolism.
- *Radiolabelled white blood cell scan.* Useful if mid-small bowel pathology suspected but not able to be found using conventional evaluations.
- *Fluoroscopic barium studies.* Small bowel follow through (SBFT) and small bowel enteroclysis can detect mucosal ulceration, or irregularities, narrowing or distension of the gut lumen, and presence of fistulae, with a sensitivity of 85–95%, and specificity of 89–94% for SBFT in patients with terminal ileal disease in CD.

ENDOSCOPY

Upper and lower gastrointestinal (GI) endoscopy remain of key importance. These comprise oesophagogastroduodenoscopy (OGD) plus full colonoscopy with ileal intubation. Biopsies are taken from each anatomical segment. Endoscopy is used to diagnose IBD, monitor progress, assess mucosal healing, and therapeutically to dilate strictured segments. In active UC, the mucosa is oedematous, hyperaemic and friable. In CD, aphthous or serpiginous ulcers may be seen, as well as erythema and 'skip' lesions, and an appearance like cobblestones.

In *small bowel video-capsule endoscopy* (SBVCE), the patient ingests the capsule, and the images are transmitted to a belt-worn recorder, allowing an ambulatory and prolonged (e.g. 8-hour) examination, which is especially useful for assessing areas where upper endoscopy or colonoscopy cannot reach. SBVCE should not be used where there are known strictures. Other contraindications include obstruction, fistulae, swallowing disorders, pacemakers and other electro-medical devices. A normal SBVCE has a high negative predictive value.

In Australia, the Health Insurance Commission has approved capsular endoscopy for children over 10 years of age with otherwise unexplained blood loss/anaemia. Any procedure (e.g. colonoscopy, barium enema) may precipitate fulminant colitis in those with severe disease.

OTHER

1. Mantoux or interferon gamma release assays (QuantiFERON Gold) to help exclude TB.

2. Urine culture (to detect urinary tract infection, which can be recurrent in CD with fistulae between gut and bladder).

Management

Short-term aims include induction and maintenance of clinical and histological remission, improvement in overall quality of life and prevention of complications. The main goals are now mucosal healing, and transmural healing, rather than just clinical healing; patients in clinical remission with steroids may have active endoscopically identified mucosal lesions in up to 70% of cases. Risk stratification based on genotype, phenotype and serology is another useful tool. The only factor that predicts prolonged remission in CD (persisting 3–4 years after initiating treatment) is complete mucosal healing. Longer-term aims include preventing relapses, normalising growth and pubertal development, maintaining bone mass and minimising the need for surgery. These therapeutic aims are based on early aggressive therapy, including the use of immunosuppressants and newer biological agents.

Earlier use of potent agents, previously considered 'third line', may be more effective than awaiting resistance to treatment. When evaluating new therapies, remember that a placebo response rate over 30% has been noted in IBD.

The Paediatric Crohn's Disease Activity Index (PCDAI) and quality-of-life measures previously have been regarded as useful in assessing response to therapies, but recently the utility of the PCDAI has been called into question, with recognition (as above) that mucosal assessment is a more appropriate mode of evaluating disease activity. The PCDAI ignores mucosal inflammation and overestimates symptoms due to comorbidities; it correlates poorly with the presence or extent of endoscopic lesions in CD.

In UC in adults, the presence of mucosal healing 1 year after diagnosis is associated with reduced need for colectomy at 5 years. In CD in adults, the presence of mucosal healing 1 year after diagnosis is associated with reduced subsequent need for corticosteroids, and is also associated with mucosal healing at 5 years. There are advantages in achieving mucosal healing with biological agents; mucosal healing during therapy with infliximab is associated with a lower risk of major abdominal surgery.

CROHN'S DISEASE (CD)

Paediatric CD is more aggressive than adult CD: it is characterised by widespread intestinal involvement, rapid early progression and a 25% rate of stricturing/penetrating disease within 4 years of presentation—25% of patients with CD first present under 16 years.

No medication alters the long-term outcome of CD. EEN is the most efficacious standard therapy for achieving *remission*. EEN leads to complete mucosal healing in three-quarters of patients in 10 weeks; this is superior to steroids, which lead to mucosal healing in only one-third of patients in the same time period.

Induction therapy for CD: exclusive enteral nutrition (EEN), steroids, biologics

EEN is the best therapeutic intervention currently available for *remission* induction. It heals mucosal disease, demonstrates more effective resolution of gut inflammation than other agents, improves nutritional status, skeletal growth and bone mass, and avoids the side effects of immunosuppression. EEN induces remission in up to 83% of new paediatric patients with CD.

EEN has a primary therapeutic effect, reducing inflammation, but also corrects malnutrition.

Nutritional interventions have been used widely in children in Europe and Japan, with steroid use diminishing accordingly. Both the European and the Japanese Societies for Pediatric Gastroenterology, Hepatology and Nutrition recommend nutritional therapy as the primary therapy for CD; this is not the case in the US, where there is resistance to committing to 8 weeks of specialised formula alone (orally or by nasogastric tube). Both elemental and polymeric diets improve scores of disease activity, with histological healing and down-regulation of pro-inflammatory cytokines. Severely malnourished patients may require overnight nasogastric tube feeds with elemental formulae or polymeric preparations; lactose-intolerant patients need lactose restriction; patients with strictures may find a low-residue diet helpful; and patients with severe terminal ileal disease should have a low-oxalate diet and decreased dietary fat.

There are now formulae with anti-inflammatory cytokines, prebiotics and probiotics, but there is insufficient evidence to support their use as yet. Total parenteral nutrition (TPN) can be used where other therapies fail, but it is more expensive, and no more effective than enteral feeding with elemental or polymeric formulae. Home TPN and home enteral nutrition are widely used in the US in patients with CD.

Despite the efficacy of EEN, **steroids** remain a first-line agent for remission in CD, **above EEN** in most practices, both adult and paediatric. *Prednisolone* is used for moderate to severe disease. *Budesonide* is an enteric-coated steroid used for targeted release in either the small intestine and right colon, or in the colon. The biological agent *infliximab* is used for refractory disease, steroid dependency or fistulising disease.

In moderate CD, corticosteroids can induce a clinical remission in around 70% of patients with small bowel disease. Steroids are given orally (prednisolone, methylprednisolone, budesonide) or intravenously (hydrocortisone, methylprednisolone).

Controlled ileal-release *budesonide* is useful in treating active ileal and ileocaecal disease and can also delay relapses. Budesonide may have fewer side effects and less adrenal suppression than prednisolone. Severe hypokalaemia and benign intracranial hypertension have been described but are rare in children receiving oral budesonide.

Steroid side effects relate to dose and duration, and can include bone loss. This can occur rapidly, within weeks of commencing treatment, and is not prevented by alternate-day treatment. Therapies used in an attempt to prevent osteopenia include calcium supplements, vitamin D and calcitriol. Their efficacy is uncertain.

Lack of response to steroids may be due to the presence of strictures or, less commonly, complications such as an abscess or fistula. Treatment may involve bowel rest (TPN in hospital or at home, or elemental diet by nasogastric infusion) or surgery.

Surgery in CD tends to be conservative, being limited to dealing with emergencies (perforation, obstruction, massive haemorrhage, toxic megacolon), relieving less urgent problems (fistulae), resecting very localised disease, strictures and preserving bowel.

Infliximab (IFX, chimeric monoclonal anti-TNF-α antibody; 75% human IgG 1 isotype) binds to soluble TNF α and its precursor, neutralising their actions, and is effective in the induction and maintenance of remission in active and fistulising CD. Pro-inflammatory cytokines such as TNFα are involved in the pathogenesis of CD. Infliximab, an anti-TNFα monoclonal antibody, neutralises these cytokines, stopping inflammation. It can induce a clinical remission and mucosal healing within weeks, with a response rate of over 80% (both clinical and endoscopic) in moderate to severely active treatment-resistant CD in patients already receiving immunosuppressives. It is given initially at 0, 2 and 6 weeks.

Its half-life is 3 weeks. The onset of benefit is 2 to 4 weeks. It can maintain remission if given every 8–12 weeks, and dosage optimised by measuring drug levels. Around 20% of patients develop antibodies (human-antichimeric antibodies [HACAs]) to infliximab, which limits its effectiveness; HACAs can be induced after one or several infusions. The clinical effect of infliximab appears to be improved when a patient is also taking one of the other immunomodulating drugs, such as AZA or 6-MP. Concurrent administration of immunomodulators also reduces the likelihood of developing HACAs.

Adalimumab (ADA, monoclonal anti-TNF-α antibody, 100% human IgG1 isotype) is also used for induction and maintenance of remission in CD. The half-life of adalimumab is 14 days. The onset of benefit is 2–4 weeks. The clinical effect is improved when taking other immunomodulating drugs.

There has been much discussion in the literature about the side effects of *TNF-alpha antibody inhibitors (TNFIs)*, reported in *adults*, although in paediatric practice side effects from steroids present a much greater problem.

For completion, reported side effects of TNFIs in *adults* can be remembered by the mnemonic **AMPLE HINTS**:

Autoimmune-like syndromes
Malignancy, especially lymphoma
Pancytopaenia/neutropenia (pregnancy should be avoided)
Liver transaminase elevation
Eczema and psoriasis

Heart failure: can be worsened by IFX
Infections: if serious bacterial infection occurs, stop, or do not start TNFIs/**I**njection site/**I**nfusion reaction: common; treat with antihistamine, steroids, slowed rate/**I**mmunisation: immunise before treatment; no live attenuated vaccine during treatment
Neurological syndromes: Guillain-Barré, optic neuritis; may be same frequency as normal population; if these occur, stop or do not start, TNFIs
Tuberculosis: increased susceptibility to TB or reactivation of TB
Surgical procedures: due to effects on wound healing, withhold drugs for 8 weeks prior)

CD maintenance: immunomodulators AZA, 6MP, MTX; biologics IFX, ADA

A mnemonic for maintenance agents in IBD is **BIAS**: **B**iologics, **I**mmunomodulators, **A**SA and **S**upplementary nutritional therapy. Local practices vary greatly in which are used. In CD, B and I are used in some institutions, whereas elsewhere A and S are used more frequently.

Immunomodulators are the first-line treatment for *maintenance* of CD *in remission*. Only these and biological agents have documented efficacy in maintenance of response and remission.

There is some evidence that the earlier these agents are started, the better: if they are commenced within 3 months of diagnosis, then there is reduced corticosteroid exposure, but no adverse effect in the rates of remission, infliximab use over time or surgery requirements.

Agents such as *6-MP* and *AZA* (which is metabolised to 6-MP, the active agent) can be used for maintenance therapy for CD, prophylaxis after surgery in CD and perianal CD. In particular, 6-MP has been shown useful as initial treatment in children with moderate to severe CD. AZA and 6-MP have a slow onset of action (up to 3–4 months) and so need to be combined with nutritional therapy or steroids until their effect is seen. Duration should be for years, as there is a high relapse rate if AZA or 6-MP are stopped within the first year. Bone marrow suppression can occur (in 2–5% of patients) at any time.

If using AZA or 6-MP, it is useful to know the patient's thiopurine methyltransferase (TPMT) status. TPMT is the enzyme that catalyses the conversion of 6-MP to 6-methylmercaptopurine (6-MMP). If TPMT activity is reduced, then 6-MP is preferentially metabolised to 6-thioguanine (6-TG). In excess, this is toxic and can cause bone marrow depression leading to leukopenia. Higher 6-MMP levels correlate with hepatotoxicity. Aminosalicylates (ASAs) and methotrexate (MTX) inhibit TPMT activity and can increase 6-TG levels.

MTX may be effective for the treatment of steroid-dependent chronically active CD if AZA or 6-MP fails (after 4 months), or if the patient is intolerant to AZA or 6-MP. MTX may be given in low-dose oral form (oral bioavailability is complete with low doses and decreases if higher doses given) or intramuscularly.

Low-dose MTX side effects include nausea (in about 40%), anorexia, stomatitis, diarrhoea, headache, dizziness, fatigue and altered mood, and can be reduced by giving supplemental folic acid therapy. Pulmonary toxicity (especially interstitial pneumonitis) can occur at any time and with any dose.

Biologics used include TNF-alpha inhibitors (TNFIs). IFX (a TNFI) can maintain remission if given every 8–12 weeks. IFX is expensive, but the introduction of 'biosimilars' has led to cost reduction. Side effects are outlined above. Other TNFIs currently used include ADA, and certolizumab pegol (humanised Fab fragment, 95% human IgG1 isotype). These aim to block destructive mucosal responses. Fatal side effects are rare but have been reported. Young male patients receiving IFX with AZA have developed hepatosplenic T-cell lymphoma; this does not occur with IFX alone (see below).

Another biologic treatment used in CD, natalizumab, has been associated with a risk of progressive multifocal leukoencephalopathy (PML).

For very severe CD, bone marrow ablation and stem cell transplantation are being investigated. Other treatments on the horizon include a number of new biological agents (abatacept, anti-IL-2 [ABT-874], visilizumab [anti-CD3], golimumab, fontolizumab).

ASAs can maintain remission in mild CD. *Supplementary enteral nutrition* also has a place in maintaining remission in CD.

ULCERATIVE COLITIS (UC)

In UC, medical management is successful in preventing relapses and surgical management is curative. *Remission* in UC can be achieved with **BASS**: **B**iologics, **A**SAs, **S**teroids or **S**urgery. Corticosteroids are used for moderate to severe disease. ASAs are used for mild to moderate disease. For acute severe colitis (ASC) or severe refractory disease, TNFIs, intravenous calcineurin inhibitors, CSA or tacrolimus (TAC) can be useful 'rescue' therapies, (palindromic mnemonic CSA ↔ ASC) avoiding immediate surgery. *IFX* is now PBS-listed in Australia for 'rescue' therapy for UC. *Maintenance of remission* in UC can be achieved with **BIAS**: **B**iologics (IFX) and **I**mmunomodulators (AZA/6-MP) for moderate to severe disease, **A**SAs for mild to moderate disease, and the other treatment modality which is **S**urgery.

Mild disease/distal colitis

Patients with mild disease look well and produce two to five stools per day. Optimal management is combined oral and rectal ASAs. Topical steroids are effective for limited rectal disease. These include prednisolone suppositories, enemas and foam enemas for progressively more extensive disease. Steroid enemas involve retaining 50–100 mL and are used as one twice a day initially, for moderate to severe disease (proctitis). As the disease settles, this can decrease to one nightly for 2 weeks or until settled fully. Topical mesalazine is also used in topical left-sided UC and this can reduce the relapse rate if used prophylactically (e.g. twice a week). The main problem with enemas is compliance.

Oral steroids may be required, but are generally ineffective for limited distal disease (procto-sigmoiditis). If there is not adequate response to these within 2 to 4 weeks, a form of enteric-coated budesonide is now available for colitis. This has limited systemic side effects.

ASAs are effective for acute mild disease and also valuable to maintain remission. Treatment is usually lifelong (for the life of the colon). Sulfasalazine comprises sulphapyridine linked to 5-aminosalicylate (5-ASA) by an azo bond, which is broken down by colonic bacteria.

The active component, 5-ASA, is effective locally in the colon. Mesalazine and olsalazine are 5-ASA formulations which do not contain the sulpha moiety. These are enteric coated and deliver the drug directly to the large bowel. The most common problems encountered with sulfasalazine are related to the sulpha part (rashes, bone marrow depression), whereas 5-ASAs can cause nephrotoxicity.

Sulfasalazine and mesalazine are first-line treatments. In acute episodes with mild to moderate extensive disease, around 80% of patients will achieve remission within 4 weeks, with oral aminosalicylates.

Maintenance of remission for mild distal colitis may include mesalazine suppositories (for proctitis), mesalazine enemas (for left-sided disease) or oral mesalazine. Topical plus oral therapy works better than oral therapy alone.

Moderate extensive disease

Patients with moderate disease have abdominal pain, rectal bleeding and urgency, are slightly unwell and tend to have static weight. They may require systemic corticosteroid therapy for a few months. Aminosalicylates are also used. A combination of steroid and 5-ASAa brings the condition under control quickly in most cases. Alternate-day steroids are not effective in remission induction. Biological agents have some benefit in inducing and maintaining remission in moderate to severe UC. IFX has been shown in adults to promote mucosal healing, and to reduce the requirement for colectomy in severe disease.

Severe disease/fulminant distal and extensive colitis/refractory disease

Children with severe disease (> 6 bloody stools per day, tachycardia, fever, ESR > 30, Hb < 100 g/L) may be very unwell, have abdominal pain and be hypoproteinaemic. Some children with severe pancolitis may have few constitutional symptoms but very severe disease. In order to induce remission, these children require topical and oral ASA plus systemic steroids, and may need parenteral steroids. If the child has 3 days of IV steroids, but still has > 8 stools per day, and a CRP over 400 nmol/L, then there is an 85% chance of needing an urgent colectomy. If the child has not improved after 3 days, treatment with cyclosporine A (CSA) or IFX should be considered, but a surgical referral and potential urgent colectomy should be planned.

Once remission has been induced, *thiopurines* (AZA and 6-MP) are *mainstays* to *maintain remission*. They are generally ineffective for induction of a remission. CSA has been used both for induction and maintenance of remission. *IFX* also has been used both to achieve induction and as a maintenance agent in steroid refractory and fulminant disease, but should not delay colectomy.

Children with fulminant colitis may have in excess of 10 bowel movements each day with continuous bleeding. The rare 'toxic megacolon' can present requiring hospitalisation for intravenous steroids, bowel rest and TPN. Medical treatments should not delay referral to the surgeons. Failure to respond to medical therapy after 5–7 days is one indication for urgent colectomy. IFX and CSA can be used as a 'rescue' treatment for severe UC to avoid emergency colectomy. If effective, this generally only postpones colectomy; despite clinical remission in around 80%, most will need colectomy within a year. IFX and CSA may allow time to educate families regarding acceptance of this treatment.

CSA is a peptide that blocks interleukin-2 production by T helper cells. Side effects of CSA are frequent, including paraesthesia in about 25% of patients, hypertrichosis, hypertension, renal insufficiency and tremors. CSA can be used only where blood levels of CSA can be determined readily.

Colectomy

Indications for emergency surgery include gastrointestinal haemorrhage (UC is the second leading cause of massive gastrointestinal blood loss in children), intestinal perforation, fulminant colitis or toxic megacolon. Emergent operative treatment usually comprises total or subtotal abdominal colectomy, with an end ileostomy, subsequent proctocolectomy and then ileoanal reconstruction or 'pouch' surgery.

Removal of the colon and rectum is curative for the intestinal manifestations of UC. Extraintestinal disease, however, continues despite colectomy. A total colectomy with endorectal removal of rectal mucosa and an ileoanal sphincter-saving anastomosis (an endorectal pull-through procedure, ERPT) with some variant of pouch reservoir, is performed commonly, and preserves continence in 90–98% of children, with an expected four to six stools per 24 hours after the first postoperative year. During this procedure, all rectal mucosa is removed to avoid the risk of malignant change. To preserve sphincter function, most surgeons leave the distal 4–5 cm of rectal muscle layer intact, and remove *only* the rectal mucosa. There is still a significant risk of inadvertent injury to the pelvic sympathetic and parasympathetic nerves responsible for sexual function.

There are several reservoir options with the ERPT, including J-, S- and W-shaped pouches fashioned from the terminal ileum. Pouchitis, presenting with loose bloody stools, urgency and frequency, develops in 30–40% of those undergoing this procedure. Pouchitis is associated with an increase in extraintestinal manifestations of UC. Treatment with metronidazole may be effective, but pouchitis can be very difficult to treat. A repeat endoscopy (pouchoscopy) in 3 months is suggested by some units.

GROWTH AND PUBERTAL DELAY

Ineffective treatment of children with CD delays puberty, decreases final adult height and often impairs catch-up growth after diagnosis. Effective therapies focus on mucosal healing and nutritional rehabilitation with uninterrupted maintenance of remission. Surgical intervention, both in UC and CD, can be associated with marked improvement in health, the onset of puberty and the reduction in need for many drugs.

Pubertal delay is thus a relative indication for surgery. Escalating therapy using biological agents or immunomodulators can be considered to maintain remission through puberty, but should be directed to achieving mucosal healing. Many adolescents are psychologically upset by pubertal delay, and many units use sex steroid therapy in these patients, through consultation with paediatric endocrinologists. In boys with IBD, testosterone for 3–6 months can have very positive effects on virilisation, growth and psychological wellbeing, although there are no controlled trials of testosterone use. In girls with IBD, ethinyloestradiol can be used for a similar period of time.

METABOLIC BONE DISEASE

Bone disease can occur in IBD as a result of malnutrition. Calcium homeostasis and bone growth are of paramount importance. Peak bone mass (PBM) is the main determining factor in the risk of developing osteoporosis later in life, and over 90% of PBM is acquired during childhood and adolescence. Calcium supplementation is effective in preventing bone disease. It is controversial as to whether bisphosphonates have any role in paediatric patients. A study in 2006 reported a prevalence of vitamin D deficiency of 35% in children with IBD, but serum 25-hydroxy-vitamin D concentration was not associated with the lumbar spine bone mineral density Z score or with serum parathyroid hormone levels. Factors predisposing to vitamin D deficiency include dark-skin complexion, winter season, lack of vitamin D supplementation, early stage of disease, more severe disease and upper intestinal tract involvement in CD.

MALIGNANT POTENTIAL

Once a child has had UC for 8–10 years, the general risk of colon cancer is 1% per year, and by 20 years may be up to 25%. After 8 years of disease, yearly colonoscopy and biopsy are recommended, with further colonoscopies if the child is symptomatic between visits.

If carcinoma is found, the treatment is colectomy. If carcinoma in situ is found, the treatment is colectomy. If dysplasia is found, colonoscopy should be repeated in 3 months and, if found again, colectomy is recommended.

If a child has continuous disease, or a frequently relapsing course, the risk of malignancy is greater than in those with less severe disease.

In IBD patients, there is an overall increased risk of lymphoma in those exposed to biological or immunomodulator therapy. There is also a rare universally fatal form of lymphoma linked to children and young adults with IBD, HSTCL, reported with combination therapy with 6-MP/AZA, and monotherapy with 6-MP/AZA, but not with infliximab alone. The risk of HSTCL is very low and should be balanced against the risk of loss of response during monotherapy with a biologic if unaccompanied by an immunomodulator.

LONG CASE: Chronic liver disease (CLD)

Liver transplant (LTx) is the standard of care for children with chronic liver failure and selected metabolic conditions. In the last decade, the rate of paediatric pretransplant mortality has declined, especially for infants under 12 months of age. Graft survival continues to improve. LTx has over 90% survival with good quality of life. CLD provides many issues for discussion. There remains a crisis in donor supply for LTx. There are improved ways to avoid graft loss while minimising consequences of immunosuppression. Several long-term complications continue to be challenging, including disease recurrence, consequences of immunosuppression (especially renal injury), development of malignancy (posttransplant lymphoproliferative disease [PTLD]), hyperlipidaemia, hypertension, as well as the issues of adolescents' transition to adult care.

The causes of CLD can be divided into three main groups: cholestatic diseases, metabolic diseases and chronic hepatitis (various forms). Other categories of disease that can require LTx include acute liver failure, oncologic diagnoses and vascular disorders.

Cholestatic diseases

EXTRAHEPATIC BILIARY ATRESIA (EHBA)

This is the most common form of liver failure in children, and the main indication for LTx (accounting for 50% of LTx in the USA and 74% of LTx in Europe). It is of unknown cause. It is more common in Asians and African-Americans than in Caucasians. In 10–15%, EHBA is associated with other anomalies: cardiac defects, polysplenia, inferior vena cava anomalies, pre-duodenal portal vein, situs inversus and malrotation.

There is destruction of extrahepatic and intrahepatic bile ducts, causing cholestasis, fibrosis and cirrhosis, with clinical correlates of jaundice and failure to thrive.

The initial treatment is the Kasai portoenterostomy, a palliative procedure, which involves removal of the fibrosed biliary tree and forming a Roux-en-Y anastomosis, which leads to biliary drainage in around 30% of affected children; it is only likely to be successful if performed before day 60 of life.

Management includes low-dose antibiotics to prevent cholangitis and nutritional support. Recurrent cholangitis, cirrhosis and portal hypertension inevitably occur, making LTx a requirement, with under 20% of affected patients surviving long term with their original, native liver.

ALAGILLE SYNDROME (ALGS)

This is an autosomal-dominant multi-system disorder (with several other names, including arteriohepatic dysplasia, and paucity of bile interlobular ducts [PBID]), which comprises intrahepatic biliary hypoplasia, plus: facial dysmorphism (wide forehead, deep-set eyes, long straight nose, prominent chin, small, low-set ears); cardiac defects (peripheral pulmonary artery stenosis, right-sided defects, septal defects); and renal (structural and parenchymal anomalies), skeletal (butterfly vertebrae) and ocular anomalies (posterior embryotoxon, causing peripheral corneal opacification). The mnemonic for features is **PBID**:

Pruritis/**P**ulmonary artery abnormalities/**P**osterior embryotoxon/**P**arenchymal renal disease, **P**UJ obstruction/**P**ancreatic insufficiency/**P**oor growth/**P**rominent forehead, chin/**P**ubertal delay/**P**remature suture closure (craniosynostosis)
Butterfly vertebrae/**B**asilar artery anomalies (and other neurovascular anomalies/ accidents)
Inverted triangle facial phenotype
Delayed gross motor milestones

ALGS is a disorder of embryogenesis. There are two genes associated with AGS: 1. the JAG1 gene on chromosome 20, mutations of which are found in 89% of cases—microdeletion of 20p12, including the entire gene, is found in 7%; and 2. the NOTCH2 gene, mutations of which comprise under 1%. The disorder presents with neonatal jaundice, cholestasis, pruritis, xanthomata and failure to thrive. Fifty per cent of patients regain normal liver function by adolescence. Medical treatment may include ursodeoxycholic acid (choleretic; increases volume of bile), cholestyramine (bile acid sequestrant), rifampicin (macrocyclic antibiotic which decreases itching) and naltrexone (opiate antagonist which decreases itching with cholestatic pruritis). Surgical treatment for pruritis or xanthomas may include partial external biliary diversion or ileal exclusion. For those who progress to cirrhosis and portal hypertension, or have intractable pruritis and poor overall quality of life, or end-stage liver failure, LTx is required (this occurs in 15%).

PROGRESSIVE FAMILIAL INTRAHEPATIC CHOLESTASIS (PFIC) DISORDERS

These are disorders of bile salt transport, related to defective canalicular transport proteins, causing substrate retention, which presents as cholestasis. PFIC 1 is due to a mutation in *ATP8B1* (on chromosome 18) which codes for FIC1; PFIC 2 is due to a mutation in *ABCB11* (on chromosome 2) which codes for the bile salt export pump (BSEP); PFIC3 is due to a mutation in *ABCB4* (on chromosome 7) which codes for the multidrug resistance protein-3 (MDR3). These conditions characterised by pruritis and jaundice. There is a low-serum gamma glutamyl transferase (GGT) in PFIC 1 and 2, and a high GGT in PFIC 3.

Metabolic disease
WATCH this is not missed (mnemonic).

Wilson disease (WD)

This is the most common cause of fulminant liver failure in children over 3 years. It is an autosomal recessive disorder of copper metabolism in which the liver cannot excrete this metal into the bile. The WD gene *ATP7B* is located on 13q14.3– q21.1, and encodes a copper-transporting P-type ATPase; there are 40 normal allelic variants, and more than 800 disease-causing mutations of this gene (see Wilson Disease Mutation Database)—this gene is needed to enable copper to attach to caeruloplasmin and to excrete copper into the bile. Initially, there is copper accumulation in the liver, then excess copper spills over into the brain (basal ganglia), kidneys, bones and cornea (Kayser-Fleischer rings represent copper deposition in Descemet's membrane of the cornea, and indicate significant copper storage in the body).

Copper also, less commonly, spills over into the lens (sunflower cataracts), kidneys (proteinuria, microscopic haematuria, Fanconi syndrome), joints (arthritis), heart (cardiomyopathy, cardiac arrhythmias) and skeletal muscle (rhabdomyolysis).

Investigation findings include low-serum copper and caeruloplasmin, and raised urinary copper. It is rare for WD to present before 3 years. Neurological features (movement disorders, or rigid dystonia) present in WD in adolescence. WD is managed with copper chelating agents (penicillamine [given with pyridoxine], trientine) and zinc (enterocyte metallothionein inducer, interferes with absorption of copper from gut); chelated copper is excreted in urine. Foods high in copper content are restricted: liver, brain, shellfish, mushrooms, chocolate and nuts. Vitamin E may be used along with chelator or zinc to consume free radicals made by excess copper. One-third of patients die if untreated.

LTx is required if the patient is unresponsive to penicillamine, or has advanced liver failure with coagulopathy and encephalopathy. WD does not recur after LTx, which provides an effective phenotypic cure, converting the copper kinetics of a homozygous child to that of a heterozygote.

Alpha-1-antitrypsin (AAT) deficiency

This is an autosomal codominant condition (one allele from each parent, each expressed equally) due to AAT allele mutations at the protease inhibitor (PI) locus. AAT is an enzyme which neutralises neutrophil elastase and prevents inflammation and tissue damage in the lung. AAT deficiency is the most common inherited cause of CLD to present in the neonatal period, the most frequent metabolic diagnosis requiring LTx, and the second most common reason for LTx in children overall. Liver disease only occurs in those with certain phenotypes (Z, M [malton] and S [iiyama]) which involve intrahepatic polymerisation of the mutated AAT. It presents with cholestasis, failure to thrive and vitamin K responsive coagulopathy in early infancy. The cholestasis usually resolves by 6 months of age.

Up to 10% of patients develop paucity of intrahepatic bile ducts, and develop jaundice and cirrhosis. In most children jaundice resolves, but cirrhosis can develop in up to 25% of patients.

Alpha-1-antitrypsin (AAT) deficiency (continued)

It is diagnosed by low-serum AAT levels (< 20 μmol/L), followed by phenotype (PI type) determination—PIZZ (homozygous AT deficiency) or PISZ (compound heterozygous). The approximate correlation between phenotype and levels is: PI*MM, 20–48 μmol/L; PI*MZ, 17–33 μmol/L; PI*SS, 15–33 μmol/L; PI*ZZ, 2.5–7 μmol/L. Note that AAT is an acute phase reactant, so normal AAT could be obtained during an inflammatory illness, in a child usually having a low AAT level. AAT is the main blood-borne inhibitor of neutrophil proteases (elastase, cathepsin G, proteinase 3).

AAT is encoded by a gene (SEREPINA1) located at 14q31–32.3. PIZZ resulting from mutation p.E342K is the most common deficiency allele. The pathogenesis of liver disease is from accumulation and retention of toxic polymerised mutant alpha-1-antitrypsin Z (ATZ) molecules in the endoplasmic reticulum (ER) of liver cells. This is entirely different from the pathogenesis of lung disease, which is due to lack of AAT and uninhibited proteolytic destruction of lung tissue. AAT augmentation therapy only works on lung disease.

No specific therapy for AAT deficiency CLD exists. AAT replacement therapy is only for the emphysema of AAT deficiency, there being no evidence that low-serum AAT levels play a role in CLD. Just over one-third of patients need a LTx, just under one-third recover and one-third get cirrhosis. After a LTx, the phenotype changes over to that of the donor, and the serum AAT level becomes normal within weeks.

Tyrosinaemia type 1

This is an autosomal recessive disorder in which there is a deficiency of fumarylacetoacetate hydroxylase (FAH), which prevents metabolism of tyrosine. Toxic metabolites accumulate and damage the liver, kidneys, heart and brain. The abnormal gene *FAH* is located on 15q23–q25. The disorder can present in infants with acute liver failure and in older children with CLD. It is diagnosed by finding succinylacetone in the urine, and increased plasma tyrosine, phenylalanine and methionine. It is detected by newborn screening.

Management of chronic tyrosinaemia includes a low-protein diet (to reduce tyrosine and phenylalanine), vitamin D and nitisinone [2-(2-**n**itro-4-**t**rifluoro-methyl**b**enzoyl)-1,3-**c**yclohexanedione (**NTBC**)], which prevents the formation of toxic metabolites, reverses biochemical and clinical effects, allows hepatic regeneration and almost eliminates the risk of hepatocellular carcinoma (HCC). If NTBC fails, LTx is required. Also, LTx is required if HCC (rising alpha-fetoprotein, liver nodularity on ultrasound, CT or MRI) is suspected.

Cystic fibrosis (CF)

See the long case on this disorder in Chapter 15, The respiratory system. This can be an indication for LTx in older children. CF liver disease does not recur after transplant.

Hereditary fructose intolerance (HFI)

This is an autosomal recessive disorder. The abnormal gene is located on 9q22.3 and codes for fructose–bisphosphate aldolase, which catalyses the cleavage of D-fructose-1, 6-bisphosphate to glycerone phosphate and D-glyceraldehyde 3-phosphate. Some cases present with neonatal hypoglycaemia and lactic acidosis. The usual presentation is fatty liver in a child who refuses to eat sweet foods (unless force fed sucrose).

The disorder can cause failure to thrive, cirrhosis, gastrointestinal bleeding, ongoing hypoglycaemia attacks later in life, vomiting, seizures, proximal renal tubular acidosis and an aversion to sweets and fruit, and is characterised by anabsence of dental caries. It is treated by avoiding fructose, and avoiding fasting,particularly during febrile episodes. Investigations may show fructosaemia, hyperbilirubinaemia, hypophosphataemia, hypermagnesaemia, glycosuria, phosphaturia, bicarbonaturia and high urinary pH. It does not require LTx, as medical treatment is successful.

Chronic hepatitis

All forms of progressive liver disease can lead to the common end point of cirrhosis with portal hypertension. Cirrhosis can be compensated or uncompensated, the latter occurring when the liver loses its synthetic function and develops complications as outlined below.

Autoimmune liver diseases (primary sclerosing cholangitis [PSC], and autoimmune hepatitis [AIH]) are the most common liver diseases in older children, but uncommon causes of liver failure. Most respond to (first-line) prednisolone or azathioprine, or (second-line) cyclosporine A or tacrolimus. LTx is reserved for failure to respond to these, or fulminant hepatic failure. AIH can recur after LTx.

With chronic hepatitis B or C, affected children are usually asymptomatic carriers who very slowly develop cirrhosis and portal hypertension (and HCC) over 20–30 years. They rarely need treatment in childhood. Hepatitis B and C can recur after LTx.

Cirrhosis is technically a histological diagnosis, usually associated with blood tests showing elevated: transaminases (**As**partate amino**t**ransferase [AST], **Al**anine amino**t**ransferase [**ALT**]), **Al**kaline **P**hosphatase (**ALP**), **G**amma **G**lutamyl **T**ransferase (**GGT**) and **P**rothrombin **T**ime (**PT**); and decreased serum albumin, calcium and phosphate (secondary to rickets) and haemoglobin.

Liver function tests (LFTs) can be divided into four categories:
1. Tests for *liver synthetic function* (albumin: synthesised exclusively in the liver; PT/international normalised ratio [INR]: clotting cascade proteins synthesised in the liver).
2. Tests for *biliary excretion* (total and direct bilirubin).
3. Tests for *cholestasis* (GGT, ALP: cholestasis means reduced or absent/stopped bile flow).
4. Tests for *hepatocellular damage* (AST, ALT: hepatic enzymes released from damaged hepatocytes into the blood stream).

Ultrasound may show echogenic liver, splenomegaly and oesophageal varices, and endoscopy may show gastric and oesophageal varices.

Complications of cirrhosis are as follows (mnemonic **HEPATIC**):

Hypersplenism
Encephalopathy/**E**sophageal varices
Portal hypertension/**P**rotein calorie malnutrition
Ascites
Thrombosis of portal vein
Infection (spontaneous bacterial peritonitis)
Coagulopathy/**C**arcinoma (hepatocellular, many years later)

History for CLD

PRESENTING COMPLAINT

Reason for current admission, length of stay in hospital, management changes that have occurred since admission, the indications for the types of investigations that have been carried out, the specialists that have been involved. In particular, look for any suggestion of incipient liver failure, and any discussion of liver transplantation as a future or current option.

PAST HISTORY (INCLUDING INITIAL PRESENTATION)

Initial symptoms (e.g. jaundice, pale stools, dark urine, gastrointestinal tract bleeding, pruritus), age at diagnosis, where diagnosed, initial treatment, response to treatment, subsequent course, doctors involved, clinics attended, previous hospitalisations, past liver biopsies, past complications of disease (e.g. haematemesis, ascites), or its treatment (e.g. rashes or marrow suppression with penicillamine in WD, or Cushingoid effects in chronic active hepatitis [CAH] treated with steroids, cyclosporine side effects in LTx patients).

GASTROINTESTINAL SYMPTOMS (INTERVAL AND CURRENT)

Appetite, nausea, vomiting, haematemesis, melaena, steatorrhoea, acholic stools, weight loss, abdominal pain.

OTHER SYMPTOMS

1. General health: lethargy, weakness.
2. Related to diagnosis: respiratory symptoms in CF, neurological problems in WD.
3. CLD complications: bruising (vitamin K deficiency), ataxia (vitamin E deficiency).

TREATMENT

Drugs, surgery, side effects of treatment, monitoring of treatment, alternative medical therapies, nutrition, fat-soluble vitamins, treatment of complications: bleeding, encephalopathy, ascites, sepsis.

SOCIAL HISTORY

Problems of chronic disease, especially in older children (e.g. behavioural problems), the effects of chronic hospitalisation, dietary restrictions, treatment side effects, effect of disease on siblings and school friends, school absence, depression.

FAMILY HISTORY

Thorough family history (include distant relatives who died in infancy of unknown causes, e.g. galactosaemia, tyrosinaemia); many diseases are autosomal recessive in inheritance (e.g. CF, WD).

Examination for CLD

Figure 8.2 shows complications (only) of CLD. For the approach to the examination for the aetiology (e.g. KF rings and neurological assessment for WD), refer to the short-case on jaundice.

Investigations

These are outlined in the Jaundice short case in this chapter. It is always worth discussing with the examiners previous investigations in which you are particularly interested, showing your understanding of the significance of each. You must also specify which investigations are important at present, which are likely to be important in future management and how often these should be checked. This may seem obvious, but is often not considered until the examiners put you 'on the spot', which is not optimal.

1. General inspection
Jaundice (note depth)
Unwell (end-stage disease)
Well (compensating at present)
Mental state (encephalopathy)
Peripheral stigmata of CLD
- Spider naevi
- Bruising, bleeding
- Scratch marks
- Xanthomata
Evidence of rickets (vitamin D malabsorption)

2. Hands
Leuconychia
Clubbing
Palmar erythema
Xanthomata (between fingers and on extensor surfaces)
Asterixis (liver failure)
Wrists: epiphyseal widening (vitamin D deficiency)

3. Head and neck
Eyelid xanthomata
Conjunctival xerosis (vitamin A deficiency)
Scleral icterus
Corneal xerosis, clouding or opacification (vitamin A deficiency)

4. Chest
Sternal deformity (vitamin D deficiency)
Rib rosary (vitamin D deficiency)

5. Abdomen
Prominent abdominal wall veins
Ascites
Splenomegaly (portal hypertension)
Hepatic bruit (HCC can have this)
Haemorrhoids

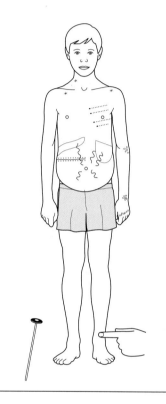

Figure 8.2 **Chronic liver disease**

Principles of management of CLD

GENERAL

Monitor weight, serum albumin, serum bilirubin (total and conjugated), prothrombin time. Psychosocial support is important.

NUTRITION

Deficiencies in nutrients are common in CLD. Patients require a high energy (120–150% of the recommended daily amount) and a moderately high protein intake (3–4 g/kg/day) for growth. Branched chain amino acid enriched formulations have been shown to be clearly advantageous in providing nutritional support and are the formulae of choice. Branched chain amino acids are metabolised in the periphery and do not require the liver for metabolism. Consider enteral feeding if the child is anorectic. Nocturnal nasogastric enteric feeding may be needed: parents can do this at home. Decreased bile flow leads to diminished intraluminal bile acids and fat malabsorption.

The provision of adequate essential fatty acids, fat-soluble vitamins (A, D, E, K), zinc, iron and calcium is important. If enteral feeding is not tolerated due to ascites, variceal bleeding or recurrent hepatic complications, TPN may be needed.

SALT AND WATER RETENTION/ASCITES

The development of ascites is a poor prognostic sign. Management is by sodium restriction (less than 2 mmol/kg/day) and salt restriction to 0.3–0.5 g/day. Aim for a negative salt balance to lose water. A loss of 100–150 mEq of salt will result in a loss of 1 L (1000 g) of water. Aim for 250 g weight loss per day. Spironolactone (aldosterone antagonist) may be used; salt-poor albumin and frusemide may be needed. An abdominal tap may be diagnostic with infected fluid, but is otherwise of little value. If acute renal failure or hepatorenal failure supervene, haemodialysis or haemofiltration may be necessary.

HEPATIC ENCEPHALOPATHY (HE)

This is classified into four types:

Type A: encephalopathy associated with acute liver failure.
Type B: encephalopathy with portosystemic bypass and no intrinsic hepatocellular disease.
Type C: encephalopathy associated with cirrhosis.
Type D: encephalopathy associated with urea cycle disorders.

There are three contributing factors:
1. Portosystemic shunting (potential neurotoxic metabolites from the gut, rather than being removed by the liver, are shunted around the cirrhotic liver).
2. Altered blood-brain barrier (changes in permeability in acute liver failure).
3. Toxic metabolites affecting the central nervous system.

There are four clinical stages of HE:
* Stage I is called the prodrome, with slow mentation, slight asterixis and minimal EEG changes.
* Stage II is the impending coma stage; with disorientation, drowsiness, easily elicited asterixis and generalised slowing on EEG.
* Stage III is called stupor, clinically very sleepy, confused, delirious, asterixis present if elicited (if patient cooperative) and EEG shows grossly abnormal.
* Stage IV includes loss of consciousness, decorticate or decerebrate posturing, asterixis usually absent and EEG shows delta waves and decreased amplitudes.

This can be difficult to detect, presenting with vague symptoms of lack of energy, drowsiness and regression in schoolwork. The mainstays of therapy are decreasing the nitrogenous load to the bowel and reducing the bacterial production of ammonia in the colon. Review precipitating factors such as infection, large gastrointestinal bleed, excessive protein intake, electrolyte imbalance and diuretics. The electrolyte imbalances include dehydration, hyponatraemia, hypokalaemia, hypoglycaemia, acidosis and alkalosis. Other precipitants include renal disease and constipation. Restrict protein (to 2 g/kg/day); consider substitution with branch-chained amino acids. Use oral lactulose and neomycin.

PORTAL HYPERTENSION, VARICES AND VARICEAL HAEMORRHAGE

Oesophageal varices inevitably develop with portal hypertension. They can be evaluated endoscopically. Some centres suggest prophylactic sclerotherapy; this is a controversial point, and most centres do not recommend it. An acute episode of variceal bleeding can be life-threatening, requiring intensive-care management, intravenous fluids and blood products, and therapy with intravenous vasopressin, octreotide or glypressin to reduce portal pressure.

Once the patient is haemodynamically stable and the diagnosis has been confirmed by endoscopy, band ligation or sclerotherapy can be performed. Should these fail, balloon tamponade with a modified Sengstaken–Blakemore tube and intravenous vasopressin for 24–48 hours are useful. Complications of balloon tamponade can include pulmonary aspiration, oesophageal rupture and suffocation.

Endoscopic sclerotherapy has been replaced by band ligation, which ablates varices successfully in 70–100% of cases, has rebleeding rates of 15–30%, has fewer complications than sclerotherapy, except for dysphagia, which is more common with band ligation.

In some children, bleeding may be controlled by insertion of a transjugular intrahepatic portosystemic stent shunt (TIPSS), which has success rates of 80–100%: complications include occlusion of stent, the development of encephalopathy and infection. TIPSS can be used to control portal hypertension in children with compensated CLD, such as in some children with CF.

Avoid splenectomy if possible. As well as the risk of infection after splenectomy, it may lead to increased bleeding from removal of good collateral vessels from the splenic capsule (azygos system) that bypass the lower oesophageal junction vessels. Haemorrhage can be exacerbated by deficiency of vitamin K dependent factors, thrombocytopenia secondary to hypersplenism and circulating fibrinolysins.

COAGULOPATHY

An adequate dose of vitamin K (2–10 mg/day) is needed. Fresh frozen plasma, cryoprecipitate and platelets (for hypersplenism) may be required during bleeding episodes.

PRURITUS

Pruritus associated with CLD may cause significant morbidity and may be intractable in children with biliary hypoplasia. Ursodeoxycholic acid is widely used and is the treatment of choice. Often more than one drug is required, including rifampicin, cholestyramine, phenobarbitone, ondansetron and naltrexone.

DRUGS

Certain drugs should be avoided in children with CLD. These include phenytoin, sulphonamides, erythromycin and paracetamol. Care is required with sedatives and opiates also.

SEPSIS

Infections are common in CLD, especially ascending cholangitis and bacterial peritonitis, and can precipitate encephalopathy, or acute or chronic liver failure.

OTHER NON-TRANSPLANTATION TREATMENT OPTIONS

There are several areas where there have been recent advances. Replacement of a deficient abnormal end product can be achieved, such as in patients with abnormal biosynthesis of bile acids, by oral administration of primary bile acids. Depletion of the substance stored is another strategy, as used in neonatal iron storage disease with chelation and antioxidant mixtures. Metabolic inhibitors may be used, such as NTBC in tyrosinaemia. Enzymes can be induced, such as with the use of phenobarbitone in Crigler-Najjar syndrome type II.

Substrates can be restricted in the diet, as with galactose in galactosaemia, or sucrose in HFI. Molecular manipulation can be achieved, such as by inhibition of polymerisation of alpha-1-antitrypsin. Future treatment may incorporate gene therapy and receptor-based targeted enzyme replacement therapy.

The following are potentially curative treatments: surgery for choledochal cyst, copper chelation for WD and immune suppression for AIH. Hepatitis B and C can be treated effectively also.

Liver transplantation (LTx)

LTx is associated with a survival of 90% at 1 year and 80% at 5 years, and can be used as treatment for a multiplicity of liver diseases, many of which were considered incurable a decade ago. Recent improvements in LTx include refinements in immunosuppression, technical advances in the transplantation process, the use of reduced, split and living related donor organs, and improved management of infectious complications.

TIMING OF TRANSPLANTATION

The timing of LTx depends upon a variety of factors and may be hastened by:

1. A history of life-threatening variceal haemorrhage.
2. The development of: (a) a hepatorenal state; (b) hepatic encephalopathy; (c) refractory ascites; (d) reduction in psychosocial development; (e) intractable pruritus; (f) severe metabolic bone disease; or (g) a diminished quality of life.
3. Decompensation.
4. Involvement of a hepatologist.

Assessment occurs in specialist liver units, with preparatory education and counselling of the child and family, a multidisciplinary team that may include a psychologist and a play therapist (especially for children under 2 years), intensive nutritional support, completion of routine immunisation (especially hepatitis A and B) before commencement of immunosuppression, and management of CLD complications.

In the US, organ allocation is assisted by the **PELD** (**P**ediatric **E**nd-stage **L**iver **D**isease) score, introduced in 2002, to enable the severity of the recipient liver disease to determine the priority list, so that the sickest children are transplanted first. The PELD score ranks children according to their likelihood of death and/or ICU admission within 3 months of listing; it is based on the INR, total bilirubin, serum albumin, age under 1 year and height less than two standard deviations from the mean for age and gender.

The PELD score is used for children up to 12 years. After this, the MELD score is used. Since this system has been introduced, fewer patients have died waiting for a transplant.

INDICATIONS FOR LTX

As noted above, indications for LTx include failure of hepatic synthetic function, poor quality of life (e.g. intractable pruritis, lethargy, anorexia, recurrent infections), intractable malnutrition or failure to thrive, refractory ascending cholangitis, hyper-ammonaemia from certain inborn errors of metabolism (IEMs), encephalopathy, oesophageal varices from portal hypertension, and hypersplenism.

Specific diseases requiring LTx, in order of decreasing frequency, include the following:

1. Extrahepatic biliary atresia (EHBA): over 50% of LTx.
2. IEMs (10–15% of LTx) include AAT deficiency, CF, galactosaemia, glycogen storage diseases (GSDs) type IA and IV, mitochondrial functional defects (e.g. defects of fatty acid beta-oxidation), some organic acidaemias, tyrosinaemia, urea cycle defects and WD.
3. Acute hepatic necrosis (around 10%).
4. Cirrhosis from CAH or primary biliary cirrhosis (under 10%).
5. Cholestatic liver disease, other than EHBA (under 5%).
6. Primary hepatic malignancy (2%).

The only absolute contraindication to LTx is irreversible extrahepatic disease (e.g. HIV, irreversible brain damage, incurable malignancy).

The following requirements must be met for a cadaveric donor for LTx:

1. Brain death prior to circulatory arrest.
2. The absence of sepsis, HBsAg and HBeAg, HIV, malignancy, drug abuse, liver or gallbladder disease, chronic hypertension.
3. Liver enzymes, serum bilirubin within three times normal values.
4. No period of hypoxia ($PaO_2 < 60$ mmHg) or hypotension (over 2 hours).
5. The absence of more than minimal pressor support to maintain normal blood pressure and peripheral perfusion.
6. To match a recipient, the suitable donor must have ABO compatibility with the recipient. Sex and human leucocyte antigen (HLA) type compatibility are not necessary.

There have been many technical innovations in the LTx process. These include reduction hepatectomy (cutting an adult liver down, in an anatomical fashion, to fit one child, which wastes some of the adult liver), followed by the development of split-LTx (one donor liver offered to two recipients, usually an adult and a child) and then living related LTx (where the left lobe [occasionally the right lobe] or left lateral segment is removed from parent/adult liver).

TRANSPLANT SURGERY PROCEDURE

The procedure itself has three main phases: 1. recipient hepatectomy, which can be complicated because of coexistent coagulopathy and portal hypertension (bleeding) and previous Kasai (adhesions); 2. the anhepatic phase, when the patient has the vascular anastomoses performed (vena cava, portal vein, hepatic artery), and then placement of the graft; 3. the neohepatic phase, where the liver graft is reperfused (cardiovascular instability can occur here, as the liver has been exposed to cold preservation techniques) and the biliary anastomosis performed—in patients with EHBA, the donor duct will be implanted into a Roux-en-Y loop, as there is no recipient biliary tree. This latter technique is also useful in small children who receive a segmental graft.

COMPLICATIONS OF LTX

Rejection occurs most often in the first 3 months after transplant; it is less common in children under 6 months and in those receiving a living donor graft. The liver allograft is an 'immunologically privileged' organ, because rejection, especially if steroid sensitive, has no adverse effect on graft survival or even function. Further, some studies show that rejection itself may benefit patient survival. It seems that some rejection may be protective of graft function: a controlled amount of immune activation seems necessary (perhaps to delete clones of the recipient's lymphocytes that can damage the graft).

Most late graft losses are related to immunosuppression: either too much leading to sepsis, posttransplant lymphoproliferative disease (PTLD), lymphomas or other de novo tumours, or too little leading to graft loss, which is often a result of non-compliance (especially in teenagers).

Chronic rejection is becoming rare, which some attribute to the increased use of tacrolimus. An increased awareness of the adverse effects of immunosuppression is channelling interest into achieving just the right amount of immunosuppression: enough to prevent damaging rejection, but without the risks of unnecessary over-immunosuppression.

Graft rejection (60%)

- Rejection is the main cause of graft dysfunction following LTx.
- Late acute rejection can occur anywhere from 1 month to several years post-LTx. It can be associated with immunosuppressant non-compliance. It presents with increased transaminases, fever, malaise or jaundice; liver biopsy shows acute cellular rejection (ACR); it responds to pulse steroids, increased calcineurin inhibitors and addition of another immunosuppressant such as mycophenolate mofetil; if unresponsive to these, treat with anti-T-cell antibody preparations.
- Chronic rejection (also known as 'ductopaenic rejection'), with the loss of over 50% of bile ducts, occurs 6 weeks to 6 months after LTx and can lead to biliary strictures, cholangitis and cholestasis. Treatment may include optimising immunosuppression, and dilatation of strictures. Severe allograft dysfunction could require retransplantation.
- AIH can develop irrespective of initial disease process. It can occur months to years after LTx. It is treated with the addition of azathioprine and prednisolone to the immunosuppressive regimen.

Infection (50%)

- Earlier infections (up to 1 month after LTx) tend to be bacterial or fungal. Intra-abdominal and line infections are the most common early causes. Bacterial and fungal infections can be secondary to technical complications such as vascular thrombosis, bile leaks and strictures.
- Fungal sepsis, especially aspergillosis, can be seen with re-operation, bowel perforation and long stays in intensive care: prophylaxis is with antifungal agents such as itraconazole and fluconazole, or newer drugs (e.g. the caspofungins) and the lipid complex formulation of amphotericin (less nephrotoxic).
- Later infections (2–6 months after LTx) tend to be viral (e.g. cytomegalovirus [CMV], Epstein-Barr virus [EBV], herpes varicella-zoster virus [HVZ]) and have been reduced by prophylactic courses of ganciclovir, acyclovir and CMV hyper-immunoglobulin. Still later infections (> 6 months) may be viral or fungal. Common respiratory viruses (adenovirus, parainfluenza, influenza) can produce necrotising pneumonitis.
- Fever in a young child in the first 12 months after LTx deserves assessment for sepsis, and depending on degree of immunosuppression, may need hospitalisation and intravenous broad-spectrum antibiotic cover.

Biliary complications (20%)

These can occur anywhere from 6 weeks to 6 years post-LTx and may present with cholangitis. There may be extrahepatic strictures (anastomosis site) or intrahepatic strictures (due to ischaemia). Treatment may include percutaneous balloon dilatation, surgical revision or retransplantation.

Hepatic vascular compromise (<10%)

This may be due to hepatic artery, hepatic vein or portal vein stenosis or occlusion. Hepatic artery thrombosis (HAT) can lead to urgent retransplantation, biliary leaks, peritonitis, relapsing septicaemia and biliary strictures. Portal vein stenosis can cause portal hypertension. Treatment may include ballooning, stenting, surgical reconstruction or retransplantation.

Posttransplant lymphoproliferative disorder (PTLD) (EBV-driven B-cell proliferation; 5–25%)

This spectrum of disease ranges from lymphohyperplasia to true lymphoma, and may occur 3–12 months post-LTx. It can present with lymphadenopathy. Risk factors include: 1. primary EBV infection after transplant; 2. young age; 3. an EBV-negative recipient of an EBV-positive donor; 4. CMV infection; and 5. significantly immunocompromised children. The evolution of PTLD can be monitored by serial EBV PCR determinations in peripheral blood: a rising EBV PCR is sensitive for PTLD.

It may be treated by decreasing or stopping immunosuppression (usually successful, but this increases risk of LTx rejection), and starting ganciclovir, acyclovir and CMV hyper-immunoglobulin (has high levels of EBV antibodies). More recent therapies include anti-CD20 monoclonal antibodies (e.g. rituximab), and injection of in vitro expanded autologous EBV-specific cytotoxic T-cells. Mortality is around 20%; this has decreased due to EBV viraemia surveillance.

De novo autoimmune hepatitis (uncommon)
- This can occur in any graft, irrespective of the original disease.
- High transaminases, positive autoantibodies and hepatitis on biopsy.
- Addition of second-line immunosuppressant required; difficult to treat.

Recurrence of primary disease (uncommon)
- Recurrence of the original disease in the graft is uncommon, because liver diseases requiring transplantation are usually congenital or developmental, and LTx is curative.
- Primary sclerosing cholangitis can recur in an almost identical form to the original disease.
- AIH and viral hepatitis also can recur.

Chronic hepatitis (uncommon)
- This is a late complication in allografts; usually diagnosed by protocol biopsies, with portal inflammation (without bile duct or vascular changes), with normal transaminases.
- Only recognised recently; the optimal treatment has yet to be clarified.

Primary non-function (PNF) (rare)
- This is rare but catastrophic; probably related to ischaemia/reperfusion injury.
- High transaminases and creatinine, coagulopathy, progress to multi-system organ failure.
- Retransplantation urgently required.

Retransplantation (Re-LTx) (10–20%)
- Not uncommon; early (< 30 days) or late (> 30 days) after the original LTx date.
- Early re-LTx usually for PNF (see above) or HAT (see previous page).
- Late re-LTx usually for chronic rejection or biliary complications.
- Decreased survival versus original LTx.

Long-term toxicities of calcineurin inhibitors (CNIs): CSA and tacrolimus

Nephrotoxicity remains the most serious complication of CNIs. The glomerular filtration rate (GFR) is the best way to monitor its development. Early renal impairment can be reversible, and the dose of CNI can be reduced, but at some stage renal impairment can become irreversible. Hypertension that requires therapy occurs in around 20–30% of LTx recipients, and can be compounded by steroid use.

Other effects include neurotoxicities and hyperlipidaemia. Some alternatives to CNIs have been used to address this problem, including the addition of either mycophenolate mofetil or sirolimus.

Bowel perforation

This is a feared complication, with high mortality. Previous abdominal surgery increases the risk. As the most common indication for LTx is EHBA with a failed Kasai, many children have a predisposing risk for perforation.

IMPROVED OUTCOMES

Improved immunosuppression has contributed to the improved outcomes of LTx. The main agents used, other than corticosteroids, are the CNIs tacrolimus (TRL) and cyclosporin (CSA). Both inhibit the production of cytotoxic T-lymphocytes and interleukin-2 (IL-2), and have similar side effects, although the former is more potent and does not cause hypertrichosis or gum hyperplasia. Levels of both TRL and CSA may be decreased by concomitant use of anticonvulsants and antituberculous drugs, and may be increased by calcium channel blockers, antibiotics (macrolides and quinolones) and antifungals.

TRL is usually combined with steroids alone, whereas CSA is often combined with a third agent, such as mycophenolate mofetil or azathioprine (AZA). TRL is interesting in that its pharmacokinetic patterns retain the characteristics of the age of the donor, not the recipient. Most children may be weaned on to a single immunosuppressive agent. Most units now focus on minimisation of long-term maintenance immunosuppression, with steroid withdrawal as the first step. Some adult LTx protocols avoid steroids entirely and use either polyclonal or monoclonal antibody therapy, instead of steroids, given with TRL or CSA.

Evaluation for complications may include serial LFTs, tissue sampling and imaging, including Doppler ultrasonography for vascular patency, MRI and percutaneous transhepatic cholangiography (PTC).

Long term, there is significant improvement in nutritional status after LTx, with weight, fat stores and muscle mass (protein) recovering within 12 months and, of more importance, maintenance of psychosocial development, normal intellectual functioning, normal (if delayed) puberty, growth spurts with normal final height and participation in age-appropriate activities. Renal dysfunction occurs in around 30% of cases. Malignancy remains a long-term concern. A further concern is the supply of available donors.

Neonatal liver transplant recipients now have similar graft and patient survival rates to older children, and normal neurodevelopmental progress.

Survival rates are very high. Post-LTx death is unusual, and most commonly associated with recurrent malignancy, sepsis, PTLD or multi-system organ failure.

LONG CASE: Malabsorption/maldigestion

Malabsorption presents as a diagnostic problem, not a specific disease. It is a state where there is inadequate digestion and/or inadequate absorption across the intestinal mucosa, related to digestive factors (e.g. pancreatic enzymes, bile) and/or absorptive factors (e.g. mucosal changes). The more common causes involve enzymes (cystic fibrosis [CF]) and mucosal surface area (coeliac disease). The presenting complaints may include failure to thrive, loose and frequent bowel motions, abdominal distension, short stature (e.g. coeliac disease), anaemia (folate, vitamin B_{12} or iron malabsorption) or chest infection (CF).

Aetiology

The common causes in the developed world include:

1. Cystic fibrosis.
2. Coeliac disease.
3. Post-gastroenteritis syndrome.
4. Giardiasis.
5. Bacterial overgrowth (usually associated with congenital gut anomalies or prior gastrointestinal surgery).

In contrast, in the developing world the most common cause of malabsorption is the combination of mucosal injury from repeated or persistent infections, plus poor hygiene and poor nutrition.

Other causes in the developed world include the following:

1. Inflammatory bowel disease (predominantly Crohn's disease [CD]).
2. Syndromic causes of exocrine pancreatic insufficiency:
   - *Shwachman–Diamond syndrome* (SDS; autosomal recessive). The abnormal gene is the Shwachman–Bodian–Diamond Syndrome (SBDS) gene located on 7q11; the SBDS protein is involved in ribosome biogenesis, stabilisation of the mitotic spindle and regulation of chromosome segregation. Features include marrow failure (various cytopenias, including cyclic neutropenia, pancytopenia), recurrent infections, increased risk for myelodysplasia and malignant transformation (especially acute myelogenous leukaemia, AML), short stature, skeletal anomalies.
   - *Johanson–Blizzard syndrome* (JBS). The abnormal gene is located on 15q15–q21.1. Features include pancreatic insufficiency due to fatty replacement, gastrointestinal anomalies (e.g. imperforate anus), deafness, unusual whorls of tissue in scalp, absent nasal cartilage, hypothyroidism. Diabetes may also occur.
3. Short bowel syndrome (SBS): residual small bowel length less than 100 cm (e.g. post-necrotising enterocolitis).
4. Chronic liver disease (CLD) with cholestasis.
5. Others: immunodeficiency syndromes, intestinal lymphangiectasia, abetalipoproteinaemia.

Infants may have congenital disorders of specific nutrient digestion or absorption/transport. These include disorders involving the following:

1. Amino acids: for example, enterokinase deficiency.
2. Fats: for example, chylomicron retention disease, intestinal lymphangiectasia; abetalipoproteinaemia.
3. Carbohydrates: congenital intestinal enterocyte brush border enzyme deficiencies or transport defects (e.g. glucose–galactose transporter deficiency, sucrase–isomaltase deficiency, lactase deficiency, microvillus inclusion disease).
4. Electrolytes, vitamins, trace elements: for example, congenital chloride diarrhoea, acrodermatitis enteropathica (zinc deficiency), selective B_{12} deficiency.

Mechanisms of malabsorption

Candidates should refresh their knowledge of the physiology of digestive and absorptive processes. These are normally divided into phases: intraluminal digestion, mucosal absorption, venous transport phase and lymphatic transport phase. Most nutrient absorption occurs in the proximal small bowel, although vitamin B_{12} and bile acids are absorbed in the terminal ileum. Malabsorbed bile acids irritate the colonic mucosa, having a detergent action that can lead to colitis and diarrhoea, especially in conditions such as CD and SBS with disorders of the terminal small bowel.

Hepatobiliary and pancreatic secretions mix with nutrients in the duodenum and jejunum to digest fat. Long-chain fatty acids are absorbed and repackaged into chylomicrons, transported sequentially via lymphatics, the venous circulation and finally the liver. Medium- and short-chain fatty acids are absorbed and transported directly to the liver via mesenteric venous blood flow.

Malabsorbed carbohydrates' osmotic properties lead to intraluminal fluid accumulation and diarrhoea, plus fermentation by ileocolonic bacteria to simple sugars, organic acids and gases (methane, carbon dioxide and hydrogen: the basis for the hydrogen breath test). Generalised malabsorption usually does not cause azotorrhoea (excessive loss of nitrogen in the stool). Hypoproteinaemia in malnourished children with malabsorption is due to deficient dietary intake and excessive intestinal protein loss (protein-losing enteropathy [PLE]).

DIGESTIVE FACTORS

1. Insufficient pancreatic enzymes (e.g. CF, SDS).
2. Lack of functioning bile salts:
   - Insufficient supply (e.g. CLD, ileal resection, coeliac disease).
   - Deconjugation (e.g. bacterial overgrowth).
3. Inadequate brush border enzymes (e.g. lactose intolerance).

ABSORPTIVE FACTORS

1. Disordered mucosal villus function:
   - Congenital defects in villus structure: for example, microvillus inclusion disease, tufting disease.
   - Reduced mucosal surface area: for example, SBS, cytotoxic drug-induced epithelial injury, malnutrition.
   - Inflammatory disorders of villus: for example, postinfectious diarrhoea (e.g. *Shigella, E. coli, Campylobacter jejuni, Giardia lamblia*), coeliac disease (gluten-sensitive enteropathy), allergic enteropathies (e.g. to cow's milk protein [CMP], soy, egg or gluten), acute infectious enteropathy, immunodeficiency syndromes, autoimmune enteritis.
2. Defective intracellular lipid transport: for example, abetalipoproteinaemia.
3. Inadequate lymphatic circulation of chylomicrons: for example, lymphangiectasia (primary, or secondary to CD), mycobacterial gut infection, radiation enteritis, forms of congenital heart disease with chronically elevated right-sided heart pressure (impeded flow from lymphatics [thoracic duct] into systemic venous circulation).
4. Abnormal water and electrolyte transport (e.g. giardiasis).

Coeliac disease/gluten-sensitive enteropathy (GSE)

GSE is a specific T-lymphocyte intolerance of gluten. It is a systemic condition, now considered the most common autoimmune disorder; the trigger is gluten, and removing that trigger resolves mucosal damage and complications. There is elevated incidence in some syndromes (Down, Turner) some endocrine diseases (type 1 diabetes mellitus [T1DM], Addison disease), and in IgA deficiency. GSE describes enteropathy in which intestinal inflammation is due to ingestion of gluten, the inclusive term for gliadin and associated prolamins (proteins with a high content of proline and glutamine), which are present in wheat (gliadin), barley (hordeins) and rye (secalins), in genetically predisposed patients. Oats contain avenin, a prolamin (hence gluten), but generally are well tolerated by children with GSE. Oats, however, can be cross-contaminated during processing with wheat, barley and rye, and so are avoided. The gluten-free diet (GFD) avoids (mnemonic **BROW**): **b**arley, **r**ye, **o**ats and **w**heat. Other cereals avoided include malt and triticale (cross between wheat and rye). Grains which are well tolerated in GSE include rice, corn and sorghum.

The gold standard in diagnosing this condition remains findings on small bowel biopsy (obtained endoscopically from the post-bulbar duodenum) of partial or complete villous atrophy, crypt hyperplasia and increased intraepithelial lymphocytes, which resolve with a GFD.

There is a strong association between coeliac disease and HLA class II genes. Most patients with coeliac disease have particular pairs of allelic variants in two genes: *HLA-DQA1* and *HLA-DQB1*. These are common: 30% of the general population has at least one of them, but only 3% of those have coeliac disease, and their *absence* effectively *excludes* the diagnosis. *HLA-DQA1* encodes the alpha chain, and *HLA-DQB1* the beta chain, of the HLA heterodimers associated with coeliac disease.

The major histocompatibility complex (MHC) class II antigens are the DQ2 heterodimer (encoded by specific *HLA-DQA1*05* and *HLA-DQB1*02* alleles) and the DQ8 heterodimer (encoded by specific *HLA-DQA1*03* and *HLA-DQB1*0302* alleles). DQ2 and DQ8 molecules present peptides derived from gliadin to intestinal T-lymphocytes (some after deamination by tissue transglutaminase [tTG; this ubiquitous enzyme normally cross-links proteins, and deaminates glutamine and proline residues in prolamins]). Activated Th1 T-cells produce pro-inflammatory cytokines that cause (probably) the gut lesions of coeliac disease.

The serological tests may be negative in patients already on a GFD, so a gluten challenge may be necessary before serology tested. An adequate challenge is two slices of wheat-based bread per day for 2 to 8 weeks.

Although celiac disease associated antibodies serology may be useful, they have yet to replace biopsy. Most cases with positive tTG IgA antibodies and endomysial antibody (EMA) IgA have coeliac disease, and are HLA DQ2- or DQ8-positive.

Testing for HLA DQ2/DQ8 is useful; a negative test excludes GSE. However, a positive test cannot be utilised to diagnose GSE, as DQ2 and DQ8 are each found in > 50% of the population.

Measurement of the serum level of total IgA to evaluate for selective IgA deficiency (which occurs in 1 in 50 patients with celiac disease) is useful for accurate interpretation, as tTG IgA and EMA IgA will not be present, so in IgA-deficient patients testing for IgG antibodies should be performed: tTG IgG or anti-deaminated gliadin-related peptide (a-DGP) IgG, the latter being a newer test where both isotypes (IgA and IgG) are highly sensitive and specific for active coeliac disease.

History

WEIGHT

Birth weight, progress of weight, timing of when weight gain started to diminish, current weight, rate of weight loss.

CHRONOLOGY OF SYMPTOMS

Age at onset of symptoms: for example, congenital villus dysfunction presents with intractable diarrhoea as neonate; coeliac disease may present between 3 and 9 months with severe diarrhoea, or later (9 months to late childhood) with moderate diarrhoea; inflammatory bowel disease is very rare before 8 years; it may present after a bout of known enteritis (e.g. *Shigella*).

FEEDING

Dietary milestones, initial feeding, age at introduction of cow's milk (CMP intolerance), age at introduction of first solids, age at introduction of first cereals and the type of cereal (gluten-containing [barley, rye, oats, wheat] in coeliac disease), age at introduction of first fruits (sucrase–isomaltase deficiency), appetite, poor feeding with irritability (iron deficiency associated with coeliac disease), parent-devised dietary restriction (attempting to avoid diarrhoea), iatrogenic dietary manipulation (decreased caloric intake and chronic non-specific diarrhoea).

STOOLS

Appearance, volume, fluidity, offensiveness, difficulty flushing stools (steatorrhoea or excess gas in stool), frequency, associated blood (CD).

SYMPTOMS OF SPECIFIC NUTRITIONAL DEFICIENCIES

Pallor (anaemia), night-blindness (vitamin A), ataxia (vitamin E), bruising (vitamin K), rashes (zinc, various vitamins). See the short case on nutritional assessment in this chapter for a comprehensive list of possibilities.

SPECIFIC DIAGNOSTIC CLUES

Chest infections (CF), susceptibility to infections (immunodeficiency states or neutropenic episodes of SDS), arthralgia or rashes (e.g. erythema nodosum, erythema multiforme in CD), delay in pubertal development (CD), travel to giardia-endemic or exotic areas (giardiasis or other infestation), day-care (giardiasis).

FAMILY HISTORY

CF, coeliac disease or other autoimmune disorders (e.g. T1DM, thyroid disorders, juvenile arthritis, autoimmune liver disease), disaccharidase deficiency, CD, infestations.

SOCIAL HISTORY

Beware of psychosocial causes of failure to thrive in the differential diagnosis.

PAST MEDICAL HISTORY

Necrotising enterocolitis (NEC) as neonate, past bowel resections or other surgery.

INVESTIGATIONS THUS FAR

The type and timing of investigations, the specialists involved, current thoughts on the diagnosis, planned future investigations.

MANAGEMENT

The current treatment approach (if any); plans for further treatment.

Examination

See the short case on nutritional assessment and suggested examinations for IBD and CLD long cases in this chapter. Start with growth parameters, weight, height and head circumference, then perform a nutritional assessment, and look for underlying IBD, CLD and any suggestions of CF or immune deficiency. Carefully check for any abdominal distension, particularly with muscle wasting, as this can occur with an enteropathy. Perform a careful perianal examination. It is not necessary to perform a rectal examination, but this should be mentioned for completeness.

Investigations

STOOL

1. Pus cells (colonic disease, e.g. CD).
2. Eosinophils (CMP intolerance).
3. Occult blood (IBD).
4. Cysts or trophozoites (e.g. *Giardia lamblia*).
5. Fat globules (CF or SDS-maldigestion [luminal] rather than malabsorption). *Note*: lubricants or ointments can produce false-positive results.
6. Fatty acid crystals (coeliac disease: malabsorption [mucosal]).
7. Reducing substances (carbohydrate maldigestion or malabsorption).
8. Faecal alpha-1-antitrypsin excretion test (FA1AT). This screens for PLE. An elevated FA1AT result suggests a mucosal disorder, as inflamed mucosa allows transudation of serum proteins. This is common in CD and occurs in coeliac disease, but *not* in CF or CLD, where there is an intraluminal maldigestive defect, which does not involve any mucosal damage.
9. Culture for pathogens (*Cryptosporidium, Yersinia*).
10. Three-day faecal fat assessment (more accurate than a qualitative stool stain).
11. Bile acids (in SBS with 40–80% ileal resection).
12. Colonic hydroxy fatty acids (in SBS with 80–100% ileal resection).
13. Ostomy output: electrolytes, osmolality (children with stomas).

BLOOD

1. Full blood count and film (anaemia, neutropenia [SDS], lymphopenia [lymphangiectasia], acanthocytosis [abetalipoproteinaemia, hypobetalipoproteinaemia, chylomicron retention disease]), megaloblastic anaemia (B_{12}, folate malabsorption).
2. Erythrocyte sedimentation rate, ESR (chronic infection, IBD).
3. Liver function tests (albumin, total protein, transaminases) (CLD, CD with PLE).
4. Vitamins: folate (serum and red cell), vitamin B_{12} (ileal disease), vitamins A, 25-OH D and E, and prothrombin time for vitamin K (fat malabsorption).
5. Minerals: calcium, magnesium, phosphate, iron, ferritin, zinc, copper, selenium.
6. Electrolytes, urea and creatinine (hydration, associated renal disease).
7. Fetal haemoglobin, HbF (SDS).
8. Pancreatic isoamylase (SDS).
9. IgA and coeliac disease serology (anti-tissue transglutaminase [tTG] IgA antibodies, EMA IgA). In addition, molecular genetic testing can be carried out: targeted mutation analysis can determine *HLA-DQA1* and *HLA-DQB1* genotypes to detect the presence or absence of coeliac disease associated alleles: *HLA-DQA1*0501, *HLA-DQA1*0505, *HLA-DQB1*0201, *HLA-DQB1*0202* and *HLA-DQB1*0302*. Over 99.9% of these alleles will be detected by this test.
10. IBD serology screening tests. None are routine, but they are included for completeness. Perinuclear anticytoplasmic antibodies (pANCAs) to neutrophil proteins may be elevated in UC. Anti-*Saccharomyces cerevisiae* (ASCA) antibodies may be present in CD (more sensitive and specific with elevated p-ANCA). Antibodies to *E. coli* (outer membrane porin C [anti-ompC] antibodies) may correlate with diagnosis of IBD.
11. Immunoglobulins (severe combined immunodeficiency syndrome and other primary immune defects).
12. HIV serology in high-risk groups.

IMAGING

1. Bone age (delay in skeletal development; abnormal in SDS syndrome with metaphyseal dysostosis; film will also show rickets).
2. Bowel contrast studies (anatomical lesions, CD).
3. Motility studies (nuclear medicine gastric emptying scan, upper gastrointestinal barium contrast study).
4. Liver scan (causes of CLD).
5. CT scan of liver and pancreas.
6. Radiolabelled Tc albumin lymphatic scan (lymphangiectasia).

SMALL BOWEL BIOPSY

This is the gold standard to diagnose villus injury. It is the standard test to diagnose coeliac disease, *Giardia lamblia*, intestinal lymphangiectasia and abetalipoproteinaemia (shows epithelial lipid). Severe villus atrophy occurs with coeliac disease and congenital microvillus inclusion disease. Less severe degrees of atrophy occur with giardiasis, immunodeficiency, allergic enteropathies and malnutrition. Biopsy can also determine mucosal enzyme deficiencies (e.g. disaccharidases).

SWEAT TEST

The standard test to detect CF.

OTHERS

Other potentially useful investigations include the following:
1. Breath hydrogen test (carbohydrate malabsorption, bacterial overgrowth).
2. Urinary catecholamines and serotonin (carcinoid, neuroblastoma: causes of secretory diarrhoea).
   Note that all these investigations can be performed as outpatient procedures. It is uncommon to need to admit a child to hospital for investigation of malabsorption, although a child with failure to thrive may require a period of hospitalisation for nutritional debilitation to resolve.

SHORT CASES

SHORT CASE: Gastrointestinal system

This is a reasonably common short case, and it is expected to be performed well. The introduction 'Examine the gastrointestinal system' is more detailed than 'Examine the abdomen', as it comprises not only abdominal but also nutritional assessment (which is a short case in itself), as well as a search for peripheral stigmata of various disease states. The most systematic method of approach, as in so many other cases, commences with inspection, followed by examining the hands, face, abdomen, lower limbs and then other systems depending on the findings. The relevant findings sought are outlined in Fig. 8.3. A more detailed listing of possible examination findings is given in Table 8.1.
   Start by introducing yourself to the patient and parent. Have the child adequately undressed for examination. Note the child's parameters and visually assess the nutritional status. Request the percentile charts, as these are always helpful and often give a good indication of the underlying diagnosis before you examine the child. A good example of this is coeliac disease, where the weight percentile chart characteristically shows a falling-off of previously adequate weight gain, at the age that gluten-containing foods were introduced to the diet.

1. Introduce self

2. General inspection
Position patient: lying, fully undressed,
    after initial inspection standing
Parameters
- Weight
- Height
- Head circumference
- Percentiles
Nutritional status
- Muscle bulk
- Subcutaneous fat
Sick or well
Pallor
Jaundice
Bruising, petechiae
Peripheral stigmata of CLD
Oedema
Tachypnoea
Involuntary movements
Access devices

3. Demonstrate fat and protein stores
Subcutaneous fat
- Mid-arm, axillae, subscapular,
    suprailiac
Muscle bulk
- Biceps, triceps, quadriceps, glutei

4. Upper limbs
Nails
Palms
Xanthomata
Asterixis
Wrists
Other joints

5. Head and neck
Face
Eyes
- Lids
- Conjunctivae
- Sclera
- Iris
- Cornea
- Lens
- Retina
Mouth

6. Abdomen – anterior aspect
Inspection
- Distension
- Scars
- Access devices
- Injection sites
- Stoma

- Herniae
- Abdominal wall veins
- Striae
Palpation, percussion, auscultation
- Abdominal tenderness
- Hepatomegaly
- Hepatic bruit (hepatoma)
- Splenomegaly (portal hypertension)
- Enlarged kidneys (polycystic
    disease)
- Ascites
- Abdominal mass
- Inguinal herniae

7. Abdomen – posterior aspect
Inspection
- Purpura on buttocks (HSP)
- Xanthomata on buttocks (CLD)
- Gluteal wasting (malnutrition)
- Perianal fissures, fistulae (IBD)
- Imperforate anus (congenital)

8. Lower limbs
Inspect
- Bowing (vitamin D deficiency)
- Erythema nodosum (IBD, chronic
    active hepatitis)
- Joint swelling (IBD)
Palpate
- Ankle
    oedema
    (CLD, PLE)

9. Other
Urinalysis
Stool analysis
Temperature
Depending on
    findings
- Neurological
    system
- Respiratory
    system
- Cardio-
    vascular
    system

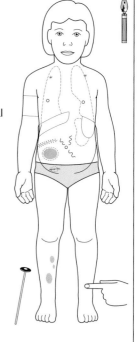

CLD = chronic liver disease; HSP = Henoch–Schönlein purpura; IBD = inflammatory bowel disease;
PLE = protein-losing enteropathy.

Figure 8.3 **The gastrointestinal system**

Table 8.1

Additional information: details of possible findings on gastrointestinal examination

GENERAL INSPECTION

Pallor (GIT blood loss, CLD, nutritional deficiencies in iron, folate, various vitamins)

Jaundice (CLD, vitamin B_{12} deficiency with ileal resection or disease)

Bruising (CLD, thrombocytopenia in hypersplenism, HSP)

Petechiae (hypersplenism in portal hypertension)

Peripheral stigmata of CLD: spider naevi, scratch marks (pruritis with cholestasis), xanthomata (cholestasis)

Oedema (CLD, PLE)

Tachypnoea, cyanosis, cough, barrel chest (CF)

Irritability (iron deficiency, coeliac disease)

Mental state (hepatic encephalopathy)

Dysarthria (Wilson)

Involuntary movements: athetosis, chorea, tremor, dystonia or myoclonus (Wilson)

Access devices (venous ports used in CF for administering antibiotics; intravenous access for total parenteral nutrition, or hyperalimentation)

Nasogastric tube

Dysmorphic features
- Alagille
- Various other syndromes

Joint swelling (IBD)

Evidence of rickets (bow legs, prominent wrists and ankles, rib rosary) (vitamin D deficiency)

Abdominal distension, scars, access devices, stoma

Skin
- Various rashes related to nutritional deficiencies
- Dermatitis herpetiformis (coeliac disease)
- Erythema nodosum (IBD, CAH)

UPPER LIMBS

Nails
- Clubbing (CLD, IBD, CF)
- Leuconychia (CLD)
- Koilonychia (iron deficiency)
- Cyanosis (CF)

Palms
- Crease pallor (anaemias)
- Erythema (CLD)
- Crease pigmentation (Addison)

Xanthomata (between fingers and on extensor surfaces)

Dark brown spots on nails, hands (Peutz–Jeghers)

Asterixis (liver failure, CO_2 retention in CF)

Wrists: palpable epiphyseal enlargement (vitamin D deficiency)

Joints: swelling (IBD)

Continued

Table 8.1 (continued)

HEAD AND NECK

Facial characteristics
- Cushingoid facies (steroid-treated IBD or CAH)
- Doll face 'cherub' (glycogen storage diseases types 1 and 3)

Eyes
- Pigmentation around eyes (2–3 mm brown–black spots in Peutz–Jeghers)
- Lids: xanthelasma (hyperlipidaemia)
- Conjunctivae: pallor (anaemias, with nutritional deficiencies, GIT blood loss [CLD, Wilson]), xerosis (vitamin A deficiency)
- Sclera: jaundice (note depth thereof)
- Iris: iritis (IBD)
- Cornea: xerosis, clouding, opacification (vitamin A deficiency), Kayser-Fleischer rings (brown/green pigmentation in limbic region, occur in Wilson disease)
- Lens: cataracts (congenital TORCH infections, steroid-treated IBD or CAH, Wilson)
- Retina: retinal pigmentation (abetalipoproteinaemia, Alagille), chorioretinitis (TORCH), retinopathy of prematurity (ex-premature with NEC)

Mouth
- Breath: hepatic fetor (liver failure)
- Lips: angular cheilosis (iron deficiency): pigmentation (Peutz–Jeghers)
- Buccal mucosa: areas of brown–black pigmentation (Peutz–Jeghers, Addison)

ABDOMEN—ANTERIOR ASPECT

Distension
- Weak abdominal muscles (protein calorie malnutrition [PCM], coeliac disease)
- Ascites (CLD, PLE, PCM)

Operative scars (Kasai, colectomy, liver transplant)

Access devices (e.g. venous port for antibiotics in CF)

Injection sites (insulin in CF with diabetes, venous port site in currently treated CF)

Stoma (colostomy, ileostomy, gastrostomy)

Prominent abdominal wall veins (portal hypertension)

Striae (Cushing's syndrome in steroid-treated IBD, CAH)

URINE, STOOL, TEMPERATURE CHART

Request inspection of
- Urine: dark (cholestasis)
- Stool: acholic (cholestasis); blood (portal hypertension)

Urinalysis
- Bilirubin (hepatobiliary disease)
- Urobilinogen (increased hepatic dysfunction)

Temperature chart (infectious hepatitis, CAH)

NEUROLOGICAL SYSTEM

Infants

Alertness (decreased in TORCH)

Choreoathetoid movements (kernicterus)

Gross motor assessment (hypertonic with TORCH)

Primitive reflexes: pathological persistence (TORCH, bilirubin encephalopathy)

Table 8.1 (continued)
Hearing: deafness (TORCH, bilirubin encephalopathy)
Older children (over 5 years)
Gait examination • Cerebellar ataxia (vitamin E deficiency) • Peripheral neuropathy (vitamin E deficiency) • Involuntary movements (Wilson) • Antalgic gait (arthritis with IBD)
Romberg sign (vitamin E deficiency)
Hold arms horizontally: wing beating tremor (Wilson)
Diminished reflexes (vitamin E deficiency)
Diminished sensation (vitamin E deficiency)
RESPIRATORY EXAMINATION
Full respiratory examination, including getting child to cough and inspecting any sputum (CF)
CARDIAC EXAMINATION
Full praecordial assessment (Alagille, congenital rubella, CF)

CAH = chronic active hepatitis; CF = cystic fibrosis; CLD = chronic liver disease; GIT = gastrointestinal tract; HSP = Henoch–Schönlein purpura; NEC = necrotising enterocolitis; PLE = protein-losing enteropathy; TORCH = toxoplasmosis, other (e.g. HIV, syphilis), rubella, cytomegalovirus, herpes (both simplex and varicella).

The height chart can indicate disease chronicity and can suggest certain diagnoses that often present as short stature, such as Shwachman–Diamond syndrome (SDS) or Crohn's disease. The head circumference is decreased in the congenital TORCH infections, which can present with poor growth and hepatomegaly.

Now, take 20 seconds or so to visually scan for those features outlined in the figure. After this, the child can be systematically examined, commencing with the hands, noting any clubbing, leuconychia or other peripheral stigmata of CLD. Move on to the head and neck, examining in particular the eyes and mouth. When examining the eyes, mention the relevance of examining the retinae, but defer actually doing it until you have completed the rest of your examination, as it is too time-consuming at this stage. This is followed by a thorough abdominal examination.

Next, inspect the lower limbs for erythema nodosum (IBD, CAH) and feel for ankle oedema (CLD). The findings noted to this point will determine whether further assessment of other systems, such as the following, is needed.

Neurological assessment

A neurological examination is appropriate in the following circumstances:

1. Any jaundice or other suggestion of liver disease in a child over 5 years (e.g. vitamin E deficiency causing cerebellar ataxia and/or peripheral neuropathy, Wilson disease causing ataxia, dysarthria, dystonia).
2. Any malabsorption or pigmentary retinopathy (e.g. abetalipoproteinaemia with vitamin E deficiency).
3. Microcephaly (congenital TORCH infections, with developmental delay).

In older children, assess the gait and then formally test the lower limbs. In infants, a gross motor developmental approach, followed by lower limb assessment, is more appropriate.

Respiratory assessment

If there is any evidence of liver disease, respiratory distress or diabetes (think of CF), a full respiratory assessment is needed, including asking the child to cough and requesting inspection of a sputum specimen.

Cardiac assessment

If there is any evidence of jaundice or hepatomegaly in an infant (pulmonary arterial stenosis in Alagille syndrome) or any suggestion of CF (for evidence of cor pulmonale), then a full praecordial assessment is warranted.

At the completion of clinical examination, request inspection of any urine or stool specimens available, as well as the urinalysis, stool analysis and temperature chart.

SHORT CASE: The abdomen

This is a common short case, but it is often failed due to several simple errors. 'Examine the abdomen' is not the same as 'Examine the gastrointestinal system', but is often interpreted as such. The other common misconception is that the abdomen can be examined with the examiner standing up: this is inappropriate, as the hand and forearm should be at the same level as the abdomen, which can be achieved only by kneeling at the bedside or sitting on a chair. The other point worth noting is that after inspection, when initially palpating, you should look not at the abdomen or examining hand but at the face of the child, as that is the only way to assess if there is any abdominal tenderness.

First have the child fully undressed. Initial inspection can be performed with the child standing, as this is the best position from which to gain an overall impression of the child's height and nutritional status, and also to assess abdominal distension. Then lie the child flat on the bed, with one pillow under the head, and, after completing an initial visual scan, sit on a chair or kneel next the bed so that the examining hand is at the same level as the abdomen for palpation.

Begin with general palpation, commencing in one or other iliac fossa and proceeding clockwise. Watch the child's face throughout, to detect any abdominal tenderness. Then palpate for the liver, noting its size, consistency, surface, edge and vertical downward movement with inspiration. Percuss in the midclavicular line, from resonant to dull, first from above, then from below, and measure the span with a ruler or tape measure (in centimetres).

Palpate for the spleen next, starting in the right iliac fossa so as not to miss massive splenomegaly. Note the movement towards the umbilicus with inspiration, and feel for the splenic notch; percuss and measure the span in centimetres.

Next, ballot for the kidneys, noting their size, and percuss for resonance above them. Percuss for ascites; if resonant to percussion to the flanks, there is no need to test for shifting dullness. If not, then check for the latter by rolling the patient away from you, waiting 20 seconds for any fluid to settle, and percussing again. Note any change in the site where the percussion note became dull. Measure this distance. Also check for a fluid thrill if there is evidence of any shifting dullness. An assistant (e.g. an examiner) is required to test for a fluid thrill.

Next, examine the inguinal regions for herniae or lymphadenopathy. Examine the genitalia: note the Tanner pubertal staging and the size of the external genitalia and, in a boy, the size, shape and consistency of the testes. If there is any mass here, then transilluminate it. After completion of palpation and percussion, auscultate over the liver, spleen, renal arteries and bowel. Finally, check the abdominal reflexes.

This completes the anterior abdominal examination. The posterior abdominal examination is also important, as many signs here may explain findings noted anteriorly (e.g. spina bifida associated with enlarged bladder or kidneys; bone marrow biopsy sites over the iliac crests, accompanying hepatosplenomegaly).

Roll the child over to inspect the posterior abdominal wall. Spring the pelvis and percuss the lumbar spine for any tenderness, and also auscultate over the kidneys for any bruits.

Next, roll the child on one side and, after asking the examiners for permission, inspect the perianal region, test for the anal wink, and mention performing a per rectal examination (you will not be expected to do this in the examination setting).

Always request the urinalysis, stool analysis and temperature chart at the completion of your examination.

Common findings in the examination setting include hepatosplenomegaly, ascites and enlarged kidneys.

In view of the large number of possibilities in this case, they are best enumerated in list form. Figure 8.4 shows several of the findings sought. For further details on the many possible signs on inspection, see Table 8.2.

The abdominal findings will determine the remainder of the general physical examination.

- If the only finding is minimal tenderness, proceed to a gastrointestinal or renal examination, depending on the site of tenderness.
- If the finding is hepatosplenomegaly, proceed to a gastrointestinal and haematological assessment.
- If the finding is enlarged kidneys, proceed with a renal examination, after requesting the blood pressure and urinalysis.
- If the finding is lymphadenopathy and splenomegaly, examine the haematological system.
- If ascites is the finding, proceed as outlined in the short-case approach to the child with oedema.
- If ambiguous genitalia is the finding, request the blood pressure, look for hyperpigmentation and then proceed as in the short-case approach to disorders of sexual development (ambiguous genitalia) in Chapter 7.

Common findings on abdominal examination and their causes are outlined in the following sections.

Hepatomegaly

The following two lists give different classifications of hepatomegaly. The first is a mnemonic (**SHIRT**) which the author has found useful. The second describes the more common findings found in three different age groups: infant, preschool (less than 5 years) and school age (5 years and over), further subdivided into jaundiced or not jaundiced. This second classification is more practical than comprehensive.

1. Introduce self

2. General inspection

Position patient: lying down (after initial inspection standing)

Rapid visual scan (take no more than 20 seconds)

Parameters
- Weight
- Height
- Head circumference

Sick or well

Pallor (chronic haemolytic anaemia, CRF, leukaemia)

Bruising (CLD, haematological malignancies)

Jaundice (CLD, chronic haemolysis)

Sallow complexion (CRF)

Nutritional status

Oedema (CLD, nephrotic syndrome, protein-losing enteropathy)

Dysmorphic features (various)

Facial characteristics
- Rodent facies (thalassaemia)
- Cushingoid facies (adrenal tumour, treated nephrotic syndrome)
- Doll face 'cherub' (glycogen storage diseases types 1 and 3)

Hemihypertrophy (Wilms' tumour, hepatoblastoma)

3. Abdomen – anterior aspect

Inspection
- Distension
- Scars
- Access devices
- Injection sites
- Stoma
- Herniae
- Abdominal wall veins
- Striae
- Genitalia

Palpation, percussion, auscultation
- Abdominal tenderness
- Hepatomegaly
- Hepatic pulsation (tricuspid incompetence)
- Hepatic bruit (hepatoma, haemangioma)
- Splenomegaly
- Splenic rub (splenic infarct)
- Enlarged kidneys
- Renal bruit (renal artery stenosis)
- Ascites
- Abdominal mass
- Inguinal lymphadenopathy (leukaemia, lymphoma)

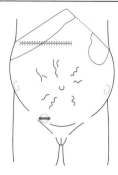

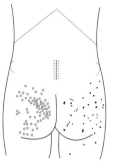

- Empty scrotum (undescended testes)
- Enlarged testis (seminoma, teratoma)
- Enlarged scrotum (hydrocoele)

4. Abdomen – posterior aspect

Inspection
- Buttocks
- Midline anomalies
- Needle marks
- Anus

Palpation, percussion, auscultation
- Pelvic tenderness on springing (ALL)
- Spinal tenderness (ALL, bone tumours)
- Renal bruit (renal artery stenosis)
- Absent anal wink (spina bifida)

5. Other

Urine inspection (dark in obstructive jaundice, haematuria in renal diseases)

Urinalysis (UTI, CRF)

Stool inspection (acholic in obstructive jaundice, melaena from bleeding oesophageal varices)

Stool analysis (CF, coeliac disease, IBD, giardiasis)

ALL = acute lymphoblastic leukaemia; CF = cystic fibrosis; CLD = chronic liver disease; CRF = chronic renal failure; UTI = urinary tract infection.

Figure 8.4 **The abdomen**

Table 8.2

Additional information: details of possible findings on inspection of abdomen

INSPECTION

Anterior aspect of abdomen

Distension, best assessed standing (ascites, coeliac disease, PCM, organomegaly)

Operative scars (e.g. Kasai, renal transplant, peritoneal dialysis, exomphalos repair)

Access devices (e.g. Tenckhoff catheter, subcutaneous venous port)

Injection sites (e.g. insulin, desferrioxamine)

Stoma (colostomy, ileostomy, ileal conduit, gastrostomy)

Herniae (umbilical, paraumbilical, inguinal, incisional)

Prominent abdominal wall veins (portal hypertension)

Striae (Cushing's)

Visible peristalsis (pyloric stenosis)

Inguinal lymphadenopathy (leukaemia, lymphoma)

Pubertal status (precocity)

External genitalia (ambiguous)

Enlarged testis (seminoma, teratoma)

Posterior aspect of abdomen

Purpura on buttocks (HSP)

Xanthomata on buttocks (cholestasis)

Buttock asymmetry (sacral tumour)

Gluteal wasting (malnutrition)

Midline anomalies related to spinal dysraphism
- Lipoma
- Midline hair tuft
- Myelomeningocele

Midline scars (repaired spina bifida, resection spinal tumour)

Needle marks over iliac crests (bone marrow biopsy site)

Perianal fissures, fistulae (IBD)

Patulous anus (spina bifida)

Imperforate anus (congenital)

Faecal soiling (habitual constipation)

HSP = Henoch–Schönlein purpura; IBD = inflammatory bowel disease; PCM = protein calorie malnutrition.

CAUSES OF HEPATOMEGALY

The mnemonic for causes of hepatomegaly is **SHIRT**:

Structural

Extrahepatic biliary atresia (EHBA), choledochal cyst, paucity of bile interlobular ducts (PBID; Alagille syndrome) polycystic disease, congenital hepatic fibrosis.

Storage/metabolic
1. Defective lipid metabolism: Gaucher disease, Niemann–Pick disease, hyperlipoproteinaemias, cholesteryl ester storage disease, carnitine deficiency, mucolipidoses.
2. Defective carbohydrate metabolism: diabetes mellitus, glycogen storage diseases (GSD types 1, 3, 4 and 6), hereditary fructose intolerance (HFI), galactosaemia, Cushing's syndrome, mucopolysaccharidoses (MPSs).
3. Defective amino acid/protein metabolism: tyrosinaemia (type 1), urea cycle enzyme disorders.
4. Defective mineral metabolism: Wilson disease (WD).
5. Defective electrolyte transport: CF.
6. Defective nutrition: protein calorie malnutrition (PCM), total parenteral nutrition (TPN).
7. Deficiency of protease: alpha-1-antitrypsin (AAT) deficiency.

Haematological

Thalassaemia, sickle cell disease (chronic haemolysis and transfusion haemosiderosis), acute leukaemia, chronic myeloid leukaemia.

Heart (congestive cardiac failure (CCF), constrictive pericarditis, obstructed IVC).

Infection
1. Viral infections: congenital rubella, cytomegalovirus (CMV) infection, coxsackievirus virus, echovirus, hepatitis (A, B, C, D and E) viruses, EB virus (EBV).
2. Bacterial infections: neonatal septicaemia, *E. coli* urinary tract infections (UTIs), tuberculosis (TB), congenital syphilis.
3. Parasitic infections: hydatid disease, malaria, schistosomiasis, toxoplasmosis, visceral larva migrans.

Inflammatory (CAH, chronic persistent hepatitis, IBD associated liver disease).

Infiltrative (histiocytosis X, sarcoidosis).

Reticuloendothelial (non-Hodgkin lymphoma, Hodgkin disease).

Rheumatological (systemic-onset juvenile idiopathic arthritis (sJIA), SLE).

Tumour/hamartoma
1. Primary hepatic neoplasms: hepatoblastoma, hepatocellular carcinoma.
2. Secondary deposits: neuroblastoma, Wilms tumour, gonadal tumours.
3. Vascular malformation/benign neoplasm: infantile haemangioendothelioma, cavernous haemangioma.

Trauma (hepatic haematoma).

Causes of hepatomegaly (practical classification)

Note that some diseases occur in both the 'jaundiced' and 'not jaundiced' lists. These are not misprints, but reflect the wide spectrum of clinical findings in these conditions.

INFANTS
Jaundiced

1. EHBA (most common).
2. AAT deficiency.
3. PBID (Alagille syndrome).
4. Metabolic: HFI, galactosaemia, tyrosinaemia, CF.
5. Choledochal cyst.
6. Infection: echovirus 11, TORCH, *E. coli* UTI.
7. Hypopituitarism.

Not jaundiced

1. Tumours.
2. Choledochal cyst. } These three are the most common.
3. Haemangioma.
4. GSD types 1, 3 and 6.
5. Lipid storage disease.
6. Congenital hepatic fibrosis.
7. CCF.
8. Metabolic: as above.

PRESCHOOL (LESS THAN 5 YEARS)
Jaundiced

1. Metabolic: AAT deficiency, HFI, CF.
2. CAH.
3. Choledochal cyst.

Not jaundiced

1. Infection: hepatitis (A, B, C and E), EBV, CMV, toxoplasmosis.
2. Metabolic: HFI, GSDs, cholesteryl ester storage disease.
3. Structural: choledochal cyst, tumours, congenital hepatic fibrosis.

SCHOOL AGE (5 YEARS AND OVER)
Jaundiced

As above, plus Wilson disease and CAH.

Not jaundiced

As above, plus Wilson disease and CAH.

Hepatosplenomegaly

The causes of hepatosplenomegaly can be seen by perusing the preceding section and the following section for diseases on both lists. In general terms, the causes are as follows:

1. Congenital hepatic fibrosis.
2. Haematological: thalassaemia.
3. Infection: EBV, TORCH.
4. Malignancy: leukaemia, lymphoma.
5. Storage diseases: Gaucher (long term), Niemann–Pick, MPSs.

Splenomegaly

A mnemonic (**CHIMPS**) is helpful to remember the causes of splenomegaly:

Cardiac
Subacute bacterial endocarditis (SBE).

Connective tissue disease
sJIA, SLE.

Haematological
Chronic haemolytic anaemias: hereditary spherocytosis (HS), glucose-6-phosphate dehydrogenase (G6PD) deficiency, beta thalassaemia major.

Infection
Viral: EBV, CMV; bacterial: SBE, typhoid; protozoal (malaria, toxoplasma)

Injury
Haematoma.

Malignancy
Leukaemia, lymphoma.

Portal hypertension
1. Extrahepatic: post-neonatal umbilical vessel catheterisation or sepsis.
2. Hepatic: the various causes of cirrhosis, congenital hepatic fibrosis.
3. Suprahepatic: Budd–Chiari syndrome.

Storage diseases
Gaucher, Niemann–Pick.

Splenic cyst or hamartoma

Renal enlargement

UNILATERAL FLANK MASS

1. Tumour
   - Renal: Wilms tumour, renal cell carcinoma, congenital mesoblastic nephroma.
   - Non-renal: neuroblastoma, adrenal cell carcinoma.
2. Hydronephrosis.
3. Hypertrophied solitary kidney.
4. Renal cyst.
5. Renal vein thrombosis.

BILATERAL FLANK MASSES

1. Polycystic kidney disease (infantile: autosomal recessive, adult type: autosomal dominant).
2. Hydronephrosis: posterior urethral valves, vesico-ureteral reflux, neurogenic bladder.
3. Tumour: Wilms, leukaemia, lymphoma, tuberous sclerosis complex (TSC).
4. Metabolic: GSD type 1 (A and B), tyrosinaemia type 1.

ASCITES

1. Hepatic: cirrhosis and portal hypertension.
2. Renal: nephrotic syndrome.
3. Gastrointestinal: protein-losing enteropathy (e.g. coeliac disease, IBD), nutritional (PCM, beriberi), intestinal lymphangiectasia.
4. Cardiovascular: right ventricular failure, constrictive pericarditis, IVC obstruction, hepatic vein obstruction (Budd–Chiari syndrome).
5. Lymphatic: acquired chylous ascites (thoracic duct obstruction by enlarged lymph nodes or neoplasms).
6. Infection: chronic tuberculous peritonitis.

SHORT CASE: Jaundice

The approach to this case depends on the child's age. In view of this, two separate diagrams of suggested approaches are included, one for the age group below 2–3 years, and one for those who are older. There is, of course, some overlap, but the author certainly found this division helpful.

A useful approach to hyperbilirubinaemia is first determining whether it is conjugated and unconjugated. If conjugated, the next question is whether the child looks sick or well. If the child looks sick, the possibilities include inborn errors of metabolism (IEMs), sepsis and liver failure. If the child looks well, the possibilities include biliary disease and hepatocellular disease.

The infant

Start by introducing yourself to the parent. Note the infant's growth parameters and any obvious dysmorphic features. Alagille syndrome can be associated with a prominent forehead, a small pointed chin and hypertelorism. Infants with a congenital TORCH infection may be small, microcephalic and neurologically abnormal, and infants with hypothyroidism can have coarse facial features and be relatively inactive.

Note if the child looks well. Children with biliary atresia usually look very well despite the serious nature of their disease. Children with congenital TORCH or UTIs or galactosaemia can look very sick.

Listen to the infant's cry, as it may be quite hoarse in hypothyroidism. Also note the infant's posturing, which may be hypertonic (with signs of upper motor unit involvement in the TORCH group). Inspect carefully for any stigmata of CLD.

The systematic general examination of the infant commences with the hands, followed by the head and neck, the abdomen, a neurological assessment, cardiac and chest examinations and, finally, interpretation of the urinalysis, stool analysis and temperature chart. This approach is outlined in Fig. 8.5. Note that the sequence outlined also includes assessing for complications of (unconjugated) hyperbilirubinaemia itself (i.e. kernicterus) or for bilirubin encephalopathy, and also examines for complications of cholestasis (if that is the underlying mechanism suspected); namely, deficiencies in the fat-soluble vitamins A, D, E and K. All but vitamin E deficiency can manifest themselves clinically in this age group.

In the examination of the abdomen, the presence or absence of hepatomegaly is particularly important. The most common four causes of an obstructive jaundice with hepatomegaly in an infant are as follows:

1. Extrahepatic biliary atresia (EHBA).
2. Alpha-1-antitrypsin (AAT) deficiency.
3. Alagille syndrome (PBID).
4. Ex-premature graduate of neonatal intensive care (multiple mechanisms).
   The other possibilities at this age include the following:
1. Endocrine/Metabolic: panhypopituitarism, galactosaemia, tyrosinaemia, HFI, CF.
2. Structural: choledochal cyst.
3. Infective: echovirus 11, TORCH.

1. Introduce self

2. General inspection
Position patient: lying, fully undressed
Parameters
- Weight
- Height
- Head circumference
Sick or well
Activity
Dysmorphic features
Posture
Peripheral stigmata of CLD
Abdominal scars
Cry

3. Hands
Leuconychia (CLD)
Clubbing (CLD)
Palmar erythema (CLD)
Xanthomata (between fingers and on extensor surfaces)

4. Head and neck
Head
Face
Eyes
- Lids
- Conjunctivae
- Sclera
- Cornea
- Lens
- Retina
Mouth
Neck

5. Abdomen
Inspect for
- Distension: ascites (CLD)
- Scars: Kasai procedures (EHBA)
- Caput medusae (CLD)
- Umbilical hernia (hypothyroidism)
- Delayed separation of umbilical cord in neonate (hypothyroidism)
Palpate and percuss
- Hepatomegaly
- Splenomegaly
- Ascites

- Auscultate liver (vascular malformation)
- Genitalia (small with hypopituitarism)
Nappy (if nappy not available, request it)
- Dark urine (cholestasis)
- Acholic stool (cholestasis)

6. Neurological
Alertness
Posture
Involuntary movements
Gross motor assessment
Primitive reflexes
Hearing

7. Cardiac
Examine praecordium for congenital heart disease

8. Chest
Auscultate for any evidence of cystic fibrosis

9. Other
Urinalysis
Temperature chart

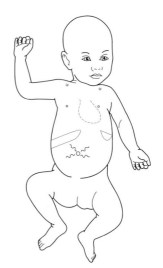

CLD = chronic liver disease; EHBA = extra-hepatic biliary atresia.

Figure 8.5 **Jaundice in infants**

Several clues can help differentiate between these. If a child is older than a few months and has no large surgical scars, it is unlikely that EHBA is the problem. Conversely, if the child has a large Kasai scar (linear scar parallel to the right costal margin), then do not mention a metabolic disease as the most likely diagnosis! If the scar is three pointed, similar to an upside-down Y or the Mercedes logo, this indicates the child has had a liver transplant; then this may have been a metabolic disease, although again EHBA is the most likely diagnosis requiring liver transplant.

If the infant looks unwell, then infectious or metabolic causes are more likely.

If the infant is only several weeks or a few months old, looks well and has acholic stools, then EHBA or choledochal cyst are the most likely diagnoses.

Associated splenomegaly can occur in chronic hepatic disease (due to portal hypertension) and in infective processes such as TORCH. Massive splenomegaly without a hard liver should lead to suspicion of a lysosomal storage disorder.

Ascites and jaundice occur with CLD.

The neurological examination is directed towards detecting underlying aetiologies, such as TORCH infection, as well as the complications mentioned earlier. Evidence should also be sought of malformations that cause hypopituitarism (e.g. septo-optic dysplasia).

In the cardiological assessment, there are several possible findings of relevance. In Alagille syndrome, there can be a congenital hypoplasia or stenosis of the pulmonary artery, and other cardiac anomalies. Other less common associations linking jaundice and cardiovascular problems include the following:

1. Polysplenia/asplenia syndromes, in which biliary atresia indistinguishable from EHBA can occur in association with dextrocardia and congenital heart disease.
2. Arteriovenous malformation of the liver, which can lead to heart failure.
3. Obstructed venous return to the right heart can cause hepatomegaly and jaundice.

In assessing urinalysis, as well as bilirubin and urobilinogen, ask whether any reducing substances are present (if the child is taking lactose in the diet) for galactosaemia, and whether there is blood or nitrites suggestive of a urinary tract infection. *E. coli* UTIs cause cholestasis and often occur in patients with galactosaemia.

The most important condition to identify early is EHBA, as its optimal treatment should be undertaken before 6 weeks of age. The examiners may therefore ask how you would investigate a child for whom this is the likely diagnosis. The following is a suggested approach.

1. Stool inspection: EHBA causes acholic stools.
2. Ultrasound of abdomen: EHBA is associated with a gall bladder less than 2.5 cm in diameter. Ultrasound can also identify choledochal cysts and exclude calculi.
3. Nuclear DISIDA scan: extrahepatic or intrahepatic biliary atresia and severe cholestasis can be indistinguishable. All are associated with lack of tracer in the gastrointestinal tract. For this test the patient should be primed with choleretic therapy with phenobarbitone and cholestyramine.

Exclude all other causes of cholestasis, as all can cause acholic stools. Investigations should include the following:

1. Blood:
   - TORCH screen.
   - Organic acids (Zellweger).
   - Amino acids (tyrosinaemia).
   - Alpha-1-antitrypsin (AAT) assay and phenotype (AAT deficiency).
   - Thyroid function tests, including TSH assay (hypothyroidism).
   - Glucose (hypopituitarism).
   - Red blood cell (galactose-1-phosphate uridyltransferase) assay (galactosaemia).
   - CF gene mutation testing (CF).

Table 8.3
Additional information: details of possible findings on jaundice examination (infant)
INSPECTION
Dysmorphic features • Alagille
Peripheral stigmata of CLD: bruising, bleeding, spider naevi
Scratch marks (pruritis with cholestasis)
Abdominal scars (Kasai)
Hoarse cry (hypothyroidism)
HEAD AND NECK
Head
Facial changes of syndromes • Prominent forehead, hypertelorism, small pointed chin (Alagille) • Down syndrome
Coarse facial features (hypothyroidism, storage disease)
Increased head circumference (extramedullary haematopoiesis in chronic haemolysis)
Microcephaly (TORCH)
Craniotabes (vitamin D deficiency)
Large posterior fontanelle (hypothyroidism)
Eyes: nystagmus (septo-optic dysplasia with hypopituitarism)
Lids: xanthelasma
Conjunctivae • Pallor (haemolytic anaemia) • Xerosis (vitamin A deficiency)
Sclerae: depth of jaundice
Cornea: xerosis, clouding, opacification (vitamin A deficiency)
Lens: cataract (galactosaemia, TORCH)
Retina • Chorioretinitis (TORCH) • Optic atrophy (septo-optic dysplasia)
Midline defects (e.g. clefts): hypopituitarism
Tongue: enlarged, protruding (hypothyroidism)
Neck: goitre (hypothyroidism)

Table 8.3 (continued)
NEUROLOGICAL
Alertness (decreased in hypothyroidism, TORCH)
Choreoathetoid movements (bilirubin encephalopathy)
Gross motor assessment • Hypertonic (TORCH)
Primitive reflexes: pathological persistence (TORCH, bilirubin encephalopathy)
Hearing: deafness (bilirubin encephalopathy)
CARDIAC
Palpate apex to exclude dextrocardia (polysplenia and asplenia syndromes)
Auscultate praecordium • Pulmonary artery stenosis (Alagille, congenital rubella)
OTHER
Urinalysis • Bilirubin (hepatobiliary disease; its absence implies unconjugated hyperbilirubinaemia) • Urobilinogen (increased in haemolysis and hepatic dysfunction) • Blood (UTI) • Nitrites (UTI) • Reducing substances (galactosaemia)
• Temperature chart (infection, e.g. UTI)

CLD = chronic liver disease; TORCH = toxoplasmosis, other (e.g. HIV, syphilis), rubella, cytomegalovirus, herpes (both simplex and varicella).

2. Urine:
   • Metabolic screen (tyrosinaemia).
3. Sweat: iontophoresis (CF).
4. Radiology: chest X-ray to identify butterfly vertebrae (Alagille).
5. Cardiac assessment: to exclude pulmonary artery stenosis (Alagille).
   If all the above are normal, or suspect biliary atresia (e.g. non-draining DISIDA scan), proceed as follows.
1. Operative cholangiogram: the 'gold standard' for diagnosing EHBA.
   If the biliary tree is normal, then:
2. Wedge liver biopsy (percutaneous): EHBA shows extrahepatic biliary obstruction, and bile duct proliferation (discriminates EHBA from other diagnoses in 80% of cases). If biliary tree is abnormal, then:
3. Kasai procedure.
   Table 8.3 gives details of the possible findings on examination of an infant with jaundice.

The older child

The examination of the older child is more like that of an adult. Again, commence by introducing yourself to child and parent. Listen to the child's voice for any evidence of dysarthria, which can occur in Wilson disease (but is very rare in children under 10 years of age). Note the child's growth parameters and whether the child looks sick or well. Look for dysmorphic features (Alagille syndrome) and any involuntary movements (Wilson disease).

1. Introduce self

2. General inspection
Position patient: lying down, fully
    undressed
Parameters
  • Weight
  • Height
  • Head circumference
  • Sick or well
Dysmorphic features
Dysarthria
Involuntary movements
Peripheral stigmata of CLD
Abdominal scars
Joint swelling

3. Hands
Leuconychia (CLD)
Clubbing (CLD)
Palmar erythema (CLD)
Xanthomata (between fingers and on
    extensor surfaces)
Asterixis (liver failure)
Wrists: epiphyseal widening (vitamin D
    deficiency)

4. Head and neck
Head
Face
Eyes
  • Lids
  • Conjunctivae
  • Sclera
  • Iris
  • Cornea
  • Lens
  • Retina
Mouth
Neck

5. Abdomen
Inspect
  • Distension: ascites (CLD)
  • Scars: liver transplant, Kasai
  • Caput medusae (CLD)
Palpate and percuss
  • Hepatomegaly
  • Splenomegaly
  • Ascites
  • Inguinal lymphadenopathy
    (infectious mononucleosis)
Auscultate liver (haemangioma,
    hepatoma)
Inspect perianal region (IBD)

Mention rectal examination for
    haemorrhoids (portal hypertension)

6. Chest
Sternal deformity (vitamin D deficiency)
Rib rosary (vitamin D deficiency)
Auscultate praecordium for pulmonary
    artery stenosis (Alagille syndrome)
Auscultate chest for any evidence of CF

7. Gait and lower limbs
Inspection
Bowing (vitamin D deficiency)
Erythema nodosum (IBD, chronic active
    hepatitis)
Joint swelling (IBD)
Gait examination (in children over
    4 years)

8. Other
Inspection
  • Urine
  • Stool
Urinalysis
Temperature chart

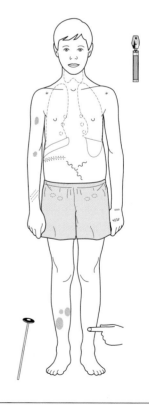

CF = cystic fibrosis; CLD = chronic liver disease; IBD = inflammatory bowel disease.

Figure 8.6 **Jaundice in older children**

Visually scan the patient for any evidence of the peripheral stigmata of chronic liver disease. Also, assess whether there is any joint swelling, particularly in an adolescent patient (IBD or CAH).

Systematic examination commences with the hands, followed by the head and neck, abdomen, heart and chest, neurological assessment and then interpretation of the urinalysis, stool analysis and temperature chart. This is outlined in Figure 8.6.

The diseases in this age group are somewhat different from those outlined in the section on the jaundiced infant. The main groups of diseases that cause hepatomegaly and jaundice are as follows:

1. *Infective*
   a. Hepatitis A, B and C.
   b. EBV.
   c. Toxoplasmosis.
   d. CMV.
2. *Metabolic*
   a. AAT deficiency.
   b. HFI.
   c. CF.
   d. Wilson disease (if child is older than 5 years).
3. *Structural*
   Choledochal cyst.
4. *Autoimmune*
   CAH.

Common causes of *chronic liver disease* include:
1. AIH.
2. WD.
3. Alpha-1 AT.
4. Structural (cyst).
5. CF.
6. Chronic hepatitis B, C.

Common causes of *acute liver failure* include:
1. Drugs/toxins.
2. Infection.
3. From A to G hepatitis.
4. HLH (haemophagocytic lymphophagocytosis).

Note that CF is the most common cause of liver disease in the 0–5 age group in Australia. There are few reports to date of Wilson disease occurring in a child under 5 years, so it is not wise to mention it early in the differential diagnosis of a 3 year old with jaundice.

Important points regarding Wilson disease are as follows:
1. Neurological problems are extremely rare in children (listed here for completeness).
2. If there is neurological disease, Kayser-Fleischer rings are usually present.
3. It may present as a psychiatric problem or with deteriorating school performance.
4. It can present early in childhood, around 5 years, as a haemolytic anaemia, which can be associated with jaundice (often in the setting of fulminant hepatic failure).
5. It is crucial not to miss the diagnosis, as it is one of the few curable causes of potentially fatal liver disease.

In the child over 10 years, CAH and Wilson disease are more likely to be seen in the examination setting. If CAH seems likely, then it is worthwhile mentioning, and examining for, autoimmune associations; namely, thyroiditis (feel for goitre), glomerulonephritis (request the blood pressure and urinalysis) and erythema nodosum (make a point of carefully inspecting the legs). In this age group, it is also worth assessing for evidence of IBD, which can be complicated by liver disease, and may be associated with arthritis and erythema nodosum, as well as uveitis.

INVESTIGATIONS

The examiners may ask what investigations you would perform. Obviously, this depends on the findings in the particular child you see, but in general it is better to assess the severity of the problem before a long differential discussion about the cause, as this is what would apply in practice. Therefore, first mention basic investigations.

Table 8.4 gives an incomplete list of some of the more important possible investigations. Table 8.5 details the possible findings on examination of an older child for jaundice.

Table 8.4	
Diagnostic investigations in the older child with jaundice	
DISEASE	**INVESTIGATIONS**
Wilson disease	Reduced serum copper (usually) and caeruloplasmin
	Elevated urinary copper excretion
	Markedly elevated liver copper content on liver biopsy (most reliable)
Chronic active hepatitis	
1. HBsAg negative	Markedly elevated serum gamma globulin (over 90% of cases)
	Positive for antinuclear antibody (75%)
	High-titre smooth muscle antibody
	Positive direct Coomb's test (75%)
2. HBsAg positive	Mildly elevated serum gamma globulin
	Negative for antinuclear antibody (95%)
	Low-titre smooth muscle antibody
	Negative direct Coomb's test
	Positive (often) HbsAb
3. HCAb positive	
Alpha-1-antitrypsin (AAT) deficiency	Pi phenotyping:
	• PiM allele; phenotype MM (normal-level A1AT)
	• PiZ allele; phenotype ZZ (5–15% of normal-level A1AT)
	• PiMZ allele; phenotype MZ (60% of normal-level A1AT)
Hereditary fructose intolerance	Fructose-1-phosphate aldolase assay on liver or jejunal biopsy specimen; genetic testing
Primary sclerosing cholangitis in IBD	Visualised on percutaneous transhepatic cholangiography (PTC) or endoscopic retrograde cholangiography (ERCP), or magnetic resonance cholangiopancreatography Ulcerative colitis + ANCA + abnormal LFTs is indication for a liver biopsy

Table 8.5

Additional information: details of possible findings on jaundice examination (older child)

INSPECTION
Dysmorphic features (Alagille)
Dysarthria (Wilson)
Involuntary movements: athetosis, chorea, tremor, dystonia or myoclonus (Wilson)
Peripheral stigmata of CLD: bruising, bleeding, spider naevi
Scratch marks (pruritis with cholestasis)
Abdominal scars (liver transplant, Kasai)
Joint swelling (IBD)

HEAD AND NECK
Head
Facial features of Alagille syndrome
Coarse facial features (hypothyroid)
Eyes
Lids: xanthelasma
Conjunctivae • Pallor (haemolytic anaemia) (Wilson)
Sclerae: depth of jaundice
Cornea • Kayser-Fleischer rings (Wilson)
Lens: cataracts (steroid-treated IBD)
Mouth
Palatal petechiae (infectious mononucleosis; unlikely in exam)
Tonsillar exudate (infectious mononucleosis; unlikely in exam)
Neck
Cervical lymphadenopathy (infectious mononucleosis)
Goitre (hypothyroidism)

GAIT AND LOWER LIMBS
Most of this section is only applicable to a child over 4 years of age, as Wilson disease does not exhibit neurological effects until later in childhood
Gait examination • Involuntary movements (Wilson) • Antalgic gait (arthritis with IBD)
Hold arms horizontally: wing beating tremor (Wilson)
Knee and ankle reflexes • Delayed return (hypothyroidism)

Continued

Table 8.5 (continued)
OTHER
Request inspection of: • Urine: dark (cholestasis)   • Stool: acholic (cholestasis); blood (portal hypertension)
Urinalysis   • Bilirubin (hepatobiliary disease; its absence implies unconjugated hyperbilirubinaemia)   • Urobilinogen (increased in haemolysis, and hepatic dysfunction)

CLD = chronic liver disease; IBD = inflammatory bowel disease.

Liver function tests (LFTs)

1. Serum bilirubin (direct and indirect): total indicates severity of jaundice; fractional determination (conjugated or unconjugated) valuable in diagnosis.
2. Serum enzymes:
   a. Transaminases (AST and ALT): indices of hepatocellular dysfunction.
   b. Alkaline phosphatase (ALP): indicates biliary tract disease.
   c. Gamma-glutamyltransferase (GGT): confers specificity to an elevated ALP, as normal GGT activity occurs in children with bone disease.
3. Serum proteins: albumin—index of liver capacity for protein synthesis.

Clotting studies

Prothrombin time (PT) is not a sensitive indicator of hepatic disease, but has prognostic value (if response to vitamin K given parenterally, good prognostic value).

Assessment for deficiency of fat-soluble vitamins

Assessment for deficiency of fat-soluble vitamins involves:

1. Serum retinol level (vitamin A).
2. Serum calcium, phosphate, ALP (vitamin D).
3. Serum vitamin E level.
4. Vitamin K assessed by PT as above.

After these have been discussed, mention appropriate investigations to clarify the diagnosis.

The single most important disease that must not be missed is Wilson disease, as it is curable. Further important diagnoses include hereditary fructose intolerance and choledochal cyst, for similar reasons.

SHORT CASE: Nutritional assessment

The simplest approach to this case comprises three successive components:

1. Assessment of growth parameters.
2. Assessment of fat and protein stores.
3. Assessment of other nutrients, systematically.

First, introduce yourself to the child and the parent. Ensure that the child is fully undressed, then stand back and inspect the child carefully. Visually scan for subcutaneous tissue and muscle bulk. Comment on the child's height and weight, request the percentile charts and interpret these. If only one measurement is given, request previous measurements to observe their progression. Work out the weight age and height age; compare these and comment. Next, if the child is underweight, work out the weight for height, to quantitate the difference in kilograms between this value and the child's actual weight.

On interpretation of percentiles, the common finding is poor weight gain, but height can also be significantly decreased by chronic disease, PCM, zinc deficiency and rickets. Head circumference can be decreased in PCM, but increased in vitamin D deficiency rickets.

1. Introduce self

2. General inspection
Position patient: fully undressed,
   standing, then lying down
Parameters
 • Weight
 • Height
 • Head circumference
 • Percentiles
 • Weight age versus height age
 • Weight for height (quantitate)
Sick or well
Nasogastric tube
Intravenous access
Posture
Skeletal deformity
Pot belly

3. Demonstrate fat and protein stores
Subcutaneous fat
 • Mid-arm
 • Axillae
 • Subscapular
 • Suprailiac
Muscle bulk
 • Biceps
 • Triceps
 • Quadriceps
 • Glutei

4. Skin
Pallor
Jaundice
Bruising
Dermatitis
Erythema nodosum

5. Head and neck
Head
Hair
Eyes: detailed examination
Mouth
Teeth
Tongue
Gums
Neck

6. Upper limbs
Palms, nails
Pulse
Wrists, forearms
Blood pressure

7. Chest wall
Rib rosary (vitamins C, D)
Sternal deformity (vitamins C, D)
Harrison's sulcus (vitamin D)

Sacral oedema (PCM, CLD)

8. Abdomen
Distension
Ascites (PCM, CLD)
Weak abdominal muscles (PCM,
   vitamin D)
Hepatomegaly (fatty infiltration with
   PCM, linoleic acid)
Hepatosplenomegaly (CLD, zinc)
Pubertal delay (zinc)

9. Gait
Full gait examination (vitamins B_1, B_6,
   B_{12}, E)
Examine back (vitamin D)

10. Lower limbs
Palpation
 • Muscle bulk
 • Ankle oedema
 • Tenderness
Neurological examination

11. Cardiovascular system
Full praecordial examination looking for:
 • Cardiomegaly (vitamin B_1,
   phosphate, selenium)
 • Cardiac
   failure
   (vitamin B_1,
   phosphate,
   anaemias)

12. Other
Urinalysis
Low specific
   gravity (CRF)
High specific
   gravity
   (dehydration)
Glucose
   (diabetes)
Stool analysis
Malabsorption
Giardiasis
Temperature
   chart
   (hypothermia
   with PCM)

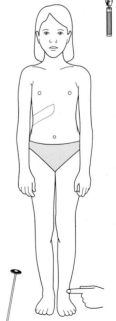

CLD = chronic liver disease; CRF = chronic renal failure; PCM = protein calorie malnutrition.

Figure 8.7 **Nutritional assessment**

After interpreting the percentile charts, demonstrate the amount of subcutaneous fat tissue by examining the skin fold thickness, between your thumb and index finger, at the mid-arm over biceps and triceps, the axillae, and the subscapular and suprailiac regions.

Demonstrate muscle bulk at the arms, thighs and buttocks, muscle wasting being best demonstrated over these areas, particularly the buttocks (glutei). In infants, poor muscle bulk can be reflected by hypotonia on picking the child up.

The next step is a systematic general examination directed at detection of various deficiencies. It commences at the hands, continues up to the head, and then essentially moves from head to toe. Figure 8.7 outlines the order of examination, and Table 8.6 at the end of this section gives additional information. Each deficiency sought is given in parentheses after the relevant physical sign.

Table 8.6
Additional information: details of possible findings on nutritional assessment
INSPECTION
Activity, awareness (PCM)
Irritability (vitamin C, iron, coeliac)
Nasogastric tube
Intravenous access for total parenteral nutrition
Posture • 'Frog leg' (vitamin C) • Bow legs (vitamin D)
Prominent wrists, ankles (vitamin D)
Rib rosary (vitamin C, D)
Harrison's groove (vitamin D)
Pot belly (PCM, coeliac, vitamin D)
SKIN
Pallor (vitamins A, B_1, B_2, B_6, B_{12}, C, E; folate, iron, copper)
Jaundice (CLD, vitamin B_{12})
Bruising (vitamins C, K)
Poor wound healing (vitamin C, PCM, zinc)
'Flaky paint' dermatitis (PCM)
Desquamation (linoleic acid, biotin)
Dry (vitamin A, linoleic acid)
Rough, scaly skin (pellagra) in sun-exposed areas (niacin)
Seborrheic dermatitis (vitamin B_2)
Eczematous scaling around mouth, elbows, knees, genitals, anus (zinc)
Waxy (vitamin B_1, in wet beriberi)
Dermatitis herpetiformis (coeliac)
Erythema nodosum (IBD)

Table 8.6 (continued)

UPPER LIMBS

Palms: crease pallor (anaemias), erythema (CLD)

Nails: leuconychia (CLD), koilonychia (iron), brittle (iron, PCM)

Pulse: bradycardia (iodine, PCM), tachycardia (vitamin B_{12}, hydration)

Wrists: palpable epiphyseal enlargement (vitamin D)

Forearms: tender (vitamin C)

Joints: swollen (vitamin C)

Blood pressure: hypotension (sodium, hydration)

Trousseau sign (calcium)

HEAD AND NECK

Frontal and parietal prominence (vitamin D)

Increased head circumference (vitamins A, D)

Soft skull (craniotabes) (vitamin D)

Fontanelle
- Large (vitamin D)
- Bulging (vitamin A)
- Depressed (hydration)
- Sutures separated (vitamin A)

Hair
- Alopecia (zinc, linoleic acid)
- Dyspigmented (PCM)
- Thinning (PCM)
- Pluckable (PCM)
- Dry (iodine)

Eyes: sunken (hydration)

Lids
- Ptosis (vitamin B)
- Blepharitis (vitamin B_2, zinc)

Conjunctivae
- Pallor (anaemias)
- Xerosis (vitamin A)
- Conjunctivitis (vitamin B_2, C)
- Bitot's spots (vitamin A)

Scleral icterus (vitamin B_2, CLD)

Cornea
- Xerosis (vitamin A)
- Cloudy (vitamin A)
- Keratomalacia (vitamin A)
- Opacification (vitamin A, zinc)
- Vascularisation (vitamin B_2)

Retina (do not need to check in exam)
- Optic neuritis (vitamin B_{12})
- Optic atrophy (vitamin B_1)

Continued

Table 8.6 (continued)
Eye movements: ophthalmoplegia (vitamin E) (do not need to check in exam)
Photophobia (vitamin B$_2$, zinc) (do not need to check in exam)
Facial nerve: percuss for Chvostek sign (calcium)
Mouth: angular cheilosis and stomatitis (iron, vitamin B$_2$, niacin)
Teeth • Caries (fluoride) • Loose (vitamin C) • Enamel defects (vitamin D)
Tongue • Glossitis, reddening and ulceration (vitamin B group) • Moisture (hydration) • Cyanosis (CHD, vitamin B)
Buccal mucosa • Reddened and ulcerated (vitamin B group) • Petechiae (vitamin C)
Gums: swollen, bleeding (vitamin C)
Contour of lower face • Prominent salivary glands (vitamin C) • Pendulous cheeks (PCM)
Neck: goitre (iodine)
GAIT AND BACK
Full gait examination, looking for: • Cerebellar ataxia (vitamin E, zinc) • Peripheral neuropathy (vitamins B$_1$, B$_6$, B$_{12}$) • Romberg sign (vitamins E, B$_{12}$)
Examine back for scoliosis, kyphosis and lordosis (vitamin D)
LOWER LIMBS
Palpate • Muscle bulk (PCM) • Ankle oedema (PCM, CLD) • Long-bone tenderness (vitamin C, phosphate) • Calf tenderness (vitamin B$_1$, selenium)
Power: decreased (PCM, vitamin C, sodium, potassium, phosphate)
Tone: decreased (PCM)
Reflexes • Decreased (vitamins B$_1$, B$_6$, B$_{12}$, E) • Increased (vitamin B$_{12}$ deficiency can cause decreased or increased reflexes) • Slowed return (iodine)
Sensation • Peripheral neuropathy (vitamins B$_1$, B$_6$, B$_{12}$, E) • Posterior column dysfunction (vitamins B$_{12}$, E)

CHD = congenital heart disease; CLD = chronic liver disease; IBD = inflammatory bowel disease; PCM = protein calorie malnutrition.

Check the skin thoroughly before examining the patient. There are numerous dermatological manifestations of many deficiencies. Some of the relevant deficiencies include marked flakiness (PCM), dryness (linoleic acid, vitamin A), bruising (vitamin C, K), pellagra (niacin) or hyperpigmented hyperkeratosis (zinc deficiency).

Examine the child's hands next. Look at the palms for crease pallor (anaemia associated with several deficiencies) or palmar erythema (CLD), and at the nails for koilonychia (iron), brittleness (iron, protein), leuconychia (CLD) or clubbing (CF, CLD, Crohn's disease).

Feel the radial pulse for bradycardia (PCM, iodine) or tachycardia (vitamin B_1, dehydration). Check the wrists for palpable epiphyseal enlargement (vitamin D), the forearms for tenderness (vitamin C) and the joints for swelling (vitamin C).

Take, or request, the blood pressure, supine and standing (sodium, dehydration), and offer to look for Trousseau's sign (cuff inflated to greater than systolic pressure for 3 minutes) at the end of the examination (calcium).

Next, examine the head and neck. Look for thinning of hair or areas of alopecia (linoleic acid, zinc), and for dyspigmentation of hair (PCM), and feel the hair for dryness (iodine) or excessive pluckability (PCM).

The eyes are the next area on which to focus, and many signs are possible here (see Table 8.6). In particular, look at the conjunctivae for pallor (iron, copper, B group vitamins, folate), or dryness and wrinkling (vitamin A), or Bitot's spots (silver plaques of desquamated epithelial cells and mucus) on the bulbar aspect (vitamin A). Look for scleral icterus (vitamin B_{12}, CLD), corneal dryness, wrinkling or clouding (vitamin A) or opacification (vitamin A, zinc). (Be aware that assessing external ocular movements [vitamin E], checking for photophobia [riboflavin, zinc], or fundoscopy for optic nerve inflammation [vitamin B_{12}] or atrophy [vitamin B_1] are not required in the exam.)

Next, percuss over the facial nerve for the Chvostek sign (calcium). Then inspect the mouth for angular cheilosis (iron, riboflavin), the gums for swelling or bleeding (vitamin C), the teeth for caries (fluoride), enamel defects (vitamin D) or looseness (vitamin C), the tongue for moistness (hydration) or glossitis (B group vitamins), and the buccal mucosa for reddening, ulceration (B group vitamins) or petechiae (vitamin C). Examine the neck for goitre (iodine).

Examine the chest for sternal deformity (vitamins C, D), or any 'rib rosary' (vitamins C, D).

Next, examine the abdomen for evidence of pot belly (weak abdominal musculature, coeliac disease), hepatomegaly (PCM, linoleic acid), hepatosplenomegaly (CLD) or ascites (PCM, CLD). Assess Tanner staging for pubertal delay (zinc, Crohn's).

Now, ask the child to walk, looking for evidence of cerebellar ataxia (vitamin E, zinc) or peripheral neuropathy (vitamins B_1, B_6, B_{12}). Check for Romberg's sign (vitamins E, B_{12}). While the child is standing up, check the back for scoliosis, lordosis or kyphosis (vitamins D, C), and look again for any evidence of bow legs or knock knees (vitamin D).

Proceed with a lower limb examination; feel for ankle oedema (PCM, CLD) and test muscle tone (decreased in PCM). Check muscle power for weakness (PCM, sodium, potassium). Tap out the knee and ankle jerks, which may be decreased (vitamins B_1, B_6, B_{12}, E), increased (vitamin B_{12}) or have slowed return (iodine). Examine sensation for peripheral neuropathy (vitamins B_1, B_6, B_{12}, E) or posterior column dysfunction (vitamins B_{12}, E).

Examine the heart for cardiomegaly (vitamin B_1, phosphate, selenium) or congestive cardiac failure (vitamin B_1, phosphate, anaemia).

Finally, request the urinalysis for specific gravity (high with dehydration, low with chronic renal failure) and glucose (diabetes), and the stool analysis for evidence of malabsorption or giardiasis.

SHORT CASE: Failure to thrive

This is a very complicated short case and fortunately uncommon. The approach outlined is essentially a nutritional assessment modified to include relevant examination for chronic diseases of the main organ systems. To prevent unnecessary duplication, only aspects not mentioned in the nutritional short case are outlined in detail.

Commence with general inspection for obvious abnormalities, such as recognisable dysmorphic syndromes, central nervous system disease (e.g. cerebral palsy [CP]), neuromuscular disease (congenital myopathies, spinal muscular atrophy), tachypnoea (cardiac, respiratory or renal [metabolic acidosis] in origin), cyanosis (congenital heart disease [CHD]) and any findings related to nutritional status. Next, request the child's parameters.

'Failure to thrive' as a term is used to describe failure of weight gain in particular, but—particularly if long-standing—may include lack of linear growth as well. If the head circumference is significantly affected, this suggests an intrauterine onset.

The percentile charts should be examined. The pattern of the height, weight and head circumference curves relative to each other may well give a valuable indication of the underlying pathology:

1. If all percentiles are equally affected, the possibilities include intrauterine TORCH infections or chromosomal abnormalities.
2. If height is most affected, possibilities include endocrinopathies and skeletal dysplasias.
3. The common pattern for malnutrition is that the weight is most affected, the height less affected and the head circumference relatively normal.

Demonstrate fat and protein stores, and then examine the skin fully; in particular, for dermatitis herpetiformis (coeliac disease), erythema nodosum (IBD) and pyoderma gangrenosum (IBD). Note any ichthyosis (Shwachman–Diamond syndrome [SDS]).

Look next at the hands, noting any clubbing (chronic lung disease, CLD, IBD, CHD) and other nutrition-related signs. Examine the structure of the hands (dysmorphic syndromes), and take the radial and femoral pulses (CHD, coarctation). Check the blood pressure (renal disease, coarctation).

Proceed to the head and neck. As well as nutrition-related signs, look for dysmorphic features, macrocephaly, scars and shunts. In the eyes, look for cataracts or chorioretinitis (TORCH), retinitis pigmentosa (abetalipoproteinaemia, SDS) and papilloedema (intracranial tumours, hydrocephalus), and check the extraocular movements (neurological disease). At the mouth, check for thrush (can occur in cell-mediated immunity defects), check the palate for a cleft, note the quality of sucking and test the gag reflex. If a bottle or breast is available, the method of feeding should be observed.

Now, move to examination of the chest. Look for sternal deformity (syndromes), hyperinflation, Harrison's sulcus, use of accessory muscles, intercostal recession (chronic lung disease), and scars of cardiac or pulmonary surgery. Palpate the tracheal position, apex beat and praecordium for thrills and heaves, percuss the chest, and auscultate the heart and lungs thoroughly to assess for chronic respiratory or cardiac disease.

Then, move on to the abdomen. Perform a full abdominal examination (see the short case on the abdomen in this chapter). The findings sought include abdominal distension (ascites with CLD, coeliac disease, PCM), prominent veins (CLD), scars of previous surgery (e.g. bowel resection with necrotising enterocolitis [NEC], Kasai procedure for biliary atresia), hepatosplenomegaly (CLD, TORCH, metabolic and haematological diseases), enlarged kidneys (polycystic kidneys, hydronephrosis), anal anomalies (syndromes), rectal prolapse (CF) and excoriated buttocks (carbohydrate intolerance).

Next, have the child stand up and walk, checking the gait for primary neurological disease, as well as for nutritional deficiencies. Examine the back for midline defects or skeletal abnormalities such as kyphoscoliosis (syndromes, cerebral palsy), and then return the child to the bed and examine the lower limbs, again predominantly to detect primary neurological disease, as well as nutritional parameters. Note that if the patient is an infant, a gross motor developmental assessment is more appropriate at this point, and this may be combined with checking the primitive reflexes.

Request the urinalysis for specific gravity (low with chronic kidney disease [CKD], diabetes insipidus), glucose (diabetes), pH (renal tubular acidosis), protein (structural kidney disease, proximal tubular disease), blood (structural kidney disease, urinary tract infection), nitrites (urinary tract infection) and bilirubin (CLD). Request stool analysis, for evidence of steatorrhoea, fat crystals (coeliac disease) or globules (CF), low pH and reducing substances (carbohydrate intolerance), or giardia (cysts or vegetative forms). Mention inspection of any vomitus for bile (obstructive bowel lesions) or blood (portal hypertension) and the temperature chart for infection, as well as watching the mother feeding the child, noting their interaction, the feeding technique and any maternal anxiety.

The examiners may ask how you would investigate the problem. If undernutrition seems possible, then a common approach would be to admit the child to hospital and document whether the child can gain weight with adequate calories, which confirms undernutrition. If the child does not gain weight despite adequate calories, then investigation for malabsorption, or for any chronic disease, would be appropriate (see the long case on malabsorption) in this chapter.

SHORT CASE: Poor feeding

This is a very similar case to failure to thrive, but the problem may be of shorter duration, such that poor somatic growth has yet to occur. The approach is essentially the same in content, with some additions, but the order is changed.

Commence with general inspection, as outlined in the previous section, and comment on parameters and percentiles. The resting respiratory rate is a guide to a cardiac or respiratory cause, and obviously abnormal posturing and movements may indicate a neurological cause (e.g. cerebral palsy, spinal muscular atrophy).

Next, watch the child feed. This will help to clarify the nature of the feeding problem: whether it is local or general and, if general, which system is affected.

Start the examination with the head, looking for local causes first, if no initial clues are apparent after inspection. If there are suggestions of specific problems, such as an infant with an alert face but paucity of movement, then 'go for the money' and 'chase' all the relevant clinical signs for the diagnosis that you suspect (in this example, demonstrate all the findings recognised in Werdnig–Hoffmann spinal muscular atrophy).

Note whether there is any regurgitation of food through the nose, or any vomiting associated with feeding. Look for local structural problems, such as cleft palate. Check the gag reflex and note the quality of sucking. If the infant is breathless, check for nostril patency by holding a shiny metal object, such as one arm of a stethoscope, immediately below the nostrils, and inspect for condensation at the point underneath. The remainder of the head examination procedure suggested for failure to thrive is appropriate here.

The remainder of the general examination can also follow the failure-to-thrive pattern; that is, assessing the cardiorespiratory system, abdomen and neurological system, as well as checking the blood pressure (renal disease), urinalysis and the temperature chart.

SHORT CASE: Weight loss—older child/adolescent

This is very similar in approach to failure to thrive, but there are numerous disorders that occur in older children that are not relevant to the infant or younger child in whom the term 'failure to thrive' is used. The commonest cause of weight loss in adolescent girls in Australia and the USA is anorexia nervosa (AN). Other conditions that tend to affect older children need to be considered, including inflammatory bowel disease (IBD), thyrotoxicosis, Addison disease, Wilson disease and various malignancies. The usual lead-in will be 'This child is thin' or 'This child has lost weight over the past [specified time period]'.

The easiest way to think about the differential diagnoses for this case is to go back to basic physiology—loss of weight can be due to any one or more of four groups:

1. Lack of caloric intake: voluntary (e.g. by desire in AN, to avoid nausea in Crohn's disease) or involuntary (e.g. PCM in developing countries, neglect, abuse, Münchausen's syndrome by proxy [a specific form of abuse], local structural craniofacial problems), or neuromuscular and neuro-developmental disorders, making intake difficult.

2. Lack of calorie utilisation, from lack of food digestion (e.g. CF, Shwachman–Diamond syndrome [SDS]) or food absorption (e.g. coeliac disease, severe Crohn's disease, short bowel syndrome [SBS]).

3. Excessive use of calories in metabolic processes. Any child with 'chronic [*fill in the organ system here—any organ*] failure' can lose weight. Hence, numerous causes can be remembered easily: CKD, chronic liver failure (CLD), chronic respiratory failure (as in CF), congestive cardiac failure (various forms of congenital and acquired heart disease), chronic immune failure (immunodeficiencies such as HIV), chronic atopic dermatitis ('skin failure'), chronic adrenocortical failure (Addison) or chronic pancreatic endocrine failure (type 1 diabetes mellitus [T1DM]). Any child with cancer will lose weight. Any child with an active inflammatory process can lose weight (e.g. juvenile idiopathic arthritis [IBD]).

4. Excessive loss of calories/nutrients/water: various causes of diarrhoea (coeliac disease), various causes of polyuria (CKD, T1DM, diabetes insipidus), various causes of vomiting (AN patients with bulimic features, subacute bowel obstruction, intracranial pathology, malignancy).

Depending on the lead-in given, as alluded to above, malignancy may need to be considered. Leukaemia, intracranial tumours and solid tumours (lymphoma, neuroblastoma, Wilms) thus all come into the differential diagnosis. The approach given in Table 8.7 includes selected findings only; the list is by no means complete. While it is unlikely that a child with a malignancy would be a short-case subject in an examination format, it is still worth learning a comprehensive approach that will be useful in day-to-day practice.

For more detailed findings in the examinations for the various systems and their disorders, refer to the relevant sections (e.g. CF, IBD, CLD, CKD, oncology). Wherever a vitamin or trace element is noted in brackets, this refers to a deficiency of this, in the context of malnutrition.

Table 8.7

Weight loss in the older child: list of possible findings on examination

1. GENERAL INSPECTION

Position patient: fully undressed, standing then lying down

Parameters
- Weight
- Height
- Head circumference
- Percentiles
- Weight age versus height age
- Weight for height (quantitate)

Sick or well

Cachectic (malignancy, AN, AIDS; none of these would be in the exam)

In pain (malignancy, IBD, JA; no patient in pain would be in the exam)

Activity, awareness (PCM)

Irritability (hyperthyroidism, PCM, iron)

Depressed affect (AN)

Pigmentation (Addison, beta thalassaemia major)

Nasogastric tube (AN)

'Raccoon eyes' (ecchymoses from neuroblastoma; would not be seen in exam)

Intravenous access port (chemotherapy in oncology patients, TPN in IBD)

Chest AP diameter increased (asthma, CF)

Pot belly (PCM, coeliac)

Posture: bow legs (vitamin D)

Hemihypertrophy (hepatoblastoma, Beckwith [e.g. with adrenal carcinoma])

2. DEMONSTRATE FAT AND PROTEIN STORES

Subcutaneous fat
- Mid-arm
- Axillae
- Subscapular
- Suprailiac

Muscle bulk
- Biceps
- Triceps
- Quadriceps
- Glutei

3. SKIN

Pallor (deficiencies various vitamins, iron, CKD, ALL)

Acrocyanosis (AN)

Jaundice (CLD, vitamin B_{12})

Yellowish hue (from hypercarotenaemia in AN)

Continued

Table 8.7 (continued)

Bruising (CLD, ALL, neuroblastoma)

Petechiae: limited to SVC distribution (vomiting in AN)

Petechiae, purpura: generalised distribution (leukaemia)

Dry (atopic dermatitis, AN)

Dermatitis artefacta (e.g. cigarette burns, other self-injury in AN)

Scaling (AN)

Excoriated acne (self-injuring AN)

Hypertrichosis: lanugo-like, fine downy-like hair (AN)

Eczematous scaling around mouth, elbows, knees, genitals, anus (zinc)

Pigmented scars (Addison)

Café-au-lait spots (NF1 with associated tumours)

Axillary freckling (NF1 with associated tumours)

Palpable non-tender subcutaneous nodules (neuroblastoma)

Dermatitis herpetiformis (coeliac)

Erythema nodosum (IBD)

Pyoderma gangrenosum (IBD)

Pretibial oedema (AN)

Necrobiosis lipoidica diabeticorum (red-brown plaques on shins, in IDDM)

4. HEAD AND NECK

Hair
- Loss of discrete areas (trichotillomania as self-injury in AN)
- Thinning (AN, PCM)
- Brittle, pluckable (AN, PCM)

Eyes: inspection (from above and from side, as well as in front)
- Exophthalmos (Graves, neuroblastoma, orbital tumour)
- Thyroid stare (hyperthyroidism)
- Blepharitis (zinc)
- Lid retraction (hyperthyroidism)
- Ptosis (intracranial tumour)
- Horner syndrome: miosis, partial ptosis, anhydrosis (neuroblastoma)
- Heterochromia (associated malignancy)
- Aniridia (Wilms)
- Conjunctival pallor (anaemias)
- Scleral icterus (CLD)
- Cataract (diabetes, AN)
- Papilloedema (intracranial tumour)
- Extraocular movements: paresis of inferior oblique; muscles of convergence—medial, superior, inferior recti; lateral rectus (intracranial tumours)
- Test for lid lag (hyperthyroidism)

Mouth: angular cheilosis and stomatitis (iron)

Tongue
- Glossitis, reddening and ulceration (vitamin B group)
- Cyanosis (CHD, CF)

Table 8.7 (continued)

Palate: scarring from self-induced vomiting (AN with bulimic features)

Buccal mucosa
- Reddened and ulcerated (vitamin B group)
- Petechiae (leukaemia, vitamin C)

Gums: gingivitis (ALL)

Teeth: erosion of enamel (AN who purge)

Contour of lower face: prominent salivary glands (AN with bulimia)

Neck
- Lymphadenopathy (lymphoma, ALL, CLL)
- Goitre (hyperthyroidism)

Full examination of cranial nerves, including motor cranial nerves (test first; for intracranial tumours)

5. UPPER LIMBS

Tremor (hyperthyroidism)

Hands
- Russell sign (calluses, scars or erosions over dorsal surface of hands, especially metacarpophalangeal joints with self-induced vomiting in AN)

Palms
- Pigmented creases (Addison, beta thalassaemia major)
- Pallor (anaemias, CKD)
- Erythema (CLD)

Nails
- Clubbing (CF, IBD, CLD)
- Bitten (AN)
- Leuconychia (CLD)
- Koilonychia (iron)
- Brittle (AN, PCM)

Fingers
- Fingertip prick marks (BSL testing in diabetes, CF)
- Hypertrophic pulmonary osteoarthropathy, HPOA (CF)

Pulse
- Bradycardia (AN, PCM)
- Tachycardia (thyrotoxicosis, phaeochromocytoma [would not be in exam], vitamin B_{12})
- Irregular (atrial arrhythmia in AN)
- Flap (hypercarbia in CF, liver failure)

Wrists: tender, palpable epiphyseal enlargement (vitamin D)

Joints: swollen (juvenile arthritis, arthropathy with IBD, CF)

Epitrochlear node enlargement (lymphoma)

Blood pressure
- Hypotension: check for postural drop (Addison, AN)
- Hypertension (CRF, phaeochromocytoma [not in exam], other neuroendocrine tumour)

Full neurological examination of upper limbs, looking for:
- Cerebellar ataxia (posterior fossa tumour)
- Peripheral neuropathy (vitamin B_{12})
- Upper motor neurone signs (intracranial tumour, spinal tumour)

Continued

Table 8.7 (continued)
6. CHEST
Full chest and cardiac examination. Findings can include:
Tachypnoea (CF, asthma, diabetic ketoacidosis, metabolic acidosis in AN)
Scars (previous cardiac surgery with CHD, lung transplant with CF, venous access port with CF, malignancy)
Chest deformity: pectus carinatum, increased AP diameter (asthma, CF)
Harrison's sulcus (CF)
Subcutaneous emphysema (with pneumomediastinum in AN)
Superior vena cava syndrome (malignancy)
Praecordium: palpate, auscultate (various forms of CHD)
Chest: ask to cough, palpate, percuss, auscultate (CF)
Sacral oedema (PCM, CLD)
7. ABDOMEN
Full abdominal examination. Findings can include:
Prominent veins (CLD with portal hypertension, malignancy)
Scars (gut surgery with IBD, hepatobiliary surgery, tumour removal)
Needle marks (diabetes mellitus, DFO in beta thalassaemia major)
Pigmented umbilicus, scars (Addison)
Venous access port, below 'bikini line' (malignancy, CF)
Distension • Ascites (malignancy, CLD) • Weak abdominal muscles (PCM, coeliac)
Striae (corticosteroid treatment in IBD, asthma, CF)
Abdominal mass (Wilms, neuroblastoma, lymphoma, germ cell tumour; would not be seen in exam) • Full examination of all aspects of a mass: location (site), size (measure), if crosses midline, consistency, surface, tenderness, mobility, relations to adjacent structures, associated bruit, venous dilatation, enlarged draining lymph nodes, percussion note, associated ascites, extension into pelvis
Hepatomegaly (hepatoblastoma, leukaemia, CCF, fatty liver: malabsorption)
Hepatic bruit (hepatoblastoma)
Hepatosplenomegaly (CLD, leukaemia)
Splenomegaly (portal hypertension in CF, CLD)
Renal mass (Wilms)
Genitalia/Tanner staging • Pubertal delay (AN, Crohn's) • Pubertal precocity (adrenal tumour, NF1 with tumour) • Testicular enlargement (ALL, testicular tumour)
Perianal disease (Crohn's)
Perianal or buttock mass (malignancy) (would not be in exam)
Rectal prolapse (CF)

Table 8.7 (continued)

8. GAIT AND BACK

Full gait examination, looking for:

- Cerebellar ataxia (posterior fossa tumour)
- Upper motor neurone signs (intracranial tumour, primary or secondary)
- Peripheral neuropathy (vitamin B_{12})
- Romberg's sign (vitamins E, B_{12})

Examine back for:
- Tenderness (spinal tumour)
- Scoliosis (NF1 with tumour; spinal tumour, neuroblastoma)
- Kyphosis and lordosis (vitamin D)

9. LOWER LIMBS

Palpation
- Muscle bulk (AN, PCM)
- Ankle oedema (CHD, hypoproteinaemia in PCM)
- Tenderness (bone tumour, primary or secondary; would not be seen in exam)

Full neurological examination of lower limbs, looking for:

- Cerebellar ataxia (posterior fossa tumour)
- Peripheral neuropathy (vitamin B_{12})
- Upper motor neurone signs (intracranial tumour, primary or secondary)

10. OTHER

Urinalysis
- Low specific gravity (CKD)
- High specific gravity (dehydration)
- Glucose (diabetes)

Stool analysis
- Malabsorption
- Giardiasis

AIDS = acquired immune deficiency syndrome; ALL = acute lymphoblastic leukaemia; AN = anorexia nervosa; AP = antero-posterior; BSL = blood sugar level; CF = cystic fibrosis; CHD = congenital heart disease; CLD = chronic liver disease; CLL = chronic lymphocytic leukaemia; CKD = chronic kidney disease; DFO = desferrioxamine; HPOA = hypertrophic pulmonary osteoarthropathy; IBD = inflammatory bowel disease; JA = juvenile arthritis; NF1 = neurofibromatosis type 1; PCM = protein calorie malnutrition; SVC = superior vena cava; TPN = total parenteral nutrition.

Chapter 9

Genetics and Dysmorphology

LONG CASE: Down syndrome

Down syndrome (DS) represents a common chromosomal disorder. The incidence has changed with the increase in the proportion of pregnancies diagnosed prenatally. In addition, the maternal age at parturition has changed, with more women over 35 giving birth; in 1986, 72% of babies with DS were born to younger mothers, whereas in 2004, 46% were born to younger mothers. However, the worldwide birth incidence of DS has not increased, but decreased from what it could have been by 2–18% per year. One in 350 pregnancies are affected, but only 1 in 1150 live births. In 2010, 95% of fetuses identified with DS were terminated. In the US, between 1989 and 2005, there was a 49% decrease between expected and observed rates, and in the UK, between 1989 and 2006, there was a 54% decrease between expected and observed rates. These trends can be attributed to the availability of prenatal testing and women preferring selective terminations. In reaction to this trend, two states in the US, North Dakota (in 2013) and Indiana (in 2016), have passed legislation to ban terminations based solely on unborn fetuses being diagnosed with DS or other causes of disability; their laws also prohibit terminations based solely on an unborn child's sex, race, colour, national origin or ancestry. Other states are expected to follow suit.

A non-invasive serum test is now available that can provide a definitive diagnosis of DS in the first trimester, with no risk to the fetus; this test detects cell-free fetal DNA (ffDNA) or RNA in maternal blood by real-time polymerase chain reaction. The impact of future testing is likely to be a further decrease in the birth incidence of DS.

Chromosome 21, now sequenced fully, has an estimated gene content of 329, including genes involved in mitochondrial energy production, folate or methyl group metabolism, brain development, neuronal loss and neuropathology. There are an increased number of associations noted with DS, including increased risk of coeliac disease and a greater awareness of comorbid psychiatric and behavioural conditions, which occur more often than in typically developing peers, but less often than in children with other forms of intellectual disability; these include autism, depression and disruptive behaviour disorders. The median age of survival in DS has improved in recent years, as have many aspects of quality of life. In 1983, average life expectancy for individuals with DS was 29 years; in 1997, it was 49 years; and currently, in 2017, it is well over 60 years.

The increased risk of developing acute leukaemias in children with DS is being investigated, as transient leukaemia (TL) and the myeloid leukaemia of DS (ML DS) offer unique models to understand better the stepwise progression of leukaemia, and of gene dosage effects mediated by aneuploidy. (Aneuploid cells have an abnormal number of chromosomes: the most common aneuploidies are trisomies; most trisomies are not compatible with life, with the exception of DS and the sex chromosomal trisomies.)

In 2015, correction of aneuploidies in human cell cultures was reported; euploid cells increased among cultured aneuploid cells when exposed to a protein ZSCAN4. This was tested on fibroblasts from DS patients; within weeks of applying ZSCAN4 to the cells, fluorescent in situ hybridisation with a chromosome 21-specific probe found up to 24% of cells had two rather than three copies; further testing with high-resolution G-banded chromosomes found 40% of cells had a normal karyotype.

Background information
DEFINITIONS

A *syndrome* is a pattern of multiple structural defects, caused by multiple defects in one or more tissues, due to a known cause. In DS, the cause is three copies of chromosome 21 (trisomy 21) in 95% of cases, translocation between chromosomes 21 and 14 in 3%, and in the remaining 2% mosaicism, with two cell lines, one being trisomy 21 and the other being normal. It is the most common chromosomal anomaly, although the epidemiology has changed because of prenatal diagnosis and selected terminations, as mentioned earlier.

DS is associated with a multiplicity of medical conditions, which are listed under Current state of health in the History section below. Details and treatment for these conditions are outlined under Management issues. Much of the management overlaps with several other sections in this book, to which cross-references are given.

History
PRESENTING COMPLAINT
Reason for current admission.

DIAGNOSIS
When made (prenatal [increased nuchal fold thickness, maternal serum screening], birth, age in days), where, problems/symptoms at birth/diagnosis (e.g. cardiovascular [CVS] symptoms [cyanosis, tachypnoea, poor feeding], gastrointestinal tract [GIT] symptoms [vomiting (duodenal atresia), delay in meconium passage], haematological concerns [transient myeloproliferative disorder], vision and hearing aspects), who gave the diagnosis, initial reaction to the diagnosis, initial investigations carried out (karyotype, full blood examination, chest X-ray, electrocardiography, echocardiography, angiography, abdominal X-ray, ultrasound, brainstem auditory evoked response, ophthalmological assessment), genetic counselling given.

INITIAL TREATMENT
1. Surgical (e.g. CVS—correction of atrioventricular canal; GIT—correction of duodenal atresia; staged reduction of omphalocele).
2. Pharmacological (e.g. diuretics) and side effects thereof.

PAST HISTORY
Indications for, and number of, previous hospital admissions. Pattern and timing of change in condition (e.g. CVS aspects—when cyanosis or heart failure developed, when

and how it was controlled; GIT aspects—when operative procedures were undertaken, duration of hospitalisation, how long until feeding was established). Episodes of infection. Other complications of disease (e.g. development of hypothyroidism, coeliac disease, obstructive sleep apnoea [OSA], seizures, leukaemia).

PAST TREATMENT

- CVS: past surgery, complications thereof, plans for further operative procedures. Past interventional catheter procedures. Medications, past and present, side effects of these, monitoring levels, treatment plans for the future. Antibiotic prophylaxis for dental procedures, maintenance of dental hygiene. Compliance with treatment. Any identification bracelet. Instructions for air travel and high altitude. Any recent investigations monitoring treatment. Any recent changes in treatment regimen, and indications for these.
- GIT: past surgery, complications thereof, plans for further operative procedures. Compliance with treatment (e.g. following diet for coeliac disease). Any recent investigations monitoring treatment. Any recent changes in treatment regimen, and indications for these.
- Hearing and vision: past ear, nose and throat surgical intervention, hearing aid placement, ophthalmological intervention, glasses.
- OSA: past adenotonsillectomy, nasal mask continuous positive airway pressure (CPAP).
- Treatments for other conditions: hypothyroidism, atlantoaxial subluxation, seizures, leukaemia, arthritis, diabetes mellitus.

CURRENT STATE OF HEALTH

Note any of the following symptoms:

- CVS disease (fatigue, shortness of breath, cough, sweating, poor feeding, recurrent chest infections; symptoms suggesting arrhythmias, such as syncope, alteration of consciousness, dizziness, palpitations, 'funny feeling' in the chest, chest pain).
- GIT disease (nausea, vomiting, change in bowel habit).
- Recurrent infection (how often, what sites [usually upper or lower respiratory tract], treatment required, any prophylactic antibiotics).
- Hearing impairment (compliance/problems with hearing aids, impacted cerumen, ventilation tubes for chronic otitis media).
- Visual impairment (development of refractive disorders, keratoconus, corneal opacities, cataracts).
- Weight concerns (obesity, non-compliance with diet, exercise, or sign of hypothyroidism).
- OSA symptoms (snoring, restless sleep, daytime somnolence).
- Skin problems (in children—seborrhoeic dermatitis, palmar/plantar hyperkeratosis, xerosis; in adolescents—folliculitis [especially back, buttocks, thighs, perigenital area], fungal infections [skin and nails], atopic dermatitis).
- Oral health (level of oral hygiene, dental caries, periodontal disease, bruxism [stereotyped orofacial movements with teeth grinding], intervention for malocclusion, non-compliance with dental recommendations).
- Respiratory problems (recurrent pneumonia due to silent aspiration).
- Orthopaedic issues (limping can be due to atlantoaxial subluxation, acetabular dysplasia with subluxing hips [not more common in DS, but may appear later], slipped femoral epiphysis, arthritis or leukaemia).

- Foot problems (hallux valgus, hammer toe deformities, plantar fasciitis, pedal arthritis).
- Joint problems (polyarticular onset juvenile arthritis-like arthropathy).
- Diabetes mellitus (increased drinking or eating, weight loss, lethargy).
- Hypothyroidism (dry skin, cold intolerance, lethargy).
- Haematological neoplasia (acute lymphoblastic leukaemia [ALL] or acute non-lymphoblastic leukaemia [ANLL] occur 10–15 times more frequently in DS, with usual symptoms of pallor, bruising, fever, hepatosplenomegaly and lymphadenopathy).
- Reproductive issues in adolescents (difficulties with menstrual hygiene, use of oral contraceptives, Depo-Provera, presentation of premenstrual syndrome [PMS] with temper tantrums, autistic behaviour episodes, seizures, sex education, desire to reproduce).
- Neurological issues (seizures [more frequent than general population, but less than other causes of intellectual impairment], strokes [due to cyanotic congenital heart disease (CHD), or moyamoya disease]).

CURRENT STATE OF BEHAVIOUR

Ask about possible comorbid psychiatric/behavioural issues:
- Symptoms of ADHD (inattention, hyperactivity, impulsivity); any treatment for these.
- Symptoms of autism (impaired social interaction, impaired communication, behaviour patterns including preferring own company, tendency to be loner, 'in their own world'), most problematic behaviours at present (e.g. rituals, anxiety, aggression, self-injury); any treatment for these.
- Other behavioural concerns: depression, conduct disorder, oppositional defiant disorder, aggressive behaviour; any treatment for these.
- Impact of these comorbid issues (on family, educational facility [e.g. special school], therapists, carers).

SOCIAL HISTORY

1. DS impact on child: level of functioning in activities of daily living (ADLs), schooling (type of school, level of support from education department, therapists, academic performance, teachers' attitudes, peer attitudes, teasing, amount of school missed and whether schooling is appropriate).
2. DS impact on parents: for example, financial situation, financial burden of disease so far, government allowances being received, marriage/partnership stability, restrictions on social life, plans for further children, genetic counselling, availability of prenatal diagnosis, contingency plans for child's future, guardianship and power of attorney issues.
3. DS impact on siblings: for example, effect of family's financial burden, whether siblings feel comfortable to bring friends home, whether siblings miss out on parental time, plans for siblings to act as guardians in future.
4. Social supports: for example, social worker, contact with DS parent support groups, any available respite.
5. Coping: contingency plans (e.g. plan if child develops severe febrile illness); parents' degree of understanding regarding health supervision issues in DS.
6. Access to local doctor, paediatrician, neurodevelopmental clinic, various subspecialty clinics attended (where, how often), other clinics attended, alternative practitioner (e.g. homeopathy) involvement.

Any other family members with DS or associated conditions. If so, could they be explained by a familial translocation?

Any delays, local doctor's attitudes, parents' understanding of the importance of immunisation.

Examination

The examination of the child with DS in a long-case setting includes a full cardiological appraisal if the child has any CVS involvement, a documentation of the dysmorphic features of DS occurring in that child, plus an assessment for the development of any of numerous associated problems that may have arisen (e.g. thyroid disease, leukaemia). In addition, an assessment of function with respect to ADLs, a developmental assessment and an impression of behaviour based on direct interaction will give a complete picture, but time constraints may preclude these being assessed adequately. The approach given in Table 9.1 deals with the physical aspects of the child with DS that are able to be assessed objectively and within the time requirements. This approach can also be used in a short-case setting.

Table 9.1
The child with Down syndrome—physical examination
A. MEASUREMENTS
Height
Head circumference
Request/plot weight
Assess percentile charts specific for Down syndrome
Calculate height velocity
Request/plot birth parameters
Request/plot parents' percentiles and ages at puberty
B. SYSTEMATIC EXAMINATION
The following is a selected listing of possible physical findings in children with Down syndrome—it does not include behavioural aspects
General inspection
Diagnostic facies
Tanner staging
Nutritional status • Obese (common after age 3; also, coexistent hypothyroidism) • Thin (commonly light for height in infancy; after age 3, unusual to be thin: consider coexistent malignancy, coeliac disease, hyperthyroidism, Crohn's disease, neglect)
Skeletal anomalies • Pectus excavatum • Scoliosis

Table 9.1 (continued)

Skin
- Cutis marmorata (extremities)
- Atopic eczema
- Hyperkeratotic dry skin (especially palmoplantar)
- Fungal infection (adolescents)
- Pustular folliculitis (adolescents)
- Vitiligo
- Seborrhoeic dermatitis

Upper limbs

Manoeuvres: palms up (to detect simian crease, clinodactyly); check for hyperextensibility (hypotonia)

Structure of fingers
- Brachydactyly (short fingers)
- Fifth finger: hypoplasia mid-phalanx with clinodactyly

Nails
- Clubbing (cyanotic congenital heart disease [CHD])

Palms
- Simian creases

Blood pressure: elevated (occult renal disease)

Joints: hyperflexibility (usual), restriction of movement (arthropathy similar to juvenile arthritis)

Head

Size: small (measure and plot on Down syndrome specific growth charts)

Shape: brachycephaly, flat occiput; facial profile (flat)

Fontanelles: late closure

Hair

- Midline hair whorl (parietal area)
- Soft, sparse hair; alopecia
- Excess skin back of neck (infant)
- Webbed neck (occasional finding)
- Low posterior hairline

Eyes

Inspection
- Examine any glasses child wears (myopia common): check vision with glasses
- Epicanthal folds
- Upward slant of palpebral fissures
- Prominent eyes (coexistent hyperthyroidism)
- Blocked tear duct (infant)
- Ptosis
- Squint
- Nystagmus

Conjunctival pallor (iron deficiency, transient myeloproliferative disorder [infant], acute myeloid leukaemia [AML], acute lymphoblastic leukaemia [ALL])

Continued

Table 9.1 (continued)

Scleral jaundice (coexistent liver disease)

Iris: Brushfield's spots (white speckling of the peripheral iris)

Cornea
- Large and cloudy (buphthalmos): glaucoma
- Keratoconus

Visual fields: field defect (cerebrovascular accident [CVA] from cyanotic CHD)

Eye movements
- Nystagmus

Ophthalmoscopy: cataracts

Nose

Small, with flat nasal bridge

Mouth and chin

Central cyanosis: various forms of CHD

Mouth: open (tendency to keep mouth open common)

Palate: short hard palate

Teeth: hypodontia, irregular placement, periodontal disease, dental caries

Tongue: prominent (small pharynx, normal-sized tongue), geographical tongue, fissured tongue

Tonsils: presence/size (can contribute to obstructive sleep apnoea [OSA]); absence (previous adenotonsillectomy for OSA)

Ears

Wearing hearing aid (hearing impairment in two-thirds of cases); check aid works and that child will wear it

Check hearing (for conductive, sensorineural or mixed loss)

Structure: small, overfolded upper helix, small/absent earlobes, low set

Eardrums: ventilation tubes, chronic serous otitis media, permanent perforation, atelectatic eardrum, tympanic membrane scarring from previous infections or tubes, middle-ear cholesteatoma

Neck

Short, pterygium colli, scoliosis, excess skin back of neck (infant), low posterior hairline, goitre (coexistent thyroid disease)

Torticollis (spinal cord compression from atlantoaxial instability)

Chest

Inspection
- Scars: repairs of congenital heart defects (atrioventricular canal, ventricular septal defect, patent ductus arteriosus, atrial septal defect, tetralogy of Fallot), repair of tracheo-oesophageal fistula, insertion of access port (for chemotherapy for ALL, AML)
- Tanner staging in girls
- Sternal deformity: pectus excavatum or carinatum

Palpate and auscultate praecordium: various forms of CHD, loud second sound with OSA, development of mitral valve or tricuspid valve prolapse, or aortic regurgitation

Table 9.1 (continued)

Abdomen

Inspection
- Scars: repairs of gastrointestinal tract anomalies (e.g. duodenal atresia, pyloric stenosis, Hirschsprung disease, omphalocele, imperforate anus), repairs of urinary tract anomalies (e.g. vesicoureteric reflux, posterior urethral valves, other obstructive uropathy), renal transplantation (e.g. dysplastic kidneys, glomerulosclerosis), operative interventions for other associated conditions (e.g. Crohn's disease)
- Prune-like appearance (prune belly syndrome)
- Tanner staging pubic hair (pubic hair tends to be straight)

Palpation
- Hepatomegaly (congestive cardiac failure [CCF])
- Splenomegaly (subacute bacterial endocarditis)
- Hepatosplenomegaly (ALL, AML)
- Enlarged kidneys (hydronephrosis)

Genitalia

Tanner stage genitalia: measure penis length and testes parameters, estimate testes volume

Penile anomalies: hypospadias (infant), corrected hypospadias

Testicular anomalies: cryptorchidism, enlarged (testicular cancer [seminoma], leukaemic deposits)

Gait, back and lower limbs

Inspection of lower limbs
- Clubbing of toes (various types of CHD)

- Gap between first and second toes wide, with plantar crease between them

- Hallux valgus

- Hammer toes

- Fungal infection of nails (adolescents)

- Pes planovalgus

Palpation: ankle oedema (CCF with CHD)

Gait—standard examination (see the short-case approach in Chapter 13, Neurology) to detect:
- Quality of gait: often 'Chaplinesque' (externally rotated hips, flexed knees (in valgus), externally rotated tibiae)
- Limp (hip dysplasia, dislocation, avascular necrosis, slipped femoral capital epiphysis)
- Hemiplegic/circumducting gait (CVA or cerebral abscess complicating cyanotic CHD)
- Proximal weakness (e.g. developmental dysplasia of hip)

Back
- Look at the back to detect short neck or neck webbing
- Bend over and touch toes to detect scoliosis

Lower limbs neurologically
- Tone (usually decreased), power (usually normal)
- Long-tract signs (quadriparesis or quadriplegia—spinal cord compression from atlantoaxial instability); hyperreflexia (spinal cord compression from atlantoaxial instability, CVA or cerebral abscess complicating cyanotic CHD)

Joints: hyperflexibility (usual), restriction of movement (arthropathy similar to juvenile arthritis)

Developmental assessment

See the short case on developmental assessment in Chapter 13, Neurology—most children with Down syndrome have developmental quotient (DQ) and later intelligence quotient (IQ) in the range 50–70

Continued

Management issues

The following directs you to most areas of management relevant in the long case.

CARDIAC DISEASE

Around 30–50% of children with DS have CVS disease, the most common being septal defects (particularly atrioventricular [AV] canal, then ventricular septal defect [VSD], then atrial spinal defect [ASD]), patent ductus arteriosus and tetralogy of Fallot; left-side defects are uncommon. These abnormalities are now more easily corrected, and are largely responsible for the increased life span of patients with DS. Cardiac disease may be entirely asymptomatic, so all neonates diagnosed with DS should have an echocardiogram after birth and again at 6 weeks.

The success rate for repair of septal defects is improving steadily: if not corrected, these conditions can lead to pulmonary hypertension, particularly if there is OSA, and shortened life span. Eisenmenger's syndrome (reversal of shunting, to cause right-to-left shunt), more common in DS than in the general population, is now rare. Children with DS under 2 years of age with cyanotic CHD have an increased risk of cerebrovascular accident (CVA); they may present with seizures or acute-onset hemiplegia. Children with DS over 2 years of age with cyanotic CHD have an increased incidence of brain abscess, the severity of which relates to the degree of hypoxia. They may present with fever, headache, seizures or focal neurological signs. Around 50% of adolescents with DS syndrome and no previously known cardiac diagnosis develop mitral valve prolapse; aortic incompetence also can develop in adolescence. These are indications for continued monitoring. Despite obesity and unfavourable lipid levels in DS, the incidence of hypertension and atheroma is low. See further discussion of cardiac disease issues in the long case in Chapter 6, Cardiology

HEARING LOSS

Between 50 and 80% of children with DS have hearing problems. This increases to 90% in adults. The hearing loss may be conductive, sensorineural or mixed. The morphology of the head and neck predispose children with DS to hearing problems: the pinnae are small (harder to localise and concentrate sound), the canals are narrow, impacted cerumen is common (may cause mild losses of 15–25 dB), and they may have conductive losses due to middle-ear fluid or structural abnormalities of the middle ear. Adolescents with DS have hearing losses in the high-frequency range, which are not seen in younger children.

Medical management for conductive loss includes treating otitis media and serous otitis media, surgical intervention with ventilation (pneumoeustachian) tubes, adenoidectomy and tonsillectomy (which also helps OSA). Some studies have questioned the effectiveness of ventilation tubes in DS, suggesting a lower cure rate, more sequelae (atelectatic eardrum, permanent perforation of eardrum, middle-ear cholesteatoma), more frequent episodes of otorrhoea, more antibiotic-resistant bacterial infection and less hearing improvement after placement of tubes. Hearing aids are underutilised in DS, mainly due to compliance problems. Cochlear implantation may be required in severely hearing-impaired infants. Other management may involve speech therapy, signing and computer-based assisted communication devices.

OPHTHALMOLOGICAL DISORDERS

Approximately 50% of children with DS have ocular impairments. These include strabismus, nystagmus, refractive errors (common between 3 and 5 years), accommodation problems (resistant to correction by glasses), congenital (or later-forming) cataracts (present at birth in 3%), blepharitis, hypoplasia of the iris, nasolacrimal duct obstruction with tearing, keratoconus and glaucoma. As well as standard visual screening, all children with DS should be assessed by a paediatric ophthalmologist by 6–12 months of age, and then yearly.

DEVELOPMENTAL ISSUES

Nearly all children with DS have a mild (IQ 50–70) to moderate (IQ 35–50) intellectual disability (ID). A small number have a severe ID, with an IQ in the 20–35 range. The IQ alone gives little clue as to function. Language milestones are slower to develop; aspects affected include articulation, expression, comprehension, phonological awareness, syntax and semantics, with reading being a relative strength. In around two-thirds of DS patients, language comprehension is equal to the mental age, but expressive language is more delayed. Gross and fine motor skills are delayed. Academic attainment is higher in mainstream schools rather than specialist schools, and is influenced also by IQ, gender (females tend to do better) and the father's role in the child's life. Self-sufficiency is determined by IQ, excitability, extent of behaviour problems (see below) and whether the parents use practical means to cope with things, showing the child what, when and why, with more showing and less talking; the level of social activity in which the child is engaged also affects self-sufficiency.

BEHAVIOURAL AND PSYCHIATRIC ISSUES

The most common behavioural issues include problems associated with ADHD-like behaviour, autism (appears in around 7% of children with DS), conduct/oppositional defiant disorder and aggressive behaviour. See the long-case discussions in Chapter 5, Behavioural and developmental paediatrics), on each of these topics, for relevant clinical aspects, and their management.

The diagnosis of autism is usually much later than in non-DS children, and parents often are reassured by various people that it is due to DS; there appear to be two groups, one where atypical behaviours appear in infancy, and the second when children have autistic regression at 3–7 years (this is a loss, or plateauing, of social and language skills). Depression is the other common psychiatric issue in DS, but tends to present beyond the paediatric age group. In those who appear depressed, thyroid function should be checked, as hypothyroidism can present in this way. Both the intellectual impairment and speech problems in DS complicate the prompt recognition of mental illness. Excluding sensory impairment in either vision or hearing, or both, should always occur before attributing new unusual behaviours to mental illness or Alzheimer's disease. In the adult population, 25% of those with DS have major depression or aggressive behaviour.

OBESITY

The well-known high incidence of obesity (> 120% of ideal body weight) in children with DS starts to develop in preschool years. Children with DS are less active, prefer indoor activities and have a lower resting metabolic rate; living at home increases the propensity to obesity compared to a residential setting, and low rates of socialisation also increase the risk. By the time teenage years are reached, the average girl weighs 133% of ideal weight and boys 124% of ideal weight. Obesity is notoriously difficult to prevent and manage in children with DS. Attempts at prevention should include decreased caloric intake, increased exercise, vitamin supplementation and weight-bearing activities (as bone density in the pelvis and spine is lower in children with DS compared to other children).

DENTAL PROBLEMS

A high level of dental hygiene should be maintained. The immunological deficiency of DS results in periodontal disease in almost all children with DS, probably due to aberrations of mouth flora. Any carious teeth should be dealt with promptly, with appropriate antibiotic cover. All DS children with CHD should be given a letter or card to show to any dentist or doctor, explaining the need for antibiotic prophylaxis for any dental or similar procedure (e.g. tonsillectomy), including the recommended doses of antibiotics. Regular visits to the dentist and routine brushing can prevent periodontal disease. Orthodontic problems occur in almost all patients with DS, but compliance with orthodontic procedures and braces can be problematic.

THYROID DISEASE

The rate of congenital hypothyroidism in DS is around 1 in 140, versus 1 in 4000 for the general population. The recommendation is thyroid screening (for thyroxine and thyroid-stimulating hormone [TSH]) at birth, 6 months and then every year thereafter. The frequency of thyroid disease increases with age, such that it eventually affects 15% of people with DS. The symptoms and signs of hypothyroidism can be difficult to differentiate from those of DS itself. Children with DS who have a normal thyroxine level, but a TSH concentration above 10 mU/L, are considered to have compensated hypothyroidism and should be treated. Treatment with thyroxine in this group often results in increased growth velocity. For further discussion of the symptoms of hypothyroidism, see the discussion in the short-case section on thyroid disease in Chapter 7, Endocrinology.

COELIAC DISEASE

The average time between the first symptoms of coeliac disease and definitive diagnosis approaches 4 years in patients with DS. The frequency of coeliac disease in DS is around 5–7%. It is sensible to screen all children with DS for coeliac disease: the Down Syndrome Medical Interest Group recommends this be done at 24 months of age, but there is yet to be consensus as to whether screening should be repeated later in life. See the short case on malabsorption for more details on screening tests in Chapter 8, Gastroenterology.

OBSTRUCTIVE SLEEP APNOEA

Obstructive sleep apnoea (OSA) is increasingly recognised in DS, and in children previously incorrectly labelled as having ADHD. OSA has also been a major contributor to pulmonary hypertension and the development of Eisenmenger's syndrome in children with DS and cyanotic CHD historically. As soon as OSA is identified, referral to an ear, nose and throat surgeon for tonsillectomy and adenoidectomy is appropriate in most cases. See the further discussion of clinical and management aspects in the long case on OSA in Chapter 15, The respiratory system.

HAEMATOLOGICAL DISORDERS (INCLUDING LEUKAEMIA)

Children with DS have an increased risk of developing leukaemia, but a decreased risk of developing solid tumours. Around 10% of newborns with DS develop a pre-leukaemic clone associated with a somatic mutation in the gene encoding for the haematopoietic transcription factor GATA1, which is on the X chromosome; this pre-leukaemia is called transient leukaemia (TL), or transient myeloproliferative disease (TMD) or transient abnormal myelopoiesis (TAM). TL is a form of self-limited leukaemia that is almost exclusive to neonates with DS, spontaneously regressing by 2–3 months. These infants must be followed up carefully, as some of them later develop myelodysplastic syndrome or, more often, megakaryoblastic leukaemia aged 1–3.

Both ALL and AML occur 10–20 times more frequently in children with DS compared to the general population. ALL and AML (most often acute megakaryoblastic leukaemia) occur with equal frequency (about 1 in 300 children with DS). In DS, AML usually occurs between ages 1 and 5 years (median 2 years). From 20–70% of patients with myeloid leukaemia of DS (ML DS) present with myelodysplastic syndrome with thrombocytopenia, followed by anaemia, developing over months. In ML DS, the presenting characteristics of these patients differ from those AML in the general population; patients with ML DS are younger than 5, have a low white cell count and do not show meningeal involvement. These patients have a better outcome than children without DS who have AML. In contrast, children with DS who develop ALL do not have a better outcome compared to their non-DS counterparts.

Chemotherapy in children with DS is associated with a higher morbidity and mortality. Anthracycline dosages are reduced in children with DS because of the increased long-term risk of cardiotoxicity in a population that may have compromised cardiac function due to CHD. For further discussion of leukaemia, see the long case in Chapter 14, Oncology. The other haematological aberrations seen in DS are neonatal polycythaemia (occurs in two-thirds of babies with DS) and macrocytosis (also in two-thirds).

Lymphomas are more common in DS, as are testicular germ cell tumours (around 50 times the risk of the general population); males with DS usually have hypogonadism and often have cryptorchidism, so orchidopexy is useful to allow early detection of tumours. The risk of other solid tumours is decreased in DS.

IMMUNOLOGICAL MANIFESTATIONS

Children with DS have increased rates of infections (especially ear and chest infections), autoimmune diseases and certain cancers, which have been attributed to immune dysfunction. The mechanism of dysfunction involves abnormal chemotaxis, deficiencies in cellular immunity, and IgG subclass deficiencies (classes 2 and 4); the latter are responsible for recurrent sinopulmonary infections. It is important to fully immunise all children with DS, and consideration should be given to serial boosters of pneumococcal vaccines.

SEIZURES

Seizures occur in around 8% of patients with DS. There is a bimodal distribution of age of onset: 40% of seizures commence by 12 months of age, and 40% commence just outside of the paediatric age group, in the third decade of life. Children with DS tend to develop infantile spasms and generalised tonic clonic seizures with myoclonus; about half of those with infantile spasms will go into remission without relapse, and there can be some restoration of development. For further discussion on seizures, see the long-case section on seizures and epilepsy in Chapter 13, Neurology.

ATLANTOAXIAL INSTABILITY (AAI)

Atlantoaxial instability (AAI) refers to excessive mobility of the articulation of the atlas (C1) on the axis (C2). The standard method to detect this has been a lateral X-ray of the neck in neutral, flexion and extension. If there is an atlanto-dens space of more than 4.5–5.0 mm, this is considered subluxation, irrespective of the presence or absence of symptoms. Around 13% of DS patients have an increased space but are asymptomatic; a further 2% become symptomatic. The symptoms and signs of spinal cord compression may include altered gait (including limp), neck pain, torticollis, loss of bladder and bowel control, hyperreflexia, hemiparesis or hemiplegia, and quadriparesis or quadriplegia.

Management of symptomatic patients involves immediate referral for stabilisation and surgical consultation. Follow-up of asymptomatic patients shows no progression to becoming symptomatic. Participation in sports does not often trigger spinal cord compromise, and there are discrepancies between guidelines and discordance between X-ray findings, symptoms and risk of spinal cord damage. Sports that are most likely to compress the neck are avoided: this includes gymnastics, boxing, diving, horseback riding and jumping on a trampoline.

ORTHOPAEDIC PROBLEMS

Apart from AAI, discussed on the previous page, there are a number of musculoskeletal problems that are more common in DS, including developmental dysplasia of the hip, acquired hip dislocation (risk related to ligamentous laxity), chronic patellar dislocation, pes planus, ankle pronation, scoliosis and degenerative joint disease (the latter two most likely related to obesity, hypotonia and premature ageing).

DIABETES MELLITUS

At least 1% of children with DS will develop diabetes. Screening is not indicated, but vigilant observation for any symptoms developing is appropriate.

CONSTIPATION

Functional constipation is not uncommon. Standard management for constipation is used. Movicol sachets are very useful. Diet does play a role; parents need to know what a healthy diet entails, and appreciate that cow's milk protein may be the cause of constipation in up to two-thirds of cases, so a diet that decreases cow's milk intake, and increases fruit juice, dried fruit, unprocessed bran and other forms of fibre, may be useful. An end point is the MACE procedure, but it can still be very difficult to perform an antegrade colonic washout in these children: some children use a colostomy bag as a missile, so much thought must be given before launching into procedures in this population.

UNPROVEN THERAPIES

Parents of children with DS are vulnerable to claims of remarkable treatment or 'improvement' with various unproven therapies. Parents need to be aware of claims of various groups, some of which are promoting a mixture of various substances (e.g. gingko, dexmethylphenidate, fluoxetine, phosphatidylcholine and folinic acid) that are entirely without any scientific evidence to support them. Polypharmacy of this type is never good.

Alternative therapies are not recommended by the Down Syndrome Medical Interest Group, due to lack of data to substantiate any of them. There are also potential dangers; for example, chiropractic manipulation should be avoided, given the risk of AAI.

LONG CASE: Turner syndrome

Turner syndrome (TS) is due to haplodeficiency (see below) of some or all genes on the X chromosome. There may be complete absence of one X chromosome or structural anomalies of one X chromosome. The consequent phenotype is variable, relating to the underlying chromosomal pattern. The classic phenotype is 45 X, but the majority of (possibly all) patients with TS demonstrate mosaicism (see below), usually with a second, normal cell line (e.g. 45 X/46 XX or 45 X/46 XY). Other cell lines can include 47 XXX. There can also be structural anomalies of the X chromosome, including rings, deletions, translocations and isochromosomes (equal length chromosome arms, from transverse division of centromere rather than the normal longitudinal division).

A Y chromosome is present in about 6% of patients with TS; an additional 3% have a marker chromosome (structurally abnormal chromosome unable to be identified by conventional cytogenetics) derived from the Y or another chromosome.

The physical signs of TS may be very subtle in childhood and adolescence. In the newborn, there may be characteristic features, such as lymphoedema of the hands and feet, nuchal folds, left-sided heart lesions, webbed neck and a low hairline. In childhood, TS should be considered in any girl with declining growth velocity (falling below the 5th centile), even if there are no obvious dysmorphic features. In adolescence, TS may cause short stature, absence of breast development by 13 years of age, or amenorrhoea with elevated follicle-stimulating hormone (FSH) levels.

TS also can present with complete phenotypic expression of X-linked recessive conditions in a female, such as haemophilia A, Duchenne muscular dystrophy or red–green colour blindness, which suggests X monosomy.

The cardiovascular lesions of TS are widespread; almost 50% of TS patients have an elongated transverse aortic arch. There is a general dilation of major arteries in adult TS patients, including the carotid and brachial arteries. Imaging studies have shown that 11% of TS patients have coarctation of the aorta, 16% have a bicuspid aortic valve (BAV), and each of these is four times more frequent in patients with webbed necks, which are now believed to be residual findings from in utero obstructed jugular lymphatics with nuchal cystic hygromas. The hygromas resolve as lymphatics open later, but the webbing remains and predicts these cardiac lesions: 37% of patients with neck webbing have a BAV versus 12% in those without webbing.

Definitions

A *syndrome* is a pattern of multiple structural defects, caused by multiple defects in one or more tissues, due to a known cause. *Mosaicism* means the presence of two or more chromosomally different cell lines, both of which derive from the same zygote. *Haplodeficiency* is presence in the cell of *one* set of genes instead of the usual *two* sets.

TS is associated with a multiplicity of medical conditions, and this leads to a large number of discussion areas in the long-case format. The relevant conditions are enumerated in the current state of health section of the history (overleaf), and in the management section. Much of the management overlaps with several sections in this book; the reader will be directed to these accordingly.

History

PRESENTING COMPLAINT

Reason for current admission.

DIAGNOSIS

When made (antenatal [ultrasound—renal anomalies, coarctation, cystic hygroma, increased nuchal fold thickness], birth [lymphoedema of hands and feet, left-sided heart problems, webbed neck, congenital glaucoma], childhood [decreased growth velocity, nail dysplasia, high-arched palate, strabismus], adolescence [pubertal delay, amenorrhoea, short stature]); where; problems at diagnosis (e.g. cardiovascular [CVS] symptoms/signs [cyanosis, tachypnoea, poor feeding, hypertension], gastrointestinal tract [GIT] symptomatology [diarrhoea, rectal bleeding]); vision and hearing aspects; loss of weight (coeliac disease, Graves' disease, inflammatory bowel disease [IBD]), weight gain (hypothyroidism from Hashimoto thyroiditis), growth delay (TS per se, coeliac disease, hypothyroidism, scoliosis); who gave diagnosis; initial reaction to diagnosis; initial investigations carried out (karyotype, full blood examination, chest X-ray, electrocardiography, echocardiography, angiography, abdominal X-ray, ultrasound, brainstem auditory evoked response, ophthalmological assessment), genetic counselling given.

INITIAL TREATMENT

1. Surgical (e.g. CVS—correction of coarctation, hypoplastic left-heart syndrome [HLHS]; urinary tract—correction of duplex system).
2. Medical (e.g. antihypertensives, growth hormone [GH], oestrogen, progesterone, calcium supplementation, vitamin D, thyroxine for hypothyroidism, gluten-free diet for coexistent coeliac disease).

PAST HISTORY

Indications for, and number of, any previous hospital admissions. Chronological progression aspects of TS: CVS problems (e.g. when hypertension developed, when and how it was controlled), urinary tract problems (e.g. frequency of urinary tract infections [UTIs], when operative procedures undertaken); ear problems (e.g. recurrent otitis media episodes); eye problems (e.g. strabismus, amblyopia); other complications of disease (e.g. hypothyroidism, coeliac disease, IBD).

PAST TREATMENT

- **CVS.** Past surgery, complications thereof, plans for further operative procedures. Past interventional catheter procedures. Medications, past and present, side effects of these, monitoring levels, treatment plans for the future. Antibiotic prophylaxis for dental procedures; maintenance of dental hygiene. Compliance with treatment. Any identification bracelet. Instructions for air travel and high altitude. Any recent investigations monitoring treatment.

  Any recent changes in treatment regimen, and indications for these. Frequency of echocardiography or cardiac MRI to screen for aortic root dilatation.
- **Growth.** When GH started (fell below 5th centile), supervised by whom (paediatric endocrinologist), dosage given (usual commencing dosage 0.05 mg/kg/day [0.1 IU/kg/day]), any combination therapy (e.g. with oxandrolone in girls aged 9–12); when oestrogen replacement therapy commenced (after age 12), when cyclic menstruation achieved.
- **Hearing.** When impairment detected, level of loss, whether hearing aids prescribed, compliance with hearing aids.

CURRENT STATE OF HEALTH

Note any symptoms of the following:

- CVS disease (symptoms suggesting dilation of root of ascending aorta): chest or epigastric pains, or 'funny feeling' in chest or epigastrium (preceding aortic dissection and rupture); symptoms of hypertension (headache); other symptoms of CVS involvement (fatigue, shortness of breath, sweating, poor feeding [infants], syncope, alteration of consciousness, dizziness, palpitations).
- Loss of weight (Graves' disease, IBD, coeliac disease, renal disease, malignancy [colon, germ cell tumours]).
- Gain in weight (obesity, non-compliance with diet, exercise, Hashimoto thyroiditis causing hypothyroidism).
- Hypothyroidism (dry skin, cold intolerance, lethargy).
- Orthopaedic problems: limp (associated developmental dysplasia of hips, juvenile arthritis, IBD-associated arthritis), back pain (scoliosis, kyphosis, lordosis, juvenile arthritis, IBD-associated arthritis).
- GIT disease: diarrhoea (coeliac, IBD), nausea, abdominal pain, rectal bleeding (IBD).
- Urinary tract problems (infection, haematuria, proteinuria).
- Hearing impairment (recurrent otitis media, recent hearing testing).
- Visual problems (development of strabismus).
- Weight concerns (obesity, non-compliance with diet, exercise, Hashimoto thyroiditis causing hypothyroidism).
- Reproductive issues in adolescents (education about advisability or otherwise of pregnancy [increased risk of maternal complications, including risk of dilatation and dissection of aorta], education about donor oocyte pregnancies, sex education, discussion of desire to reproduce).
- Psychosocial/behavioural issues: being bullied, unsatisfactory peer interactions, ADHD-like symptoms (inattention, hyperactivity, impulsivity), immature behaviour, anxiety, depression; any treatment for these.

SOCIAL HISTORY

- TS impact on child: schooling (type of school, level of support from teachers, therapists, academic performance, teachers' attitudes, peer attitudes, teasing, amount of school missed and whether it is appropriate).
- TS impact on parents: for example, financial situation, financial burden of disease so far, government allowances received, marriage/partnership stability, restrictions on social life, plans for further children, genetic counselling, availability of prenatal diagnosis, contingency plans for child's future, guardianship and power of attorney issues.
- TS impact on siblings: for example, effect of family's financial burden, siblings missing out on parental time.
- Social supports: for example, contact with TS parent support groups.
- Coping: contingency plans (e.g. parents' degree of understanding regarding health supervision issues in TS).
- Access to local doctor, paediatrician, paediatric endocrinologist, neurodevelopmental clinic, various subspecialty clinics attended (where, how often), other clinics attended.

Any other family members with associated autoimmune conditions.

IMMUNISATIONS
Any delays, local doctor's attitudes, parents' understanding of importance.

Examination

The examination of the child with TS in a long-case setting includes a full cardiological appraisal if the child has any CVS involvement, a documentation of the dysmorphic features of TS occurring in that child, plus an assessment for the development of any of numerous associated problems that may have arisen (e.g. thyroid disease, coeliac disease). The approach given below deals with the physical aspects of the child with TS that are able to be assessed objectively and within the time requirements. This approach can also be used in a short-case setting.

Growth parameters are assessed first: measurements and manoeuvres are given below.

MEASUREMENTS

Measure height and the lower segment (LS); that is, from the pubic symphysis to the ground. Calculate the upper segment (US) by subtracting the LS from the total height. Work out the US:LS ratio. Normal values (in normal children) are 1.7 at birth, 1.3 at 3 years, 1.0 at 8 years and 0.9 at 18 years. If the US:LS ratio is increased, it suggests short lower limbs (e.g. hypothyroidism). If the US:LS ratio is decreased, it suggests a short trunk (e.g. scoliosis) or a short neck.

Measure the child's arm span, and compare this to the total height. The normal child's values (arm span minus height) are: −3 cm from birth to 7 years, 0 cm from 8 to 12 years, +1 cm (girls) and +4 cm (boys) at 14 years. An apparently long arm span can be seen with a short neck, or trunk.

Measure the head circumference and weight.

Plot the available measurements on TS-specific percentile charts, and calculate the height velocity. Check the birth parameters and plot these. Plot the parents' percentiles and ages of puberty. After all these parameters have been evaluated, proceed with the manoeuvres below, or commence a systematic head-to-toe examination and slot in the manoeuvres along the way as relevant.

MANOEUVRES

With each manoeuvre, stand opposite the child and demonstrate, so that she will mirror your movements. The skin should be evaluated concurrently with inspecting from front, back and side. Note any pigmented naevi, any scars (keloid common).

1. Inspect from in front

- Screen for carrying angle: have the child hold her arms by her side, with the palms forwards. This angle can be increased in TS.
- Screen for short limbs: have the child touch the tips of the thumbs to the tips of the shoulders. If the thumbs do not reach the shoulders, there may be middle-segment (mesomelic) limb shortening, found in TS and the associated Leri–Weill dyschondrosteosis (caused by abnormalities of the same SHOX gene—the haplodeficiency [loss of one allele] which contributes to the TS stature).

1. Inspect from in front (continued)
- Screen the hands. Have the child hold the palms up: look for short mid-phalanx of fifth finger, Madelung deformity (congenital subluxation or dislocation of head of ulna with radial deviation of hand). Turn the hands over (palms down) and check the nails (e.g. hyperconvex).
- Screen for short metacarpals by having the child make a fist and look for shortened third, fourth or fifth metacarpal.

2. Inspect from the side
The child should be standing with her arms by her side. Note whether there is micrognathia. Note the shape of the back, for lordosis or kyphosis. Note how far the upper limbs reach. If the limbs are short, the fingers may only reach the proximal thigh; if the trunk is short, the fingers may reach the knees.

3. Inspect from the back
Examine for scoliosis. Have the child bend forwards and touch the toes, to determine whether any scoliosis is structural.

COMPLETING THE EXAMINATION
Formal physical examination flows well if commenced at the hands, working up to the head and then downwards—essentially a head-to-toe pattern. Table 9.2 gives a selected listing of possible physical findings in children with Turner syndrome. It does not include behavioural aspects (see later in this case).

Table 9.2
The child with Turner syndrome: physical examination
A. MEASUREMENTS
Height
Lower segment (LS)
Calculate upper segment (US) by subtracting LS from height
Calculate US:LS ratio
Arm span
Head circumference
Record weight
Assess percentile charts
Calculate height velocity
Record birth parameters
Record parents' percentiles and ages at puberty
B. MANOEUVRES
• Arms by side with palms forwards (to detect cubitus valgus over 15 degrees between extended supinated forearm to upper arm) • Thumbs on shoulders, to detect short limbs: can detect middle-segment shortening • Palms up: to detect short mid-phalanx of fifth finger; Madelung deformity (congenital subluxation or dislocation of head of ulna with radial deviation of hand) • Make a fist (to detect short third, fourth, fifth metacarpal) • Look at the back to detect short neck or neck webbing • Low hairline • Bend over and touch toes (to detect scoliosis)

Continued

Table 9.2 (continued)
C. SYSTEMATIC EXAMINATION
Sitting up is the preferred position for the commencement of the systematic examination—the following is a selected listing of possible physical findings in girls with Turner syndrome
General inspection
Diagnostic facies
Tanner staging • Delayed
Nutritional status • Obese (coexisting undertreated hypothyroidism) • Poor (coexisting inflammatory bowel disease [IBD], cancer)
Skeletal anomalies • Broad shield-like chest with widely spaced hypoplastic, and/or inverted nipples • Pectus excavatum • Scoliosis • Kyphosis
Skin • Lymphatic vascular malformations: congenital lymphoedema, residual swelling over hands and feet, dorsal aspect • Haemangiomata • Pigmented naevi
Upper limbs
Structure • Short mid-phalanx fifth finger • Short third, fourth, fifth metacarpal • Madelung deformity
Nails • Dysplastic • Hyperconvex, deep-set
Pulse • Radiofemoral delay (coarctation of aorta)
Blood pressure: elevated (essential hypertension, coarctation of aorta, renal disease)
Joints: swelling, decreased range of movement (coexistent juvenile idiopathic arthritis [JIA])
Eyes
Inspection • Epicanthal folds • Ptosis • Squint
Sclerae • Icterus (coexistent liver disease) • Blue
Cataracts
Fundi • Hypertensive retinopathy

Table 9.2 (continued)

Mouth and chin
Central cyanosis: partial anomalous pulmonary venous return (PAPVR), hypoplastic left heart (neonate)
Narrow maxilla/high-arched palate
Teeth: caries (risk of SBE)
Micrognathia
Ears
Wearing hearing aid (hearing impairment common): check aid works and that child will wear it
Check hearing (for conductive, sensorineural or mixed loss)
Structure: malformed, rotated
Eardrums: ventilation tubes, chronic serous otitis media, permanent perforation, atelectatic eardrum, tympanic membrane scarring from previous infection
Neck/hairline
Pterygium colli
Short
Scoliosis
Low hairline
Chest
Inspection • Shield-like broad chest • Sternal deformity: pectus excavatum or carinatum • Scars: repaired left-sided heart lesions (coarctation, aortic stenosis, aortic root dilatation) • Tanner staging breasts: delay • Wide-spaced, hypoplastic, inverted nipples
Palpation • Praecordium (e.g. for CHD)
Auscultation • Praecordium (e.g. for CHD)
Abdomen
Inspection • Scars: gonadectomy, IBD surgery, removal of tumour (e.g. gonadoblastoma, neuroblastoma) • Tanner staging pubic hair: delay
Palpation • Hepatomegaly (e.g. CCF from CHD) • Splenomegaly (e.g. SBE) • Hepatosplenomegaly (e.g. coexistent neuroblastoma) • Enlarged kidneys (e.g. hydronephrosis)
Genitalia
Tanner staging: delayed

Continued

Table 9.2 (continued)
Gait, back and lower limbs
Inspection of lower limbs • Feet: short metatarsals • Oedema of dorsa of feet • Clubbing of toes (various types of CHD)
Palpation: ankle oedema (CCF with CHD)
Joints: swelling, decreased range of movement (coexistent JIA)
Gait—standard examination screening for: • Limp (e.g. developmental dysplasia of hip [DDH], coexistent JIA) • Proximal weakness (e.g. DDH)
Back • Scoliosis • Kyphosis • Lordosis • Decreased range of movement (coexistent JIA)

SPECIFIC COMPLICATIONS AND ASSOCIATIONS

The mnemonic **TURNER ULLRICH'S** helps recall most of these:

Thyroiditis and other autoimmune disease (juvenile idiopathic arthritis [JIA], coeliac disease)
Undermineralised bone
Root of aorta dilatation risks (BAV, aortic stenosis, aortic coarctation, hypertension)
Neck short, webbed/**N**ails hyperconvex/**N**ormal intelligence (but impairments in memory, maths, spatial perception, goal-setting, goal-attainment, attention span)
Endocrine deficiency (pubertal failure, short stature)/**E**ye findings (epicanthic folds, strabismus, ptosis, congenital glaucoma)/**E**ars (unusual shape, rotation)
Reproductive technology assistance (egg donor programs)

Ulcerative colitis/Crohn's disease
Left-sided heart problems/**L**inear growth deficiency
Lymphoedema/**L**ymphatic malformations (e.g. cystic hygroma)
Renal anomalies (hydronephrosis)
Infertility
Cancer risks (gonadoblastoma, neuroblastoma, colonic carcinoma)
Hearing loss/**H**ypertension/**H**epatic cirrhosis
Skeletal (DDH, Madelung)/**S**pine (scoliosis, kyphosis, lordosis)

Management issues

The following directs you to most areas of management relevant in the long case.

CARDIOVASCULAR DISEASE

Up to 60% of TS patients have some form of cardiovascular disease/malformation. Cardiac disorders are the sole source of increased mortality in TS. Patients with TS are at increased risk of aortic root dilation and rupture. Cardiac findings in TS may include left-sided heart defects that can present in infancy, such as bicuspid aortic valve (BAV)

(50%), coarctation of the aorta (30%), aortic stenosis (10% of those without BAV) or mitral valve stenosis (under 3%). Systemic hypertension is common in TS and is a risk factor for aortic dilatation (as are BAV, aortic stenosis, aortic regurgitation and obesity).

Aortic root dilatation can occur in up to 9% of patients. Aortic dissection and rupture have been reported rarely: there is one report of a 4-year-old patient dying from aortic rupture. The symptoms for aortic dilation are chest or epigastric pains, often misinterpreted as being of pulmonary or gastrointestinal origin.

Some patients with aortic dilation have had no risk factors. All TS patients must be screened for aortic root dilation. MRI may be more useful than echocardiography in delineating aortic pathology: MRI can detect aortic coarctation or dilation missed by echocardiography. Abnormalities of the aortic valve may not be seen on a neonatal echocardiogram, so that repeated echocardiograms or MRIs every year are essential. If a TS patient later becomes pregnant (through oocyte donation), this significantly increases the risk of aortic dissection or rupture. Patients with TS should have echocardiograms at least every 5 years throughout life.

Around 50% of patients have a particular angulation of the aortic arch termed 'elongated transverse arch'; of itself, it has no significance clinically, but there is concern that it could represent an abnormal aortic wall, with a tendency to dilation and perhaps dissection. A dissecting aortic aneurysm usually has risk factors (BAV, other aortic valve anomalies, coarctation or dilatation of aorta, hypertension) although a few cases do not have known risk factors; it may be the vasculopathy of TS itself that may predispose to dissection. The International Turner Syndrome Aortic Dissection Registry was established to study this problem.

Up to 40% of TS patients have hypertension, usually idiopathic, but cardiac or renal causes must be excluded. Once identified, hypertension must be aggressively treated. Blood pressure should be measured at all routine follow-up visits.

Less commonly seen cardiovascular diagnoses include mitral valve prolapse (5–15%), partial anomalous pulmonary venous drainage (PAPVD), which often involves the left upper pulmonary vein (13%), persistent left superior vena cava (13%), ventricular septal defect (VSD) (< 5%) and atrial septal defect (ASD) (> 5%).

Hypertension occurs in around 25% of girls, and a higher percentage of adults, with TS; hypertension is a risk factor for aortic dilation and dissection. It has been noted that some babies with TS have an unusual resting tachycardia, that starts in utero, and the occurrence of impaired sympathovagal tone infers that there could be a problem with autonomic regulation of the cardiovascular system in TS. Many patients with TS have nocturnal hypertension, such that 24-hour monitoring may be helpful.

Beta blockers have been used for hypertension, and have been used to reduce the rate of aortic dilation in Marfan syndrome; recently, angiotensin receptor blockers (ARBs) have been used for this in Marfan syndrome and were found to be superior to beta blockers in reducing aortic dilation; but there is insufficient data on the use of ARBs at present to make any recommendations.

Monitoring for aortic dilatation should include measuring the aorta (at the end of systole), at three levels: 1. the annulus, at the hinge point of the valve; 2. at the level of the sinuses of Valsalva perpendicular to the ascending aorta long axis; and 3. at the ascending aorta, 10 mm above the sino-tubular junction. There are tables of aortic diameter as a function of body surface area.

Electrocardiographic findings can include conduction and repolarisation abnormalities, right-axis deviation (especially with PAPVD), T wave anomalies, accelerated AV conduction and QTc prolongation.

Ongoing follow-up should be with one type of imaging, either echocardiography or MRI. Echocardiography is usually sufficient in infants and younger children; but in older adolescents and adults, its use may be limited due to an abnormally shaped chest, or obesity. Pregnancy in TS should be considered only after a full cardiac evaluation. Extreme exercise should be avoided. Patients should have MedicAlert bracelets outlining their aortic disease.

Cardiac anomalies are more common with a 45 X karyotype, and more common in patients with lymphoedema. Prophylaxis for endocarditis is important, particularly as dental malocclusion occurs in TS, and these patients may require dental procedures. Those requiring cardiac surgery may develop keloid, another predisposition in TS. Ankle oedema may occur due to lymphoedema rather than a cardiac cause.

LYMPHATIC ABNORMALITIES

In TS fetuses that do not survive, there are often cardiovascular and lymphatic abnormalities found; fetuses with cardiac failure almost always have obstructed jugular lymphatics with nuchal cystic hygromas. In TS girls who survive, there is often peripheral oedema and webbed neck, which are the residua of fetal lymphoedema and cystic hygromas, respectively. The newborn lymphoedema usually resolves by 2 years, although it may reoccur at any age, particularly when growth hormone or oestrogen are commenced, as these both can cause salt retention. Support stockings and elevation may be required. 'Decongestive physiotherapy' has been recommended, comprising skin and nail care, massage for manual lymph drainage, compression bandaging and exercise. These patients should avoid any vascular surgery or diuretics. There is a National Lymphoedema Network in the US, which provides useful information for families, at www.lymphnet.org.

GROWTH

From the age of 2 years, growth should be plotted on TS-specific growth charts. GH treatment should be started as soon as the child falls below the 5th centile on the normal female growth charts (or the 95th centile on the TS-specific growth charts). The earlier GH treatment is started, the longer the duration of treatment can be, until oestrogen is commenced, which then leads to growth plate closure.

Between the ages of 9 and 12, oxandrolone has been given with GH to improve skeletal maturity, but the drawbacks are potential masculinising effects and potential risk of hepatotoxicity.

GH increases the rate of growth without increasing bone age. Increases in final height of 15 cm have been described if there were at least 6 years of GH therapy, and oestrogen was delayed. The advantages and disadvantages must be covered fully in discussion with the parents. When GH is commenced, it can lead to enlargement of naevi and recurrence of lymphoedema. The approved doses are 4.7–9.3 mg/m^2/week (0.16–0.32 mg/kg/week) in Australia.

INDUCTION OF PUBERTY

More than 90% of girls with TS have gonadal failure; however, up to a third may undergo spontaneous puberty and around 3% will have spontaneous menses. Oestrogen therapy is essential for the physical, emotional and psychosexual changes of puberty, and should be commenced around 12 years of age, and no later than age 14; otherwise, adequate uterine size may not be achieved. Pelvic ultrasound can be done before starting oestrogen to check uterine size. The recommended preparation is oestradiol valerate, commencing at 0.5–1 mg on alternate days, increasing the dosage 6–12 monthly until feminisation is complete, which usually takes 2–3 years. Bone density needs to be checked around the time of late puberty to ensure that adequate bone mineralisation has occurred. A progestin such as medroxyprogesterone acetate can be added when vaginal spotting occurs, or after 2 years of treatment with oestrogen, to enable regular withdrawal bleeding to occur.

During treatment, height, weight, Tanner staging and blood pressure should be checked, and blood should be taken for serum FSH and oestradiol levels every 3–6 months.

RENAL AND URINARY TRACT ANOMALIES

Around 30–60% of patients with TS have congenital renal anomalies, particularly horseshoe kidney (10%) and double-collecting systems (20%). Only a small minority develop any renal impairment: there are reports of hypertension, urinary tract infection, hydronephrosis, focal segmental glomerulonephrosis and membranoproliferative glomerulonephritis (MPGN). Follow-up ultrasound examinations of the renal tract are recommended every 5 years.

HEARING LOSS

This is common, with most girls with TS having recurrent otitis media, which can lead to scarring and conductive hearing loss, even in early childhood. This is related to the morphology of the head and neck in TS: the palate is high-arched and there is Eustachian tube dysfunction. Commonly, these patients have tympanostomy tube placement for recurrent otitis media, and adenoidectomy and tonsillectomy for airway problems, although adenoidectomy can adversely impact on palatal function, and negatively influence quality of speech.

There is a progressive sensorineural loss characterised by a sensorineural dip at a frequency of 1–2 kHz and high-frequency loss (above 8 kHz), due to anomalies of the outer hair cells of the lower middle coil of the cochlea; this can present as young as 6 years of age. This is more frequent in patients with 45 X or 45 X/46 Xi (Xq) karyotype. Some children will need hearing aids, but hearing loss is progressive, and eventually at least 25% of adults with TS will require hearing aids because of this sensorineural complication.

OPHTHALMOLOGICAL DISORDERS

Approximately 16% of children with TS have ptosis. Other ocular findings include hypertelorism, epicanthal folds, upward-slanting palpebral fissures, strabismus (25–35%), hyperopia (farsightedness) (25–35%), amblyopia (due to the preceding two), blue sclerae and cataracts. Red–green colour blindness occurs in around 8%. In addition to standard visual screening, all children with TS should be assessed by a paediatric ophthalmologist yearly.

OBESITY

There is an increased incidence of obesity (> 120% of ideal body weight) in children with TS. Attempts at prevention should include decreased caloric intake, increased exercise, vitamin supplementation and weight-bearing activities (as bone density is lower in children with TS compared to other children).

THYROID DISEASE AND AUTOIMMUNITY

The incidence of Hashimoto thyroiditis (leading to hypothyroidism) is increased in TS after the age of 10 years; the incidence of hypothyroidism is around 10–30% in later childhood, rising to 50% in adults. Patients with structural defects of the X chromosome have increased susceptibility to autoimmune disorders, including Hashimoto thyroiditis and Graves' disease, IBD, myasthenia gravis and MPGN. The recommendation is thyroid screening every year from the age of 10 years (for thyroxine and TSH, and for anti-thyroid antibodies). The symptoms and signs of hypothyroidism can be subtle. Once identified, hypothyroidism should be treated promptly. For further information about the symptoms of hypothyroidism, see the discussion in the short-case section on thyroid disease in Chapter 7, Endocrinology.

CRANIOFACIAL/DENTAL PROBLEMS

A narrow maxilla/palate occurs in over 80% of cases. Dental crowding is frequent, as is micrognathia (it occurs in 70%). There is an increased prevalence of distal molar occlusion, early eruption of secondary teeth, thinner enamel and root resorption that can lead to tooth loss. Growth hormone treatment can alter craniofacial proportions. A high level of dental hygiene should be maintained.

All TS children with CHD should be given a letter or card to show to any dentist or doctor, explaining the need for antibiotic prophylaxis for any dental or other surgical procedure, including the recommended doses of antibiotics. Regular visits to the dentist and routine brushing are important. Orthodontic evaluation is recommended around 8–10 years of age.

GASTROINTESTINAL DISEASE: COELIAC DISEASE, IBD AND HEPATIC EFFECTS

The frequency of coeliac disease in TS is around 5%. It is sensible to screen all children with TS for coeliac disease, from mid-childhood, regardless of presence or absence of symptoms, repeating the screening every 2 years. See the short case on malabsorption in Chapter 8, Gastroenterology, for more details on screening tests.

IBD (especially Crohn's disease) is around two to three times more common in TS than in the general population. Either IBD or coeliac disease can present with poor weight gain or a range of gastrointestinal symptoms, and should be considered in these scenarios.

Elevation of serum hepatic enzyme levels occurs in 40–80% of TS patients, and is associated with up to a five-fold increase in cirrhosis in adult life. The aetiology of this is uncertain.

OSTEOPOROSIS

Osteopenia occurs commonly in TS. Peak bone mass attainment is inhibited in adolescents with TS, even with treatment: GH and oestrogen replacement improves, but does not normalise, bone mineralisation. To attempt to optimise bone mineral density, oestrogen should be used with adequate exercise, calcium and vitamin D.

PSYCHOSOCIAL ASPECTS

Adolescents with TS are at increased risk for a number of behavioural abnormalities, including anxiety, depression, significant shyness, social isolation and poor self-esteem. Many of these girls demonstrate social immaturity for their age, and they often need support in becoming independent and in interacting with others socially (particularly with males). Girls with TS may be the subjects of teasing and bullying at school: once identified, this situation must be dealt with promptly and decisively by teachers and parents. Meeting with other girls with TS and their families is very beneficial, and offers valued support for these girls and their parents. Patients with TS are not at any increased risk of significant mental health problems.

EDUCATION

Children with TS are known to have problems in four domains: visual–spatial organisation deficits (poor sense of direction); difficulty with socialising (not 'getting' subtle social clues); difficulty with problem-solving (difficulties with mathematics); and problems with fine motor coordination. Educational and vocational training need to take these specific difficulties into account, as these problems persist into adulthood and throughout life. As a group, despite variable learning difficulties, girls or women with TS often excel at verbal skills, and many adults with TS have university degrees.

SHORT CASES

SHORT CASE: The dysmorphic child

This case potentially covers more clinical ground than any other and requires a very structured routine, quite similar to that used for the short-stature examination, except that many children with conditions that make them dysmorphic are of normal height, or may be tall (e.g. Sotos, Marfan). A systematic head-to-toe approach gives one or two differential diagnoses for each of the selected signs listed: these are merely examples, not the most frequent or important findings. This approach looks at each anatomical structure in turn (e.g. eyebrow, eyelid, conjunctiva, sclera, iris, pupil, lens, retina) and asks whether it appears normal or abnormal.

If any finding appears abnormal, it is noted and may need checking later against reference values (e.g. if you suspect hypertelorism, take the outer canthal, inner canthal and interpupillary measurements and then compare these to standard percentile charts). The three areas in the examination that provide the most clues in the diagnosis of a dysmorphic child are often assessments of the head (concentrating on the face), heart and hands.

Definitions

Patterns of morphological defects include sequences, syndromes and associations. Most often, the term 'syndrome' is used in a broader sense than its true meaning. The definitions of relevant terms are as follows:

1. A *sequence* is a pattern of structural defects caused by a single problem in morphogenesis (e.g. early amnion rupture sequence, Pierre Robin sequence due to hypoplasia of the mandible before 9 weeks' gestation).
2. A *syndrome* is a pattern of multiple structural defects, caused by multiple defects in one or more tissues, due to a known cause (e.g. Down syndrome).
3. An *association* is a pattern of structural defects that are statistically related; that is, a non-random occurrence in at least two people of multiple anomalies not due to a sequence or syndrome. The classic example is the **VACTERL/VATER** association:

Vertebral anomalies
Anal atresia with/without fistula
Cardiac anomalies (e.g. VSD)
Tracheo-
Esophageal fistula with oesophageal atresia
Renal anomalies (urethral atresia with hydronephrosis)
Limb anomalies (polydactyly, humeral hypoplasia, radial aplasia and proximally placed thumb)

Examination

The lead-in will always be very clear in directing the candidate to what examination is required. One possible lead-in could be 'This girl looks different to other family members. Please examine her to determine a cause' or 'This girl has short stature. Please examine her to find a cause'. The approach outlined here is a blueprint for one method that can work and has proved successful in the examination. While it is true that 'spot diagnosis' short cases are best avoided, it is worth having a reproducible approach, as so many unusual-looking children will be encountered by a paediatrician or a general practitioner during his or her working life.

Listen to the child's age in the lead-in. Introduce yourself to the child and parent. Ask the child which grade he or she is in at school and note whether the response seems age-appropriate (intellectual impairment is a feature of numerous syndromes). Do not overlook the child's sex when discussing differential diagnoses. It would be embarrassing to talk about Turner syndrome when assessing a boy.

Stand back and look for evidence of an obvious diagnosis (e.g. Down syndrome). Look at the face, noting any dysmorphic features suggesting any of the well-recognised syndromes (e.g. craniofacial syndromes). Note the morphology of the eyes (microphthalmia in Hallermann–Streiff; proptosis in Crouzon, Pfeiffer; hypertelorism in Apert, Crouzon, Pfeiffer, Saethre-Chotzen; iris colobomata in CHARGE). Note if the child has a hearing aid (deafness can occur in Treacher Collins, CHARGE, fetal rubella effects, Waardenburg syndrome), and look at the ears (displaced and malformed in Goldenhar, Treacher Collins) and the jaw. Look for midface hypoplasia (Apert, Crouzon, Pfeiffer, Saethre-Chotzen). Note any facial asymmetry (Beckwith-Wiedemann, Goldenhar). Check the size of the jaw from the side (micrognathia with Robin sequence, Hallermann–Streiff). Look for any neck swelling (e.g. cystic hygroma). Note whether sick or well, and whether there is any stridor, tachypnoea at rest, tracheal tug or use of accessory muscles (e.g. craniofacial syndromes with upper airway obstruction).

Note any particularly unusual body habitus (e.g. Marfanoid in Marfan, homocystinuria; eunuchoid in Klinefelter), obvious disproportion (skeletal dysplasias), obvious asymmetry (e.g. Beckwith-Wiedemann) or abnormal posturing (e.g. hemiplegia in homocystinuria complicated by a CVA due to thrombotic tendency).

Visually assess the pubertal status (hypogonadism can occur in many syndromes; e.g. Down, Prader–Willi, Fanconi pancytopenia, Noonan).

Explain what you are doing as you proceed. Ask for the height and offer to measure the patient yourself: stand the child against a wall, position the head and heels appropriately, and record the height. If the child is short or tall, then the upper segment:lower segment ratio and arm span are worth doing, but in a child of normal stature these additional measurements are not needed, unless there is the impression of disproportion. The lower segment (LS) is the distance from the pubic symphysis to the ground. The upper segment (US) is calculated by subtracting the LS from the total height. Work out the US:LS ratio—normal values are 1.7 at birth, 1.3 at 3 years, 1.0 at 8 years and 0.9 at 18 years.

If the child is short, then proceed as per the short-stature short-case approach (see Chapter 7, Endocrinology). If the child is tall, then proceed as per the tall-stature short-case approach (also in Chapter 7). If the child has obvious disproportion, then proceed with manoeuvres (p. 363). If the child seems to have normal proportions, then proceed with a head-to-toe systematic examination, starting with a careful examination of the face.

FURTHER MEASUREMENTS

Measure the head circumference (HC). HC can be increased in syndromes with hydrocephalus (e.g. X-linked hydrocephalus) or macrocephaly (e.g. Sotos). HC is decreased in the many syndromes with microcephaly (e.g. Seckel). The course adopted by the tape measure being placed around the skull can accentuate the abnormal skull shapes in cases of craniosynostosis (e.g. Apert, Crouzon).

Request the weight. Obesity occurs in many syndromes (e.g. Prader–Willi, Bardet–Biedl), while a slim habitus (aesthenia) can occur in others (e.g. Marfan). Request percentile charts and progressive measurements (if not given), and calculate the height velocity. Request birth parameters (for intrauterine and chromosomal causes: numerous chromosomal syndromes have intrauterine growth retardation as a component).

After all these parameters have been evaluated, either: 1. proceed with the manoeuvres below, particularly if the child is very short, or has obvious skeletal anomalies or clearly disproportionate short stature; or 2. commence a systematic head-to-toe examination, and slot in the manoeuvres along the way, should they appear relevant. The order adopted is unimportant; it is the demonstration of a comprehensive approach that is required.

MANOEUVRES

Inspect from in front

Note any gross structural anomalies of the upper or lower limbs, such as limb deficiency (e.g. in early amnion rupture sequence, Holt–Oram), or aplasias of any long bones (e.g. radial aplasia in VACTERL association or in thrombocytopenia absent radius [TAR] syndrome), contractures (e.g. distal arthrogryposis syndrome) or pterygia of axilla, antecubital and popliteal areas (e.g. Escobar multiple pterygium syndrome). Next, a set of manoeuvres can be performed that very rapidly screens for a number of syndromes: most of these are relevant for short children. With each manoeuvre, stand opposite the child and demonstrate, so that he or she will mirror your movements.

Screen for asymmetry (irrespective of whether tall or short): have the child put the palms together with the arms out straight, and stand with the legs together. Asymmetry occurs in Russell–Silver syndrome. It may also occur as a result of hemihypertrophy in several syndromes; for example, Beckwith-Wiedemann (B-W), Klippel-Trénaunay-Weber (KTW), neurofibromatosis type 1 (NF1) and congenital hemihypertrophy (CH). This manoeuvre may also detect approximation of shoulders (absent clavicles in cleidocranial dysostosis).

Focus on the upper limbs first, then evaluate the lower limbs: look at the knees, for any bowing (e.g. in hypochondroplasia), look at the feet for talipes equinovarus and the toes for their number (e.g. polydactyly in Ellis–van Creveld) and structure (syndactyly, and/or broad malformed distal hallux in Apert).

Screen for carrying angle: have the child hold the arms by his or her side, with the palms forwards. This angle can be increased in Turner or Noonan syndromes. Also, restriction of elbow extension may be detected (e.g. hypochondroplasia).

Screen for short limbs: have the child touch the tips of the thumbs to the tips of the shoulders. If the thumbs overshoot, there is proximal segment (rhizomelic) limb shortening. If the thumbs do not reach the shoulders, there might be either middle-segment (mesomelic) or distal-segment (acromelic) limb shortening, or alternatively the limbs may be bent (camptomelic). Thus, this manoeuvre should detect proximal segment shortening (e.g. achondroplasia), middle-segment shortening (e.g. Langer mesomelic dysplasia) or distal-segment shortening (e.g. acromesomelic dysplasia).

Screen the hands: have the child hold the palms up. Look for simian crease (Down syndrome) and clinodactyly (Russell–Silver syndrome). Note the structure of the fingers (e.g. short with hypochondroplasia), their number (e.g. polydactyly in Ellis–van Creveld) and any syndactyly (e.g. Apert syndrome). Turn the hands over (palms down), note the structure of the hand (e.g. trident deformity in achondroplasia) and check the nails (e.g. hypoplastic in Ellis–van Creveld, hyperconvex in Turner).

Screen for short metacarpals: have the child make a fist, and look for shortened third, fourth or fifth metacarpal (e.g. Gorlin syndrome), first metacarpal (proximally placed thumb; e.g. in diastrophic dysplasia) or all metacarpals (e.g. in Poland anomaly).

Screen for joint laxity (relevant if short or tall): check the degree of wrist extension and whether the child can appose the thumb to the radius (e.g. hypermobility in Ehlers–Danlos, osteogenesis imperfecta or Marfan). If the child is tall or of normal height, check for arachnodactyly by having the child wrap the fingers of one hand around the other wrist. Check whether there is complete overlap of the distal phalanx of the fifth finger on the distal phalanx of the thumb (the 'wrist sign'). Then check whether the thumb can project from beyond the ulnar border of the hand when the thumb is apposed to the palm when making a fist ('the thumb sign'). Arachnodactyly occurs in Marfan syndrome.

Inspect from the side

The child should be standing with the arms by his or her side. Note whether there is a prominent forehead (e.g. achondroplasia), flat occiput (Down), proptosis (e.g. syndromes with craniosynostosis, NF1), micrognathia (e.g. Pierre Robin sequence) or prognathism (e.g. achondroplasia). Note how far the upper limbs reach; if the limbs are short, the fingers may only reach the proximal thigh; if the trunk is short, the fingers may reach the knees. Note the shape of the back, for lordosis (e.g. achondroplasia), thoracolumbar kyphosis (e.g. achondroplasia) or crouched posture (e.g. diastrophic dysplasia).

Inspect from the back

Examine for scoliosis (and any kyphosis, which should have been noted already). Have the child bend forwards and touch the toes to determine whether any scoliosis is structural. Scoliosis can occur in dozens of syndromes, including many skeletal dysplasias, several trisomies and a number of popular examination syndromes (fragile X, Marfan, NF1, Noonan).

Do explain what you are doing as you proceed, so that the examiners will be aware of the significance of the manoeuvres.

SKIN

The skin should be evaluated concurrently with inspecting from the front, back and side. Note any altered pigmentation: café-au-lait spots may occur with NF1 and Russell–Silver; hypopigmented areas can occur in tuberous sclerosis.

- Freckling occurs in xeroderma pigmentosum and Noonan Syndrome with Multiple Lentigines (NSML, previously called **LEOPARD** syndromes, the acronym standing for **L**entigines, **E**CG changes, **O**cular hypertelorism, **P**ulmonary stenosis, **A**bnormal genitalia, **R**etardation of growth, **D**eafness.) Small brown to blue–black macules occur in Peutz–Jeghers syndrome. Whorls of pigmentation occur in incontinentia pigmenti.
- Note any vascular malformations (e.g. Sturge-Weber, Klippel–Trénaunay–Weber), telangiectasia (e.g. ataxia-telangiectasia, Osler's haemorrhagic telangiectasia syndrome), or telangiectatic erythema in butterfly distribution over the malar area (e.g. Bloom, Cockayne). Ichthyotic skin can occur in CHILD syndrome (acronym for Congenital Hemidysplasia, Ichthyosiform erythroderma, Limb Defects). Alopecia or sparse hair may be noted in CHILD and Cockayne syndromes, as well as incontinentia pigmenti. The above are merely a small sample of the vast number of skin disorders within syndromal diagnoses.

COMPLETING THE EXAMINATION

Formal physical examination flows well if commenced at the hands, working up to the head and then downward—essentially a head-to-toe pattern. Table 9.3 lists a small number of sample findings sought at each point.

Finally, summarise your findings succinctly and give a brief differential diagnosis, placing the most likely diagnosis first.

Table 9.3

Dysmorphic child: measurements, manoeuvres and systematic examination

A. MEASUREMENTS

Height

If short, tall or disproportionate:

Lower segment (LS)

Calculate upper segment (US) by subtracting LS from height

Calculate US: LS ratio

Arm span

Head circumference

Request weight

Assess percentile charts

Calculate height velocity

Request birth parameters

Request parents' percentiles and ages at puberty

B. MANOEUVRES

- Hands and feet together, to detect asymmetry (e.g. Russell–Silver), hemihypertrophy (e.g. Beckwith-Wiedemann [B-W], McCune–Albright, Proteus) and unilateral growth arrest (e.g. homocystinuria with CVA)—this also detects approximation of shoulders (absent clavicles in cleidocranial dysostosis), genu valgum (e.g. homocystinuria), genu recurvatum (e.g. Marfan), and pes planus (e.g. Marfan)
- Arms by side with palms forwards, to detect cubitus valgus (e.g. Turner, Noonan; over 15 degrees in girls; over 10 degrees in boys)
- Thumbs on shoulders, to detect short limbs: can detect if proximal, middle or distal segment shortening
- Palms up, to detect simian crease (e.g. Down, Seckel), clinodactyly (e.g. Russell–Silver, Down, Seckel)
- Make a fist, to detect short fourth metacarpal (e.g. Turner, FAS)
- Check extensibility for hyperextensibility (e.g. Marfan) and for limitation of extension (e.g. homocystinuria)
- Look at the back to detect short neck (e.g. Noonan, Klippel–Feil), or neck webbing (e.g. Turner, Noonan)
- Low hairline (e.g. Noonan, Klippel–Feil)
- Bend over and touch toes, to detect scoliosis (e.g. Noonan, Klippel–Feil)

C. SYSTEMATIC EXAMINATION

Sitting up is the preferred position for the commencement of the systematic examination—the following is a selected listing of possible physical findings in children with dysmorphic features

General inspection

Diagnostic facies
- Dysmorphic syndromes (e.g. Russell–Silver, Down, Turner, Noonan, FAS)

Disproportionate stature
- Skeletal dysplasias (e.g. achondroplasia)
- Connective tissue disorders (e.g. osteogenesis imperfecta)

Tanner staging
- Advanced (e.g. McCune–Albright)
- Delayed (e.g. Noonan)

Nutritional status
- Obese (e.g. Prader–Willi, Bardet–Biedl)
- Poor (e.g. Marfan, homocystinuria)

Continued

Table 9.3 (continued)
Skeletal anomalies • Asymmetry (causes of hemihypertrophy: B-W, NF1) • Pectus excavatum (e.g. Marfan, Noonan) • Scoliosis (e.g. Noonan, Klippel–Feil)
Skin • Vascular malformations (e.g. Klippel-Trénaunay-Weber [KTW], Sturge-Weber) • Hypopigmented macules (e.g. tuberous sclerosis) • Café-au-lait spots (e.g. NF1, Fanconi anaemia, Russell–Silver)
Upper limbs
Structure • Clinodactyly fifth finger (e.g. Russell–Silver, Shwachman–Diamond) • Short fourth metacarpal (e.g. Turner, FAS) • Trident hand (e.g. achondroplasia) • Polydactyly (e.g. Bardet–Biedl) • Contractures (e.g. distal arthrogryposis)
Nails • Short (e.g. cartilage hair hypoplasia) • Hyperconvex (e.g. Turner) • Hypoplastic (e.g. FAS)
Palms • Simian creases (e.g. Down)
Wrists • Splaying (e.g. X-linked hypophosphataemic rickets) • Contractures (e.g. 'classic arthrogryposis')
Pulse • Radiofemoral delay (e.g. coarctation of aorta with Turner, NF1)
Elbows • Contractures (e.g. 'classic arthrogryposis')
Blood pressure: elevated (e.g. coarctation of aorta with NF1, Turner, renal artery stenosis with NF1, phaeochromocytoma with NF1)
Head
Size • Small (e.g. TORCH, numerous syndromes) • Large (e.g. Sotos, X-linked hydrocephalus)
Shape • Frontal bossing (e.g. achondroplasia)
Consistency: craniotabes (e.g. X-linked hypophosphataemic rickets)
Fontanelle • Large (e.g. Russell–Silver, X-linked hypophosphataemic rickets) • Bulging (e.g. X-linked hydrocephalus with raised ICP)
Hair • Sparse (e.g. hypohidrotic ectodermal dysplasia, progeria) • Greasy (e.g. precocious puberty with NF1)

Table 9.3 (continued)
Eyes
Inspection • Prominent (e.g. Crouzon) • Microphthalmos (e.g. CHARGE, fetal rubella effects) • Hypertelorism (e.g. Noonan, Williams) • Epicanthal folds (e.g. Noonan, Williams, Turner, Down) • Ptosis (e.g. Noonan) • Squint (e.g. Williams, Prader–Willi, septo-optic dysplasia [SOD]) • Nystagmus (e.g. SOD)
Conjunctivae: pallor (e.g. Fanconi pancytopenia)
Sclerae • Icterus (e.g. Alagille) • Blue (e.g. osteogenesis imperfecta)
Iris • Aniridia (e.g. Wilms' tumour, aniridia, genital anomalies, retardation syndrome [WAGR]) • Coloboma (e.g. WAGR, CHARGE) • Brushfield's spots (e.g. Down, Zellweger) • Pale blue (e.g. fragile X, Angelman) • Heterochromia (e.g. Waardenburg, KTW) • Stellate (e.g. Williams)
Cornea • Large and cloudy (buphthalmos): glaucoma (e.g. WAGR, fetal rubella effects, Marfan, NF1) • Keratoconus (e.g. Noonan)
Visual fields: field defect (e.g. brain tumour with NF1)
Eye movements • Nystagmus (e.g. SOD, WAGR, Chédiak-Higashi) • Lateral rectus palsy (e.g. Möbius sequence)
Cataracts (e.g. rubella, WAGR)
Lens dislocation: Marfan (goes up), homocystinuria (goes down)
Fundi • Papilloedema (e.g. hydrocephalus with raised ICP) • Optic nerve hypoplasia (e.g. SOD) • Chorioretinitis (e.g. TORCH)
Nose
Midface hypoplasia (e.g. FAS)
Anosmia (e.g. Kallmann)
Mouth and chin
Central cyanosis: various forms of congenital heart disease (CHD)
Midline defects • Cleft lip (repaired): cleft lip sequence • Cleft palate (repaired): cleft lip sequence

Continued

Table 9.3 (continued)
Teeth • Hypodontia (e.g. incontinentia pigmenti, Williams) • Irregularly placed (e.g. Down, Crouzon) • Late eruption (e.g. incontinentia pigmenti, progeria)
Tongue • Enlarged (e.g. B-W, Pompe's disease) • Ptosed (e.g. Pierre Robin sequence) • Prominent (e.g. Down: small pharynx, normal-sized tongue)
Facial hair or acne (e.g. precocity with NF1)
Micrognathia (e.g. Pierre Robin sequence)
Ears
Low set (e.g. Turner, Noonan, Treacher Collins)
Posteriorly rotated (e.g. Russell–Silver)
Malformed (e.g. CHARGE, Treacher Collins, B-W)
Hairline
Low (e.g. Turner, Noonan)
Neck
Pterygium colli (e.g. Klippel–Feil, Turner, Noonan)
Short (e.g. Klippel–Feil, Noonan, CHARGE)
Scoliosis (e.g. Klippel–Feil)
Chest
Inspection • Scars: repair of tracheo-oesophageal fistula (e.g. VACTERL, CHARGE), repair of diaphragmatic hernia (e.g. Marfan, DiGeorge [22q11]) • Tanner staging in girls, for precocity (e.g. McCune–Albright) or delay (Turner)
Nipples • Wide-spaced (e.g. Turner, several trisomies) • Hypoplastic (e.g. Poland anomaly)
Chest wall • Sternal deformity: pectus excavatum or carinatum (e.g. Marfan, Noonan) • Small thoracic cage (e.g. several skeletal dysplasias)
Palpation • Praecordium (e.g. for CHD)
Auscultation • Praecordium (e.g. for CHD)
Abdomen
Inspection • Scars: repair of duodenal atresia (e.g. Down), repair of Hirschsprung (e.g. Down, Waardenburg), removal of tumour (e.g. WAGR, adrenal tumour in B-W), repair of inguinal herniae (e.g. Marfan), repair of omphalocele (e.g. B-W) • Prune-like appearance (prune belly syndrome) • Tanner staging pubic hair, for precocity (e.g. McCune–Albright) or delay (Klinefelter, Noonan)

Table 9.3 (continued)

Palpation
- Hepatomegaly (e.g. Shwachman–Diamond, storage diseases)
- Splenomegaly (e.g. storage diseases)
- Hepatosplenomegaly (e.g. various storage diseases)
- Enlarged kidneys (e.g. polycystic kidneys, hydronephrosis)

Auscultation
- Hepatic bruit (e.g. haemangioma, hepatocellular carcinoma associated with B-W)
- Renal artery stenosis (e.g. NF1)

Posterior aspect
- Midline scar (e.g. spina bifida repair)

Genitalia

Tanner staging genitalia
- Measure penis length
- Measure testes parameters; estimate testes volume
- Advanced stage (e.g. NF1)
- Delayed stage (e.g. Noonan)

Penile anomalies
- Micropenis (e.g. Prader–Willi)
- Hypospadias (e.g. Noonan)

Testicular anomalies: cryptorchidism (e.g. Noonan)

Gait, back and lower limbs

Inspection of lower limbs
- Lower limb bowing (e.g. X-linked hypophosphataemic rickets)
- Proximal, middle or distal shortening (e.g. bony dysplasias)
- Oedema of dorsa of feet (e.g. Turner)
- Clubbing of toes (various types of CHD)

Palpation: ankle oedema (CCF with CHD)

Gait—standard examination screening for:
- Long-tract signs (e.g. X-linked hydrocephalus; brain tumour with NF1)
- Ataxia (e.g. ataxia-telangiectasia)
- Proximal weakness (e.g. myopathies, developmental dysplasia of hip)

Back
- Scoliosis (e.g. various skeletal dysplasias, NF1)
- Kyphosis (e.g. achondroplasia)
- Focal spinal shortening (e.g. various skeletal dysplasias)
- Midline scar (spina bifida)
- Spinal tenderness (X-linked hypophosphataemic rickets)

Lower limbs neurologically
- Long-tract signs (e.g. brain tumour with NF1)

B-W = Beckwith-Wiedemann; CCF = congestive cardiac failure; CHD = congenital heart disease; FAS = fetal alcohol syndrome; ICP = intracranial pressure; KTW = Klippel-Trénaunay-Weber; LS = lower segment; NF = neurofibromatosis; SOD = septo-optic dysplasia; TORCH = intrauterine infections with toxoplasmosis, other (e.g. syphilis, HIV), rubella, cytomegalovirus, herpes (both simplex and varicella); US = upper segment; VSD = ventricular septal defect; WAGR = Wilms' tumour, aniridia, genital anomalies, retardation syndrome.

SHORT CASE: Body asymmetry and hemihyperplasia

The term hemihyperplasia refers to asymmetric and (typically) unilateral overgrowth of the head, face, trunk, limbs and digits, and may involve viscera, hence can be part, or parts, of one half of the body, or one entire half of the body (including all tissues and organs of that half). The term 'simple hemihyperplasia' refers to unilateral enlargement of one limb. The term 'complex hemihyperplasia' refers to involvement of half of the body, including at least one upper limb and one lower limb, and where affected parts may be ipsilateral or contralateral; for example, a child can have hemihyperplasia affecting the head, upper limb and lower limb, on one side, but hemihyperplasia of the tongue.

There are many causes of hemihyperplasia but only a few causes of hemihypoplasia. Isolated hemihyperplasia (IH) [MIM%235000] is due to a mutation at chromosome 11p15, and is associated with an increased risk of embryonic tumours in childhood, especially Wilms tumour. IH used to be known as 'hemihypertrophy', but the name has changed to reflect the pathology of increased cell number rather than increased cell size.

Hemihyperplasia occurs in a number of 'overgrowth syndromes' which include Beckwith-Wiedemann syndrome (BWS) [MIM #130650], which shares IH's predisposition to embryonic tumours, and also in a number of other conditions which do not have that predisposition, such as neurofibromatosis type 1 (NF1) [MIM#162200], which predisposes to a different group of tumours, Proteus syndrome [MIM#976120] (which was, apparently, the diagnosis in John Merrick, the 'Elephant Man'), which predisposes to a less serious group of tumours (yolk sac tumour of testis, parotid adenoma, ovarian cystadenoma, papillary adenoma of epididymis), and Klippel–Trénaunay–Weber syndrome (KTW) [MIM%14900] which does not predispose to tumours at all.

In an examination format, children with Beckwith-Wiedemann syndrome (BWS) [MIM #130650] are not infrequently encountered, as is the case with children with Russell–Silver syndrome (RSS) [MIM #180860]; BWS can cause hemihyperplasia, RSS can cause hemihypoplasia. These conditions have exactly opposite epimutations at the same region (the imprinting control region) on distal chromosome 11p15.5; BWS is an overgrowth syndrome, which, in 10–15% of cases, has DNA *hyper*methylation at the same site where RSS has DNA *hypo*methylation. The only other common cause of hemihypoplasia is hemiplegic cerebral palsy.

The most important aspect of the child with hemihyperplasia is monitoring for the appearance of embryonic tumours, particularly Wilms tumour; less frequently hepatoblastoma, adrenal carcinoma, gonadoblastoma and neuroblastoma, which can occur in both IH and BWS. Children with hemihyperplasia are routinely scanned by ultrasound for intra-abdominal tumours, every 3 months until 8 years of age, which is the schedule for BWS.

The causes of hemihyperplasia can be conveniently divided into three groups based on presence or absence of skin markers, for ease of recall, but also for prognostic significance with respect to tumour development; one group has vascular malformations, one group has café-au-lait spots (although Proteus syndrome overlaps both groups) and the other group has neither. It is the latter group who have increased risk of embryonic tumour development, not those with vascular anomalies nor those with café-au-lait macules.

Vascular birthmark related group (no increased risk of embryonic tumours):

1. **Klippel–Trénaunay–Weber** syndrome (**KTW**) [MIM %149000] includes a triad of vascular malformations, abnormal lymphatics and hemihyperplasia; venous malformations in KTW are slow flowing. Children with KTW tend to have localised hypertrophy rather than generalised hemihypertrophy.

2. **Parkes Weber syndrome** (**PKWS**) [MIM #608355] includes micro-AVFs (arteriovenous fistulas) associated with skeletal and soft tissue overgrowth; the AVFs in PKWS are fast flowing, and involved limbs are pinker and warmer than in KTW.

3. **Sturge-Weber syndrome** (**SWS**) [MIM 185300] is a phakomatosis, characteristically comprising facial capillary malformations (termed 'port wine stains' [PWSs] or 'port wine birthmarks' [PWBs]) in trigeminal nerve distribution, with ipsilateral leptomeningeal [pial] angiomas involving occipital and parietal lobes leading to calcification, cortical necrosis; this can result in hemiparesis, epilepsy, developmental delay and glaucoma (see SWS long/short cases on this).

4. **PIK3CA-related segmental overgrowth** includes: (a) **CLOVES** (congenital lipomatous asymmetric overgrowth [trunk], lymphatic, capillary, venous and combined type vascular malformations, epidermal naevi, skeletal/spinal anomalies) [MIM #612918], which is due to a mutation in the gene PIK3CA which is sited at 3q26.32; and (b) **M-CM** (macrocephaly-capillary malformation) [MIM #602501].

5. **Proteus syndrome** [MIM #176920] is named after the 'polymorphous' Greek God who could adopt any shape; it is due to a mutation in the AKT1 gene, on chromosome 14q32.3, and leads to asymmetrical and disproportionate excessive growth of any tissue or body part.

Cafe au lait macules (no increased risk of embryonic tumours, except neuroblastoma in NF1) occur in:

1. **Neurofibromatosis type 1** (**NF1**) [MIM #162200], National Institutes of Health (NIH) criteria: two or more of: (a) six or more café-au-lait macules > 5 mm greatest diameter in prepubertal children and > 15 mm diameter in postpubertal people; (b) two or more neurofibromas of any type, or one plexiform neuroma; (c) freckling in the axillary or inguinal region; (d) optic glioma; (e) two or more Lisch nodules (iris hamartomas); (f) distinctive osseous lesions such as sphenoid dysplasia or tibial pseudoarthrosis; and (g) a first-degree relative with the NF1. These criteria apply to children 4 years and over (see long/short cases on NF1 in Chapter 13, Neurology).

2. **Proteus syndrome** [MIM #176920]. See paragraph above, mnemonic overleaf.

3. **Russell–Silver syndrome** (**RSS**) [MIM #180860]; cause of hemi*hypoplasia*, includes significant intrauterine growth retardation, triangular-shaped, small face, blue sclera (in infancy), micrognathia, broad forehead, frontal bossing, but normal head circumference (although 'pseudohydrocephalic' appearance), asymmetry of upper limbs and lower limbs, fifth finger clinodactyly, developmental delay and hypospadias. Children with RSS have increased risk of tumours: Wilms, craniopharyngioma, hepatocellular carcinoma and testicular seminoma.

Other causes have neither of these skin findings. These include:

1. **Beckwith-Wiedemann syndrome** (**BWS**) [MIM #130650].

2. **Isolated Hemihyperplasia** (**IH**) [MIM #235000].
   Both BWS and IH have the same cytogenetic location at 11p15, and increased risk of embryonal tumours, especially Wilms tumour, BWS having a four-fold higher risk than IH; the epigenotypes in children with IH and Wilms tumour are not the same as the epigenotypes in those children with BWS and Wilms tumour.

3. **Hemifacial hyperplasia** [MIM 133900] is an entity that does not involve trunk or limbs, but just the head, with asymmetric, unilateral overgrowth of bones of the facial skeleton (from frontal bone down to inferior border of mandible, and from the pinna of the ear across to the midline, with enlargement of all the tissues in this anatomical region).

Mnemonics for IH, BWS, RSS and Proteus syndrome are below; for SWS and NF1, see the SWS and NF1 short cases and long cases in Chapter 13, Neurology.

ISOLATED HEMIHYPERPLASIA: **HEMIS**

Hemihyperplasia of spine, limbs, hands, feet
Embryonal tumours
Muscle hypertrophy in affected areas, **M**yelomeningocele
Intellectual impairment: seen in 20%
Spine involvement: **S**coliosis, myelomeningocele

BECKWITH-WIEDEMANN SYNDROME (BWS): **BECKWITH EMG**
(Exomphalos-Macroglossia-Gigantism syndrome)

Blastomas (gonado-, hepato- and nephro-blastoma) (Wilms)/**B**lood count high in
  neonates (polycythaemia)/**B**one age advanced first 4 years
Eyes: prominent/**E**ar lobe: linear fissures, creases
Craniofacial anomalies/**C**apillary vascular malformation central forehead/**C**ardiac
  disorders: **C**ardiomegaly (isolated), **C**ardiomyopathy (focal), **C**ardiac hamartoma
Kidneys enlarged
Wilms tumour
Indentation posterior rim helix/**I**slet cells excess, **I**nsulin high (pancreatic hyperplasia)
Tumours: adrenal carcinoma, embryonal cancers, gonadoblastoma, hepatoblastoma,
Hepatomegaly/**H**ypoglycaemia (early infancy)

Exomphalos (also called omphalocele)
Macroglossia/**M**acrosomia/**M**uscle mass increased/**M**etaphyseal flaring/**M**alocclusion
  (**M**andibular: **M**axilla relative position: prognathism due to mandibular
  overgrowth, maxilla less prominent)/**M**etopic ridge/**M**icrocephaly (mild)
Gigantism/**G**enito-urinary: large ovaries, hyperplastic uterus, bicornate uterus,
  clitoromegaly, hypospadias, undescended testes

RUSSELL–SILVER SYNDROME: **RUSSELL**

Retrognathia/micrognathia/**R**enal: Wilms tumour, renal anomalies/**R**efractive errors
Uniparental (maternal) disomy of chromosome 7 in 10%/**U**rethral valves
  (posterior)
Small stature (prenatal onset)/**S**mall face/**S**mall fifth finger with clinodactyly
Skin: cafe au lait/**S**clera blue/**S**houlders: **S**prengel's deformity/**S**eminoma/**S**yndactyly
  second and third toes/**S**low development (delay)/**S**weating: excessive
Eleven, chromosome number (11p15.5)/**E**pigenetic alterations: DNA
  hypomethylation at H19/IGF2-imprinting control region/**E**sophageal reflux,
  Esophagitis/**E**ndocrine: fasting hypoglycaemia aged 10 months to 3 years
Linear growth decreased, growth hormone deficiency/
Liver: hepatocellular carcinoma/
Large fontanelle/**L**imb asymmetry

PROTEUS SYNDROME: **PROTEUS HEAD VARIABLE**

Ptosis, **P**alpebral fissure downslant, **P**ectus excavatum, **P**alate (cleft, submucous)

Renal: enlargement, hydronephrosis, cysts, haemangiomata

Ophthalmological: macrophthalmia; microphthalmia; nystagmus; strabismus; cataract/**O**pen mouth

Tumours: ovarian adenoma, parotid adenoma, yolk sac tumour of testis/**T**hyroid enlargement/**T**hymus enlargement

Elongation head and trunk

Uneven growth pattern: normal at birth, features appear over first year; progress throughout childhood; hamartomata growth completed by puberty; normal adolescent somatic growth, final height normal

Skin: thickened; café-au-lait macules/**S**ubcutaneous tumours (epidermal naevi, lipomas)

Hyperpigmentation (skin)/**H**eart: Hypertrophic cardiomyopathy (HOCM); conduction defects/**H**ead: enlarged; craniosynostosis/**H**yperostoses: skull, facial bones, jaw, external auditory canal, nasal bridge, alveolar ridges

Enlarged genitals (testes and penis)

Absent fat (regional)

Dolichocephaly/**D**epigmentation of skin/**D**ermoids (epibulbar)/**D**eep venous thrombosis (DVT)/**D**islocated hips/**D**igits: enlarged, clinodactyly

Vascular malformations: capillary, lymphatic, venous (esp. thorax, upper abdomen)/**V**ertebral dysplasia and enlargement (mega-spondylo-dysplasia)/**V**algus deformities of feet

Atrophy: muscles

Renal enlargement

Intellectual impairment in 20%

Angulation defects: knees

Back: scoliosis, kyphosis, spinal stenosis

Lipoma/**L**ipomatosis (abdominal and pelvic)/**L**ong face/**L**ung cysts

Epidermal naevi

Examination procedure

In this short case, first confirm the presence of the body asymmetry, perform measurements and manoeuvres, and then look for underlying causes, and associated findings of those conditions, including checking the blood pressure for hypertension. There may be hemihyperplasia affecting the entire body, or there may be hemihypoplasia. The former has several causes, but the key aspect is checking for associated tumours, which happen in BWS and in IH. The latter only has two causes likely relevant for examination purposes: RSS and hemiplegic cerebral palsy. Hence, establishing the growth percentiles early should sort out whether this is likely to be RSS with hemihypoplasia, as children with RSS are short, or BWS with hemihyperplasia, as children with BWS typically are tall.

In many of the causes of hemihyperplasia, there are skin findings that narrow the differential quickly. And in the case of hemihypoplasia due to hemiplegic cerebral palsy, there will be posturing and quality of movement that differentiates these children from other children with body asymmetry.

Start by introducing yourself to the parent and the child. Note the child's level of consciousness, quality of movement and any obvious asymmetry of movement (as in hemiplegic cerebral palsy). Ensure that the child is adequately undressed so as not to miss any vascular birthmarks, café-au-lait macules or subcutaneous tumours. Stand back and look for any skin findings such as vascular birthmarks over the face (SWS), over the trunk or limbs (KTW or PKWS), or café-au-lait macules (NF1, Proteus). Note the growth parameters, ask for height and weight plotted on percentile charts, and mention you will measure the head circumference yourself later. Tanner staging can be appropriate if any suggestion of precocity (precocious puberty can occur in patients with adrenocortical tumours [IH, BWS] and in NF1).

The next step can be performing the manoeuvres. First get the child (if the child is cooperative) to stand with hands and feet together to demonstrate asymmetry and to see whether it is at the upper limbs and lower limbs, or just affecting upper limbs or just affecting lower limbs. Then the child can stand with the palms exposed, which allows a different perspective on any difference in hand or finger sizes.

Next, turn your attention to the child's back, get the child to bend over and touch their toes, to look for scoliosis (can occur in IH, NF1, Proteus [hemihyperplasia], or hemiplegic cerebral palsy [hemihypoplasia]). At this point, so you do not forget, it may be worth asking for the blood pressure; this can be elevated with Wilms tumour or with adrenocortical tumours, both of which can occur in IH and BWS, or in several conditions in patients with NF1 (neuroblastoma, coarctation of the aorta, renal artery stenosis, phaeochromocytoma and essential hypertension).

A gait examination can be next (if the child is old enough to cooperate; if not, a gross motor developmental assessment can be substituted), focusing on aspects that could help diagnose hemihyperplasia affecting lower limb length, as the child will have trouble clearing the ground if walking normally, and like the child with hemiplegic CP, there may be circumduction, again, to clear the ground walking with a lengthened limb.

Next the child can lie on an examining couch, so the lower limbs can then be formally measured, both for length and for circumference. Lower limb length (called 'leg length', although 'leg' is from [usually] knee to foot) is the distance from the anterior superior iliac spine (ASIS) to the medial malleolus of the ankle, with the tape measure passing across the knee on the medial side. Measure the circumference of each thigh, measured at the same distance (depends on size of child; say 15 cm for adolescent) on each limb from a major landmark (say patella).

Once this is done, measure the upper limbs for length and circumference. Upper limb length (called 'arm length', although 'arm' is [usually] from shoulder to elbow) is the distance from the acromion to the distal ulnar prominence, with the tape measure passing over the olecranon process. Next measure the mid-upper arm circumference of each arm, at approximately the midpoint between the olecranon process and the acromion, again measuring at the same distance (depends on size of child; say 15 cm for an adolescent) on each limb from a major landmark (say olecranon process).

If there is any suggestion of a neurological problem, or scoliosis, noted during the gait examination, then the lower limbs and upper limbs should be examined neurologically. Otherwise, move on to evaluate the child's head. Look for asymmetry of the head (hemifacial hyperplasia, KTW) and measure the head circumference (may be increased with NF1, may be decreased with BWS; KTW can cause either macrocephaly or microcephaly).

Look at the eyes next, as several of the causes have eye involvement; look for any dysmorphic features, note if they are prominent (due to relative infraorbital hypoplasia in BWS, or enlargement in Proteus, or proptosis in NF1), any nystagmus (Proteus) and check with the ophthalmoscope for cataracts (KTW, Proteus) or any suggestion of glaucoma (SWS, KTW).

Look at the ears for signs of asymmetry, and specifically for BWS (linear creases over lobes, indentations of posterior rim helix). Next look in the mouth for palate inequality (IH), macroglossia (BWS), hemihyperplasia of tongue (which can be ipsilateral, or contralateral to hemihyperplasia of the limbs).

Next turn your attention to the upper limbs. If not already done, measure each upper limb to demonstrate and quantify asymmetry. Look for any skin conditions (CAL macules [NF1, Proteus, RSS], axillary freckling [NF1], vascular malformations [KTW, PKWS]).

Check the hands for any abnormalities of finger number or structure (polydactyly, oligodactyly and syndactyly can all occur in KTW; clinodactyly and simian creases occur in RSS). Check the blood pressure if not already requested or done. Hypertension can occur from several pathologies in neurofibromatosis (coarctation, renal artery stenosis, phaeochromocytoma, neuroblastoma), or in adrenal cortical tumours which can occur in IH or BWS patients.

The cardiorespiratory system can be assessed for evidence of chest asymmetry, pectus excavatum (NH-1, Proteus) and cardiac findings of BWS (cardiomegaly, cardiomyopathy), or Proteus (HOCM, arrhythmias), or NF1 (pulmonary stenosis, coarctation of aorta).

The abdomen should be inspected for any fullness reflecting underlying masses, and for any umbilical scars of exomphalos repair (BWS), and then palpated for any evidence of embryonal tumours of the liver, kidneys (Wilms) or adrenal glands (each can occur in IH, BWS; Wilms tumour and hepatocellular carcinoma can each occur in RSS also). The genitalia can be inspected next for any hemihypertrophy involving them or for hypospadias or undescended testes (BWS). The pubertal status should be commented upon, if any precocity (precocious puberty with NF1, adrenocortical tumour with IH, BWS). The testes should be palpated for undescended testes and for gonadoblastoma (IH, BWS).

This completes the examination. Relevant imaging and appropriate genetic testing for your differential list can be mentioned.

Chapter 10

Haematology

LONG CASES

LONG CASE: Haemophilia

The last few years have seen several major advances in the management of haemophilia (both haemophilia A and haemophilia B), including the development of extended half-life (EHL) products (for both recombinant factor VIII [rFVIII] and recombinant factor IX [rFIX]), introduced into widespread clinical practice in 2015, which can lead to less frequent infusions, longer lasting protection from bleeds, less problems with inhibitors (EHL products having less immunogenicity), and better quality of life. Genotyping has become very important in assessing the severity, and pattern, of bleeding, prediction of inhibitor development, and assisting individualisation of therapy (e.g. low inhibitor risk patients getting standard/classical therapy, versus high inhibitor risk patients getting 'early prophylaxis'; see below).

The World Health Organization (WHO), the World Federation of Hemophilia (WFH) and various national haemophilia foundations (in Australia, the US, Canada and many European countries) uniformly recommend that prophylaxis with an intravenous factor replacement for at least 46 weeks per year through *adulthood* is the standard of care. In children, the first prospective randomised controlled trial in the US assessing the progression of arthropathy in children (under 30 months) treated (until 6 years old) with prophylaxis (rFVIII 25 IU/kg every other day) versus on-demand treatment (rFVIII 40 IU/kg initially, then 20 IU/kg at 24 and 72 hours post-joint bleed) showed an 83% reduction in risk for joint damage on MRI.

The establishment of an international network of specialised Haemophilia Treatment Centres (HTCs) in developed countries has decreased the morbidity and mortality of haemophilia. There still is no international consensus regarding the optimal age to commence prophylaxis. It is recognised that the most cost-effective strategy is to start therapy early to protect joints. It is clear that children with no or few joint bleeds who start prophylaxis early (mean age 3 years) have a better musculoskeletal outcome. Prophylaxis decreases joint bleeds, decreases joint damage on MRI scanning and is the current standard of care for haemophilia. In developing countries, the high cost has precluded primary prophylaxis being adopted. Those with severe haemophilia may die before adulthood, but in developed countries the life expectancy for a child with severe haemophilia is now normal, whereas patients who are already adults have a life expectancy approximately 10 years less than males without haemophilia.

Discussion issues in the long-case setting may include the potential appropriate use of the newer EHL rFVIII preparations (e.g. rFVIII FC fusion protein [rFVIIIFc], or PEGylated full-length rFVIII [PEG-rFVIII]), or FIX preparations (e.g. rFIX FC fusion protein [rFIXFc]) as prophylactic replacement (the rationale, benefits, barriers, the terminology of various subgroups of prophylaxis, including primary [determined by age or first bleed], secondary, short-term, full dose, partial), the timing of placing of central venous access devices (CVADs) and the optimal management of joint disease.

Recombinant clotting factor concentrate is available to all patients with haemophilia. This has effectively eliminated the risk of transfusion-related viruses.

Background information
DEFINITIONS

Haemophilia A is factor VIII (FVIII) deficiency, and accounts for 80–85% of haemophilia. Haemophilia B is factor IX (FIX) deficiency, which accounts for 15–20% of haemophilia. Clinically, it is not possible to distinguish between them. Both are X-linked recessive conditions.

FVIII and FIX are both inactive precursors which become activated with vascular injury. FVIII is a protein cofactor, whereas FIX is a serine protease zymogen, which only functions with FVIII present as a cofactor. When they are activated, FVIIIa and FIXa combine as the tenase complex; this in turn activates factor X (FX). In both forms of haemophilia, patients are lacking the ability to activate FX normally, which decreases the ability to produce thrombin and fibrin.

The FVIII (F8, OMIM*300841) gene is at the telomeric end of the long arm of the X chromosome, at band Xq28. It is a large gene, 186 kilobases (kb) long, and it has 26 exons. Over 2000 mutations (missense, nonsense, splicing, and small or large deletions and insertions) have been described in the F8 gene. Mutations occur throughout the gene, with some concentration around exon 14.

The most prevalent gene defect seen in severe haemophilia A is an intron 22 inversion (int22), which accounts for 40–45% of all mutations. An inversion affecting exon 1 is present in around 5% of patients with severe haemophilia A. Over 200 smaller deletions have been described, which generally involve reading frame shifts, and non-functional gene products. Large deletions comprise 15% of haemophilia A; these result in truncated transcripts that are non-functional. Children with larger deletions and nonsense mutations are at higher risk of developing FVIII inhibitory antibodies, and are less likely to respond to immune tolerance therapy. Most of FVIII is synthesised in the liver endothelial cells and is immediately linked to von Willebrand's factor (vWF) on entering the circulation; this prevents enzymatic degradation of factor FVIII until it is required for coagulation.

The FIX (F9, OMIM*300746) gene is on the X chromosome at band Xq27. The gene is 33 kb long. FIX is synthesised in the liver and released into the circulation in inactive form.

Over 1000 mutations have been described in the F9 gene. Molecular defects described include: large gene deletions, frameshift mutations and nonsense mutations (all of these types of defects cause severe disease); and also missense mutations (which can cause mild, moderate or severe disease, depending on their site and the particular substitutions made). In contrast to haemophilia A, severe haemophilia B is frequently due to missense mutations.

Over 60% of cases have a positive family history; over 30% are spontaneous mutations. Diagnosis is based on prolonged activated partial thromboplastin time (aPTT), FVIII or FIX assay, and DNA analysis; the latter allowing prenatal and carrier diagnosis.

DISEASE MANIFESTATIONS

The severity and the frequency of bleeding complications are a reflection of the residual activity of FVIII or FIX:

- *Severe haemophilia* corresponds to < 1% FVIII or FIX clotting activity: this accounts for approximately 70% of type A and 50% of type B cases. These children are predisposed to having spontaneous bleeding into joints, muscles and deep organs, including central nervous system bleeds. Without preventative treatment, these children have two to five spontaneous bleeding episodes each month. The usual age of diagnosis is within the first year of life.
- *Moderately severe haemophilia* means 1–5% of FVIII or FIX clotting activity: these children rarely have spontaneous haemorrhages, but may have significant haemorrhage with mild or moderate trauma. The usual age at diagnosis is before 5 years.
- *Mild disease*, infers > 5%–40% of FVIII or FIX clotting activity: these children may have bleeding with trauma or surgery. Some carrier females, who have low levels of these factors, may present clinically with gynaecological or obstetric haemorrhage.
- Around 10% of carriers have FVIII or FIX clotting activity lower than 35%.
- Individuals with more than 30% FVIII or FIX clotting activity usually do not spontaneously bleed and may not need supplemental clotting factor in the setting of minor surgery.

AGE-RELATED PRESENTATION

Birth to 4 weeks

1. Bleeding following circumcision (infants of known carriers should not be circumcised until testing for FVIII/FIX rules out haemophilia).
2. Bleeding from heel puncture or other blood-taking.
3. Central nervous system haemorrhage.
4. Cephalhaematoma.

4–6 months

1. Large haematomas following immunisation (intramuscular injections).
2. Palpable subcutaneous ecchymoses.

6–24 months

1. Gingival haemorrhages when teething.
2. Bleeding from oral mucosa (e.g. from small lacerations of the frenulum or tongue).
3. Increased bruising once becoming ambulatory.

3–4 years

Joint and muscle haemorrhage become problematic.

COMPLICATIONS

Haemarthrosis

1. Repeated haemarthroses can result in destructive arthritis, joint instability and ankylosis. Released from red cells, haemoglobin deposited in the joint space activates an inflammatory response. With each bleed, an inflammatory synovitis, thickening the synovium; eventually this process can destroy cartilage and bone. With prophylaxis now the standard, severe arthritis has become very uncommon in children.
2. The commonest joints affected are the knees, followed by the elbows, ankles and shoulders. The most important joints, in terms of maintaining mobility with age, are the ankles.

Neurological problems
Intracranial haemorrhage
1. One of the more common causes of death.
2. Survivors may have severe neurological deficits: see the later discussion.

Haemorrhage into vertebral canal
1. Rare; 75% are extramedullary and 25% intramedullary.
2. Presents with severe neck or back pain, followed by ascending paralysis.

Peripheral nerve compression
1. External compression or traction from intramuscular bleeds.
2. Nerves affected and relevant muscles often affected: femoral (iliopsoas), ulnar and median (forearm flexors), sciatic (glutei).

Life-threatening haemorrhages
Retropharyngeal
1. Usually associated with pharyngitis.
2. Presents with dysphagia and drooling.
3. Can be diagnosed by lateral neck X-ray.

Retroperitoneal
1. Can have the loss of a large volume of concealed blood.
2. May be spontaneous or from trauma.
3. Diagnosed by ultrasound or CT scan.

Intracranial
As above (neurological).

History
Ask about the following.

PRESENTING COMPLAINT
Reason for current admission.

PAST HISTORY
1. Initial presenting symptoms, diagnosis (when, where, how), subsequent management, progress of disease, hospitalisation details.
2. Complications of the disease (e.g. neurological deficits, joint disease) or its treatment (e.g. inhibitor formation; impact inhibitors have on patient, including on quality of life and number of bleeds).
3. Previous elective surgery or dental procedures (their management and outcome).
4. Outpatient clinics attended (where, how often).
5. Past treatments used (e.g. FVIII, FIX, desmopressin [DDAVP], prothrombin complex concentrate). The majority of young children should have only received recombinant clotting factor concentrate.
6. Age when parents started administering FVIII, FIX.
7. Age of self-administration.
8. Age of venous access port placement.
9. Recent change in symptoms or management.
10. Approach to the management of painful procedures.

CURRENT STATUS

1. Average number of bleeds per year, common sites involved (e.g. knee, elbow), 'target joint' (most patients with significant joint disease will typically develop one joint that is more affected by recurrent bleeds), any common precipitants (e.g. sport), treatment required (type of concentrate), usual outcome, where usually managed (home or hospital), who gives infusions (patient or parent), prophylaxis regimen, details of venous access port use.
2. Ongoing symptoms of joint disease (e.g. pain, stiffness), neurological disease (e.g. weakness from peripheral nerve compression, hemiplegia from intracranial bleed).
3. Management of bleeds away from home (school, on holidays, overseas).

SOCIAL HISTORY

1. Disease impact on patient (e.g. avoidance of participation in sports such as rugby and football), self-image, schooling (attendance, performance, teacher awareness of, and attitudes towards, the disease and its treatment, peer interactions). Most patients with haemophilia are encouraged to participate in sports; there is some evidence that participation in sports reduces the incidences of bleeding episodes in boys on prophylaxis.
2. Disease impact on parents (e.g. marriage stability, fears for future, financial considerations [medical treatment, awareness of benefits available], modification of holiday plans).
3. Disease impact on siblings (e.g. sibling rivalry, hostility, genetic implications for girls).
4. Social supports (e.g. social worker, extended family). Parents of paediatric patients with haemophilia are eligible for the government funded carer's payment.
5. Coping; for example, who attends with the patient, confidence with management, degree of understanding of the disease, expectations for the future, understanding of the prognosis.
6. Access to hospital, local doctor, paediatrician, haematologist, orthopaedic surgeon, rheumatologist.

FAMILY HISTORY AND GENETIC ASPECTS

Other boys with haemophilia, more children planned, prenatal diagnosis (and subsequent management for positive result), carrier detection in girls (normal factor VIII/factor IX level does not exclude a female being a carrier of haemophilia).

IMMUNISATION

Routine, associated bleeding, hepatitis B.

Examination

The salient findings to be sought in the haemophilia long case are as follows.

GENERAL INSPECTION

1. Position patient standing, undressed to underpants.
2. Parameters: weight, height, head circumference (subdural bleed).
3. Visually scan skin for bruises (number, size, age), joints for swelling and posture for evidence of neurological sequelae (e.g. hemiparesis [intracranial bleed] or foot drop [lateral popliteal palsy]).
4. Unwell (e.g. severe bleed) or well.
5. Pallor (anaemia from large bleed, e.g. retroperitoneal).

6. Jaundice (hepatitis).
7. Vital signs: respiratory rate (e.g. pulse [anaemia], blood pressure [hypotension from bleeding], urinalysis [blood]).
8. Distress due to painful bleed.

DIRECTED EXAMINATION FOR DISEASE EXTENT AND COMPLICATIONS

1. Full skin examination, for distribution of bruises, including mucous membranes (mouth, tongue).
2. Full joint examination for evidence of arthropathy, focusing on the range of movement of affected joints, associated muscle wasting, any supportive devices (wheelchairs, splints, orthotic devices), gait.
3. Full neurological examination for any evidence of intracerebral or intravertebral haemorrhage, or peripheral nerve lesions. Best commenced with gait examination, followed by examination of the motor system.
4. Abdominal examination for liver and spleen size (liver disease), or tenderness (gastrointestinal or retroperitoneal bleed).

Available treatment modalities

FACTOR CONCENTRATES: STANDARD HALF-LIFE (SHL)

Recombinant DNA-engineered FVIII and FIX are the treatments of choice. (Previously, concentrates were made by refining cryoprecipitates and removing some of the fibrinogen. Their multi-donor source meant that concentrates carried the greatest risk of transmission of various infections [e.g. HIV, hepatitis C virus].) The Australian Government supplies recombinant factor VIII (rFVIII) and factor IX (rFIX) for all patients with haemophilia:

- Available rFVIII preparations are: Advate (octocog alfa; recombinant antihaemophilic FVIII [rAHF]; Baxter); Recombinate (octocog alfa; rAHF; Baxter); Kogenate FS (octocog alfa; Bayer).
- Available rFIX preparations are: BeneFIX [nonacog alfa; Pfizer]; Rixubis [nonacog gamma; Baxalta].

FACTOR CONCENTRATES: EXTENDED HALF-LIFE (EHL)

There are a number of new extended half-life factor concentrates; the Food and Drug Administration (FDA) in the US approved three products which became available in 2015: two new FVIII preparations and one FIX product. There are three approaches to manipulating the clotting factor molecules, each of which involves adding a protein to the relevant factor to prolong its half-life, with the FIX preparations increasing it three- to five-fold, whereas the FVIII preparations are increased around 1.5-fold. As well as prolonging half-life, so far these preparations have not induced any clinically important inhibitors.

EHL FVIII preparations

1. Fc-IgG fusion protein: recombinant factor VIII-FC fusion protein (rFVIIIFc) (FDA approved).
2. PEGylated/glycoPEGylated proteins: N8-GP; BAY 94-9027; PEG-rFVIII (the latter FDA approved). 'PEGylated' means having added strands of poly ethylene glycol.

EHL FIX preparations

1. Fc-IgG fusion protein: recombinant factor IX-FC fusion protein (rFIXFc) (FDA approved).
2. PEGylated/glycoPEGylated proteins: N9-GP (Nonacog beta pegol, a glycoPEGylated recombinant factor IX; also called PEG-rFIX).

3. Recombinant albumin-fusion protein: rFIX-FP (recombinant albumin has a long physiological half-life).

EHLs have the potential for patients having: a longer duration with blood levels of > 1% factor, less frequent infusions, less ports, less visits to hospital, less immunogenicity leading to less inhibitors, less joint disease and a better quality of life. All the EHLs activate and increase regulatory T-cell epitopes, induce tolerance in vivo, and are not immunogenic themselves.

PHARMACOKINETIC (PK) PROFILES: PERSONALISED THERAPY

The newer EHL preparations were extensively evaluated regarding their pharmacokinetic (PK) characteristics compared with the PK responses of the previously/currently available SHL preparations, to confirm bioequivalence, before they were able to be licensed.

PK profiles are affected by age, genotype, von Willebrand's factor (vWF) activity levels, clearance mechanisms and thrombophilia factors. PK responses are very useful in designing individual prophylaxis (PK-guided prophylaxis). The dose of factor required to keep FVIII/FIX greater than or equal to 1% varies from patient to patient. Optimal prophylaxis can be modelled based on the patient's individual PK and their bleeding pattern.

Regarding the FVIII trough level, and level of protection against bleeds, one small study of 34 patients showed that: if the trough is kept above 1%, then 44% patients were bleed-free; if the trough is kept above 5% then 76% patients were bleed-free; if the trough is kept above 15%, then 94% patients are bleed-free; and if the trough was above 30%, then 100% of the 34 patients were bleed-free. The WFH recommends the trough should be above 15%. The question is: what is more important, dose interval or trough?

In a graph of per cent factor level (on the y-axis) versus time (on the x-axis), the peak range (from the plasma factor peak level following infusion down to trough level) can prevent activity-related bleeds, the extent of the area under the curve determines prevention of subclinical bleeding, and the trough level determines prevention of spontaneous bleeds.

There is an option of selecting longer intervals between infusions with maintaining trough levels comparable to standard acting factor products, or leaving intervals as they are, currently and increasing the trough levels above 15%, to 20% or even 30%. The current approach used widely is to keep the trough level above 1%, which effectively protects about 75% of patients. However, if cost was no object, aiming for 15–30% factor levels would effectively protect 99–100% of patients. Unfortunately, these products are very expensive.

PK responses to the factor concentrates are quite individualised. An optimal pre-determined plasma clotting factor level can be reached by checking PK responses to dosage given. Checking PK responses involves a large number of blood tests, which cannot be taken from a venous access port, but must be taken from a peripheral vein. This is very traumatic for younger children, so management that involves comprehensive PK information is not favoured in infants or preschool children.

ANTIFIBRINOLYTICS

Epsilon-aminocaproic acid (EACA) and tranexamic acid are useful ancillary agents. These inhibit clot lysis by the fibrinolytic system. They are commenced in conjunction with factor replacement therapy or DDAVP (see overleaf), and continued for up to 14 days. They are particularly important in the management of oral haemorrhage, as saliva contains fibrinolytic enzymes. They are useful for tooth extractions and for uterine, gastrointestinal and intraocular bleeding, but are not recommended in haemarthrosis or haematuria, as in both their use may be associated with excessive fibrin deposition, possibly causing joint or renal tract damage/obstruction respectively. Antifibrinolytics are not given with prothrombin concentrates due to the risk of potentiating thrombosis.

DESMOPRESSIN (1-DEAMINO 8-D ARGININE VASOPRESSIN: DDAVP)

This is a synthetic analogue of vasopressin that raises the FVIII level by up to five times in normal subjects and seven times in some mild haemophiliacs, but has no effect in patients with severe disease. The mechanism is not fully understood.

It can be given intravenously (0.3 µg/kg in 50 mL saline over 20 minutes, peaks at 30–60 minutes) or by intranasal spray (150–300 µg, peaks at 60–90 minutes). Tachyphylaxis may occur after several doses. Complications include facial flushing, hyponatraemia (especially in infants; contraindicated in children under 2 years) and thrombosis (rare). Fluid restriction and urine output monitoring are important considerations. It is best for use in controlled situations such as elective minor surgery.

CORTICOSTEROIDS

Prednisolone has been used for haematuria, sometimes in conjunction with factor replacement. Brief courses (1–4 weeks) of steroids have been used for joint bleeds.

FRESH FROZEN PLASMA (FFP)

This contains all the clotting factors. Its use is limited by volume; 20 mL/kg can be given over 6 hours, followed by 10 mL/kg every 6 hours for maintenance. Harvested from one donor, FFP can be used for coagulopathy secondary to liver failure.

Management
TREATMENT OF ACUTE HAEMORRHAGE
1. Control of specific bleeding problems
Clotting factors

The dose of FVIII or FIX required to achieve haemostasis varies with the severity of the bleed. One unit of FVIII or FIX is the amount that is present in 1 mL of 'pooled' normal plasma. One unit per kilogram of recombinant FVIII increases the activity of FVIII by approximately 2%. The standard factor VIII half-life averages 8–12 hours. Standard FIX has a longer half-life of 12–18 hours, and one unit per kilogram of recombinant FIX increases plasma levels by approximately 0.8%. The target replacement has aimed traditionally for 50% correction for the plasma levels for most haemorrhages, but 100% correction for major haemorrhages (intracranial, head and neck, intraabdominal).

FVIII replacement guide

1. Minimal bleeds: first aid, antifibrinolytics if indicated. The need for factor VIII replacement should be assessed recognising the occasional difficulties with intravenous cannulation, particularly in young children.
2. Moderate bleed (e.g. joint, muscle, small oral mucosal or tongue laceration or bleed, epistaxis, gastrointestinal or genitourinary): 20–40 units/kg, given 12–24-hourly, usually for 3 days. Frequent repeated doses may be required if bleeding does not settle.
3. Severe bleed (life-threatening haemorrhage [e.g. major trauma], retropharyngeal, retroperitoneal, intracranial, large oral mucosal bleeds): 50–75 units/kg initially, followed by repeat doses of 25–40 units/kg every 12 hours until bleeding has ceased, or continuous infusion (especially intracranial bleeds, trauma).
4. Generally, haemarthroses and soft tissue bleeds require 1–3 infusions, whereas serious bleeds, such as areas with peripheral nerves at risk (e.g. psoas), retropharyngeal or

retroperitoneal bleeding, may require prolonged treatment, including continuous infusions of factor VIII.

5. The formula for dosage is:

$$\text{required international units}$$
$$= \text{bodyweight (kg)} \times \text{desired factor VIII rise (\%)} \times 0.5$$

FIX replacement guide

rFIX doses are 2–3 times the doses for rFVIII listed above. The formula for dosage is:

$$\text{required international units}$$
$$= \text{bodyweight (kg)} \times \text{desired factor IX rise (\%)} \times 1.1$$

(under age of 12 years), *or* × 1.4 (greater than or equal to 12 years).

2. Other treatments

Musculoskeletal bleeds also benefit from (mnemonic **RICES**):

Rest/immobilisation
Ice
Compression of the affected part
Elevation of the affected part
Splinting

In addition to antifibrinolytics (EACA, tranexamic acid) and replacement therapy in oral or nasal mucous membrane bleeding and dental extractions, children should remain nil by mouth if they have oral or tongue bleeds/lacerations.

ANALGESIA

Haemarthrosis can be very painful. Temporary immobilisation in a splint, with infusion of FVIII and wise use of simple analgesics, such as paracetamol or codeine, which are free of any aspirin or other non-steroidal anti-inflammatory drugs (NSAIDs), may be sufficient. The only NSAIDs which may be used are COX-2 inhibitors (e.g. celecoxib, meloxicam). Narcotic analgesia should be avoided. Joint aspiration, under FVIII cover, may be needed to stop the pain (rarely in childhood).

RESTORING NORMAL FUNCTION

Physiotherapy should be initiated as soon as pain has diminished. Immobilisation should ideally not exceed 24–48 hours, and then static followed by active exercises should be introduced. Depending on the chronicity of the joint problem, FVIII cover may be required to prevent physiotherapy-induced haemorrhage. The use of ultrasound may help to restore function after a large soft-tissue bleed.

PREVENTION OF IATROGENIC PROBLEMS

With medical procedures, apply pressure for 10 minutes after any injection (e.g. venepuncture or SC injection). Immunisations can be given without clotting factor concentrate cover, but a small-gauge needle and deep SC injections are recommended, rather than intramuscular injections. The injection site should be compressed for 10 minutes after the injection. For lumbar puncture (LP), give enough clotting factor to raise the level to 50%, 30 minutes before the LP.

COMPLICATIONS OF MEDICAL TREATMENT
Analgesic abuse

This tends to be more of a problem in the adult haemophiliac population, but is well recognised in adolescents. Avoidance of addictive drugs is extremely important; this area should be considered in any adolescent.

CHRONIC PROBLEMS
Neurological sequelae

Intracranial haemorrhage is one of the more common causes of mortality and morbidity. Between a third and half of affected children die; and of the survivors, half have neurological sequelae, including convulsions, and motor and cognitive impairment. All patients with any neurological symptoms or signs need appropriate imaging (CT or MRI) to diagnose small intracerebral bleeds early. The sequelae may require use of anticonvulsants, physiotherapy, occupational therapy, speech therapy and prolonged rehabilitation.

Joint involvement and synovectomy

Haemophilic arthropathy proceeds through many stages, with a cycle of haemarthrosis from inflammatory changes with erosion of cartilage and bone to proliferative chronic synovitis (highly vascular tissue) and increased haemarthrosis. Hypertrophied synovium causes destruction of cartilage, narrowing of the joint space, bone resorption and cyst formation, resulting in anatomical joint instability and chronic pain. Disuse leads to osteoporosis. Abnormal epiphyseal growth will occur, followed by atrophy of local muscles and further joint instability. Finally, the joint becomes immobile, with repeated bleeding, leading to fibrous and bony ankylosis of large joints or complete destruction of small joints.

Haemophilic arthropathy can be staged radiographically:

Stage 1 Soft-tissue swelling due to haemorrhage into joint
Stage 2 Overgrowth of epiphysis
Stage 3 Joint disorganised
Stage 4 Cartilage destroyed, joint space narrowed
Stage 5 Fibrous contracture, loss of joint space, loss of joint

MRI gives the best assessment of synovial hypertrophy, and can give additional information particularly in Stage 2, demonstrating erosion, cysts and joint effusions.

The optimal treatment to prevent this cycle is prophylaxis (see below), which is associated with a significant reduction in the average number of haemarthroses per year and in the rate of joint deterioration. When children are started on prophylactic replacement therapy to keep plasma factor levels above 1%, this effectively changes severe disease to moderate disease, and if it is commenced in children between 1 and 3 years of age, joint destruction will not occur.

Prompt treatment of any breakthrough bleeding and intensive physiotherapy are also important. Brief courses of oral corticosteroids (1–4 weeks) may be given in cases of severe synovitis as well, to decrease the synovium, but their beneficial effect is temporary. As mentioned previously, the only NSAIDs regarded as safe in haemophilia patients, are COX-2 inhibitors, as they may be used without any associated risk of bleeding.

If a joint remains chronically enlarged despite optimum medical therapy, synovectomy may be considered, preferably non-surgical. The rationale for synovectomy is that removing synovium decreases bleeds, thus reducing ongoing joint damage. An alternative is isotopic or chemical synovectomy (synoviorthesis), where the synovium is ablated by intra-articular injection of yttrium-90 (or colloidal P32 chromic phosphate; or rhenium-186, erbium-169 or radioactive gold) or chemical agents (oxytetracycline chlorhydrate, osmic acid, hyaluronic acid, rifampicin). Radioactive agents have better results in the long term, with more rapid rehabilitation. Short-term results are very good with either mode of treatment.

Complications of synovectomy can include re-bleeding, long periods of rehabilitation, long-term ankylosis and the potential requirement for total joint replacement (arthroplasty). Arthroplasty has very good short-term effects; the most common joints on which it is performed are the knees, hips, shoulders and, less often, the elbows or ankles.

SPECIFIC DISCUSSION AREAS

Home treatment

This is the cornerstone of modern management. The two forms of treatment are prophylactic (regular injections to prevent bleeds) and symptomatic (when a bleed has just started). Prophylactic treatment is the optimal therapy.

CVADs or 'ports' are placed to enable institution of home treatment at an early age, which avoids repetitive and difficult venepuncture. Most parents have a mobile phone so that they can be contacted when a bleed occurs at school and administer treatment without delay.

Home-based treatment means that these patients do not spend a lot of time in hospital, and there is the potential for 'de-skilling' of doctors with regard to the management of haemophilia.

Prophylaxis

This is the standard approach for most boys with severe haemophilia. There are a number of types of prophylaxis; the specific terminology used is as follows.

Primary prophylaxis

Primary prophylaxis is the ongoing regular infusion of FVIII from early childhood, before significant joint bleeding is established, to prevent most bleeding episodes. This is usually started after the first significant joint bleed (often at around 12 months of age) and is typically given through a venous access port (see the next page). In neonates who have intracranial bleeding, prophylaxis is best started as soon as possible (i.e. without waiting until after a first major joint bleed), implanting a venous access port during the hospital admission for the presenting intracranial bleed (in one of the author's patients, this included a [successful] burr hole at age 4 days for a subdural haematoma with midline shift, a 'blown' pupil and incipient coning).

Recombinant FVIII is given three times a week, at a dose of 25–40 units/kg. Prophylaxis has led to a marked decrease in the number of bleeds suffered by these children. The age at which prophylaxis is started is an independent predictor for the development of arthropathy; the earlier it is started, the less joint disease will occur, irrespective of the variables of dose and infusion intervals used at the start of treatment before the age of 3 years. The increased cost of prophylaxis would be offset by the decrease in later interventions such as synovectomy and the avoidance of significant arthritis in the adult years.

Primary prophylaxis can be determined either by age, starting long-term continuous (52 weeks a year) treatment before 2 years and before any clinically evident joint bleeds, or by first joint bleed, starting long-term continuous (52 weeks a year) treatment before the onset of joint damage.

The advantages of primary prophylaxis include: the prevention of haemarthroses, chronic joint disease, and pain; less school interruption (and higher academic achievement in mathematics and reading); increased participation in physical activities; and less frequent hospital visits.

The disadvantages include the port requirement in younger children, the increased number of injections, the increased usage of products, the possible earlier development of inhibitors, and the requirement for a compliant patient and family. rFVIII is provided as 250 IU, 500 IU, 1000 IU, 1500 IU, 2000 IU, 3000 IU and 4000 IU glass vials, so the dose is rounded up to the nearest number of bottles (i.e. dose divisible by 250).

Prophylaxis will not prevent all bleeds. It should be continued indefinitely.

Secondary prophylaxis

This refers to a specified period of regular infusions of FVIII after joint bleeding has been established. It is used for particular events such as surgical procedures or strenuous activities. Secondary prophylaxis is less successful in arresting recurrent joint bleeds.

Full-dose prophylaxis

This refers to infusion of FVIII at least 2–3 times a week, or FIX at least 1–2 times weekly, for a minimum of 46 weeks per year.

Partial prophylaxis

This is defined as 3–45 weeks of prophylaxis per year. *Short-term prophylaxis* refers to short-term treatment to prevent bleeding. *On-demand therapy* means treatment given when bleeding occurs.

Central venous access devices (CVADs or 'ports')

CVADs allow easier access, with minimal discomfort (use of local anaesthetic cream), improved home treatment, and parent and patient acceptance. Negative aspects include the need for hospitalisation for insertion (usually 3–5 days) and significant risk of infection, given that the port is accessed 150 times a year. There is no lower age limit for CVADs. One port can last longer than 5 years. If a port is infected, attempted sterilisation with antibiotics may succeed, but once the port has been infected two or three times it is unlikely to be able to be salvaged. The usual infective agent is *Staphylococcus epidermidis*, although gram-negative organisms are not uncommon. The other complication of CVADs is thrombosis, which can occur in around 50% of cases by 4 years.

Elective surgery and continuous infusion of replacement factors

Before any elective surgical procedures, all patients with haemophilia should be assessed for inhibitors (see the next section) and to establish the optimum intervals of factor infusion. This comprises evaluation of increase in FVIII or FIX level per unit of FVIII or FIX per kilogram and the biological half-life of the factor in that child. It must be ensured that there are sufficient quantities of FVIII or FIX available on the day of surgery and for the week after. In general, for all surgical procedures, a dose to bring the patient's level to 100% can be given at induction for the procedure.

The use of continuous infusions of FVIII makes surgery safer and easier. A preoperative dose of 50 units/kg is followed by an infusion at a rate of 3 units/kg per hour to maintain a constant plasma level of factor VIII. The standard half-life of FVIII is 8–12 hours. FVIII is stable for 24 hours after reconstitution (longer than the product information states), provided that it is not diluted with other fluids. A syringe driver should be used for administration, as factor VIII adheres to plastic bags. The exact regimen for clotting factor concentrate infusion will depend on the nature and extent of surgery.

When a CVAD is placed (usually the first surgical procedure undergone by these children), most units give continuous FVIII or FIX for 3–5 days, then access the CVAD for the first time postoperatively at 7 days.

Inhibitors and immune tolerance induction (ITI)

After treatment with FVIII or FIX concentrates, patients can develop antibodies against FVIII or FIX, which are called inhibitors. Inhibitors are polyclonal IgG antibodies, usually directed against functional epitopes of FVIII or FIX. These develop in 20–30% of patients with severe haemophilia A, in 5–10% with moderate-mild disease, although in only 1–4% of those with haemophilia B.

Of those with haemophilia A, some 35–50% are termed 'low responders', where the antibody circulates at low levels and no major anamnestic response occurs. The remaining patients are 'high responders', and do show an anamnestic response to FVIII infusion.

Low responders may benefit from infusions at a greater dose or from more frequent infusions. Patients with high-responding inhibitors typically will not respond to standard clotting factor concentrate. These patients may require 'bypassing' agents, such as activated recombinant coagulation factor VII (rFVIIa; eptacog alfa [activated]; NovoSeven RT [Novo Nordisk]), or prothrombin complex concentrate (PCC) and activated PCC (APCC), for the treatment of bleeding. Two doses of rFVIIa are equivalent to one dose of APCC, although some patients respond better to one agent than the other. The recommended dose of rFVIIa is 90–120 micrograms/kg given every 2 hours until bleeding stops (for an acute bleed), or for at least 24 hours for major surgery (including total hip and knee replacement). rFVIIa enhances the generation of thrombin on platelets activated by the initial thrombin formation, and the formation of a firm fibrin plug that is resistant to premature fibrolysis. rFVIIa is expensive.

Inhibitors: low- versus high-risk patients

There are both genetic and environmental aspects that contribute to whether a patient is at low risk or high risk to develop inhibitors. Genetic factors which portend low risk include: mild to moderate haemophilia, negative family history, white (Caucasian) origin, genetic missense mutation, testing negative for interleukin (IL) 10 134, negative for TNF alpha A2, but positive for cytotoxic T-lymphocyte-associated protein 4 (CTLA4)-318 T (CTLA4 downregulates the immune system). An environmental factor associated with low risk is receiving early prophylaxis. Genetic factors which portend high risk include: severe haemophilia, positive family history, African origin, genetic null mutation, testing positive for IL10 134, positive for TNF alpha A2, but negative for CTLA4-318 T. Environmental factors associated with high risk include intensive treatment and early on demand-based treatment.

Immune tolerance induction (ITI)

ITI, also called tolerisation, refers to eradicating inhibitors by manipulating the immune system through recurrent exposure to regular infusions of FVIII or FIX. In Australia, ITI is overseen by the Tolerisation Advisory Committee (TAC) of the Australian Haemophilia Centre Directors' Organisation (AHCDO). There is controversy over the ideal dosing, interval and product choice. Many patients can be tolerised on a regimen of rFVIII, in a dose of 100 units/kg 3 times a week (coordinated by TAC). An international study which compared high-dose 200 units/kg/day infusions of FVIII with 50 units/kg, 3 times a week, had to be stopped due to the high rate of intercurrent haemorrhages. Cases which have a strong family history of haemophilia, or multidomain gene deletion, have a higher failure risk, so a higher dose or a plasma-derived factor may be used. The advantages of ITI include better control of bleeds and reduced use of expensive products. The disadvantages include increased use of FVIII in some cases, and a success rate of up to 80%.

Occasionally, switching to new concentrate can induce inhibitor formation; in these children, the inhibitor may vanish when the newer product is ceased. Prior to ITI, high responders are advised to avoid FVIII products so that inhibitor levels can decrease, and this can prevent anamnestic rise.

Inhibitors to FIX are less common; around a third of patients achieve successful immune tolerance. As many as half of all haemophilia B patients with inhibitors can have allergic reactions to FIX. In those with genetic predisposition to inhibitor development, the first 20 treatments should be in hospital anticipating possible anaphylaxis. Patients with FIX inhibitors treated with PCC or APCC are likely to get an anamnestic immune response, as PCC and APCC contain FIX. Hence ITI must be considered very carefully in these patients.

Rituximab, a monoclonal antibody directed against CD-20 positive cells, is being evaluated for those who fail to respond to ITI. Occasionally, immune modulation with steroids, or cyclophosphamide (to inhibit antibodies), IV immunoglobulin, plasmapheresis or protein A adsorption (to remove antibodies) have been considered.

Risks associated with sporting activities

The National Hemophilia Foundation (NHF) in the US has a rating system for activities, based on what is known about their risk to patients with bleeding disorders. These are set out in their guide, 'Playing it safe: bleeding disorders, sports and exercise'. The activities are given a numerical rating from Category 1, which is 'Safe' through to Category 3, which is 'Dangerous':

- Category 1 (safe) activities include: non-contact sporting activities, like swimming, snorkelling, fishing, hiking, stationery bike at the gymnasium, golf, archery, Frisbee throwing.
- Category 1.5 (safe to moderate risk) activities include: bicycling, certain cardiovascular training exercises (rowing machine, treadmill, circuit training), Pilates and weightlifting.
- Category 2 (moderate risk) activities include: sports with excess strain on particular parts of the body, such as bowling, running, jogging, skipping rope, indoor rock-climbing, rollerskating, cross-country skiing, rowing, tennis and yoga.
- Category 2.5 (moderate to dangerous risk) activities include: sports with some contact or which are fairly vigorous, such as basketball, martial arts, baseball, softball, horseback riding, ice skating, downhill skiing, snowboarding, canoeing, kayaking, waterskiing, jet skiing, surfing, gymnastics, cheerleading, football (soccer, rugby), volleyball.
- Category 3 (dangerous) activities include: trampoline, boxing, BMX racing, motorcycling, motorcross racing, rodeo, power lifting, wrestling, outdoor rock-climbing, lacrosse, competitive diving, football (gridiron), hockey.

It is a myth that avoidance of strenuous activity prevents bleeding: only about 7% of recreational or sporting accidents lead to bleeding in an otherwise well child. Affected boys should be encouraged to participate in age-appropriate sporting activities with their schoolfriends, the only exceptions being those where there is a definite risk of head injury (e.g. martial arts, boxing, rugby). A good level of physical fitness may help to reduce the number of joint bleeds.

Immunisation

Routine immunisations should be given to haemophiliac children. The risk of bleeding is minimal if pressure is applied over the injection site for at least 10 minutes.

Dental care, including extractions

Prevention of periodontal disease and caries is important, as these predispose to gum bleeding; excellent oral hygiene is a necessity. Ideally, teeth should be brushed twice daily. Dental floss is recommended. Orthodontic assessment in early adolescence should occur to detect any overcrowding, which can lead to periodontal problems. Injections by dental surgeons may be done with factor cover (to 20–40%). For dental extractions, input of a haematologist is recommended; a combination of tranexamic acid (15–25 mg/kg, 8-hourly) and FVIII replacement to 30–60%, given at least 4 hours and 1 hour, respectively, may be used, with the former continued for 5–10 days. Repeat doses of FVIII are seldom used. Dental intervention in children with inhibitors also needs planning input of a haematologist.

Genetic counselling

Diagnosis at a DNA level allows the abnormal gene to be identified and marked, and its inheritance to be traced. Carrier detection and prenatal diagnosis require only the ability to recognise the abnormal gene. Most families of patients with haemophilia can have DNA analysis to elucidate the carrier status of females, prenatal diagnosis (on chorionic villus biopsy at 11–14 weeks) and linkage analysis to trace the origin of the abnormality. Mutation analysis may be performed initially on an affected male. First-degree females can be offered cascade carrier testing; if carrier status is confirmed, then an FVIII level should be performed. The gender of the fetus can be elucidated by testing for Y-chromosome-specific polymerase chain reaction (PCR) in maternal blood beyond 7–9 weeks' gestation, or by ultrasound from 11 weeks' gestation.

Preimplantation genetic diagnosis (PGD)

This can involve whole gene amplification (WGA) and preimplantation genetic haplotyping (PGH) of embryos. PGD is the detection of genetic information in an embryo fertilised in vitro by taking a blastomere at the preimplantation stage (day 3) of development to find embryos that are not affected by a serious genetic disorder—in this case, haemophilia. It is an alternative to prenatal diagnosis (PND) and termination of affected pregnancy for couples at risk of having a pregnancy affected by a serious genetic disorder.

Progress

Cures for both haemophilia A and B have occurred with orthotopic liver transplantation (performed for liver failure). Newer EHL concentrates, and utilisation of pharmacokinetics, were discussed earlier. Other novel approaches to management include the following.

ALN-AT3 (N-acetyl-galactosamine-conjugated RNA interference against anti-thrombin III) is a 'small interfering' or 'silencing' RNA (siRNA), which inhibits gene expression, targeting antithrombin III mRNA in the liver and prevents it being synthesised. SC injection of ALN-AT3 leads to a dose-dependent 'knockdown' of AT III of up to 86%. AT III lasts over 2 months, which enables once-monthly SC injections. AT III knockdown increases thrombin generation by 350%, enhancing whole blood clotting.

ACE 910 is a bispecific antibody, which is factor VIII-mimetic, substituting factor VIII co-factor activity, leading to factor IXa-catalysed factor X activation, just as FVIII does, which restores thrombin production. Annualised spontaneous bleeding rates are markedly reduced with the use of ACE 910. This is considered a breakthrough therapy.

Concizumab is a monoclonal anti-tissue factor pathway inhibitor (TFPI) antibody, which has a procoagulant effect, evidenced by elevated D-dimers and prothrombin fragment 1 + 2, enhancing thrombin production, in a concentration-dependent manner. It can be given subcutaneously.

LONG CASES

LONG CASE: Sickle cell disease (SCD)

The last decade has seen improved morbidity and mortality due to many advances in the management of sickle cell anaemia (SCA) (OMIM#603903), which occurs in around 1 in 400 African American people, 1 in 36 000 Hispanic people and 1 in 123 000 Caucasian people. Newborn screening is now widespread, prophylactic therapy programs have expanded and there are coordinated care programs including hydroxyurea (HU) treatment (decreases painful crises and the requirement for transfusions), and cure through haematopoietic stem cell transplantation (HSCT), for which there are clear indications. The two main pathophysiological processes are haemolytic anaemia and vaso-occlusion. These are secondary to deoxygenation of the haemoglobin S (Hb S) molecule, which has a hydrophobic valine residue replacing a hydrophilic glutamic acid at position 6. This acid is prone to aggregating into a polymer, which causes a distortion of the red blood cell to a 'sickle' shape, rigid and crescentic. Triggers for polymerisation include hypoxia and acidosis. Sickle cells block the microvasculature, and can adhere to vascular endothelium, causing hyperplasia of the intima and slowed blood flow. The consequent deleterious effects of SCA can involve most organ systems.

The rate of sickling is related to the concentration of deoxy-Hb S: it takes only seconds—and if the cell is rammed through the capillaries, it becomes reoxygenated and the polymers of Hb S depolymerise. The cell shape lags behind, and repeated hypoxic stress will alter the cytoskeleton of the cell and cause an irreversibly sickled cell. SCD represents an inflammatory process with abnormal granulocyte and monocyte activation. Organ damage in SCA can develop throughout childhood, starting with splenic and renal changes in infancy, and continuing through to pulmonary and neurological involvement with vasculopathy in older children and adolescents.

Although the condition is less common in Australia than in the US, Canada or the UK, children suffering from it do tend to appear in the examination setting. Because of their relative infrequency, candidates (and consultants) may find management of these children challenging, although over recent years there has been a change in the demographics in Australia with increased migration of families from Africa.

Background information
BASIC DEFECT

SCA is due to homozygosity for the genetic point mutation (a single nucleotide change, GAT to GTT), whereby glutamic acid is replaced by valine at position 6 on the β-globin chain (abbreviated as Glu6Val) of the haemoglobin heterotetramer: the resulting haemoglobin is Hb S. Deoxygenated Hb S polymerises, is denatured and releases toxic oxidants, distorting (sickling) the red cell shape. Red blood cells containing Hb S travel through the circulation undergoing a continuous cycle of oxygenation and deoxygenation. The ongoing formation of polymers of Hb S, leads to these inflexible proteins damaging the erythrocyte membrane. The erythrocytes become dehydrated, leading to greater adherence to endothelial cells and shortened red cell survival. Sickled red cells have difficulty negotiating the capillary beds. They block vessels (intermittent vaso-occlusive episodes, leading to ischaemia) and are destroyed prematurely (haemolysis). In the homozygous state (Hb SS disease) there is no Hb A, and over 90% Hb S. In the heterozygous state, red blood cells contain 30–45% Hb S.

The gene has a wide geographical distribution, including equatorial Africa, the US, the Caribbean, Italy and Greece, the Near and Middle East, and India, especially areas with endemic malaria; sickle cell trait is protective against malaria. The β-globin gene cluster is on chromosome 11. The beta S gene is flanked by distinct haplotypes that are associated with specific ethnic groups of particular geographical regions, which may determine disease severity. They are named after the places where their initial identification occurred.

Of the various haplotypes, CAR (Central Africa Republic) has the lowest level of Hb F, and worst clinical severity with three times the usual risks of stroke, chronic lung disease, renal failure, leg ulcers and a higher risk of death in young adulthood. CAR leads to more severe disease than the Benin haplotype, which in turn is more serious than the Senegal haplotype.

There are many sickling haemoglobins, which are double substitution variants, meaning these haemoglobins have both the typical sickle cell mutation (Glu6Val), and an additional amino acid substitute in the same beta globin chain. These include:

- Hb S Antilles (Glu6Val + Val23Ile), Hb S Cameroon (Glu6Val + Glu90Lys).
- Hb S Oman (Glu6Val + Glu121Lys), Hb S Providence (Glu6Val + Lys82Asp).
- Hb S South End (Glu6Val + Lys132Asn), Hb S Travis (Glu6Val + Ala142Val).
- Hb Jamaica Plain (Glu6Val + Leu68Phe), Hb C Harlem (Glu6Val + Asp73Asn).

Hb C is important when coinherited with Hb S, (Hb SC disease), or coinherited with beta-thalassaemia (Hb C-β-thalassaemia), as the presence of Hb C leads to fewer symptoms than Hb SS (except for two particular complications which occur more frequently in Hb SC, the first being vascular retinopathy [proliferative sickle cell retinopathy, PSCR], and the second being avascular necrosis of the femoral head).

There is an inverse relationship between the level of Hb F and clinical severity. Children with high Hb F have mild disease. The percentage of Hb F is the most important predictor of early mortality in patients with SCD. In unaffected children, Hb F comprises 5% of total haemoglobin by 3–6 months of age, and less than 1% in adults. SCD patients can have Hb F levels between 1% and 20%; those with the genetic mutation for hereditary persistence of Hb F (HPFH) may have Hb F levels between 30% and 40% of total haemoglobin.

Definitions

The term 'sickle cell anaemia' (SCA) typically refers to homozygosity for the sickle cell gene, (Hb SS), although some consider the term SCA to include sickle-β^0-thalassaemia (Hb Sβ^0), which is clinically very similar to Hb SS. The term 'sickle cell disease' (SCD) is a more general one that includes compound heterozygous states such as sickle cell/haemoglobin C disease (Hb SC), sickle cell-β^+-thalassaemia (Hb Sβ^+) and other sickling disorders.

There are two groups of sickle cell syndromes:

1. Sickle states, which are relatively benign (e.g. sickle cell trait, Hb AS).
2. Sickle cell diseases (SCDs), which present a variety of problems. These include: SCA, Hb SS; sickle β^0-thalassaemia (β-thalassaemia without production of any β globin); sickle haemoglobin C disease (Hb SC); and sickle β^+-thalassaemia (β-thalassaemia with decreased [not absent] production of β-globin).

Patients with sickle β^0-thalassaemia and sickle β^+-thalassaemia have clinical features that are more like SCD than thalassaemia, because the sickle β-globin predominates as a result of inadequate production of normal β-globin.

Patients with untreated Hb SS or Hb Sβ^0 typically have a haemoglobin level of 6–9 g/dL, and a reticulocyte count of 10–25%, and have clinically severe disease.

Patients with untreated Hb SC typically have a haemoglobin level of 9–12 g/dL, and a reticulocyte count of 5–10%, and less severe disease than Hb SS or Hb Sβ^0.

Patients with untreated Hb Sβ^+ typically have a haemoglobin level of 10–13 g/dL, and a reticulocyte count of 2–10%, and less severe disease again than Hb SC.

Diagnosis

Haemoglobin electrophoresis is the most common technique used in the diagnosis of haemoglobinopathies. The diagnosis of SCD requires demonstration of the presence of significant amounts of Hb S by high-performance liquid chromatography, isoelectric focusing, or cellulose acetate or citrate agar electrophoresis, and the lack of a normal β-globin gene (HBB) on molecular genetic testing. Targeted mutation analysis can detect the HBB mutations Glu6Val (for Hb S), Glu6Lys (for Hb C), Glu121Gln (for Hb D-Punjab) and Glu121Lys (for Hb O-Arab), the large number of β-thalassaemia mutations, and various other specific haemoglobin variants. HBB sequence analysis may be used if targeted mutation analysis is uninformative, or as the initial test to detect mutations associated with β-thalassaemia variants.

In North America, and increasingly throughout Europe (especially Mediterranean countries) and Africa, newborns are screened for the presence of SCD. The WHO has requested 50% of its member states to establish SCD control programs by 2020, as the United Nations has noted SCD to be a global public health concern.

The most common method used for newborn screening is electrophoresis and high-performance liquid chromatography (HPLC). When initial testing detects a haemoglobinopathy, the result is confirmed within 6 weeks by another complementary method; for compound heterozygotes (e.g. Hb SC, SD or SO), a repeat test is sufficient. Newborns with Hb F levels higher than Hb S levels could have any of: homozygous sickle cell (Hb SS), S β^0-thalassaemia or S β^+-thalassaemia with a low level of Hb A; these can be difficult to distinguish in the neonatal period when 95% of total haemoglobin is Hb F, and molecular testing may be needed. Additional testing is performed again at 1 year of age, once Hb F levels have fallen, to determine if there is coexisting thalassaemia, which is important for genetic counselling.

Sickle cell trait

Clinically benign, the major significance is genetic counselling. Growth and development are normal. Haemoglobin and reticulocyte counts are normal, and red cells are normocytic and normochromic. Affected people may have acute splenic infarction if exposed to significant hypoxia (e.g. exposure to altitudes above 3000 metres). Also, renal sickling with spontaneous haematuria can occur. Partners of heterozygotes need screening to exclude haemoglobinopathies, which may lead to a child being born with a sickle disease.

Sickle cell anaemia (SCA): clinical course

The course of SCA is one of ongoing haemolysis episodically punctuated by 'crises', which are clinical events that may be acutely painful or even life-threatening. Any crisis may be precipitated by **ACIDOSES** (mnemonic: **A**cidosis, **C**old, **I**nfection, **D**ehydration, **O**xygen lack, **S**tress, **E**levated temperature, **S**port [exercise]). Types of crises are sequestration crisis (especially affects infants), aplastic crisis, vaso-occlusive (infarctive) crisis and, least commonly, haemolytic crisis.

Suggestions of more aggressive treatment for more aggressive haplotypes have been made, considering potential curative therapy such as HSCT.

Effects of α-thalassaemia

Hb SS patients with α-thalassaemia have a larger number of painful events (in extremities/back/abdomen/head) but fewer acute anaemic events (this does not include splenic sequestration).

Major complications

Vaso-occlusion and haemolysis are the main pathological processes in SCD. The organs most commonly affected are the spleen, brain, kidneys and lung. Accordingly, the most lethal complications (and common ages affected) are splenic sequestration (under 5 years), overwhelming sepsis due to functional asplenia (under 3 years), stroke (median 5 years) and acute chest syndrome (ACS, usually 2–4 years). Most significant complications are common after 1 year of age. In the first year of life, complications can include dactylitis, splenic sequestration and sepsis. SCD also is characterised by hypercoagulability (which increases the risk of vaso-occlusive complications), and immune dysregulation.

SICKLE CELL is a mnemonic for major vaso-occlusive complications:

Sequestration (spleen and liver)
Infection
Cerebrovascular accidents (CVAs)
Kidney disease
Lung disease (ACS, pulmonary hypertension)
Eye disease

Crises (painful, infarctive)
Erection (priapism)
Limb effects (bone infarcts, marrow necrosis, osteomyelitis and aseptic necrosis)
Leg ulcers

There are a number of other aspects which can be remembered as **H**s and **A**s:

Haemolysis and anaemia (chronic)
Haemolytic crisis
Haemolysis due to transfusion
Hand–foot syndrome (dactylitis)
Hepatobiliary and abdominal involvement
Hyperviscosity due to transfusion
Aplastic crisis
Anaesthetic considerations
Alloimmunisation and autoimmunisation with transfusion
Accumulation of iron due to transfusion

The following sections are set out in this order.

Painful crises (or vaso-occlusive pain events [VOE]) and ACS are the most common sickle-cell related complications in Hb SS, Hb SC and β-/sickle thalassaemia patients. The risks of these begin in the first year of life; both are vaso-occlusive events.

SPLENIC SEQUESTRATION CRISIS

1. This is the most severe crisis in those under 5 years of age. It occurs in 10–30% of children with Hb SS, most commonly between 6 months and 3 years. Splenic involution tends to occur by 5 years of age in children with Hb SS and Hb Sβ⁰-thalassaemia, so sequestration is infrequent after that age. Splenic involution is delayed in children with Hb SC and Hb Sβ⁺-thalassaemia, so sequestration can occur in older patients with these. The use of hydroxyurea and chronic transfusion therapy can delay splenic involution in those with Hb SS and Hb Sβ⁰-thalassaemia, and lead to sequestration in older children.

2. Sequestration results from acute entrapment of a large volume of blood in the spleen (trapping of erythrocytes within splenic sinusoids)—often a large fraction of the circulating blood volume.

3. Children with SCA get rapid splenic enlargement (at least 2 cm increase in spleen size from baseline) with an acute fall in haemoglobin of greater than 2 g/dL, and with a raised reticulocyte count. They present with sudden collapse, shock, profound anaemia and abdominal fullness due to the massive splenomegaly. This often occurs during an acute infection.

4. It is life-threatening: it can be fatal within 30 minutes. Hypovolaemic shock can be treated with an initial transfusion of packed red blood cells (PRBCs). If further transfusions are required, these are given more slowly due to the risk of autotransfusion of sequestered blood which could cause hyperviscosity.

5. If the child is older (e.g. over 2 years), consider splenectomy in susceptible patients. If under 2 years of age, a chronic transfusion program may be needed.

6. There is a tendency for recurrence: up to 50% of children have a second episode, usually within 2 years. Elective splenectomy is generally recommended in patients presenting with the first episode of splenic sequestration.

INFECTION: OVERWHELMING SEPSIS

1. This particularly affects children under 3 years of age, as a result of poor development of immune response to polysaccharide antigens, complicated by early loss of splenic function (this 'autosplenectomy' occurs in 60% by 2 years, and 90% by 5 years).

2. Pathogens are most commonly *Streptococcus pneumoniae* (pneumococcus)—various serotypes—and occasionally *Haemophilus influenzae* type B. Other pathogens include meningococcus, and other *Streptococci*, *Salmonella* and fastidious gram-negative organisms, such as DF-2 (*Capnocytophaga canimorsus*) after a dog bite.

3. Prevention is by immunisation against pneumococci, *Haemophilus* and meningococcus. Prophylactic penicillin is recommended until the age of 5 years, as it decreases the incidence of pneumococcal bacteraemia by 84%. Many units continue penicillin prophylaxis throughout childhood.

4. If children with Hb SS or sickle β⁰-thalassaemia present febrile, after clinical assessment it is prudent to take blood for a full blood count, blood cultures, plus type and cross-match if pale, the spleen is enlarged, or there are neurological or respiratory symptoms. Then treat with ceftriaxone or cefotaxime (or vancomycin if in an area with a high prevalence of resistant pneumococci). Other investigations for sepsis (e.g. other cultures, CXR) and coexisting complications depend on presentation.

5. The case fatality rate is up to 30%.

CEREBRAL INFARCTION (CEREBROVASCULAR ACCIDENT)

1. Central nervous system involvement, manifesting as an overt cerebrovascular accident (CVA), is seen in up to 11% of children with Hb SS; the peak ages between 2 and 9 years, with the median ages between 5 and 8 years. CVA is less frequent in those with Hb SC or Hb Sβ⁺-thalassaemia.

2. CVA particularly affects internal carotid (ICA), anterior cerebral (ACA) and middle cerebral (MCA) arteries. Overt strokes are due mostly to occlusive cerebral arterial vasculopathy, although some may involve SCA's haemoglobin deoxygenation and polymerisation in the microcirculation and venous system, and some may involve Hb SS membrane procoagulant. Permanent sequelae can result (e.g. hemiplegia).

3. Transient ischaemic attacks (TIAs) may predate completed strokes, and warrant emergent neuroimaging.

4. CVAs can happen in conjunction with other SCD complications, including aplastic crises, ACS or priapism.

5. Acute treatment of an overt stroke involves transfusion; initial exchange transfusion is associated with less risk of recurrent stroke.

6. Without treatment, CVA recurs in 50–70% within 3 years; it can be progressive.

7. MRI and MR arteriography are useful in evaluating the timing, location and extent of the ischaemia or infarction, and the state of the vessels.

8. Haemorrhage into infarcted areas (from bleeding from delicate vessels from neovascularisation), or ruptured aneurysm (in the contralateral circulation from compensatory increased blood flow) with subarachnoid haemorrhage, can occur as early as 4 years of age and cause further neurological deficits.

9. The recommended treatment after cerebral infarction has been long-term transfusion (TX) therapy maintaining Hb S levels below 30%; this lowers the risk of recurrence to 10–20%. Recently the TWiTCH trial studied patients switched over from chronic TX to high-dose hydroxyurea (HU) and found HU to be non-inferior to chronic TX, with equal prevention of strokes whether HU or chronic TX is used.

10. For prevention, many units recommend chronic TX or high-dose HU for at-risk children. They may be detected by transcranial Doppler (TCD). Studies that have shown that high blood flow velocity through the ICA (over 200 cm/min) clearly increases the probability of arterial occlusive stroke. TCD studies have been used in many countries for over 30 years, and are available in most Australian centres in 2017. Abnormal TCD indicates a stroke risk of around 10% each year for the 3 years after the test. The STOP trial (Stroke Prevention Trial in SCA) demonstrated that chronic TX reduced the rate of initial stroke in children with abnormal TCD by 92%, and the TWiTCH trial showed that chronic TX and HU had similar efficacy in stroke prevention. Yearly TCD is recommended for children with SCA.

11. Subsequent stroke can occur after cessation of TX therapy after 30 months. This was shown by the follow-up STOP2 trial. Treatment (whether TXs or HU) should be continued indefinitely.

12. Up to 50% of patients with SCD may have some degree of cerebrovascular disease by 14 years of age.

13. Silent cerebral infarction (SCI) is well recognised, occurring in up to 37% of children with Hb SS and Hb $S\beta^0$-thalassaemia, identified by MRI appearances in the absence of clinical motor or sensory deficits. SCI leads to cognitive impairment, learning difficulties and increased risk of overt stroke. Risk factors for SCI include low Hb and elevated systolic blood pressure.

14. Acute silent cerebral ischaemic events (ASCIEs) are more recently recognised lesions; some are transient, some progress to SCIs.

KIDNEY INVOLVEMENT AND HYPERTENSION

1. Hyposthenuria (the inability to concentrate urine) is due to chronic sickling in the region of the loop of Henle (microvascular ischaemia induced by sickle cell, with obliteration of the vasa recta of the kidney medulla; the medulla provides an environment that predisposes to the risks of erythrocyte sickling and vaso-occlusion, as it is hyperosmolar, acidic and hypoxic). This often has occurred by the age of 1 year.

2. This leads to an obligatory urine output of up to 2 L/m^2/day in infants, up to 4 L/m^2/day in adults, and associated nocturia, enuresis, and puts patients at risk of rapid dehydration.

3. Other renal sequelae include renal ischaemia-induced papillary necrosis and medullary interstitial fibrosis, renal tubular acidosis, impaired potassium excretion, microscopic and macroscopic haematuria, proteinuria and nephrotic syndrome, focal glomerulosclerosis and renal insufficiency. It can be difficult to identify early kidney disease because patients with SCD can hypersecrete creatinine at their proximal tubules which masks deterioration in glomerular filtration rate (GFR) before elevation of creatinine occurs. Patients with even modest elevations in creatinine should be considered to have renal impairment, to allow timely intervention.

4. Proteinuria indicates glomerular disease; to decrease this, angiotensin-converting enzyme (ACE) inhibitors and angiotensin receptor blockers may be prescribed. At the time of writing (2017), studies of losartan in SCD were ongoing.

5. In adulthood, hypertension, ineffective erythropoiesis, renal osteodystrophy and end-stage renal disease (ESRD) can supervene, requiring top-up transfusion, recombinant human erythropoietin, haemodialysis, peritoneal dialysis or renal transplantation. Between 4 and 18% of people with SCD develop chronic renal disease; the median age for this is 23 years.

6. Hypertension screening is vital. The BP should be measured regularly in children with SCD, as hypertension increases the risks of stroke, microalbuminuria, hospital admission and mortality in those with SCA. Normal BP is below the 90th centile of blood pressure measurements for that patient's age, sex and height, systolic (SBP) or diastolic (DBP). Pre-hypertension refers to BP measurements between the 90th and 95th centiles, and hypertension refers to BP measurements above the 95th centile. Stage 1 hypertension means 95th to 99th centiles plus 5 mmHg, and Stage 2 hypertension refers to above the 99th centile plus 5 mmHg. In most patients with Hb SS, the BP is typically lower (systolic, diastolic and mean) than in healthy controls.

LUNG DISEASE: ACUTE CHEST SYNDROME (ACS) AND PULMONARY HYPERTENSION (PH)

1. Acute pulmonary disease with new respiratory symptoms (fever, cough, sputum production, dyspnoea, hypoxia), and new infiltrates on CXR.

2. May be due to pulmonary infarction or infection: for example, bacterial (*Haemophilus influenzae*, *Staphylococcus aureus*, *Klebsiella pneumoniae*, *Mycoplasma pneumoniae*, pneumococcus, *Chlamydia pneumoniae*, *Legionella pneumophila*, TB, *Cryptococcus*) or viral (respiratory syncytial virus, parvovirus, adenovirus, influenza, cytomegalovirus), or both; it can be difficult to distinguish between them. Definite aetiology is not established in 65–70% of cases with pneumonia. ACS can also be caused by rib or sternal infarction.

3. Pulmonary fat embolism (PFE) is the second most common cause of ACS. Marrow infarcts during a vaso-occlusive crisis (VOC) can generate fat emboli, which cause a marked inflammatory response in the lung. Secretory phospholipase A2 (sPLA2) is an inflammatory mediator that liberates free fatty acids and causes the acute lung injury with PFE. In children with VOC and elevated sPLA2, blood transfusion may prevent the development of ACS.

4. ACS is most common in the 2–4-year age group and declines with increasing age. Hb F seems to protect those under 2 years. Incidence is related to genotype: it is more common in Hb SS and Hb S β^0-thalassaemia than in Hb SC or Hb S β^+-thalassaemia. Lower haematocrit also reduces incidence.

5. Repeated episodes of ACS are associated with the development, in adulthood, of chronic restrictive lung disease, pulmonary hypertension, cor pulmonale, hypoxia, osteonecrosis at multiple sites and myocardial infarction.

6. Treatment involves the following: avoidance of hypoxia; judicious use of intravenous rehydration, analgesia, prevention of atelectasis (with incentive spirometry if possible), antibiotics (for all with fever, and most without), transfusion with packed cells (to increase the oxygen carrying capacity), exchange transfusion for clinical deterioration or hypoxia, or those unresponsive to other therapies. Transfusion risks include viral disease transmission, acute hyperviscosity and alloimmunisation. In adults, hydroxyurea treatment leads to a significant reduction in ACS.

7. It is the single largest contributor to mortality in children under 2 years.

8. Asthma is common in patients with SCD. Presenting symptoms can be similar between ACS and asthma. Optimal management of the asthma or asthma-like component of SCD can decrease the risk of ACS.

9. Pulmonary arterial hypertension (PAH) may affect up to 10–30% of children, but the prognosis is far better than in affected adults. Mentioned here for completion, PAH is important to detect in adults as it is associated with early mortality. It is yet to be elucidated whether screening in childhood is beneficial. In adults, echocardiography is used to screen for PAH, with a tricuspid regurgitant jet velocity (TRJV) above 2.5 m/s being indicative of higher pulmonary artery pressure; however, there is a high false-positive rate when echo findings are compared to right heart catheterisation.

EYE INVOLVEMENT: PROLIFERATIVE SICKLE RETINOPATHY (PSR) AND VITREOUS HAEMORRHAGE

Sickle retinopathy is due to retinal arterioles being plugged by sickled red cells; the consequent ischaemia leads to vascular tissue factors being released, which stimulate angiogenesis. Neovascular tissue bleeds readily, and can lead to traction forces developing between the vitreous and the retina. Lesions may be non-proliferative (e.g. intraretinal haematoma) or proliferative, with tufts of new vessels extending along the retina or into the vitreous. These forms can be seen as early as 5 years of age. There are five stages of PSR: Stages I and II describe arteriolar occlusion and vessel remodelling; Stage III describes neovascularisation and formation of 'sea fans' (pre-retinal neovascular formations, bright red if viable, white if auto-infarcted); Stage IV describes vitreous haemorrhage; and Stage V retinal detachment. The latter two stages are more common with Hb SC disease. Laser photocoagulation is used. On occasion, vitrectomy may be needed for severe vitreous haemorrhage.

CRISES (VASO-OCCLUSIVE CRISES [VOC]; INFARCTIVE CRISES)

Vascular occlusion in SCA involves both microvascular occlusion (mostly in the bone marrow, causing acute painful episodes or 'crises') and macrovascular occlusion (the vessels affected by this [obstructed and injured] are the vulnerable vascular beds in the brain, spleen, lung, eye and heart). Crises and ACS involve components of bone marrow ischaemia and necrosis, embolisation and inflammation. Over 90% of hospital admissions of adults with SCD are for treatment of painful crises.

A 'vaso-occlusive phenotype' is described, comprising the markers of coinherited alpha thalassaemia trait, higher white blood cell count, lower Hb F, higher iron stores (iron overload), and vessel flow resistance associated with deoxygenation.

Reiterating, the three most dangerous complications are **S**equestration (**s**pleen), **S**epsis (especially *Streptococcus*) and **S**troke (**s**ilent or overt).

ERECTILE PROBLEMS: PRIAPISM

1. Painful failure of penile detumescence can occur as early as 3 years old, and up to 90% boys with SCA will have an episode by 20 years old. When it first occurs,

boys should urinate, drink water and have a warm shower. Oral pseudoephedrine, along with analgesics, can be given at home (**pr**iapism/erection is a **pre**dominantly **para**sympathetic, so it can be treated with the **s**ympathetic drug p**s**eudoephedrine).

2. 'Stuttering' priapism often occurs: the development of erections lasting 1–2 hours. Priapism lasting for over 3 hours is a medical emergency. It is caused by obstruction between the corpora cavernosa and the spongiosa, followed by sickling within the corpora cavernosa, particularly in adolescents.
3. If the child cannot urinate, this indicates involvement of the corpora spongiosa.
4. Priapism may resolve within a few hours or last more than 24 hours, with extreme pain.
5. Management is medical initially, with analgesia, IV hydration, oxygen, sedation, warmth and pseudoephedrine (if not taken already) or other vasoactive drug.
6. If medical treatment is unsuccessful after 12 hours, surgical intervention is required (e.g. corpora cavernosa aspiration and irrigation—the earlier performed, the better).
7. Priapism may cause a fibrotic corpora cavernosa, penile atrophy and impotence.
8. Previous treatments no longer recommended (either shown to be ineffective or fraught with complications) include acute blood transfusion (ineffective), exchange transfusion (can cause stroke) and surgical shunts (impair future erectile function).
9. In patients with SCD and stuttering priapism, available treatments include hydroxyurea, PDE-5 esterase inhibitors, alpha-adrenergic agents, chronic transfusion therapy and chronic hormonal therapy, but there is a lack of data on functional outcomes. Consultation between the haematologist and a urologist is a sound consideration.

LIMB (BONE AND JOINT) INVOLVEMENT, INCLUDING AVASCULAR NECROSIS (AVN)

1. Painful episodes usually occur after the age of 3 years.
2. Pathology includes infarction of bone marrow, cortical bone and periarticular tissues.
3. It may present with limitation of movement and swelling.
4. Osteomyelitis may occur, particularly under 5 years of age, with *Salmonella* as the pathogen in over half the cases.
5. Differentiating between infarction and infection can be hard; bone scans may help.
6. Infarcts are most commonly seen in the long bones, spine, sternum and ribs.
7. Vaso-occlusion of the vessels supplying the head of the femur can lead to AVN of the femoral head; this may be seen by 5 years of age, presenting with knee or hip pain, and may require NSAIDs, physiotherapy or surgery (core decompression done at Ficat Stage I or II of AVN of hip). The pain is worse with walking, associated with limitation of movement, and is relieved by rest. It can be bilateral in 40–80% of cases. AVN can occur also in the proximal humerus, affecting the shoulder joint.
8. The SCD genotypes most at risk of developing AVN in younger patients are Hb SS-α-thalassaemia and Hb Sβ^0-thalassaemia.

LEG ULCERATION

This is secondary to chronic haemolysis and anaemia, and more common in males. Ulcers are less common if α-gene deletion, elevated total Hb and elevated Hb F.

Features which predispose to ulcer formation include severe anaemia, infection and trauma. Deeper ulcers can be complicated by osteomyelitis. Infected ulcers can be treated with systemic or topical antibiotics, and wound care specialists consulted for optimal dressings.

HAEMOLYSIS AND ANAEMIA (CHRONIC)

Sequelae include poor growth, delayed puberty and pigmented gallstones.

HAEMOLYTIC CRISIS

This is not common and is associated with a rise in the reticulocyte count (which differentiates this from aplasia) and the bilirubin level. A 'haemolytic phenotype' is described, comprising the markers of high lactate dehydrogenase (LDH), low Hb and high reticulocyte count. Patients with the highest level of haemolysis are at increased risk for PAH.

HAEMOLYSIS RELATED TO TRANSFUSION THERAPY

Haemolysis that occurs during or after blood transfusion is immunologically mediated. Delayed haemolytic transfusion reactions (DHTRs) can happen between 1 and 4 weeks post-transfusion, due to IgG alloantibodies, leading to worsening anaemia, increased red cell antibodies (positive direct antiglobulin [Coomb's] test) and increased antibodies in serum (positive indirect antiglobulin test). DHTRs can also lead to hyperhaemolysis where patients haemolyse their own red cells in addition to transfused red cells.

HYPERVISCOSITY

Red cell transfusion increases haematocrit, and increased blood viscosity can be a problem which should be avoided as it can precipitate a VOC.

HAND–FOOT SYNDROME (DACTYLITIS)

1. Infants as young as 3 months may present with painful swollen hands and feet due to symmetric infarction of red marrow and associated periosteal inflammation involving metacarpals, metatarsals and phalanges. Patients may be misdiagnosed with rheumatological disorders.
2. Dactylitis may be the first sign of diagnosis. Initial X-rays show swelling only; but after a few days, periosteal elevation and areas of osteoporosis and sclerosis may be seen.
3. It is rare after 3 years of age, as the haematopoietic tissue in hands and feet is later replaced by fatty tissue.
4. Treatment is by pain relief and hydration.

HEPATOBILIARY AND ABDOMINAL INVOLVEMENT

1. Infarction within the spleen, mesenteric lymph nodes or liver.
2. It may present with signs of acute abdomen, with generalised abdominal pain and distension, with vomiting and diminished bowel sounds. X-ray is consistent with ileus. Management is conservative, with IV fluids and nasogastric aspiration.
3. Hepatic sequestration crisis can occur, with sickled cells held up in the liver.
4. Hepatocellular necrosis can occur, with hepatic failure.
5. Less serious hepatobiliary complications include cholelithiasis (pigmented bilirubinate gallstones, found in 10% of children aged 2–4 years with SCD), cholecystitis, and cholestasis (intrahepatic). Surgical management of these is the same as in those without SCA, with great care taken to avoid complications after general anaesthesia, such as ACS (see Anaesthetic considerations).

APLASTIC CRISIS

1. This is due to compromise of the compensatory response (increased red cell production) to ongoing haemolysis.
2. In SCA, red cell survival is only 10–20 days. If infection develops, patients may have red cell aplasia for 10–14 days. Causes include parvovirus B19, pneumococci, streptococci, *Salmonella* species and EB virus.

3. Cases present with pallor, tachypnoea, tachycardia and weakness.
4. White cell and platelet counts are normal; reticulocytes are decreased or absent.
5. Management is with transfusion (packed cells or exchange).

ANAESTHETIC CONSIDERATIONS

1. Both ACS and VOEs can complicate general anaesthesia (GA), attributed to changes which increase deoxyhaemoglobin polymerisation including altered pH, temperature, blood volume, blood flow and oxygenation. Hence, intraoperative attention must be paid to prevent acidosis, hypothermia, hypovolaemia, hypotension and hypoxia.
2. Postoperative complications can include atelectasis and respiratory splinting, which may be prevented by adequate analgesia, and incentive spirometry. ACS can occur, especially in thoracic or intraabdominal procedures, and/or if there is over-hydration. Postoperative supplemental oxygen should be given until patients are fully alert and breathing normally.

ALLOIMMUNISATION AND AUTOIMMUNISATION

Alloimmunisation describes an immune response where the patient's (recipient's) immune system mounts a response against the donor's erythrocytes, which are seen as foreign antigens. This process can limit the ability to find appropriate donor blood for future transfusions.

Autoimmunisation describes an immune response where the patient's (recipient's) own red cells become immunogenic; these typically occur in patients who already have a number of alloantibodies. Strict phenotypic matching of the Rh blood group system red cell antigens (C, c, D, E, e) and of minor group antigens (Duffy, Kell, Kidd), between donor and recipient, may decrease the frequency of alloimmunisation.

ACCUMULATION OF IRON (TRANSFUSION HAEMOSIDEROSIS)

The transfusion of red cells equates to the transfer of iron; as a rough rule of thumb, 1 mL of red cells contains 1 g of iron. Transfused blood contains iron which bypasses the usual control mechanisms for iron regulation, and particularly tends to accumulate in the heart, pancreas and the liver. Chelation therapy may be needed using desferrioxamine parenterally or deferiprone orally. MRI can estimate iron stores fairly accurately, enough to replace liver biopsy in the management plan. See the thalassaemia long case in this chapter for more on iron overload.

History

Ask about the following.

PRESENTING COMPLAINT

Reason for current admission.

PAST HISTORY

1. Age and mode of presentation (e.g. screening as a newborn, dactylitis as an infant, sequestration as a toddler, painful crisis as a schoolchild).
2. The progress of the disease, hospitalisation details, complications experienced (e.g. aplasia, sepsis, stroke), outpatient clinics attended.
3. Past treatment used (e.g. intravenous rehydration, analgesia, bicarbonate).
4. Recent changes in symptoms or management.

CURRENT STATUS

The nature and number of crises per year (e.g. bone, abdominal or chest pain), the usual precipitants (e.g. infection), treatment required (e.g. analgesia with narcotics, transfusions), the usual outcome.

Ongoing symptoms of complications: directed questioning regarding chronic haemolysis and anaemia (e.g. pallor, lethargy, poor growth, jaundice), neurological deficits (e.g. developmental progress), medications (e.g. prophylactic penicillin for hyposplenism) and management of crises when away from home (e.g. on holidays, travel to remote areas).

SOCIAL HISTORY

1. Disease impact on patient: effects of hospitalisations, behaviour, school attendance, self-image (e.g. short stature, leg ulcers, delayed puberty), peer group anxieties, narcotic abuse in older children.
2. Disease impact on parents: for example, financial considerations (medical treatment, awareness of benefits available), modification of holiday plans.
3. Disease impact on siblings: for example, sibling rivalry, genetic implications (screening for occult disease).
4. Social supports: for example, social worker, extended family.
5. Coping: for example, level of understanding of the disease by the parent (awareness of risks of sepsis, ability to palpate spleen to detect sequestration) and the patient (understanding of precautions to take with risks of hypoxia, high altitude, exposure to cold, and of the necessity for penicillin prophylaxis); any problems with analgesic abuse.
6. Access to the local doctor, paediatrician, hospital, tertiary centre of excellence.

FAMILY HISTORY

Ethnic origin, consanguinity of parents, other affected members, infant deaths in the family, plans for further children, genetic counselling.

IMMUNISATION

Routine, pneumococcal vaccine, meningococcal vaccine, hepatitis B vaccine.

Examination

The following outlines the main features sought in a long case with SCD; this approach would be adequate for a short-case examination.

GENERAL INSPECTION

1. Position patient: standing, fully undressed and then lying down.
2. Parameters: height, weight, head circumference, percentiles.
3. Tanner staging (delayed).
4. Racial origin (e.g. African).
5. Well or unwell (e.g. sepsis, painful crisis).
6. Skin: pallor (aplastic crisis, haemolytic crisis), jaundice, scratch marks (haemolysis).
7. Joint swelling: periarticular infarction.
8. Posture: for example, hemiparesis (cerebral sickling), restricted movement (bony infarction).
9. Dysphasia (cerebral sickling).
10. Abdominal distension (sequestration crisis).
11. Vital signs: respiratory rate (e.g. pneumonia), pulse (anaemia), BP (hypotension from bleeding), urinalysis (low specific gravity, blood, white cells).

DIRECTED EXAMINATION FOR COMPLICATIONS

Upper limbs

1. Screen joints for swelling.
2. Palpate bones for tenderness.
3. Neurological assessment.

Head and neck

1. Check eyes for visual field defects (cerebral infarction), conjunctival pallor, scleral icterus and proliferative retinopathy.
2. Examine the motor cranial nerves, especially noting whether there is an upper or lower motor neurone lesion of the seventh nerve (for localisation of damage in hemiplegia).
3. Check mouth for hydration.

Chest

Full examination of praecordium and lung fields for evidence of cardiac murmur, cardiac failure, pulmonary infarction or infection.

Abdomen

Full examination, noting any distension, tenderness or organomegaly.

Lower limbs

1. Inspect for ulcers (ankles).
2. Screen joints for swelling.
3. Palpate bones for tenderness.
4. Assess neurologically, commencing with gait examination for evidence of hemiplegia (or limp with joint involvement).

Management

Common management issues are as follows:

1. Management of acute complications.
2. Chronic transfusion therapy—prevention of primary manifestations.
3. Hydroxyurea—prevention of crises.
4. Avoiding known precipitants.
5. Elective surgery.
6. Complications of medical treatment.
7. Chronic problems.
8. Specific discussion areas.

1. MANAGEMENT OF ACUTE COMPLICATIONS

Acute transfusion therapy—simple transfusion and exchange transfusion

The efficacy of transfusion to treat acute complications of SCD is now proven. Exchange transfusion is preferred for four scenarios: acute chest syndrome; acute cerebrovascular accident/stroke; acute multi-organ failure; and in preparation for elective surgery. Exchange transfusion will be preferable in scenarios where there is a higher pre-transfusion haemoglobin, or when fluid overload or hyperviscosity are concerns. The exchange transfusion can be performed manually or can be automated; automated exchange transfusion is termed 'erythrocytapheresis' and is haematocrit and volume controlled, and Hb S can be decreased to a chosen level. Erythrocytapheresis can reduce the degree of transfusion-associated iron overload.

Simple transfusion can be used for sepsis (early use is preferable), sequestration (splenic or hepatic) and anaemia (aplastic episode or acute symptomatic).

Complications of transfusion can include infection, transfusion-related acute lung injury, transfusion-associated circulatory overload, (rarely) mismatched blood and, in the SCD population, alloimmunisation (a discrepancy in red cell antigens between the African American SCD population and the donor population; 30% develop antibodies), DHTR, hyperhaemolytic syndrome (if this occurs, the Hb level ends up lower than the pre-transfusion Hb, and erythropoietin, immunoglobulin and corticosteroids may be needed to resolve this).

Acute crises—supportive measures

All children should be admitted to hospital when having a crisis. Antibiotics are used for suspected infection; the ambient ward temperature should be moderately high. In suspected infarction/sickling, where the situation does not warrant acute transfusion therapy, then double maintenance intravenous fluids are given (5% dextrose is used, as it is isotonic and decreases propensity for sickling). If there is pulmonary involvement, oxygen therapy may be given. In severe sickling episodes, as outlined above, blood transfusions can be used to reduce the percentage of Hb SS to around 40–50%, which may prevent further sickling.

In cases with cerebral sickling, exchange transfusion can be performed. Adequate analgesia must be given (e.g. paracetamol, aspirin, codeine). Narcotic analgesia (e.g. morphine infusion) may be needed, but the risk of addiction must be considered (see Issues of adolescence). Adequate analgesia is important to limit the effects of vaso-occlusion. Ongoing pain can lead to sympathetic stimulation and ongoing restriction of blood flow, and perpetuate vaso-occlusion. Some units give bicarbonate during a crisis as prophylaxis against acidosis.

2. CHRONIC TRANSFUSION THERAPY—PREVENTION OF PRIMARY MANIFESTATIONS

The aim of chronic red blood cell transfusion therapy is, in the first instance, to keep the percentage of Hb S below 30% and suppress reticulocytosis. Chronic transfusion therapy is disease-modifying, and usually comprises monthly transfusions of PRBCs, which decreases the level of anaemia and suppresses the amount of Hb S in the blood. The following is a list of current indications for chronic transfusion therapy, at the time of writing (2017). Chronic transfusion and chelation therapy is an established therapy for primary and secondary prevention of overt stroke; hydroxyurea at maximum tolerated doses recently has been shown to be non-inferior to transfusion therapy in primary stroke prevention in children with SCD and high TCD velocities.

There are seven main indications for chronic transfusion—two associated with strokes, two with the pulmonary vasculature and three with chronic conditions—as follows:
1. Stroke prevention in patients with abnormal transcranial Doppler studies (high TCD velocities).
2. Prevention of stroke recurrence.
3. Pulmonary hypertension.
4. Recurrent episodes of pulmonary/acute chest syndrome.
5. Chronic pain refractory to all other treatment modalities.
6. Chronic kidney disease.
7. Chronic end-organ damage (other than kidney).

Complications of chronic transfusion therapy include iron overload, alloimmunisation and infection. It is recommended that extended matching of red cell antigens should be performed and blood products should be leukoreduced (white cells removed), to prevent alloimmunisation and transfusion reactions.

3. HYDROXYUREA—PREVENTION OF PRIMARY MANIFESTATIONS

Hydroxyurea (HU) remains the only approved medication in the management of SCD. It induces production of fetal haemoglobin (Hb F), decreasing sickling and increasing red cell survival, it lowers the white cell count, and its metabolism releases nitric oxide, which is a vasodilator. Treatment with HU leads to lower rates of acute painful crises, fewer episodes of ACS, less frequent transfusion requirements and improved survival.

HU is now established as being equivalent in efficacy to chronic transfusion therapy in stroke prevention, demonstrated by the TWiTCH study. Another study, the BABY HUG trial evaluated HU in younger children 9–18 months, to see if it could preserve splenic or renal function, but unfortunately there was no difference between HU and placebo in its co-primary endpoints, although secondary assessment indicated HU decreased need for transfusion, frequency of ACS, dactylitis, and other painful events. The several mechanisms of action of HU involve increasing the percentage of Hb F, which protects against sickling (increased intracellular Hb F dilutes Hb S and inhibits polymerisation), reducing the white blood cell count that may be involved in the sickling process, increasing red blood cell hydration, and decreasing the expression of red cell adhesion molecules. HU can ameliorate the course of SCA to resemble the milder sickle cell–Hb C disease.

HU may cause bone marrow suppression; patients need to be monitored carefully during the initiation of treatment and as the dose of HU is increased. Recommended testing before commencing HU includes full blood count and film, quantitative HbF level, urea and electrolytes, liver function tests, and in older female adolescents and adult females, pregnancy should be excluded. There has been concern that long-term exposure to HU in young patients may cause secondary malignancies.

Potential indications for HU include acute vaso-occlusive complications (painful events, dactylitis, ACS), severe disease on laboratory testing (low Hb, low Hb F, high WBC, high LDH), organ dysfunction (brain—increased transcranial Doppler velocities, silent MRI or MRA changes consistent with CVA, or prophylaxis against stroke; lungs—hypoxaemia; kidneys—proteinuria). Sometimes parents will request it after having read about it on the internet, and in some families an older sibling may be receiving it. Families need to know that it takes 6–12 months of therapy and monthly blood tests before an optimal dosing regimen can be established; treatment will fail without good compliance.

HU was developed as an anti-cancer drug. Its side effect profile is quite benign; acutely, it can cause mild abdominal discomfort, it can cause hyperpigmentation and melanonychia, and in around 1 in 1000, it can lead to renal or hepatic drug-related toxicity. It can depress all three cell lines; if neutrophils drop significantly (ANC < 1000 per microlitre), or Hb drops below 7.0 g/dL, or reticulocytes drop below 80 K per microlitre, or platelets drop below 80 K per microlitre, then stop HU until counts recover, and then recommence at a decreased dose. Its long-term risks are largely unknown; theoretical risks based on animal studies (potential teratogenicity or cancer development) have not come to fruition in humans.

4. AVOIDING KNOWN PRECIPITANTS

Knowledge of the common precipitants of crises allows guidelines to be drawn up. Patients should avoid the following:

1. Dehydration, to which they are prone because of their fixed hyposthenuria. Encourage the patient to drink plenty of fluids, especially during viral illnesses or in hot weather. During any infection, dehydration is anticipated and early hydration is instituted.

2. Infection with encapsulated bacteria. Prophylactic penicillin may be given, as well as immunisation against pneumococcus, *Haemophilus influenzae* type b and meningococcus.
3. Vascular stasis. Tight clothing (e.g. fashion jeans, cycling pants) and tourniquets when in hospital must be avoided.
4. Cold temperatures, either environmental (e.g. getting caught in the rain, swimming in rivers, cold baths, washing the car or doing the laundry [adolescents]) or related to ice-cold food or drinks.

Remember, *any* crisis may be precipitated by **ACIDOSES** (mnemonic: **A**cidosis, **C**old, **I**nfection, **D**ehydration, **O**xygen lack, **S**tress, **E**levated temperature, **S**port [exercise]).

A sequestration crisis may not necessarily be prevented by the above measures, but parents can be taught to palpate for splenic enlargement and seek medical attention more rapidly.

5. ELECTIVE SURGERY

Exchange transfusion may need to be undertaken before elective surgery. The other points worth noting are the avoidance of tourniquets, avoidance of preoperative dehydration and ensuring the administration of oxygen with any general anaesthetic agent. Close collaboration with the anaesthetic and surgical teams is critical. See the earlier section on anaesthetic considerations.

6. COMPLICATIONS OF MEDICAL TREATMENT

Analgesic abuse is a well-recognised complication in adolescents, so narcotic analgesia is best avoided except when absolutely necessary.

Chronic transfusion programs, which are occasionally needed (see later), can be associated with haemosiderosis, as in thalassaemic patients, and consequently the large number of related complications (see the long case on thalassaemia in this chapter).

Recent chronic transfusion regimens involve elective red blood cell apheresis (where the patient's red cells are removed at the same time as the patient has a red blood cell transfusion). This reduces the percentage of haemoglobin S and also reduces the need for iron chelation therapy. Other complications of transfusion therapy, such as transmission of HIV and hepatitis C, are infrequent.

7. CHRONIC PROBLEMS
Related to intravascular sickling

The most severe problems are neurological sequelae, commonly hemiplegia, which may require extensive rehabilitation, physiotherapy, and occupational and speech therapy. Hemiplegia may be recurrent, causing progressive damage, and may warrant chronic transfusion therapy. In adults, chronic failure of various organs (e.g. liver, kidney) is not infrequent, but this tends not to occur in children.

Related to susceptibility to encapsulated organisms

Parents need to be instructed to seek medical help if the child develops a significant fever (e.g. above 38.5°C). At the hospital, these children should have blood cultures taken, and consideration should be given to admission, and to intravenous or oral antibiotics.

This problem is lifelong, but is more common in infants. However, adolescents in particular must be reminded that the risk remains, as compliance can be difficult in this age group.

Related to chronic haemolytic anaemia

Chronic ankle ulceration is common in adolescent and adult patients, and is due to inadequate healing (a result of anaemia) of minor traumatic lesions. Management may include complete bed rest (immobilisation), debridement with proteolytic enzymes (or crushed papaya, as used in Jamaica), clean dressings, antibiotics, oral zinc sulfate or pinch skin grafting.

Pigmented gallstones can occur from as early as 3 years old. Stones are usually small and multiple, and can block the cystic and bile ducts, or be associated with acute or chronic cholecystitis. May require laparoscopic cholecystectomy.

Many units prescribe folic acid to prevent superimposed folate deficiency.

8. SPECIFIC DISCUSSION AREAS

Education

Given that parents assimilate a limited amount of information regarding SCA at any one time, the essential facts should be delivered and reinforced incrementally during the course of regular follow-up. Parents need to be taught about contingency plans for dealing with any of the following: fever, sudden pallor, abdominal distension, jaundice, recurrent pain (musculoskeletal, chest, abdomen), neurological symptoms (CVAs), swelling of hands and feet, and respiratory distress. A MedicAlert bracelet is advisable. The family should be taught home management of pain, and given guidelines about when to contact their doctor. The importance of routine immunisation, plus immunisation against pneumococcus, meningococcus and influenza, cannot be overemphasised. Penicillin therapy and folic acid therapy should be stressed also.

Discussion of the child's involvement in appropriate sporting activities is important, while the need for adequate hydration, avoidance of temperature extremes and good dental hygiene must be stressed.

Most patients with SCA know the names of their medications, and their regimens, by the age of around 10 years. Also, they should understand the basics of the pathophysiology.

Issues of adolescence

Problems include poor self-image (especially related to delays in both the adolescent growth spurt and sexual maturation), inability to predict onset, complications, difficulty planning an uncertain future, depression and the realisation of their own mortality. Drug addiction is another concern: adolescents should devise an appropriate pain management plan that explores non-addictive analgesics, but fear of addiction should not lead to denial of narcotics for severe pain.

Pregnancy

This should be discussed with all adolescent female patients. Pregnancy is a possible indication for a transfusion regime, because pregnancy is associated with an increased risk of infarctive crises, urinary tract problems and neonatal morbidity. In terms of contraception, combined oral contraceptives are not recommended, as they may increase the risk of vaso-occlusive episodes. Intrauterine devices may be associated with the risk of pelvic sepsis, infertility or menorrhagia. This leaves progesterone-only contraceptives or barrier methods as the most appropriate options.

Genetic counselling

Parents need to be aware of the 1 in 4 risk of recurrence, and not assume that the next three children will be normal. Siblings need to be screened at the time of diagnosis of the child with Hb SS. Parents should be given the option of antenatal diagnosis by chorionic villus biopsy at 9 weeks, and if the fetus is an Hb SS homozygote, termination may be undertaken if desired. Neonatal testing and the resultant improved outcome can be discussed with the parents should they opt for more children irrespective of the risk of an affected infant.

Neonatal screening—preventing early mortality: penicillin, immunisation, education

Neonatal screening for early detection of Hb SS (and related haemoglobinopathies), coupled with comprehensive medical management (immunisations, prophylactic penicillin), has decreased the mortality from sickle haemoglobinopathies. Universal screening would identify newborns with all forms of SCD, and initiate the trifecta of preventative strategies: 1. prophylactic penicillin, given twice daily, from early infancy to at least 5 years; 2. vaccination against encapsulated organisms; and 3. education of children with SCD and their parents regarding importance of urgent medical attention for fever, pallor and splenic enlargement.

Retrospective studies have shown previous mortality rates of up to 30% in the first 5 years for patients with Hb SS disease. The three greatest risks to the young patient are acute splenic sequestration, aplastic crisis and overwhelming sepsis.

Sepsis has been reported in up to 30% of patients and in some areas is associated with a mortality rate of almost 50%. Commence regular penicillin at 3 months, with immunisation against pneumococcus, *Haemophilus* and meningococcus at 18–24 months, and boosters at 3–5 years. Patients with Hb SC or sickle/β-thalassaemia, at same risk, require the same approach. The most important feature in preventing early mortality is parental education. Due to their protective high Hb F levels, the first 3 months of life are asymptomatic in affected babies. Splenic dysfunction can occur by 3 months, so penicillin prophylaxis is usually begun around 1 or 2 months of age. For children under 3 years, the usual treatment is phenoxymethylpenicillin 125 mg orally twice a day; over 3–5 years the dose is 250 mg orally twice a day. Children with Hb SC or with Hb Sβ-thalassaemia may not develop hyposplenism until much later than those with classic SCA, so these children may not start taking penicillin until 4 or 5 years of age.

Pain

Sickle cell pain is secondary to tissue damage. 'Severe painful crisis' infers treatment at a hospital with parenteral opioids for 4 hours or longer. There are three useful groups of medications with which candidates should be familiar: non-opioids (e.g. paracetamol, NSAIDs), opioids (e.g. morphine, meperidine) and adjuvants (e.g. antiemetics, antihistamines, laxatives).

Haematopoietic stem cell transplantation (HSCT)—potential cure

In 1999, the first unrelated cord blood cell transplant was used to cure a 12-year-old boy of SCA. He had some graft-versus-host disease, which responded to prednisolone, and was free of crises and no longer required any transfusions after the procedure. Umbilical cord blood (UCB)—the blood remaining in the placenta after the birth of a child—contains early and committed haematopoietic progenitor cells in sufficient numbers for transplantation.

There have been many successful reports of UCB transplantation in SCD from a related donor, the 2-year disease-free survival rate being 90%. Outcomes after UCB transplantation from sibling donors are similar to those after bone marrow transplantation (BMTx); see overleaf. Cryopreserved placental stem cell banks, which collect and store UCB for families who might benefit from UCB transplantation, are established in many countries.

Bone marrow transplantation (BMTx) is the best-established curative procedure, and the most conventional application of HSCT, but its risks can outweigh its advantages. These include the risk of infertility, graft-versus-host disease, worsening of sickle-related vascular disease, other complications of conditioning for transplantation (e.g. side effects of any of busulfan, cyclophosphamide, cyclosporine, methotrexate, anti-thymocyte globulin [ATG] or prednisolone), and a short-term mortality of 10%.

Given that the average life span of an SCA patient is over 60 years, this must be carefully weighed against the risks of BMTx, also knowing that other treatment modalities are improving rapidly. After BMTx, event-free survival among children with SCA has been around 85%.

Indications for BMTx have included recurrent ACS, CVA and recurrent severe vaso-occlusive crises. Graft rejection occurs in 10–15%. Only 10% of children with Hb SS fulfil criteria for BMTx, and only 20% of those have a suitable donor. The best results have been achieved following transplantation from HLA-identical sibling donors. BMTx is a consideration for a child on a long-term transfusion regimen, with HLA-identical siblings. Contraindications have included sero-positivity for HIV, lack of compliance with medical care, severe lung disease, severe renal impairment, severe neurological impairment, acute hepatitis, or severe portal fibrosis or cirrhosis.

The indications for HSCT relate to patients 16 years old or younger with SCD, with an HLA-identical sibling bone marrow donor, with one or more of the following (mnemonic: **STAR IS BORN**):

Stroke, central nervous system (CNS) haemorrhage or a neurological event lasting longer than 24 hours, or an abnormal cerebral magnetic resonance imaging (MRI) scan, cerebral arteriogram or MRI angiographic study and impaired neuropsychological testing

Transfusion requirement, but with red blood cell (RBC) alloimmunisation of more than two antibodies during long-term transfusion therapy

ACS, with a history of recurrent hospitalisations or exchange transfusions

Recurrent vaso-occlusive pain—three or more episodes per year for 3 years or more—or recurrent priapism

Impaired neuropsychological function and abnormal cerebral MRI scan

Stage I or II sickle lung disease

Bilateral proliferative retinopathy and major visual impairment in at least one eye

Osteonecrosis of multiple joints, with documented destructive changes

Respiratory disease—see **S** above

Nephropathy (moderate-severe proteinuria or GFR 30–50% of the predicted normal value)

Cure through stem cell transplantation

There are several reports of patients having been cured by stem cell transplantation, using healthy tissue-matched siblings as donors, without requiring any chemotherapy to 'prepare' the bone marrow.

Transition to adult care and prognosis

At the time of writing (2017), almost all children with SCD, who are born in developed countries, are able to reach adulthood. The transition to adult medical management is a time of increased risk for morbidity and mortality, partially due to the ongoing pathological processes of chronic end-organ injury, and partially due to the imperfect interface between the parent-supervised paediatric care coordinated within highly organised SCD centres, and the adult clinics which patients now attend by themselves. The life span for SCD now exceeds 60 years. The life span for those with Hb SC and Hb Sβ+thalassaemia is the same as for the general population.

Therapies being investigated

These include: induction of fetal Hb (Hb F) (e.g. inhibitors to protein Bc111a [a Hb F cell quantitative trait locus which suppresses fetal globin gene expression in adult cells]); antioxidants therapy (e.g. glutamine); replenishment of NO stores (e.g. arginine); prevention of Hb S polymerisation (e.g. 5-HMF); decreased adhesion to endothelium (e.g. GMI-1070, prasugrel); changing inflammatory responses (e.g. regadenoson); gene therapy is likely to be an available treatment eventually, but progress has been slow so far due to inadequate gene transfer, and low gene expression. Research accelerated after the identification of a locus control region (LCR), which is necessary for transcriptional activity of the globin cluster. Research is focusing on gene therapy to inactivate the Hb S gene, or its messenger RNA, increase the expression of the Hb F gene, or utilise genes that produce inhibitors of Hb S polymerisation. As this area of research is constantly advancing, refer to https://clinicaltrials.gov.

LONG CASES

LONG CASE: Thalassaemia—β-thalassaemia major (β-TM)

The thalassaemias are the most common single-gene diseases in the world. They are disorders of haemoglobin synthesis, classified according to the globin chain, which is ineffectively produced. Therefore β-globin gene mutations lead to β-thalassaemia, and α-globin mutations lead to α-thalassaemia. β-thalassaemia major is particularly prevalent in countries around the Mediterranean Sea and the Middle and Far East, and, with population migration, it is found throughout the world. Many components of management are just as relevant in other types of thalassaemia, or thalassaemia-like disorders (e.g. homozygous haemoglobin Lepore, β-thalassaemia haemoglobin Lepore double heterozygotes or haemoglobin-E β-thalassaemia). The anaemia can be corrected by blood transfusion, but ongoing transfusions have adverse effects including iron overload.

Background information
BASIC DEFECT (β-THALASSAEMIA MAJOR)

1. Decreased synthesis of the β-globin chain of haemoglobin.
2. Normal synthesis of the α chain of haemoglobin, leading to the accumulation of unstable aggregates within the red blood cells, resulting in ineffective erythropoiesis and haemolysis. In patients with concomitant α-thalassaemia, the symptoms of haemolysis may be ameliorated.
3. Hypochromic microcytic anaemia (*note*: the mean cell volume may be in the normal range for children, but abnormal for that child). The number of reticulocytes is less than expected for the degree of the anaemia. Diagnostic blood film features include target cells, anisocytosis, poikilocytosis, schistocytosis, basophilic stippling and erythroblastosis.

GENETICS

1. Autosomal recessive; β-globin gene on the short arm of chromosome 11, in a region that contains the embryonic- and fetal-globin genes. The expression of these globin

genes is controlled by the LCR, a major regulatory region containing a series of hypersensitive sites that interact with a variety of transcription factors.

2. The frequency of the gene in Greek Cypriots is 0.2; in Italians and Lebanese, 0.04.

3. By 2002, over 200 different molecular defects were known, mostly involving single nucleotide substitutions or oligonucleotide insertions/deletions, which inactivate the β gene expression by various mechanisms. Some mutations silence the β-globin gene (from mRNA modification at the splicing or cleavage steps; or from RNA mutations, causing abnormal translation of the gene to a globin chain product, mostly caused by premature termination codon), resulting in β^0-thalassaemia; others reduce β-globin output, resulting in β^+-thalassaemia (either by DNA transcriptional mutations at the promoter site, or from mRNA modification at the splicing or cleavage steps). Depending on the residual β-globin production, β^+-thalassaemia may be silent, mild or severe. β^0-Thalassaemia mutations are usually severe. If a single β-globin gene is affected, then the resulting phenotype depends on whether there is partial or absent gene expression. If partial, then this is silent carrier status; if absent, then this is the β-thalassaemia trait. Should both β-globin genes be affected, then the phenotype is more severe, depending on the degree of gene expression, and on the relative imbalance of the globin chains. It is termed 'thalassaemia intermedia' if the genotype is β^+/β^+, but thalassaemia major if the genotype is β^0/β^0. The resultant imbalance between the excessive α chains and the diminished β chains leads to unpaired globin chains, which can precipitate and cause premature death (apoptosis) of red cell precursors in the bone marrow, this being called 'ineffective erythropoiesis'.

DIAGNOSIS

1. Usually not clinically evident until the child is 6–12 months old.
2. Definitive diagnosis is by haemoglobin electrophoresis: HbA is absent or minimal, HbF is elevated and HbA2 may be raised. The percentage of fetal haemoglobin is the most important laboratory parameter.
3. Molecular genetic testing methods may be based on ancestry such as targeted analysis for pathogenic variants or, if there is no high-risk ancestry and targeted analysis does not show a pathogenic variant, single-gene testing by sequence analysis of HBB or gene-targeted duplication/deletion analysis of HBB.
4. There is a screening program provided in Australia based on the detection of microcytosis in females of child-bearing age, and testing their partners to confirm their status.

MAJOR COMPLICATIONS

Excess erythropoiesis (causing bone marrow expansion)

1. Bony changes to face: maxillary overgrowth, protrusion of teeth, separation of orbits, frontal bossing, chronic sinusitis and impaired hearing.
2. Bones (general): cortical thinning and risk of fractures. Most adult patients get osteopenia and osteoporosis, with backache, scoliosis, fractures and other spinal deformities. Males who are diabetic and have pubertal delay are most at risk for osteoporosis. DXA (dual-energy X-ray absorptiometry) assesses for bone density.
3. Spinal cord compression (vertebral expansion).
4. Lymphadenopathy (especially mediastinal).
5. Hepatosplenomegaly.

Iron overload (causing parenchymal organ toxicity)

This is transfusional or from increased iron absorption. Free iron is toxic to cells, so iron is normally complexed to proteins; in plasma, iron is bound to transferrin, which transports it to the cells. Remember the basics of iron metabolism: an average adult has 4 g of iron in his/her body; of this, two-thirds is in haemoglobin in erythrocytes. Each day, 25 mg of iron is needed for erythropoiesis, although the majority is recycled iron by macrophages from old red cells.

The diet usually provides 1 or 2 mg absorbable iron daily; intestinal absorption regulates total body iron. The formula for transfusional iron input is:

$$\text{volume of packed red cells} \times \text{haematocrit of the unit} \times 1.08$$

A packed red blood cell unit (of around 250 mL) contains around 180–200 mg of iron. For most patients transfusional iron input approximates 0.3–0.5 mg/kg/day.

Iron not bound to transferrin (which includes labile plasma iron [LPI] and non-transferrin bound iron [NTBI]) is toxic to the endocrine organs, the liver and the heart, where myocyte damage can lead to arrhythmias and cardiac failure. Cardiac toxicity is the main cause of death related to iron overload in thalassaemia.

The goal of chelation is to prevent organ toxicities. Chelation can reverse some already developed toxicities, such as cardiac complications, but the endocrinopathies are generally irreversible. After transfusion of 10–20 red cell units, iron overload may have occurred sufficient to require chelation. After transfusion of 50–100 red cell units, iron overload may have occurred sufficient to cause organ dysfunction.

There is a significant difference between the iron overload in TM and that in SCD. Patients with TM have ineffective erythropoiesis and increased iron absorption, even if they are not transfused. Patients with SCD have effective erythropoiesis but do not develop increased iron absorption unless transfused. Inflammation (which is part of SCD, but not TM) increases hepcidin secretion, decreases iron absorption and keeps iron in the reticuloendothelial system. Iron-induced cardiac and endocrine disorders are fair more common in TM than in SCD. Transfusion requirements are higher in TM (starting at 3–6 months, every 2–4 weeks) than SCD (starting later in life and less frequently). TM is associated with a higher prevalence of disease-specific iron overload than SCD: cardiac disease occurs in 20% of TM (versus 0% of SCD); growth failure occurs in 27% of TM (versus 9% of SCD); and endocrine failure occurs in 37% of TM (versus 0% of SCD). There is also a difference in oxidative stress levels between the two diseases. Inflammation in SCD causes more elevated levels of the anti-oxidant gamma-tocopherol, which causes less tissue peroxidation and injury than occurs in TM.

Endocrine failure (in order of frequency)

1. Short stature: growth is usually normal until about 12 years, but no pubertal growth spurt occurs: two-thirds of these children are below the 10th height percentile at 21 years. A possible pituitary or hypothalamic defect. Growth hormone level may be normal or raised.
2. Delayed puberty: gonadotropin levels are normal until puberty, but then no increase occurs. Hypogonadotrophic hypogonadism can be treated with hormonal therapy and aggressive iron chelation, to preserve fertility.
3. Oestrogen/testosterone deficiency.
4. Hypothyroidism.
5. Diabetes mellitus.
6. Hypoparathyroidism.
7. Osteopenia and osteoporosis can occur in adults; bisphosphonate therapy may be used.

Cardiac involvement

1. Cardiomyopathy from myocardial iron deposition, hypertrophy, dilatation, degeneration of myocardial fibres; unbound iron generates toxic oxygen metabolites; higher risk for myocarditis; occasional pulmonary hypertension.
2. Pericarditis: first attack usually after 10 years of age.
3. Arrhythmias (ventricular/atrial) can occur. Risk increased after 150–200 units of blood.
4. Congestive cardiac failure: once this develops, the mortality is 90% within 12–18 months. Cardiac function can be reversed by aggressive chelation. Treatment may include ACE inhibitors, digoxin, diuretics and a low-salt diet, in addition to chelation therapy. If refractory to medical treatment, heart transplantation is an appropriate consideration.
5. Measurement of liver iron correlates best with total body iron and predicts the threshold for risk for moderate complications (levels of hepatic iron 7–15 mg/g dry weight), or for risk of cardiac disease and early death (levels over 15 mg/g dry weight). The gold standard is liver biopsy. There are two non-invasive procedures that give results that correlate well with biopsy: liver iron concentration by MRI, and liver iron concentration by the superconducting quantum interference device (SQUID) technique—which is expensive and has limited availability. Ferritin over 2500 micrograms/L can help predict cardiac disease.
6. Measurement of cardiac iron loading by MRI can predict risk for cardiac disease, but cannot be validated with biopsy specimens, as can occur with the liver. Iron deposits shorten MRI T2* decay time (T2* is a relaxation parameter, representing the half-life of tissue darkening; cardiac T2* is measured in milliseconds, and the worse it is, the lower the value of T2* would be): if cardiac T2* is > 20 ms, this is normal; if cardiac T2* is 10–20 ms, there is a moderate to severe cardiac iron load; and if cardiac T2* is < 10 ms, there is severe cardiac iron load and risk of death.
7. Heart disease is the cause of death in 70% of transfusion-induced iron-overload patients. Cardiac iron removal can be achieved with chelation with deferasirox (DFS).

Hepatic involvement

1. Inflammation, cirrhosis and hepatic fibrosis: the risk for this is increased after 7 years of treatment.
2. Liver function tests may be abnormal, but it is rare to see symptoms of cirrhosis. If hepatic enzyme levels are increased four- to five-fold, then there is a possibility of hepatitis and liver biopsy may be needed.
3. Common cause of morbidity and early death; worsened by coexistent hepatitis C virus (HCV).
4. If HCV is suspected, liver biopsy is needed and the HCV RNA PCR should be checked. Image to exclude hepatocellular carcinoma. Curative treatment is available.

Chronic haemolysis

Gallstones are present in 50–70% of patients by around 15 years of age. Consider cholecystectomy only if biliary colic or obstructive jaundice occurs. At the time of splenectomy, consider ultrasound of the gall bladder and cholecystectomy if calculi are present. Appendicectomy at this time may be appropriate, because these patients are at risk of *Yersinia* infection, which can mimic appendicitis and might lead to surgery at a time when an operation should be contraindicated.

Alloimmunisation

Chronic transfusion can lead to anti-RBC antibodies, alloantibodies and autoantibodies developing. The rate of alloimmunisation is between 3 and 37%, and the rates are higher if there is ethnic disparity between donor and recipient, or if the spleen is already removed. It has been recommended that extended RBC phenotyping is done before transfusions are initiated. There is evidence that matching for Rhesus and Kell antigens can halve the alloantibody rate.

Hypercoagulable state

There is an increased risk for thrombosis for patients with β-thalassaemia major and for patients with haemoglobin-E/β-thalassaemia. Increased risk occurs in those who are transfused infrequently and in those who are splenectomised. The mechanism involves increased platelet activation, elevated endothelial adhesion protein levels and activation of coagulation cascade by damaged red cells (these have disrupted membranes, exposing negatively charged lipids, such as phosphatidylserine, on the surface of the cell, which are thrombogenic). Deep venous thrombosis, pulmonary embolism (mostly asymptomatic) and cerebral ischaemia have been described.

Infection

There is an increased risk of infection, particularly *Yersinia*, in iron-overload patients; patients may be splenectomised.

History

Ask about the following.

PRESENTING COMPLAINT

Reason for current admission.

FAMILY HISTORY

Consanguinity of parents, other affected members, neonatal deaths in family, plans for further children, genetic counselling.

SPECIFIC COMPLICATIONS

The current status of the following complications (mnemonic **THALASSAEMIA**):

Tanner stage (pubertal delay)
Heart (cardiomyopathy)/**H**aematopoiesis (extramedullary)/**H**ypercoagulable
Anaemia
Liver/**L**ong tracts (neurological involvement)/**L**eg ulcers
Appearance (thalassaemic facies, pigmentation)
Sugar diabetes
Short stature
Arrhythmias
Eye/**E**ndocrine
Metabolic (hypocalcaemia)/**M**alocclusion
Iron overload/**I**cterus/**I**nfection/**I**atrogenic (DFS, DFO side effects)
Adenopathy and hepatosplenomegaly

PAST HISTORY

1. Ethnic origin.
2. Diagnosis (age, where, how).
3. Age at insertion of first venous access port; age at first transfusion and at commencement of iron chelation with DFS or DFO.
4. Number of transfusions per year.
5. Previous hospitalisations (other than routine transfusions), previous surgery (e.g. splenectomy), medications given (e.g. penicillin with splenectomy, vitamin C), local centre of excellence where patient cared for.

SOCIAL HISTORY

1. Disease impact on patient: for example, effects of hospitalisations, behaviour, school performance, amount of school missed, self-image, pubertal anxieties, peer group anxieties, stigma of 'bad blood', adolescent denial, poor compliance, anxiety, 'live for today' approach, concerns about developing relationships, wanting a family.
2. Disease impact on parents: for example, marriage stability, financial considerations (family income; if receiving DFO, cost of this plus pump), dealing with non-compliance and teenage rebellion.
3. Disease impact on siblings: for example, sibling rivalry.
4. Social supports: for example, extended family, Australian Thalassaemia Association and state thalassaemia societies, social worker, financial benefits obtained (e.g. Child Disability Assistance Payment).
5. Coping: for example, compliance, degree of self-management, perception of the disease and its rate of progression, future plans, career thoughts.

Examination

See the short case on thalassaemia in this chapter.

Standard management principles

BLOOD TRANSFUSION

1. Regular transfusions every 4–6 weeks.
2. Timing of first transfusion usually at haemoglobin (Hb) < 60 g/L. Venous access ports are placed for chronically transfused patients if transfusions start at a very young age.
3. Maintain Hb > 100 g/L (range 100–150 g/L; e.g. pre-transfusion Hb about 95 g/L, post-transfusion 140 g/L, with a mean of about 120 g/L). This level is enough to suppress endogenous erythropoiesis and compensatory marrow hyperplasia, while avoiding unnecessary iron overload.
4. Use packed cells, or filtered red blood cells, negative for hepatitis B, C and HIV (phenotyped filtered red cells).
5. Watch for reactions at the time of transfusions.
6. Pre-transfusion investigations: group and cross-match (genotype); full blood count (for haemoglobin level and reticulocyte count, and to assess for hypersplenism); initial viral serology for hepatitis B, C (± G: research units), cytomegalovirus (CMV), toxoplasmosis, Epstein-Barr virus, HIV; assessment for alloantibodies. The red cell genotype determines all the important red cell groups, including Duffy and Kell. Antibody screening at the time of cross-match is to detect any irregular alloantibodies.
Whenever the child is seen (at monthly transfusion and at regular outpatient review), an assessment of the transfusion requirements is needed, looking at the pre-transfusion Hb and transfusion interval.

If the child needs more frequent transfusions than previously, the considerations include the following:

1. Development of hypersplenism (± decreased platelet and white cell counts).
2. Development of red cell antibodies.
3. Concurrent gastrointestinal blood loss.
4. Use of 'old' blood.

CHELATION WITH DEFERASIROX (DFS)

Transfusional iron overload can be prevented with appropriate iron chelation. Oral chelator therapies are used in preference to the previous 'gold standard' of SC desferrioxamine (DFO, Desferal). DFO had been used for many years, but its disadvantage of requiring SC or IV administration has led to it being superseded by deferasirox (DFS, Exjade [Novartis]), an oral medication given once per day, which can prevent iron overload.

1. Deferasirox (DFS) was the first oral agent approved for use in the US. It is a tridentate chelator; two molecules of DFS are needed to bind one atom of iron.
2. It is supplied as a dispersible tablet to be dissolved in water or juice. It has a long half-life (up to 16 hours) and so can be given once daily. The recommended initial daily dose is 20 mg/kg. For patients who are already well controlled and receiving DFO, the starting dose of DFS is half that of DFO; hence DFS 20 mg/kg is equivalent to DFO 40 mg/kg.
3. The response to DFS depends on the transfusion requirements; for patients with a lower transfusional iron intake, it is effective in decreasing liver iron stores, but it is ineffective in some patients with higher transfusional iron intake.
4. DFS is effective in removing myocardial iron, which is associated with a concomitant decrease in total body iron. Iron levels can be quantified in a non-invasive manner using cardiac MRI to measure myocardial T2*, which is a measure of magnetic relaxation, and it shortens when the particulate stored iron interrupts the magnetic microenvironment, so that as T2* falls, the risk of left ventricular dysfunction increases.
5. The side effects of DFS include gastrointestinal problems (nausea, vomiting, abdominal pain), skin rashes, elevated transaminases, cataracts and audiotoxicity.
6. As with DFO, pre-chelation evaluation may include clinical photography, bone X-rays, ferritin level, full blood count, liver function tests, thyroid function tests, fasting blood glucose level, tests of the hypothalamic–pituitary (HP) axis, calcium, phosphate and magnesium, audiovisual assessment (audiometry; slit-lamp examination) and baseline electrocardiogram.
7. Avoidance of red meat and cereals should be recommended, as above.
8. Patients who are compliant with iron chelation therapy should have a life expectancy of more than 50 years, as above.

CHELATION WITH DESFERRIOXAMINE (DFO)

DFO (Desferal) requires SC or IV administration, but remains widely used worldwide.

1. Start when ferritin level is around 1000–2000 µg/L (before 3–4 years) or at preschool age. DFO was previously standard therapy. It has high molecular weight (MW), is poorly absorbed from the gut and so is given parenterally, aiming for negative iron balance.
2. The DFO molecule has six binding sites and wraps itself around the iron nucleus.
3. Dosage for DFO is 20-30 mg/kg for young children, increasing to 40 mg/kg after age 6 years, SC over 8–10 hours, 6 days per week.
4. Side effects of DFO include local irritation and hypotension if given too quickly intravenously. More severe effects were originally described when doses in the range 100–200 mg/kg/day were used. These included problems with vision (cataracts,

night blindness, reduction of visual fields, decreased visual acuity, and pigmentary retinopathy) and hearing (sensorineural deafness). Other side effects described have included bone abnormalities (pseudorickets, metaphyseal changes, flat vertebral bodies) and altered renal function. At doses less than 50 mg/kg/day, these effects are not often seen.

5. Pre-chelation evaluation may include clinical photography, bone X-rays, ferritin level, full blood count, liver function tests, thyroid function tests, fasting blood glucose level, tests of the HP axis, calcium, phosphate and magnesium, audiovisual assessment (audiometry; slit-lamp examination), baseline electrocardiogram.

6. Avoidance of red meat and cereals should be recommended.

7. Patients who are compliant with iron chelation therapy should have a life expectancy of more than 50 years.

8. DFO treatment is suspended if the patient has sepsis, as DFO promotes *Yersinia enterocolitica* gastroenteritis.

SPLENECTOMY

1. The main indication is hypersplenism, usually evidenced by increased transfusion requirements. Another indication is a 'large spleen', causing discomfort.

2. Most authorities recommend the use of pneumococcal and meningococcal vaccines (given before splenectomy) and prophylactic penicillin.

3. Consideration should also be given to gall bladder ultrasound for calculi, with a view to the possible need for cholecystectomy, which can be performed at the same time as splenectomy. Appendicectomy can be performed at the same time.

4. If a patient with a splenectomy is febrile, blood cultures should be taken and treatment instituted with intravenous antibiotics in hospital or oral antibiotics at home.

5. Some units suggest splenectomy only if transfusion requirements > 180–200 mL/kg/year.

IMMUNISATION

Routine; it should include hepatitis B plus pneumococcal vaccine (before splenectomy, and boosters every 5 years), meningococcal vaccine (splenectomised) and influenza vaccine.

Common management issues

Although the previous section is headed 'Standard management principles', much is not 'black and white', but 'grey'. This section touches on some of these areas.

WHEN TO START TRANSFUSIONS?

This is really a clinical decision. There is no specific haemoglobin level, but if the level is below 50 g/L, there needs to be a good reason not to transfuse. Careful assessment in the first 2 months after diagnosis is needed, and treatment with folate. If there is any failure to thrive, significant anaemia or (especially) cardiac compromise related to anaemia, then transfusion should probably be instituted.

WHICH TRANSFUSION REGIMEN?

The aim of transfusion is to correct anaemia and achieve marrow suppression to decrease myeloproliferation. Usually, a level of between 100 and 150 g/L is desirable, but this depends on the individual patient. Some patients with a haemoglobin level of 110 g/L will have multiple nucleated red cells and will need to be transfused to over 120 g/L, whereas in other patients 110 g/L may suffice. If the patient presents quite late (e.g. at

3 or 4 years of age) with splenomegaly, on occasion splenectomy can be offered first, which may cause a rise in the haemoglobin and defer the need to start transfusion therapy. Most children require transfusion every 4 weeks. Children requiring multiple transfusions from an early age have venous access ports placed.

WHEN TO CHELATE?

Chelation should start when the child can tolerate the treatment. If this is DFO, this is when the child is large enough for the parents to manage needles. Another indicator is a rising ferritin level. By 3–4 years of age, most patients have been transfused for 2 years. These children may have ferritin levels over 2000 µg/L. Some haematologists commence chelation when the ferritin level reaches 1000 µg/L.

HOW TO CHELATE?

Deferasirox (DFS) is the preferred agent. It is taken orally, as a dissolvable tablet, and has been shown to remove iron from the heart. Previously, using DFO, some units chelated daily for the first 6 months, then allowed one day off per week. Thus most patients had chelation therapy 6 days a week, by SC infusion, over 8–10 hours each day, via a portable pump. When the child is having regular transfusion therapy, some units add desferrioxamine to the blood being transfused, whereas other centres are averse to this idea for reasons of potential lack of sterility. Recommended dosage depends on age and ferritin.

ARE THERE ALTERNATIVE CHELATORS?

There are three iron chelators used in thalassaemia. DFS is now the preferred therapy. DFO is the previous standard therapy. Another oral chelator, deferiprone (DFP, Ferriprox), has been available for some time, but is not approved for use in the USA. DFP has only two binding sites: three molecules are needed to bind one iron atom. It has low MW and is readily absorbed from the gut; however, it can penetrate other cells and interfere with iron-requiring enzyme systems. DFP is used predominantly in countries where the effects of haemosiderosis outweigh the risks of DFP. The side effects of DFP can include neutropenia and agranulocytosis (idiosyncratic, but reversible), arthropathy (affects mainly large joints; usually reversible), zinc deficiency, gut symptoms and fluctuations in liver function. Other iron chelators are being developed, including deferitrin (DFT) and pyridoxal isonicotinoyl hydrazone (PIH); both are orally active tridentate iron chelators.

CURATIVE THERAPIES: HAEMATOPOIETIC STEM CELL TRANSPLANTATION (HSCT)

A definitive cure is either a BMTx from a HLA-identical sibling, or a cord blood transplantation from a related donor. BMTx is the most conventional form of HSCT that can cure β-thalassaemia. There appear to be three clinically important variables in patients under 16 that are predictive of the success of BMTx. If there is 1. no significant liver enlargement, 2. no liver fibrosis and 3. adherence to the regular high-quality iron chelation, there is around 90% event-free survival. The rate decreases as the risk factors increase.

The enthusiasm for this mode of treatment varies between countries. Some countries prefer to wait for breakthroughs in genetic engineering or a HbF switch mechanism; whereas in Italy, BMTx is quite popular but has a 10% mortality rate related to infection or acute graft-versus-host reaction.

The donor must be fully compatible (usually a sibling who is normal or heterozygous). It is not justified to offer any mismatched or matched unrelated donor transplantation. This treatment modality should be discussed with the parents of any child with thalassaemia, so that they are aware of this option in the future.

Cord blood-derived stem cell transplantation (CB-SCT) also can cure thalassaemia major. UCB, the blood remaining in the placenta after the birth of a child, contains early and committed haematopoietic progenitor cells in sufficient numbers for transplantation. There have been many successful reports of UCB transplantation in β-thalassaemia from a related donor, the 2-year disease-free survival rate being 79%. Outcomes after UCB transplantation from sibling donors are similar to those after BMTx.

It is worth remembering that the myeloablative therapy that is involved in the conditioning regimen for HSCT has the associated risks of chronic graft-versus-host disease (GVHD), cancer and, in particular, sterility; whereas with optimal compliance and supportive therapy, young adults with thalassaemia can have children themselves naturally.

CHELATION AFTER BONE MARROW TRANSPLANTATION

Post-stem cell transplantation there remains the iron accumulated over the previous years of transfusion therapy. If the patient has a high enough haemoglobin, then phlebotomy can be effective in removing this excess iron. Many patients receive their stem cell transplant from a donor with thalassaemia trait, and their haemoglobin level may not reach a level that allows phlebotomy. In these patients, chelation therapy may be needed for several months.

GENE THERAPY

The first report of transfusion independence following gene therapy was for a patient with $\beta^E\beta^0$-thalassaemia in 2007; an SIN (self-inactivating) LV (lentivirus)-based β^{T87Q} vector was used, and a transduction efficiency of 30% reported. That patient had busulfan conditioning for myeloablation, and then 3.9×10^6 CD34+ cells/kg of haematopoietic stem cells which had been gene-transduced.

It took 2 years to become transfusion independent and 5 years later this had been maintained. Trials are ongoing with lentivirus vectors in multiple research sites; other vectors include retrovirus vectors (RV) and foamy virus vectors (FV). Other newer technologies include the use of induced pluripotent stem cells (iPSC), and gene editing.

FETAL HAEMOGLOBIN (Hb F) AUGMENTATION: HU, r-HuEPO, SCFAs

Hydroxyurea (HU), which is a ribonucleotide reductase inhibitor, can induce production of fetal haemoglobin (HbF). HU has been reported to eliminate transfusion requirements in some children with severe β-TM with specific mutations. Some studies have used *recombinant human erythropoietin (r-HuEPO)* by itself or with HU. HU is a very cost-effective treatment, and an ideal option for millions of people in developing countries who do not have access to safe transfusion and chelation. *Short-chain fatty acids (SCFAs)* can be Hb F inducers; these include: *arginine butyrate*, which can increase the total Hb by more than 3 g/dL in β-TM, and can decrease the duration of days spent as an inpatient in hospital by three quarters; and *sodium phenylbutyrate*, which can increase total Hb in 50% of those with β-TM.

HEPATITIS C

For patients who are positive for hepatitis C (HCV), there is curative therapy available, and although it is very expensive, the Australian Government has seen fit to list these new direct-acting antiviral agents (DAAs) on the Pharmaceutical Benefits Scheme (PBS). The DAAs include: *single agents*: daclatas**vir**; riba**vir**in; sofosbu**vir**, the *duo* of sofosbu**vir** + ledipas**vir**; the *combination* of paritapre**vir** + ritona**vir** + ombitas**vir** + dasabu**vir**; and the latter *combination* with the addition of ribavirin. Response to treatment can be monitored by HCV titres. Some units recommend 6-monthly liver ultrasound studies, and even yearly liver biopsies, to look for hepatocellular carcinoma.

PRENATAL DIAGNOSIS (PND)

There are over 200 different molecular defects of the haemoglobin subunit β (HBB) gene known for β-thalassaemia. Within given communities, there are a dozen or so common molecular defects.

Targeted mutation analysis uses a number of PCR-based procedures, such as reverse dot blot analysis or primer specific amplification using a set of probes or primers complementary to the most common mutations in that particular community, to detect common mutations. If this fails to identify the mutation, then mutation scanning or sequence analysis can be used. Prenatal diagnosis and PGD (see below) can be performed only in at-risk pregnancies where the mutation is known.

If the parents already have an affected child, then prenatal identification of HLA compatibility with an unaffected fetus enables collection of placental blood at delivery and future cure with cord blood transfusion. If the fetus is affected but there is an older sibling who is unaffected and HLA compatible, then the parents may continue the pregnancy with a plan for a later BMTx.

PREIMPLANTATION GENETIC DIAGNOSIS (PGD)

Although this is unlikely to be a major discussion point in the paediatric long case, this area of technological advancement, which can involve whole gene amplification (WGA) and preimplantation genetic haplotyping (PGH) of embryos, leads to the ethical question of creating matched siblings suitable for haematopoietic stem cell transplantation, utilising PGD along with HLA testing (PGD-H).

PGD is the detection of genetic information in an embryo fertilised in vitro, by taking a blastomere at the preimplantation stage (day 3) of development to find embryos that are not affected by a serious genetic disorder—in this case, thalassaemia. It is an alternative to prenatal diagnosis (PND) and termination of affected pregnancy for couples at risk of having a pregnancy affected by a serious genetic disorder.

FOLLOW-UP

For the preschool child, some units recommend monthly pre-transfusion outpatient clinic reviews. For older children, an outpatient review is warranted on a 6-monthly basis, monitoring the child's growth in particular. In terms of investigations, some units recommend the following:

1. A check of the ferritin level (the degree of iron overload) every 3–6 months. Once receiving chelation, if ferritin levels are 2000 µg/L, this suggests non-compliance. Levels over 3000 µg/L may warrant liver MRI (for iron content; MRI images darken at a rate proportional to the iron concentration) and hospital admission for continuous intravenous DFO once or twice a month.
2. Blood tests every 6 months for calcium, magnesium, phosphate (hypoparathyroidism), liver function (hepatitis or hepatic fibrosis), thyroid function (hypothyroidism), urea, electrolytes and creatinine (renal dysfunction from DFO). If ALT is elevated, repeat in one month: if still up, check for hepatitis A, B, C or G, or CMV or Epstein-Barr virus (EBV). If ALT is elevated for 3 months, consider liver biopsy and hepatitis viral titres by RNA analysis. HIV serology should be checked as well.
3. Yearly assessments for DFS or DFO toxicity (audiometry and slit-lamp examination) and of growth and pubertal status (bone age and, over the age of 14, tests of the HP axis). By the age of puberty, essentially all of these patients attend endocrine

outpatient clinics. The boys usually require supplementation with testosterone preparations, and the girls low-dose oestrogens and progestogens. Screening for the development of diabetes mellitus includes testing for glycosuria and performing glucose tolerance tests. Approximately 50% of patients will have an abnormal glucose tolerance test by 10 years of age.

4. Yearly cardiac assessment, with a gated blood pool scan in children over 10 years to assess the left ventricular ejection fraction (at rest and during exercise), has been a preferred cardiac investigation. Some units recommend annual ECG, Holter monitoring and cardiac stress testing. Myocardial siderosis can be assessed using T2* MRI, as on the previous page. Cardiac iron overload has been the cause of most deaths in β-thalassaemia major.

5. Annual dental examination is useful. Dental procedure antibiotic prophylaxis in splenectomised patients is important. Reminding these patients to take their antibiotics is another important point in follow-up.

6. Other points regarding clinic follow-up include the discussion of any emotional or social problems.

PROGNOSIS

A favourite question is: 'What do you tell the parents of a child newly diagnosed with thalassaemia major?' The answer should include telling the parents the following:

- The child is very likely to need transfusions.
- A wait-and-see approach regarding the need for, and frequency of, transfusions should be adopted.
- A cure by HSCT, or genetic engineering, may be possible (after discussing the more standard treatment options).
- Current treatment modalities allow patients to reach adulthood. Better treatments are constantly being developed and cure is possible by stem cell transplantation.
- Regular erythrocyte transfusions plus adequate iron chelation has improved the prognosis of β-thalassaemia dramatically over the last three decades.

Compliance with chelation therapy is important. Teenage rebellion is often a problem and is difficult to manage, but must be addressed in adolescents with chronic disease. Patients who are compliant with their recommended therapy have a 50% chance of surviving into their thirties, but non-compliant patients only have a 10% chance of being alive at 30 years. The main cause of death remains cardiac disease, caused by iron overload. Improved imaging techniques to monitor for cardiac iron accumulation, and better compliance with chelation, with the increased availability of effective oral iron chelators, have led to improved survival and quality of life.

THE ISSUE OF FURTHER CHILDREN

Parents can be angry that they have not 'beaten the odds', if they already knew the 1 in 4 risk, and had assumed, incorrectly, that the next three children would be normal. This raises the issue of further children and prenatal diagnosis.

SUMMARY

In discussing your management, as well as being familiar with the above-mentioned areas, it is worthwhile asking the examiners for results of relevant investigations, such as the ferritin level, liver function tests, the most recent chest X-ray and ECG, and the latest eye and hearing checks, as this is what you would need to know in practice. Of course, appropriate interpretation of this information is expected, if it is requested.

SHORT CASES

SHORT CASE: The haematological system

The usual introduction involves assessment for anaemia or bruising.

First, note the child's sex (haemophilia and glucose-6-phosphate dehydrogenase deficiency [G6PD] are X-linked), nationality (thalassaemia is more common in children of Asian or Mediterranean descent, and SCA is more common in African children), growth (short with some syndromes, SCA or chronic kidney disease [CKD]) and any dysmorphic features (Fanconi anaemia, Blackfan–Diamond red cell aplasia, thrombocytopenia absent radius [TAR]; see later).

Check, and comment on, the growth parameters. The head circumference may be increased with a subdural haematoma from non-accidental injury (NAI), which may present with unexplained bruising. Weight may be decreased in children with a nutritional deficiency as the basis of their anaemia. Note pubertal status (delay in SCA, thalassaemia).

Assess whether the child looks sick or well. Patients with acute lymphoblastic leukaemia (ALL), CKD, or purpura due to meningococcaemia look unwell. Patients with SCA may be in pain if a recent crisis has occurred. Infants with NAI may be wary of any attempts to get close. Note any pallor (various causes of anaemia).

Note any abnormal posturing suggesting hemiplegia, which can complicate haemophilia or SCA.

Visually scan the joints for swelling, which can occur in haemophilia, SCA, Henoch–Schönlein purpura (HSP), ALL, inflammatory bowel disease (IBD) such as Crohn's disease, or juvenile idiopathic arthritis (JIA): the latter two can present with anaemia. Also note any abdominal distension (due to hepatosplenomegaly) and needle marks on the abdomen (DFO therapy).

Examine the skin for petechiae, purpura and ecchymoses. If any of these are present, make a thorough assessment of their distribution (e.g. purpura on buttocks in HSP, fingertip-shaped bruises in NAI). In the case of purpuric areas, note whether they are raised and/or tender (vasculitic) or flat and/or non-tender (platelet deficiency or dysfunction). Note any jaundice or scratch marks (haemolysis), haemangiomas (which can cause a consumptive coagulopathy) or cigarette burns. Also look for the cutaneous manifestations of systemic lupus erythematosus (SLE) and peripheral stigmata of chronic liver disease (CLD), which can be associated with a coagulopathy.

The remainder of the examination is best commenced at the hands, working up to the head and then downwards.

Look at the nails for koilonychia (iron deficiency), leuconychia (CLD), clubbing (CLD, congenital heart disease [CHD]) and splinter haemorrhages (subacute bacterial endocarditis [SBE]). Inspect the palms for crease pallor (suggests haemoglobin level below 70 g/L) or palmar erythema (CLD). Note the pulse rate (anaemia).

Moving up the forearm, examine the epitrochlear nodes bilaterally. Then request, or take, the BP for evidence of hypertension (as the result of CKD, haemolytic uraemic syndrome [HUS], or as the cause of microangiopathic haemolytic anaemia [MAHA]) or hypotension (acute blood loss, cardiomyopathy from iron overload) or increased pulse pressure (anaemia). Then examine the axillary nodes bilaterally.

Next, examine the head and neck, followed by the chest wall, spine, abdomen, gait, lower limbs and heart. This is outlined in Figure 10.1.

A mnemonic that may be useful for outlining the order of the examination is the 11 Ss: Sex, Syndrome, Size, Structure (hands), Scone (head), Sternum, Spine, Spleen (abdomen), Stand (gait and lower limbs), SBE (heart) and Stool.

1. Introduce self

2. General inspection
Position patient: standing, undressed;
   then lying down

3. Upper limbs
Structure
Joint swelling
Nails
Palms
Pulse
Epitrochlear nodes
Blood pressure
Axillary nodes

4. Head and neck
Face
Ears
Eyes (include fundoscopy)
Nose
Mouth
Tongue
Gums
Palate
Throat
Neck (lymph nodes)

5. Chest wall
Spider naevi (CLD)
Supraclavicular nodes
Skeletal tenderness:
• Sternum
• Clavicles
• Shoulders
• Spine (ALL, NAI)

6. Abdomen
Distension
Splenomegaly
Hepatomegaly
Enlarged kidneys
Genitalia
Inguinal lymph nodes
Pelvis (spring)
Buttocks

7. Lower limbs and gait
Inspect
Palpate
Gait
Neurological
Joints

8. Cardiovascular system
Full praecordial examination

9. Other
Urinalysis
Stool analysis
Temperature chart

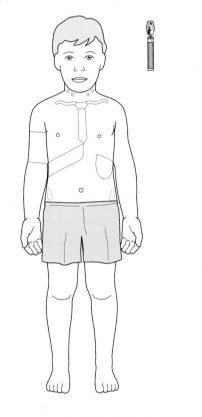

ALL = acute lymphoblastic leukaemia; CLD = chronic liver disease; NAI = non-accidental injury.

Figure 10.1 **The haematological system**

At the completion of the examination, request results of stool analysis for blood, urinalysis for blood, protein, fixed low specific gravity (CKD) or infection, and the temperature chart for infection.

An alternative approach is based on assessing the three cell lines first, by looking at skin and mucous membranes: 1. the red cell line for deficiency (signs of anaemia) or excess (plethora from polycythaemia); 2. the white cell line for deficiency or excess (gingivitis, infected skin lesions); and 3. platelet deficiency (signs of bruising).

After this, examine the three main areas of interest:

1. First, all the lymph nodes (lymphadenopathy with ALL, AML, lymphoma) and the abdomen (hepatosplenomegaly, or abdominal masses, from ALL or AML infiltrates, or extramedullary haematopoiesis).
2. Next, the musculoskeletal examination (skeletal tenderness at sternum, clavicles, ribs, spine, pelvis and tibiae [leukaemic infiltrates, SCA]; joint tenderness, swelling or decreased range of movement [ALL, AML, SCA, IBD, HSP, JIA]).
3. Finally, dysmorphic features.

This approach thoroughly assesses one system at a time and is easy to remember. The only disadvantage is that it does not flow quite as smoothly as the 'Ss' approach.

A comprehensive listing of findings not listed above is given in Table 10.1. Which of the findings listed is relevant depends on the particular case involved.

Table 10.1
Additional information: comprehensive listing of possible findings in the haematological examination
GENERAL INSPECTION
Well or unwell (DIC, ALL, meningococcaemia)
Sex (haemophilia, G6PD deficiency in males)
Race • Thalassaemia in Mediterraneans, Asians • SCA in African Americans, Jamaicans, Middle Easterners
Syndrome (Fanconi, Blackfan–Diamond, TAR)
Thalassaemic 'chipmunk' facies
Parameters: height, weight, head circumference, percentiles
Pubertal status: delayed (thalassaemia, SCA)
Nutritional status
Posture: hemiplegia (haemophilia, SCA)
Skin • Pallor • Petechiae, purpura, ecchymoses (ALL, AML, aplastic anaemia, ITP) • Pigmentation (thalassaemia) • Jaundice, scratch marks (haemolysis, CLD) • Cavernous haemangiomas (can cause Kasabach Merritt syndrome; MAHA) • Cigarette burns (NAI) • SLE rashes • CLD stigmata • Subcutaneous nodules (ALL) • Small angiomata (HHT) • Eczema (Wiskott–Aldrich syndrome) • Infected lesions (immune deficiency, ALL, AML)
Joint swelling (haemophilia, HSP, SCA, leukaemia, IBD, JIA)

Table 10.1 (continued)

UPPER LIMBS

Structure of:
- Forearms (TAR)
- Thumbs (Fanconi, Blackfan–Diamond)

Joint swelling (JIA)

Nails
- Koilonychia (iron deficiency)
- Leuconychia (CLD)
- Clubbing (CHD, CLD)

Palms
- Crease pallor (anaemia)
- Crease pigmentation (thalassaemia)
- Erythema (CLD)

Pulse: tachycardia (anaemia)

Epitrochlear nodes

BP
- Hypertension (CKD, HUS or as cause of MAHA)
- Hypotension (acute blood loss, cardiomyopathy)
- Raised pulse pressure (anaemia)

Axillary nodes

HEAD AND NECK

Face (thalassaemic facies, syndromal, Cushingoid, SLE)

Ears
- Abnormal structure (Fanconi)
- Discharge (Wiskott–Aldrich syndrome)

Eyes
- Squint (Fanconi, sixth cranial nerve palsy with intracranial bleed)
- Ptosis (Fanconi)
- Nystagmus (Fanconi, intracranial bleeding)
- Conjunctival pallor
- Scleral icterus
- Subconjunctival haemorrhage
- Cataracts (DFO or corticosteroid therapy)

Fundoscopy
- Retinal haemorrhage (ALL, AML, NAI)
- Roth spots (SBE)
- Papilloedema (raised intracranial pressure with ALL, AML, NAI)
- Proliferative retinopathy (SCA)
- Retinopathy from DFO

Nose: evidence of epistaxis

Mouth: angular cheilosis (iron deficiency)

Tongue
- Pale atrophic (iron deficiency)
- Raw, beefy (B group vitamin deficiency)
- Red spots (HHT)

Continued

Table 10.1 (continued)

Gums • Hypertrophy (ALL, AML) • Inflammation (ALL, AML)
Palate: petechiae
Tonsils • Hypertrophy (ALL, AML) • Exudate (EB virus)
Neck: enlarged cervical nodes (viral infections, lymphomas, ALL, AML)
ABDOMEN
Distension (due to hepatosplenomegaly)
Needle marks on abdomen (DFO treatment)
Splenomegaly • Haemoglobinopathies • Malignancy (ALL, AML) • Infection (SBE) • Osteopetrosis • Storage diseases • Congenital spherocytosis
Hepatomegaly: as above, plus hepatitis and Wilson's disease (decrease in clotting factors I, II and V)
Enlarged kidneys (ALL)
Adrenal mass (neuroblastoma)
Genitalia • Tanner staging (delay with thalassaemia, SCA) • Testes: enlarged (ALL, HSP: orchitis or bleeding) • Penis: priapism (SCA, ALL, CML)
Inguinal nodes
Spring pelvis (bony tenderness)
Posterior iliac crests (bone marrow aspiration site)
Buttocks (HSP rash)
Perianal region: fissures, fistulae (IBD)
LOWER LIMBS AND GAIT
Inspection • Joint swelling (see above) • Ulcers (SCA) • Erythema nodosum (IBD)
Palpate: tibial tenderness (ALL, NAI)
Stand: Rombergism (vitamin B_{12} deficiency)
Walk • Antalgic gait (haemophilia with haemarthrosis, ALL, SCA) • Ataxic gait (vitamin B_{12} deficiency) • Hemiplegic (haemophilia with intracranial bleed, SCA with cerebral sickling)

Table 10.1 (continued)

Depending on above findings, further examination of:
- Joints
- Peripheral nervous system
- Central nervous system

CARDIOVASCULAR SYSTEM

Full praecordial examination, looking for evidence of:
- SBE
- Cardiac surgery (fragmentation anaemia with artificial valves)
- Congenital heart disease (associated with bruising; syndromes)
- Cardiomyopathy (transfusion haemosiderosis with thalassaemia or SCA)
- Cardiac failure (anaemia)

OTHER

Urinalysis
- Blood (haemophilia, SCA, HUS)
- Haemoglobin (intravascular haemolysis)
- Urobilinogen (haemolysis)
- Protein (renal disease)
- Specific gravity (SCA, CKD)

Stool analysis: blood (HSP, IBD)

Temperature chart

Hess test can be offered in older child if relevant

SELECTED SYNDROME FINDINGS

Blackfan–Diamond red cell aplasia

- Turner syndrome-like phenotype
- Bone deformities
- Ocular abnormalities
- Abnormal ears
- Cleft lip
- Abnormal thumbs (bifid, double or triphalangeal thumbs)
- Talipes

Fanconi anaemia

- Short stature
- Café-au-lait spots
- Pigmentation at groin, trunk and axilla
- Small head
- Squint, ptosis, nystagmus
- Abnormal ears
- Abnormal hands (aplastic, hypoplastic or supernumerary thumbs; syndactyly; decreased number of carpal bones; occasionally, absent radius)
- Small genitalia

Thrombocytopenia absent radius (TAR) syndrome

- Radius absent, but thumbs present

Continued

Table 10.1 (continued)
Dyskeratosis congenita
• Male (usually) • Nail ridging and atrophy • Pigmentation (brown–grey) with telangiectasia and atrophy, at head, neck, shoulders, chest • Mucous membrane leucoplakia • Sparse hair • Hyperkeratosis of palms and soles
Wiskott–Aldrich syndrome
• Eczema (severe) • Ear discharge, other infections (middle ear, chest, skin) • Immune deficiency, decreased IgM, infections (middle ear, chest, skin) • Thrombocytopenia, small platelets

ALL = acute lymphoblastic leukaemia; AML = acute myeloid leukaemia; CHD = congenital heart disease; CLD = chronic liver disease; CKD = chronic kidney disease; DIC = disseminated intravascular coagulation; G6PD = glucose-6-phosphate dehydrogenase deficiency; HHT = hereditary haemorrhagic telangiectasia; HSP = Henoch–Schönlein purpura; HUS = haemolytic uraemic syndrome; IBD = inflammatory bowel disease; JIA = juvenile idiopathic arthritis; MAHA = microangiopathic haemolytic anaemia; NAI = non-accidental injury; SBE = subacute bacterial endocarditis; SCA = sickle cell anaemia; SLE = systemic lupus erythematosus; TAR = thrombocytopenia absent radius.

After presenting your findings, you may be asked by the examiners which investigations you would perform. Depending on the presenting problem, a suggested plan is given below.

Anaemia

The full blood examination and film is the most useful investigation. The classification based on the size and appearance of the red blood cells is well known and can be very useful. The three most commonly described morphologies are as follows.

1. MICROCYTIC

The most common cause of this is iron deficiency. Other causes include thalassaemia minor and chronic inflammation.

2. NORMOCYTIC

This group can be subdivided into two groups, based on the reticulocyte count:
1. A low-reticulocyte response occurs most commonly with transient erythroblastopenia of childhood. Other causes include aplastic crises and Blackfan–Diamond anaemia.
2. A high reticulocyte count occurs with bleeding or haemolysis. Haemolysis can be classified by extrinsic or intrinsic causes.

Extrinsic causes

1. Mechanical injury to red cells (e.g. small vessel disease in HUS, or in disseminated intravascular coagulation [DIC]; or larger vessel disease, such as poorly epithelialised prosthetic cardiac valves).
2. Chronic kidney or liver disease (CKD or CLD).
3. Haemolysis mediated by antibodies, including autoimmune haemolytic anaemia (e.g. warm antibody type in Epstein-Barr virus infections, cold antibody type in mycoplasma infections) and isoimmune haemolysis (e.g. incompatible transfusions).

Intrinsic causes

1. Membrane abnormalities (e.g. hereditary spherocytosis).
2. Enzyme abnormalities (e.g. G6PD).
3. Haemoglobin disorders (e.g. SCA).

3. MACROCYTIC

This can occur with folate or vitamin B_{12} deficiency.

Bleeding

This may be due to abnormalities of blood vessels, platelets or the coagulation system. The useful screening investigations include the following:

1. A full blood count and film, noting the haemoglobin level (associated anaemia, e.g. in aplastic anaemia or ALL), the white cell count (e.g. leucopenia in aplastic anaemia, blast forms in ALL), any thrombocytopenia and also the platelet size (large in Bernard–Soulier syndrome).
2. The prothrombin time, which assesses the extrinsic coagulation system.
3. The partial thromboplastin time, which assesses the intrinsic coagulation system.
   In bleeding associated with vascular defects, the above tests will be normal.
   Although mentioned in some texts, a bleeding time should not be done in children. It is painful, unable to be standardised and there are now better tests for von Willebrand's disease. These include:

1. Platelet aggregation studies with ristocetin (an antibiotic that causes von Willebrand's factor [vWF] to bind to platelets and activate them). These studies reflect both plasma and platelet vWF.
2. vWF antigen (VIII-related antigen).
3. vWF activity (ristocetin cofactor).
4. vWF factor multimer analysis.

SHORT CASE: Thalassaemia

This case involves demonstrating the complications of extramedullary haematopoiesis, iron overload and chelation (DFO or DFS) therapy.

The mnemonic **THALASSAEMIA** helps list the important areas to examine:

Tanner stage (pubertal delay)
Heart (cardiomyopathy)/**H**aematopoiesis (extramedullary)/**H**ypercoagulable
Anaemia
Liver/**L**ong tracts (neurological involvement)/**L**eg ulcers
Appearance (thalassaemic facies, pigmentation)
Sugar diabetes
Short stature
Arrhythmias
Eye/**E**ndocrine
Metabolic (hypocalcaemia)/**M**alocclusion
Iron overload/**I**cterus/**I**nfection/**I**atrogenic (DFO, DFS side effects)
Adenopathy and hepatosplenomegaly

Initial inspection should include assessment of growth parameters (usually short, head circumference often increased [due to skull bossing], pubertal status delayed), colour (pigmentation from melanin and iron deposition, pallor from anaemia, jaundice from haemolysis), whether the child has any respiratory distress (e.g. anaemia or cardiomyopathy causing congestive cardiac failure [CCF], or massive splenomegaly causing marked increase in intraabdominal pressure), and a description of any obvious bony abnormalities associated with the 'chipmunk facies'. Note any obvious stigmata of CLD. Figure 10.2 outlines the salient clinical features sought in the thalassaemia short-case examination.

Commence a general systematic examination by looking at the hands for fingertip prickmarks (blood sugar level testing) and periungual pigmentation, and at the palmar creases for pallor or pigmentation, and look carefully (if not done already) for any more subtle stigmata of CLD. Take the pulse (bradycardia with untreated hypothyroidism, irregularity with arrhythmias, pulsus alternans with CCF).

Examine the head, looking at the conjunctivae for anaemia and the sclerae for icterus. Check for cataracts and retinopathy from DFO or DFS toxicity. Check the mouth for dental malocclusion secondary to maxillary hyperplasia, and the gum margins for hyperplasia (which may not be apparent in the well-transfused patient).

Feel the neck for goitre, secondary to iron deposition.

Examine the cardiovascular system fully; in particular, for evidence of cardiomyopathy and pericarditis. Next examine the abdomen; inspect for distension (e.g. from organomegaly, or ascites with CLD), injection sites (from DFO and/or insulin) and any splenectomy scar. Palpate for hepatosplenomegaly, percuss for ascites and assess Tanner staging.

Inspect the lower limbs for injection sites on the thighs (insulin), the peripatellar fossa for increased pigmentation and check for ulcers on the lower leg. Palpate for ankle oedema (CCF, CLD) and bony tenderness (fracture, bony expansion). The gait should then be examined, followed by neurological assessment of the lower limbs on return to the bed, looking for evidence of long-tract signs secondary to vertebral bony expansion and cord compression. Also check the ankle jerks for delayed relaxation, from hypothyroidism. Following this, examine the back for lordosis and bony tenderness. Request the urinalysis for glucose.

If time permits, assess for hypocalcaemia secondary to hypoparathyroidism by testing for Trousseau's and Chvostek's signs, and check the hearing for sensorineural deafness due to DFO or DFS toxicity, or bony expansion and compression of the eighth cranial nerve.

Figure 10.3 lists the normal haemoglobins and shows haemoglobin synthesis during prenatal and postnatal development.

SHORT CASE: Lymphadenopathy

The mnemonic **MATCHES** (see below) covers many causes of lymphadenopathy. Three versions of this are given: the *first* lists causes of *cervical* lymphadenopathy; the *second* lists causes of *generalised* lymphadenopathy; and the *third* lists *all causes* together, both regional and generalised. The third list is very 'busy', with generalised causes identified with an asterisk (*), and causes of cervical lymphadenopathy identified with *[Cx]*.

Obviously, any of the causes of generalised lymphadenopathy can cause cervical or other regional lymphadenopathy; these mnemonics are simply to make it easier to hone in on likely pathology in the presentation of *(specifically)* cervical lymphadenopathy or to adopt a broader short-case approach if the presentation is generalised.

1. Introduce self

2. General inspection

Position patient: standing, adequately exposed; then lying down

Parameters
- Height
- Weight
- Percentiles

Tanner staging

Well or unwell

Colour
- Pigmentation
- Pallor
- Jaundice

Facial features
- Frontal bossing
- Parietal bossing
- Chipmunk facies
- Maxillary overgrowth
- Dental malocclusion
- Prominent malar eminence
- Broadened nasal bridge
- Mongoloid eye slant
- Epicanthal folds

Abdominal distension

3. Hands

Fingertip pricks

Palmar creases

Peripheral stigmata of CLD

Pulse

4. Head and neck

Eyes
- Conjunctival pallor
- Scleral icterus
- Cataracts (DFO)
- Retinopathy (DFO)

Teeth: dental malocclusion

Neck: goitre

5. Heart

Full praecordial examination: cardio-myopathy, CCF, haemic murmurs

Chest: pulmonary oedema

6. Abdomen

Distension

Splenectomy scar

Injection sites: DFO, insulin

Hepatosplenomegaly

Tanner staging

7. Lower limbs and gait

Leg ulcers

Ankle oedema

Bony tenderness

Gait examination: long-tract signs

Delayed ankle jerk relaxation

Back examination: lordosis, tenderness

8. Other

Urinalysis for glucose

Chvostek's and Trousseau's signs (hypoparathyroidism)

Hearing (sensorineural deafness from DFO)

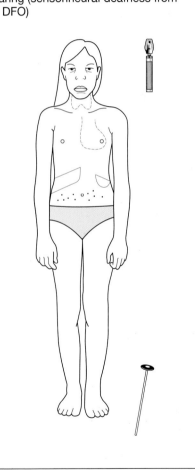

CCF = congestive cardiac failure; CLD = chronic liver disease; DFO = desferrioxamine.

Figure 10.2 **Thalassaemia**

Human Hemoglobins			
Stage in Development	Hemoglobin	Structure	Proportion in Normal Adult (%)
Embryonic	Gower I	$\zeta_2\varepsilon_2$	—
	Gower II	$\alpha_2\varepsilon_2$	—
	Portland I	$\zeta_2\gamma_2$	—
Fetal	F	$\alpha_2\gamma_2$	<1
Adult	A	$\alpha_2\beta_2$	97–98
	A_2	$\alpha_2\delta_2$	2–3

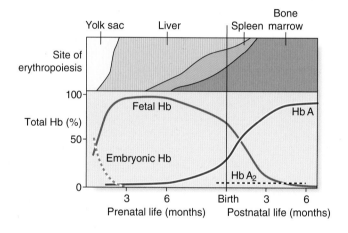

Figure 10.3 Haemoglobin switching

Source: Emery, A.E.H., Turnpenny, P.D. & Ellard, S. (2007). *Emery's Elements of Medical Genetics* (13th ed.). London: Elsevier/Churchill Livingstone. Table 10.1 and Figure 10.2. After Huehns E.R. & Shooter E.M. (1965). Human haemoglobins. *Journal of Medical Genetics*, 2, 48–90, with permission.)

Causes of cervical lymphadenopathy

MAIS complex (*Mycobacterium Avium-Intracellulare-Scrofulaceum*)/**M**alignancy (lymphoma [non-Hodgkin], rhabdomyosarcoma)/**M**ucocutaneous lymph node syndrome (Kawasaki syndrome)

Atopic dermatitis

Tonsils: hypertrophy with upper respiratory tract infection (URTI)/**T**eeth: caries

Cat-scratch disease (*Bartonella henselae*)/**C**hlamydia trachomatis

HSV (gingivostomatitis)/**H**odgkin disease

EBV (Epstein-Barr virus)

Streptococcus A

Causes of generalised lymphadenopathy

Malignancy (neuroblastoma, leukaemia, lymphoma [non-Hodgkin])/**M**easles
/**M**edications (e.g. phenytoin, isoniazid, allopurinol)

ALL/**A**ML/**A**denovirus/**A**utoimmune (JIA, SLE)

TB/**T**oxoplasma gondii/**T**yphoid (salmonella typhi)

CMV (cytomegalovirus)/**C**oxsackie virus/**C**occidioidomycosis

HIV/**H**erpes viruses: **H**HV-6 (roseola infantum); **H**VZ/**H**epatitis A, B, C/**H**odgkin
disease/**H**istiocytosis X

EBV (Epstein-Barr virus)/**E**xanthemata (rubella, roseola, measles)/**E**nteroviruses/
Endocrinopathies (Graves, Addison)/**E**ndocarditis

Staphylococcus/**S**ystemic viral infections (most common)/**S**arcoidosis/**S**torage
diseases (Gaucher, Niemann-Pick)/**S**erum sickness/**S**epticaemia/**S**yphilis

Causes of lymphadenopathy (cervical *[Cx]* or generalised *)

MAIS complex *[Cx]* (mycobacterium avium-intracellulare-scrofulaceum)/**M**alignancy*
(neuroblastoma, leukaemia, lymphoma [non-Hodgkin's], rhabdomyosarcoma *[Cx]*)/
Mucocutaneous lymph node syndrome (Kawasaki) *[Cx]*/**M**easles*/**M**edications*
(e.g. phenytoin, isoniazid, allopurinol)

ALL*/**A**ML*/**A**topic dermatitis *[Cx]*/**A**denovirus*/**A**utoimmune* (JIA, SLE)

TB* (tuberculosis, tubercle bacillus, mycobacteria tuberculosis)/**T**oxoplasma gondii*/
Teeth: caries *[Cx]*/**T**yphoid* (salmonella typhi)

CMV* (cytomegalovirus)/**C**at-scratch disease *[Cx]* (*Bartonella henselae*)/**C**hlamydia
trachomatis [Cx] **C**oxsackie virus*/**C**occidioidomycosis*

HIV*/**H**erpes viruses: **H**HV-6 (roseola infantum)*/**H**SV (gingivostomatitis)
[Cx]/**H**VZ*/**H**epatitis A, B, C*/**H**odgkin's disease*/**H**istiocytosis*/**H**idradenitis
suppurativa (axillary adenopathy in obese)

EBV* (Epstein-Barr virus; infectious mononucleosis)/**E**xanthemata* (rubella, roseola,
measles)/**E**nteroviruses*/**E**ndocrinopathies* (Graves, Addison) **E**ndocarditis*

Streptococcus A *[Cx]*/**S**taphylococcus*/**S**ystemic viral infections* (most
common)/**S**arcoidosis*/**S**torage diseases* (Gaucher, Niemann-Pick)/**S**erum
sickness*/**S**epticaemia*/**S**yphilis*

Lymphadenopathy: a *very* abbreviated list:

MAIS, **A**LL, **T**B, **C**MV, **H**IV, **E**BV, **S**trep

Background information
CERVICAL LYMPHADENOPATHY

The distribution of the lymph nodes in the neck includes a *horizontally* positioned circle of nodes at the junction of the head and the neck, which are fairly superficial, and two *vertically* positioned groups of nodes. The vertical main chain of deep cervical nodes, situated around the internal jugular vein, drain the deeper structures, and are found beneath the sternocleidomastoid muscle (SCM). There is also a more superficial vertical group which follow the external jugular vein and are situated at the anterior and posterior borders of the SCM.

Two of the deep cervical nodes of the jugular chain are specifically named: the jugulodigastric (JD) or tonsillar node, near the angle of the jaw; and the jugulo-omohyoid (JO) or lingual node, which is above the inferior belly of the omohyoid adjacent to the internal jugular vein (see Fig. 10.4) Have a system to include all the node groups and be aware of their respective drainage areas. The approach is important; as a rule, neck nodes are best examined from behind the patient.

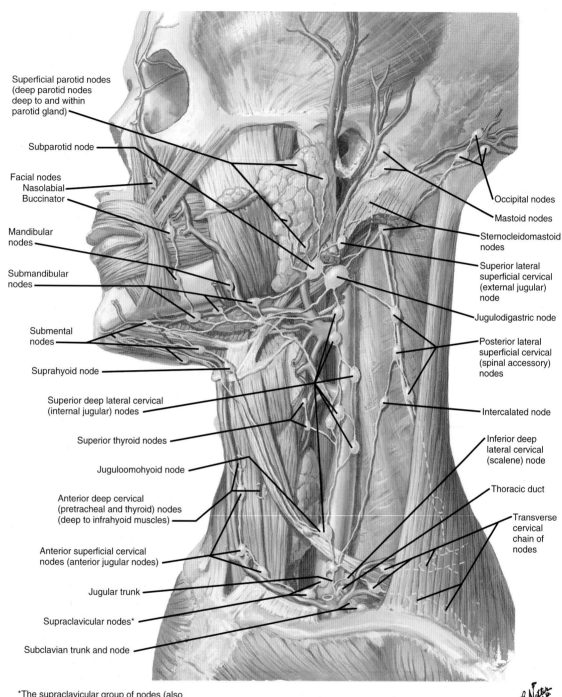

Superficial parotid nodes
(deep parotid nodes
deep to and within
parotid gland)

Subparotid node

Facial nodes
Nasolabial
Buccinator

Mandibular
nodes

Submandibular
nodes

Submental
nodes

Suprahyoid node

Superior deep lateral cervical
(internal jugular) nodes

Superior thyroid nodes

Juguloomohyoid node

Anterior deep cervical
(pretracheal and thyroid) nodes
(deep to infrahyoid muscles)

Anterior superficial cervical
nodes (anterior jugular nodes)

Jugular trunk

Supraclavicular nodes*

Subclavian trunk and node

Occipital nodes

Mastoid nodes

Sternocleidomastoid
nodes

Superior lateral
superficial cervical
(external jugular)
node

Jugulodigastric node

Posterior lateral
superficial cervical
(spinal accessory)
nodes

Intercalated node

Inferior deep
lateral cervical
(scalene) node

Thoracic duct

Transverse
cervical
chain of
nodes

*The supraclavicular group of nodes (also
known as the lower deep cervical group),
especially on the left, are also sometimes
referred to as the signal or sentinel lymph
nodes of Virchow or Troisier, especially when
sufficiently enlarged and palpable. These
nodes (or a single node) are so termed because
they may be the first recognized presumptive
evidence of malignant disease in the viscera.

Figure 10.4 Lymph vessels and nodes of the head and neck

Source: Netter, F.H. (1997). *Atlas of Human Anatomy* (2nd ed.). East Hanover, N.J.: Novartis. Plate 66.

However, children prefer being examined from the front, so they can see what is happening more readily. Therefore, initially, have the child sitting on their parent's lap, or for older children in a chair, or on the side of the bed/examining couch. Talk to the child and explain you just need to gently feel their neck, asking if anywhere is sore, approaching from the front (face to face); after this, ask to palpate again by approaching from behind the child.

One suggested order is as follows:

1. Start palpation with the *suboccipital* nodes at the base of the skull (drain posterior aspect of scalp), then the *postauricular* (mastoid) nodes which lie over the mastoid process (drain scalp and ear), then the *preauricular* nodes immediately in front of the ear (drain external ear, conjunctivae, eyelids, skin of cheek and temporal aspect of scalp), then the *parotid* nodes, which lie over the parotid gland (drain the parotid gland, gums, middle ear, external ear, temporal scalp, forehead, midface).

2. Next, check the *submandibular* nodes halfway between the tip and the angle of the mandible (drain the upper respiratory tract and oropharynx, including upper lip, gums, buccal mucosa, anterior two-thirds of the tongue, and submaxillary gland, as well as the nose, conjunctivae and face), and then the *submental* nodes, which are in the midline behind the tip of the mandible (drain the tip of the tongue, teeth, lower lip, floor of mouth, skin of cheek and chin). This completes the 'horizontal circular' group.

3. Now move on to palpating the vertical groups, one side at a time, starting with the anterior triangle of the neck (anterior to the SCM), ideally with the head position controlled by the examiner having one hand behind the occiput), and then the posterior triangle (posterior to the SCM). The nodes being examined are the *superficial cervical* nodes which are distributed along the external jugular vein, and can be felt along the anterior and posterior borders of the SCM muscle (anterior triangle nodes drain parotid and lower part of the ear; posterior triangle nodes drain scalp, neck, skin of arms and chest wall), and the *deep cervical* nodes which are deep to the SCM muscle.

4. The *deep cervical* nodes drain tonsils and adenoids, palate, paranasal sinuses, nasal cavities, nasopharynx, tongue, larynx, thyroid, oesophagus and all the other lymph nodes of the head and neck. To relax the SCM muscle to optimise feeling the deep nodes, the best position is for the child's head to be flexed forwards and inclined towards the side being examined; this position also works for optimising palpation of *submental* and *supraclavicular* nodes (see below).

5. Take note of the *tonsillar* (JD) node, one of the upper group of deep cervical (jugular) nodes, which is near the angle of the jaw, in the angle between the inferior border of the jaw and the anterior border of the SCM muscle (drains pharynx, palatine tonsil, tongue). Continue to palpate downwards to the *lingual* node (JO), so called because it drains the tongue.

6. There is a further collection of nodes along the anterior aspect of the neck, including the *infrahyoid* nodes, *pre-laryngeal* nodes, *pre-tracheal* nodes and *post-tracheal* nodes, although it is infrequent to encounter these.

7. Next palpate the *supraclavicular* nodes, (both sides drain anterior chest and mediastinum, retropleural lymphatics; the left-sided node also drains intraabdominal and pelvic organs, retroperitoneal lymphatics; the left-sided node is also called Virchow's node). Supraclavicular lymphadenopathy is always of significance, as

lymph from the right upper body travels to the right lymphatic duct, which then drains into the right subclavian vein, traversing the right subclavicular nodes on the way; lymph from the remainder of the body travels to the thoracic duct, which drains into the left subclavian vein, traversing the left supraclavicular nodes on the way.

Examine one side at a time; it can be disconcerting to children having an adult stranger putting both hands around their throats simultaneously. Examine all nodes from the front, then examine them all from behind the child.

ASPECTS OF A LYMPH NODE/LUMP/SWELLING

Should an enlarged node or group of nodes be encountered, the next question is to confirm these are lymph nodes, and thus to specify the anatomical site, and the physical characteristics of the node(s), and any associated pathological findings.

All the aspects of examining any lump or swelling should be covered, as there are differential diagnoses for lymph nodes in regional areas, particularly the neck.

Two mnemonics are given here, one based on two letters, **S** and **T**, the other based on an acronym reflecting the wide spectrum of differential diagnoses: **SPECTRAL**.

The characteristics, based on **S** and **T** are:

Inspection: **S**ite, **S**ize, **S**ides (edges), **S**hape, **S**ymmetry, **S**hine (colour), **S**urface, **S**urroundings

Palpation: **T**enderness, **T**emperature, **T**ethering (mobility), **T**ransmitted pulsation, **T**wo-finger separation (expansile pulsation with aneurysm), **T**hrill (from vascular lesion), **T**ension (consistency), **T**ap (for fluctuation), **T**ransfer contents (reducibility; disappears with pressure, but can reappear with opposing force applied), **T**ransient compressibility, **T**ongue attachment (moves with poking out tongue (thyroglossal cyst), **T**racheal attachment (move up and down with swallowing: thyroid swellings); and finally, of occasional relevance:

Percussion (resonant means air present)

Auscultation (for bruits or bowel sounds [herniae])

The additional aspects to the examination of a lump are:
* *Associated pathology*. In the case of lymph nodes, indications of the primary pathology, whether it be indicating localised conditions (such as streptococcal pharyngitis) or generalised illnesses (such as EBV causing splenomegaly, hepatomegaly).
* The other aspects are local effects (such as a mass compressing and/or displacing the carotid sheath, or trachea or oesophagus) which includes: checking for contiguous disease (malignant masses in the lower cervical region can extend to the upper thorax); examining the lungs, particularly percussing (from behind) and auscultating the supraclavicular fossa (for upper lobe pathology).

SPECTRAL ASPECTS TO A LUMP/SWELLING

Site (can describe with respect to fixed anatomical landmark, such as a bony prominence)/**S**ize (measure in cm)/**S**ides (edges)/**S**hape/**S**ymmetry (pathological nodes usually distributed asymmetrically)/**S**urface (smooth? irregular?)/**S**urroundings

Palpation (specific features of some swellings; e.g. collar-stud MAIS abscess has narrowing between lymph node and pus collection, prior to discharging)/**P**ercussion/**P**ulsatility (transmitted pulsation from a vascular lesion, or lesion on artery)

Edge/**E**xpansibility (specific form of pulsation, found by placing fingers on each side of a swelling, to see if they move away from each other, with each heartbeat, in three planes, as with an aneurysm)

Colour (e.g. red with acute pyogenic infection, cellulitis; purple over MAIS lymphadenitis)/**C**onsistency: soft (unlikely significant pathology), rubbery (classically lymphoma feels like this), firm or hard (possible malignancy or granulomatous disease)/**C**ompressibility

Tenderness/**T**emperature (using back of hand)/**T**ethering (mobility)/**T**hrill (from vascular lesion)/**T**ap (fluctuance is tested for by grasping the lump between the finger [usually either index or middle] and the thumb, and then tapping the central aspect of the lump with the other hand [usually with the index finger]; any resultant fluid thrill is perceived by the finger and thumb); fluctuance indicates fluid-filled swellings, such as lymphatic malformations (such as cystic hygromas), or liquid pus within an abscess/**T**ransfer contents (reducibility; disappears with pressure, but can reappear with opposing force applied)/**T**ransillumination (using pen torch, or auroscope light with attached ear speculum, applied to each side of swelling; lymphatic malformations [especially cystic hygromas] can transilluminate brilliantly)

Resonance (to percussion)/**R**elations (anatomical relations, which can be compressed by swelling)/**R**educibility (disappears with pressure, but can reappear with opposing force applied)

Auscultation/**A**ttachments: to underlying tissues (fixation); to tongue (moves upwards with protrusion of tongue [thyroglossal cyst]; to trachea (moves up and down with swallowing: thyroid swellings); so, attached to **t**issues, **t**ongue or **t**rachea

Local effects (e.g. torticollis, compression of neighbouring structures). Acute inflammation in a mass of inflamed nodes can cause reflex sternocleidomastoid muscle spasm, leading to torticollis with head tilt and restricted neck movement. Large masses can cause compression of local anatomical structures by swelling; this can include vascular malformations/hamartomatous swellings of lymph or blood vessels, enlarging secondary to bleeding, thrombosis or infection, which then can compress the trachea; or haemangiomata, which also can compress the trachea. Some lymphatic malformations can deform the expected configuration of the head and neck, to make the head appear displaced; cystic hygroma is the classic example of this

Lymph nodes draining the area

Physical characteristics of normal nodes

Normal lymph nodes number around 600 in the body. It is normal to be able to palpate cervical, axillary and inguinal nodes in perfectly well children but the size should be less than 1 cm in the greatest diameter.

Most lymph nodes in most regions of the body are under 1 cm in their longest diameter, and have a soft consistency. Lymph nodes occur in groups, superficial nodes lying in the SC tissues, deep lymph nodes being situated beneath muscle fascia or within body cavities.

Physical characteristics of pathological nodes

Acute inflammation (acute lymphadenitis) causes a red, hot, tender, swollen lymph node. There may be secondary torticollis (wry neck), due to reflex spasm of adjacent muscles, especially the sternocleidomastoid muscle, such that any movement of the neck is painful, whether active or passive.

Acute lymph node abscess presents as a red, hot, tender swollen node which can be fluctuant, has been enlarging over a few days, and which may point, and then discharge pus. These are often seen in children between 6 months and 3 years of age.

Atypical MAIS (subacute) lymphadenitis causes swollen nodes with purple skin discolouration overlying them, with low-grade inflammation, they tend to be soft, they may be matted and they are often not tender. There can be an underlying collar-stud, 'cold' abscess (although cold means normal body temperature). These typically present in a 1–2-year-old child, for 1–2 months. If a lymph node drains spontaneously, or develops a fistulous tract, this infers a MAIS infection particularly if it takes a few weeks to form, whereas a fast-developing abscess that drains suggests either staphylococcus aureus or streptococcus pyogenes.

Reactive hyperplastic nodes present with swelling, are non-tender and can be up to 3 cm in length, although if nodes of this size are noted, excisional biopsy is often the management planned, if these are present for 4–6 weeks. Reactive hyperplasia typically occurs with common upper respiratory tract infections.

Neoplastic (malignant) diseases typically cause rubbery, firm or stony nodes, which are usually neither tender nor discoloured. Lymphoma and chronic leukaemias tend to cause firmer nodes than leukaemia. However, haemorrhage within such a node can cause tenderness and/or discolouration; immunologic stimulation and certain malignancies can also cause tenderness, so presence or absence of tenderness is not very discriminatory. Malignant nodes can be shotty and discrete in early stages, becoming fixed to underlying structures or matted together by the time the diagnosis is made. Primary lymph node tumours, often in cervical nodes, include Hodgkin's and non-Hodgkin's lymphoma. Secondary lymph node tumours, again often in cervical nodes, include neuroblastoma, thyroid tumours or nasopharyngeal tumours.

Differential diagnosis of cervical nodes

There are a large number of swellings in the neck which can be mistaken, initially, for lymph nodes. Some of these are developmental conditions, related to remnants of embryological structures. Some are lateral, some are midline. The most characteristic ones should be readily identified, although uncommon.

LATERAL NECK LUMPS OTHER THAN LYMPH NODES

Branchial cyst

This is derived from 2nd and 3rd branchial clefts and is situated beneath the middle third of the sternocleidomastoid muscle. It transilluminates, as it is full of milky cholesterol-containing fluid, and has been described in the past, as feeling like a half-empty hot water bottle. Branchial cysts can extend to the base of the skull, lie over the carotid sheath, and can get infected, which is why they are excised.

Cystic hygroma

These are a macrocystic lymphatic malformation; also termed 'cystic lymphangioma'; a hamartoma of the jugular lymphatic sacs. There are two types: simple and complex. A simple cystic hygroma is on one side of the neck, usually situated over the anterior triangle, brilliantly transilluminable, fluctuant (full of lymph), and of variable size; these lesions can increase in size rapidly, if there is internal haemorrhage, or they become infected, and compress vital structures such as the trachea. Complex cystic hygromas are less common, but can infiltrate neighbouring structures (including oropharynx, larynx, mediastinum and pleura), causing upper airway obstruction, which can necessitate emergent treatment such as intubation and tracheostomy placement.

Vascular tumours

If these are deep enough, they do not seem obviously vascular in nature, at first glance, as they do not appear red as they do when as superficial as 'strawberry' birth marks. There are two types worth mentioning.

1. *Infantile haemangioma (IH)* would only be a relevant differential in an infant, as these lesions grow rapidly until 80% of their full growth by 12 weeks of age under a few months, if it was a deep lesion, so not readily identifiable by the 'strawberry' colouring. Several characteristics should make it fairly straightforward to differentiate this from a lymph node: palpation for thrill (as it is a vascular lesion), and for transient emptying/filling; and *auscultation* as any haemangioma can have a bruit.
2. *Kaposiform haemangioendothelioma (KHE)* can look like an IH, but more rapidly growing, with the ability to cause Kasabach Merritt syndrome (KMS, which comprises a vascular tumour, consumptive coagulopathy, microangiopathic haemolytic anaemia and thrombocytopaenia; can lead to cardiac failure, so look for tachypnoea and hepatomegaly, if KMS suspected).

Sternomastoid tumour

This can be a relevant differential only in a neonate, particularly aged *2–3 weeks old*, who presents with a lump in the vicinity of, and in line with, the sternocleidomastoid muscle. On closer examination it can be found to be within the sternocleidomastoid muscle itself. It is typically *2–3 cm long*, non-tender and very firm, and it may be associated with a degree of angulation of the head, and/or with plagiocephaly, so the baby's head should be examined for this.

Recurrent parotitis with sialectasis

These can occur in a child aged *2–4 years old*, can impersonate mumps or preauricular lymphadenitis, and is associated with episodes of unilateral parotid swelling which is tender, and produces purulent fluid from the parotid duct, when pressure is applied over it; these episodes last *2–4 days*, but can be quite recurrent occurring on and off for years, but generally has resolved by 10 years.

MIDLINE NECK LUMPS OTHER THAN LYMPH NODES
Thyroglossal cyst

This derives from remnants of the thyroglossal duct, which traces the embryological migratory path of the thyroid gland from the foramen caecum in the floor of the pharynx, to its final position in front of the trachea, which is in the midline of the neck. There can be an associated fistula, from which saliva, mucus or pus can appear. The classic diagnostic finding is the cyst moving up when the tongue is protruded; get the child to open the mouth, then lightly hold the cyst between thumb and index finger, and then get the child to poke out their tongue. The other useful sign is getting the child to swallow while the lesion is palpated from behind; if attached to the hyoid, it will move up and down when the child swallows some water.

These cysts are translucent when transilluminated. When infected, they tend to develop cellulitis that spreads horizontally more than vertically. Over two-thirds of these cysts are located very close to, attached to or just below, the hyoid bone; others can be found at midline positions; submental, suprasternal or lingual. When infected, these lesions can impersonate acute bacterial submental lymphadenitis. Treatment is excision of the cyst and the duct remnants, including removing the middle third of the hyoid.

Ectopic thyroid

Like the thyroglossal cyst, this can be found anywhere along the migratory path of descent of the thyroid gland from the foramen caecum to the front of the trachea. Ectopic thyroid feels softer than thyroglossal cyst. On occasion, this aberrant tissue is the only thyroid tissue in the body, so there should always be a thyroid isotope scan performed before any consideration of removing this, once its nature has been ascertained, so as not to remove the only functioning gland. The back of the tongue should be inspected to detect a lingual thyroid. If the ectopic tissue is the only thyroid tissue, then it is preserved, but divided into two, with each half positioned deep to the strap muscles.

Dermoid cyst

These derive from embryonic remnants, ectodermal cells which detach along lines of fusion, or in the midline, so they may be in a similar position to a thyroglossal cyst. Unlike many cysts, these do not transilluminate because they are filled with thick, cheesy, opaque, sebaceous fluid. Dermoid cysts do not move with swallowing or tongue protrusion, as they are not attached to the hyoid. They generally grow slowly, are often spherical and are not tender.

IMPORTANT POINTS

The main differential diagnoses for swollen cervical nodes are inflammatory processes and neoplastic processes. Searching for the underlying cause is the next step. The first thing is to examine all the other lymph nodes, but then to focus on the main suspects in the head and neck. Check for upper respiratory tract infection, dental infection, pus on tonsils or retropharyngeal abscess. Check the abdomen for enlargement of liver, or spleen, any other masses of adrenal origin (neuroblastoma), or para-aortic lymph nodes (lymphoma). It is also worth checking the BP as hypertension can be caused by neuroblastoma (which can also arise in sympathetic ganglia) which readily spreads to lymph nodes. A more detailed approach is given below.

Once it is established these are cervical lymph nodes, there are two options: either look for local primary sites; or examine all the other lymph node areas, to decide whether the process is more widespread and part of generalised lymphadenopathy. If the latter approach is adopted, then the order, after checking the neck, flows well if examining next for *epitrochlear* nodes and then *axillary* nodes, followed by abdominal examination for evidence of hepato- or splenomegaly or any other mass (intraabdominal [para-aortic] lymphadenopathy), including *inguinal* and *subinguinal* lymph nodes, and finally *popliteal* lymph nodes, although these are palpated largely for completion, as it will already be apparent whether there is generalised lymphadenopathy.

Epitrochlear lymphadenopathy

These nodes are usually not palpable, so when they are, invariably there is some pathology. The epitrochlear nodes drain the ulnar/medial aspect of the hand and the forearm.

Axillary lymphadenopathy

The axillary lymph nodes are situated along neurovascular bundles of the walls of the axilla, running to a central node and thence to an apical node superiorly; the walls of the axilla comprise anteriorly, the pectoralis major, posteriorly the subscapularis, teres major and latissimus dorsi, medially the ribs, intercostal muscles and serratus anterior, and laterally, the neck of the humerus and coracobrachialis, with the apex at the lateral border of the first rib.

The axillary nodes drain the arms, chest wall and the breasts. There are five main groups of nodes: the *anterior* (pectoral) group (drain the anterolateral abdominal wall, above the umbilicus); the *posterior* (subscapular) group (drain the back from level of iliac crests and above); the *lateral* group (lying along the axillary vein; drain the upper limb); the *central* group situated in axillary fat (drain above-mentioned groups); and the *apical* group (drain all other axillary nodes).

The examination is best performed with the child sitting up. The pectoral muscles need to be relaxed to enable adequate palpation of the axilla. This is achieved by lifting the child's arm and, while supporting the child's forearm with your own, gently push your fingers high into the axilla (your finger pulps positioned so as to roll over the nodes) and lower the child's arm, and gently explore the axilla with your fingertips, using your left hand to examine the child's right axilla, (supporting the child's right forearm with your own right forearm), and vice versa. Palpate the medial wall, then turn your hand 90 degrees to palpate anteriorly and posteriorly.

Inguinal lymphadenopathy

The nodes of the groin comprise two groups, *inguinal* and *subinguinal*. The former lie along the inguinal ligament (drain external genitalia, perineum, anus, gluteal region, lower abdominal wall), the latter consist of a superficial group which follows the course of saphenous vein (drain skin/SC tissues of leg and foot) and a deep group which is medial to the femoral vein and follow its course (drain lower limbs).

The examination of the groin is best performed with the child lying on their back on the bed, with slight flexion at the hips. Always ask about tenderness and always wear gloves if examining the draining areas (genitalia, perineum and anal region).

Brief list of typical causes for typical locations of nodes

- *Cervical*: 1. oropharyngeal/scalp infection (viral [usual URTI pathogens, EBV, CMV, HSV, HHV-6], streptococcus, staphylococcus, mycobacteria [TB, MAIS]); 2. cat-derived: cat-scratch disease; toxoplasmosis; 3. Kawasaki disease; 4. dental caries (infectious disease of dental hard tissues, decalcification of inorganic parts of tooth, then breakdown of organic matrix, dietary carbohydrate-modified, saliva-regulated).
- *Supraclavicular*: 1. (a) left side: intraabdominal malignancy; (b) right side: intra-mediastinal malignancy or infection; 2. lymphoma; 3. TB.
- *Epitrochlear*: 1. hand or arm infection; 2. cat-scratch disease; 3. lymphoma.
- *Axillary*: 1. arm or chest wall infection or malignancy; 2. animal related: cat-scratch disease; brucellosis; 3. lymphoma/leukaemia.
- *Abdominal*: 1. malignancy; 2. TB; 3. mesenteric adenitis from *Yersinia enterocolitica*, group A streptococcus or measles.
- *Inguinal*: 1. lower limb suppurative infection; 2. perineal/genito-urinary/venereal infection; 3. malignancies (rhabdomyo- and nonrhabdomyo-sarcoma; Hodgkin's and non-Hodgkin's lymphoma, neuroblastoma).
- *Popliteal*: foot or leg infection.

Examination procedure

After the preliminary observations of whether the child appears well or unwell, check the growth parameters of head circumference, weight and height. Unwell children may have infective or infiltrative conditions. Children with Kawasaki disease are remarkably irritable. Underweight children may have immune deficiencies, chronic diseases or malignancy. Overweight children may have hidradenitis suppurativa (axillary adenopathy in the obese).

Check the vital signs: fever and tachycardia may accompany infective or infiltrative diagnoses; BP may be elevated with certain tumours and connective tissue disorders with renal involvement; or decreased with sepsis or Addison disease; pulse pressure may be widened in hyperthyroidism; respiratory rate may be elevated with infective or infiltrative conditions.

Note any pallor (e.g. ALL), ecchymoses, purpura or petechiae (e.g. ALL, AML). Scan the skin; children with atopic dermatitis often have lymphadenopathy. Stand back and look for any asymmetry in the head and neck, and quickly scan for goitre. Examine all the lymph node groups as described above. If there are two groups of nodes enlarged, then it is considered generalised.

It would be prudent to examine next for hepatosplenomegaly if you have not already checked for this by including an abdominal examination.

If the finding is *cervical nodes only*, the head and neck need to be examined thoroughly. The ears, nose and throat must all be examined with the auroscope, including making a careful inspection of the teeth and gums. If any teeth appear carious, then wear gloves to palpate them for tenderness. Look at the external aspects of the eyes, for conjunctivitis (which can occur with Kawasaki disease, Parinaud's oculoglandular syndrome [with preauricular lymphadenopathy] or leptospirosis), and for Horner's syndrome, which can occur with neuroblastoma.

Inspect and palpate the scalp for any infected areas (which may be hiding under the hair, such as tinea capitis, or a kerion). Examine the skin for any local lesions (such as herpetic infections [HSV I or II, HVZ], cat-scratch disease's papular lesions on hands/fingers [*Bartonella henselae*], any inflamed areas, reddened, cellulitic, or purulent from staphylococcal or streptococcal infection; any generalised rash [rubella classically causing suboccipital lymphadenopathy; Kawasaki disease can have many types of rash; SLE causes a malar rash]) or discolouration over the nodes themselves (purplish discolouration classic for MAIS).

Examine the chest for any evidence of asthma (for underlying Churg–Strauss syndrome, or diffuse pulmonary Langerhans cell histiocytosis) or histoplasmosis (from inhaling fungal spores, *Histoplasma capsulatum*).

Examine the abdomen, for hepatosplenomegaly (**M**alignancy [neuroblastoma, lymphoma], **A**LL/AML, **T**oxoplasmosis, **C**MV, **C**onnective tissue disorders, **H**IV, **E**BV, **S**yphilis).

Examine the musculoskeletal system looking for: skeletal tenderness at sternum, clavicles, ribs, pelvis, tibiae (tibial infiltrates); joint tenderness; swelling; or decreased range of movement (ALL, AML, JIA).

After presenting your differential diagnosis, present your management plan, including which investigations should be done, and whether excisional lymph node biopsy is appropriate, knowing that in 80% of cases, the biopsy does not reveal a condition that is treatable.

Prompt node biopsy if: concerning history: night sweats, weight loss, fever for over a week, pallor, bruising; concerning examination: site; supraclavicular or lower cervical nodes; multiple sites of adenopathy; characteristics: size > 1 cm if neonatal onset, > 2 cm increasing in size or not decreasing with antibiotics; fixed nodes, which are not tender; lack of ENT infectious symptoms or signs; concerning initial investigations: abnormal full blood count and blood film, persistently elevated ESR/CRP (can be higher in Hodgkin's than in infection) although treated with antibiotics, or abnormal CXR (hilar adenopathy, or mediastinal masses). A mnemonic for this is **EXCISE**:

Enlarged beyond 1 cm neonatal, 2 cm (and growing), in older; enlarged in many sites
X-ray (CXR) abnormal: mediastinal nodes
Concerning (**C**ancer, **C**hronic inflammatory, **C**onnective tissue) symptoms: night sweats, loss of weight/**C**ervical (deep, lower) node/**C**RP persistently up despite treatment (like ESR)
Immobile (fixed)
Supraclavicular nodes
ENT symptoms and signs absent/**E**SR persistently up despite treatment (like CRP)

Investigating lymphadenopathy

In the same order as the **MATCHES** acronym, investigations can be remembered as:

Malignancy; useful investigations: *FBC, film, ESR, CRP, CXR* (mediastinal masses: anterior or middle: lymphoma [Hodgkin's or non-Hodgkin's]; posterior: neuroblastoma); *excisional biopsy, bone marrow biopsy* (ALL, AML); **M**AIS: *excisional biopsy*
ALL, AML: *FBC and film, bone marrow biopsy*
Toxoplasmosis: *serology*
Cat-scratch disease (*Bartonella henselae*): *serology/***C**hlamydia trachomatis: *serology, culture, nucleic acid probe after amplification*
HSV (gingivostomatitis): *HSV cell culture and PCR for HSV DNA/***H**odgkin's disease: *FBC, film, CXR, excisional biopsy*
EBV (Epstein-Barr virus): *serology: EBV viral capsid antigen (VCA) IgM, EBV VCA IgG, EBV nuclear antigens (EBNA): EBV EBNA-1 IgG; EBV EBNA IgM;*
Streptococcus A: *culture, serology*

Chapter 11

Neonatology

SHORT CASE: The neonatal examination

A thorough perinatal examination is the most commonly performed systematic assessment in paediatric practice. All medical undergraduates, graduates and paediatric postgraduates should be able to perform a thorough 'baby check'. If there is ever a shortage of children with impressive signs around examination time, there is always a ready supply of neonates in level 2 nurseries, ideally suited to having a comprehensive baby check performed. The examination is standard irrespective of the gestation of the infant, although the interpretation of neurobehavioural findings requires a thorough knowledge of the variations between different gestational ages. The gestational age can be assessed by the Ballard method; this is indicated where the gestational age is in doubt, but is fairly complicated and not covered in this section. The object of this section is to provide a framework for the perinatal examination that is easy to remember. Only a limited sample of possible findings is given here, as a comprehensive discussion could double this book's extent. Entire books can be, and have been, devoted to the examination of the newborn.

In hospital practice, ideally three checks are performed. An initial screening check is performed in the delivery room, assessing the baby's adaptation to the extrauterine environment. This includes assessing the Apgar scores at 1 and 5 minutes, noting any life-threatening conditions, obvious dysmorphic features (e.g. Down syndrome), gross congenital anomalies (e.g. neural tube defects), any birth injuries and counting the umbilical cord vessels, making sure there are two arteries and one vein.

The second check should be the later comprehensive examination, within the first 24 hours of life. This is the check that must be done, irrespective of the introduction, in a neonate. The order of the examination is variable, depending on what the baby is doing at the time. Generally, babies are quieter at the beginning of the examination, so always auscultate the heart first, before palpating anywhere else and disturbing the baby. The check may be approached in a somewhat opportunistic fashion: if the baby's eyes are open when first approached, check the eyes and red light reflexes (with the ophthalmoscope set at +10); if the baby yawns or cries with a wide-open mouth, take your torch and check the pharynx. Do not palpate or move the baby until the cardiorespiratory auscultation is complete: crying does not interfere very much with the remainder of the check.

After listening to the heart, listen to the chest and then palpate the abdomen and the femoral arterial pulsations in particular. Then re-inspect, checking the baby from head to toe, but leave the less pleasant aspects until later (such as checking the mouth and palate with a spatula, checking the red reflex when the baby will not open his or her eyes, checking the hips). A detailed approach is given below.

A third check is required. This may be done in hospital on day 5, but is usually performed by the local doctor at 5–10 days of age. This examination should repeat the comprehensive examination, but with particular emphasis on the following:

- The cardiovascular system, particularly the heart and pulses for any evidence of cyanosis, murmurs, left-sided obstructive lesions or failure.
- The central nervous system, fontanelles and sutures.
- The skin, for jaundice, evidence of dehydration (skin turgor) or rashes.
- The umbilical cord, for any signs of infection (omphalitis).
- The abdomen, for any masses previously overlooked.
- Repeating the hip examination.

At this examination, the urine and stool outputs are noted and growth parameters are repeated as well, checking for adequate weight gain and feeding.

Inspect: growth, colour, respirations, posture, movements, cry

The initial thorough examination commences with inspection. Note the baby's weight, length, head circumference and nutritional status (muscle bulk, fat). Note the colour (peripheral cyanosis is common) and the respiratory rate (normal being 40–60 breaths per minute; periodic breathing is normal) and depth (retraction indicates some respiratory distress). Causes of tachypnoea include primary respiratory disorders (e.g. hyaline membrane disease, transient tachypnoea of the newborn, meconium aspiration, congenital pneumonia, pneumothorax), space-occupying lesions (e.g. diaphragmatic hernia, congenital cystic lung lesions) or non-respiratory systems: cardiac (e.g. shunts, left-heart obstructive lesions, myocardial disease, arrhythmias), metabolic (e.g. hypoglycaemia), infective (e.g. septicaemia) or haematological causes (e.g. anaemia, polycythaemia). Stridor may be noted with upper airway obstruction. It may be purely inspiratory if the obstruction is extrathoracic, and may involve expiration if intrathoracic. The causes are usually divided into site, intraluminal (e.g. meconium, mucus, blood or milk), intramural (e.g. subglottic oedema from overenthusiastic tracheal suctioning) or extramural (e.g. vascular ring). For more details, see the short case on stridor in Chapter 15, The respiratory system.

Posture, quality of movement and nature of cry are noted. The gestation of the infant must be considered with respect to posture. Normal full-term neonates usually lie with their hips abducted and slightly flexed, their knees flexed and their upper limbs adducted, with flexion at the elbow and clenching of the fists (not tight), with fingers covering the thumb.

Term babies with significant hypotonia may lie with their hips and thighs in the 'frog's legs position' (see the floppy infant case in Chapter 13, Neurology). Babies with serious intracranial pathology may lie with extended necks (opisthotonic posture), obligate flexion of thumbs or scissored lower limbs. Very premature infants (less than 30 weeks) normally have minimal flexor tone, like a rag doll; by 34 weeks, flexor tone appears in the lower limbs, and by 36 weeks in the upper limbs as well. A formal gestational assessment should be undertaken if the gestation is in doubt and the infant seems hypotonic, so as not to overinterpret normal findings of prematurity.

Normal movements may include alternating movements in all limbs, myoclonic jerks when asleep (sleep myoclonus) and jaw tremors when crying. Paucity of movement can occur in neuromuscular diseases (see the floppy infant case in Chapter 13, Neurology).

Involuntary movements can include tremulousness or 'jitters' (which can be stopped by gentle pressure) and seizures (may be subtle, tonic or more often focal, irrespective of the underlying pathology, and cannot be stopped by pressure, clearly differentiating them from jitters). Jitters can occur with hypoglycaemia, hypocalcaemia, sepsis and neonatal abstinence syndrome (NAS). Seizures can be due to neonatal encephalopathy (formally termed hypoxic ischaemic encephalopathy), intracranial haemorrhage, meningitis, metabolic causes (hypoglycaemia/hyponatraemia/hypocalcaemia/hypomagnesaemia; hypernatraemia/hyperammonaemia; kernicterus, various inborn errors, pyridoxine deficiency), developmental brain disorders and NAS, or can be idiopathic.

Asymmetric movement can occur secondary to cerebral malformations or intrauterine cerebrovascular accidents, or with birth injuries such as intracranial haemorrhage, or brachial plexus lesions such as Erb (C5,6) and Klumpke (C8,T1) palsies. Remember the myotomes of the upper limbs by the children's nursery rhyme 'five, six, pick up sticks [flex biceps], seven, eight, lay them straight [extension predominantly due to C7]'.

The cry is noted. A high-pitched cry goes with cerebral irritation, as in neonatal encephalopathy or meningitis. A hoarse cry can occur with upper airway obstruction and a cat cry occurs with the uncommon cri du chat syndrome (chromosome 5p-syndrome).

Remember that you have to be opportunistic while a baby is settled. Do not examine the eyes or pharynx before other aspects of the examination that require a quiet baby. A suggested head-to-toe examination procedure is given below. The baby will determine in which order this occurs, however.

Systematic examination: head to toe
HEAD, NECK AND UPPER LIMBS

Initial inspection should detect any dysmorphic features. The head is examined for any traumatic injuries (abrasions, depressed fractures, haematomata or lacerations) and swellings (central [caput succedaneum] or to one [or both] side[s], stopping at suture lines [cephalhaematomata]). Fontanelles and sutures are palpated to assess size. They may be widened with increased intracranial pressure, as with hydrocephalus, or narrowed (or undetectable) and immobile with craniosynostosis.

The anterior fontanelle is highly variable in its shape and size. The head circumference (HC) must be measured, ideally with a paper (non-stretching) tape measure, around the head at the widest point: at term, the normal range is 32–37 cm. A useful rule of thumb is HC (cm) = height/2 + 10.

Next, the eyes are checked (if the baby allows this at the time), including red light reflexes. Make sure that the eyes are examined. Even a baby who refuses to open the eyes at all (even on parental report) should have the corneas visualised (forcibly) to exclude glaucoma (which causes them to appear enlarged and very hazy). The nose is inspected. The metal condensation test can show bilateral nasal patency. A shiny pink lesion in the nostril can be a frontal lobe encephalocele (not mucus, so do not try to suck it out—the author has seen an encephalocele being assaulted with a suction catheter for several minutes in just such a case). The lips, gums, tongue, palate and oropharynx must be thoroughly assessed, including using a torch and spatula. A submucous cleft can easily be missed if direct inspection is not performed. The size of the tongue is also noted: macroglossia can be a clue to hypothyroidism or to Beckwith syndrome.

The size and structure of the chin are noted. Micrognathia (mandibular hypoplasia) can occur separately or as part of the Pierre Robin sequence. At this point, the suck can be checked by placing the little finger in the baby's mouth. The rooting reflex does not need to be tested. The ears are then checked for symmetry and positioning: deviations in each can occur with several syndromes.

The neck is then inspected for redundant skin posterolaterally, or 'web neck' (Noonan and Turner syndromes), and checked for any masses (e.g. lymphatic malformation or 'cystic hygroma') or fistulae (e.g. branchial), asymmetry (transient as in persistent fetal posturing; permanent as in the maldeveloped cervical vertebrae of Klippel–Feil syndrome) and range of movement (torticollis from sternocleidomastoid fibrosis/tumour).

Check the hands, forearms and arms from a dysmorphic viewpoint (see the case on the dysmorphic child in Chapter 9, Genetics and dysmorphology).

CARDIORESPIRATORY SYSTEM

The conditions that must not be missed include coarctation (and other critical left-sided obstructive lesions such as hypoplastic left-heart syndrome, critical aortic stenosis and aortic interruption) and pulmonary hypertension, as evidenced by an active right ventricle (the presence of which, beyond day 3, may be associated with a significant systemic-to-pulmonary shunt, or an obstructed left-heart lesion, as above). A warm stethoscope helps to keep the infant quiet during auscultation. Localise the apex by auscultation. Note the heart rate (normal is 120–160 beats per minute). A murmur on day 1 can be due to a closing ductus arteriosus. This should disappear over the following days. Murmurs due to valvular lesions and vessel abnormalities (e.g. coarctation) will be present on day 1 also.

Septal defects are unlikely to be heard on day 1, as there is minimal pressure differential between the left and right sides. As pressure changes occur (right ventricular pressure dropping, and left ventricular pressure increasing) the left side becomes dominant, and left-to-right shunts due to ventricular and atrial septal defects become audible after a few days. The second heart sound may be loud, and single or closely split, with pulmonary hypertension. After thorough auscultation, including all sites of possible radiation of any murmurs, listen to the chest. Finally, palpation of the femoral arteries and comparison with the brachial pulses is crucial to allow detection of the obstructed left-heart problems noted above.

ABDOMEN AND GENITALIA

After inspection, gentle palpation for any masses or organomegaly is performed. The normal liver edge may be felt 1–2 cm below the costal margin in the midclavicular line, with the baby supine. The liver span at birth is around 2–2.5 cm. The kidneys may be easily palpable, especially the left one. Remove the nappy to check the groin, the genitalia and the anus. Any swelling in the groin is abnormal (e.g. indirect inguinal hernia).

In male babies, the scrotum is prominent, and should contain both testes (which should be of similar size). Hydrocoeles are common but often transient. Note the position of the urethral orifice (to detect epi- or hypospadias).

In female babies, the labia majora are prominent, and mucosal tags are frequent. There may be creamy vaginal discharge, replaced by day 3 with bleeding (pseudomenses). The labia should be spread to exclude imperforate hymen or other abnormalities (e.g. cysts of vaginal wall).

Ambiguous genitalia may represent virilised females (e.g. congenital adrenal hyperplasia [CAH], aromatase deficiency), inadequately virilised males (e.g. testicular defects, disorders of androgen production or action) or chromosomal defects. Take particular note of the phallus size, the position of orifices, labioscrotal fusion, pigmentation (CAH) and whether any gonads are palpable. For more detail, see the short case on ambiguous genitalia in Chapter 7, Endocrinology. The baby's anus must be evaluated for patency and position.

HIP EXAMINATION

The hip examination is most important—to detect developmental dysplasia of the hip (DDH, previously called congenital dislocation of the hip [CDH]). DDH can be difficult to detect on just one examination, even for very experienced clinicians, as the femoral head could be enlocated on that occasion. Thus, examination of the hip should be re-performed after the initial assessment. Asymmetric skin creases in the buttocks may occur with DDH, but are not a reliable sign of this. Similarly, unilateral DDH can be accompanied by a weaker femoral pulse to palpation on the affected side, but this is uncommon.

There are two standard manoeuvres:

1. **Ortolani's test** is to reduce a posteriorly dislocated femoral head. The middle finger is placed over the greater trochanter, with the hips and knees flexed to 90 degrees, the baby lying on a firm surface. With the knee in the palm, the thigh is gently abducted while the thigh is brought forward to enlocate the femoral head, which should (may) produce a 'clunk' of relocation.

2. **Barlow's test** is to detect whether the femoral head can be dislocated. The pelvis is fixed with one hand (with the thumb over the pubic symphysis, and the other four digits behind the coccygeal area). The other hand firmly holds the thigh and adducts it gently downwards: in DDH, the head dislocates over the posterior lip of the acetabulum, with an accompanying 'clunk'.

To remember which test is which, **O**rtolani's **O**pens **O**ut the lower limbs, **B**arlow's **B**umps **B**ack the femoral head. You need remember only one of these, the other being the opposite. Often, these manoeuvres will detect a 'click' or 'snap', which is ligamentous or muscular in origin and usually of no significance if the hip feels otherwise stable. If the clinical examination is equivocal, or normal but there is a history of breech presentation, or a first-degree relative with DDH or significant oligohydramnios, hip ultrasound is indicated at 6 weeks.

LOWER LIMBS

The lower limbs are checked for their length and shape. The feet are checked for postural and structural variations. Talipes calcaneovalgus is usually due to postural deformity secondary to intrauterine pressure. If full inversion can be achieved such that the sole is aligned vertically, the talipes is postural. Talipes equinovarus may be postural, or structural with muscle wasting. If full eversion is achieved, with the forefoot abducted and the little toe touched to the tibia (thus apposing the dorsum of the foot to the shin), the problem is probably postural.

NERVOUS SYSTEM AND SPINE

After having inspected for posture, symmetry and quality of movement, check the palmar grasp, pull the baby to sitting position, and note tone, degree of head control and head lag. Next, the baby can be positioned supine along the forearm, with the hand, palm upwards, supporting the neck and head and lifting the head gently. This support is transiently withdrawn by suddenly dorsiflexing the hand, eliciting the Moro (startle) reflex in a gentle fashion. The Moro reflex may demonstrate asymmetry of limb movement (e.g. with brachial plexus injury) or of facial expression (e.g. facial nerve palsy), or may be absent with significant intracranial pathology. If there are any concerns in any of the above areas, tap out the deep tendon reflexes.

The baby is then held in ventral suspension (normal being a convexity), and the spine is inspected carefully for abnormal curvature (e.g. scoliosis from vertebral anomalies), midline birthmarks, masses, pits or tufts of hair (e.g. diastematomyelia). Sacral or sacrococcygeal pits and sinuses are common and of no clinical importance. The anus can be inspected at this time if previously omitted.

The Galant (truncal incurvation) reflex can then be checked by stroking down one side of the spine from the neck to the coccyx; the spine should curve towards that side. The Galant reflex gives some indication of segmental integrity from T2 to S1.

Next, the stepping and walking reflexes can be tested. A supported baby will make walking movements when the feet are placed on a firm surface. The baby may then have the dorsum of each foot placed against the underside of a ledge, and will normally step up on to the ledge.

This completes the neurological assessment. Testing of deep tendon reflexes is not required unless there are specific concerns, as above.

SKIN

Many benign, transient rashes may affect neonates and often worry new parents. The most common rash noted in the first days of life is erythema toxicum neonatorum, appearing on any part of the body except the palms and soles as erythematous macules, usually with a central white or yellow papule. These 'pustules' are sterile, containing eosinophils. Milia are pinhead-sized white papules on the nose, forehead and cheeks, containing keratogenous material. Miliaria is due to obstructed eccrine sweat glands, usually seen on the forehead, scalp and skin folds.

Several pigmented lesions are common, especially the Mongolian spot, a blue–grey area over the lumbosacral region seen in most Asian and African American babies, which can be mistaken for a bruise initially. Multiple café-au-lait macules (CALMS) occur in neurofibromatosis and several other syndromal diagnoses. Hypopigmented macules occur in tuberous sclerosus.

Vascular birthmarks are common, and there are two distinct types:

1. **Vascular malformations**, which are always present at birth (e.g. trigeminal distribution 'port wine stain' in Sturge-Weber syndrome, with accompanying angiomatous malformation of the brain) and will grow in proportion to the rest of the body. See later this chapter for a short case on vascular birthmarks.

2. **Haemangiomata** (e.g. 'strawberry naevus'), which (usually) are not present at birth, and will grow out of proportion to the rest of the body for 24 weeks, then involute slowly, with 50% gone by 5 years. Haemangiomata are of concern in certain areas: for example, near the eyes (can block vision, causing amblyopia), ears (can block ear canal causing 'auditory amblyopia') or 'beard' region (may indicate underlying laryngeal involvement), and may need to be treated with corticosteroids or laser therapy. This is more likely an issue at the 6-week check. See later this chapter for a short case on vascular birthmarks.

To reiterate, unpleasant aspects of the baby check may be best left until last, but must not be forgotten. These include the inspection of the palate (using spatula and torch), checking the hips (some babies seem to hate this), the Moro reflex and checking the eyes if this was not possible earlier.

Why 3 and 5 are the most useful numbers in neonatology

- **3.5 kg**: average **weight** of a term baby
- **35 cm**: average **head circumference** of a term baby
- **50 cm**: average **length** of a term baby
- **7.35–7.45**: normal range for **pH** in arterial blood
- **35–45 mmHg**: normal range pCO_2 in arterial blood
- **135–145 mEq/L**: normal range for serum **sodium**
- **3.5–4.5 mEq/L**: normal range for serum **potassium**
- **3.5 mm**: size (internal diameter) of **endotracheal tube** used to intubate term baby
- **35–40 cm H_2O**: pressure at which **blow-off valve** operates **in most resuscitaire devices** (bag and mask) to prevent pressures above 35–40 cm H_2O being transmitted to baby causing pneumothorax
- **350 µmol/L: serum bilirubin level (SBR)** above which, historically, exchange transfusion was considered, to prevent kernicterus (actually it is 342 µmol/L, which is 20 mg/dL in the older pre-SI units, and led to the coining of the term **vigintiphobia** [fear of the number 20]; this pre-dated phototherapy)
- **35 weeks'** gestation: gestational age (really applies to 34–35 weeks, but close enough)
  - **under which** almost all babies will need (at least some) **nasogastric feeding**
  - **under which** excessive **oxygen** can still be **toxic to retinae**
  - **over which apnoea of prematurity stops** being a problem
- **35–60 breaths per minute**: range for normal **respiratory rate** (close enough; most references say around 40–60 breaths per minute)
- **135–160 beats per minute**: range for normal **heart rate** (close enough; most references say 140–160 beats per minute when awake, but can be 100–120 when asleep; some babies have a resting pulse rate below 100 when asleep, which is termed 'baseline bradycardia', being a normal variant)
- **30 WCC × 10^9**: highest white cell count in normal neonatal full blood count in first 24 hours of life

Complications of prematurity

The mnemonic for complications of prematurity is: **PREMATURITY**

Patent ductus arteriosus (PDA)

Respiratory distress syndrome (RDS; surfactant deficiency, hyaline membrane disease [HMD])

Encephalopathy: from bleed (periventricular, intraventricular, intracranial haemorrhage [PVH, IVH, ICH] or ischaemia [periventricular leukomalacia, PVL])

Metabolic immaturity (hypoglycaemia, hypocalcaemia, hypomagnesaemia)

Apnoea of prematurity

Thermoregulatory immaturity (importance of neutral thermal zone [NTZ])

Umbilical line requirement for those under 28 weeks

Retinopathy of prematurity

Infection/**I**mmunological immaturity

Transient anaemia (anaemia of prematurity)

Yellow (jaundice)

SHORT CASE: The 6-week check

The procedure for the examination of the infant at the 6-week check is essentially the same as for the perinatal examination. By 6 weeks, most term infants should be able to smile responsively (spontaneous smiling occurs later, from 6 weeks to 5 months), and some primitive reflexes have been fully incorporated (stepping and walking reflexes). The baby is now able to lift the head momentarily when prone (usually by 3 weeks) and can hold the head in line with the trunk when held in ventral suspension.

The key areas to re-examine include growth parameters, particularly weight gain (normally 150–200 g per week), head circumference (e.g. to exclude hydrocephalus), cardiovascular system (murmurs and femoral pulses) for defects that may not have been apparent at discharge from hospital (e.g. septal defects, coarctation), hip examination (you can never examine the hips too often, as DDH can still present late), and eye examination to exclude cataracts or causes of leucocoria (white eye) that may have been overlooked or more difficult to detect in the earlier examination, and to check the ability to fix and follow to the midline (normally occurs by 5 weeks). If there is any jaundice, biliary atresia must be borne in mind, and direct and indirect bilirubin levels checked. Other, new problems may have arisen (e.g. nappy rashes, haemangiomata, umbilical granulomata). As with the neonatal examination, leaving the unpleasant parts until the end can be a good idea. The 6-week check is also a good time to discuss the importance of upcoming immunisation.

SHORT CASE: Vascular birthmarks

Occasionally in an examination, but more commonly in real life, one can encounter an infant, usually a newborn, with a facial vascular birthmark, and the first question to decide is: is this a vascular malformation or a haemangioma? If it is a vascular malformation, is it associated with any relevant syndrome. There are five which are easily recalled: three have Weber in the name (Sturge-Weber syndrome [SWS], Parkes-Weber syndrome [PKWS], and Klippel-Trénaunay-Weber [KTW] syndrome), the other two are Proteus syndrome (PS), and cerebral cavernous malformations (CCM) [MIM 116860] which includes hyperkeratotic cutaneous capillary-venous malformations (HCCVMs).

If it is a haemangioma, is it localised (and is it superficial or deep) or is it segmental? If the latter, is it associated with any relevant syndrome (there are two that are associated with haemangiomata: with facial haemangioma, the PHACE syndrome, and with perineal haemangiomata, the PELVIS syndrome). If it is not segmental but localised, note if it is over an area that could cause significant impairment: those near the eye can cause amblyopia, those near the ear can cause an auditory equivalent of amblyopia, those near the nose can cause nasal obstruction, those near the mouth can cause feeding issues, and those in the 'beard' distribution can be associated with underlying intra-tracheal haemangiomata.

The next question is whether there are lesions elsewhere. In the case of vascular malformations, signs to seek include hemihyperplasia (see the short case on body asymmetry in Chapter 9, Genetics and dysmorphology). In the case of haemangiomata, are there multiple lesions involving only the skin (such as in eruptive neonatal haemangiomatosis) or are there lesions within internal organs (specifically brain, eyes, lungs and the gastrointestinal tract)? The short case examination should therefore involve not only inspection and palpation, but auscultation. It is possible to detect vascular bruits with lesions in the brain, liver or spleen. A child with this is unlikely to be encountered in the examination, as they are usually very unwell, but as very atypical conditions present to very typical doctors, it is worth mentioning for completion.

Candidates should also be aware of Kasabach-Merritt syndrome (previously called, inappropriately, haemangioma-thrombocytopaenia syndrome) which occurs only with a small number of very rapidly growing vascular tumours; it does not occur with large haemangiomas, as was previously believed. It comprises a vascular tumour (usually either a **Ka**posiform haem**a**ngioendothelioma, or a tufted angioma, **c**onsumptive coagulopathy, **m**icroangiopathic haemolytic anaemia and **t**hrombocytopaenia, [**Kasabach-Merritt**]). These lesions, in addition to significant local growth, can cause cardiac failure, so in any pale infant with petechiae and what appears to be a fast-growing haemangioma, this diagnosis should be considered, and is a further reason to auscultate another area: the heart for a gallop rhythm. The author had a neonatal patient exactly like this, with what seemed to be a fast-growing haemangioma of the upper limb, until one day the baby developed marked pallor and some petechiae, and had a gallop rhythm; the Hb level was below 40, the platelet count below 20, the patient required platelet and blood transfusions, and later laser treatment, and plastic surgery including skin grafting.

Describe the lesion in a similar fashion to how one would describe any lump or swelling; obviously a haemangioma truly is a swelling, whereas vascular malformations such as a port wine stain birthmark are macular skin lesions, but the 'swelling' approach is largely applicable here as well.

To refresh the memory of the many aspects of any swelling, there are inspection aspects (start with S), palpation aspects (start with T), plus auscultation; some aspects are unnecessary (such as percussion) but most are relevant.

The relevant characteristics are: on *inspection*: **s**ite, **s**ize, **s**hape, **s**ides (edges), **s**hine (colour), **s**urface, **s**urroundings; on *palpation*: **t**enderness, **t**emperature, **t**ethering (mobility), **t**ransmitted pulsation, **t**hrill (from vascular lesion), **t**ension (consistency), **t**ransient emptying/filling; and *auscultation* (for bruit; any haemangioma can have a bruit, but if a swelling looks more like a venous malformation, but has a bruit, there could be an underlying arteriovenous malformation [AVM]). The final aspect is *associated pathology*: in the case of haemangiomata, indications of underlying syndromes (PHACES, PELVIS) or particular subgroups (segmental, multiple); in the case of vascular malformations, other underlying syndromes (SWS, PKWS, KTW, PS, CCM). Further examination is guided by the type of lesion.

For **haemangiomata**, after scanning all the skin to check for multiple lesions, examine the head (for bruits), then the abdomen (specifically liver for bruits), and then the cardiorespiratory system (for heart rate [may be taking propranolol] or for signs of failure, such as gallop rhythm, or crackles, for the remote possibility of a Kasabach-Merritt syndrome; *not* specifically for stridor in the short case examination [unless the child is in hospital because awaiting a bronchoscopy] because with any intra-tracheal haemangioma, as soon as stridor has been recognised, there is usually an urgent bronchoscopy and definitive treatment, at that time, for any intratracheal haemangioma, and the signs are gone).

For **vascular malformations**, after scanning all the skin to check for multiple lesions, stand back and look for any asymmetry (in particular, look for hemihyperplasia [can occur in PKWS or in KTW]). If there is facial involvement with port wine stain (PWS) capillary malformations in the distribution of the trigeminal nerve, then examine the child as per the Sturge-Weber short-case approach: do not forget to examine the eyes for glaucoma or field defects, and do not forget to examine the gait for signs of hemiplegia on the side opposite to the facial PWS. If there is no facial involvement of PWSs, but there is asymmetry, examine the child as per the hemihyperplasia (body asymmetry) short case looking for features consistent with PKWS or KTW. If there are both facial PWSs and asymmetry, follow the Sturge-Weber approach and then add in relevant aspects of the hemihyperplasia approach.

Haemangiomata—associated conditions: **PHACES association** (OMIM#606519) and **PELVIS association**

PHACES association is a neurocutaneous condition, comprising segmented facial or scalp haemangiomata, and extracutaneous anomalies of the cerebrovascular, cardiovascular and ocular systems, plus posterior fossa brain malformations and ventral developmental defects, set out as an acronym. Over 85% of patients are female.

Posterior fossa brain malformation (Dandy-Walker syndrome, cerebellar hypoplasia, developmental delay, seizures)

Haemangiomata of face/scalp (large, complex, segmented, > 5 cm diameter; can be subglottic)

Arterial malformations (aneurysms [including aorta {see below}, internal carotid, subclavian, cerebral arteries], moya-moya phenomenon, arterial stenoses)

Cardio-aortic anomalies (ventricular septal defect [VSD], patent ductus arteriosus [PDA], coarctation of the aorta, congenital aneurysms including ascending aorta and aortic arch, steal syndrome)

Eye anomalies (microphthalmia [ipsilateral to haemangioma], Horner syndrome, cataract, optic atrophy)/**E**ndocrine: lingual thyroid/hypothyroidism (congenital)

Sternal anomalies (clefts, pits)/**S**upraumbilical abdominal raphe (ventral developmental defects)

PELVIS association (also known by alternate acronyms SACRAL and LUMBAR) is a neuocutaneous condition, comprising segmental haemangiomata in the perineal/pelvic region (lumbosacral, buttock and perineal/nappy area), and extracutaneous anomalies of the spine (spinal dysraphism), genitourinary system and anorectal region (including imperforate anus). The haemangioma may be difficult to diagnose as it can appear macular, telangiectatic or mottled reddish-blue ('livedoid').

Perineal segmented haemangioma
External genitalia anomalies
Lipomeningocele
Vesicorenal anomalies
Imperforate anus
Skin tag

Chapter 12

Nephrology

LONG CASES

LONG CASE: Chronic kidney disease (CKD)

There has been much progress in the last few years in paediatric nephrology. Most paediatric renal transplants (RTx) come from live-related donors (usually a parent or grandparent), as these enable better long-term outcomes (graft survival 5 years in 75–80% versus 65% for deceased donor transplant). Barriers to transplantation are being overcome through strategies including paired kidney exchange (see RTx section), selective use of ABO-incompatible RTx, and desensitisation for children with elevated levels of donor-specific HLA antibodies. Infants with genetic causes of end-stage kidney disease (ESKD) can have a pre-emptive RTx (without prior dialysis) from a member of their family, avoiding the morbidity and mortality associated with dialysis.

Chronic kidney disease (CKD) is divided into six stages (CKD 1–5, 5D), the first stage having a normal glomerular filtration rate (GFR) and the sixth stage requiring renal replacement therapy (RRT) by dialysis and/or RTx. The stages in between describe mild, moderate and severe reductions in renal function. RTx is the treatment of choice for ESKD. Many of the multiple long-term problems of CKD involving growth and neurocognitive development are improved with RTx.

The management of paediatric CKD now has incorporated fully the findings of the landmark ESCAPE trial (**E**ffect of **S**trict Blood Pressure **C**ontrol and **A**CE [Angiotensin-Converting Enzyme] Inhibition on the **P**rogress of CRF in Pediatric Patients), published in the NEJM in October 2009. This proved that intensified blood pressure (BP) control (keeping ambulatory BP < 50th centile) in children aged 3–18 years with CKD Stages 3–5, delayed progression of kidney disease. All children received ACE inhibition at a standard dose, so additional medications such as calcium channel blockers were used to achieve BP targets. BP control improved 5-year renal survival by 35% in children with CKD.

Technical progress has been made towards improved renal supportive therapy for those requiring RRT. Proposed alternatives to dialysis include: a wearable system, termed the 'Human Nephron Filter (HNF)', which has a biocompatible nano-membrane with a solute clearance profile superior to haemodialysis; a bioartificial kidney, which contains a renal tubule-cell cartridge and can deliver some functions of a normal kidney that dialysis does not provide; the 'Vincenza wearable artificial kidney (VAK)', which is a wearable form of peritoneal dialysis; and cellular therapies, utilising stem cells to repair or regenerate damaged kidney tissue.

Prenatal programming of renal disease is now well recognised. Being born with low birth weight (from IUGR [intrauterine growth restriction], small for gestational age [SGA] or from being born prematurely) increases the risk of CKD in adulthood.

It is postulated that an adverse intrauterine environment decreases the final number of nephrons; hence the job for the paediatrician is to identify children at risk, avoiding nephrotoxic drugs (e.g. aminoglycosides, non-steroidal anti-inflammatory drugs [NSAIDs]), obesity counselling starting in the neonatal period (other risk factors should be discussed with parents of IUGR/SGA or premature babies to minimise exposure to smoking and to encourage healthy diet) and monitoring blood pressure to prevent hypertension, early recognition of proteinuria (and treatment with ACE inhibitors or angiotensin blockers) and obesity.

Genetic aspects of adult and paediatric CKD have been discussed widely. In adults, genes associated with CKD include the gene ACTN4 (actinin alpha 4), which encodes for a non-muscle alpha actinin isoform; mutations in this gene are associated with an inherited form of focal segmental glomerulosclerosis (FSGS). Another associated gene is UMOD (uromodulin), which encodes for uromodulin, the most abundant protein in urine; mutations in this gene are associated with medullary cystic kidney disease-2 (MCKD2), familial juvenile hyperuric nephropathy and with CKD in the general population by genome-wide association.

In children, mutations in the genes (NPHS1, NPHS2) encoding for the proteins nephrin and podocin in the slit diaphragm between podocyte foot processes result in congenital nephrotic syndrome and FSGS respectively.

Mutations in at least 11 different genes have been identified in children with juvenile nephronophthisis (NPH), with all these genes encoding for proteins in primary cilia of renal epithelial cells; hence NPHs are now termed 'ciliopathies'.

The infantile form of NPH causes ESKD by 4 years; the mutated gene is NPHP2. The juvenile form of NPH causes ESKD by around 13 years; the mutated genes are NPHP1, NPHP4, NPHP5, NPHP6, NPHP7, NPHP8, NPHP9, NPH11 and NPH1L. The adolescent form of NPH causes ESKD by around 20 years. Other genetic kidney disorders now recognised as ciliopathies are autosomal dominant polycystic kidney disease (ADPKD, mainly affects adults, rarely children) and autosomal recessive polycystic kidney disease (mutated gene is PKDHD1 and encodes the protein 'fibrocystin/polyductin', which maintains [normal] tubular architecture), which affects neonates, and requires RTx.

Children with CKD often appear in the long-case section of the clinical examination, most having end-stage renal disease (ESRD), and requiring renal supportive (dialysis) or (transplant) therapy to survive. The principles of management should be well understood, and the candidates should be fully conversant with treatment modalities such as automated peritoneal dialysis (APD; also called continuous cycling peritoneal dialysis, CCPD), continuous ambulatory peritoneal dialysis (CAPD), haemodialysis, RTx and the commonly used immunosuppressive drugs and biological agents.

Background information
AETIOLOGY

1. Glomerulonephritis: 30%.
2. Malformation (structural) of kidney/urinary tract: 30%.
3. Hereditary nephropathies (e.g. nephronophthisis, cystinosis): 20%.
4. Others (e.g. haemolytic uraemic syndrome [HUS], nephrotoxins): 20%.

Causes can be divided into congenital and acquired. Congenital nephropathies and maldevelopments of the urinary tract tend to cause 'delayed' ESRD, by 5–15 years, with a protracted course of (perhaps subclinical) CKD, causing poor growth. Acquired conditions (rarer in infancy and early childhood) tend to progress faster, affected children having previously had normal growth before their illness. In general, congenital causes equate with groups 2 and 3, and acquired causes with groups 1 and 4.

At present, the most common form of glomerular disease causing ESRD is focal segmental glomerulosclerosis. In some populations, around 30% of patients with sporadic forms of the disease have mutations in the gene encoding for podocin. However, in African American populations with FSGS, detection of mutations is uncommon. Other causes of ESRD are systemic lupus erythematosus (SLE), rapidly progressive glomerulonephritis, IgA nephropathy, Henoch–Schönlein purpura nephritis and mesangiocapillary glomerulonephritis.

Hereditary nephropathies are numerous (over 50 types at present).

There are two important points to remember:

1. *Structural* problems tend to cause salt- and water-losing forms of CKD.
2. *Glomerular* disease tends to cause oliguria, salt retention and hypertension.

Many children have dysplastic disease (structural), which leads to polyuric renal failure, so they may drink large amounts of fluid, and do not have any problems with oedema or hypertension.

This is quite different to adults with CKD, most of whom are oliguric or anuric. Irrespective of the original cause of kidney damage, once CKD supervenes, there is relentless progression towards kidney failure, but the rate of this is quite variable. Risk factors for rapid decline include lower levels of kidney function at presentation, higher levels of proteinuria, and hypertension. Increased protein in urine causes injury to tubular cells, which leads to interstitial inflammation and fibrosis; in patients with CKD, blocking the RAS decreases proteinuria and slows the deterioration to ESKD. Systemic hypertension causes intraglomerular hypertension, which leads to glomerular hypertrophy and injury; intensified BP control slows progression of renal failure.

Glomerular filtration rate (GFR) and clinical correlates

In general, *asymptomatic* CKD is correlated with a *GFR > 30 mL/min/1.73 m^2* and *symptomatic* CKD with a *GFR < 30 mL/min/1.73 m^2*, but this depends on the cause of CKD. For example, children with FSGS and nephrotic syndrome are symptomatic with significantly reduced quality of life at minor reductions in GFR. At a GFR below normal (normal being 100–120 mL/min/1.73 m^2) but > 30 mL/min/1.73 m^2, serum creatinine is usually up to 0.2 mmol/L (this depends on the size of the patient). This corresponds to the group of children with CKD who are monitored regularly (for their growth, development, BP, serum creatinine, evidence of renal bone disease and estimated GFR) and may receive specific treatment for their specific diagnoses (e.g. cysteamine for cystinosis).

They may also require antihypertensive agents, sodium supplements, bicarbonate supplements, calcitriol and phosphate binders. However, most of this group will progress to ESKD. Clinical problems usually are not evident until *GFR < 25–30 mL/min/1.73 m^2*.

At a *GFR 30–15 mL/min/1.73 m^2*, usually serum *creatinine* level is *0.2–0.8 mmol/L*, depending on the size of the child. This corresponds to a group who require medical manipulation, but not yet dialysis or transplantation. In children in this group who are undiagnosed, symptoms develop (e.g. anorexia, fatigability) and finally bring the child to medical attention.

At a *GFR < 15 mL/min/1.73 m²*, usually serum *creatinine is > 0.8 mmol/L* in older children, but small children may require RRT at creatinine levels of 0.35–0.5 mmol/L. This group requires dialysis or RTx. If the *GFR is < 5 mL/min/1.73 m²*, symptoms such as nausea, vomiting and oedema become severe, and, without treatment, pericarditis, bleeding diatheses and uraemic encephalopathy will supervene. The new staging is as follows:

- *Stage 1*: normal or increased GFR (≥ *90 mL/min/1.73 m²*), with some evidence of kidney damage.
- *Stage 2*: mildly decreased GFR (*60–89 mL/min/1.73 m²*); the emphasis is on prevention of disease progression.
- *Stage 3*: moderately decreased GFR (*30–59 mL/min/1.73 m²*); the emphasis is on prevention of disease progression, plus managing complications.
- *Stage 4*: severely decreased GFR (*15–29 mL/min/1.73 m²*); the emphasis is on treating complications, and preparing for dialysis or transplant.
- *Stage 5*: very little GFR left (*< 15 mL/min/1.73 m²*); dialysis imminent.
- *Stage 5D*: *RRT* required.

ESKD refers to the time when medical management is insufficient and renal supportive/replacement therapy is needed (dialysis or transplant).

AIDE-MÉMOIRE FOR GFR

An easy way to remember these stages is to think of two numbers: 30 and 15 (mL/min/1.73 m²). Thus:

- GFR > 30: monitor (Stages 1, 2 and 3); each stage 30 below the previous.
- GFR 15–30: medical manipulation (Stage 4); symptomatic.
- GFR < 15: RRT imminent/commenced (Stages 5 and 5D); waiting for a transplant.

Useful calculations

CALCULATION OF GFR

The estimated GFR (eGFR) can be approximated by an empirically derived formula, the Schwartz formula, based on the relationship between muscle mass and serum creatinine:

$$eGFR = 40 \times height\ (cm)/serum\ creatinine\ (micromol/L)$$

The calculation for a child who is 120 cm tall and has a serum creatinine level of 200 micromol/L would be: eGFR = 40 × 120/200 = 24.

This child's GFR would be 24 mL/min/1.73 m². Note that this formula is less useful in children under 2 years. Also, the Schwarz formula is not valid for patients with abnormal body proportions or markedly reduced muscle mass, and can overestimate GFR at lower levels of GFR. It is not valid in children with acute renal failure or where renal function is not stable.

GFR also can be measured by DTPA (Tc99m **d**iethylene **t**riamine **p**enta-acetic **a**cid) clearance, or by iohexol plasma disappearance.

ASSESSMENT OF RATE OF EVOLUTION OF RENAL FAILURE

The use of the reciprocal of creatinine to measure this has fallen out of favour. A graph was plotted of the reciprocal of the serum creatinine (on the vertical axis) against time (on the horizontal axis) for 1 year; at least five measurements over that time were needed, and the patient had to be stable (no development of hypertension, urinary tract infections or such like) for it to be more accurate. This was thought to give the rate of decline of renal function, and the stage at which a given child will develop ESRD could be determined by extrapolating the graph to where it intersected the time axis.

History

PRESENTING COMPLAINT

Reason for current admission.

PAST HISTORY OF UNDERLYING KIDNEY DISEASE

Initial diagnosis (when was kidney disease diagnosed; when was the chronic nature clarified; where; what were the presenting symptoms; initial investigations—which tests, e.g. MCU, MAG3, DTPA, DMSA, renal biopsy, cystoscopy; aetiology), number of hospitalisations, sequence/tempo of development of complications (growth failure, anaemia, bone disease) and their management.

CURRENT SYMPTOMS

Essentially, this is an extensive systems review, relating to CKD:

1. General health (e.g. tiredness, coping at school, sports, poor exercise tolerance).
2. Urinary (e.g. polyuria, nocturia, anuria, bed wetting).
3. Gastrointestinal (e.g. anorexia, nausea, vomiting, abdominal pain, diarrhoea).
4. Neurological (e.g. headache, paraesthesiae, seizures, confusion).
5. Cardiovascular (e.g. hypertension, cardiac failure symptoms: dyspnoea, oedema).
6. Growth (e.g. monitoring weight, height, causes attributed to poor growth).
7. Skin (e.g. itching [from microscopic subcutaneous calcium deposits], bruising).
8. Skeletal (e.g. bone pain, muscle cramps, muscular weakness).
9. Fluid intake, particularly need for night-time drinks.

FAMILY HISTORY

Other members of the immediate family affected (e.g. siblings), renal problems (e.g. nephronophthisis, polycystic kidney disease, cystinosis), deafness (e.g. Alport syndrome).

CURRENT MANAGEMENT

Current diet, medications, dialysis routine, management problems, present treatment in hospital, usual treatment at home, sequence of prior treatment changes, use of growth hormone, erythropoietin, drug side effects (e.g. steroid effects), diet, compliance, degree of self-management (e.g. with CAPD), future treatment plans (e.g. 'living related donor' [LRD] transplant, home haemodialysis), usual follow-up (by whom, where, how often, routine investigations done), use of identification bracelet, use of alternative therapies or medications.

SOCIAL HISTORY

- Disease impact on child; for example, amount of school missed, limitations on lifestyle, body image, self-esteem, peer reactions, future plans, education, career, educational difficulties related to development and/or time lost from school.
- Impact on family; for example, financial considerations such as the cost of frequent hospitalisations, drugs (especially post-RTx if not eligible for [in Australia] a Health Care Card, a problem for those > 16 years of age), special feeds (low-phosphate, high-calorie, low-protein, designed for renal patients; in Australia, Kindergen is on the Pharmaceutical Benefits Scheme [PBS] and is useful for infants, but other feeds such as Suplena and Nepro have to be bought from the hospital and can be expensive), pumps and disposables (many children are on nasogastric feeds, or feeds via gastrostomy overnight), surgery (RTx), treatment for other affected children, parents' worktime lost, transport, private health insurance.

- Parents, other family members, as potential kidney donors; who will be the donor and what they understand about their own potential morbidity; financial considerations.
- Impact on siblings; for example, sibling as kidney donor, sibling rivalry, sibling neglect.
- Benefits received, social supports; for example, social worker, extended family, Kidney Health Australia, dialysis and renal transplant associations.
- Discussion on transition from paediatric to adult renal services by 18 years of age. (In Australia, dialysis machines and disposables are provided by the government.)
- Compliance with and understanding of medications by child/family.

UNDERSTANDING OF DISEASE

Both the child's and the parents' understanding. Ask about the degree of previous education (e.g. in hospital, by local paediatrician) and contingency plans (e.g. who to contact first when child unwell).

Examination

See the short case on renal examination in this chapter. Some of the findings mentioned there will be of no relevance to the case you see, but the framework should be helpful.

Management

The main goal is for the child to have as normal a life as possible, free of uraemic symptoms, and able to be involved with the usual activities of daily living. The candidate should avoid getting 'bogged down' in the acute management of electrolyte problems and should discuss issues such as bone disease, growth including use of rhGH, development and psychosocial issues (especially schooling in chronic patients, transition). Discuss schooling in particular, as children on dialysis often miss key parts of their education (especially maths) and have major problems at school later, often with some acting-out behaviour. Ask about schooling during haemodialysis treatment for children on in-centre haemodialysis.

In patients with lesser degrees of CKD, discuss slowing of progression, such as controlling hypertension, excluding urinary tract infections, obstruction, use of angiotensin-converting enzyme (ACE) inhibitors and/or angiotensin receptor blockers (ARBs) in patients with proteinuria with an aim to reduce proteinuria as close to normal as possible by increasing medications as tolerated.

The candidate should recognise that CKD and ESKD are not synonymous.

The management of CKD can be divided into over a dozen main areas, comprising the following, organised within the mnemonic **URAEMIA FACTS**:

Uraemic complications (includes monitoring for development of neuropathy, encephalopathy; measuring serum urea and creatinine)
Renal replacement therapy (dialysis, RTx)
Acid–base status
Electrolytes and fluids: this includes serum potassium; this is very important, but the candidate should not go directly to this unless the child is already on dialysis; it is usually not the most important problem in CKD; also includes salt and water balance (including hypertension).
Mineral and bone disease
Intake: nutrition/**I**mmunisation/**I**mmunosuppression
Anaemia

Family disruption/**F**inancial burden
ADHD/**A**nxiety/**A**ffective disorders (e.g. depression)
Cardiovascular/**C**ognitive effects/**C**ompliance (with treatment) issues
Therapeutic burden of care
Stature (growth)/**S**leep disturbance/**S**ocial/**S**chool

The examiners expect the candidate to be familiar with the standard management of all these areas. The following presents discussion in order of priority and chronicity, not in the order of the mnemonic.

ELECTROLYTES AND FLUIDS 1—CONTROL OF SERUM POTASSIUM

Hyperkalaemia

The potassium [K$^+$] level should be kept in the normal range. This is usually not difficult, as renal excretion of K$^+$ remains fairly satisfactory in CKD. If the level rises above 5.0 mmol/L, dietary K$^+$ restriction and administration of sodium polystyrene sulphonate may be adequate temporarily. However, if there is an acute rise in [K$^+$] level (e.g. with intercurrent bacterial infection or haemolysis) above 7.0 mmol/L, this is poorly tolerated, and more acute intervention is needed.

The treatment of acute hyperkalaemia (serum [K$^+$] level above 7.0 mmol/L) should be known by all candidates. Note that dosages have deliberately been omitted, as it is unwise to try to quote doses in the examination unless you are absolutely conversant with the particular drug used. It is always safer to say that you would look up the dosage, based on weight or surface area.

Treatment of acute hyperkalaemia

1. Salbutamol, given nebulised (same doses as in asthma) or intravenously, works quickly and lasts a couple of hours. This is the easiest treatment to give in a paediatric service.
2. Calcium gluconate 10%, or calcium chloride 10% (cardioprotective) intravenously over 2–5 minutes, with electrocardiographic monitoring. This modifies myocardial cells' action potential and protects for around 30 minutes.
3. Sodium bicarbonate intravenously over 30 minutes. Alkalosis shifts K$^+$ into cells. The effect lasts 2 hours.
4. An intravenous infusion of 50% dextrose with soluble insulin over 30 minutes. This shifts K$^+$ into cells. The effect lasts 2 hours.

5. Sodium polystyrene sulphonate orally in 70% sorbitol (or in water), or rectally in 1% methylcellulose suspension (or 20% sorbitol). This binds K^+ with ion exchange resin. This takes 1–2 hours to take effect, and lasts 4–6 hours.
6. Acute dialysis.

The above measures are temporary only. If chronic hyperkalaemia cannot be managed with dietary restriction and oral sodium polystyrene sulphonate, definitive treatment (dialysis and eventually transplant) is needed.

ELECTROLYTES AND FLUIDS 2—CONTROL OF SALT AND FLUID BALANCE

Be careful here not to mix up CKD with ESKD. Most children with ESKD, regardless of cause, require restriction.

In CKD (but not ESKD), there are two main groups to consider: those who require fluid restriction, a low-salt diet, diuretics and dialysis for fluid overload; and those who waste salt and water well into the disease process, requiring a high fluid intake (often waking for fluids at night), and require salt supplementation and intravenous hydration if vomiting with intercurrent illnesses. The former group commonly have a glomerular cause for their CRF and the latter group a structural cause, with tubular dysfunction and decreased concentrating ability. Consideration of the history (e.g. salt craving), examination (blood pressure, weight, oedema) and urinary sodium excretion help determine into which group the child falls.

Salt and fluid restriction

This is required for the majority of patients with ESKD and for some with advanced CKD. However, note that all patients with ESKD are thirsty (because hyperosmolarity makes anyone thirsty, even if there is increased intravascular volume), and that all ESKD patients drink too much, leading to problems with oedema, hypertension and increased weight. Candidates should recognise this problem, but know that in practice it is unwise to confront the patient, as it is unhelpful (although some children will admit to drinking too much). The diet should have no added salt, but not be so restrictive that the child stops eating.

High salt and fluid intake

Some children, particularly those in whom CKD is caused by congenital renal disease, have high output problems and require high fluid intake and salt supplementation. The amount given is guided by parameters such as urinary sodium excretion and weight. This is not a common problem in ESKD, as most children retain sodium and water, although a few continue to have a large urine output.

Hypertension

Tight control of hypertension is important to slow progression of CKD. Hypertension is common in oliguric forms of CKD (e.g. chronic glomerulonephropathies, reflux nephropathy, HUS). Fluid overload is the main cause of the hypertension in advanced CKD, so that when a child is finally on dialysis, antihypertensive agents (optimally) should not be needed, as dialysis should be able to manage fluid overload. If a patient is oedematous (i.e. fluid-overloaded), blood pressure cannot be controlled.

In children being medically managed, before needing dialysis, salt restriction and antihypertensive drugs can be used. The drugs used ideally will slow progress to renal failure, and block the RAS: ACE inhibitors (e.g. ramipril, lisinopril) or ARBs (e.g. irbesartan). Other drugs used have included diuretics, and calcium channel blockers (e.g. amlodipine). Less frequently used drugs include beta blockers (e.g. atenolol, metoprolol, propranolol) and prazosin (alpha$_1$ post-synaptic blocker). Different nephrologists have different preferences for the order in which various drugs are tried.

One suggested general plan is as follows:

1. No-added-salt diet.
2. ACE inhibitors (e.g. lisinopril, an easy-to-use tablet that can be dissolved and dose titrated for small children) or ARBs (e.g. irbesartan). They can cause hyperkalaemia, which limits their use in children with severe reductions in GFR or ESRD.
3. Diuretics (e.g. frusemide); these lose effectiveness once 70% of renal function is lost.
4. Calcium channel blockers (e.g. nifedipine, amlodipine, diltiazem).

Acute hypertensive crisis

The following may be useful:

1. For the conscious patient:
   a. Clonidine (central sympatholytic action; given orally).
   b. Nifedipine (calcium channel blocker, given orally).
   c. Minoxidil (vasodilator, given orally).
   d. ACE inhibitors (given orally).
2. For hypertensive encephalopathy (all given intravenously):
   a. Clonidine (central action).
   b. Labetalol (alpha and beta blocker).
   c. Nitroprusside (vasodilator).
   d. Diazoxide (vasodilator).
   e. Hydralazine (vasodilator).

Differentiate between CKD and ESKD. Hypertension in ESKD is fluid overload until proved otherwise, and in compliant patients it is manageable with dialysis to remove fluid. Antihypertensive administration makes fluid removal on haemodialysis more difficult because of vasodilation.

CKD may require diuretics (e.g. glomerulonephritides), but reflux nephropathy is usually better controlled with nifedipine, or with ACE inhibitors (again, remember to beware of hyperkalaemia here). Amlodipine is an easy drug to use for longer-term control of blood pressure, as a 5-mg tablet can be dissolved in water and then the required dose given. Breaking a nifedipine tablet turns it into a shorter-acting agent, so it is difficult to titrate the dose in small children.

Remember that tight control of hypertension can decrease the rate of decline of renal function. The ESCAPE study used a fixed dose of ramipril, but added non-ACE inhibitor antihypertensives to achieve the target BP measurements in both groups. Anti-RAS antihypertensives are preferred. Be sure to know the side effects of any drug that you mention in your presentation. For completion, here is a more comprehensive list of antihypertensives that can be used in children:

- Alpha and beta blocker: labetalol (IV)—also available orally.
- ACE inhibitors: 'prils'—benazepril, captopril, enalapril, fosinopril, lisinopril, quinapril + enalaprilat (IV). Lisinopril is easy to use, as a tablet can be dissolved in water and then the required dose administered as a liquid.
- Angiotensin receptor blockers: 'sartans'—irbesartan, losartan.
- Beta blockers: 'olols'—atenolol, bisoprolol, esmolol (IV), metoprolol, propranolol.

- Calcium channel blockers: diltiazem + 'dipines'—amlodipine, felodipine, isradipine, nifedipine, nicardipine (IV).
- Central alpha agonist: clonidine.
- Diuretics: hydrochlorothiazide, chlorthalidone, frusemide (loop diuretic), spironolactone, triamterene, amiloride. Note that the latter three may be associated with hyperkalaemia because of their site of action.
- Dopamine 1 receptor agonist: fenoldopam (IV).
- Peripheral alpha agonists: 'azosins'—doxazosin, prazosin, terazosin.
- Vasodilators: hydralazine (IV, IM), minoxidil, sodium nitroprusside (IV).

ACID–BASE BALANCE

Acidosis in CKD is caused by an inability to excrete acids (approximately 2–3 mEq/kg of H^+ ions produced from metabolism, daily) and an inability to retain bicarbonate. In advanced CKD and ESKD, metabolic acidosis is mainly related to problems with ammonium ion production and titrable acidity. Despite this, alkaline bone salts acting as buffers keep the plasma bicarbonate level stable at levels of between 14 and 18 mEq/L.

Acute severe acidosis is preferably treated by dialysis, as the patients are often fluid-overloaded and hypertensive, such that intravenous sodium bicarbonate administration would not be optimal.

For chronic acidosis, management includes administration of alkali (2–3 mEq/kg/day), which can be given as sodium bicarbonate tablets or liquid (1 mL of 8.4% sodium bicarbonate solution is equivalent to 1 mmol).

If acidosis is intractable, treat with dialysis.

Patients with ESKD on dialysis will not need bicarbonate supplements, as dialysis alone corrects acidosis.

CKD-MINERAL AND BONE DISORDER (CKD-MBD)

CKD-MBD is caused by the kidneys being unable to excrete phosphate, or to make $1,25(OH)_2 D_3$. Dysregulation of $[Ca^{2+} - PO_4^{3-} - 1,25(OH)_2 D_3]$ metabolism leads to the parathyroid glands being stimulated and secondary hyperparathyroidism develops.

Bone disease (previously termed renal osteodystrophy, or renal rickets with hyperparathyroidism) can be detected histologically within 6 months of the onset of ESKD, in almost all patients. It is due to a combination of lack of $1,25(OH)_2$ vitamin D_3 (calcitriol), secondary hyperparathyroidism and acidosis leading to the use of alkaline bone salts as buffers. Secondary hyperparathyroidism is invariably present once there is a 50% reduction in GFR; serum parathyroid hormone (PTH) levels are inversely correlated with renal function. Histological descriptions include a spectrum from high-turnover disease (osteitis fibrosa) to low-turnover disease (osteomalacia and adynamic lesion of bone), but there are no clear clinical correlates.

Clinical features tend to be fairly non-specific, and may include muscle weakness, bone pain, bone deformity and growth restriction. Bone deformities can lead to slipped epiphyses, bow legs or knock knees. Dental anomalies may occur, including defective enamel and malformed teeth, especially in those with congenital renal disease.

Soft-tissue calcification can occur if serum phosphorus and calcium levels are too high. This can involve ischaemic necrosis of skin, muscle or subcutaneous tissues (termed 'calciphylaxis', or calcific uraemic arteriopathy [CUA]), and occasionally visceral calcification (e.g. pulmonary involvement, causing restrictive lung disease). Phosphate is a powerful vessel toxin by itself, or via its effects on PTH or through increasing fibroblast growth factor 23 (derived from bone, a regulator of phosphate metabolism), which then suppresses $1,25(OH)_2 D_3$ production by the kidney.

It is now recognised that effective management of CKD–MBD significantly affects the development of cardiovascular disease. Altered $[Ca^{2+} - PO_4^{3-} - 1,25(OH)_2 D_3]$ metabolism is a non-traditional risk factor that can perpetuate cardiovascular disease.

A major objective of managing bone disease is preventing pain and deformity. Assessment includes measurement of serum $[Ca^{2+}]$, serum $[PO_4^{3-}]$, serum $[1,25(OH)_2 D_3]$ serum alkaline phosphatase (SAP) and PTH levels, and taking bone X-rays. SAP is used to monitor the success of treatment. Radiologically, the findings of renal osteodystrophy include widened growth plates, with fraying and cupping of metaphyses (renal rickets), plus subperiosteal bone resorption and osteopenia (secondary hyperparathyroidism).

The rachitic components are best seen at the ends of rapidly growing bones (e.g. proximal tibia, distal femur) and the hyperparathyroid components on the radial aspects of the second and third digits. Delay in skeletal maturation also occurs. The overall plan of management is as follows.

Control of serum phosphate

This is important, as hyperphosphataemia can lead to a rapid decline in renal function. It is best to correct the hyperphosphataemia before trying to increase the serum calcium level. Phosphate control starts with dietary phosphate restriction. A low-phosphate diet is recommended (avoiding ice-cream, milk, dairy). Calcium carbonate (e.g. Caltrate, or Cal-Sup chewable) or sevelamer hydrochloride (non-calcium-based) can be used as a phosphate binder, but needs to be given with food to be effective.

Data from the International Pediatric Peritoneal Dialysis Network, on 900 children, showed that around half of them had PTH five times the upper limit of normal. Dietary restriction alone is inadequate. Involvement of a dietician early could improve this. Phosphate binders are needed earlier than in adult patients with CKD. Unfortunately they taste unpleasant, but are needed with every meal.

Phosphate binders can be increased in dosage until the calcium level is also returning towards normal. Sevelamer hydrochloride, which is much more expensive than calcium carbonate, is indicated where phosphate levels cannot be controlled with calcium carbonate without causing hypercalcaemia.

Calcium supplementation

The preparation of choice is calcium carbonate, which acts as a phosphate binder as well (as mentioned above). Note that when used as a calcium supplement, it is better given between meals. The serum calcium is not restored to normal until after the hyperphosphataemia is under control, because of the risk of metastatic calcification if hyperphosphataemia persists.

Vitamin D supplementation

This is usually given as $1,25(OH)_2 D_3$ (calcitriol), once a day, but can be given as 'pulse' therapy 2–3 times a week. Serum PTH is used to monitor treatment, aiming for PTH to be twice the upper limit of normal. Higher levels indicate healing and the risk of overshooting, with resultant hypercalcaemia. Lower levels of PTH are associated with adynamic bone disease, with reduced bone turnover. Serum alkaline phosphatase can also be used to monitor treatment. The main problem with management is non-compliance. In patients receiving haemodialysis, IV forms of vitamin D analogues can be given to improve compliance and decreased number of oral medications needed; these include paricalcitol (a synthetic vitamin D analogue) and doxercalciferol (vitamin D_2). A recent Cochrane review in 2015 noted that bone disease, evaluated by PTH changes, is improved by all vitamin D preparations.

X-ray bones annually

Once a year: 1. check bone age; and 2. X-ray hips, knees and ankles (weight-bearing joints are usually the most severely affected).

STATURE (GROWTH)

There are many factors that can adversely affect growth in CKD:

1. Deficient caloric intake: a most important factor in infants and young children.
2. Salt wasting: another important factor in infants and young children.
3. Disease onset (e.g. CKD from infancy [congenital renal diseases] leads to an attained height of –3 Height Standard Deviation Score [SDS] at 3 years of age— probably one-third of reduction in height occurs in the first 3 months of life, as most children with CKD have normal birth weights and lengths).
4. Disease type (e.g. cystinosis, or nephrotic syndrome requiring high-dose cortico-steroids, may lead to particularly poor growth).
5. Abnormalities in insulin-like growth factor-1 (IGF-1) and IGF-binding proteins (IGFBPs, especially IGFBP-3).
6. Growth hormone resistance, secondary to point 3 above.
7. Poor protein synthesis and low-protein turnover.
8. CKD-mineral and bone disorder (MBD) (previously termed renal osteodystrophy).
9. Glucose intolerance (on steroids).
10. Acidosis.
11. Polyuria (decrease in extracellular volume).
12. Infection.
13. Associated genetic diagnoses.

Over a third of children with CKD have a height below the 3rd centile, or a median height standard deviation score (HtSDS) below –1.88. There is a significant correlation between GFR and height, and a still stronger correlation between age and height. The lower the GFR, the lower the height percentile, and the younger the child, the more severe the growth restriction. Given that one-third of the body's growth occurs in the first 2 years, it is understandable that infants and younger children with CKD have a different group of determinants of growth than older children. In infants, and younger children, growth is mainly determined by nutrition, so treatment needs to focus on optimising this, maximising caloric intake to 80% of requirements. In older children, growth is largely determined by growth hormone and its mediator, insulin-like growth factor-I (IGF-I). It is recommended that all children with HtSDS < 3rd centile, or height velocity standard deviation score < –2 SD, should be treated with recombinant human growth hormone (rhGH); see overleaf for details.

As noted above, growth problems are worse if the disease-causing CKD dates from (before) birth. These children may have several problems, especially sodium wasting, leading to significant undernutrition in the first 2 years of life. Growth problems are also significant around puberty.

Each case may have several factors operating. Optimum nutrition, monitoring of bone disease, correction of acidosis and anaemia, avoidance of high-dose steroids and provision of adequate salt (especially in young children) may improve growth. Poor growth can have a devastating effect on the child's self-image and cause severe problems (e.g. being teased at high school). It may be the major issue in some cases.

Recombinant human growth hormone (rhGH)

Supraphysiological doses of recombinant human growth hormone (rhGH) are very effective in increasing height velocity: for example, in one study, from a baseline median of 4.1 cm/year to 9.2 cm/year after 12 months, and to 6.6 cm/year after 2 years of treatment. (The reduced GH-stimulating effect in the second year is also seen in children with idiopathic GH deficiency.) RhGH is used in children with CKD and a GFR below 30 mL/min/1.73 m^2, whose height is below the 25th centile for age, or whose height velocity is below the 25th centile for bone age. The maximum dose is 28 units/m^2 per week. If growth velocity fails to increase to at least the 50th centile for bone age, rhGH may be discontinued. Prepubertal patients respond particularly well to rhGH.

Mechanism

CKD causes decreased renal clearance of IGFBP-3, which binds 95% of insulin-like growth factors (IGF). IGFBP-3 increases and binds to IGF-1, decreasing available, free, active IGF-1, and hence causing uraemic GH resistance and growth impairment. RhGH is safe and effective in CKD, in patients with ESKD on dialysis (although slightly less effective) and in growth-restricted paediatric allograft recipients. RhGH should be continued until epiphyseal closure or renal transplantation occurs. Potential complications of rhGH therapy include hypercalciuria, aseptic necrosis of the femoral head, pseudotumour cerebri and suggestions of possible (although no evidence for this) induction of malignancy. The last of these, if correct, could be a consideration for those who have received cytotoxics, or have ESKD from Wilms tumour.

Intake: nutrition

The diet in CKD is a difficult therapy problem and depends on the stage of CKD. If CKD is advanced and dialysis is imminent, protein restriction may be used to keep urea at acceptable levels. Protein intake is no longer reduced to slow the progression to ESKD, as it has now been shown that it does not work in children, and there is a risk of reduced growth. Also, ACE inhibitors are effective and better tolerated than the previously recommended diet. Optimum nutrition is needed for these children with nutritional and growth failure, who are anorectic too.

A further problem is the intake of milk in infants. Milk has a high phosphate content and hyperphosphataemia is deleterious to renal function, so milk intake should be limited. Infant formulae can be used with added calories (e.g. polyjoule) and salt, or special formulae designed for renal patients (with high calories, and with low-phosphate and high-salt content).

Different units have different philosophies on diet. Candidates should learn (and understand) the regimen used by their training hospital and be able to discuss this.

Children with CKD have an inadequate intake of energy. Energy supplementation aims to raise this intake to the recommended daily allowance (RDA) calculated at mean weight for age. This can be achieved by adding glucose polymer to feeds, oral or flavoured supplements, but avoiding standard energy supplements (e.g. Ensure, Osmolyte), as these have high protein and phosphate content unsuitable for CKD. For infants, standard infant formulas can be supplemented with Polyjoule and Calogen (a long-chain fatty acid preparation).

In some children, volume constraints will limit the amount of nutritional supplementation that can be given. For younger children with structural disease, nutrition can be optimised by supplemental feeding (e.g. overnight by gastrostomy, or nasogastric feeding), as volume overload is not a problem. Should fluid restriction be necessary, high-calorie supplements (e.g. Suplena, Nutrison Energy Plus or Nepro) can be used for overnight feeds. If overnight feeds are not tolerated because of coexistent gastro-oesophageal reflux, fundoplication may be needed.

The general principle is to encourage a normal, balanced diet, in order to maximise growth potential, while correcting electrolyte and acid–base imbalances by medications where needed. Nutritional supplementation by itself does not lead to catch-up growth, but does allow stabilisation of growth rates.

Anaemia

This is mainly due to lack of erythropoietin. Other contributing factors include: increased red blood cell destruction; blood loss (nose, gut, skin); decreased erythropoiesis by uraemic toxins; marrow suppression by drug treatment; poor intake of protein, iron and vitamins; defective utilisation of iron; inadequate dialysis; co-existing systemic disease; uncontrolled hyperparathyroidism; and chronic inflammation. Anaemia can be alleviated by giving r-HuEPO (SC), aiming for a haemoglobin level of 110–120 g/L. Patients probably should be transfused when the haemoglobin drops below 60 g/L, to avoid the risk of cardiac decompensation. For maximum efficiency of r-HuEPO, a child needs to be iron-replete. In most children pre-dialysis or on peritoneal dialysis, this can be achieved with oral iron therapy. Children on haemodialysis usually require iron supplements intravenously, to maximise their response to r-HuEPO. The aim should be that the ferritin level should exceed 100 µg/L and the transferrin saturation should exceed 20%.

Recombinant human erythropoietin (r-HuEPO)

Erythropoietin increases the terminal differentiation of erythroid progenitor cells, increases cellular haemoglobin synthesis and increases reticulocyte release from bone marrow. Several symptoms previously attributed to uraemia are definitely improved by r-HuEPO, including fatigue, poor exercise tolerance, anorexia, pruritis, uraemic bleeding, sleep disturbance, cold intolerance and cognitive dysfunction (typical problems being difficulties staying on task, concentrating, poor short-term memory and suboptimal performance at school).

The benefits of r-HuEPO are improved overall wellbeing, increased energy levels, increased exercise tolerance, improved school attendance, increased physical activity and improved overall cognitive functioning. Other improvements have included regression of ventricular hypertrophy and normalisation of impaired brain-stem auditory evoked responses.

The avoidance of transfusions, with their attendant risks of sensitisation and transmission of infective agents, and the amelioration of anaemia, are the main advantages of using r-HuEPO. Disadvantages include the cost and the potential side effects of r-HuEPO: hypertension, hyperkalaemia (remember that the first symptom of hyperkalaemia is death), iron deficiency and vascular access thrombosis.

R-HuEPO can be given intravenously (IV) or subcutaneously (SC). Previously, it was given intraperitoneally (IP), but this increased the risk of peritonitis. It may be given SC, twice a week, if the haemoglobin level is below 100 g/L. This is continued until the Hb level is around 110 g/L, at which stage once a week is enough. The child's B_{12}, folate and iron status should also be checked.

There are three forms of r-HuEPO:

- Epoetin alfa (Eprex): this can be given 2–3 times per week as SC injection, or in those on haemodialysis, given IV on dialysis days, although the IV route is less effective than the SC route.
- Darbepoetin alfa (Aranesp): this can be given SC or IV, has a longer half-life, and so needs to be given only weekly or less frequently (fortnightly or even monthly). The main problem with this is pain at the injection site.
- Epoetin beta (Neorecormon): this can be given once weekly, but can be required more frequently. Its advantage is being less painful SC than darbepoetin.

Suboptimal responses (persistent anaemia) occur with several conditions: iron deficiency, aluminium intoxication, blood loss, hyperparathyroidism, inflammation and infection, or the dose being too low or not administered correctly. If there is such a response, check the ferritin, iron and total iron-binding capacity (TIBC) and transferrin saturation (iron/TIBC).

If there is iron deficiency (transferrin saturation of < 20% is the most useful indicator), replacement oral iron is given. If the oral preparation is insufficient to replete iron stores, then an IV iron preparation (such as IV iron polymaltose, or IV iron sucrose) may be warranted; this is a common problem in haemodialysis and peritoneal dialysis patients. Also, check PTH levels to exclude hyperparathyroidism, as increased PTH causes some resistance to hormone action.

Renal support and replacement

Dialysis

Dialysis is only waiting for a transplant. Occasionally, parents are not aware of this, so make a point of assessing their understanding of this point. Dialysis only provides around one-tenth the clearance function of normal kidneys.

Dialysis is commenced when the complications of CKD can no longer be managed by medical therapy. It is usually started when the GFR is below 15 mL/min/1.73 m^2.

Indications include inability to control the main management headings (electrolytes, hypertension, oedema, acidosis, bone disease) and uraemic symptoms not corrected by treatment with r-HuEPO. Other considerations include availability of donors. Some children can have a transplant as their initial renal replacement therapy, this being known as a 'pre-emptive transplantation' (PET) (see later in this section). Overall, it is an individual clinical decision for each child. It is better if the child is still fairly stable and reasonably well, when first started on dialysis, rather than waiting until he or she becomes very ill.

A child may be excluded from the transplant program if there are congenital malformations with very poor functional prognosis. Infants under 6 months may be excluded for technical reasons, including size (usually, a child must weigh at least 10 kg to receive an adult kidney). It is a joint decision made by the doctor, child and parents.

The modality of dialysis varies—haemodialysis, CAPD or automated peritoneal dialysis (APD; also known as CCPD). Most young children are started on peritoneal dialysis unless this is specifically contraindicated; most patients in the long-case setting thus will be on home-based peritoneal dialysis (although more and more children, especially adolescents, are on inpatient haemodialysis). CAPD uses gravity to instil prefilled bags of dialysate into the peritoneal cavity three or four times a day. It has the advantages of not causing any pain and providing continuous dialysis. CAPD is a simple portable procedure and is relatively cheap. Disadvantages include no days off, the requirement for repeated connections and disconnections, and the attendant risk of peritonitis (usually from *Staphylococcus aureus* or *Staphylococcus epidermidis*).

APD involves use of an automated cycler for overnight instillation and drainage of dialysate fluid. APD has the advantages of only one connection and disconnection between the cycler and the peritoneal catheter per day, and hence less risk of infection, and decreased time demands on the family. It does interfere with the child's social life, especially for teenagers. APD in the form of CCPD is performed nightly and then fluid remains in the peritoneal cavity during the day. Most children need an additional bag change in the late afternoon for optimum dialysis.

Children are admitted to hospital, have a peritoneal (e.g. Tenckhoff) catheter inserted and are trained (along with their parents) in the management of APD and CAPD, usually for 3 weeks. All get cyclers, but they need to know CAPD for holidays or machine breakdowns. The volume of dialysis fluid instilled into the peritoneal cavity on each occasion is usually between 40 and 60 mL/kg (this partly depends on the child's tolerance). In CAPD, bags are changed three or four times a day. The bag sizes are 500 mL, 1000 mL, 1500 mL and 2000 mL. In APD, there are a variable number of bags overnight, 5–8 cycles, and fluid dwells in the abdomen during the day.

The available solution strengths (different glucose concentrations) are 1.5%, 2.3% and 4.25%. Which one is used depends on the amount of fluid one wishes to remove. Of all dialysis modalities, CCPD is associated with the best growth, the best control of anaemia and the best patient tolerance. When started on dialysis, the child is usually put on the transplant program.

Common complications of APD or CAPD include peritonitis, exit-site and catheter-tunnel infections, and catheter blockage. To treat peritonitis, which occurs in about 1 in 8 patient months, or three times every 2 years, the standard IP antibiotics are cephazolin and gentamicin. Antibiotics are added once daily to fluid that dwells in the abdomen all day. The insertion of catheters can be covered with antibiotics. If the child develops abdominal pain and the fluid becomes cloudy, a culture of peritoneal dialysis fluid should be obtained and intraperitoneal antibiotics commenced. Antibiotic treatment may be altered once the culture result is available. Catheter life varies, averaging about 9 months.

Haemodialysis (HD) takes 5 hours, 3–4 times a week. In the US, haemodialysis accounts for 35% of children on dialysis. It is usually undertaken in a tertiary renal centre, and access is via a central venous double- lumen catheter designed for HD, or via an arteriovenous fistula. Central venous haemodialysis catheters are percutaneously inserted for acute HD and the short term, or inserted like Hickman catheters for the longer term. Infection and obstruction are the main catheter problems. Fistulae and vein grafts are used in long-term HD patients if the child has suitable veins. A schoolteacher and a play therapist are essential to support children on haemodialysis.

Renal transplantation (RTx)

RTx is the treatment of choice for ESKD. The donor is usually a relative ('living related donor') who has a compatible blood group. To expand the donor pool, the **paired kidney exchange** has been developed, where a recipient with an incompatible live donor can be matched with another pair, compatible to their needs, through a national database. The pairs then exchange/swap donor kidneys, so each has a live donor transplant. Alternate mechanisms to expand the donor pool include utilising ABO-incompatible transplants, and desensitisation in patients with elevated donor-specific HLA antibodies.

There is no longer a lower age limit for transplantation. In infants under 1 year of age, an adult living related donor is the ideal donor. As regards adolescents, it has become clear that: 1. suboptimal graft survival is largely related to non-adherence to immunosuppressive regimens, leading to late acute rejection; and 2. the longer adolescents spend on dialysis the more likely their grafts will fail, such that pre-emptive grafts (see below) are recommended, as they give a 50% decrease in the risk of graft failure. RTx is particularly beneficial in terms of cognitive development and growth.

Once the RTx is performed, the usual medications treating CKD are stopped and the immunosuppressants are started. The latter must be continued indefinitely; in adolescence, issues with compliance can be the single greatest threat to graft survival. LRD grafts are preferable to cadaveric donor (CD) grafts (also called deceased donor [DD] grafts), as they give a better rate of patient survival at 5 years (95% for LRD, versus 80% for CD) and of graft survival at 5 years (up to 95% for LRD, versus 65% for CD: less difference with newer immunosuppressives such as tacrolimus). The allograft half-life (time for half of the transplanted kidneys from a particular cohort to be lost) for a LRD graft is more than 25 years, versus 16 years for a CD graft. Adult kidneys can be used, even in children under 5 years of age. The use of LRDs has increased steadily; now around 60% of RTx in children have used LRD allografts. Over 80% of LRD allografts come from a parent.

Pre-emptive transplantation (PET) is where children have a transplant as their initial renal replacement therapy, if there is a living related donor. PET is performed before reaching ESRD and dialysis, and has become increasingly popular, with around 30% of transplants in the US being PETs. Recipients of PETs have improved patient and allograft survival.

The initial work-up for transplantation includes adding the name of the child to the cadaveric waiting list and sending blood, monthly, to the blood bank. The average waiting time for RTx in Australia is around 2.5 years: all children have a priority rating, which operates once they have been on dialysis for more than a year, so that children are waiting around 18 months for a cadaveric transplant.

Blood grouping and tissue typing are done on suitable family members if an LRD is considered, this being increasingly the case. Donors must be ABO blood group compatible; otherwise pre-formed isohaemagglutinins interact with renal vascular endothelium, leading to loss of the graft. HLA matching clearly is beneficial in LRD transplants, although there is less evidence for its importance in cadaver donor grafts. HLA matching does improve the outcome of second or subsequent transplants.

Pre-transplant immunisation is very important. Varicella vaccination should be given before RTx if possible, while pre-transplant viral surveillance for serological evidence of any prior exposure to cytomegalovirus, herpes simplex virus, hepatitis B, hepatitis C, HIV and Epstein-Barr virus is essential, although currently only prevention of CMV disease is possible by using prophylactic valganciclovir therapy. Work-up also involves assessing the bladder for vesicoureteric reflux and outlet obstruction.

Recipients must weigh at least 10 kg, which can be a problem. For example, in a very small 2-month-old infant with ESKD, transplant would be preferable to dialysis, so if there is a related donor available, the best plan would be to supplement the child's caloric intake (such as by nasogastric tube) and 'feed up' the child to 10 kg.

IMMUNOSUPPRESSIVE THERAPY

A major problem with transplantation is the need for long-term immunosuppressive therapy, with the associated risk of opportunistic infection and an increased risk of malignancy later in life. Corticosteroids are still used. The most common standard treatment used comprises prednisone, mycophenolate mofetil (MMF) and tacrolimus.

There has been a rapid expansion in the number of newer immunosuppressants. The following agents may be used to prevent graft rejection. They are arranged as the **ABC** of immunosuppression (**A**ntiproliferatives, **B**iologicals, **C**alcineurin blockers) for mnemonic purposes only. The main side effects are listed.

Antiproliferatives

1. Mycophenolate mofetil (MMF) is an antimetabolic agent that interferes with purine metabolism in B- and T-lymphocytes. It is metabolised to mycophenolic acid, which blocks conversion of inosine monophosphate (IMP) to guanosine IMP; this blocks synthesis of guanosine nucleotides, which decreases proliferation of T- and B-lymphocytes. It is more effective than azathioprine (AZA) in preventing acute rejection in the first year posttransplant, and has similar toxicities to AZA. It is also used to treat refractory rejection.

   Notable side effects (mnemonic for MMF side effects: **MMG**):

   Myelosuppression, increased risk of infection
   Malignancy (haematological especially lymphoma, occurs in 0.6% versus 0.3% for AZA)
   Gut effects (diarrhoea [30%], bleed [3%], perforation [rare])

2. Sirolimus (SLM) is a product of *Streptomyces hygroscopicus*. It forms a complex with FK binding proteins in lymphocytes, which interrupts second messenger signalling, leading to blockage of cytokine-mediated proliferation of T- and B-cells. With the combination of sirolimus and CSA, there is a synergistic effect that allows a lower dose of CSA to be given. Sirolimus is not nephrotoxic, and has no adverse effect on blood pressure. There is a competitive drug interaction with CSA and sirolimus, such that sirolimus should not be given within 4 hours of CSA. Sirolimus is an alternative to CSA or tacrolimus, as it has less nephrotoxicity, but it is also less potent than either of these; thus there is a slightly higher rate of rejection early.

Grapefruit and grapefruit juice (CYTP3A4 inhibitor) should be avoided as they lead to elevated SLM levels. Side effects include mouth ulcers, hypercholesterolaemia, pneumonia and rash. Notable side effects (mnemonic **HT LIMUS**):

Hyperlipidaemia/Hypercholesterolaemia/Hypertension/Hepatic necrosis (rare)
Thrombocytopaenia

Leucopenia and increased infection risk/**L**ymphoedema/**L**ung fibrosis (rare)
Intestinal: diarrhoea, abdominal pain/**I**nflammatory: stomatitis, pancreatitis
Malignancy (especially skin)/**M**uscle: rhabdomyolysis increased risk with statins
UV light: limit to avoid skin cancer
Slow wound healing

Biological agents

- Monoclonal antibodies:
  - Basiliximab is a chimeric human/murine antibody directed against the CD 25 antigen (the interleukin-2 [IL-2] receptor alpha chain on the surface of activated T-cells), which causes IL-2 receptor blockade. It is used instead of ATG (see below), together with CSA, MMF and prednisone, for prevention of rejection. It has almost no side effects. As long as serum basiliximab levels are kept above 0.2 micrograms/mL, it completely blocks the interleukin-2 receptor.
  - Daclizumab is a humanised antibody directed against the alpha chain of the IL-2 receptor. Adding this to CSA, AZA and prednisone therapy reduces acute allograft rejection. It has almost no side effects.
- Polyclonal IgG antibodies:
  - Thymoglobulin, an antilymphocyte antibody, is rabbit-derived. It blocks many T- and B-cell receptors which causes cell dysfunction, lysis and prolonged lymphocyte suppression. Targets for thymoglobulin include: T-cells: CD3, CD4, CD8, CD28, CD 58; B-cells: CD5, CD28, CD58, CD152; Antigen presenting cells: HLA-DR, CD40, CD58, CD80, CD86. Side effects are allergic reactions, serum sickness, neutropenia, thrombocytopenia and increased propensity to infections.

    Fever, chills, arthralgia and dyspnoea can occur, but are decreased with pre-treatment with high-dose steroids, antihistamines and antipyretics. Thymoglobulin is used in the treatment of rejection.

    Thymoglobulin also can be used to prevent rejection, especially in patients likely to suffer acute tubular necrosis (ATN) posttransplant, so that tacrolimus does not have to be started immediately (which could increase the risk of prolonged ATN). Side effects are generally mild: nausea, vomiting, headache. Thymoglobulin can be used in cases of acute rejection, when there is a failure to respond to steroids, as an alternative to TAC.

The calcineurin inhibitor tacrolimus (TAC) is a fungus-derived macrolide. It inhibits lymphokines derived from T-cells, including IL-2, IL-3, IL-4 and gamma interferon, and clonal expansion of helper and cytotoxic T-cells; it is very potent as a T-cell immunosuppressor. Tacrolimus is effective in inducing graft tolerance. Its side effects include nephrotoxicity, neurotoxicity and infection, plus lymphoproliferative disease. It may induce diabetes mellitus; it also increases the risk of BK virus infection.

Noteworthy side effects can be remembered as a mnemonic: **TACROLIMUS**:

Tremor/**T**ingling (neurotoxicity)
Alimentary (diarrhoea, constipation, nausea, vomiting, anorexia)/**A**naemia
Cancer risk increased
Renal toxicity (includes irreversible vasculopathy, interstitial fibrosis, tubular damage)
Osteoporosis
Lymphoproliferative disease/**L**ow Phosphate
Increased: blood pressure, [K⁺], [creatinine]
Magnesium low
Urea high
Sugar diabetes

Grapefruit and grapefruit juice (CYTP3A4 inhibitor) should be avoided as they lead to elevated TAC levels. TAC is not to be given with antilymphocyte treatments.

Trough blood levels are checked with any dosage alteration; the target levels decrease gradually over time; initial target levels are 5–15 ng/mL for the first month, decreasing to a target of 3–7 ng/mL at 6 months. TAC can be used in cases of acute rejection, when there is a failure to respond to steroids, as an alternative to thymoglobulin.

Management

The above agents can be divided into two groups:
• Induction therapy agents: biological (thymoglobulin, basiliximab, daclizumab).
• Maintenance therapy agents: steroids, TAC, MMF, sirolimus.

Prednisone, TAC, MMF and basiliximab have become the standard immunosuppressive agents. Quadruple regimens are preferred in many centres, especially in the US. Candidates should be familiar with the side effects of the above treatments.

After transplantation, children usually remain in hospital for a week to 10 days, after which they are reviewed regularly (daily for the first month or so). Rejection episodes occur, but are relatively uncommon with the currently used group of immunosuppressant agents. Clinical features of rejection include tenderness over the graft and fever (although this sign is less useful in tacrolimus-treated patients), and laboratory findings of a rising serum creatinine level and leukocytosis.

In most children now, rejection is suspected because of a rising creatinine and is confirmed on renal biopsy. High-dose intravenous steroids are usually effective, but thymoglobulin may be required. Some units use cotrimoxazole prophylaxis against pneumocystis for 6 months.

Most units now use valganciclovir, the prodrug of ganciclovir, as prophylaxis for CMV. If treatment of CMV is needed, then IV ganciclovir is given for 2 weeks. Prophylaxis against CMV disease is used in many units for 3 months in all renal transplants except donor CMV-negative to recipient CMV-negative. Others use it for donor CMV-positive to recipient CMV-negative or when giving ATG, where there is an increased risk of CMV disease. If treatment (as opposed to prophylaxis) for CMV is needed, then IV ganciclovir can be given for 2 weeks.

At each outpatient visit, check growth and blood pressure (hypertension can occur in up to 85% of transplant recipients), and look for signs of opportunistic infection and side effects of drugs (e.g. Cushing's syndrome from steroids, abdominal pain and diarrhoea from MMF). Check the skin and all lymph nodes (skin cancer and lymphomas can be seen in paediatric transplant recipients). Take blood to check renal function and for a full blood count. If the serum creatinine level is rising, think of the following possibilities: rejection, infection, obstructed blood supply to graft, or obstructed ureter or nephrotoxicity if taking TAC. It can be particularly difficult to decide between rejection and calcineurin inhibitor toxicity. Blood glucose should be checked when taking TAC.

The main issues posttransplant can be divided into short term (at time of transplant and next few months), which comprise problems of rejection and infection, and long term, comprising decrease in renal function (50% renal survival at 15 years), malignancies (particularly lymphoma and skin cancer; in Queensland, 50% of post-renal transplant patients get skin cancer, squamous cell carcinoma or basal cell carcinoma, in their early twenties, and rarely, this can be fatal, so applying adequate sunscreen, wearing hats and avoiding sun are very important to prevent these) and cardiovascular disease (long-term effects of left-ventricular hypertrophy, hypertension and hypercholesterolaemia lead to cardiovascular diseases [e.g. stroke, ischaemic heart disease] being more common).

ALLOGRAFT LOSS

1. **Chronic rejection (or chronic allograft nephropathy)** is the most common cause: incomplete understanding of mechanism; presumed combination of immunological and non-immunological mechanisms, non-compliance, drug toxicity and recurrent disease; risk increased by multiple acute rejection episodes; late acute rejection. No effective therapies yet available.
2. **Acute rejection** (second most common cause). Complete rejection reversal can be achieved in around two-thirds of patients, but reversal is less likely with an increased number of rejections, increased age of the recipient and late (over 12 months post-RTx rejection) rejection episodes.
3. **Vascular thrombosis** (third most common cause). The risks are decreased by use of calcineurin inhibitors or thymoglobulin on day 0 to 1, and increased by peritoneal dialysis pre-RTx, cadaver donors under 5 years of age, recipients under 2 years of age or repeat RTx recipients.
4. **Recurrent disease.** See the list below. FSGS is a particular problem, and the most important, as most lose their grafts quickly. Children with FSGS are twice as likely as all other diagnostic groups (below) to have primary ATN requiring dialysis post-RTx. If it does recur once, there is an 80% chance it will recur in any subsequent RTx.

RECURRENCE RATES IN TRANSPLANTS (HISTOLOGICAL RECURRENCE)

1. Membranoproliferative glomerulonephritis (MPGN) type II: 100%.
2. Membranoproliferative glomerulonephritis (MPGN) type I: 70%.
3. Henoch–Schönlein purpura (HSP): 55–85%.
4. IgA nephropathy: 25–45%.
5. Focal segmental glomerular sclerosis (FSGS): 25–30%. FSGS is the most important, as most lose their grafts quickly, though some patients may respond to plasma exchange with or without rituximab.
6. Haemolytic uraemic syndrome (HUS): 12–25%. Most children with recurrent HUS associated with Factor H mutations lose their grafts with recurrent disease.
7. Systemic lupus erythematosus (SLE): 5–40%.

Histological recurrence does not correlate with clinical recurrence, the latter being much rarer. Recurrence also can occur in oxalosis, cystinosis (but no adverse effect on graft function) and congenital nephrotic syndrome.

SOCIAL PROBLEMS

Although mentioned last, often these are the most important discussion points in the long case. Ensure that a full social history is taken, and that the social circumstances have at least been thought over before you confront the examiners. Knowing all the side effects of calcineurin inhibitors but not knowing if the family have their own transport or receive the Child Disability Allowance will cause you to fail the long case.

Schooling is a particular problem. There are well-known neurocognitive comorbidities including lower IQ, impaired executive functioning and poor memory, sleep problems, school refusal, absenteeism, specific learning disabilities, and behavioural issues related to ADHD symptomatology. ESKD patients may go to school, but do not seem to learn as much as other children (components of low self-esteem, and depression may contribute) and tend to miss school for no good reason. This may all add up to poor school performance. How well the family copes is extremely important.

DISEASE BURDEN

The management of CKD involves a particularly large number of medications, a challenging medication dosing schedule, a variety of unpleasant medication routes including injections, and infusions, a need for regular monitoring of BP and urine, and a need for multiple blood tests, dietary requirements, and the need for dialysis, and immunosuppression post-RTx. It is not surprising that there can be associated psychological and psychiatric issues, such as depression.

The candidate should explore the areas of family disruption, the financial burden of the disease, whether this has impacted adversely on siblings (who may feel neglected, less important), whether the parents are together, how much this has impacted on the parent's work, and gain an impression of the impact on the family. Exploring the child's feelings about school may uncover bullying, and associated anxiety. It is often these aspects which are the discussion points of the long case.

Compliance with medications is a real problem, particularly with adolescents. A significant proportion (around 25%) of grafts lost from rejection are associated with non-compliance/non-adherence.

The author had a renal long case in the exam, and was asked about the child's schooling, family, financial burden, transport issues, and nothing about any of the 'medical' issues. This is not an uncommon scenario.

CARDIOVASCULAR DISEASE (CVD)

Children with CKD have a lower long-term survival rate than the general population. This is largely attributable to CVD. The prevalence of adverse cardiovascular events in ESKD is around 25% for the 0- to 4-years age group, and around 36% in the 15- to 19-years age group. These events include arrhythmias and cardiomyopathy. Hypertension is found in over half of paediatric patients in the early stages of CKD and occurs in three-quarters by the time they require dialysis or RTx. Masked hypertension is a particular problem, where the BP is measured as normal in the clinic, but is elevated outside of the clinic.

The other risk factors for CVD, which are less 'traditional', include anaemia, the abnormal $[Ca^{2+} - PO_4^{3-} - 1,25(OH)_2 D_3]$ metabolism, chronic inflammation, and oxidant stress. In these children, managing the BP, lipids and anaemia may be vitally important, as well as exercise, statins, ACE inhibitors and angiotensin receptor antagonists.

MINOR ISSUES
Congestive cardiac failure

This is usually related to fluid overload. Management includes normalising blood pressure, maintaining haemoglobin above 90 g/L, salt restriction and cautious use of diuretics and dialysis. Cardiomyopathy is not uncommon and generally resolves posttransplant. It is related in part to nutrition.

Drugs

Many drugs require reduced dosage in CKD. It is impossible to remember them all, so it is safest to simply use a reliable pharmacology reference to look up any drug that is being considered. A brief list of commonly used drug groups that require decreased dosage in CKD is as follows:

- Aminoglycosides: in renal failure, gentamicin should not be given as a single daily dose—dose reductions and/or increased intervals between doses are required; in haemodialysis patients, gentamicin is given post-dialysis.
- Other antibiotics: some cephalosporins; some penicillins; sulphonamides.
- Digoxin; thiazide diuretics; paracetamol; phenobarbitone.

OTHER ISSUES
Genetic counselling

In children with hereditary nephropathies, genetic counselling is a very important and necessary component of the overall management.

Monitoring

The examiners may ask what follow-up you would recommend for your long-case subject. A brief checklist to consider is as follows:

1. Routine check of growth, blood pressure, oedema.
2. Electrolytes, bicarbonate, creatinine, urea, calcium, phosphate, alkaline phosphatase.
3. Haemoglobin, white cell count, platelet count.
4. Cholesterol, triglycerides, uric acid.
5. Bone X-rays: hips, knees, ankles, hands.
6. Chest X-ray.
7. Calculated GFR.
8. Follow-up by dietician, social worker, occupational therapist, especially for adolescent issues, and in younger children, development.

LONG CASE: Nephrotic syndrome

Recognition of the key role of the podocyte in preventing proteinuria, resulting from discovering various gene mutations as the causes of many forms of steroid-resistant nephrotic syndrome, has been associated with significant advances in the understanding of the pathophysiology of nephrotic syndrome in recent years. This process started with the discovery, in 2006, that the cause of congenital nephrotic syndrome of the Finnish type (CNF1; OMIM#256300) is a mutation of a protein named nephrin, coded for by the gene NPHS. Nephrin is located within the visceral glomerular epithelium, at the slit diaphragms, which are membranes that bridge filtration pores between neighbouring podocytes. The slit diaphragm is attached to the cell cytoskeleton by adaptor proteins, including podocin and CD2AP. Podocytes are known to regulate integrity and survival of glomerular epithelial cells.

It is recognised now that several diseases, both acquired and inherited, are due to defects in podocytes, affecting the slit diaphragm, which is essentially a multi-protein signalling complex. The phenotype FSGS can be caused by defects in the gene/proteins: NPHS2/podocin, located at the slit diaphragm; CD2AP/CD2AP, located near the slit diaphragm; TRPC6/TRPC6 (which affects calcium flux) located at the podocyte; and ACTIN4/alpha actinin 4 (which affects the actin cytoskeleton) located at the podocyte.

Other genetic aetiologies of albuminuric glomerular disease include: genes affecting the podocyte nuclear proteins (WT1 [Wilms' tumour suppressor gene]; mutations of WT1 can cause: isolated nephrotic syndrome [NPHS4; OMIM#256370]; Denys–Drash syndrome [OMIM#194080]; **WAGR** syndrome [**W**ilms tumour, **A**niridia, **G**enitourinary anomalies and mental **R**etardation] OMIM#194072); genes affecting type IV collagen at the glomerular basement membrane (GBM; COL4A5, mutations of which cause Alport syndrome [OMIM#301050]); other genes affecting the GBM (LAMB2 which causes Pierson syndrome [OMIM#609049]); and transcription factor regulating podocyte genes (LMX1B, mutations of which cause nail–patella syndrome [OMIM#161200]).

Autosomal recessive nephrotic syndrome is an inherited form of FSGS due to mutations in the gene NPHS2 situated on chromosome 1q25–q31, which codes for podocin; it has early onset, minimal changes on early biopsy, FSGS on later biopsy, rapid progression to ESKD, but rare recurrence after RTx; it can present as familial FSGS with later onset, adolescent or adult. Podocin mutations occur in some 10–30% of sporadic steroid-responsive nephrotic syndrome in some populations.

Knowing there is a genetic cause allows avoidance of steroid therapy, as steroids cannot help if there is a podocin mutation. Also, patients with genetic mutations are less likely to have recurrences in their disease, should they develop ESKD and require a RTx. In congenital nephrotic syndrome, for example, now there can be directed early nephrectomies, dialysis and renal transplantation, rather than wasted time trialling steroids and experiencing side effects without benefit.

Children with nephrotic syndrome often appear in the examination. Those chosen as long-case subjects are unlikely to have uncomplicated idiopathic nephrotic syndrome (INS), but may present with therapeutic dilemmas, difficult-to-control disease or significant side effects from drug treatment.

Background information
DEFINITION

Nephrotic syndrome (NS) is characterised by four components:

1. Proteinuria above 40 mg/m^2/hour (or 1 g/kg/24 hour) *or* urinary protein ratio more than 200 mg/mmol creatinine.
2. Hypoalbuminaemia (serum albumin less than 25 g/L).
3. Hypercholesterolaemia (serum cholesterol over 200 mg/dL [5.17 mmol/L]) (not essential for diagnosis).
4. Oedema.

The primary abnormality is proteinuria. The other features are secondary to this. Other characteristic findings include the following:

- Hypocalcaemia (ionised fraction normal): below 2.25 mmol/L (9.0 mg/dL).
- Hyperkalaemia: over 5.0 mmol/L.
- Hyponatraemia: below 135 mmol/L.
- Hypercoagulability (decreased partial thromboplastin time [PTT]).

The most common causes of INS are: minimal change disease (MCD), FSGS, and mesangial proliferative glomerulonephritis (MesPGN).

- **MCD** accounts for 80–90% of all forms of NS in childhood.
- **Focal segmental glomerulosclerosis (FSGS)** is the most common progressive glomerular disease in children, and the second most common cause of ESRD (the most common cause being congenital renal anomalies). Several different genetic forms are known, some autosomal recessive (putative genes NPHS2, and WT1) and some autosomal dominant (putative genes TRP6, and ACTIN4). FSGS can be idiopathic (some genes not discovered yet) or secondary to post-infectious glomerulonephritis, obstructive uropathy, reflux nephropathy or systemic diseases (e.g. sickle cell disease [SCD], SLE).
- **Mesangial proliferative glomerulonephritis (MesPGN)** is usually idiopathic, but can be due to chronic infection (bacterial or viral), SCD, SLE, renal transplant or bone marrow transplant. Idiopathic forms of MesPGN may be associated with IgM or C1Q deposition on immunofluorescence, and are then referred to as IgM or C1Q nephropathy. It remains unclear whether MesPGN is a forerunner of FSGS in some patients.
- INS is further subdivided into (cortico-) Steroid-Sensitive NS (SSNS) and (cortico-) Steroid-Resistant NS (SRNS).
- Other causes of NS include gene mutations, membranous nephropathy and SLE.
- **Membranous nephropathy** can be idiopathic, or due to SCD, SLE, drugs such as NSAIDs, or captopril, toxins such as heavy metals or infections such as hepatitis B or C.
- **SLE.** This can cause FSGS, MesPGN or membranous glomerulonephritis, but the typical histology is of a diffuse proliferative GN with typical immunofluorescent findings. Clinically, SLE is more likely to present with haematuria and acute nephritis, rather than a nephrotic syndrome.

These are the only diagnoses likely to come into the differential diagnosis of NS. Some textbooks give the impression that each type of glomerulonephritis has one particular type of presentation. Note that *any* clinical picture can be caused by *any* histological picture, which can have *any* clinical outcome.

MINIMAL CHANGE DISEASE (MCD)

MCD tends to affect younger children (2–5 years), and more often boys (until puberty, then the sex incidence is equal). The proteinuria is due to changes in the integrity of the glomerular filtration barrier, which comprises three layers: *fenestrated endothelium* (cells have multiple openings [fenestrae], measuring 70–100 nm in diameter, which stop macromolecules passing from plasma into the renal tubule); the *glomerular basement membrane (GBM)* (contains negatively charged heparan sulfate proteoglycans, which block passage of anionic macromolecules, such as albumin); and the *visceral epithelium*, which is made up of podocytes and slit diaphragms. Filtration of albumin is limited by charge, whereas the filtration of IgG is not limited by charge, but by size, as circulating IgG is mainly neutral or cationic.

MCD occurs due to an immune-mediated, T-cell derived permeability factor which changes the permeability of the podocytes, altering an electrostatic glomerular barrier (removal of anionic charge), and permitting albumin and other negatively charged proteins to pass through.

MCD characteristically shows fusion/effacement of epithelial foot processes on electron microscopy (although this is characteristic of all proteinuric states if 'nephrotic'). MCD is associated with loss in the urine of low-molecular-weight anionic proteins (e.g. albumin), but some higher molecular weight proteins such as IgG are also lost.

Clinically, hypertension and haematuria occur in 10% of children with MCD, but are transitory. Most children (80–90%) with INS respond to corticosteroids (SSNS). Up to 90% of children relapse, of whom 50% have a frequently relapsing course or become steroid dependent (see below). Children may have one or more episodes per year for many years, and sometimes into adult life. Approximately 50–70% of those with SSNS achieve permanent remission by 5 years, 80% remit by 8 years, and 85% remit by 10 years. The mortality rate for SSNS is very low (0.7%). SRNS usually means a need for renal biopsy and genetic testing. SRNS requires immunosuppressive treatments. Steroid resistance is more likely in infancy, and in adolescence (> 12 years). If an affected child does not respond by complete or partial remission by 5 years, there is a 50% chance of progressing to ESKD.

GLOMERULONEPHROPATHIES OTHER THAN MCD

The other glomerulonephropathies tend to present in older children (6–15 years), with a variable sex ratio depending on the particular condition. Generally, in this group there tends to be a greater leakage through the glomerular filtration barrier, and higher molecular weight proteins may be lost. Clinically, haematuria is often present, and hypertension may also occur. If there is reduced renal function, then consideration of rarer causes of NS may be appropriate. Most of this group does not respond to steroids. In particular, FSGS is often the finding in a child who has SRNS.

DEFINITIONS USED IN INS

- **Remission**: urinary protein excretion less than $4 \text{ mg/m}^2/\text{hour}$, or no trace of protein on urine dipstick, or protein:creatinine ratio below 0.02 g/mmol for three consecutive days.
- **Relapse**: recurrence of proteinuria as defined in definition of INS, or 2+ or more on dipstick for three consecutive days.
- **Frequent relapsers**: children with two or more relapses within the first 6 months of initial response, or more than four relapses in 12 months.
- **Corticosteroid dependence**: two consecutive relapses while on prednisone or within 2 weeks of ceasing prednisone.
- **Corticosteroid resistance**: failed response after 8 weeks of 2 mg/kg/day prednisone.
- **Cyclosporine (CSA) dependent**: relapses when CSA is tapered or stopped; it refers to the group of steroid-dependent children who achieve remission with CSA.

DIFFERENTIATING BETWEEN MCD AND OTHER GLOMERULONEPHROPATHIES

In practice, in children with uncomplicated NS, initial differentiation is not crucial, as they are all given a trial of steroids. Ultimate prognosis seems to depend on steroid response rather than selectivity of proteinuria or biopsy findings.

Complications of NS

INFECTION

Children with NS have increased susceptibility to infection with encapsulated bacteria (e.g. pneumococcus, *Haemophilus*, *Escherichia coli*), including cellulitis, peritonitis and urinary tract infections. This is due to multiple factors, including urinary loss of immunoglobulin (IgG), loss of factors B and D of the alternate complement activation path, loss of transferrin, altered T-cell function, impaired ability to make antibodies, loss of opsonising factors (specifically, increases the risk to encapsulated organisms) plus the burden of steroid therapy or other immunosuppressive drugs, and mechanical factors such as oedema and ascites. Peritonitis occurs in 2–6% of patients. The risk is further increased by decreased mesenteric blood flow and increased coagulability (see below), with decreased flow and sludging causing microinfarction. In peritonitis, signs of peritoneal irritation are almost always present, and are not masked by steroid therapy. Other infections seen include septicaemia, meningitis, cellulitis and urinary tract infection.

With pneumococcal polysaccharide vaccination now widespread, *Streptococcus pneumoniae* is less common and gram-negative organisms, such as *E. coli* and other coliforms, more common. Viral infections can include varicella, particularly in those receiving immunosuppressive therapy; again, increased uptake of varicella vaccine is making this less common.

COMPLICATIONS OF TREATMENT

Steroids often cause Cushingoid effects, but poor growth is the most serious complication. Medications used as steroid-sparing agents (cyclophosphamide [CPA], cyclosporine [CSA], tacrolimus [TAC], levamisole [LVS], ACE inhibitors, mycophenolate mofetil [MMF] and rituximab [RTX]) have significant potential side effects.

OEDEMA

For years, the theory has been that children with *rapid* onset of INS develop loss of oncotic pressure: fluid moves from the intravascular space to the interstitium, resulting in hypovolaemia (the 'underfill' mechanism). In these patients, infusion of albumin with administration of a loop diuretic (e.g. frusemide) has been given, leading to increased excretion of salt and water loss. Plasma volume is decreased in children during the initial phase of a relapse. Children with *chronic* nephrotic syndrome, however, may have increased or normal plasma volume (the 'overfill' mechanism: with salt and water retention, increasing the intravascular volume with hydrostatic 'push' into the interstitium). In these patients, diuretics alone can be given (e.g. frusemide, together with spironolactone).

ACE inhibitors (e.g. enalapril) have been used in children with SRNS to reduce proteinuria, raise serum albumin and reduce oedema. It is now believed that rather than being due to the oncotic pressure theory, oedema is due to a primary defect in sodium excretion; also, vasopressin excess occurs. Anasarca (generalised, massive oedema) can lead to the following: difficulty walking, from severe scrotal or vulval oedema; respiratory distress, from pleural effusions and/or severe ascites splinting the diaphragm; and tissue breakdown with cellulitis. This can be treated successfully with infusing salt-poor albumin followed by frusemide (see the later section on management).

THROMBOSIS AND EMBOLISM

NS can be associated with hypercoagulability, due to increase in plasma fibrinogen and clotting factors II, V, VII, VIII, IX, X and XIII (due to increased hepatic synthesis), decreased plasma antithrombin III and decreased protein S (latter two lost in urine), platelet abnormalities (thrombocytosis, increased aggregability), increased blood viscosity, decreased blood flow and hyperlipidaemia. In some cases of nephrotic syndrome due to SLE, the antiphospholipid syndrome has been implicated; this involves persistently raised antibodies against membrane anionic phospholipids (such as anticardiolipin antibody, and antiphosphatidylserine) or their associated plasma proteins (e.g. beta-2 glycoprotein I [apolipoprotein H]). This leads to increased risk of major vessel thrombosis, usually venous (risk around 2–5%). Most commonly, this involves renal veins or sagittal sinuses, but can occur in deep vessels of the limbs, the pulmonary artery, the inferior vena cava, the femoral/iliac artery, the pulmonary venous system, the cerebral arteries, the meningeal arteries, the mesenteric veins and the hepatic veins.

Thromboembolic complications include pulmonary embolism. Bilateral renal vein thrombosis can present with acute renal failure. Infants with congenital nephrotic syndrome are at particular risk of renal vein thrombosis. Thrombosis is more common in children with SRNS.

The likelihood of thrombosis is further increased by any co-existing illness leading to fluid loss, and by haemoconcentration, from vomiting or diarrhoea, from diuretic use and from immobilisation and the presence of indwelling catheters. Irrespective of cause, the first line of treatment is low-molecular-weight heparin; if the thrombosis extends, then it may need thrombolytic drugs (e.g. tissue plasminogen activator)—it then may need warfarin until the nephrotic syndrome resolves. Aspirin therapy has been discussed, as it can prevent arterial thrombosis, but it cannot prevent venous thrombosis and thus its routine use is not recommended.

HYPERLIPIDAEMIA AND CARDIOVASCULAR DISEASE RISK

Hyperlipidaemia is reversed quite quickly in SSNS, in 4–6 weeks, and is not usually a clinical concern. Concerns for cardiovascular sequelae include exposure to corticosteroids, hypertension, hypercoagulability and anaemia (erythropoietin-responsive anaemia has been reported in NS). In children with unremitting NS, persistent hyperlipidaemia raises concerns, reflecting adult NS experience of increased risk of coronary heart disease, and the rare reports of myocardial infarction in children with NS.

In adults, HMG-CoA-reductase inhibitors are used successfully to limit hyperlipidaemia and its complications. These drugs have been used in children, but adequate safety and efficacy data have yet to emerge.

GROWTH DISTURBANCE

This is noted particularly in congenital nephrotic syndrome, and is thought to be due to urinary loss of IGF-binding protein, decreasing the levels of IGF-I and IGF-II, and decreasing IGF-receptor mRNA. The use of recombinant human GH (rhGH) in treatment is as yet unproven. Growth disturbance can be compounded by use of corticosteroids. Children with SRNS unresponsive to other therapies may also grow poorly.

HYPOCALCAEMIA

This is due to loss of vitamin D-binding protein in the urine. It can lead to bone demineralisation in the long term.

HYPOTHYROIDISM

Due to loss of thyroid-binding protein in the urine, this is a common problem in children with congenital nephrotic syndrome.

NEGATIVE NITROGEN BALANCE

Loss of protein in urine, plus poor appetite and nausea contribute to poor intake.

END-STAGE KIDNEY DISEASE (ESKD)

Only a small minority of children presenting with NS develop ESKD. The group most likely to do so have steroid-resistant FSGS. Around 8–10% of this group will ultimately develop ESKD. Rarely, children who were initially steroid responsive become steroid resistant and progress to ESKD.

History

PRESENTING COMPLAINT

Reason for current admission.

CURRENT SYMPTOMS

1. General health (e.g. anorexia, weight gain, lethargy, poor height gain).
2. Oedema (e.g. periorbital or ankle swelling, ascites).
3. Urinary (e.g. haematuria, oliguria, concentrated urine).
4. Other (e.g. infections, abdominal pain, hypertension).

PAST HISTORY

Initial diagnosis (when, where, presenting symptoms, initial investigations, established aetiology, initial treatment), number of episodes per year (usual precipitants, usual treatment), number of hospitalisations, sequence of complications, management. Differentiate between congenital nephrotic syndrome (commences within the first 3 months of life) and patients with SRNS, who usually present later in life.

MANAGEMENT

Current diet, medications, management problems, present treatment in hospital, usual management at home, home urine testing, the sequence of prior drugs used, drug side effects (e.g. steroid effects), compliance, future treatment plans (e.g. introduction of steroid-sparing drugs) and usual follow-up (by whom, where, how often).

SOCIAL HISTORY

Disease impact on child (e.g. amount of school missed, body image), impact on family (e.g. financial considerations, such as the cost of frequent hospitalisations), social supports.

UNDERSTANDING OF DISEASE

By child and by parents.

Examination

See the short cases on oedema and renal examination in this chapter.

Management

INVESTIGATIONS

Any child with NS should probably have the following tests.

Urine

Urinalysis, including looking for cellular casts, which do not tend to occur in MCD but may well occur in other glomerulonephropathies (note that hyaline or waxy casts are common in MCD). Microscopic haematuria is usually transitory in SSNS, but may persist in SRNS.

Blood

1. Urea, creatinine and electrolytes (renal function is usually normal in MCD; may be abnormal in other glomerulonephropathies).
2. Albumin and total protein levels (to evaluate severity).
3. Serum complements C3 and C4 (low with MesPGN, SLE; normal in MCD).
4. Full blood examination. The haemoglobin level is normal in MCD. If anaemia is present, this suggests other diagnoses.
5. Hepatitis B and C serology (hepatitis B is associated with membranous nephritis; hepatitis C is associated with MesPGN).

Renal biopsy indications

Note that renal biopsy should be reserved for those with very atypical features. It is not a routine requirement. There is probably no indication for biopsy before commencing non-steroid agents if the child is completely responsive to prednisone (i.e. proteinuria absent for over 3 days).

Indications are as follows:

1. Age under 1 year.
2. Nephritic features (haematuria, hypertension), raised creatinine/renal impairment.
3. Persistent abnormal serum complement level (low C3).
4. Steroid resistance.
5. Older children, particularly among African Americans, where FSGS is more common.

Other tests

Another test that is often mentioned is the 24-hour urinary protein estimation. This is not very useful, as it is almost impossible to perform accurately and does not add to the diagnosis (although it may be useful in non-MCD forms of NS or in non-nephrotic proteinuric states). Demonstration of steroid responsiveness may require the simpler test of the urinary protein:creatinine ratio (normal ratio less than 0.02 mg/micromol). Serum cholesterol and triglycerides are often requested, as is protein electrophoresis, but they do not aid diagnosis or management. Antinuclear antibody (screening for SLE) is not necessary in younger patients with uncomplicated NS.

Treatment

1. CORTICOSTEROIDS

The mainstay of therapy remains steroids. Protocols vary between different units; it is wise to learn the regimen of your own teaching hospital. There is good data that, in the first episode of NS, when oral prednisone is given for 4–6 weeks and then on alternate days for 6–8 weeks or more (increase in benefit up to total course of prednisone of 7 months), fewer children relapse than those who are given 'standard therapy' of daily prednisone for 4 weeks (2 mg/kg/day or 60 mg/m^2/day) and then alternate daily for 4 weeks. This standard therapy leads to remission within an average of 2 weeks in those with INS. There is good evidence that increasing the total dose of prednisone during the first episode and increasing duration results in fewer children relapsing by 12–24 months.

Around 50–70% of children relapse after 8 weeks of therapy, with the relative risk of relapse falling by 13% for each month that the initial duration of therapy is extended beyond 8 weeks. In subsequent episodes, prednisone can be used until remission occurs for more than 3 days, and then alternate-daily prednisone, considering other agents when the toxicity of the steroids exceeds the side effects of other agents. Most children will grow quite well on alternate-day steroids until they go into puberty, when growth slows.

The Kidney Disease: Improving Global Outcomes (KDIGO) guidelines recommended for SSNS, daily prednisolone for 4–6 weeks, then alternate-day weaning for 2–5 months. There is some evidence that it is cumulative dose which determines response, rather than the length of treatment.

Infrequent relapsers

For this group, prednisolone 60 mg/m^2/day is used until 3 days clear of (or trace only of) protein on dipstick, followed by shortened weaning by alternate-day regime.

Frequent relapsers

There are three main approaches to managing these children. The first option is low dose second daily prednisolone, the second is 'prophylactic' steroids, and the third is a non-steroid (steroid-sparing) agent.

Prophylactic steroid therapy requires a reliable parent who knows when to commence extra steroids, to switch/increase to daily dose (from alternate-daily, to daily, at the same dose) whenever their child develops an intercurrent infective illness, such as an upper respiratory tract infection (URTI), and continue this daily dose for 1 week. This approach has been shown to be successful, reducing the risk of relapse during an intercurrent infection by around 60%.

Steroid-sparing agents used in this group include CPA, LVS and RTX.

Steroid-dependent NS

The three main steroid-sparing agents used for this group are CPA, LVS and RTX. CPA is being used less often than previously because of concerns regarding infertility and potential for malignancy developing long term.

A tiered approach to treatment

Generally, the order of approach would be: first-line treatment with steroids, as above; then, second line treatment with TAC, or CPA, or LVS. Most of the second-line drugs (TAC, LVS) are given for 12 months. Should one second-line agent be ineffective or complicated by unacceptable side effects, then another second-line agent can be tried. If there are relapses on TAC, then MMF can be added. If there are frequent relapses despite TAC and MMF, then RTX should be considered.

2. (A) CORTICOSTEROID-SPARING AGENTS/OTHER DRUGS FOR SSNS

The main agents that can claim success in NS (mnemonic **CLAIM**), including the three main steroid-sparers CPA, TAC and LVS, are as follows:

CPA: 2 mg/kg/day for 8-12 weeks)/**C**alcineurin inhibitor: tacrolimus (TAC: 0.1 mg/kg/day in two divided doses)
Levamisole (2.5 mg/kg alternate daily for 12–24 months)
ACE inhibitors
Immunisation with pneumococcal vaccine
Mycophenolate mofetil (MMF: 25 mg/kg/day in divided doses for 12–24 months)/**M**onoclonal antibody: B-cell depleting: rituximab (RTX)

- CPA has significant side effects, short term (e.g. bone marrow suppression, risk of viral infections such as varicella, measles) and long term (e.g. gonadal toxicity and risk of carcinogenesis); mnemonic **CPA**: **C**ancer risk/**C**ystitis (haemorrhagic; rare); **P**ancytopenia/**P**ostpones immunisation schedule; **A**zospermia/**A**lopecia (uncommon). However, it offers the chance of prolonged remission off therapy, with 36% of children with frequently relapsing SSNS remaining in remission at 5 years. Less useful in steroid-dependent patients.
- CPA given for 8 weeks and cyclosporine A (CSA) given for 6–9 months were equally effective in maintaining remission in randomised controlled trials while CSA is being given. However, the effect of CSA is not sustained, while that of CPA is. CSA is no longer used due to cosmetic side effects of gingival hyperplasia and hypertrichosis; TAC is used in its place, as it has no such cosmetic side effects.
- TAC can cause nephrotoxicity, hypertension, hyperkalaemia and hypomagnesaemia, and it can cause diabetes mellitus. There is a risk of relapse on stopping TAC. See the long case on CKD in this chapter for the side-effect details mnemonic.
- Levamisole (LVS) is an antihelminthic drug and immunomodulator, enhancing cellular immune responses in certain conditions with depressed immune function. LVS may help maintain remission in SSNS, is well tolerated and has few side effects (neutropenia, rarely vasculitis, liver toxicity, convulsions), and these are all reversible on withdrawing the drug. Side effects of rash, vasculitis and arthralgia can occur after about 2 years of treatment, so treatment is usually stopped at 2 years. It decreases the steroid requirement by 50%, and the relapse rate by 50%. There is a risk of relapse on stopping LVS.
- ACE inhibitors reduce glomerular hyperfiltration. Also, from the ESCAPE trial (see the long case on CKD in this chapter), it is known now that intensified blood pressure control (keeping blood pressure below the 50th centile) in children aged 3–18 with CKD, using high-dose ACE inhibition with ramipril at a fixed dose, delayed progression of kidney disease. Adverse effects include hypotension and cough.
- Immunisation as per schedule for pneumococcal vaccination of immunocompromised children: heptavalent conjugated pneumococcal vaccine (7vPCV) in children under 5, and polysaccharide pneumococcal vaccine (PPV23) in children 5 or older. Normal immunisation schedule is interrupted by steroid and other immunosuppressive therapies.
- MMF is used for SSNS, largely on the basis of observational data. A single underpowered RCT demonstrated no significant difference in efficacy between MMF and CSA, but there was considerable imprecision in the results. Its side effects include gastrointestinal effects (diarrhoea and abdominal pain), and haematological abnormalities, but its side effect profile is preferable to that of CSA. MMF is not nephrotoxic. It is less effective than TAC, but can be used alongside it.
- Rituximab (RTX) is a biological agent which depletes B-cells for 6 to 9 months. It can produce prolonged remissions in steroid-dependent patients on multiple immunosuppressants, or in frequently relapsing disease after unsuccessful trials of standard treatment or intolerable adverse effects. It has been successful in treating SSNS and SRNS. There are concerns about the increased susceptibility to infections, which can be significant.

Indications for commencing steroid-sparing agents

1. Failure to respond to steroids (depends on pathology—only CSA and ACE inhibitors have been shown to reduce proteinuria significantly in RCTs).
2. Unacceptable steroid side effects (e.g. reduced height gain).
3. SSNS (only if side effects are unacceptable).
4. Relapses with hypertension or thrombosis (only if frequent relapser or steroid dependent).

Poor compliance is not an indication, as monthly intravenous methylprednisolone can be given. One notable (relative) contraindication for the use of CPA is lack of varicella antibodies. While a patient is taking these drugs, the full blood count must be checked regularly to detect development of marrow suppression (e.g. neutropenia).

2. (B) STEROID-RESISTANT NEPHROTIC SYNDROME (SRNS)

In children who are steroid resistant, the choices are different to the above. Agents that have been shown to be effective in RCTs are TAC and ACE inhibitors. In RCTs, there was no significant difference in efficacy between CPA and prednisone alone, so CPA is not recommended for SRNS. Some children respond to MMF or to RTX. Intravenous methylprednisolone is commonly used with a calcineurin inhibitor in an attempt to achieve complete or partial remission. Patients who fail to achieve complete or partial remission usually progress to ESKD. Thus, it is important to try therapies to achieve complete or partial remission, but without excessive medication-related toxicity.

3. ANTIBIOTICS

Some units administer prophylactic daily penicillin, to avoid pneumococcal infection to children in relapse. However, other units feel that vaccination against pneumococcus is successful enough to not warrant penicillin, the use of which could increase the risk of infection with more serious organisms. *Haemophilus* can be a problem if children are not fully immunised. If a child with a relapse of nephrotic syndrome develops bacterial infection, most units now recommend broad cover for both gram-positive and gram-negative organisms, such as a third-generation cephalosporin (e.g. cefotaxime), which may cover penicillin-resistant pneumococcus, and coliforms, plus ampicillin to cover for *Enterococcus*.

4. IMMUNISATIONS

Live viral vaccines should be avoided in patients taking high-dose corticosteroids or any immunosuppressive agents. Pneumococcal, *Haemophilus* and varicella vaccines are recommended, as above, because of the increased risk of infection with these pathogens.

5. SEVERE OEDEMA (ANASARCA)

Children with MCD with massive oedema (e.g. pleural effusions, ascites, scrotal or labial oedema) can receive intravenous concentrated (20%) albumin (1 g/kg infused over 4 hours) with intravenous frusemide (1 mg/kg) after the first hour of albumin. Note that albumin infusions can cause circulatory overload, hypertension and acute pulmonary oedema in patients with impaired renal function, or if MCD is not the cause of the oedema. In the latter case, giving a diuretic may precipitate renal compromise.

Albumin infusions should be used only when the child is very troubled by severe oedema symptomatically. They should not be used simply because albumin is very low, and should not be monitored by a rise in albumin.

6. HYPERTENSION

A minority of children with NS will have hypertension. Agents of choice are ACE inhibitors or ARBs, as these delay deterioration in renal function that can occur with ongoing proteinuria in a minority of children with steroid-sensitive nephrotic syndrome, but in more children with steroid-resistant nephrotic syndrome.

7. DIET

No added salt. No fluid restriction, except when very oedematous and diuretics are required. High biological value protein. Dietary and fluid restrictions are generally not required in children in remission. However, they should maintain an adequate calcium and vitamin D intake. As obesity is a common side effect of steroid therapy, families should be encouraged to put in place a healthy eating regimen, with adequate exercise to prevent excessive weight gain.

8. IN-HOSPITAL MANAGEMENT

When these children are admitted, important observations include fluid balance chart, twice-daily weight and 4-hourly temperature, pulse, respirations and blood pressure.

9. ACTIVITY

There is no need for bed rest or any restriction of activity.

10. PROGNOSIS

The best prognostic indicator in NS is steroid sensitivity. Of children with SSNS, 60–80% will relapse, and 60% of them have five or more relapses. Most children ultimately 'lose' the nephrotic syndrome towards adolescence (non-relapse rate 84% at 10 years). There are fewer relapsers if children are aged over 4 at presentation (remission occurs within 7–9 weeks of the start of corticosteroid treatment) and there is no microhaematuria.

In children with steroid-resistant FSGS, many progress to ESKD if they do not achieve complete or partial remission with non-corticosteroid therapies and ultimately need renal transplantation. FSGS recurs in around 25% of renal allografts. For children with genetic causes for NS, immunosuppressive treatment is less likely to be effective, transplantation is the definitive treatment and the original disease rarely recurs in the graft. However, sometimes children develop an immunologically based nephrotic syndrome (e.g. development of antibody to nephrin in congenital nephrotic syndrome) in the transplanted kidney.

SHORT CASE: Renal examination

A short-case approach to a renal examination is useful both in the long-case setting, for cases with CKD, and in the short-case setting for children with haematuria, proteinuria or other symptoms referable to the urinary tract.

Start by introducing yourself, and try to gain an impression of the patient's mental status (for encephalopathy, due to uraemia, or depression, due to chronic illness); note the child's age to assess any delay in pubertal development.

Stand back and observe whether the child looks sick or well. Look at the growth parameters and percentile charts, and note the nutritional status (visually scan for muscle bulk and subcutaneous fat) and pubertal status (Tanner staging). Note any dysmorphic features (several malformation syndromes involve the genitourinary system). Look for any evidence of rickets (CKD) or hemihypertrophy (association with Wilms tumour).

Look at the skin, for sallow complexion (CKD), pallor (anaemia of CKD or HUS), and periorbital or peripheral oedema. Also note any jaundice (hepatorenal syndrome), bruising (CKD), uraemic 'frost' (CKD) or scratch marks (pruritis with CKD), although it is unlikely that patients who are that sick would participate in the examination. Note any hirsutism (steroids), hypertrichosis/gum hypertrophy (cyclosporine [CSA]) or Cushingoid features (steroids for transplant or nephrotic syndrome).

There may be other peripheral signs, such as nearby bags of peritoneal dialysis fluid (CKD), and a visible peritoneal dialysis catheter (CKD), arteriovenous fistula, subclavian or jugular venous catheter. Look for evidence of previous dialysis access (particularly in renal transplant patients); in the neck for subclavian or internal jugular dialysis catheters, in the arms for previous fistulae and in the abdomen for previous peritoneal dialysis catheters (both the incision and exit sites of the catheter). Also look for scars of previous or current transplants. Most transplants are in the right or left iliac fossae and are easily palpated beneath a 'hockey stick' scar. However, in small children there may be a central abdominal incision and the kidney may be palpated bimanually, usually to the left of the scar.

After initial inspection, a systematic examination can be performed, starting with the hands, followed by checking the blood pressure, and then examining in turn the head and neck, chest and abdomen, and finally the gait and lower limbs. This suggested order is outlined in Figure 12.1. Details of findings sought at each step are outlined in Table 12.1.

The urinalysis may be requested at any stage (e.g. before laying hands on the patient), but it must not be forgotten.

SHORT CASE: Hypertension

This is an infrequent case, and as such often 'stumps' the candidate. The lead-in can take several forms; for example, 'This child has hypertension; examine her/examine her for complications/examine her for the cause'. The approach given here includes both causes and complications, and may need modification depending on the introduction.

It is essentially an extended cardiovascular examination. Likely cases would be renal artery stenosis with bruits, NF1, or infantile polycystic kidneys with large kidneys, liver, portal hypertension and previous portosystemic shunts. Remember that the vast majority of young children with chronic hypertension have a renal cause for their hypertension. The most common are reflux nephropathy (usually proteinuria) and renal artery stenosis (usually bruits).

Begin by introducing yourself to the child and asking his or her name, age and school grade, noting any irritability (hypertensive encephalopathy), dysphasia (intracerebral bleeding) or difficulty hearing your speech (deafness with Alport syndrome, or with congenital rubella). Any suggestion of developmental delay should be further assessed (previous cerebrovascular accident or congenital rubella).

Commence the general inspection with assessment of the growth parameters. Children with CKD, syndromal diagnoses (e.g. Turner's syndrome) or other systemic disease, such as neurofibromatosis type 1 (NF1) or Cushing's syndrome, are often short.

Children with congenital rubella (and associated renal artery stenosis) and some with NF1 may have small head circumferences, whereas others with NF1 may have large head circumferences. NF1 is associated with renal artery stenosis, phaeochromocytoma, coarctation of the aorta and neuroblastoma, all of which can cause hypertension. Weight is important in Cushing's syndrome. Truncal obesity with buffalo hump, loss of supraclavicular hollow and striae suggest this diagnosis.

While inspecting for growth parameters, note any asymmetry of limb size (hemihypertrophy with Wilms tumour) or posture (hemiplegia from intracerebral bleed), and look for obvious scoliosis (NF1).

Note any syndromal features (e.g. webbed neck in Turner's syndrome) and, in infants, the typical 'ex-premmie' appearance of the neonatal intensive-care graduate (umbilical arterial catheterisation leading to renal arterial thrombosis).

Look at the skin for pallor or sallow appearance (CKD), purpura (Henoch–Schönlein purpura, haemolytic uraemic syndrome, CKD), plethora (Cushing's syndrome), flushing and sweating (phaeochromocytoma), hirsutism (congenital adrenal hyperplasia [CAH], Cushing's syndrome), hyperpigmentation (CAH), café-au-lait spots or freckling (NF1), or depigmented macules (tuberous sclerosis with renal angiomyolipoma).

Note the facial characteristics. In particular, look for the moon face, hirsutism and acne of Cushing's syndrome, the heliotrope rash of dermatomyositis, the butterfly rash of SLE, the periorbital oedema of nephrotic syndrome and, in girls, the syndromal findings of Turner's syndrome (e.g. webbed neck, low hairline). Also note any asymmetry, either of facial movement—especially smiling (seventh cranial nerve palsy)—or facial structure (hemihypertrophy associated with Wilms tumour).

After inspection, take the BP reading yourself, in both arms. Make sure you use the right cuff size and the correct technique. The recommended cuff bladder width is 40% of the circumference of the midpoint of the upper limb, midway between the olecranon and the acromion. The cuff bladder must cover at least 80% of the circumference of the arm. The BP should be measured with the cubital fossa at the level of the heart, the arm being supported, with the stethoscope placed over the brachial arterial pulse, medial and proximal to the cubital fossa, inferior to the lower edge of the cuff. Note that current normative BP tables include height percentiles, age and gender, as BP depends on all these variables. A taller child will have a slightly higher BP than a shorter child of the same sex and age. Reference to the appropriate tables is essential. Note also that the fifth Korotkoff sound is used to define diastolic BP.

A rough rule of thumb is that an adult-sized cuff is appropriate in a normal-sized 6-year-old or older child. A thigh cuff can be used in large obese teenagers. Take particular note of the size (width) of the cuff supplied and, if it is too small, request a more appropriate cuff size. Question the values given if these were obtained with the same incorrectly sized cuff.

Note that most children and adolescents with BP levels at or above the 95th centile for their age and sex are overweight. Body size is the most important determinant of BP in childhood and adolescence. If the child has both diastolic and systolic BP above the 95th centile, there will be an underlying cause, usually renal disease. In children under 12 months of age, systolic BP is used to define hypertension.

Request the values for the lower limbs, or measure these yourself (make sure that you have practised this, as the exam is not the best place to start).

1. Introduce self
Assess mental state (encephalopathy)
Position patient: sitting up

2. General observations
Sick or well
Growth parameters
- Height (short with CRF)
- Weight (thin with CRF, obese with steroids)
Tanner staging (delay with CRF)
Nutrition
- Muscle bulk (poor in CRF)
- Subcutaneous fat (poor in CRF)
Skin
- Sallow (CRF)
- Pallor (CRF, HUS)
- Jaundice (hepatorenal syndrome)
- Bruising, petechiae (CRF)
- Scratch marks (CRF)
Valgus deformity of knees (CRF)
Hemihypertrophy (Wilms' tumour)
Tachypnoea (with acidosis in CRF)
Peritoneal dialysis catheter, bag
Arteriovenous fistula
Nasogastric tube
Gastrostomy

3. Upper limb
Pulse: tachycardia (dehydration, cardiac failure with CRF)
Hands/nails (vasculitis)
Nails: brown lines (CRF)
Palms: crease pallor (CRF, HUS)
Wrists
- Flaring; tender (CRF)
- Shunt (CRF)
Asterixis (CRF)
Blood pressure
Arms: proximal myopathy (CRF, steroids)

4. Head and neck
Face (e.g. hirsute)
Eyes (e.g. cataract)
Hearing (impaired)
Mouth (e.g. dry)
Neck (e.g. JVP)

5. Chest
Rib rosary
Praecordium
Lung fields

6. Abdomen
Inspect
- Intervention (e.g. CAPD)
- Scars
- Swelling
- Tanner stage
Palpate
- Musculature
- Tenderness
- Kidneys
- Lymph nodes
- Genitalia
Percuss bladder
Auscultate

7. Lower limbs and gait
Inspection
Palpation
Gait examination
Reflexes
Hips

8. Urinalysis
Blood
Protein
Specific gravity
Nitrites
pH
Glucose
(various)

9. Temperature chart
Fever (e.g. infection, transplant rejection)

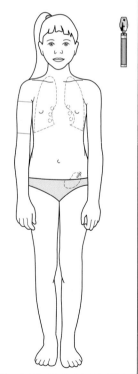

CAPD = continuous ambulatory peritoneal dialysis; CRF = chronic renal failure; HUS = haemolytic uraemic syndrome; JVP = jugular venous pressure.

Figure 12.1 **Renal examination**

Table 12.1

Additional information: details of possible findings on renal examination

HEAD AND NECK

Face
- Malar flush (SLE)
- Hirsute (Cushing's syndrome, CSA)
- Periorbital oedema (nephrosis)
- Hearing aid (Alport syndrome, aminoglycoside toxicity)

Eyes
- Aniridia (Wilms' tumour)
- Anaemia (CKD, HUS)
- Jaundice (hepatorenal syndrome)
- Band keratopathy (hypercalcaemia)
- Cataract (steroids)
- Uraemic retinopathy (CKD)
- Retinitis pigmentosa (nephronophthisis)

Hearing: impaired (e.g. aminoglycosides, Alport syndrome)

Mouth
- Dry (hydration)
- Uraemic breath (CKD)

Neck
- Jugular venous pressure raised (cardiac failure with CKD); measure at 45 degrees
- Cervical adenopathy (e.g. CMV, lymphoma, if immunosuppressed)

CHEST

Anterior aspect

Rib rosary (CKD)

Examine praecordium for:
- Cardiomegaly (fluid overload, CKD cardiomyopathy)
- Murmurs (anaemia)
- Pericarditis (CKD)
- Cardiac failure (fluid overload)

Posterior aspect

Sacral oedema (nephrosis)

Examine lung fields for pleural effusion (nephrosis) and pulmonary oedema (fluid overload)

ABDOMEN

Inspection

CAPD catheter

Other intervention, often related to congenital anomalies
- Ureterostomy
- Vesicostomy
- Ileal conduit
- Colostomy/ileostomy (e.g. related to imperforate anus)
- Nephrostomy or pyelostomy (e.g. related to sacral agenesis)

Continued

Table 12.1 (continued)
Scars (e.g. transplant [current or previous renal transplant has central abdominal scar in younger children, and scar in either iliac fossa for older children], CAPD)
Swelling (ascites due to CAPD fluid, or nephrosis)
Prune belly appearance (triad syndrome)
Tanner staging (delay with CKD)
Palpation • Abdominal wall musculature (lacking in triad syndrome) • Tenderness (peritonitis) • Kidneys (e.g. enlarged with polycystic disease, hydronephrosis) • Transplanted kidney (also measure, note consistency, tenderness) • Lymph nodes (enlarged with CMV or lymphoma, from immunosuppression)
Genitalia • Tanner stage of testes (delay with CKD) • Cryptorchidism (e.g. triad syndrome)
Percussion: bladder (for urine retention)
Auscultate • Renal arteries (renal artery stenosis) • Transplanted kidney (arterial stenosis)
LOWER LIMBS AND GAIT
Inspection • Muscle bulk (poor in CKD) • Flaring at ankles (CKD bone disease)
Palpation: ankle oedema (nephrosis, cardiac failure)
Stand and re-inspect: valgus deformity at knees (CKD bone disease)
Gait • Foot slapping (peripheral neuropathy with CKD) • Limp (slipped femoral epiphysis from CKD)
Squat: proximal weakness (CKD, steroids)
Return to bed • Reflexes (decreased with peripheral neuropathy of CKD) • Hip movement (slipped femoral epiphysis from CKD)

CAPD = continuous ambulatory peritoneal dialysis; CMV = cytomegalovirus; CKD = chronic kidney disease; CSA = cyclosporine; HUS = haemolytic uraemic syndrome; SLE = systemic lupus erythematosus.

The remainder of the examination can commence at the hands, as in a standard cardiovascular examination; in particular, feeling the radial and femoral pulses simultaneously, looking for coarctation, as evidenced by diminished strength of femoral pulsation. Then work up to the neck for jugular venous pressure and carotid pulses. The examination of vision, fundoscopy and hearing are best left until after abdominal examination, but scanning the face and head for signs such as conjunctival pallor is valid at this stage. After this, examine the heart, lungs and back. When examining the abdomen, it may be worth checking with the examiners that there is no contraindication to deep palpation, particularly if there is flushing or sweating, as palpation of a phaeochromocytoma can cause an acute hypertensive crisis. This need not be asked if the signs clearly suggest another diagnosis, such as renal disease (this is only a theoretical consideration, as it is very unlikely that a patient with this tumour would be in the examination, but it is a point worth noting in practice). Next, check the vision and hearing, and then the gait.

The urinalysis is an essential part of the examination of the hypertensive child. It is valid to request the result of this before anything else, as it may direct the examination (and renal causes are by far the commonest) and will also prevent it being overlooked and the case consequently being failed.

The relevant findings sought at each point are listed in Table 12.2, and the suggested order of approach is outlined in Figure 12.2.

Table 12.2
Additional information: details of procedure and possible findings in the hypertension short case
INTRODUCTION
Irritability (encephalopathy)
Dysphasia (CVA)
Hearing impairment (Alport syndrome, congenital rubella, aminoglycoside toxicity)
GENERAL INSPECTION
Parameters • Height (short with CKD, Cushing's syndrome, NF1, congenital rubella; with CAH, tall early, short later) • Weight (obese with Cushing's syndrome) • Head circumference • Percentiles
Request urinalysis (protein, blood, casts, specific gravity)
Pubertal status • Advanced (CAH) • Delayed (Turner's syndrome)
Posture: hemiplegia (CVA)
Symmetry: hemihypertrophy (Wilms tumour)
Scoliosis: NF1, spina bifida

Continued

Table 12.2 (continued)

Skin
- Pallor (CKD, HUS)
- Purpura (HSP, HUS, CKD)
- Plethora (Cushing's syndrome)
- Flushing, sweating (phaeochromocytoma)
- Pigmentation (CAH)
- Café-au-lait spots (NF1)
- Axillary freckling (NF1)
- Depigmented macules (TS with renal involvement)

Facial characteristics
- Moon face (Cushing's syndrome)
- Acne, hirsutism (Cushing's syndrome, CAH)
- Butterfly rash (SLE)
- Periorbital oedema (nephrotic syndrome)
- Findings of Turner's syndrome (webbed neck, low hairline)
- Asymmetrical smile (seventh cranial nerve lesion)
- Hemihypertrophy (Wilms tumour)
- 'Ex-premmie' appearance (UAC causing renal artery thrombosis)

Wears glasses (Alport syndrome, medullary cystic disease, congenital rubella, NF1)

Wears hearing aid (Alport syndrome, congenital rubella, aminoglycoside toxicity)

Tachypnoea (pleural effusion with nephrotic syndrome, BPD in ex-premmies, LVF secondary to hypertension)

HEAD

This is best examined after chest and abdomen, unless obvious clues on inspection

Face: as under 'General inspection', above

Eyes
- Conjunctival pallor (CKD)
- Cataracts (Cushing's syndrome, congenital rubella)
- Leave testing vision and fundoscopy until later

Ears
- Low set or hypoplastic (congenital renal dysplasia)
- Hearing can be left until later

Facial nerve palsy due to hypertension

CHEST

Full praecordial examination for sequelae of hypertension
- Palpate for heaving apex, cardiomegaly
- Listen for: loud S2 (aortic); prominent S3 or S4; systolic murmur (coarctation)

Lung fields
- Percuss for hyperinflation (ex-premmie infants with BPD), pleural effusion (nephrotic syndrome)
- Listen for radiation of murmurs (coarctation), crackles (LVF).

BACK

Inspection
- Midline scars (spina bifida)
- Sacral agenesis (renal anomalies)
- Buffalo hump (Cushing's syndrome)
- Scoliosis (NF1): get child to bend forwards to check this

Table 12.2 (continued)

Palpation
- Sacral oedema (renal disease, CCF)
- Spinal tenderness (Cushing's syndrome)
- Renal angle tenderness (nephritis)

Auscultation for renal arterial bruits (renal artery stenosis)

ABDOMEN

Inspect

Anteriorly
- Distension (ascites with renal disease)
- Dialysis catheter (CKD)
- Striae (Cushing's syndrome)
- Scar of renal transplant
- Tanner staging (CAH)

Posteriorly
- Midline scar (repaired myelomeningocele)
- Sacral agenesis (associated renal anomalies)
- Buttock purpura (HSP)

Palpate

Kidneys
- Bilateral enlargement (polycystic disease, hydronephrosis)
- Unilateral enlargement (polycystic disease, Wilms tumour, hydronephrosis, dysplastic kidneys, renal vein thrombosis, trauma)
- Tenderness (glomerulonephritis, pyelonephritis)

Suprarenal areas: mass (neuroblastoma)

Liver and spleen: enlarged (connective tissue diseases, congenital hepatic fibrosis associated with polycystic kidneys)

Bladder (after micturition): enlarged (posterior urethral valves, neurogenic bladder, obstructive uropathy)

Percuss

For ascites (nephrotic syndrome); over any masses to determine whether retroperitoneal

Auscultate

Bruits (renal arterial in renal artery stenosis, abdominal coarctation)

VISION AND HEARING

Visual acuity decreased in Alport syndrome, congenital rubella

Visual fields: hemianopia (intracranial bleed), constricted peripheral fields (medullary cystic disease)

Fundoscopy
- Papilloedema (raised ICP)
- Hypertensive retinopathy
- Perimacular degeneration (Alport syndrome)
- Retinitis pigmentosa (medullary cystic disease [nephronophthisis])

Hearing
- Loss with Alport syndrome, aminoglycoside toxicity
- Do Rinne and Weber tests to confirm sensorineural loss

BPD = bronchopulmonary dysplasia; CAH = congenital adrenal hyperplasia; CCF = congestive cardiac failure; CVA = cerebrovascular accident; HSP = Henoch–Schönlein purpura; HUS = haemolytic uraemic syndrome; ICP = intracranial pressure; LVF = left-ventricular failure; NF1 = neurofibromatosis type 1; SLE = systemic lupus erythematosus; TS = tuberous sclerosis; UAC = umbilical artery catheterisation.

1. Introduce self

2. General inspection
Position patient: standing, fully
    undressed; then lying down
Well or unwell
Growth parameters
Request urinalysis
Tanner staging
Posture
Symmetry
Scoliosis
Skin
Facies

3. Blood pressure
Check the cuff size
Take the blood pressure in all four limbs

4. Upper limbs
Pulses
- Tachycardia (CCF)
- Absent (coarctation, Takayasu's
  arteritis)
- Pulsus alternans (CCF)

Nails
- Clubbing (SBE)
- Splinter haemorrhages (SBE)
- Brown lines (CRF)

Palms
- Sweaty (phaeochromocytoma)
- Pale creases (CRF)
- Pigmented creases (CAH)

Wrists
- Widened (renal osteodystrophy)

5. Neck
Jugular venous pressure (CCF)
Carotid pulse (may be absent with
    Takayasu's arteritis)
Carotid bruits (Takayasu)
Webbed neck (Turner's)
Buffalo hump (Cushing's)

6. Head
Face
Eyes
Ears
Facial nerve

7. Chest
Full praecordial examination, for
    sequelae of hypertension

8. Back
Inspect
Check for scoliosis

Palpate
Auscultate

9. Abdomen
Inspect
Palpate
- Kidneys
- Suprarenal area
- Liver
- Spleen
- Bladder

Percuss for ascites
Auscultate for renal artery bruits,
    abdominal coarctation

10. Vision and hearing
Visual acuity
Visual fields
Fundoscopy
Hearing

11. Gait and lower limbs
Gait examination
Walk normally, on outsides of feet
    (Fog's test), run, hop
Lower limbs
- Weak femorals (coarctation)
- Examination
  for long-tract
  signs due to
  intracranial
  bleed

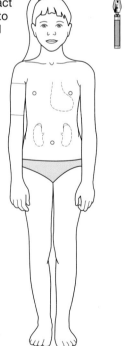

CAH = congenital adrenal hyperplasia; CCF = congestive cardiac failure; CRF = chronic renal failure;
SBE = subacute bacterial endocarditis.

Figure 12.2 **Hypertension**

SHORT CASE: Oedema

This short case is not infrequent and requires a rapid assessment of several major systems to determine the aetiology. Oedema can have the following causes:

1. Renal; for example, nephrotic syndrome or CKD.
2. Liver; for example, chronic liver disease (CLD).
3. Cardiac; for example, congestive cardiac failure (CCF).
4. Bowel; for example, protein-losing enteropathies, including inflammatory bowel disease (IBD) and cystic fibrosis (CF).
5. Nutrition; for example, protein calorie malnutrition (PCM).
6. Local causes; for example, lymphadenopathy causing leg oedema; lymphatic malformation; vascular malformation; abnormal deep veins (e.g. absent valves; very rare). If asymmetrical swelling, then it will likely be a local, structural problem, involving vessels, lymphatics or veins.

Each of these conditions deserves initial consideration.

This is one case where it is reasonable to request the urinalysis and blood pressure results before beginning to examine the patient, as these may well direct the candidate along a renal path (see the short case on renal examination in this chapter). If the urinalysis and blood pressure are unhelpful (i.e. normal), then a careful appraisal is necessary to detect other groups of causes.

A suggested way to approach this case is first to assess the extent of the oedema, and then to look for the cause.

Begin by asking the child to stand up (in underwear only) and inspect for periorbital oedema, findings of CKD (e.g. sallow complexion, pallor, skeletal changes of renal osteodystrophy), CLD (e.g. jaundice, spider naevi) and CCF (e.g. raised jugular venous pressure), Cushingoid features of steroid-treated glomerulonephritis (especially idiopathic nephrotic syndrome [INS]), and nutrition and abdominal swelling from ascites. Also inspect from the side for ascites and kyphoscoliosis (osteodystrophy) and from the back for scoliosis (osteodystrophy) and buttock rash (Henoch–Schönlein purpura).

Next, demonstrate the distribution of the oedema. This can be done starting at the feet and working up (child lying down initially), or by starting at the head and working down (child standing up). The following abnormal signs should be sought:

1. Ankle oedema: press over the anterior tibiae for one minute (remember: one finger, one spot, one minute).
2. Ascites: shifting dullness, fluid thrill.
3. Sacral oedema: press over sacrum for one minute.
4. Pleural effusion: percuss the posterior chest wall.
5. Periorbital oedema: inspect.

Note that the time you spend palpating for oedema can give you the opportunity to re-inspect the child and comment on whether there are any (previously overlooked) signs of CKD (e.g. transplant scar), CLD (clubbing, leuconychia, palmar erythema, caput medusae) or bowel disease (e.g. clubbing, erythema nodosum, joint swelling with IBD).

After demonstrating the extent of the oedema, proceed to examine for the aetiology. A suggested order is as follows: hands, blood pressure (if not yet requested), face, chest, abdomen and urinalysis (again, if not already requested). Figure 12.3 outlines the findings sought at each stage of the examination procedure.

At the completion of the case, summarise succinctly, give a brief differential diagnosis and suggest which investigations you think are appropriate.

1. Introduce self

2. General observation
Position patient: standing
Periorbital oedema
Pale sallow complexion (CRF)
Jaundice (CLD)
Cushingoid (steroids for GN)
Nutritional status
Spider naevi (CLD)
Tachypnoea (CCF, CRF, pleural
   effusions)
Rickets (osteodystrophy)
Ascites: inspect from side as well
Kyphoscoliosis (osteodystrophy)
Buttock purpura (HSP)

3. Request
Blood pressure (CRF, various GNs)
Urinalysis (proteinuria with GNs)
Weight chart
Stool chart (IBD, other protein-losing
   enteropathies)

4. Demonstrate distribution of oedema
Ankle and leg oedema
Ascites
Sacral oedema
Pleural effusions
Periorbital oedema

5. Upper limb
Hands
  • Clubbing (CLD, IBD, CF)
  • Leuconychia (CLD)
  • Pulse: rapid (CCF)
  • Palmar crease pallor (CRF)
  • Palmar erythema (CLD)
  • Joint swelling (IBD)
  • Wrist flaring (osteodystrophy)
Arms
  • Spider naevi (CLD)
  • Muscle bulk: poor (PCM, CRF,
    CLD)
  • Subcutaneous fat: poor (as
    above)

6. Head and neck
Neck
JVP: elevated (CCF)
Face
Moon face, hirsute (steroids)
Malar flush (SLE causing GN)
Eyes
Scleral icterus (CLD)
Conjunctival pallor (CRF)

Mouth: uraemic foetor (CRF)
Tongue: glossitis (nutritional deficiency)

7. Chest
Palpate
  • Rib rosary (osteodystrophy)
  • Cardiomegaly (CCF, CRF)
Auscultate
  • Flow murmur (CCF)
  • Gallop rhythm (CCF)
  • Crepitations (CCF)

8. Abdomen
Palpate
  • Hepatomegaly (CCF, CLD)
  • Splenomegaly (CLD)
  • Nephromegaly (polycystic
    disease, hydronephrosis)
  • Inguinal lymphadenopathy (if leg
    oedema only: local cause)
  • Scrotal oedema
Demonstrate ascites
Inspect
  • Buttock purpura (HSP)
  • Perianal disease (IBD)
Stool analysis

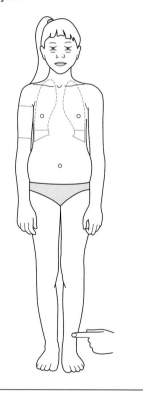

CCF = congestive cardial failure; CF = cystic fibrosis; CLD = chronic liver disease; CRF = chronic renal failure; GN = glomerulonephritides; HSP = Henoch–Schönlein purpura; IBD = inflammatory bowel disease; PCN = protein calorie malnutrition.

Figure 12.3 **Oedema**

Chapter 13

Neurology

LONG CASE: Cerebral palsy (CP)

Cerebral palsy (CP) remains the leading cause for disability, in the paediatric age group, affecting development and function. The prevalence of 2 in 1000 has been unchanged for over 40 years, despite technological advances in neonatal and paediatric care; there are multiple competing influences, such as kernicterus decreasing, but survival of extremely premature babies increasing, and with more multiple births secondary to assisted reproduction (twins over 2.5 kg having a higher risk of CP compared to singletons). There is a higher prevalence of CP among babies born premature (such as 'ex-premmie' graduates of NICUs [neonatal intensive care units]), babies born post-term, beyond 42 weeks, and babies born small for gestational age (SGA). Children with CP often participate in both long- and short-case examinations. The following is a very brief listing of some of the major issues raised in the CP long case, plus a short-case approach.

Background information

CP is a static encephalopathy—a non-progressive disorder of motion and/or posture, secondary to an insult in the developing brain. This excludes active degenerative progressive disorders. CP really is an 'umbrella' term, encompassing a number of types and subtypes of non-progressive brain lesions which can occur from the fetal or neonatal period up to the age of 3 years; some authorities use the terminology 'CP syndromes' as opposed to just 'CP' to delineate the types and subtypes. Despite its static nature, the peripheral manifestations of various forms of CP may seem to progress, and can mimic progressive central nervous system pathology.

CLASSIFICATION

CP is classified according to the clinical type of neuromotor dysfunction:
1. Spastic (subgroups: hemiplegic [unilateral involvement], diplegic [disproportionate lower extremity involvement] and quadriplegic [total body involvement]).
2. Dyskinetic (extrapyramidal; subgroups: choreoathetoid, dystonic).
3. Ataxic.

4. Hypotonic.
5. Mixed (subgroups including spastic–athetoid, ataxic–spastic).

These groups are well delineated by 5 years of age. There is overlap between the types, with regards to clinical signs.

Spastic diplegia is the most common subtype, and the underlying pathology is periventricular leukomalacia in most cases. Spasticity classically develops between 6 and 18 months. The most commonly affected muscles are the paraspinal muscles, hip flexors and adductors, hamstrings, gastrocnemius and soleus. Muscle spasticity and contractures can lead to bone and joint changes. There is also a group of hereditary spastic paraplegias (SPGs), including X-linked, autosomal dominant and autosomal recessive forms, such as SPG1 (spastic paraplegia 1, X-linked, located at Xq28, gene L1CAM, MIM#303350) and SPG2 (located at Xq22.2, gene PLP1, MIM#312920). Spastic hemiplegia is usually secondary to an infarct in the distribution of the middle cerebral artery. Spastic quadriplegia, or total body involvement CP, with bilateral cerebral infarction and multicystic encephalomalacia, can occur secondary to an hypoxic ischaemic insult in the late third trimester. Spastic quadriplegic CP can also be inherited, and there is considerable genetic heterogeneity (e.g. CPSQ1 [cerebral palsy, spastic quadriplegic, 1, located at 2q31.1, gene GAD1, MIM#603513]; CPSQ2 [located at 9p24.3, gene KANK1, MIM#612900]; these are just two of many genetic forms). Dyskinetic CP can be the result of an acute profound hypoxic insult in the third trimester, such as cord prolapse, ruptured uterus or massive antepartum haemorrhage; dyskinetic CP also may occur secondary to bilirubin encephalopathy/kernicterus, where there may be associated sensorineural deafness. Ataxic CP can be genetically determined in 50% cases (e.g. cerebral palsy, ataxic, autosomal recessive [OMIM%605388], located at 9p12–q12, gene CPAT1).

CAUSES

In around one-third of cases, the underlying aetiology is unknown. Known causes can be classified into three groups:

1. *Prenatal problems*; for example, cerebral malformations, intrauterine TORCH infection (toxoplasma, other [e.g. syphilis], rubella, CMV, herpes [simplex or varicella] or HIV infection), toxins (e.g. drugs), placental insufficiency, fetal coagulation and autoimmune disorders, cerebrovascular accidents, trauma or chromosomal anomalies.
2. *Perinatal problems*; for example, neonatal encephalopathy, hypoglycaemia, toxins (e.g. kernicterus from hyperbilirubinaemia), viral (e.g. HSV) encephalitis, bacterial (e.g. early onset Group B streptococcus) meningitis, prematurity (babies born before 28 weeks' gestation have 50 times the risk of CP compared with babies born at term; mechanisms can include intraventricular haemorrhage and periventricular leukomalacia).
3. *Postnatal problems*; for example, head trauma (accidental or non-accidental), hypoxic insult (from near-drowning, choking or poisoning), cerebrovascular accident, toxic encephalopathy (e.g. lead), meningitis or hypoglycaemia.

Epidemiological studies show that in 90% of cases, the cause of CP could *not* be intrapartum hypoxia. In the remaining 10%, intrapartum signs consistent with hypoxic damage may have had maternal or intrapartum origins. Recommendations have been made that the term 'birth asphyxia' should not be used, as it is inappropriate and inaccurate. Rather, the terms 'antenatal hypoxia' and 'intrapartum hypoxia', concerning correct timing of damaging hypoxia, should be used. Similarly, the term 'hypoxic ischaemic encephalopathy' is used loosely, in situations where hypoxia and ischaemia have not been proved; it should not be used in this manner. The term 'neonatal encephalopathy' is preferred, as it does not apportion aetiological liability to any particular pathology. Within the 10% minority, it is recognised that placental infarction, and tight nuchal cord, are each associated with spastic quadriplegic cerebral palsy. An Apgar score less than, or equal to, 3 at 5 minutes is associated with increased risk of CP, as is chorioamnionitis.

Criteria have been developed defining acute intrapartum events sufficient to cause permanent neurological impairment:

1. Evidence of metabolic acidosis in the fetal umbilical arterial cord or early neonatal blood (pH less than 7.00; base deficit greater than, or equal to, 12 mmol/L).
2. Early onset of moderate to severe neonatal encephalopathy in infants of 34 weeks' gestation or more.
3. Spastic quadriplegic or dyskinetic types of CP.

Prevention of premature birth would decrease the incidence of CP; antenatal magnesium sulfate in women at high risk of preterm birth (before 34 weeks of gestation), may reduce cerebral palsy (but not mortality rate) in preterm infants born under 34 weeks' gestation.

DIAGNOSTIC ASSESSMENT

CP remains a clinical diagnosis, despite all the technology available today. Clinical findings should include delayed motor milestones, abnormal muscle tone (can be hypo- or hypertonic), hyperreflexia, and absence of regression or of a more specific diagnosis. A thorough history and physical examination should be all that is required to make the diagnosis; rarer conditions that may be treatable or progressive must not be missed; however, a routine laboratory 'work-up' to exclude CP 'impersonators' is difficult to justify, given their rarity. There are a number of conditions that can masquerade as CP as they evolve, but many are subjects of small case series or single case reports. Some units would include blood tests for thyroid function, lactate, pyruvate, organic and amino acids, chromosomes and other tests, depending on the clinical scenario.

Neuroimaging is more useful than any single pathology test; MRI will show abnormalities in about 90% of patients with CP, delineating pathology, helping determine whether injury was prenatal, perinatal or postnatal in onset, and helping exclude treatable causes, such as hydrocephalus, hamartomata or tumours. In premature babies, MRI finds abnormalities in 99% of cases, especially periventricular leukomalacia. Data from studies where 1384 children with CP underwent neuroimaging showed the rarity of underlying disorders: previously unsuspected metabolic disorders totalled 4%, and genetic disorders 2%.

EEGs are only worthwhile if the patient has had fits, to determine classification of any epilepsy syndrome; they are not useful in determining the aetiology of the child's CP.

Exclusion of other diagnoses is important, as some of these unsuspected 'impersonators' of CP may be amenable to treatment (e.g. hydrocephalus can be treated with a shunt, subdural haematomata can be drained [the chance of finding a surgically treatable lesion by imaging CP patients is 5%], dopa-responsive dystonia responds to dopamine supplementation, hypothyroidism responds to thyroxine). Inborn errors of metabolism can impersonate CP, but a family history of neurological problems or unexplained infant deaths would point to a metabolic disorder, as would neurodevelopmental regression or significant vomiting, hypoglycaemia or worsening seizures. There are several types of genetically determined 'familial spastic paraplegias', as mentioned above. Progressive disorders should be ruled out clinically; if not screened for, they come to light with the passage of time, when a salient aspect becomes apparent. Examples of notable rare CP mimics include the following (4 **M**s: **M**etabolic, **M**uscular dystrophies, **M**itochondrial disorders, **M**alformation syndromes):

- *Metabolic conditions.* Treatable conditions should not be missed. Example: glutaric acidaemia type 1; mutation in the gene encoding glutaryl-CoA dehydrogenase (GCDH); alters catabolism of amino acids lysine, hydroxylysine and tryptophan; can impersonate dyskinetic CP; treatable—low-protein (low lysine and tryptophan) diet (avoiding milk, cheese, dairy, meat, poultry, fish, dried beans and legumes, nuts, peanut butter), special low-protein formula, supplements: riboflavin and L-carnitine.

  Other metabolic conditions are not treatable but have a different prognosis to CP. First example: Lesch–Nyhan syndrome (X-linked deficiency of hypoxanthine guanine phosphoribosyl-transferase, HGPRT); patients eventually self-mutilate, and diagnosis is made. Second example: Sjögren–Larsson syndrome (mutation in gene coding for fatty aldehyde dehydrogenase); patients eventually develop ichthyosis, and diagnosis is made.
- *Muscular dystrophies* (e.g. Becker muscular dystrophy; eventually proximal myopathy and Gowers' sign, and calf hypertrophy).
- *Mitochondrial disorders* (e.g. Leigh syndrome; eventually developmental regression becomes apparent).
- *Malformation syndromes.* Example 1: Miller–Dieker lissencephaly syndrome (MDLS), chromosome 17p13.3; subtle dysmorphic findings (e.g. wrinkled skin over glabella, downward-slanting palpebral fissures) are eventually noticed. Example 2: Rett syndrome; eventually acquired microcephaly, hand-wringing and hyperventilation become apparent.

Candidates should be familiar with the *Gross Motor Functional Classification System, (GMFCS)* which is widely used to clarify questions about walking:

Level I: Ambulatory in all settings
Level II: Walks without aides, but has limitations in community settings
Level III: Walks with aides
Level IV: Mobility requires wheelchair or adult assist
Level V: Dependent for mobility

Candidates should also be familiar with the *Manual Ability Classification System, (MACS)* which is widely used to clarify questions about functional ability of the hands:

Level I: Handles objects with ease.
Level II: Handles most objects; some limitations in ability and speed of achievement.
Level III: Handles objects with difficulty, needs help preparing and/or modelling activities.
Level IV: Handles limited number of easily manipulated objects, in adapted situations.
Level V: Does not handle objects, severely limited ability for simple actions.

The other classification system used widely is the *Communication Function Classification System (CFCS)* to clarify questions about communication in CP:

Level I: Effective sender and receiver with unfamiliar and familiar partners.
Level II: Effective but slower paced sender and/or receiver with unfamilial and/or familiar partners.
Level III: Effective sender and receiver with familiar partners.
Level IV: Inconsistent sender and/or receiver with familiar partners.
Level V: Seldom effective sender and receiver even with familial partners.

Strength is best measured using the British Medical Research Council scale. For testing grip strength, the Jamar dynamometer is useful, and handheld dynamometry can be used for other muscle groups.

Children with CP are more likely to have associated conditions in the following decreasing order of frequency: intellectual impairment (around 50%); epilepsy (around 45%); speech and language disorders, with additional oromotor deficits (around 40%); ophthalmological defects (around 30%); hearing impairment (around 10–15%). Children with right-sided hemiplegia are more likely to have impaired language function due to left hemisphere injury. Intellectual impairment is more likely in the presence of epilepsy, an abnormal EEG or an abnormal neuroimaging study.

Most children with CP are born with the condition, but abnormal features may not be noted for months; most are diagnosed by 3 to 5 years. Serial developmental assessment of six motor milestones, in one study, was better at predicting CP than any single milestone; these were: roll prone to supine (average age 5.1 months); roll supine to prone (average 5.7 months); sit with support (range 4 to 7 months); sit without support (range 6 to 9 months); crawl (range 6 to 9 months); and cruise (range 9 to 11 months). Delays in four of these were considered 'worrisome', meaning concerning, and predictive. Another report noted increased risk of CP if, at 4 months, there was inability to support weight on forearms, inability to sit supported with head erect, lack of interest in surroundings and not responding socially. The finding of abnormal general movements can also help predict development of CP; this can be measured by a classification system (Prechtl), which is reported to have 100% sensitivity and 98% specificity. Also, in premature babies with abnormal cranial ultrasounds, abnormal synchronised general movements and lack of typical, normal, fidgety movements may anticipate CP. A good assessment tool for babies at high risk of CP is the Hammersmith Infant Neurological Examination (HINE), which assesses babies between 2 and 24 months with a scoring system which can be correlated with the GMFCS system.

Diagnosis of CP before 12 months, however, despite these various assessment systems, remains fraught with uncertainty due to the plasticity of the newborn brain; infants can be seen who have apparently clear-cut signs of CP that then resolve by the age of 1 or 2 years. The 'ideal' diagnostic age for CP, according to some authorities, may be 5 years, as the clinical picture will be clear by then, and also this enables exclusion of progressive conditions.

For each child with CP, the above areas (classification, cause) should be defined, as well as functional severity and prognosis. The long-case presentation should address the major problems 1. as the parent sees them and 2. as the various caregivers (e.g. doctors) see them; the interpretations may be quite different.

It is advisable to cover areas that were of interest to the examiners when they took the history and examined the child (ask 'What did the examiners ask about? What areas did they examine?').

History
PRESENTING COMPLAINT
Reason for current admission.

CURRENT SYMPTOMS/FUNCTIONING
1. Intellectual abilities (or present developmental status), current placement regarding education, domestic situation, employment.
2. Behaviour (e.g. hyperactivity), affect (e.g. depression).

3. Vision (e.g. cortical visual impairment, strabismus, myopia, hemianopia).
4. Speech, hearing and communication problems (e.g. expressive or receptive dysphasia, dysarthria, athetoid movements, use of aids such as communication boards and computers).
5. Activities of daily living (e.g. bathing, cleaning teeth, combing hair, dressing, writing and other hand usage, toileting, menses).
6. Feeding and nutrition (e.g. sucking and swallowing ability, tube feeds, gastrostomy, gastro-oesophageal reflux, aspiration, failure to thrive).
7. Seizures (e.g. type, duration, frequency, usual treatment including side effects, compliance and drug levels, last seizure).
8. Mobility (e.g. walking ability ['community', 'household' or 'non-functional' ambulator], gait pattern, wheelchair mobility), skeletal problems (e.g. kyphoscoliosis, lumbar lordosis, spondylolisthesis, hip subluxation and dislocation, pseudoacetabulum formation, contractures, unequal leg length), abnormal posturing.
9. Other problems: urinary incontinence, constipation, management of menses, chest infections, pressure sores.

BIRTH HISTORY

1. Maternal past history of miscarriages or infertility.
2. Pregnancy: hyperemesis, hypertensive disease of pregnancy, teratogenic medications, placental problems, clinical evidence of, or exposure to, infection (e.g. TORCH), quality of fetal movements, gestational age.
3. Delivery: presentation (e.g. breech, face), instrumental delivery, Apgar score, resuscitation required, birth weight, need for oxygen, nursery care.
4. Neonatal period: respiratory distress, feeding difficulties, seizures, hyperbilirubinaemia (phototherapy or exchange transfusion), intraventricular haemorrhage (IVH), periventricular leukomalacia (PVL), hydrocephalus, retinopathy of prematurity (ROP).

DEVELOPMENTAL HISTORY

Age at which milestones achieved (including quality of attainment: e.g. bottom shuffling, bunny-hopping, gross motor development, early hand preference in fine motor development).

FAMILY HISTORY

Any family history of CP (e.g. familial spastic paraplegia).

MANAGEMENT

Recent management in hospital, usual treatment at home, daily routine, frequency of therapies, (e.g. physiotherapy, occupational therapy, speech therapy), usual doctors seen (e.g. local doctor, local paediatrician, subspecialists such as orthopaedic surgeon, neurologist), compliance with treatment, alternative therapies tried (e.g. acupressure, patterning).

SOCIAL HISTORY

Impact on parents and siblings, disruption to family routine, family financial considerations (e.g. private health insurance, visits to multiple specialists, cost of hospitalisations, surgical procedures, aids, home modifications, drugs, benefits received, such as Child Disability Allowance), social supports (social worker, extended family, respite care, involvement of the Cerebral Palsy Alliance [CPA], self-help groups), legal proceedings surrounding perinatal care.

Parents' and siblings' understanding; degree of education regarding CP; question of resuscitation.

Important signs in examination of the child with CP

The procedure outlined below can be used for a long- or short-case examination. When presented in the long case, the examination of the child with CP should convey to the examiners an overall picture of the patient (e.g. 'a profoundly intellectually impaired microcephalic girl with spastic quadriplegia') as the initial introduction.

In the short-case context, a wide number of introductions may be given; for example, 'not walking', 'not developing as well as his siblings', 'has unusual movements', 'has a limp', 'wears out the tips of his shoes', 'has back arching', or more directed introductions such as 'This boy has cerebral palsy; please assess him for complications', or 'This girl was premature; please assess her for complications of prematurity'.

In the case of a child with hemiplegic CP, the lead-in may more likely be 'Please examine this boy's gait' or 'Please examine the peripheral nervous system'.

See the short case on hemiplegia in this chapter for a suggested examination procedure.

In each case, the initial 1–2 minutes spent standing back and inspecting should identify CP as the most likely problem and direct the examination accordingly.

GENERAL OBSERVATIONS

1. Dysmorphic features (e.g. chromosomal anomalies).
2. Parameters: head circumference (often obvious microcephaly), weight (often failing to thrive), height (usually decreased), progressive percentile charts.
3. Posture (e.g. fisting, increased extensor tone, asymmetric tonic neck reflex [ATNR], hemiplegic, quadriplegic).
4. Movement: (a) involuntary (e.g. choreoathetoid movements, dystonic spasms, seizures); (b) voluntary (e.g. immature gait pattern with wide base, up on toes, arms out for balance; hemiplegic, diplegic gaits; note posturing of arms when walking).
5. Asymmetry (e.g. hemiatrophy: look at the size of the thumbnails and the great toenails for subtle clues to asymmetry).
6. Behaviour (e.g. lack of interaction with environment, crying).
7. Eye signs (e.g. squint, nystagmus).
8. Bulbar signs (e.g. dysarthria, drooling).
9. Interventions (e.g. nasogastric tube, gastrostomy tube, scars of orthopaedic procedures).
10. Clothing (e.g. nappies in child over 4 years old).
11. Peripheral aids (e.g. wheelchair, splints, orthoses).

DEMONSTRATION OF SIGNS OF CP

1. If possible, perform a standard gait examination.
2. If the child cannot walk, but can crawl, look for abnormal crawling:
    a. Those with spastic diplegia or quadriplegia—buttock crawling and 'bunny-hopping' (jumping while on knees).
    b. Those with hemiplegia—asymmetrical crawl.
3. Gross motor '180° manoeuvre', incorporating primitive reflexes:
    a. Lying supine (assess position adopted, e.g. ATNR).
    b. Pull to sit by hands (to assess head lag and grasp).
    c. Sitting (assess sitting ability, then lateral propping).
    d. Hold up vertically, under axillae (to detect increased extensor tone, scissoring, automatic walking).

    e. Tilt sideways (to assess head righting).

    f. Ventral suspension (to detect excessive extensor tone).

    g. Parachute reflex (to detect asymmetry).

    h. Place prone (to detect back arching).

4. Inspect carefully for tendon release scars.
5. Palpate muscle bulk in each muscle group.
6. Tone: as above, plus assessment of upper and lower limbs, and evaluation of contractures (e.g. tight hip adductors, and tendo Achilles).
7. Power: voluntary movement, functional power (grasp of toys, cloth cover test).
8. Reflexes: the head should be held in the midline (e.g. by an examiner) so that an ATNR does not give a false impression of unilateral hypertonia; note whether there is any crossed adductor reflex, spread of reflexes, clonus or upgoing plantar responses.

COMPLICATIONS OF CP

1. Measure the head (for microcephaly, or macrocephaly due to hydrocephalus).
2. Check the vision, visual fields and extraocular movements (for myopia, squint).
3. Check the hearing (for sensorineural deafness).
4. Check the ears (for chronic serous otitis media).
5. Ask to check the gag reflex (bulbar dysfunction).
6. Look at the teeth (for dental caries).
7. Look at the back (for kyphoscoliosis).
8. Inspect and auscultate the chest (for chest infection).
9. Palpate the abdomen (for constipation).
10. Examine the hips (for dislocation).
11. Screen nutritional status (demonstrate fat and protein stores).
12. Perform a functional assessment for activities of daily living (e.g. offer cup, spoon, fork, knife, comb, toothbrush; ask the child to put on a piece of clothing).

Investigations

The examiners may ask which investigations you would think appropriate in the particular child you have seen. While this depends on the type of CP the child has, the following brief list may be helpful:

1. Brain imaging (MRI) may show abnormalities in some 90% of patients with CP. It may show the basis of CP (e.g. gross malformations, hydrocephalus, intracranial calcification from congenital infection). It may suggest the timing of the aetiology (e.g. cortical dysplasias develop around 12–20 weeks' gestation; periventricular leukomalacia around 28–34 weeks' gestation; cortical and subcortical gliosis and atrophy in parasagittal watershed areas in term babies with intrapartum hypoxia) or show unexpected degenerative disorders (e.g. one of the leucodystrophies).
2. TORCH screen (including HIV), in infants, for intrauterine infection.
3. Urinary metabolic screen (various inborn errors of metabolism).
4. Chromosomes (various anomalies).
5. Lumbar puncture in dyskinetic CP, to diagnose the treatable genetic condition, glucose transporter 1 deficiency syndrome, especially if there are associated refractory seizures (see next page).

Management

The management of CP is multifaceted and complex. It is beyond the scope of this section to give a comprehensive account of the various treatment modalities used. Rather, a list of the main treatment areas and issues is presented, as a framework around which to base further reading.

ROLE OF THE GENERAL PAEDIATRICIAN

The general paediatrician (the candidate) should coordinate and oversee the various caregivers involved in the management of the child with cerebral palsy. A multidisciplinary team is needed, including a social worker, occupational therapist, physiotherapist, speech therapist, orthopaedic surgeon and psychologist.

Information would routinely be requested when a child is transferred to the care of the local paediatrician looking after the child (which is how candidates should view themselves). As part of the management discussion, it is quite valid for the candidate to request information to clarify aspects of the past history, such as the neonatal notes, results of any investigations (e.g. imaging or metabolic studies) performed and summaries of previous hospital admissions. In any child with dyskinetic CP, an important condition to consider is glucose transporter 1 deficiency syndrome (GLUT1-DS; mapped to 1p34.2), as it is a treatable neurometabolic condition (responds to ketogenic diet); this should be excluded, particularly if there is a coexistent refractory seizure disorder and developmental delay. The diagnosis is made by lumbar puncture: there is hypoglycorrhachia (CSF glucose < 2.2 mmol/L), and a CSF:plasma glucose ratio below 0.4.

GENERAL NURSING CARE

Children with CP may require tube feeds, have trouble with gastro-oesophageal reflux requiring aggressive therapy, be very irritable, need attention to skin for pressure sores, tend to soil well into childhood (requiring attention to toileting) and may dribble. They can constitute a significant workload for the parent at home and for the nursing staff in hospital.

PHYSIOTHERAPY, OCCUPATIONAL THERAPY, SPLINTS/ORTHOSES

These are important in maintaining range of movement and function of trunk and limbs, and preventing contractures. Physiotherapists and occupational therapists enable the child to perform the activities of daily living (ADLs) as well as his or her potential allows. They can evaluate whether there is a problem in the areas of dressing, washing, toileting, feeding, positioning, methods of carrying and lifting (which vary with the different types of CP), mobility aids, and whether the furniture and bathroom fittings at home are appropriate. As much as possible, therapeutic manoeuvres can be built into everyday activities (e.g. handling/feeding/playing in younger children; in older children, simple activities such as lying prone watching television for those with hip flexion contractures).

Serial casting is useful for reversing ankle/foot equinus in younger children. Over 2–6 weeks, the calf muscle is stretched gradually, with the foot and ankle held in position by a below-the-knee plaster.

Orthoses (splints) act as exoskeletons, assist with position and function, and may prevent contractures developing. Soft orthoses may be made from high-density foam, neoprene or lycra (e.g. more for low tone, good for flexed knees). Hard orthoses include solid (fixed) ankle–foot orthoses (AFOs), hinged (articulated) AFOs (allow dorsiflexion); in-shoe orthoses (e.g. supramalleolar orthoses [SMOs]); dynamic movement orthoses (DMO) suits.

The selection of orthoses is aided by computerised gait evaluation in gait laboratories (see overleaf). The ankle–foot orthosis (AFO) is the most commonly used orthosis. It may prevent ankle deformity and improve gait pattern.

Splinting is of great value in the prevention of contractures. Muscles kept in a normal position for the majority of the day will grow normally. Night splinting is beneficial.

THREE-DIMENSIONAL (3-D) GAIT ANALYSIS: COMPUTERISED GAIT LABORATORIES

Examination of gait in CP patients in gait analysis laboratories can detect primary movement problems, differentiating them from secondary or coping manoeuvres. Assessment of the complex gait deviations, which occur in three planes of motion, can direct an interdisciplinary team's clinical decisions as to the best course of treatment. This may be orthopaedic surgical intervention, or treatment that may be of more direct benefit than surgery, including orthotics, botulinum toxin A (BTX-A) therapy (see below) or physiotherapy.

Optical/reflective markers are placed at specific anatomical landmarks/limb segments, and as the child walks the 3-D location is detected by multiple infrared cameras. Gait analysis usually includes clinical lower limb examination, videotaped walking, measurement of limb segment motion (kinematics), and measurement of forces and moments causing that motion (kinetics). This includes 3-D joint motion at ankle, hip and knee; joint mobility; joint angular velocities; joint powers; gait parameters such as step, stride length and cadence; synchronised dynamic electromyography (EMG); ground reaction forces and foot pressure analysis. Children walk on a force plate to assess the amount of power generated. The energy cost of walking is also assessed: oxygen consumption, respiratory function and heart rate can be measured with a portable telemetric system. Most units have specific referral criteria, which may include being ambulatory (with or without aids) for at least 10 steps, being at least 4 years old, cooperative and at least 100 cm tall.

MANAGEMENT OF SPASTICITY

In 2010, the American Academy of Neurology (AAN) released an evidence-based review of pharmacological treatments for childhood spasticity due to CP, where a multidisciplinary panel reviewed relevant literature from 1966 to 2008. In the case of localised/segmental spasticity that warrants treatment, the AAN recommendation was that botulinum toxin A (BTX-A) is effective and generally safe in reducing spasticity in the upper and lower extremities, but there is conflicting evidence regarding functional improvement, and severe generalised weakness can occur; there is insufficient data to support or refute BTX-A use to improve motor *function*. There is insufficient data to support or refute other medications used for the same indication (and these are not discussed further): phenol, alcohol and BTX type B. In the case of generalised spasticity that warrants treatment, the AAN recommendation was that diazepam could be considered for short-term treatment, and also tizanidine may be considered; but, again, there is insufficient data to support or refute other medications used for the same indication: dantrolene, oral baclofen or continuous intrathecal baclofen. The latter is discussed because patients who have received this treatment may present in the examination, so a candidate should have some knowledge of the side effects.

Botulinum toxin A (BTX-A)

BTX-A is a neurotoxin produced by *Clostridium botulinum*, given by intramuscular (IM) injection, and taken up by endocytosis at cholinergic nerve terminals at the motor endplate, preventing release of acetylcholine from these terminals, which leads to a prolonged, reversible relaxation of skeletal muscle. There are seven serotypes (A–G) of botulinum toxin; types A, B and F have been used clinically. BTX-A causes local paralysis in the injected muscle with an onset within 1–3 days of the IM injection. Duration of action is 3–6 months, by which time motor nerves generate new neuromuscular junctions by terminal sprouting, and there is then a clinical return of spasticity (from 12–16 weeks in most patients). Injections then may be repeated.

BTX-A injected locally, is well established as the standard treatment for reducing hypertonicity of muscles in children with spastic CP. The indication for use is dynamic contracture in the absence of a fixed deformity. Muscles typically targeted include the gastrocnemius–soleus complex, the tibialis posterior (to relieve equinovarus), the hamstrings (to relieve crouch gait), the adductors (improves positioning and perineal access for hygiene), the rectus femoris (to relieve flexed stiff knee gait) and the iliopsoas (to relieve dynamic deformity of hip flexion during gait). Decreased spasticity in the iliopsoas and adductors may modify the natural history of subluxation or dislocation of the hip. BTX-A is useful for correcting gait abnormalities and for reducing the need for orthopaedic surgery. BTX-A may be used in the upper limbs as well as the lower. It may decrease muscle spasm after soft-tissue releases.

BTX-A is well tolerated, but there are several potential side effects. BTX-A can diffuse intra-axonally and across fascial planes, causing distant side effects. Side effects can be gait-related, including deterioration in walking, local weakness, unsteadiness, increased falls, and fatigue. Other side effects have included aspiration pneumonia (impaired pharyngeal function from systemic spread of small amounts of BTX-A), local pain, worsening of strabismus, dysphagia, muscle atrophy, global weakness, and incontinence of urine and faeces. Drug interactions include non-depolarising muscle relaxants and aminoglycosides, causing potentiation of neuromuscular blockade. Other disadvantages include the cost and need for repeated injections. The neuromuscular junctions that are blocked are the same as those that cause meaningful movement. BTX-A may reveal underlying weakness or cause weakness by 'overcorrection', and 6 weeks later there will be a return of strength/function, but without the presenting problem. There have been very rare reports of intermittent tetraparesis after treatment. It may be used for relief of rigidity, but the effects in the extrapyramidal forms of CP are not so dramatic.

The majority of patients using BTX-A for treating spasticity demonstrate objective improvement in tone and function. Kinematic parameters of gait are improved in lower limb spasticity. Integrated multilevel BTX-A has a similar effect to a medical rhizotomy.

Intrathecal baclofen (IT-BLF)

Baclofen is an analogue of gamma-aminobutyric acid (GABA), which inhibits monosynaptic and polysynaptic reflexes, reducing gamma efferent activity. In view of its severe side effects, it is only used in spasticity unresponsive to any other treatment. In view of the paucity of data to support this treatment, it may well become of historical interest only. There are many and varied side effects, several related to the mode of delivery: an implantable drug-delivery pump system for continuous infusion. Significant complications include central side effects such as apnoea, respiratory depression, bradycardia, hypotension and sedation, mechanical complications including pump or side-port failure, catheter kinks, extrusions or dislodgement, cerebrospinal fluid fistula, local infection and meningitis; also, rapidly progressive scoliosis has been reported. There have been a few studies evaluating IT-BLF's performance, one showing improvement in pain and in sleeping, initially, and subsequently improvement in mobility and social interaction; another study showed IT-BLF to decrease tone and spasms, and improve comfort.

Selective dorsal rhizotomy (SDR)

This has been widely used to treat spasticity in children with diplegic CP, but never shown to improve functional outcome conclusively. SDR involves intraoperative stimulation of lumbar nerve rootlets, monitored with EMG: the nerves that cause increased tone are cut. SDR decreases spasticity, but does not affect selective motor control, weakness, poor balance or fixed deformities. There are reports that SDR combined with physiotherapy and occupational therapy leads to greater functional motor improvement, compared to physiotherapy and occupational therapy alone. A report described children aged 4 to 10 years who had significant improved function with SDR plus physiotherapy, versus physiotherapy alone.

Other treatments

Oral diazepam has been used for generalised spasticity as outlined above; side effects can include sedation, drowsiness, hypersalivation and weakness. There have been some positive reports that physical training in CP increases aerobic power and isokinetic muscle strength, and that movement and swimming programs improve baseline vital capacity and water-orientation skills. It is likely that more research will be conducted in these areas. Other therapeutic options in the management of spasticity include repetitive magnetic stimulation and the use of gabapentin (which has proven useful in adults). Deep brain stimulation (DBS) has been used in adults with dyskinetic CP, using an electrode to stimulate part of the globus pallidus; this may be effective but there are no conclusive studies.

ORTHOPAEDIC PROCEDURES

Single-event multilevel surgery (SEMLS)

Multilevel orthopaedic surgical procedures for gait are performed at tertiary centres. The plan is based on comprehensive 3-D gait analysis. There are two surgeons and two operative teams. Generally, 6–16 soft-tissue/bony procedures are undertaken, with postoperative epidural anaesthesia for up to 5 days and a total hospital stay of 7 days. Subsequently, there is community rehabilitation and review at 3, 6, 9 and 12 months in the 3-D gait laboratory. SEMLS allows correction and prevention of deformities, and has positive benefits as regards cosmesis. Procedures performed may include hip adductor tenotomies (help prevent hip subluxation and allow easier attention to perineal hygiene), hamstring releases (relieve knee contractures), lengthening of the tendo Achilles (correcting equinus deformity), and surgery to correct valgus deformity of the foot.

Surgical procedures for spastic hip displacement

The natural history of hip displacement in CP is enlocation at birth, but with displacement occurring at 4–8% per annum. Displacement is easily missed on clinical examination, but easily detected and monitored by X-ray. There are preventative procedures (soft tissue), reconstructive procedures (osteotomies) and salvage procedures. These may be performed in the setting of SEMLS. The procedures available are as follows:

- *Preventative (soft-tissue surgery)*: adductor longus release, gracilis release, adductor brevis release, iliopsoas lengthening, obturator neurectomy (anterior branch only).
- *Reconstructive (redirectional osteotomies)*: femoral varus derotation osteotomy, pelvic osteotomy, combined femoral and pelvic osteotomy with or without open reduction.
- *Salvage*: excision of proximal femur, valgus osteotomy, interpositional arthroplasty, replacement arthroplasty, arthrodesis.

These procedures lead to significant improvements in function, including improved walking speed.

Other orthopaedic procedures

Upper limb surgery may be offered to correct a flexion–pronation deformity of the wrist, to achieve a better functional position; however, usually only cosmetic improvement is achieved, with little gain functionally, largely because of associated cortical sensory loss. Some children will require surgery for scoliosis (e.g. placing of Luque rods).

GASTROINTESTINAL (GIT) PROBLEMS: DYSPHAGIA AND NUTRITIONAL ISSUES

Up to two-thirds of children with CP have disorders of GIT motility. Significant GIT symptoms include constipation (delayed colonic transit, especially of proximal colon, poor muscle tone, inadequate feeding, prolonged immobility), swallowing disorders (especially dysfunction of the oral and/or pharyngeal phase of swallowing, from corticobulbar dysfunction), vomiting and/or regurgitation (delay in gastric emptying, abnormal oesophageal motility, gastro-oesophageal reflux disease [GORD]), abdominal pain (due to GORD-associated oesophagitis or constipation) and respiratory symptoms due to chronic pulmonary aspiration, secondary to GORD. GIT symptoms are not related to specific types of CP.

Children with CP often fail to thrive, due to GORD and/or impairment of swallowing. Work-up for GORD may include endoscopy and biopsy, pH studies, barium studies and nuclear medicine milk scan. Endoscopy results: usually around 40–50% will show oesophagitis, 40–50% will be normal, and the remainder may have H pylori, Barrett's oesophagus or eosinophilic oesophagitis. Management of GORD may include acid suppression (proton pump inhibitors, or H_2-antagonists), and antireflux surgery. There is no evidence to support efficacy in GORD for prokinetic agents or thickened feeds. Nissen fundoplication is uncomplicated in about 70%; complications can include gagging/retching, dumping, bloating and cyclic vomiting. In around 3%, a 're-do' is needed.

Patients with CP who have fundoplication have similar rates of aspiration pneumonia to patients with CP who have gastrojejunal feeding tubes (both around 15%) and similar mortality.

Those children with impaired swallowing and poor nutrition may require assessment and therapy by a dietician (assessing diet and increasing calories), speech therapist (altering consistency of food), physiotherapist (positioning during feeding), as well as nasogastric tube feeding, gastrojejunal feeding tube and placement of a gastrostomy. Post-gastrostomy placement, there is usually improved weight, height and skin fold thickness and a decrease in chest infections, but no change in hospitalisation rates.

RESPIRATORY PROBLEMS

Lung disease is common in CP, and multifactorial in aetiology. Sleep-disordered breathing is also well recognised, but underdiagnosed and undertreated until recently. In addition to assessing for GORD (see above), aspiration can be assessed with video-fluoroscopy, the lungs can be assessed with a helical CT scan, and any sleep disorder with a sleep study. Occasionally, bronchoscopy may be undertaken to investigate for aspiration. Management plans are required for mealtimes (establish with assistance of therapy team plus dietician), for dental hygiene and for hypersalivation, as well as a chest management plan, including positioning (feeding and sleeping), physiotherapy to improve mucociliary clearance, inhalations of normal or hypertonic saline, or bronchodilators, and, using sputum culture as a guide, antibiotics, which may involve a single course, rotating courses or prophylactic antibiotics, depending on the circumstances; nebulised antibiotics can also be useful. Other aspects of management that can contribute to respiratory wellbeing may include scoliosis surgery, management of upper airway obstruction and obstructive sleep apnoea (OSA) (with surgery or nasal CPAP; see the long case on OSA in Chapter 15, The respiratory system), management of lower airway obstruction (with bimodal positive airway pressure [BiPAP] or CPAP) and oxygen support.

EXCESSIVE SALIVATION (SIALORRHOEA)

Anticholinergic drugs (e.g. glycopyrrolate) have been used for excessive drooling with some success, but can have unpleasant side effects, such as urinary retention, constipation, blurred vision, headache, drowsiness, dizziness and behaviour changes.

BTX-A injections into the parotid and/or submandibular salivary glands under ultrasound localisation have been used for severe drooling, with success in small case series. Ongoing excessive salivation may lead to consideration of operative intervention. Three procedures have been tried:
1. Transplanting the salivary ducts to the back of the pharynx.
2. Excising one of the salivary glands.
3. Section of the chorda tympani nerve.

Unfortunately, none of these procedures has any lasting benefit, and the incidence of dental caries increases after such surgery.

SPEECH THERAPY

Anarthric or dysarthric speech and other oral-motor dysfunctions are common, due to bilateral corticobulbar dysfunction in many children with CP, with articulation problems and decreased speech intelligibility. Many children have limited social interactions and may have difficulty developing the linguistic skills to advance their speech abilities. The management of dysarthria, dysphasia and drooling requires assessment and treatment by an experienced speech pathologist.

SOCIAL IMPLICATIONS

This is a major discussion point. Behaviour disorders in the child (e.g. attention deficits, depression from realisation of disability) are common. The siblings may be neglected inadvertently. There may be several significant burdens on the parents: emotional, physical and financial (e.g. hospitalisations, electric wheelchairs, home aids, home modifications, computer and communication devices). Inordinate amounts of time may be spent on the activities of daily living (ADLs), including feeding the child, physiotherapy and occupational therapy, and administering medications, with the parent/carer not having time for anyone else. Marriages may break up from the strain of managing a chronic disabling disorder such as CP.

It is vital to give parents the opportunity to detail their problems, offering to organise a social worker to discuss these, and encouraging the use of respite care. Ask the mother how much time is spent on the child's needs each day. The examiners will know the answer, having asked this themselves to ascertain the candidate's understanding of the implications of care in CP.

SLEEP PROBLEMS

Around a quarter of children with CP have sleep problems, including frequent night waking, OSA, difficulty getting to sleep or a sleep pattern that is socially challenging for the family. Melatonin can be useful to help a child get to sleep, and maintain fewer night wakenings and longer duration. Other medications that have been used include the melatonin agonist ramelteon, and antihistamines, but these lacks supportive research.

SEIZURES

The management of seizures in CP follows the same general approach as that of other seizure disorders. See the long-case approach to recurrent seizures in this chapter.

COGNITION/LEARNING AND COMMUNICATION

The risk of associated cognitive and learning difficulties varies with the type of CP. Those with quadriplegic CP have the highest risk of cognitive impairment and those with hemiplegic CP have the lowest risk. In children with movement impairment hindering their verbal communication, augmentative and alternative communication systems are available. Aided formal communication systems include communication boards and books, where pictures and symbols are used to communicate specific messages, and electronic devices of varying complexity, some allowing the person to communicate with recorded speech; unaided formal communication systems include key word signing (Makaton vocabulary), and informal communication systems include facial expression, eye contact, vocalisations, body language and gestures, to convey feelings, wants and needs.

VISUAL IMPAIRMENT

A large number of children with CP have a squint (30%). Decreased visual acuity is common in spastic quadriplegia, and visual field defects are common in hemiplegic CP. There is increased incidence of nystagmus, optic atrophy and refractive errors. Referral to an ophthalmologist is necessary. Management may include spectacles for refractive errors. For squint, which may cause permanent amblyopia after the age of 6 years, patching the good eye may be required. Surgical rearrangements of extraocular muscle actions to achieve parallel eye axes may well be needed. Educational aids will also be very important.

If the best-corrected acuity is less than 3/60, the child will require use of braille and teaching by methods not involving sight. 'Blind' means acuity of less than 6/60, not correctable by glasses. In 'partially sighted' children (i.e. acuity between 6/24 and 6/60), large print and magnifying aids will be useful.

HEARING IMPAIRMENT

Management depends upon the degree of hearing loss. Mild loss—that is, 25–45 decibel (dB) loss—does not necessarily require intervention. Moderate loss (45–65 dB) requires some treatment with otological intervention or the fitting of a hearing aid. Severe loss (65–85 dB) always requires amplification to hear speech. Profound loss (over 85 dB) requires special education for the deaf, as there is insufficient hearing for any useful communication.

Intervention by an ear, nose and throat specialist may be necessary for conductive causes amenable to surgical intervention (e.g. suction myringotomy and insertion of ventilation tubes, tympanoplasty). For provision of hearing aids and information regarding auditory training facilities, referral to a competent audiology centre—for example, in a large teaching hospital, or the Australian Hearing Service—is appropriate.

DENTAL ISSUES

Children with CP are at high risk for dental problems, including malocclusion due to altered forces on the oromotor muscles, poor (difficult to achieve) dental hygiene, because of oral aversion or hyperactive gag reflex, or care for their teeth simply given less priority because of all nutrition is given by gastrostomy, and nothing is taken orally. In these patients who neither bite or chew, there is a high rate of gingivitis and calculus deposition. It is prudent for these children to regularly see a paediatric dentist who specialises in children with disabilities.

PAIN

This is a common complaint, which can be very challenging in the non-verbal child with severe CP. The most common sites of pain seem to be gastrointestinal (constipation,

GORD), and orthopaedic/musculoskeletal (scoliosis, hip dislocation, patella alta); other possibilities include: neuromuscular—muscle spasms; head and neck—migraine, raised intracranial pressure, glaucoma, corneal abrasions, tooth abscess, temporomandibular joint pain; urological—urolithiasis, bladder spasm; skin—boils, decubitus ulcers. A thorough history (e.g. temporal association with feeding, or nappy changes) and thorough general examination (e.g. inspecting the mouth with a torch and spatula to find tooth abscesses) may find the cause, but often empirical interventions are tried before the patient is eventually free of discomfort.

SCHOOLING

Many children with CP have some degree of intellectual impairment, as well as physical disabilities. Many require special educational assistance to maximise their potential. Most states, regions or areas have their own centres that are designed to assist in all aspects of management of CP (e.g. Choice, Passion, Life [CPL], Cerebral Palsy Alliance [CPA]).

INTERVENTION PROGRAMS—ORTHODOX

Most orthodox-trained therapists aim to enhance the child's quality of life and to give the parents realistic expectations of outcome. This goal begins from the early intervention stage, encouraging parents to modify how they handle their child to allow the full use of the child's motor abilities, and giving advice and support at all levels of developmental experience, in the home, child care, kindergarten, preschool, school, university and/or workforce settings. The main practice in Australia is based on facilitation techniques, with training in motor functional activities following the developmental sequence from head control to walking. This aids posture and movement control, towards eventual independence, recognising that those who are going to walk will usually do so by 7 years of age.

INTERVENTION PROGRAMS—LESS ORTHODOX/UNORTHODOX

There is no evidence that any specific intervention significantly changes the course of the motor disorder in CP. There are no convincing studies that show that outcomes from any 'unorthodox' therapies have any advantage over the outcomes from orthodox therapies, as practised by paediatric rehabilitation units in tertiary/teaching centres of excellence.

Unfortunately, none of the unproven methods has been shown to be effective in any well-designed randomised double-blind controlled trial. Despite this, many parents will try 'alternative' therapies; proponents of some may exhibit messianic zeal regarding their favoured therapy. A sensible approach to adopt is not to criticise these parents for doing so, as long as the child is not harmed in any way. One should explain to the family that there is no proof that these methods work better than more conventional treatment. The inadvertent engendering of false hope should be discouraged.

DRUGS

Anticonvulsants for children with seizures are the only drugs that are consistently of use.

PROGNOSIS

A few 'rules of thumb' are worth knowing when parents ask about prognosis; most parents ask whether their child will walk. While unlikely to be an active discussion issue with a patient in a long case, examiners may ask hypothetical questions such as how to approach answering the parents' concerns when the concept of permanent neurological damage has been mentioned. Children with hemiplegic or diplegic CP usually walk; those with quadriplegic CP rarely walk; those with the dyskinetic subtype are more difficult to predict. Most children who can sit independently by 2 years will walk, but most children who cannot sit by 4 years are unlikely to walk. Of children with spastic hemiplegia or spastic diplegia variants, 95% will reach GMFCS level I–II; of children with spastic quadriplegia or dyskinetic variants, 25% will reach GMFCS level I–II. In terms of life span, only the most profound degrees of CP are associated with a decreased life expectancy. If a child cannot lift the head to prone, and requires tube feeding, the median survival is around 17 years. Adults with CP, based on a population-based cross-sectional study, have increased rates of asthma, emphysema, stroke, hypertension, heart disease, arthritis and arthralgia, compared to those without CP.

LONG CASE: Dystrophinopathies—Duchenne muscular dystrophy (DMD)

DMD (MIM#310200) is the most common childhood muscular dystrophy and is at the most severe end of a spectrum of muscle diseases caused by mutations in the dystrophin gene (dystophinopathies) on the X chromosome.

The natural (untreated) history of DMD comprises:

- Mean age of diagnosis 5 years.
- Delayed motor milestones, mean age of walking 18 months, proximal skeletal muscle weakness and waddling gait with difficulty climbing stairs; motor regression ensues, with patients wheelchair-bound by 12 years.
- Decline in respiratory function and cardiomyopathy.

Becker muscular dystrophy (BMD; MIM#300376) is a less severe form of dystrophinopathy, with later-onset skeletal muscle weakness. In contrast to DMD, wheelchair dependency can occur at any point between the third and seventh decade. Life expectancy is far higher, with the median age at death > 67 years. Cardiomyopathy can paradoxically be severe, presumably related to greater stress placed on ventricular function by a greater capacity to exercise. Rarely cardiac transplantation may be indicated.

There is a third clinically important dystrophinopathy, where cardiac muscle is primarily affected. Dystrophin-associated dilated cardiomyopathy (DCM; MIM#302045) is a distinct entity where males present between 20 and 40 years of age with cardiac failure; female carriers of dystrophin mutations are also at risk of this DCM.

Boys with DMD are often subjects for the long-case examination. Genetic counselling and prenatal diagnosis are likely discussion areas in the management of the DMD long case.

Background information: genetics of DMD

DMD is an X-linked recessive disorder, due to mutations (often deletions) in the dystrophin gene on the X chromosome (Xp21.2). It has a frequency of 1 in 3600–6000 male births. Dystrophin (MIM*300377) is the largest known human gene comprising 2.6 million base pairs (79 exons) coding for a large, rod-like 427-kD protein containing 3685 amino acids located at the inner surface of the muscle cell membrane (sarcolemma). Dystrophin is part of the dystrophin-associated protein complex (DAPC), which spans the muscle membrane, linking the muscle cytoskeleton (specifically actin) and the extracellular matrix (see Fig. 13.1). Dystrophin reinforces the sarcolemma and shields the DAPC from proteases. Absence of dystrophin destabilises the DAPC, making the muscle membrane vulnerable to damage from shearing stresses culminating in the degeneration of muscle fibres. Dystrophin is virtually undetectable on immunohistochemical stains in the muscle of DMD patients.

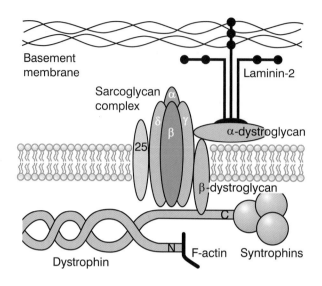

Figure 13.1 Subsarcolemmal cytoskeleton

Redrawn from: Isaacs, D., Roberton, D. & South, M. (2007). *Practical Paediatrics* (6th ed.). London: Churchill Livingstone, p. 609, Figure 17.3.4.

Almost all males with DMD have identifiable mutations in the dystrophin gene. Around two-thirds of patients have deletions involving one or multiple exons with a disruption of the reading frame resulting in a prematurely truncated protein product. Around 10% have duplications of one or more exons of the gene and the remaining 25% have point mutations or other small rearrangements, including intronic deletions, insertions of repetitive sequences and splice site mutations. Generally, out-of-frame mutations (alter the reading frame) cause lack of dystrophin resulting in DMD, and in-frame mutations (don't alter the reading frame) cause abnormal but partially functional dystrophin resulting in BMD.

Molecular genetic testing of DMD can confirm the diagnosis of a dystrophinopathy without the need for muscle biopsy in most patients with DMD or BMD. There is a high incidence of new mutations, and two-thirds of new patients have no positive family history.

In addition to skeletal, smooth and cardiac muscle, dystrophin is also expressed within the central nervous system (CNS). The clinical manifestations of an absent or reduced CNS dystrophin expression are variable and can include a static encephalopathy and cognitive deficits.

MOLECULAR TESTS FOR DMD

With current techniques, efficiency of mutation detection approaches 100%, which allows precise evaluation of the carrier status of female members of the family:

1. Microarray-based comparative genomic hybridisation (array CGH) can detect large deletions and duplications in any exon of the dystrophin gene by analysing copy number variations (CNVs) relative to the level in reference DNA. CGH is unable to detect aberrations that do not cause CNVs, and is limited in its ability to detect mosaicism; CGH is only able to detect unbalanced chromosomal anomalies (i.e. it cannot detect reciprocal translocations, inversions and ring chromosomes that do not affect copy number). There are two areas within the gene where there are frequently found CNVs (deletions and duplications), at exons 2–20 and at exons

44–53. Dystrophin mutations detected by array CGH still have to be confirmed using multiplex ligation-dependent probe amplification (MLPA).

2. Next-generation sequencing-based (NGS-based) targeted gene analysis in MLPA-negative patients can detect point mutations and sequence variants, including small deletions or insertions and splice site mutations.

3. Muscle biopsy-based approaches utilising protein and RNA-based analyses in combination with direct cDNA sequencing increase the mutation detection frequency to almost 100%.

4. Prenatal diagnosis is available by chorionic villus biopsy or amniocentesis. The mutation of the index case and carrier status of the mother would need to be known.

RECENT ADVANCES

In the last decade advances in medical care have shifted the natural history of this disease and affected patients may reach their fourth decade (a significant advance on the previous life expectancy). Research into DMD has continued to accelerate, with a number of different treatment strategies being developed, but most of these are still at the experimental stage in animal models or early human trials.

Newer experimental therapies include:

1. *Gene therapy* trials using new-generation adenovirus carriers known as 'stealth' or 'gutted' vectors (containing no original viral genes) are being developed to overcome the obstacle of the immune system, the problem being preexisting T-cell immunity to dystrophin being present even before the therapy is started.

2. *Exon skipping* is a suggested alternative strategy to replace the defective dystrophin gene in DMD patients. Exon skipping involves regular intravenous administration of an anti-sense oligonucleotide compound (e.g. eteplirsen, drisapersen), which causes specific exon skipping while messenger RNA splicing is occurring; this aims at restoring the open reading frame to produce partially functioning dystrophin, thereby converting DMD into BMD.

3. *Utrophin upregulation* involves a protein related to dystrophin, which can substitute or compensate for it if made in sufficient amounts.

4. *Ataluren* (previously PTC 124) has been developed for the 10–15% of DMD patients who have nonsense (stop) mutations as their aetiology; it has been designed to permit ribosomal read-through of nonsense mutations, effectively bypassing the mutation and completing the translation process to protein production; preliminary animal experiments demonstrated some production of dystrophin.

   A double-blind, placebo-controlled trial published in late 2015 showed some benefit, enabling patients who could walk 300–400 m on the 6-minute walking test (6MWT) before taking ataluren, to gain an additional 47 m distance in their subsequent 6MWT; no patient taking ataluren lost ambulation, but four patients receiving placebo treatment did lose ambulation. The European Medicines Agency has approved its use and it is available and subsidised in several European jurisdictions. It is not yet available in Australia.

5. *Creatine monohydrate* has been trialled to increase muscle strength; it was found to improve grip strength of the dominant hand, and to increase fat-free mass, but there was no change in ADLs or any functional improvements.

6. *Stem cell therapy* remains under investigation.

7. *Myostatin inhibition* in animals using antibodies to myostatin caused increased muscle mass and strength.

8. *Oxandrolone*, the anabolic steroid, increases skeletal muscle myosin synthesis, and is being further investigated.

9. *Idebenone*, an anti-oxidant, was trialled in DMD patients not on steroids at enrolment; it reduced decline in respiratory function, and further study is ongoing.

History

Ask about the following.

PRESENTING COMPLAINT

Reason for current admission.

CURRENT PROBLEMS

1. Functional abilities with ADLs (e.g. dressing, writing, toileting); aids required (e.g. splints, supportive prostheses, computer-assisted communication/learning).
2. Mobility (e.g. long leg braces, wheelchair use, school and home access).
3. Home modifications required (e.g. ramps, bathroom fittings, specialised beds and mattresses).
4. Transport needs (e.g. van with hoist).
5. Scoliosis (e.g. progression, any planned surgery).
6. Joint contractures (AFOs, night splints).
7. Respiratory problems (e.g. symptoms of respiratory failure at later stage, sleep-disordered breathing, non-invasive ventilation).
8. Cardiac symptoms (e.g. arrhythmias, symptoms of cardiac failure).
9. Gastrointestinal problems (e.g. constipation, incontinence, gastro-oesophageal reflux, vomiting).
10. Difficulties with micturition.
11. School (e.g. any access problems, educational problems, any help needed or provided with toileting; attitudes of class teacher, principal, fellow students).
12. Behavioural/psychological problems (e.g. attention deficit hyperactivity disorder [ADHD], obsessive compulsive disorder [OCD], anxiety, depression, aggression).

PAST HISTORY

1. Initial diagnosis: when, where, presenting symptoms (e.g. late walking, tendency to fall, method of rising after fall, any ability to jump [boys with DMD often are unable to jump, whereas children with BMD may be able to], clumsiness, muscle cramps, learning delay, cognitive impairment, global or gross motor developmental delay).
2. The time period between onset of symptoms and diagnosis.
3. What investigations were undertaken to make the diagnosis.
4. Stages of deterioration (e.g. age at which the child lost the ability to climb stairs, stand from the floor or walk independently). Recognised stages include: 'early ambulatory' (boys show signs including Gowers' manoeuvre, waddling gait, walking on toes; steroids started); 'late ambulatory' (walking difficult, more trouble with stairs, difficulty getting off floor; steroids continuing); 'early non-ambulatory' (need for wheelchair, upright posture is maintained; physiotherapy focus shifts to upper limbs; respiratory decline may commence); 'late non-ambulatory' (increased need for technology, equipment, adaptations, non-invasive ventilation).
5. Number of hospitalisations.
6. Development of complications (e.g. scoliosis, cardiac failure) and their management.
7. Surgical procedures (e.g. release of contractures).
8. Commencement of steroids: timing, side effects.

CURRENT MANAGEMENT

Present treatment in hospital, usual treatment at home (including physiotherapy, exercise, breathing exercises, medications taken), future treatment plans (e.g. surgical procedures), usual follow-up (by whom, where, how often), alternative therapies tried (e.g. acupuncture, naturopathy).

SOCIAL HISTORY

1. Impact on child (e.g. difficulties at school, poor job prospects, limitations on lifestyle, body image, self-esteem, peer reactions).
2. Impact on family (e.g. parental coping, difficulties between mother and father, genetic implications for further children; financial considerations, such as cost of wheelchairs, home modifications, transport, hospitalisations, private health insurance; physical burden of helping children in and out of wheelchairs, cars, bed, bath).
3. Benefits received.
4. Social supports (e.g. social worker, DMD Family Support Group provided by the Muscular Dystrophy Association, visits to school by occupational therapist and community liaison nurse from hospital muscle clinic to meet class and teachers).

FAMILY HISTORY

Other known family members with DMD, other males with developmental delay or late walking.

UNDERSTANDING OF DISEASE

By the child, by the family (e.g. parents, grandparents, siblings) and by teachers. Ask about the degree of previous education (e.g. in hospital, by local paediatrician) and contingency plans (e.g. what to do when child develops a respiratory infection, sick day management for steroids).

At the completion of the history, think about what particular problems this family is experiencing at the moment, from the viewpoints of the child, the parents and the attending physicians. These three perspectives may be quite different.

Examination

GENERAL INSPECTION

Describe the resting posture (undressed). If the child can still stand, describe the standing posture. Usually, this includes findings of small interscapular muscle bulk, small proximal upper limb musculature, abnormal anterior axillary fold (atrophic sternal head of pectoralis major), lumbar lordosis, some internal rotation of the femurs (due to muscle imbalance), small thighs with preservation of vastus lateralis, but prominent calves (pseudohypertrophy) and equinus deformity of the feet. If in a wheelchair, describe the child's posture, and also comment on the chair itself (that is, whether it is appropriate or needs some adjustments). Note whether the respiratory rate is raised (for intercurrent respiratory infection or cardiac failure). Also note the child's demeanour, apparent mood, intelligence and ability to communicate.

GAIT

Ask the child to walk normally. Focus on each component of the gait in turn, starting at the feet (foot drop due to weak tibialis anterior, inversion due to relatively strong tibialis posterior and weak peroneals, heels off ground partly due to tightened tendo Achilles, higher step to gait than normal).

Next, inspect the knees (weakened quadriceps leading to knee-locking gait, where the knee is snapped back into extension quickly for stability) and then the hips (weakened hip flexors require rotation of the upper body to enable the leg to swing forwards; weakened hip abductors, the gluteus medius, cause tilting of the pelvis down on the unsupported side with each step during walking—Trendelenburg's gait; weakened hip extensors, the gluteus maximus and hamstrings, lead to a forward pelvic tilt and marked lordosis to maintain the centre of gravity). Overall, the gait also has a wide base and the appearance of waddling.

Proceed with the other components of a full gait examination, including asking the child to run, hop, jump, squat and rise, walk upstairs, step on to a stool or chair, and do a sit-up and a push-up.

Boys with DMD can walk well on their toes, but are unable to walk on their heels, and if they try they end up inverting the feet. On squatting, these children are slow to return to standing, need to extend the knee before the hip, and lean on their thighs to assist extension at the hip.

Of particular importance is the demonstration of Gowers' manoeuvre. The boy is asked to lie supine on the floor and then to get up. Gowers' manoeuvre includes first rolling over to be prone (cannot sit up because of weak neck and spine flexion), then on to the knees, then on all fours (hands and feet) and then 'climbing up' the legs to stand. Timing how long it takes to arise from the floor is useful to monitor deterioration over time. See Fig. 13.2.

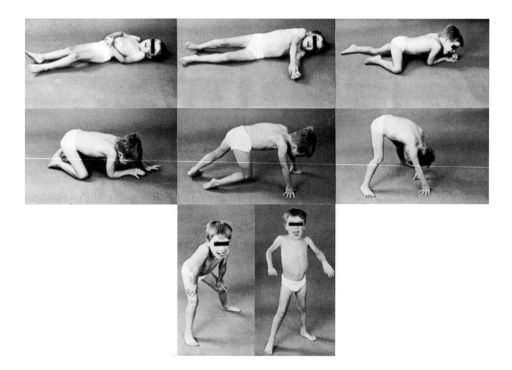

Figure 13.2 **The Gowers' sign in a patient with DMD, illustrating the sequence of manoeuvres required to rise from the supine position**

(With permission from Williams 1982.). Isaacs, D., Roberton, D. & South, M. (2007). *Practical Paediatrics* (6th ed.). London: Churchill Livingstone, p. 610, Figure 17.3.5.

MUSCLE POWER

All the muscle groups should then be tested and graded according to the Medical Research Council scale; that is, 3 = full range against gravity, 4 = full range against resistance, 5 = normal.

Begin by testing against gravity. If this is attained, then test with resistance, but if it is failed, test with gravity removed. An example is the examination of the hip movements. First, testing against gravity: hip flexion (lying supine), hip abduction and adduction (lying on side) and hip extension (lying prone with legs over the end of the bed). If extension is possible, then assess the gluteus maximus specifically by testing with the knee bent (if the knee is extended, this tests hamstrings as well). If the patient is unable to move against gravity, test with gravity removed, testing hip abduction and adduction (lying supine), hip extension and flexion (lying on side).

After comprehensive assessment of muscle power, check for tone and reflexes (knee jerks often lost) and contractures, especially at the ankles, knees and hips.

The usual pattern of weakness in DMD includes, initially, proximal lower limb and truncal weakness, neck flexor weakness, and later proximal upper limb weakness, and distal muscle weakness. Boys with DMD continue to gain strength and achieve new motor skills until around 6 years of age.

REMAINDER OF EXAMINATION

The rest of the examination should comprise a full neurological assessment. Examine the back, noting the details of any scoliosis, and perform a full evaluation of the cardiorespiratory system, for evidence of respiratory insufficiency, respiratory infection, tachycardia (which may represent pre-clinical cardiac involvement), arrhythmias, cardiomyopathy, cardiac failure).

Also, an impression of any degree of intellectual impairment is important. Note any overt ADHD or ASD behaviours, as these are more common in DMD than in the general population. Remember that intellectual involvement is static, whereas motor weakness is progressive.

In any child with a neuromuscular problem, presenting as a short case, localisation of the weakness will aid in diagnosis. In proximal weakness, the differential diagnosis includes muscular dystrophy (DMD or BMD), myopathy and anterior horn cell disorders (spinal muscular atrophy [SMA]). Examination should include looking for myotonia and fasciculations. If the weakness is distal, then a neuropathy is more likely. Sensation should be assessed, with joint proprioception, two-point discrimination and vibration most likely to be affected. The ulnar and common peroneal nerves (at the fibular neck) should be palpated for nerve thickening. In disorders of the neuromuscular junction such as autoimmune myasthenia gravis and congenital myasthenic syndromes, fatiguability is the pathognomonic feature. Examining the child following exercise (e.g. star jumps, stairs) can unmask weakness, and asking the child to sustain an upward gaze for at least 3 minutes can reveal ptosis.

Management

The management of a child with DMD is very complex and has much relevance to managing other chronic conditions, particularly other neuromuscular diagnoses such as SMA.

A team approach is appropriate in the management of DMD. A hospital-based team would usually comprise a neurologist, geneticist, respiratory physician, cardiologist, orthopaedic surgeon, physiotherapist, occupational therapist, orthotist, clinical nurse coordinator and social worker.

The local paediatrician's (i.e. the candidate's) role, in the case of a child under the care of a muscle clinic team, includes keeping in full contact with the team regarding changes in medical care, being available to coordinate overall medical care and dealing with any problems that arise between clinic visits, such as managing intercurrent infections. Perhaps the general practitioner or paediatrician should be the principal adviser/counsellor, although this is seldom the case: the candidate may have views on this issue.

The main management areas will now be described below.

MEDICAL MANAGEMENT
Corticosteroids

Glucocorticoids remain (as of 2017) the *only* medication currently available that can slow down the decrease in muscle strength and function in DMD. Moderate-dose steroids are very useful when boys are still walking, to improve motor function. The time of commencement of steroids has been controversial. Previously, recommendations were to wait until identifying a plateau in the child's motor development, once that plateau was identified, steroids were commenced. They were not recommended for children still gaining motor skills, especially under 2 years. More recently this approach has been challenged with suggestions that starting earlier may be more appropriate. These patients need close monitoring, adjusting dose and timing to avoid unwanted side effects, especially weight gain.

Prednisone is effective in achieving the following: delay in disease progression; prolongation of ability to walk; maintenance of strength and function in the arms and hands; delay in, or prevention of, development of scoliosis; and preservation of respiratory function by attenuating fibrosis of the diaphragm. It also prevents, or at least slows, progressive cardiac dysfunction. The precise mechanism by which prednisone exerts a therapeutic effect is unknown, but it is hypothesised that it is via a stabilising effect on muscle membranes. Prednisone is immunosuppressive, and also has direct effects on muscle cells. It can modulate proteolysis and calcium handling, increase myogenesis and inhibit apoptosis. A dose of 0.75 mg/kg per day (maximum dose 30–40 mg per day) can increase muscle strength within 10 days of commencement, and this effect can be maintained for 2 years, as long as the child continues to take it. The recommended schedule is daily (morning) steroid dosing, although other regimens have been used, including 10 days on, 10 days off, alternate daily doses or weekly high doses (5–10 mg/ kg per week; *Lancet* guidelines by Bushby et al. [2010]). Side effects include weight gain, reduced linear growth, pubertal delay, Cushingoid features, hypertension, osteoporosis with consequent long bone and vertebral compression fractures, hyperglycaemia, easy bruising and usually transient behavioural problems. The side effects can preclude its ongoing use, although dose reductions (down to 0.3 mg/kg per day), alternative dosing regimens or nighttime dosing may overcome these problems.

Another steroid that is as effective as prednisolone in maintaining muscle strength and function is *deflazacort*, a methyloxazoline derivative of prednisone. Deflazacort (DFZ) also enhances cardiac and pulmonary function and attenuates the development of scoliosis, including when ambulation is lost. DFZ treatment has been shown to improve left ventricular systolic function. The recommended dose for deflazacort is 0.9 mg/kg per day (maximum dose 36–39 mg per day).

DFZ may cause less severe adverse side effects (e.g. less weight gain) than prednisone. DFZ is not freely available in Australia, but is used on a case-by-case basis by some neuromuscular specialists.

Monitoring steroid therapy includes:

1. Assessing benefits: timed muscle function tests, pulmonary function tests; note the age when independent walking is lost.
2. Assessing risks: look for steroid side effects (Cushingoid appearance, weight gain, decreased linear growth, pubertal delay, acne, behavioural change, back pain due to vertebral compression fractures). The dose of steroid can be reduced by a quarter to a third, if side effects are difficult to tolerate. Steroid treatment should not be given up on, until other regimes have been explored.
3. Ensuring patients have a medical alert bracelet, such as MedicAlert (www.medicalert .com.au) or Emergency ID (www.emergencyid.com.au), to identify their diagnosis of DMD in case they need emergency anaesthesia, and it should also note whether they are receiving steroids, to avoid adrenal crisis from abrupt withdrawal thereof.

REHABILITATION MANAGEMENT: PHYSIOTHERAPY, OCCUPATIONAL THERAPY AND ORTHOTICS

The maintenance of muscle extensibility, and the avoidance of joint contractures, are achieved by stretching, guided by physiotherapists and occupational therapists. Stretching at least 4–6 times a week is recommended. Particularly important areas to stretch are hips, knees and ankles, and later on in the progress of the disease stretching of the fingers, wrists, elbows and shoulders.

Night splinting, using custom-made ankle–foot orthoses (AFOs), can assist control of contractures in the ankle. Powered wheelchairs with or without standing function are used once ambulation becomes untenable. Resting hand splints may be needed for tight long flexors of the fingers.

Physiotherapy details

1. Physiotherapy to encourage walking and avoid joint deformity is very important. Serial casting to reduce ankle contracture is an additional strategy to AFOs.
2. Stretches for contractures (e.g. flexion contractures at knees, hips, elbows, wrists, fingers); to minimise contractures, daily passive range-of-motion exercises of all joints of upper and lower limbs.
3. Exercises for strength (against gravity or resistance). Once the muscles are very weakened, these have little effect.
4. Chest physiotherapy for respiratory problems; teaching effective coughing. The use of inspiratory and expiratory exercises against resistance has increased over the last decade (motivational breathing exercises/incentive spirometry/manual assisted coughing techniques are used to open the alveoli). Negative pressure exsufflation (cough assist) devices have been shown to be of value in maintaining respiratory health but are expensive.

Occupational therapy details

1. A very important function is prescribing specifications for equipment (e.g. wheelchairs).
2. Home visits and visits to the school (meetings with teaching staff, and question and answer sessions with the affected boy's class). These visits are very valuable.
3. Advice regarding aids to ADLs (e.g. getting in and out of wheelchairs, bed, bath or cars).
4. Aiding posture: avoidance of certain positions (e.g. postural scoliosis, flexion), orthoses (e.g. arm supports).
5. Assessment and advice on installation of ramps for adequate mobility at home. Assess the need for lifting machines (dependent on the strength of the caregiver at home), modifications to home (e.g. bathroom access).

Equipment details

1. Wheelchairs: generally, a manual type is used from around 9 years of age, and a powered type from 11 years. An appropriate vehicle is required for transport (e.g. between home and school). New-generation wheelchairs have been developed, including one that has gyroscopic electronic sensors, and the ability to switch between four wheels and two to go through sand, up and down stairs and over kerbs, as well as a standing function to tackle high counters and allow eye-level interaction with standing adults.
2. Inclined standing board, to stretch tendo Achilles.
3. Prone board.
4. Standing desks, or lying on inclined prone board.
5. Swivel feeders (make forearms essentially weightless).
6. Hoists: mobile, fixed and fitted to car.

ORTHOPAEDIC SURGERY

In addition to dealing with scoliosis (see next section), orthopaedic procedures include:
1. Management of long bone fractures with internal fixation, if ongoing ambulation is threatened by the site of the fracture; boys with DMD have decreased bone density compared to the general population, and increased risk of sustaining fractures.
2. Elongation of tendo Achilles if still walking, although it may appear that weakness is the main problem inhibiting walking, not contractures per se. Immobilisation post-surgery may also hasten loss of muscle strength.
3. Tendo Achilles tenotomies, tibialis posterior transfer (either or both of these if wheelchair-bound).

SCOLIOSIS MANAGEMENT

If boys with DMD do not receive corticosteroids, there is a 90% chance they will develop progressive scoliosis. Steroid treatment delays the onset of, and decreases the risk of, scoliosis. When boys are still ambulatory, clinical observation for scoliosis is sufficient, only performing spinal X-ray once scoliosis is apparent. When boys are wheelchair dependent, spinal X-rays should be done as a baseline, and subsequently at least once a year; 12 monthly if the Cobb angle of the curve is less than 15°, and 6 monthly if over 15°. A proper seating system in the wheelchair is very important, supporting spine and pelvis symmetry and spinal extension. Attention to good posture is very important, avoiding asymmetrical contractures when still ambulatory.

Scoliosis commonly develops around 13–15 years, usually in the thoracolumbar region, becoming most apparent after loss of walking, when in a wheelchair, and rapidly progresses during the pubertal growth spurt. This adversely affects respiratory function, appearance, body image, posture, feeding, sitting and comfort. The advent of corticosteroid treatment, leading to prolonged walking and increased truncal muscle strength, has also led to a reduced incidence and severity in scoliosis. Bracing does not prevent progression, but may have a place in patients who refuse spinal surgery or where such surgery is contraindicated.

Criteria for surgical spinal fusion include:
1. Before the primary curve becomes greater than 20–25% if not receiving steroids, or greater than 40% if receiving steroids.
2. Progressive curve.
3. Substantial growth capacity remaining.
4. Patient physically, and emotionally, fit for surgery.

5. Vital capacity has not gone below 50% predicted for height, although some units use the value 30%, but the risks are greater; surgery should occur in a tertiary centre.
6. Cardiac function, as demonstrated on echocardiography, must be satisfactory.

The surgery comprises insertion of metal rods (e.g. Harrington–Luque rods or Luque rods for segmental spinal stabilisation), which may be accompanied by facet joint arthrodesis using autogenous bone from spinous processes.

An important area is fitness surgery. Adequate presurgical assessment of respiratory function is essential. Postoperatively, early mobilisation should be undertaken to prevent deterioration in function while confined to bed. The occupational therapist helps to accommodate ADLs to increase sitting height (increased shoulder and elbow height) and rigid spine.

In any surgical procedure, neuromuscular depolarising agents such as succinylcholine must be avoided.

BONE HEALTH

There are three reasons why boys with DMD have poor bone health: decreased mobility, weakness and steroids. There is an increased risk of vertebral and long bone fractures with prolonged steroid use. However, immobilisation of fractures should be avoided in DMD. This is an additional burden on bones adversely affected by lack of mobility; these boys already have decreased bone density. Corticosteroids increase the already present risk of vertebral compression fractures, which can be asymptomatic. It is prudent to recommend sunshine, a balanced diet, adequate vitamin D and calcium.

Current recommendations are for annual screening investigations:

- Calcium, phosphate, magnesium.
- Alkaline phosphatase.
- 25-hydroxyvitamin D (25OHD).
- PTH.
- Urine (calcium for hypercalciuria; sodium; creatinine).

Spine X-ray, bone age and dual-energy X-ray absorptiometry (DXA) scanning for bone mineral density may also be indicated. Daily supplementation of all boys with 1000 IU vitamin D and 600 mg calcium is recommended. If there is a vertebral fracture, intravenous bisphosphonates are appropriate. Oral bisphosphonates remain controversial. Standing and weight bearing, where possible, for 30 minutes a day has also been recommended.

PUBERTAL DELAY

Delay in the onset of puberty is almost universal in patients on long-term steroid therapy. Suppression of the hypothalamic–pituitary (HP) axis is the purported mechanism. Testing of hormonal status (FSH, LH and sex steroids) with testosterone replacement, if indicated, is best managed in consultation with an endocrinologist. Advancing puberty, if delayed, has the psychosocial benefit of improving self-esteem (one less point of difference with peers) and may play a role in improving bone density and accelerating linear growth.

RESTRICTIVE LUNG DISEASE (RLD) AND NON-INVASIVE VENTILATION (NIV)

1. RLD is secondary to weakness of the diaphragm, chest wall and abdominal musculature. In teenage years, this is associated with worsening respiratory reserve and sleep hypoventilation, episodes of REM-sleep-related hypoxaemia and OSA.
2. Patients tend to have recurrent chest infections, which should be treated aggressively, as they can tip these boys into overt respiratory failure. They may also require inhaled treatment (nebuliser or pressurised metered dose inhaler with spacer)

with bronchodilators, mucolytics or antibiotics. They must not be exposed to tobacco smoke. They should be fully immunised, including receiving yearly influenza vaccine.

3. They may develop cor pulmonale secondary to hypoxia, due to ventilatory difficulties and ventilation–perfusion inequalities associated with scoliosis.

4. Monitor with regular (6-monthly) pulmonary function tests (PFTs), including forced vital capacity (FVC) and maximal inspiratory and expiratory pressure, the former reflecting diaphragmatic strength, the latter reflecting the strength of the chest wall and abdominal muscles, correlating with the ability to cough and clear secretions. FVC predicts the development of hypercapnia and survival. When the FVC falls below 50%, this is the time to consider non-invasive ventilation (NIV; see below). Other useful aspects of respiratory monitoring used to attempt to predict respiratory failure are: peak cough flows (PCFs), which measure the capacity for mucociliary clearance; maximum expiratory mouth pressure (MEP), which can measure effective cough capacity; and maximum inspiratory mouth pressure (MIP) testing, which can indicate the need to consider starting NIV. All these tests can be carried out after the age of 5 years. Sleep studies (overnight polysomnography) should be done when the patient is first in a wheelchair, or when he first exhibits symptoms of sleep-disordered breathing (SDB) or hypoventilation.

5. Symptomatic respiratory failure can supervene, with hypoventilation, hypercapnoea (e.g. restless at night, somnolent by day, morning headaches, anorexia at breakfast, nausea, general malaise, fatigue, poor concentration at school, and cyanosis possibly occurring during meals or on transfer from the wheelchair). Untreated, hypercapnoea can prove fatal within a year. Symptoms can resolve with nocturnal ventilatory support, such as BiPAP, a mode of positive pressure ventilation.

6. In the last decade, domiciliary NIV has been proven effective in relieving symptoms of OSA and hypercapnoea, improving quality of life and prolonging survival. A compact portable ventilator is used, with a snugly fitting face or nose mask; the requirement for a good face or lip seal on the mask or nasal/oral orthotic interface cannot be overemphasised. NIV corrects hypoventilation and OSA, and with cough assist devices, has extended average survival to the mid-twenties, and occasionally to the fourth decade. There is now a widely held view that withholding NIV from hypercapnoeic patients with DMD is unethical. The benefits of NIV at night, may lead, within a couple of years, to a decision about daytime support and then 24-hour ventilation.

7. Decisions about whether or not to go into long-term 24-hour ventilation have to be made in consultation with the respiratory physician, the parents and the teenage boy, with the decision based on patient and family preference. Some units point out that waiting for daytime hypercapnoea/ventilator failure, until suggesting daytime NIV, is unsafe, as it exposes the patient to the risk of a rapid deterioration should he be exposed to a minor viral respiratory tract infection. Education and early discussion of options are the keys.

8. Volume ventilators may be used when vital capacity is below 40% of normal. These use a soft plastic nasal or face mask (for connection to the airway), with Velcro head and chin straps to hold them in position. The ventilator can fit on a ventilator tray on the bottom of a powered wheelchair.

9. Eventually, a tracheostomy may be appropriate, as masks may cause skin irritation due to constant skin pressure. A Passy–Muir valve can allow air through the vocal cords and improve voicing. The respiratory support area remains a major current issue in management of DMD.

10. NIV use in DMD is usually considered if the patient has symptoms (e.g. fatigue, morning headache) and any of the following: $PaCO_2$ of 45 mmHg or more; nocturnal oxygen saturation of below 88% for 5 minutes consecutively; maximal inspiratory pressure below 60 cm H_2O, or FVC below 50% predicted. Long-term NIV has been shown to reduce respiratory tract infections and hospital admissions in children with neuromuscular disorders.

11. The main determinant of operative risk in DMD is respiratory function.

12. The usual cause of death in most texts and journals has usually been given as RLD, but in patients who are already receiving non-invasive ventilation, the main determinant of survival is cardiac status. Of patients receiving NIV who died under the age of 30, over half died of cardiomyopathy. Overall, in DMD, the median age of death was 22 years in 2005; the mean age of survival has increased from 19 years in 2000 to over 30 years in 2016, mainly due to NIV and corticosteroids.

CARDIAC DISEASE

Cardiac phenotype is a major determinant of survival in DMD, with some studies indicating it as the main determinant. Ninety per cent of patients with DMD (or BMD) have subclinical or clinical cardiomyopathy. ECG findings can include short PR interval, tall R waves in the right precordial leads, and deep, narrow Q waves in the left precordial leads.

Cardiac arrhythmias may occur, including premature atrial or ventricular contractions, and sinus tachycardia. Persistent tachycardia is a common early cardiac finding, before overt clinical involvement occurs.

Cardiomyopathy usually develops after 10 years, affecting one-third of patients by 14 years, around the time when patients become non-ambulatory, and present in the majority of patients by adulthood (18 years). The first symptoms are typically dyspnoea and palpitations on exertion, the first signs being tachycardia.

Heart failure from loss of contractility and increased ventricular size is common. Cardiac involvement is the cause of death in 20% of patients with DMD (and 50% of patients with BMD). Ventricular remodelling can occur in patients with DMD (or BMD) if treated early enough with an ACE inhibitor such as lisinopril or perindopril (or angiotensin II receptor blockers [ARBs] such as losartan, if intolerant of ACE inhibitor) and/or a beta blocker, such as metoprolol or carvedilol. If there is overt heart failure, digoxin and diuretics may be needed. This treatment can lead to normalisation of left ventricular size and systolic function. Arrhythmias occurring may warrant periodic Holter monitoring.

Ongoing research still is assessing whether ACE inhibitors and beta blockers should be given prophylactically to patients with DMD to prevent cardiac deterioration. Although the optimal time to commence therapy is not agreed upon, it is agreed that early therapy is superior to late therapy. Treatment with ACE inhibitors or beta blockers typically is commenced when cardiac imaging shows ventricular dysfunction, the left ventricular ejection fraction (LVEF) is below 55% and fractional shortening (FS) is under 28%, or there is dilatation of the left ventricle.

Without aggressive treatment, DCM can be rapidly progressive after onset in the teenage years, and cause death from cardiac failure within 2 years. In patients with mild BMD with limited clinical skeletal muscle involvement, or in patients with DMD-related DCM, cardiac transplantation can be offered in cases with severe dilated cardiomyopathy. The clinical outcomes after heart transplantation in DMD patients are similar to those of non-DMD patients who have non-ischaemic cardiomyopathy. It is important to treat coexisting nocturnal hypoventilation (which aggravates cardiac dysfunction) with NIV.

Around 8–10% of carriers develop DMD-related cardiac disease, which can occur in the absence of muscle weakness.

Surveillance for cardiac disease should commence at diagnosis with a baseline assessment, and include, as a minimum, an ECG and an echocardiogram, and these should be repeated every 2 years until 10 years of age, and then annually. Some units also recommend yearly Holter monitoring and cardiac MRI to assess for cardiac abnormalities.

GASTROINTESTINAL AND ORAL ASPECTS

Dysphagia can occur in later stages, and may present with the sensation of food getting stuck, weight loss, longer time taken to complete meals or meals associated with choking, coughing, drooling or tiredness. Videofluoroscopic studies may be needed. Aspiration pneumonia may occur and necessitate gastrostomy placement. Other common gastrointestinal features are constipation, gastro-oesophageal reflux and problems with air swallowing due to ventilator usage leading to gastric and intestinal bloating. Laxatives and proton pump inhibitors are prescribed. Oral and dental care is important; special individually made adaptive devices for dental hygiene become important as upper body (upper limbs and neck) strength diminishes.

NUTRITIONAL ISSUES

These can involve failure to thrive or obesity, depending on the phase of the patient's condition. Failure to thrive can be a presenting complaint initially. Obesity can supervene in the late ambulatory phase, due to lack of mobility, and this is exacerbated by steroid therapy. There can be significant weight loss again after spinal surgery, and in the late teenage years, when chewing and swallowing difficulties become more problematic, with meals taking much time to complete, and episodes of choking on food.

The involvement of dieticians, and of speech and language therapists, is crucial to avoid obesity (ideally, this should be in place prior to commencement of steroids), obtain correct dietary advice, observe mealtimes, organise swallowing fluoroscopy, and discuss nutritional supplementation, feeding aids and gastrostomy insertion. Constipation is common, and patients often have spurious diarrhoea. Management with diet and aperients can obtain good results, with a rigid, well-supervised regimen.

URINARY PROBLEMS

Incontinence is uncommon, but frequent enough to be a feature of DMD and not a coincidence. It may be contributed to, or increased by, toileting avoidance. In addition to treating coexisting constipation as above, it is managed with anticholinergic agents (e.g. penthienate bromide). Nephrolithiasis may also be increased in DMD.

ANAESTHETIC ISSUES

Anaesthesia poses a significant risk to all patients with dystrophinopathies. Malignant hyperthermia-like reactions can occur (which can lead to hyperkalaemia, rhabdomyolysis and cardiac arrest), as can anaesthesia-induced rhabdomyolysis (AIR) (elevated K^+ or creatine kinase [CK] without hyperthermia). Depolarising muscle relaxants (suxamethonium chloride; also called succinylcholine) and inhalational agents (halothane, isoflurane, sevoflurane) should be avoided. For this reason, as well as the fact that they are on corticosteroids, patients with dystrophinopathies should have a medical bracelet such as a MedicAlert (www.medicalert.com.au) or Emergency ID (www.emergencyid.com.au).

Other potential complications related to anaesthesia in DMD include increased risks of upper airway obstruction, atelectasis, hypoventilation, respiratory failure, problem with weaning off ventilation, heart failure and cardiac arrhythmias. The American College of

Chest Physicians (ACCP) produced, in 2007, a consensus statement on the management of DMD patients undergoing anaesthesia.

SPEECH AND LANGUAGE MANAGEMENT

Boys with DMD often have speech and language problems, learning disorders, and difficulties with short-term verbal memory and phonological processing. Referral to a speech pathologist is very useful if any of these arise, and exercises for improved articulation may be needed in some boys. For older affected patients, there can be difficulties related to use of the ventilator, and some, with more limited speech, may require speech-generating devices (SGDs, also called voice output communication aids [VOCA]).

PSYCHOSOCIAL

1. Education of parents, patient and school. Clarification of misinformation from other sources requires multiple informative sessions with the various disciplines involved in the comprehensive management of these patients. The school must be informed about DMD. Regular feedback is needed to ensure that no misunderstandings occur. Other family members (e.g. siblings, grandparents, aunts, uncles and cousins) often are very much involved emotionally and may be inadvertently neglected.
2. Expectation of a grief reaction to the diagnosis and its implications. Preparatory explanation to parents of probable feelings such as guilt, anger and depression. Explanation regarding any misapprehensions or strange beliefs about the nature of the illness.
3. As with many chronic diseases, the incidence of depression and affective disorders is higher in children and adolescents with DMD and needs to be screened for.
4. Ensuring sufficient social supports, both from professionals (such as social workers) and non-professionals (such as other affected patients, families of other patients and groups such as the Muscular Dystrophy Association [MDA], Montrose Therapy and Respite Services [Qld] or Northcott [NSW]). The MDA provides parents' groups and a useful handbook that deals with the home situation, recreational activities, education and vocational possibilities. There are excellent sites on the internet, listed overleaf. With the National Disability Insurance Scheme being rolled out, patient support organisations are playing an increasingly important role in connecting patients and families with case coordinators and service providers.
5. Informing about financial assistance measures, such as any government benefits (which may assist directly with the child's care, transport costs, accommodation costs and provision of aids). The illness places a very large financial burden for home modification (such as ramps, bathroom modification, lifting machines) on the family.
6. Discussion of treatment difficulties (such as non-compliance), seeking other opinions, and understanding and acceptance of alternative therapies sought by parents.
7. A major point is helping the family to determine how various people (especially the affected son) are to be informed. The paediatrician may not be the person who will help most, but he or she does have responsibility to ensure that it is done adequately. The consequences of failure in this aspect of management may include: parents who will not discuss the disease with their son, siblings, teachers or each other; one parent (usually the father) who withdraws from reality; and help being refused (because the parents believe that the child will be cured by divine intervention).

8. Useful websites:
   - TREAT-NMD Neuromuscular Network, www.treat-nmd.eu/diagnosis-and -management-of-DMD (international consensus on the medical care of DMD; excellent resource for candidates)
   - The Diagnosis and Management of Duchenne Muscular Dystrophy, www.dmd -guide.org (an online guide for parents, an excellent resource)
   - Muscular Dystrophy Queensland, www.mdqld.org.au
   - Montrose Therapy & Respite Services, www.montrose.org.au
   - Northcott, www.northcott.com.au
   - Australasian Neuromuscular Network, www.ann.org.au
   - Australian Neuromuscular Diseorders Registry, www.nmdregistry.com.au
   - Action Duchenne (UK), www.actionduchenne.org
   - Duchenne Family Support Group (UK), www.dfsg.org.uk
   - Parent Project Muscular Dystrophy (US), www.parentprojectmd.org

SCHOOLING, CAREER PROSPECTS, LIFESTYLE

1. Most children with DMD are integrated into a normal school, or may attend a special unit in a regular school. Special schools are less often required.
2. Dystrophin is expressed in the brain (role not known). Boys with DMD have a decrease in IQ of 1 standard deviation (around 15 IQ points) compared with unaffected siblings. Thus, the mean IQ is around 85, and a higher percentage have intellectual impairment (around 20–30% have an IQ below 70). Encephalopathy is static, unlike muscle disease. A problem is underestimating the abilities of DMD patients (and disabled people generally).
3. The outlook for work is poor.
4. Some children, or young adults, can have what they feel is a fairly reasonable lifestyle, such as those pursuing courses of tertiary education, working in quadriplegic workshops or working with computers.
5. Sex education is a very valid area, which should not be ignored. Often, these patients can be quite ignorant of sexual matters, and education, such as group sessions discussing sexuality in disabled people, can be very useful.
6. Special accommodation needs should be addressed, such as the need for wide doors, special fittings and the availability of lifting hoists, as these may represent an enormous financial burden to the family.

CARRIER FEMALES

Although most DMD carrier females are asymptomatic, up to 20% have some degree of weakness, and around 50% have elevated serum CK levels. As 8–10% of carrier females do have cardiac involvement, they should be assessed for dilated cardiomyopathy at least every 5 years from the age of 16 years. Mothers should be advised to seek cardiac review with ECG and echocardiogram.

Sisters should be assessed if symptoms suggest this. Genetic testing is not recommended for sisters until they have reached adulthood, so that they can be appropriately counselled.

GENETIC COUNSELLING

1. All families with an affected boy with DMD should receive genetic counselling.
2. Recent advances allow improved detection of carriers and prenatal diagnosis in families with a child known to have DMD.
3. A female is defined an obligate carrier if she has an affected son and at least one other affected male relative in a pedigree that corresponds to X-linked recessive inheritance.

4. Mothers of isolated DMD patients are possible carriers, as are non-obligate carrier females related to affected males. Analysis of pedigrees and DNA analysis may clarify carrier status.
5. One-third of DMD patients represent new mutations. Effective genetic counselling will increase this proportion.
6. Some countries now perform newborn screening for DMD.

LONG CASE: Seizures and epileptic syndromes

Seizures are among the numerous problems of many long-case patients. In the past decade, significant advances in the understanding of epilepsy neurogenetics have occurred. Two-thirds of all epilepsies are genetic in origin. 'Genetic' does not equate with 'hereditary' as many genetic aetiologies arise de novo. Ninety-nine per cent of epilepsies are sporadic and have polygenic influences. Only 1 per cent are familial epilepsies due to a single gene. It is increasingly apparent that most epilepsy-related genes demonstrate phenotypic heterogeneity. As an example, SCN1A mutations can occur in association with the severe Dravet syndrome or with much the less severe generalised epilepsy with febrile seizures (GEFS)+ syndrome. Most epileptic clinical syndromes demonstrate genetic heterogeneity. An example of this is early infantile epileptic encephalopathy (EIEE), which has 35 different genetic causes (named EIEE1 to EIEE35) according to Online Mendelian Inheritance in Man (OMIM). Recently terminology has been revised; older terms (idiopathic, symptomatic, cryptogenic) are no longer in favour; recommendations have been made to replace 'benign' with 'self-limited', and 'complex partial' has been replaced with 'focal dyscognitive'. The newer International League Against Epilepsy (ILAE) terminology changes are somewhat at variance with OMIM terminology, so candidates need not jettison older terminology quite yet; mnemonics here involve whichever terminology makes them easier to remember. The definitions of various types of status epilepticus have been updated by the ILAE. The last decade has seen an increased number of newer anti-epileptic drugs (AEDs) used, and although most have preferable side effects to older AEDs they have, overall, similar efficacy to the older drugs. A third of patients with epilepsy continue to have seizures refractory to AEDs. Surgical treatment of epilepsy has improved with over half of all operated patients becoming seizure free. The points outlined in this section may apply to any child with recurrent seizures.

Background information

A 'seizure' is a paroxysmal clinical episode that results from an excessive hypersynchronous discharge of neurons; the term 'epilepsy' is used when recurrent unprovoked seizures occur. Recurrent febrile convulsions do not signify epilepsy.

Candidates should be familiar with the classification of epileptic seizures according to seizure type (ILAE). The ILAE has revised terminology and concepts for the organisation of the epilepsies. Generalised epileptic seizures are 'now considered to originate at some point within, and rapidly engage, bilaterally distributed networks'. Focal epileptic seizures are 'now considered to originate within the networks limited to one hemisphere, which may be discretely localised or more widely distributed'. The word 'focal' has replaced the previous term 'partial'. The term 'syndrome' will be restricted to a group of clinical entities that are reliably identified by a cluster of electroclinical characteristics. Previous groupings of underlying causes (genetic, structural/metabolic or unknown) have been expanded to six headings proposed by the ILAE: genetic, structural, metabolic, immune, infectious and unknown. Electroclinical syndromes are defined as 'a complex of clinical features, signs and symptoms that together define a distinctive recognisable clinical disorder'.

Currently recognised aetiological groupings are listed below, giving some examples, using the ILAE group headings.

Genetic causes include chromosomal abnormalities (e.g. Angelman's, Down, Klinefelter [XXY], Miller–Dieker [Del 17p], Pallister Killian [tetrasomy 12p], Wolf-Hirschhorn [Del 4p]) and gene abnormalities. At the time of writing (2017) there are 37 known genes, mutations of which can cause epilepsy, listed on the ILAE website. These include: calcium channel (CACNA1A, CACNB4); potassium channel (KCNQ2, KCNQ3, KCNT1) and sodium channel (SCN1A, SCN1B, SCN2A) genes; GABA receptor (GABRA1, GABRD, GABRG2) genes; and the genes for fragile X syndrome (FMR1) and Rett syndrome (MECP2).

Structural (distinct pathological) causes can be remembered with a mnemonic **MTV-H**:

Malformations (malformations of cortical development [MCDs], focal cortical dysplasia [FCDs])
Tuberous sclerosis complex (TSC)/**T**umours/**T**rauma
Vascular malformation/**V**ascular accident (stroke, haemorrhagic or ischaemic)
Hippocampal sclerosis (HS)/**H**ypothalamic hamartoma (HH)/**H**ypoxic ischaemic encephalopathy (HIE)

Aetiologies for structural pathologies can be genetic or acquired or both.

Metabolic causes include the seven listed in the ILAE's epilepsy diagnosis manual (in alphabetical order): biotinidase and holocarboxylase deficiency (both respond to biotin); cerebral folate deficiency (responds to folinic acid); creatine disorders (respond to creatine); folinic acid responsive seizures (respond to pyridoxine with folinic acid); glucose transporter 1 (GLUT 1) deficiency (responds to the ketogenic diet); mitochondrial disorders; pyridoxine-dependent epilepsy/PNPO (pyridoxine 5'-phosphate oxidase) deficiency (the former responds to pyridoxine, the latter [PNPO] deficiency responds to pyridoxal-5-phosphate [PLP]).

Immune causes (immune-mediated CNS inflammation) include Rasmussen syndrome (seizures, evolving hemiparesis, treatment includes AEDs, immunosuppression and neurosurgical intervention [hemi-disconnection]) and several rare antibody-mediated conditions including coeliac disease, epilepsy and cerebral calcification syndrome.

Infectious causes include meningitis, encephalitis, cerebral tuberculosis, cerebral toxoplasmosis, cerebral malaria, HIV, subacute sclerosing panencephalitis (SSPE) and neurocysticercosis.

Epilepsies of unknown cause include febrile infection related epilepsy syndrome (FIRES), a post-infectious condition associated with intractable status epilepticus after a febrile illness; prognosis is very poor: there is high mortality, and survivors have severe residual neurocognitive impairment.

Selected currently recognised electroclinical syndromes by age of onset are listed in the next section, using ILAE grouping and reorganised to simplify recall, listing causes including (if known) the chromosome location, gene, mechanism and salient clinical features. The ones that are asterisked are worth knowing in detail. These are thumbnail summaries, attempting only to give an overview, with some mnemonics using OMIM rather than ILAE terminology, and newer alternate names included (e.g. 'self-limited' [ILAE-proposed newer names] versus 'benign' [still-used OMIM terminology]).

NEONATAL PERIOD

Mnemonic **OBE**: **O**htahara, **B**FNS, **E**ME

Ohtahara syndrome (EIEE with suppression burst). Causes include cerebral malformations such as: **Aic**ardi syndrome (mnemonic **AIC**): **A**genesis corpus callosum, **I**nfantile spasms, **C**horioretinal lacunae [holes], (MIM%304050, sited at chromosome Xp22); linear sebaceous naevus syndrome (MIM#163200); porencephaly; hemimegaloencephaly; focal cortical dysplasia; and cerebral dysgenesis. Genetic causes are many, with significant heterogeneity, in EIEE: EIEE 1 through to EIEE 35 listed in OMIM at time of writing; the genes involved include STXBP1 (EIEE4; MIM#612164), which has a very broad range of phenotypes of epileptic encephalopathy from Ohtahara to Dravet. EIEE phenotypes also can be seen in other genetic conditions including: GLUT1 deficiency syndrome 1 (GLUT1DS1, MIM#606777; glucose transport defect affecting blood–brain barrier—sited at 1p34.2, the gene SLC2A1 encodes the GLUT1 transporter); glycine encephalopathy (MIM#605899); and males with MECP2 mutation (MIM#300673). Ohtahara syndrome can be considered an age-dependent reaction to an insult, and can be seen as the start of a continuum, which can progress, in 75%, to West syndrome and thence to Lennox-Gastaut syndrome. Clinically: tonic spasms (forward flexion), last 1–10 seconds, often in clusters up to 100 times per day, EEG shows burst suppression; 50% mortality rate within weeks or months; survivors have severe cognitive/neurological deficits; no treatment is consistently effective. AEDs found helpful on occasion have included: trials of vitamins, vigabatrin, levetiracetam, chloral hydrate, and epilepsy surgery if surgically resectable lesions found.

BFNS (benign familial neonatal seizures; ILAE-proposed name: self-limited FNS) and BNE (benign neonatal epilepsy; ILAE-proposed name: self-limited NE); these have the same aetiology. Chromosomes/gene: BFNS1: 20q13.33/KCNQ2 (MIM#121200); BFNS2: 8q24/KCNQ3 (MIM#121201); BFNS3: pericentric inversion of chromosome 5 (MIM%608217); BFNS, autosomal recessive (MIM269720). Onset day 4–7, brief, various features (apnoea, deviation of head/eyes, tonic–clonic, autonomic changes), remit in days to months, normal intelligence long term. If they need treatment, acutely, phenobarbitone, benzodiazepines or phenytoin can be used, and preventatively, levetiracetam, valproate or carbamazepine.

EME (early myoclonic encephalopathy). Multifactorial. Commonest causes: inborn errors of metabolism (IEMs); for example, non-ketotic hyperglycinaemia, Menkes disease, Zellweger syndrome and methylmalonic acidaemia. It is essential to exclude treatable metabolic causes early, and particularly pyridoxine-dependent epilepsy or PNPO (pyridoxine 5′-phosphate oxidase) deficiency, the former responding to pyridoxine, the latter (PNPO deficiency) responding to pyridoxal-5-phosphate (PLP).

Genetic causes include mutations in the genes ERBB4 (MIM*600543; MIM#609304 EIEE3) and SCN1A (MIM*182389). Onset is usually before day 10, with the clinical triad: myoclonus (randomly shifting, fragmentary), then focal fits, then tonic (infantile) spasms; devastating psychomotor developmental regression; all have bilateral pyramidal signs. Work-up should include metabolic testing and neuroimaging. No treatment is consistently effective. Vitamins can be tried (biotin, folinic acid, pyridoxine, pyridoxal phosphate); the ketogenic diet may help in non-ketotic hyperglycinaemia.

The investigations to exclude metabolic causes, with which candidates should be familiar, are numerous; the mnemonic **BACCALAUREATES** contains most of these:

Biotinidase (biotinidase deficiency)
Ammonia
Copper (low in Menkes)
Caeruloplasmin (low in Menkes)
Acylcarnitines (carnitine acylcarnitine translocase deficiency)
Lactate (elevated in mitochondrial disease)/**L**iver function tests
Amino acids
Urate (low in molybdenum cofactor deficiency)
Renal function tests
Electrolytes (includes calcium and magnesium)
Alpha amino-adipic semialdehyde (alpha ASA) (urine test; elevated levels in pyridoxine-dependent epilepsy, molybdenum cofactor deficiency and sulphite oxidase deficiency)
TORCH screen/**T**ogether (paired) tests: CSF/plasma amino acids (which include serine and glycine, to diagnose serine biosynthesis disorders, and glycine encephalopathy), CSF/plasma glucose and lactate (for glucose transporter type 1 deficiency syndrome)
EEG (burst suppression in various: [normal under 28 weeks], term asphyxia, meningoencephalitis, malformations, Ohtahara ARX mutation, pyridoxine-dependent epilepsy, pyridoxine 5′-phosphate responsive epilepsy, Menkes, mitochondrial glutamate SLC25A22 mutation, glycine encephalopathy, molybdenum cofactor deficiency, sulphite oxidase deficiency, purine synthesis disorder)
Sugar (glucose)/**S**ialotransferrin (congenital disorders of glycosylation [CDG])/**S**uccinylpurines (adenylosuccinate lyase deficiency [ASLD])/**S**ulphites (urine) (positive test in sulphite oxidase deficiency, and molybdenum cofactor deficiency)

INFANCY

Mnemonic refers to Dr West, who described the condition in his son: **MB, MB, MD, West**. Candidates should have knowledge of the asterisked conditions discussed in this case.

Malignant migrating partial seizures in infancy (MMPSI). Two patients described with mutations affecting KCNT1 (at 9q34.3; MIM#614959; EIEE14), and one case with 47 XYY syndrome. Clinical: onset average 3 months, multifocal seizures (tonic and/or clonic, can be autonomic features), frequent (almost continuous) seizures, associated psychomotor/regression, quadriplegia, prognosis dire, may die by 12 months.
Most AEDS are ineffective. Some helpful AEDs tried include: combination of stiripentol, clobazam and levetiracetam; combination of phenytoin and levetiracetam and acetazolamide; vitamins, ketogenic diet, rufinamide and potassium bromide, and acetazolamide by itself for apnoeic seizures.
Benign familial infantile seizures (BFIS) and non-familial infantile seizures (Fukuyama-Watanabe-Vigevano syndrome); ILAE-proposed name is self-limited familial infantile epilepsy and non-familial infantile epilepsy. Chromosome/gene mutations include: BFIS1: 19q (MIM%601764); BFIS2: 16p11/PRRT2 (MIM#605751; accounts for over 90% of cases); BFIS3: 2q24.3/SCN2A (MIM#607745); BFIS4: 1p36.12–p35.1 (MIM%612627); 20q13.33/KCNQ2; 8q24.22/KCNQ3. Clinically the familial and non-familial forms are almost identical, as aetiology involves similar

genes but non-familial forms occurring de novo: onset average 5 months, focal, brief (under 3 minutes), diurnal seizures, in clusters of 5–10 daily (first fit being longer) for 1–3 days, recur in 1–3 months, familial cases have longer fits; altered consciousness, motor arrest, unilateral clonic seizures, automatisms. Familial form, chromosomes: 2q24, 16p12–q12, 19q12–13.1.

Myoclonic epilepsy in infancy (MEI). A generalised epilepsy. Onset between 6 months and 3 years; myoclonic jerks may be spontaneous or reflex (to photic, auditory, somatosensory stimuli); usually head nodding, upper limbs flinging outward; duration brief (1–2 seconds); consciousness often intact; responds well to AEDs (valproate).

Benign familial neonatal–infantile seizures; ILAE-proposed name: self-limited familial neonatal–infantile seizures. Chromosome/gene: 2q23–24/SCN2A. This is a sodium channelopathy, the gene being a sodium channel subunit gene; onset between day 2 and 7 months; focal seizures; can resolve by 12 months.

Myoclonic encephalopathy in non-progressive disorders. Causes: chromosomal syndromes: PAW: Prader–Willi (MIM#176270), Angelman's (MIM#105830), Wolf-Hirschhorn (MIM##194190; chromosome 4p16.3 deletion): mnemonic WHirschhorns: Warrior Helmet (facies), intellectual impairment, restricted growth, small head, closure defects (clefts [lip/palate], coloboma of iris, cardiac [ASD, VSD]), hypertelorism, high forehead, high arched eyebrows, ocular findings (protruding eyes, epicanthic folds), retrognathia, nose (beaked, widened, skeletal [scoliosis, kyphosis, dislocatable hips, talipes]); gene disorders: Rett (MIM#312750); structural brain disorders, developmental (cerebral malformations) or acquired (ischaemic encephalopathy); metabolic: non-ketotic hyperglycinaemia; unknown (about one-fifth). Onset range day 1–5 years; average 12 months; preexisting encephalopathy; repetitive long periods of myoclonic-absence status epilepticus; frequent startle episodes; severe cognitive deficits. AEDs of choice: benzodiazepines, valproate, ethosuximide, ACTH.

Dravet syndrome (severe myoclonic epilepsy of infancy [SMEI]); MIM#607208; EIEE6. Chromosome/gene: 2q24.3/SCN1A (MIM*182389; sodium channel voltage-gated type 1 alpha polypeptide; same gene as affected in GEFSP2, FEB3A, FHM3); 80% have this mutation, 95% de novo. Other genes associated: 5q34/GABRG2 (a GABA receptor subunit gamma-2 gene); 5q34/GABRA1 (a GABA receptor subunit alpha-1 gene; mutations of this gene also cause EIEE19); 9q34.11/ STXBP1 (syntaxin-binding protein; syntaxin is involved in synaptic vesicle fusion; mutations of this gene also cause EIEE4); 19q13.11/SCN1B; 2q24.3/SCN2A; 1p36.33/GABRD; 15q26.1/CHD2; 5p12/HCN1; 1p13.3/KCNA2. Carriers for the SCN1A gene are relatively unaffected or have GEFS+ (see overleaf). Onset average 6 months; can present in status (hemiclonic, general or febrile); can have hemimotor status (but involve other side next time) plus focal dyscognitive (pallor, automatisms, absence), in clusters, often head turn and flexed upper limbs, mainly myoclonic by 4 years; can have atypical absence seizures, atonic seizures, non-convulsive status; 25% have visual-induced seizures. Exclusionary features: spasms (if patients have spasms, or tonus, then the diagnosis is not Dravet and must be reassessed). Precipitants: hyperthermia, water (bathing), light, CBZ; frequent fits until 12 months, multiple seizure types between 1 and 4, mainly myoclonic by 4; most have normal development initially, but after 12 months, developmental/neurocognitive regression. Ataxia and pyramidal signs evolve. IQ outcome poor, fits may continue. AEDs used (suggested sequence): first try valproate, then topiramate, then clobazam, then levetiracetam, then stiripentol (chemically unrelated to other AEDs, approved in Europe for Dravet syndrome as an adjunct to valproate and clobazam). Cannabidiol might decrease seizure frequency in children with treatment-resistant epilepsy; an open label trial published December 2015 in *The Lancet* showed a median reduction in monthly motor seizures of 36.5% in a group with treatment-resistant epilepsy which included 33 patients (20% of study group) with Dravet syndrome. Avoid sodium channel blockers which can aggravate seizures (mnemonic **CR FLOP**): **C**arbamazepine, **R**ufinamide, **F**osphenytoin, **L**amotrigine, **O**xcarbazepine and **P**henytoin; also avoid vigabatrin and tiagabine, as these can increase myoclonic seizures. Dravet syndrome was the first epilepsy to have a gene test commercially available; test the child and parents. Expensive, but stops the need to do other tests (for mitochondrial disorders and so on) and affects the parents' decision to have further children. Some girls with Dravet-like phenotypes can have mutations in the gene PCDH19 on Xq22.1 (MIM*300460), causing EIEE9 (MIM#300088); mutations of this gene also can cause GEFS+ (see below).

West *syndrome**. Epileptic encephalopathy with multiple causes: *structural* (developmental cerebral malformations; genetically determined conditions such as tuberous sclerosis complex [TSC], Aicardi syndrome, lissencephaly; acquired causes such as cerebral ischaemia [pre-, peri- or postnatal], cerebrovascular accidents, intrauterine infections); *chromosomal* abnormalities (Down, Miller–Dieker lissencephaly Syndrome [MDLS, MIM#247200]); *gene* abnormalities leading to various numbered forms of EIEE (mutations in: ARX [associated with several phenotypes associated with seizures such as EIEE1 {MIM#308350} and lissencephaly {MIM#300215}], CDKL5 [EIEE2 {MIM#300672}], STXBP1 [EIEE4 {MIM#612164}] SPTAN1 [EIEE5 {MIM#613477}]); *metabolic* disorders (which are rare but very important as potentially treatable, such the creatine disorder, cerebral creatine deficiency syndrome 2, also known as GAMT [guanidinoacetate methyltransferase] deficiency {MIM#612736}, for which treatment is available: a combination of creatine monohydrate, L-ornithine, sodium benzoate and protein/arginine-restricted diet, which can decrease plasma guanidinoacetate levels). It may respond to creatine supplementation (around 80% symptomatic: cerebral ischaemia [pre-, peri- or postnatal], chromosomal anomalies, cerebral malformations, tuberous sclerosis [TS], infections [congenital or acquired, e.g. TORCH, pertussis, meningitis]; 20% idiopathic). Onset average 5 months, comprises epileptic (infantile) spasms (which are an age-dependent reaction to an insult), EEG changes of hypsarrhythmia, and in many, developmental regression. Spasms occur in clusters of up to 30 per day, with each cluster having 20–150 spasms, these being short (2 seconds or less), usually fairly violent, bilateral tonic flexor 'jack-knife' or 'salaam spasms', on arousal or awake states, and Moro-like extensor spasms. The prognosis is related to the cause. It is worth considering a trail of pyridoxine and/or pyridoxine 5′-phosphate oxidase (PNPO) to exclude pyridoxine-dependent epilepsy/PNPO deficiency, if there is a previous history of neonatal or focal seizures. AEDs of choice are ACTH, steroids or vigabatrin. If TS is the cause, then vigabatrin is first line; if non-TS, then ACTH or prednisolone are first line.

CHILDHOOD
Mnemonic **FEEL BALANCE**

Febrile seizures plus (FS+)* (can start in infancy): also called *GEFS+ (generalised epilepsy with FS+)*. Chromosomes/genes/OMIM reference GEFSP1 to GEFSP9:

GEFSP1: 19q13.11/SCN1B (MIM#604233); GEFSP2: 2q24/SCN1A (MIM#604403); GEFSP3: 5q34/GABRG2 (MIM#611277); GEFSP4: 2q24 (MIM%609800); GEFSP5: 1p36.33/GABRD (MIM#613060); GEFSP6: 8p23–p21(MIM%612279); GEFSP7: 2q24.3/SCN9A (MIM#613863); GEFSP8: 6q16.3–q22.31 (MIM%613828); GEFSP9: 16p11.2/STX1B (MIM#616172). The term 'GEFS' describes a family of conditions, a familial epilepsy syndrome, not a patient. Can be simple febrile seizures (which typically occur between 6 months and 6 years; this component is generally self-limiting, predictably remitting by puberty), febrile seizures older than 6 years, absences, temporal lobe epilepsy (TLE), myoclonic-astatic epilepsy and SMEI. Phenotype guides treatment and prognosis, not finding mutation.

Early onset childhood occipital epilepsy (Panayiotopoulos type); also called Panayiotopoulos syndrome. No known genetic causes yet, at time of writing (2016), but this and other epileptic syndromes can occur in siblings and families. Onset range 1–14 years, peak 4–5 years; autonomic symptoms (especially emetic: nausea, retching, vomiting; others include pallor, mydriasis, hypersalivation and incontinence); consciousness and speech preserved at onset; behaviour change (ictal: restlessness, terror); syncope-like unresponsiveness and loss of tone; unilateral eye deviation; often prolonged (5–10 minutes), can lead to autonomic status, may end with hemiconvulsions or generalised convulsions. Interictal EEG multifocal, high-amplitude, sharp and slow-wave complexes. Prognosis benign: 25% have one seizure only, 50% have 2–5 only. AEDs rarely needed. (Mnemonic for features: **PaNaylOToPoULoSSS**: **Pa**llor, **Na**usea, **y**, **I**ncontinence, **O**cular: mydriasis, **To**ne lost, **P**rolonged duration, **o**, **U**nilateral eye deviation, **L**imited to under 14 years, **o**, **S**alivation [hypersalivation], **S**yncope-like, **S**tatus common.)

Epilepsy with myoclonic-atonic (previously astatic) seizures (EM-AS, also called Doose syndrome, or Myoclonic-Atonic Epilepsy [MAE]). This is an epileptic encephalopathy. Chromosomes/genes: 3p25.3/SLC6A1 (encodes a GABA transporter) (MIM#616421) 19q13.11/SCN1B (MIM*600235); 2q24.3/SCN1A (MIM*182389) and 1p34.2/SLC2A1 (encodes a facilitated glucose transporter) (MIM*182389). Family history of febrile seizures in 50%, epilepsy in a third. Onset 6 months to 6 years, with peak 2–4 years, more common in boys. In two-thirds, febrile and afebrile GTCSs occur initially, months before myoclonic-atonic; all patients have symmetrical myoclonic jerks followed immediately by loss of tone (post-myoclonic inhibition); can also have pure atonic or absence, and non-convulsive (myoclonic-atonic) status (the latter being a frequent feature). A third will have status epilepticus at some stage. This condition is **not** associated with tonus, so if this is a component the diagnosis should be questioned.

EEG. photic stimulation can precipitate myoclonic-atonic seizures; non-convulsive status causes repetitive 2–3 Hz spike-wave pattern, can be continuous or discontinuous; increased epileptogenicity in sleep. Prognosis varies: 50% eventually seizure free, normal development; other 50% usually symptomatic or part of other syndromes, continue to have seizures and neurocognitive deterioration, with ataxia, dysarthria and language problems. AEDs of choice: valproate, lamotrigine, levetiracetam; occasionally clonazepam, clobazam or nitrazepam. The ketogenic diet has worked better than any AEDs for some patients; a modified Atkins diet can also be helpful. Glucose transport disorders need to be excluded. Note contraindicated AEDs: carbamazepine, vigabatrin and phenytoin.

Late-onset childhood occipital epilepsy (Gastaut type). Phenotype of 'benign (self-limiting) childhood seizure susceptibility syndrome'; often family history of epilepsy or migraine. Onset range wide (15 months to 19 years), peak average 8–9 years; pure occipital seizures, with visual hallucinations (usually small multicoloured circular patterns, compared to 'fuzzy' confetti, or sequins), blindness or a combination; short (few seconds to 3 minutes), frequent, often diurnal; non-visual features may include deviation of eyes with ipsilateral turning of head, eyelid blinking, eyelid closure; consciousness preserved; interictal EEG shows occipital paroxysms. AED of choice: carbamazepine. Secondary GTCS can occur if not treated. continuous spike-and-wave during sleep (CSWS) (see below) can exist as a comorbidity.

*Benign epilepsy with centrotemporal spikes (BECTS)**. ILAE-proposed name: self-limited epilepsy with centrotemporal spikes (ECTS); also called childhood epilepsy with centrotemporal spikes, benign Rolandic epilepsy (after region involved; lower part of central gyrus of Rolando) and centralopathic epilepsy (MIM%117100; chromosome 11p13). BECTS is the most common epileptic syndrome. Other chromosomes/genes: 16p13.2/GRIN2A; 22q12/DEPDC5; onset 3–14, peak age 8–9 years, resolution by 13; nocturnal orofaciobrachial focal seizures, short (1–3 minutes), involving the vocal tract, with oropharyngolaryngeal guttural sounds ('chuggers' and 'gluggers'), and hemifacial sensorimotor symptoms that spread to the tongue, mouth and face, causing hypersalivation and speech arrest; consciousness preserved; secondarily GTCSs in 50%.

Occur during non-REM sleep, around sleep onset or just before waking, especially 5–7 a.m., in boys more than in girls (3:2). EEG: interictal CTS. Neurodevelopmental disorder can lead to learning disabilities and behaviour problems. AEDs may not be needed if seizures are infrequent. If frequent or secondary GTCS, AEDs used: carbamazepine, levetiracetam. History of febrile seizures in 5–15%; can be history of Panayiotopoulos syndrome; EEG has features in common with three other conditions: ECTS/CSWS/LKS (see later this section); these are all focal epilepsies with speech disorder; CSWS and LKS are associated with cognitive impairment; MIM#245570 is epilepsy, focal, with speech disorder and with or without mental retardation (FESD) due to a mutation in the GRN2A gene on 16p13.2, and includes all the above three conditions. If there is any cognitive impairment, should also be checked for fragile X syndrome.

Absence, myoclonic—epilepsy with myoclonic absences (EMA). No definite genetic causes clearly defined, although one case report describing an altered SYNGAP1 gene as the aetiology; there is a family history in a fifth of patients. Onset range 1–12 years, peak 7 years, affects boys more often (70%) than girls (30%); seizures comprise rhythmic myoclonic jerks (shoulders, arms, legs), with tonic contraction, usually unilateral; impairment of consciousness, short (8–60 seconds), frequent (several times a day, every day). Over 75% have other seizure types, GTCS or atonic, which may portend a poor prognosis. EEG generalised or multifocal spike and slow wave; around 50% have decreased cognition prior to absences, although 50% of the normal (prior) patients develop cognitive and behavioural impairment as well, giving a total of 70% having a learning disability eventually. Often hard to treat; half the patients have seizures as adults, some develop other forms of epilepsy (e.g. LGS, juvenile myoclonic epilepsy [JME]). AEDs tried: valproate plus ethosuximide or lamotrigine, clonazepam, acetazolamide.

Lennox-Gastaut syndrome (LGS)*. Causes: genetic de novo mutations are anticipated to be discovered as causes of presently unexplained cases; similar to those for West syndrome. Most cases relate to a preexisting neurological disorder, including (70%) cerebral malformations, genetic disorders including Aicardi syndrome, lissencephaly and TSC, acquired brain injuries (pre-, peri- or postnatal), diffuse encephalopathies; 10–30% derive from West syndrome, being the third part of an encephalopathic continuum (mnemonic **OWL**): **O**htahara to **W**est to **L**GS. Onset range 1–8 years, peak 3–5 years. Sudden falls often first sign. LGS is an age-specific epileptic encephalopathy. Seizure semiology: three main types (mnemonic **TAA**): **T**onic, **A**bsence (atypical), **A**tonic, with polymorphic intractable seizures—tonic (symmetrical, brief [2–10 seconds]), atypical absences (clouding of consciousness, tone changes, myoclonic jerks), atonic (sudden brief [1–2 seconds] loss of postural tone); other seizure types can occur (e.g. GTCS), and most will have status epilepticus at least once (types of status: absence, [atypical, which can last weeks and mimic confusion tonic]; tonic [which carries risk of apnoea]). Behaviour problems are typical and can mimic ADHD and ASD, and include aggression, personality disorder and eventually psychosis. Learning problems, impaired language and impaired cognition are usual. Head injuries can occur secondary to drop attacks or tonic seizures, causing subdural haemorrhages. Ictal EEG may show paroxysmal fast activity (around 20 Hz), and flattening, in tonic seizures, whereas atypical absences are associated with slow activity (< 2.5 Hz) Prognosis is very poor: 80–90% have seizures into adult life. AEDs used: valproate (beware hepatic failure, acute haemorrhagic pancreatitis) is the first agent tried usually; AEDs with proven efficacy against drop attacks in LGS include lamotrigine, topiramate and rufinamide; clobazam is also used. Other useful treatments here include ketogenic diet, and surgical treatments (corpus callosotomy, focal cortical resection and vagus nerve stimulation). Treatment mnemonic 2**V**s, 2**C**s, 2**R**s (2VCRs), + 2**L**s + **T**opiramate + **K**etogenic diet: **V**alproate, **V**agus nerve stimulation, **C**lonazepam, **C**orpus callosotomy, **R**ufinamide, **R**esection of focal cortex, **L**amotrigine, **L**evetiracetam, **T**opiramate. Note also several contraindicated AEDs; carbamazepine, oxcarbazepine, gabapentin, pregabalin, tiagabine (so, in LGS avoid 2 'carbs' and 3 with 'gab/a' in name).

Absence—childhood absence epilepsy (CAE)*. Susceptibility conferred by several genes; termed 'ECA' (epilepsy, childhood absence) by OMIM. Chromosome/gene: ECA1: 8q24 (MIM%600131); ECA2: 5q31.1/GABRG2 (MIM#607681); ECA4: 5q34/GABRA1 (MIM#607681); ECA5, 15q11–q12/GABRB3 (MIM#612269); ECA6: 16p13/CACNA1H (calcium channel subunit) (MIM#611942). Onset range 2–10 years, peak 5–7 years, more in girls; very frequent (dozens per day) absences; brief (under 20 seconds); abrupt loss of consciousness; may be automatisms. Hyperventilation for 3 minutes (easily done using a pinwheel being blown repetitively and continuously by the child) will precipitate seizures in over 90%. Associated features can include very subtle myoclonic movements affecting the eyes, eyebrows, eyelids at the start of episodes; two-thirds of children have non-stereotyped automatisms. EEG ictal 3 Hz generalised high-amplitude spike and spike/slow wave. Avoid misinterpreting atypical age presentations: when early onset (< 4 years), exclude glucose transporter disorders (e.g. GLUT1 deficiency); when older onset (> 8 years), consider juvenile absence epilepsy or juvenile myoclonic epilepsy. Prognosis excellent: under 10% go on to have GTCSs in adolescence. AEDs of choice: ethosuximide, valproate, lamotrigine. Note contraindicated AEDs: most others; that is, carbamazepine, oxcarbazepine, phenytoin, phenobarbitone—

ones with 'gab/a' in their name, such as pregabalin, vigabatrin, gabapentin and tiagabine (so, in CAE avoid 2 'carbs', 2 'phens' and all 'gab/as'). Can withdraw AEDs over 6 months after 2–3 years of being seizure free. Remission usual by 12 years. One-sixth of patients later are found to have juvenile myoclonic epilepsy.

Nocturnal—*autosomal dominant nocturnal frontal lobe epilepsy (ADNFLE); also called epilepsy, nocturnal frontal lobe [ENFL]).* Chromosome/gene/OMIM: ENFL1 : 20q13.33/CHRNA4 [encodes nicotinic acetylcholine receptor (nAChR) subunit] (MIM#600513); ENFL2: 15q24 (MIM%603204); ENFL 3: 1q21.3/CHRNB2 (MIM#605375); ENFL4: 8p21/CHRNA2 (MIM#610353); ENFL5: 9q34.3/KCNT1 (MIM#615005); 22 q12.2–q12.3/DEPDC5 (MIM*614191); 8q13.1/CRH (MIM*122560). Onset range infant to adult; average 9–11 years; 85% have seizures before 21 years; frequent (almost nightly) clusters of short (20–50 seconds) hyperkinetic motor seizures with dystonic posturing; may be aura; may be thrown out of bed; consciousness preserved; may be precipitated by movement, sound; often misdiagnosed as OSA, night terrors, nightmares, parasomnia. AEDs of choice: carbamazepine, levetiracetam, clobazam, lamotrigine, topiramate.

CSWS—*epileptic encephalopathy with continuous spike-and-wave during sleep (CSWS).* Chromosome/gene: 16p13.2/GRIN2A is a known genetic cause, the same as in many patients with BECTS and LKS. Also, 50% have preexisting problem (e.g. cerebral malformations); problem is CSWS causing neurocognitive regression rather than the seizures. Onset of seizures range 2–12 years, peak 4–5 years, EEG finding of CSWS, which correlates with encephalopathy developing, has onset 1–2 years after seizures, with a peak of 8 years; seizures may be nocturnal unilateral motor seizures, diurnal absences or atonic; regression of IQ, language, behaviour and psychological state; deficits depend on spike localisation. Frontal lobe targeting leads to disinhibition, aggressiveness, inattention, cognitive decline, psychosis (frontal lobe dementia); temporal lobe involvement causes expressive aphasia. Motor problems: ataxia, hemiparesis, dyspraxia. Treatment: spike suppression; similar to approach in LKS treatment (see below). EEG and clinical remission occurs in second decade, including improvement in psychological wellbeing, but not back to normal.

Epileptic encephalopathy, including *Landau–Kleffner syndrome (LKS)**; also called acquired epileptic aphasia. Chromosome/gene: 16p13.2/GRIN2A is a known genetic cause, the same as in many patients with BECTS and CSWS. Onset range 2–8, peak 5–7 years; normal prior development or isolated language delay; regression in receptive and expressive language abilities, auditory agnosia (cannot identify sounds in environment, e.g. dog barking), global aphasia; seizures tend to be mild, infrequent, nocturnal, resolving by 15 years. EEG: focal/bilateral slow spike-wave foci over temporal regions; can be continuous, unilateral or bilateral synchronous; NREM sleep accentuates EEG abnormalities. AEDs used: valproate with lamotrigine, ethosuximide, clonazepam, clobazam, levetiracetam; if unsuccessful, then ACTH or prednisolone; if intractable deterioration, surgical treatment with multiple subplial intracortical transections can succeed. Prognosis: earlier onset imparts worse prognosis.

ADOLESCENCE–ADULT

Mnemonic **Juvenile TAPE**

Juvenile *absence epilepsy (JAE).* Susceptibility conferred by several genes; termed 'EJA' (epilepsy, juvenile absence). Chromosome/gene: EJA1: 6p12–p11/EFHC1

(MIM#607631); EJA2: 3q27.1/CLCN2 (MIM#607628); 5q34/GABRG2 (MIM#607681); 19p13.13/CACNA1A (MIM*601011). Onset range 8–20 years, average 9–13 years; absences similar to CAE, severe, frequent, short (4–30 seconds); GTCS and myoclonic jerks commence up to 10 years after absences start. Ictal EEG: 3–4 Hz generalised polyspike wave discharge; lifelong, but good control in 80% with AEDs valproate and lamotrigine; control of absences generally means control of GTCSs.

Juvenile *myoclonic epilepsy (JME)*, also called Janz syndrome.* Susceptibility conferred by several genes; termed 'EJM' (epilepsy, juvenile myoclonus). Chromosome/gene: EJM1: 6p12.2/EFHC1(MIM#254770); EJM2: 15q14/CHRNA7 (MIM%604827); EJM3: 6p21/BR2 (MIM#608816); EJM4: 5q12–q14 (MIM%611364); EJM5: 5q34/GABRA1 (MIM#611136); EJM6: 2q23.3/CACNB4 (MIM#607682); EJM7: 1p36.33/GABRD (MIM#613060); EJM8: 3q27.1/CLCN2 (MIM#607628); EJM9: 2q33–q36 (MIM%614280); microdeletions (e.g. 15q13.3). Onset range 8–25 years, typically around 12–18 years; myoclonic jerks typically occur within an hour of waking (often drop their breakfast cereal bowl), with GTCSs appearing some months after jerks, and absence episodes also can occur, which are usually subtle; a third have all three types of seizure (myoclonic, GTCS, absence); precipitants include fatigue, sleep deprivation, photosensitivity, psychologic stress. EEG: 3–6 Hz polyspike wave discharge, photosensitive. Probably lifelong treatment needed; control achieved in around 90% of patients. It is lifestyle dependent: if taking medication but awake all night, will fit; patients with this can drown in the surf. AEDs of choice: valproate, levetiracetam. Note contraindicated AEDs: all the 'gab/a' ones (vigabatrin, gabapentin, pregabalin, tiagabine), plus phenytoin and two 'carbs' (carbamazepine, oxcarbazepine).

Temporal *lobe–other familial temporal lobe epilepsies.* A genetic form of epilepsy involving the temporal lobe is termed 'familial focal epilepsy with variable foci' (FFEVF): 22q12.2–q12.3/DEPDC5 (MIM#604364).

Autosomal *dominant partial epilepsy with auditory features (ADPEAF).* Also called autosomal dominant lateral temporal lobe epilepsy (ADLTLE) or epilepsy, familial temporal lobe (ETL). Chromosome/gene: ETL1: 10q23.33/LGI1 (MIM#600512); ETL2: 12q22–q23.3 (MIM%608096); ETL3: 4q13.2–q21.3 (MIM%611630); ETL4: 9q21–q22 (MIM%611631); ETL5: 8q13.2/CPA6 (MIM#614417); ETL6: 3q25–q26 (MIM%615697); ETL7: 7q22.1/RELN (MIM#616436); ETL8: 11q13.2/GAL (MIM#616461); ETL1 was the first non-ion channel familial epilepsy described; onset peak teenage years; mainly simple auditory hallucinations (humming, ringing); also may be visual, olfactory, vertiginous; infrequent nocturnal GTCSs. AEDs: carbamazepine, levetiracetam. Prognosis excellent.

Progressive *myoclonus epilepsies (PME).* This is a group of rare, genetic disorders (mainly autosomal recessive); details beyond this section. Examples: Unverricht–Lundborg disease (commonest PME); mitochondrial encephalopathy with red ragged fibres (MERRF); all causes have devastating neurocognitive morbidity. Not very age specific.

Epilepsy *with generalised tonic–clonic seizures alone (EGTCSA)*.* Also called epilepsy, idiopathic generalised (EIG). OMIM lists genetic causes of EIG numbered EIG1 through to EIG14 at time of writing (2016). Onset range 5–40 years, peak 11–23 years; probably lifelong, with 80% relapsing if off AEDs. AEDs used: valproate, levetiracetam, lamotrigine, topiramate, phenobarbitone.

LESS-SPECIFIC AGE RELATIONSHIP

These include:

- Familial focal epilepsy with variable foci (childhood to adult) (mentioned previously, involving temporal lobe).
- Reflex epilepsies. These can be sensory-evoked or stimulus sensitive. Sensory stimuli include flashes of light, removal of light, touch, hot water and music. Stimulus activities include simple causes such as undergoing a particular movement, or more complex such as calculating during mathematics. Two well-described types are startle epilepsy (onset range 1–16 years), and reading epilepsy (onset range 12–19 years).
- PME (see earlier).

Distinctive constellations include the commonest form of epilepsy, *mesial temporal lobe epilepsy with hippocampal sclerosis (MTLE with HS)**. The cause is unknown, although many have an early childhood history of febrile convulsions, head injury, meningoencephalitis or hypoxic insults. This is the commonest epileptic syndrome. Simple focal seizures commence with an ascending epigastric aura, a 'welling up' from the stomach; impaired ability to speak, but retained ability to comprehend conversations, last 1–2 minutes; can progress to complex with automatisms, restlessness or motor arrest, staring, head deviation (when early, to side of lesion; when later, can be to contralateral side and precede [infrequent] secondary GTCS), dystonic posturing, autonomic features, lasting 2–3 minutes; complex partial status epilepticus involves ongoing disturbance of consciousness, also called dyscognitive or psychomotor status. High-resolution MRI shows hippocampal sclerosis. Interictal EEG may show focal spike/sharp and slow complexes in a third, thus it may well be normal in two-thirds. Prognosis is variable. AEDs used are carbamazepine and levetiracetam. Neurosurgical treatment is available if AEDs fail, with anterior temporal lobe resection with hippocampectomy having a success rate of 60% of patients seizure free; however, 10% get no benefit and 10% get worse (e.g. neurosurgical complications).

SUMMARY

Candidates should have knowledge of the asterisked conditions discussed in this case. In the context of the exam, epilepsy is symptomatic of the underlying problem and represents one aspect of management problems. The candidate should have an approach to the management of epilepsy.

Advances in understanding clinical and molecular genetics continue to accelerate. It is well established that genetic predisposition to epilepsy (excessive neuronal membrane excitation) is often related to ion channel dysfunction or disorders of synaptic transmission. Dysfunction of ion channels has been demonstrated in several monogenetic epilepsies. Genetic heterogeneity is apparent in several monogenetic epileptic channelopathies, as seen earlier in this case: benign neonatal–infantile convulsions can be caused by sodium or potassium channelopathies; familial GEFS+ can be due to a sodium channel or a GABA receptor channel disorder.

Channelopathies cause seizures that are worse at night/when sleeping, but there is currently no explanation for this.

SCN1A-RELATED SEIZURE DISORDERS

Of the various channelopathies, candidates should be very aware of the sodium channel alpha 1 subunit gene SCN1A, as mutations in this gene are responsible for a spectrum of seizure disorders, with varying phenotypes, the severity even varying within the same family. Of the myriad mutations described, around 40% are truncation mutations, 40% are missense mutations and the remainder are splice site mutations or deletions. These phenotypes are not specific for SCN1A-related seizure disorders, and some features refer to those within the family rather than a particular patient.

Commonly associated phenotypes: febrile seizures (FS); GEFS+; Dravet syndrome (SMEI); and three that are not in the ILAE list mentioned earlier—severe myoclonic epilepsy, borderline (SMEB), intractable childhood epilepsy with generalised tonic–clonic seizures (ICE–GTC) and infantile partial seizures with variable foci (also called severe infantile multifocal epilepsy).

Less commonly associated phenotypes include myoclonic-astatic epilepsy (Doose syndrome), Lennox-Gastaut syndrome, epileptic spasms and 'vaccine-related encephalopathy and seizures'. The latter is important; so-called 'vaccine encephalopathy' is not caused by vaccine but, rather, is a genetically determined disease, where the vaccine is merely a trigger: it is no more a cause than light 'causing' photosensitive epilepsy, or fever 'causing' GEFS+.

As can be seen from the ILAE listing, among the genetically determined epilepsies, defects are recognised in the following:

- **Voltage-gated ion channels.** Sodium (GEFS+, severe myoclonic epilepsy of childhood, benign neonatal–infantile convulsions), potassium (neonatal seizures), chloride (generalised epilepsies), calcium (absence epilepsy).
- **Ligand-gated ion channels.** GABA receptors (GEFS+, absence epilepsy, juvenile myoclonic epilepsy), ACh receptors (autosomal dominant [AD] nocturnal frontal lobe epilepsy).
- **Non-ion channel genes.** Temporal lobe epilepsy with auditory features (LGI1).
- **Pre-synaptic protein-coding genes.** PRRT2 (most frequent cause of BFIS); STXBP1 (can cause Ohtahara or Dravet), SNAP25 (codes for protein which is part of the pre-synaptic fusion machinery, and interacts with STXBP1 protein.
- **Genetic epilepsies** with simple inheritance (usually quite benign) are now well recognised but are relatively rare: AD syndromes of early infancy (benign familial neonatal, neonatal–infantile and infantile; three different ages of onset; three different genes), AD nocturnal frontal lobe epilepsy, AD partial epilepsy with auditory features and familial temporal lobe epilepsies. In contrast, most common epilepsies have quite complex inheritance.

A very important disorder that can cause atypical epilepsy, particularly difficult to treat absences with onset under 4 years, is glucose transporter 1 deficiency syndrome (GLUT1-DS); this is a treatable neurometabolic condition and so must not be missed. Diagnosis is usually achieved by evaluating CSF:serum glucose ratios (samples taken at the same time), although gene testing can be undertaken in research centres. There is typically hypoglycorrhachia (CSF glucose < 2.2 mmol/L) and a CSF:plasma glucose ratio below 0.4.

Treatment is with the ketogenic diet. Most patients with GLUT 1-DS will require treatment with a ketogenic diet (classical or modified) until early adulthood.

The spectrum is widening, with the condition being associated with paroxysmal movement disorders, genetically determined epilepsies such as epilepsy with myotonic atonic absences (Doose syndrome), and migraine.

Status epilepticus (SE)

The ILAE has recently revised the definition and classification of SE (www.ilae.org): 'Status epilepticus is a condition resulting from either the failure of the mechanisms responsible for seizure termination or from the initiation of mechanisms, which lead to abnormally prolonged seizure (after time point t 1). It is a condition which can have long-term consequences (after time point t 2), including neuronal death, neuronal injury and alteration of neuronal networks, depending on the type and duration of seizures'. Time point t 1 refers to the point beyond which the seizure is considered 'continuous seizure activity', and time point t 2 to the point after which damage can occur, leading to long-term consequences. The classification refers to four axes: those of semiology, aetiology, EEG correlates and age. Semiology refers to the clinical description: whether motor symptoms predominate ('convulsive SE') or not ('non-convulsive SE' [NCSE]). Aetiology is divided into 'known' (further subdivided into acute [e.g. encephalitis], remote [e.g. post-encephalitic], progressive [e.g. brain tumour], and 'SE in defined clinical syndromes') and 'unknown'. EEG patterns in SE are not specific, with a lack of evidence-based criteria; ILAE suggests terminology of EEG patterns to be related to location (generalised, lateralised, bilateral independent, multifocal), name of pattern (e.g. periodic discharges, rhythmic delta activity), morphology (e.g. sharpness, polarity), time-related features (e.g. onset, dynamics [evolving, fluctuating]), modulation (stimulus-induced or spontaneous), and effect of intervention (medication) on EEG. The age axis is divided into neonatal (0 to 30 days), infancy (1 month to 2 years), childhood (> 2 to 12 years), adolescence and adulthood (> 12 to 59 years), and elderly (60 years and over). The operational dimensions are noted for: tonic–clonic SE (t 1 = 5 min., t 2 = 30 min.), focal SE with impaired consciousness (t 1 = 10 min., t 2 ≥ 60 min.), and absence SE (t 1 = 10–15 min., t 2 = unknown). Overall, around 50% of patients with SE do not have epilepsy, but have acute or remote CNS or systemic diseases.

Of patients with known epilepsy syndromes, there is a propensity towards getting SE in several. The following are selected examples: children with Ohtahara, West or Lennox-Gastaut syndromes may have tonic SE; children with Dravet syndrome, progressive myoclonic epilepsies or juvenile myoclonic epilepsy may have myoclonic SE; children with Panayiotopoulos syndrome may have autonomic SE; children with Landau–Kleffner syndrome may have aphasic SE, and children with juvenile absence epilepsy may have absence status.

The management of SE may be discussed. Candidates should be familiar with the standard protocol in their own tertiary paediatric centre, and with the relevant country's advanced paediatric life support/resuscitation courses' algorithms for SE. As a rule, benzodiazepines are first line, usually midazolam, lorazepam or diazepam; how they are given depends on where they are treated: outside hospital (buccal midazolam or IM midazolam are very useful) or as inpatients (IV midazolam or lorazepam or diazepam). These work well in both convulsive SE and NCSE; rapid cessation of NCSE with benzodiazepines is expected. If benzodiazepines do not stop the seizure within 5 minutes, then next is phenobarbitone (can be given IM outside hospital) or phenytoin (given IV in hospital). Paraldehyde is available in a limited number of facilities, and can be very useful, both outside and inside hospital, as it can be given PR, IM or IV and does not have the degree of respiratory depression that the above medications do. A further dose of benzodiazepines may be given, but if this is unsuccessful, then thiopentone, or propofol, with general anaesthesia. A simple mnemonic for this sequence is the 5 **P**s: **P**ams (benzodiazepines include diaze**pam**, loraze**pam** and midazolam), **P**henobarbitone, **P**henytoin, **P**araldehyde, **P**entone (as in Thio-pentone) or **P**ropofol. See below for further discussion of management of prolonged seizures.

Ketogenic diet (KD)

The KD is often considered in children with refractory seizure disorders, several of which are frequently encountered in long-case scenarios: benefit has been reported in syndromes (Dravet, Doose, Lennox-Gastaut, Rett, West), metabolic disorders (GLUT1 deficiency, pyruvate dehydrogenase deficiency [PDHD]), and TSC. There has been less well documented, but suggested, benefit in Landau–Kleffner, subacute sclerosing panencephalitis (SSPE) and some mitochondrial disorders. Overall, KD can lead to up to 10% of patients being seizure free, it decreases seizure frequency by 50% in 50% of patients who are prescribed it, and in a third, it decreases seizure frequency by 90%. It is essential to exclude any underlying disorders of fat metabolism or fatty acid transportation and oxidation, before considering KD, thus it is *contraindicated* in: coronary artery disease, carnitine and CoA disorders: short-, medium- and long-chain acyl dehydrogenase deficiencies (SCAD, MCAD and LCAD); carnitine deficiency, carnitine palmitoyltransferase (CPT I or II) deficiency, carnitine translocase deficiency; and medium- and long-chain 3 hydroxyacyl-CoA deficiencies. It is also contraindicated in pyruvate carboxylase deficiency, beta-oxidation disorders and porphyria. It is avoided with liver disease, cardiomyopathies, GORD and bulbar dysfunction (because of aspiration risk), dyslipidaemia and failure to thrive. When initiating KD, hypoglycaemia can occur rarely. However, once receiving ongoing KD, carbohydrates are avoided, and other medications must be sugar-free (e.g. vitamin preparations, analgesics, antibiotics) as unexpected introduction of carbohydrates and abolition of ketosis can precipitate seizures. If KD has no effect within 3 months, it is usually considered unsuccessful and is weaned.

History

The history of any seizure disorder depends on the description of the event by an eyewitness, with some input from the child, particularly with simple partial seizures. One must remain alert to the differential diagnoses, which are broad but more commonly include syncope (e.g. breath-holding spells), behavioural, parasomnia and postures of spasticity in children with cerebral palsy.

For each type of seizure the child has, the following must be established. The classification of the seizure type (e.g. generalised tonic–clonic seizures [GTCS], absence, atonic) is determined from the history, taking into account the points below. Always ask the age of onset for each seizure type.

1. Any prodromal symptoms (e.g. irritability, pallor). The setting in which the events occur (e.g. from sleep, during exercise, when ill, when sleep-deprived). Any precipitating factors (seizure triggers): tiredness, lack of sleep, fever, infectious illness, hot water, having a hot bath, change of dosage or type of anticonvulsant, intake of other substances (in adolescents), falls or blows to the head, movements, sensory stimuli such as flashing lights, television, computer games, patterns (e.g. stripes), elimination of central vision or fixation, sounds, music, startling by sudden noises or touch, reading, calculating, decision-making, playing chess. Reflex seizures are consistently elicited by a particular stimulus. The term 'catamenial' refers to seizures that increase in relation to the menstrual cycle, whether perimenstrual, periovulatory or luteal (oestrogens generally are proconvulsant, and progesterones anticonvulsant). Adolescent girls may be asked about this.

2. Any aura (e.g. a specific psychic or sensory symptom, as distinct from a prodromal symptom). This includes running to the parent for comfort. This is applicable to children with partial seizures.

3. Initial cry or scream.

4. Initial localising signs (e.g. twitching of one hand).

5. Description of all the manifestations (motor and autonomic) of the seizure (e.g. eyes 'rolling back', altered awareness, cyanosis, jerking movements of limbs, urinary and/or faecal incontinence).

6. The duration of the seizures—the range (e.g. between 5 and 20 minutes) and the 'usual' time (e.g. 5 minutes). Any episodes of status epilepticus (duration > 30 minutes).

7. The frequency of the seizures—range (e.g. none for 6 weeks to 6 in a day) and the 'usual' (e.g. once every 3 weeks).
8. Time of occurrence of seizures (e.g. on waking, or on going to sleep).
9. The date and time of the last seizure.
10. Postictal events (e.g. sleeping, confusion, headache, vomiting, Todd's paralysis).
11. Presence of neurological dysfunction (other than seizure).

The past history of the seizures—in terms of number of hospital admissions, previous anticonvulsants used and why they were changed, any previous complications of seizures or their treatment, and whether febrile convulsions occurred at a younger age—should be covered thoroughly. The past history of possible aetiological factors (epilepsy risk factors), such as prematurity, cerebral infection, head injury or other neurological insult, should be sought. Note any family history of seizure disorders or other neurological problems in the immediate or extended family (e.g. familial GEFS+).

The details of any anticonvulsant therapy must be known, including the dose, efficacy, when levels were last taken, what they were, recent dosage changes and any current side effects. Common symptoms raised by parents that are often blamed on medication include drowsiness, cognitive slowing and poor behaviour.

Obtain an outline of how the parents manage when the child is having a seizure, what contingency plans exist for a prolonged seizure, their criteria for seeking hospital treatment, any medications given by them acutely at home (e.g. rectal diazepam), how long it takes to get the child to hospital in an emergency and what restrictions are placed on the child because of the seizures (e.g. swimming). Remember to evaluate the parents' understanding of seizures; for example, in terms of prognosis, chances of remission and complications. Are the parents afraid of the child dying? Are there steps of overprotectiveness, including sleeping in the parents' bed, or excessive social restrictions? An assessment of the child's schooling progress is important. Compliance with treatment must be discussed.

Finally, remember to take a full social history, including any benefits the child is receiving (e.g. Child Disability Assistance Payment), social supports (e.g. Epilepsy Association) and the impact of the disease on the child, schooling, parents and siblings. An enquiry into social isolation or bullying at school can be revealing. If the patient is an adolescent, this involves a whole range of new issues, including compliance, effects on career prospects, driver's licence, and menstrual and reproductive issues. Mental health issues often come to the fore with the high rates of teenage depression and anxiety seen.

Examination

This is outlined in the short-case section on recurrent seizures in this chapter.

Investigations

The extent of investigation depends on the clinical picture. The following is an incomplete list of some of the more commonly used investigations.

ELECTROENCEPHALOGRAM (EEG)

An EEG is performed to look for interictal focal slowing or epileptiform activity—that is, spike or sharp wave (localised or generalised). On some occasions the EEG may capture s typical event. However, epileptiform activity on the EEG does not equate with the diagnosis of epilepsy unless a typical event is captured during the recording. An EEG provides collateral information. Interictal epileptiform discharges (IEDs) are found in association with epilepsy. Their yield can be increased by activation methods such as sleep, sleep deprivation, hyperventilation and photic stimulation. Children with epilepsy should have an EEG performed and this may be helpful in making the diagnosis, particularly which epilepsy syndrome is present (e.g. CAE). However, it should be noted that children with epilepsy may well have normal EEGs (in up to 50% of cases) and, conversely, non-epileptic children may show 'epileptiform activity' on their EEGs (3–5% of children).

Certain patterns are well recognised and expected to be known (e.g. BECTS with centrotemporal spikes). Interictal EEG provides valuable information in these epileptic syndromes: BECTS, CAE, JME, LGS, and Panayiotopoulos syndrome (PS) and some focal epilepsies.

Video/EEG monitoring is often reserved for when there are diagnostic issues (Is this epilepsy?) or management issues (What is the epilepsy syndrome?). It may be particularly useful in assessing a child who has a confusing or unconvincing history of 'funny turns', or possibly several seizure types. It may aid in assessing conditions such as atonic seizures (e.g. documenting the period of lost muscle tone, and the risk of head injury). Replaying the videotape to the parents may help them to appreciate aspects of their child's attacks that had not been noted, and allow many questions to be answered, based on what is seen. Video/EEG is indicated in children with medication-resistant epilepsy. It can guide further investigation and management, such as a presurgical evaluation.

BIOCHEMICAL EVALUATION

A blood glucose level taken at the time of the seizure may detect a treatable metabolic cause, particularly in younger children. Serum calcium and magnesium should also be checked in someone presenting for the first time with an unexplained generalised seizure. An ECG is valuable to help exclude risk of an arrhythmia, such as a prolonged QT syndrome as a cause of syncope-seizure.

Other tests that may be useful in certain patients include serum electrolytes and metabolic evaluation (urine for amino acids, organic acids, acylcarnitine, acylglycines and mucopolysaccharides). In neonates, the mnemonic **BACCAULAUREATES** (see earlier section on neonatal seizures) includes most causes of symptomatic seizures.

IMAGING: STRUCTURAL

Brain-imaging studies by either MRI or CT scanning may be indicated in the following circumstances. The present gold standard is MRI. Thin cuts can identify atrophy of the hippocampus, developmental anomalies (e.g. cortical dysplasia), and low-grade tumours. Three-dimensional fluid attenuation inversion recovery (FLAIR) sequences, and voxel-based analyses of numerous contrasts, can detect very subtle abnormalities of the cortex:

1. Focal seizures, except for BECTS, which is diagnosed on clinical and EEG features that are characteristic enough to make MRI/CT scanning unnecessary. However, a scan should be done if atypical features are present.
2. Focal EEG findings (again, except for those of BECTS).
3. Abnormal neurological signs (particularly focal signs).
4. Developmental delay.
5. Seizures that are difficult to control.

IMAGING: FUNCTIONAL

Functional neuro-imaging modalities have become more widely used over the last decade. These modalities can help to accurately localise seizure onset without invasive means. They include:

1. Positron emission tomography (PET) scanning, which assesses cerebral metabolism (mnemonic: **PET** checks **MET**abolism), using fluorodeoxyglucose. PET shows a

decreased metabolic rate of the epileptogenic area during the interictal period. It is especially useful in identifying TLE.

2. Single-photon emission computed tomography (SPECT) scanning, which evaluates cerebral perfusion, using hexamethyl-propyleneamine oxime (HMPOA) or iodoamphetamine or technetium-labelled Ceretec. There is interictal hypoperfusion, but ictal intense hyperperfusion at onset, with depression of perfusion after seizure. (Mnemonic for **SPECT**: **S**eizure [area] **P**erfusion **E**valuated by **C**eretec with **T**echnetium.) SPECT is ideally performed during a seizure to demonstrate regional hyperperfusion.

3. Functional MRI allows regional localisation of primary language, motor and visual cortical areas, measuring brain activity by detecting changes in blood flow.

4. Magnetoencephalopathy (MEG) MRI describes functional neuroimaging which maps brain activity by recording of magnetic fields caused by electrical currents within the brain by magnetometers.

Common management issues

The number of potential issues is enormous. This section addresses a small number of selected areas that may be quite relevant in the type of patients seen in the examination.

INCREASING FREQUENCY OF SEIZURES AND INTRACTABLE EPILEPSY

If the seizures seem to be worsening in duration or frequency, or are changing in nature (such as the appearance of a different type of seizure), the overall management needs to be reconsidered. There are several important areas to question.

Question the diagnosis

There are a number of conditions that can mimic epilepsy, such as syncope, breath-holding attacks and psychogenic non-epileptic seizures (PNES). Structural causes that are as yet undiagnosed (e.g. brain tumour) can present with seizures. Neurodegenerative conditions may present with seizures. The most common group to have PNES are epileptic patients.

Concentrate carefully on the history for any suggestion of developmental regression. Physical examination may detect features of neurodegenerative conditions (e.g. macrocephaly, macular degeneration) or structural causes (e.g. focal neurological signs).

Question the medication

The dose may be wrong, the drug may be wrong or adverse drug interactions may be occurring. The dosage may be too low, usually related either to non-compliance or to 'outgrowing' the dosage given (weight increase). The drug may not be the most appropriate choice for the types of seizure the child has (see later in this case), or a drug appropriately chosen for one seizure type may worsen, or even 'unmask', another type of seizure (e.g. carbamazepine can worsen absence seizures). Insufficient numbers of medications may have been trialled.

Question an intercurrent problem

Intercurrent problems can include electrolyte imbalances consequent on drug side effects (e.g. hyponatraemia as a complication of carbamazepine, via the syndrome of inappropriate antidiuretic hormone secretion) or intercurrent infections (e.g. urinary tract infection).

Are there unrecognised precipitating factors?

The patient may have become increasingly exposed to unrecognised precipitants such as drugs, television, computer or video games.

Is this form of epilepsy commonly a treatment problem?

Certain types of epilepsy are notoriously difficult to control; examples are Lennox-Gastaut syndrome and infantile spasms.

ADVICE TO PARENTS (AND SCHOOLTEACHERS)
Management during a seizure

Lay the child on the side. Do not put things in the child's mouth. Move away any nearby objects to avoid the child hurting him- or herself. Have a time plan: for example, if a seizure lasts longer than 5 minutes, call an ambulance.

EVERYDAY CHILDHOOD/ADOLESCENT ACTIVITIES: SAFETY CONSIDERATIONS
Strategies to avoid drowning

1. No swimming alone. Swimming pools, and dams should be fenced off.
2. No bathing alone for younger children. Turn taps off before get in bath. No unattended buckets of water.
3. Showers rather than baths for older children (with the bathroom door open and someone nearby). Shower curtains rather than glass screens. Retractable taps to avoid head injury. Never lock the bathroom door from inside.
4. No diving or surfing if JME, avoid scuba diving. but tandem parachute diving is acceptable. Wear lifeboat if boating or fishing.

Strategies to prevent burns

1. Put guards in front of fires and heaters; use of: microwaves (rather than stoves or conventional ovens), stove barriers, anti-spill mugs, insulated plastic (rather than metal) kettles that switch off automatically.
2. Avoidance of: handheld hair dryers, electric irons, accessible bar heaters, open fires, hotplates, barbeques, cigarettes, cigars, pipes, lighting matches when alone (avoiding the latter four also to prevent fires), temperature-controlled hot water supply, spas, heaters.
3. Always run cold water before hot.

Strategies to avoid significant/traumatic injuries

1. No climbing ladders or similar pursuits with a risk of falls (avoid rock climbing without harness and experienced company, avoid flying fox).
2. Wear helmet (and protective armguards, elbow guards and knee pads if skateboarding), if riding bicycle, scooter, horse; also use of helmets for drop attacks (as in atonic seizures).
3. Stair barriers, or avoid accommodation with stairs. Avoid top bunk bed. Avoid standing close to road awaiting buses, taxis or trams or to edges of platforms awaiting trains. Use rubber mats in bathrooms to avoid slipping.

Strategies to avoid suffocation

1. Sleep without pillow or use firm, porous pillow. Sleep on a wide bed with a firm mattress and fitted sheet.
2. Use monitor/alarm system, or intercom, to alert parents/carers if nocturnal seizures.

Strategies to avoid abrasions, bruising or cuts

1. Toughened, tempered or reinforced glass is preferred to normal glass for doors and windows, or application of safety film to preexisting glass. Minimise sharp objects in house (knives, scissors stored with sharp edges pointed downwards).

Strategies to avoid medication-related problems

1. Adolescent females taking AEDs, who are sexually active, should take folate 5 mg per day, as AEDs increase risk of neural tube defects in their offspring (valproate 2%, carbamazepine 1%).
2. Medications often have significant interactions with other medications, plus non-proven therapies; need to have any new therapies (e.g. over the counter) discussed with prescribing paediatrician/neurologist before starting any.

Avoid overprotection

Allow participation in normal sports and school activities. There is no contraindication to body-contact sports. Some neurologists prefer to encourage participation in non-contact sports such as tennis and athletics.

Driver's licence

The rules vary in different states and different countries. Commonly, the recommendation is that a conditional licence is granted if the patient has had no seizures in the previous 2 years; however, guidelines are now more tailored to individual circumstances and the type of epilepsy. The single greatest motivator for compliance with medication in adolescence is wanting to be able to drive.

Avoid known precipitants

For example, in photosensitive epilepsy, avoid sitting close to the television in a dark room, and wear sunglasses outside, particularly in cars and buses, when sunlight dappling through trees combined with sitting in a moving vehicle can be a problem.

Rationale for treatment

Parents should have the reasons for recommending treatment explained to them, covering fully both the benefits and the possible side effects of whichever drug is chosen. Issues such as the morbidity and generally low mortality of epilepsy should be discussed.

Probable duration of treatment

All parents will want to know about this. A rough guide is that medication may generally be stopped when the child has been free of seizures for 2 years, depending on the syndrome. If the child had an abnormal physical examination or abnormal EEG, the treatment could be stopped later (e.g. at 3–4 years) but this should be after discussion between the treating doctor and carer.

Remember that a number of factors are associated with an increased probability of seizure recurrence, once medications are stopped. The epilepsy syndrome itself is the best guideline. Other factors include abnormal neurological signs, mixed types of seizures, focal seizures (excluding BECTS) and seizures that were originally difficult to control.

Genetic counselling

Parents often want to know whether there is a risk that their other children could develop the same condition. Accurate diagnosis is essential: if the problem is a known monogenetic problem, the risk can be predicted accurately, but for most clinically (not molecularly) diagnosed epilepsies, an estimate only is available. Overall, the risk to siblings of generalised epilepsies is around 10%, the risk to siblings of focal epilepsies is around 5%, and the risk to siblings of febrile seizures is around 8%. Most genetic epilepsies are benign.

ANTICONVULSANT MEDICATIONS

General aims

Monotherapy is the goal: one drug, given in the correct dosage for the child's body weight, with drug levels checked initially (if applicable) to confirm the adequacy of the dose when a steady state has been achieved (after five times the half-life of the drug). Many anticonvulsants need to be started at a low dosage and then gradually increased, until the appropriate dose is reached over 1–2 weeks. In the case of lamotrigine, the process is usually over several months.

If one drug, given at the correct dosage and within the therapeutic range of serum levels, is unsuccessful in controlling the seizures, the next most appropriate agent can be started. Only after the first drug has reached steady state should it be slowly withdrawn. The reality in long-case patients is often polypharmacy, hopefully rational polypharmacy.

Which drugs can have serum levels measured?

The candidate should know which drugs can have serum levels measured, but also recognise the limitations of such levels. A drug can be at the recommended range, but the patient still has fits and/or side effects; this is not an adequate 'therapeutic' drug level, as it is not providing adequate therapy. A level is only 'therapeutic' if there are no fits and no side effects. Of the 'older' AEDs, carbamazepine (CBZ), phenytoin (PHT) and phenobarbitone (PB) all have recommended 'optimal' ranges of serum drug levels, which may be useful in monitoring therapy. Valproate (VPA) is an exception: levels can be measured, but they do not correlate with efficacy or toxicity and so are unhelpful (except in suspected non-compliance, where a level of zero may confirm this suspicion). The same applies to the benzodiazepines (BDZs). Of the newer drugs, serum levels are important only for lamotrigine, topiramate and zonisamide.

Which drug is preferable in which type of seizure?

Table 13.1 is an incomplete list of epilepsy syndromes and the useful drugs in each. Table 13.2 is an incomplete list of types of seizure and useful drugs in each.

What side effects are likely?

It is beyond the scope of this book to list all the side effects of the commonly used anticonvulsants. Behavioural and cognitive effects are among the most common side effects reported in children. Candidates should be familiar with the acute toxicities (e.g. drowsiness, nystagmus and ataxia with carbamazepine and phenytoin), acute idiosyncratic reactions (e.g. skin manifestations such as Stevens–Johnson syndrome/toxic epidermal necrolysis [SJS/TEN]), chronic toxicities (e.g. various effects on the haematological system, bones, connective tissue, cosmetic effects and teratogenic effects) and drug interactions, both between anticonvulsants (e.g. CBZ lowers PHT levels, VPA increases PB levels) and with other drugs (e.g. erythromycin increases CBZ levels). Patients carrying HLA-B*15:02 are at much higher risk of developing CBZ-induced SJS/TEN; this has been described in certain Asian countries (China, India, Malaysia, Thailand) only. Patients carrying HLA-A*31:01 are at much higher risk of developing CBZ-induced hypersensitivity syndrome (HSS) or maculopapular exanthema (MPE); this has been described in Caucasians, Japanese, Korean and Chinese patients and patients of mixed origin. It is recommended that genetic testing for HLA-B*15:02 and HLA-A*31:01 be done in appropriate patients before considering commencing CBZ.

ARE ANY OF THE NEWER AEDS LIKELY TO BE OF USE HERE?

Of the several newer AEDs introduced over the last decade or so, the efficacy is yet to be established. Remember that, unlike other new drugs where RCTs can compare

Table 13.1	
Selected epilepsy syndromes and examples of drugs used	
EPILEPSY SYNDROMES	**TREATMENT (DRUGS, DIET, SURGERY)**
West syndrome/epileptic spasms	First line: if not caused by TSC: **ACTH, prednisolone**; if these fail, try VGB
	First line: if caused by TSC: **VGB** (monitor: for field cuts, get ERG 3 monthly); if fails try ACTH, prednisolone
	Other options: ketogenic diet, VGB, VPA, CLZ, TPM, surgery
Dravet syndrome (SMEI)	**VPA + CLB + stiripentol** effective. Other options: TPM, LEV, (cannabidiol). (**Avoid CBZ, OXC, PHT, LTG, PGB, TGB, VGB, GBP**)
Doose syndrome (MAE)	**VPA, LTG, LEV**, CLZ, CLB, NZP, TPM, ESM, ketogenic diet, modified Atkins diet, steroids (non-convulsive status) (**Avoid CBZ, PHT, VGB**)
Lennox-Gastaut syndrome	**VPA, LTG, RFM, TPM**, CLZ, CLB, LEV ketogenic diet, vagus n. stimulation, surgery (**Avoid CBZ, OXC, PGB, TGB, GBP**)
Childhood absence epilepsy (CAE) or other absence syndromes such as juvenile absence epilepsy (JAE)	**ESM, LTG, VPA**, CLB, CLZ, LEV, TPM, ZNS. (**Avoid CBZ, OXC, PHT, PGB, TGB, VGB, GBP**)
Benign epilepsy with centrotemporal spikes (BECTS)	**CBZ, LTG, LEV, OXC, VPA**, CLB, GBP, LCM, PHB, PHT, TGB, VGB, ESL
Landau–Kleffner syndrome (LKS)	**VPA + LTG**, ESM, CLZ, CLB, LEV, ACTH, prednisolone, multiple subpial subcortical transection
Juvenile myoclonic epilepsy (JME)	**LTG, LEV, VPA, TPM**, CLB, CLZ, ZNS (**Avoid CBZ, OXC, PHT, PGB, TGB, VGB, GBP**)
Symptomatic focal/partial epilepsy	**CBZ, VPA**, LTG, CLB

ACTH = adrenocorticotropic hormone; CBZ = carbamazepine; CLB = clobazam; CLZ = clonazepam; ESL = eslicarbazepine acetate; ESM = ethosuximide; GBP = gabapentin; LCM = lacosamide; LEV = levetiracetam; LTG = lamotrigine; NZP = nitrazepam; OXC = oxcarbazepine; PGB = pregabalin; PHB = phenobarbitone; PHT = phenytoin; RFM = rufinamide; TGB = tiagabine; TPM = topiramate; VGB = vigabatrin; VPA = valproate; ZNS = zonisamide.

to placebo, new AEDs are commenced by adding them onto treatment to which the patients are refractory. Long-term adverse effects may not be known as yet. Initial enthusiasm for previous 'newer' AEDs were dampened by realisation that vigabatrin (VGB) caused persistent visual field constriction in a third of patients, and cerebral MRI abnormalities; retigabine caused bluish discolouration; and felbamate could lead to aplastic anaemia. Enthusiasm for levetiracetam initially has been tempered by studies showing little significant advantage over older drugs, other than less adverse effects. Around 30% of patients will keep having seizures despite AEDs; adding a second or third only leads to freedom from seizures in a further 14%. Variables which influence choice of AED are epilepsy syndrome/seizure type, patient aspects (genetic background, age, gender, comorbidities) and drug availability in many countries.

Eslicarbazepine acetate (ESL)

A prodrug to eslicarbazepine (the active metabolite of OXC), used as adjunct in refractory focal-onset seizures, member of the dibenzazepine family of AEDs (CBZ, OXC), different to CBZ in that it lacks a toxic epoxide; lower incidence of side effects of rash, of hyponatraemia or of cognitive and psychiatric changes. Half-life 13–20 hours; given once daily.

Table 13.2	
Selected seizure types and examples of AEDs used	
SEIZURE TYPE	**AEDS**
Generalised tonic–clonic	First line: CBZ, LTG, OXC, VPA; Adjunctive: CLB, LTG, LEV, TPM [**Avoid: if absence or myoclonic CBZ, OXC, PHT, PGB, TGB, VGB, GBP**]
Tonic or atonic	First line: VPA; Adjunctive: LTG Other: RFM, TPM [**Avoid CBZ, OXC, PGB, TGB, VGB, GBP**]
Absence	First line: ESM, LTG, VPA Other: CLB, CLN, LEV, TPM, ZNS [**Avoid CBZ, OXC, PHT, PGB, TGB, VGB, GBP**]
Myoclonic	First line: LEV, VPA, TPM Other: CLB, CLZ, PIR, ZNS [**Avoid CBZ, OXC, PHT, PGB, TGB, VGB, GBP**]
Focal	First line: CBZ, OXC, LTG, LEV, VPA Adjunctive: CLB, GBP, TPM Other: ESL, LCM, PHT, PGB, TGB, VGB, ZNS
Convulsive status	Hospital: first line: benzodiazepines (BZDs): buccal or IV midazolam, IV diazepam, IV lorazepam; IV phenobarbitone, IV phenytoin Out-of-hospital: buccal midazolam, rectal diazepam, IV lorazepam
Refractory convulsive status	IV midazolam, thiopental sodium

ACTH = adrenocorticotropic hormone; CBZ = carbamazepine; CLB = clobazam; CLZ = clonazepam; ESL = eslicarbazepine acetate; ESM = ethosuximide; GBP = gabapentin; LCM = lacosamide; LEV = levetiracetam; LTG = lamotrigine; LZP = lorazepam; NZP = nitrazepam; OXC = oxcarbazepine; PGB = pregabalin; PHB = phenobarbitone; PHT = phenytoin; RFM = rufinamide; TGB = tiagabine; TPM = topiramate; VGB = vigabatrin; VPA = valproate; ZNS = zonisamide.

Gabapentin (GBP) (infrequently used)

This incorporates GABA into the cyclohexane ring; it is taken up into neurons. For intractable partial seizures, there is a 25% response rate. It has no specific interaction with other AEDs. Side effects are drowsiness, dizziness, diplopia, weight gain and behavioural change.

Lacosamide (LCM)

This affects voltage-gated sodium channels by selectively enhancing slow inactivation, but without any effect on fast gating, has a good safety profile and has minimal drug interactions. It has been used in refractory epilepsies of various causes, with focal/partial-onset epilepsies and in juvenile myoclonic epilepsy. Adverse effects can include dizziness, drowsiness, diplopia, blurring of vision, headache and prolongation of the PR interval. Other AEDs affecting sodium channels must be avoided (CBZ, OXC, PHT, ZNS).

Lamotrigine (LTG)

LTG stabilises pre-synaptic neuronal membranes, inhibits excitatory neurotransmitters (especially glutamate and aspartate) by blocking sodium channels. It is used as an add-on treatment for partial and generalised seizures. Around 25–33% of patients have a 50% reduction in intractable partial seizures.

It has a pharmacokinetic interaction with sodium valproate (VPA): elimination of LTG is prolonged if it is given with VPA, doubling the half-life. There is a pharmacodynamic interaction with VPA:LTG and VPA are a good combination, leading to greater efficacy than LTG with other agents, although there is a small chance of upper limb tremor, which stops on lowering the dose of either.

The most serious side effect is a skin rash, which can include Stevens–Johnson syndrome; this is increased by concomitant use of VPA. Care should be used with the combination of VPA and LTG: lower dosage and slower escalation rates are used. Other side effects of LTG: insomnia, double vision, blurred vision, dizziness, ataxia and drowsiness.

Levetiracetam (LEV)

This is unrelated to other AEDs chemically. The mechanism of action is via altering intraneuronal calcium (ion) levels, by partial inhibition of N type calcium currents and by decreasing calcium ion release, from intraneuronal stores. LEV also binds to synaptic protein 2A (SV2A), which is involved in vesicle fusion and neurotransmitter exocytosis. It has been used in intractable symptomatic partial/generalised seizure disorders, including LGS, symptomatic and idiopathic epilepsies, photosensitive epilepsy and myoclonus (epileptic and non-epileptic). Advantages of **LEV** include the following: **L**aboratory tests (e.g. drug levels) not needed; **E**xcellent pharmacokinetics, excellent safety profile; **V**ersatile (most types of epilepsy treated), very fast onset. Side effects include blurred vision, sleepiness, dizziness and poor coordination. Behavioural symptoms have been reported in up to around 40% of paediatric patients, including agitation, anxiety, apathy, depersonalisation, depression, emotional lability, hostility, hyperactivity, nervousness, neurosis and personality disorder.

Oxcarbazepine (OXC)

Indications are as for CBZ. There are fewer interactions with other drugs with OXC than with CBZ. Dose-related, idiosyncratic and chronic toxicity side effects are all less than for CBZ. Hyponatraemia has been described where OXC has replaced CBZ therapy, with Na level < 135 mmol/L in 26.6% and Na < 125 mmol/L in 2.6%; clinical symptoms of hyponatraemia have been described.

Rufinamide

This blocks voltage-dependent sodium channels, and has efficacy against: drop attacks in LGS; focal seizures; and secondarily generalised tonic–clonic seizures (GTCS). Its levels are increased by valproate.

Stiripentol

This increases GABA-ergic transmission, and in combination with clobazam and valproate is one of the few medications that has efficacy against refractory GTCS in Dravet syndrome (severe myoclonic epilepsy in infancy [SMEI]). It inhibits several other AEDs.

Tiagabine (TGB) (rarely used)

This blocks GABA uptake in glial cells and neurons, via a specific transport system (keeps GABA at receptor), and increases GABA in extracellular fluid and GABA-ergic mediated inhibitors in the brain. It is used for simple partial, complex partial and secondary generalised seizures. It has faster onset than VGB. Side effects are dizziness, tiredness and non-specific 'nervousness'.

Topiramate (TPM)

This is an example of polypharmacy in one drug. A sulfamate-substituted monosaccharide, it blocks seizure spread (similar to carbamazepine [CBZ] and phenytoin [PHT]), blocks glutamate receptors, increases GABA and weakly inhibits carbonic anhydrase. It has minimal interaction with other AEDs. It has no effect on CBZ, phenobarbitone (PB), PHT or VPA, but some of these AEDs (CBZ, PB, PHT) are enzyme inducers and can decrease serum concentration of TPM. TPM is used for simple partial, complex partial and secondarily generalised seizures. Side effects are drowsiness, cognitive dysfunction (in 10%) with word-finding difficulties, dizziness, weight loss, renal stones and acute glaucoma. TPM needs to be introduced slowly, over 4–8 weeks.

Vigabatrin (VGB)

An irreversible inhibitor of GABA transaminase, VGB increases the availability of GABA. Around 50% of patients have a 50% reduction in intractable partial seizures. It remains the drug of choice for West syndrome/infantile spasms, when caused by tuberous sclerosis, despite great concern involving the risk of some loss of peripheral visual fields, which can be irreversible despite cessation of the drug when detected. Side effects: sedation and fatigue, weight gain, agitation and hyperkinesis.

Zonisamide (ZNS)

A sulphonamide which inhibits the zinc enzyme carbonic anhydrase. This is unrelated to other AEDs chemically. Its main mechanism of action is inhibiting T-calcium currents in the thalamus; it also blocks sodium channels, disrupts coordinated neuronal firing, decreases seizure spread, and also has effects on GABA, glutamate, serotonin, dopamine and acetylcholine. It is useful for absence epilepsy and juvenile myoclonic epilepsy for refractory focal/partial seizures. Its side effect profile includes hyperchloraemic metabolic acidosis, nephrolithiasis, pancreatitis, muscle pain/weakness, mood changes and concentration difficulties. Its long half-life of 63 hours allows once daily dosing; the half-life is decreased by concomitant use of PHT, CBZ, PHB or VPA, to 27–46 hours.

Sodium channel blockers

The AEDS which act this way include a number of AEDS such as eslicarbazepine acetate, lacosamide, lamotrigine, oxcarbazepine, carbamazepine and phenytoin. If these are combined, their CNS side effects are increased. Predictably, sodium blocking drugs should not be given to children with epilepsies due to sodium channelopathies (e.g. Dravet) as these worsen the situation by increasing the insult to the sodium channels.

WHAT TO TRY IN INTRACTABLE SEIZURES?

In patients with intractable seizures all aetiologies should be considered, including metabolic (trial of pyridoxine). The ketogenic diet can be a valuable alternative, particularly in younger children. Any child with intractable focal epilepsy should be considered for surgery (see below).

SURGICAL TREATMENT

Surgical treatment of epilepsy is now safe and effective for those with epilepsy that is medically refractory and surgically remediable, with an emphasis towards 'the sooner the better' in children. Most adult surgical work has been carried out involving the temporal lobe. In children, extratemporal cases are of similar frequency.

About 1 in 7 patients with epilepsy are refractory to AEDs. Of these, 1 in 4 will be candidates for surgery. The commonest pathologies are focal gliosis, low-grade tumours and focal cortical dysplasia. Less frequent are conditions such as Sturge-Weber syndrome (SWS), tuberous sclerosis (TSC) and hemimegaloencephaly. Contraindications include any of the primary generalised epilepsies (PGEs), any neurodegenerative or neurometabolic disorder.

Before surgery is even considered, an adequate trial of AEDs, including the newer AEDs if appropriate, is undertaken. If truly intractable, the localisation of the site of seizure initiation is detected using methods including clinical assessment, video-EEG monitoring, neuropsychology (to assess the functional importance of the site of onset: left-sided function includes verbal IQ and memory, right-sided function includes performance IQ and visual memory), CT, MRI, SPECT, PET, functional MRI and invasive monitoring. Electrical-stimulation mapping can be performed intra- or extraoperatively to identify eloquent cortex in relation to epileptogenic areas.

Ictal SPECT (commonly using Tc99m HMPAO [technetium-99m hexamethyl-propylene amine oxime]) pre-operatively requires availability of the isotope at the bedside, to be quickly injected at the start of any seizure activity.

Useful coregistration techniques, in surgery work-up, include MRI coregistered with 18F-fluorodesoxyglucose PET, EEG-functional MRI and EEG magnetoencephalopathy.

Non-invasive testing to decrease surgical morbidity includes memory functional MRI (predicts postoperative memory loss) and tractography of optic radiations (predicts visual field deficits).

The Wada test, which comprises anaesthetising each hemisphere to evaluate memory, may still occasionally need to be performed in children over 5. It determines (mnemonic: **WADA**): **W**hich hemisphere is dominant for language, to see if the other side can maintain memory function, after **A**mytal sodium injection into internal carotid, **D**ysfunctional hippocampus identified and **A**mnesia avoided as complication. It would only be done if it was unclear which side of the brain contained language function, if there were investigations that were discordant, or if psychological testing suggests significant risk to memory or hippocampal disease is bilateral; the Wada test is not infallible, and a positive test result does not guarantee intact memory postoperatively.

Examples of the types of surgery undertaken are as follows:
1. Seizures secondary to focal cerebral lesions: lesionectomy or partial lobectomy.
2. Seizures secondary to hemimegaloencephaly or to SWS or other large unilateral pathology: hemispherectomy.
3. Atonic seizures (drop attacks): corpus callosotomy.

Overall mortality from focal resective surgery is very low. A higher mortality rate is seen with hemispherectomy, particularly if under 1 year of age. Morbidities, depending on the site of surgery, include hemiparesis (1–5%), visual field defects (1–5%), language dysfunction (1–3%) and global amnesia (1%).

In well-selected patients, seizure freedom can be seen in up to 80% of tumour cases, and patients with other focal pathologies can be 50–70% seizure free.

Some centres offer vagal nerve stimulation (VNS) to those intractable patients who are not candidates for surgery. The success rate is around a 50% reduction in seizures in over 50% of patients, but less than 5% get complete cessation of seizures. The VNS device is a battery-powered electrical pulse generator (batteries last three years) implanted under the skin in the left chest, attached to electrodes that are wrapped around the main trunk of the left vagus nerve. The device is programmed, via a computer and a handheld 'wand', to stimulate the vagus at various frequencies (usually for 30 seconds each 5 minutes). Exposure to powerful magnets (e.g. MRI, hair trimmers, loudspeakers) can interfere with the stimulator or electrode leads. There should be similar precautions to those with cardiac pacemakers.

MANAGEMENT OF THE PROLONGED SEIZURE
At home

In patients with neurological abnormalities (e.g. CP) and a history of unprovoked status epilepticus (particularly if at an isolated address), prolonged seizure can be treated with early administration of rectal diazepam, or buccal or nasal midazolam, while awaiting the ambulance.

In ambulance/at hospital

Having checked that the airway is secured, giving high flow oxygen, checking breathing and circulation, and checking the blood glucose, if the seizure has already gone on for longer than 5 minutes, an intravenous loading dose of phenobarbitone or phenytoin would be an appropriate next step. Once the infusion of either of these drugs is complete, if the seizure continues, then that medication has failed, and the next step in the treatment algorithm should be followed. There are many versions of an 'ideal approach'; candidates should be conversant with that used at their teaching hospital.

A suggested 'ideal' time course for treating a seizure at presentation (assuming immediate vascular access achieved) is as follows:

- Initial minute: intravenous (IV) midazolam or diazepam or lorazepam; if no access, intramuscular (IM), intranasal (IN) or buccal midazolam.
- 5 minutes: repeat IV midazolam or diazepam or lorazepam.
- 10 minutes (still fitting): intravenous phenytoin or phenobarbitone infusion over 20 minutes, (with ECG monitoring if use phenytoin); if no access, repeat IM, IN or buccal midazolam.
- 20 minutes: (still fitting, still no access) PR Paraldehyde diluted 50:50 in normal saline.
- 25 minutes (still fitting, phenytoin or phenobarbitone infusion almost complete): contact anaesthetist/intensivist/emergency physician (if not already done) to prepare for intubation (rapid sequence induction with thiopentone or propofol).
- 30 minutes (still fitting): rapid sequence induction with thiopentone or propofol.

The underlying cause for the prolonged seizure must be thoroughly investigated. Investigations may include CT or MRI scanning, with or without lumbar puncture. A common end point for a resistant prolonged seizure is for the child to be anaesthetised, while investigations continue, and treated (antibiotics, aciclovir, dexamethasone, plus continued anticonvulsants) to cover serious underlying pathology.

MANAGEMENT OF THE FIRST NON-FEBRILE SEIZURE

The chances of further seizures occurring after a single seizure, at 5 years of age, are as follows:

1. In neurodevelopmentally normal children, with a normal EEG: 25%.
2. In children with mild neurological problems: 70%.
3. In those with severe neurological problems (e.g. CP): 90%.

Different seizure types have different risks of recurrence. BECTS, for example, is associated with a very high chance of recurrence (90% will have a second seizure). After a first epileptic seizure, EEG abnormalities are associated with an increased risk of seizure recurrence.

PSYCHOSOCIAL ISSUES

The management of psychosocial issues is of particular importance in children with recurrent seizures. The key point in managing this area is clear communication and providing information to the family. The following points cover issues where education will resolve most of the difficulties.

Parents

The parents of an epileptic child often have concerns in the following areas:

1. Fear of brain damage.
2. Being uncomfortable with the label/stigma of 'epilepsy'.
3. False beliefs that the cause relates to themselves (e.g. 'stress' during pregnancy).

4. Equating an EEG with a treatment modality such as electroconvulsive therapy.
5. Difficulty accepting the need for medication: ambivalence (forgetting to give medications); the belief that the need for drugs equates with, or causes, 'intellectual disability/retardation'; and suddenly stopping the medication when the supply is used up.

Children

Children with seizures not uncommonly have significant psychosocial problems. Their concerns include the following:
1. Fear of dying or being injured during a seizure.
2. Fear of loss of control, loss of friends or loss of continence.
3. Overprotection, inappropriate restrictions and the 'vulnerable child' syndrome.

Other issues of concern to parents and doctors are actions that demonstrate significant underlying worries and conflicts in the child: denial, psychogenic non-epileptic seizures (PNES), and self-induced seizures.

LONG CASE: Spina bifida (SB)/myelomeningocele (MMC)

Neural tube development is disrupted by maternal folate deficiency; 70% of all cases of neural tube defects (NTDs) are preventable by maternal folate supplementation which provides adequate periconceptual folic acid. Since 2006, there has been an annual worldwide decrease in folic acid preventable spina bifida (SB) and anencephaly cases, attributable to the worldwide programs of folic acid fortification of wheat and maize flour. This has been further improved by more countries requiring fortification of both wheat and maize flour and setting fortification levels high enough to increase a woman's daily average requirement of folic acid to 400 μg. Not only does folate supplementation reduce the incidence substantially, but it also decreases the severity of NTDs should they still occur.

In September 2009, mandatory folic acid fortification was introduced into Australia, requiring Australian millers to add folic acid to wheat flour for bread-making purposes. Current recommendations include folic acid supplementation 1 month before conception and through at least the first 8–12 weeks of pregnancy. All women contemplating pregnancy should ingest a daily multivitamin containing 0.5 mg folic acid. If there is a family history of NTD, one needs to advise that 5 mg is taken. It has been suggested that NTDs are not due to folate deficiency per se, but due to enzymatic abnormalities involving metabolic processes that depend on folate and its metabolites, tetrahydrofolate and 5-methyltetrahydrofolate, abnormalities that could be overcome with folate supplementation.

Neural tube closure is believed to occur in five separate sites within the first 28 days of gestation: NTDs result from failure of closure at one site or failure of two sites to meet, between day 17 and day 28, when the mother may not be aware she is pregnant. Each site may be controlled by separate genes and influenced by differing external factors.

Known environmental influences implicated in the development of NTDs include the following problems in the first-trimester pregnant mother (mnemonic **NTDs causing NTDs**):

Nutritional causes (pregestational low folate [as above]; pregestational high BMI [> 29] increases risk 1.5- to 3.5-fold)

Temperature elevation (pregestational, from fevers or saunas; increases risk up to twofold)

Diabetes (pregestational high blood sugar levels; increases risk 2- to 10-fold) or **D**rugs (AEDs, particularly sodium valproate and carbamazepine; increase risk to 1–2%)

Known genetic causes are far rarer than those mentioned, but are important. Chromosomal causes include the trisomies 13, 18 and 21. There are three major gene pathways which are associated with NTDs: folate 1-carbon metabolism (FOCM) genes (more than 40 genes have been investigated); cilia-related genes (this includes Meckel syndrome type 1 [MSK]; location: 17q22; gene: MKS1; MIM#249000; other genes associated include MKS3, RPGRIP1L, TMEM216, CEP290, CC2D2A, B9D1 and B9D2, all of which are needed for normal ciliogenesis), and PCP (planar cell polarity) pathway genes, variations in which lead to susceptibility to NTDs (MIM#182940): VANGL1 (on 1p13.1), VANGL2 (on 1p23.2), CCL2 (on 17q12), CELSR1 (on 22q13.31), FUZ (on 19q13.33), and T (on 6q27). Other monogenic causes include Waardenburg syndrome type 1 (location: 2q36.1; gene: PAX3; MIM#193500); and Joubert syndrome type 1 (location: 9q34.3; gene: INPP5E; MIM#213300). The total number of affected children with these genetic aetiologies is small in terms of the population burden.

Advances in prenatal diagnosis allow identification of myelomeningocele (MMC) as early as the first trimester. In specialised centres in the US, in-utero repair of fetal MMC (fMMC) has been performed at 18–25 weeks; this can theoretically reverse hindbrain herniation, decrease the need for postnatal ventriculo-peritoneal shunting due to hydrocephalus, and prevent late loss of function due to tethering. By 2009, over 400 fMMC repairs had been performed worldwide. The MOMS (Management Of Myelomeningocele Study) trial ran from 2003 until 2010. The results answered the question of whether prenatal or postnatal closure was preferable: fetal surgery has been shown to decrease the risk of death or placement of a shunt, in the first 12 months of life, and to increase cognitive development and motor abilities at 30 months. The trial was stopped earlier than planned because of these positive results. The American College of Obstetricians and Gynaecologists (ACOG) advises fetal surgery should only be undertaken in units with the required specialised expertise including intensive care facilities and multidisciplinary teams of treating physicians and surgeons. The risks associated with fetal surgery include higher risk of premature delivery, and of pulmonary oedema; obstetric complications may include dehiscence of hysterotomy site and placental abruption.

A child with MMC provides a good example of an examination case with an enormous number of potential problems and management issues. To organise assessment of the child, history-taking and management issues may be structured as follows:

1. How does this child function in day-to-day life (i.e. a brief outline of the child's practical problems)? This will make clear how the disability affects the child's life.
2. What medical problems are relevant in this child?

History
CURRENT HISTORY
How does this child function?

1. *Mobility.* Type, aids, therapy.
2. *Incontinence care*
   a. What is the program for urinary incontinence (e.g. intermittent catheterisation, pads, pants, penile appliances, artificial sphincter, Mitrofanoff procedure [appendicovesicostomy])?
   b. What is the program for bowel care (e.g. regular toileting, laxatives, suppositories, enemas, transanal irrigation devices/system [e.g. Peristeen], Malone Antegrade Continence Enema [MACE])?
3. *Education.* What type of schooling does the child have (e.g. regular school, special class, special school)? What particular problems are there with learning?

4. *Developmental problems.* Related to age (e.g. awareness of disability, making friends, self-esteem, adolescent problems of identity, independence, sexuality, employment). How independent is this child in self-help skills such as bathing, dressing and feeding?

SPECIFIC MEDICAL PROBLEMS

1. *Hydrocephalus.* Does this child have a shunt? Are there any problems with the shunt?
2. *Cognitive aspects.* Are there learning disabilities? Are these related to attentional deficits, difficulties with memory, executive skills, ability to organise? Are there any medications being taken (e.g. stimulants)?
3. *Urinary system.* Infections, operations, any concerns on routine tests (reflux, kidney damage), any medications (antibiotics, anticholinergics).
4. *Bowel management.* Faecal incontinence impairing independence, time taking to manage, effective irrigants, any medications (laxatives), any operations (MACE).
5. *Orthopaedic problems.* Feet and hips (e.g. deformity, pressure areas, problems with splints, callipers, crutches or wheelchairs); spine (see below).
6. *Other significant medical complications.* The 6 **S**s: ask about (a) **S**pine (scoliosis, kyphosis) and **S**keleton (bone health: decreased bone mineral density; fracture propensity); (b) **S**leep-disordered breathing; (c) **S**kin: pressure ulcers, burns, latex allergy; (d) **S**enses: sight and hearing; (e) **S**ize: growth and development—precocious puberty, growth hormone (GH) deficiency, short stature, obesity; (f) **S**eizures.
7. *Issues of adolescence.* Problems with motivation; transition to adult care.

PAST HISTORY

This should include: 1. pregnancy and birth history; 2. antenatal screening; 3. the family history of neural tube defects, including anencephaly; 4. diagnosis; 5. initial management (counselling, understanding of the condition and expectations for the child); 6. early management; and 7. complications (infections, hospitalisations, operations).

SOCIAL HISTORY

Ask about the impact on: 1. the child (e.g. restricted opportunities, fewer friends, teasing, depression, poor motivation); 2. schooling and social integration (poor mobility limits opportunities, time in hospital, missing school, learning difficulties); 3. the family (extra time spent with child, effect on siblings, marriage and finances).

WHAT ASSISTANCE DOES THE FAMILY RECEIVE?

Community supports include community nurse, community therapy, respite care, social worker, Spina Bifida Association and the Crippled Children's Society (now called the Victorian Aids and Equipment Program). After the age of 16, catheters can be accessed via the Commonwealth Continence Aids Payment Scheme (CAPS).

CHILD'S ADAPTATION TO DISABILITY

Ask what he or she thinks about him- or herself (self-esteem), friends, achievements, hopes for future.

Examination

See the separate short case on MMC later in this chapter.

Management

Entire books have been written on almost every aspect of MMC. This section gives a skeleton outline of the more common and important issues raised. Every child with MMC has a unique set of problems, the emphasis of each case being more individualised than the major texts would suggest. The problems tend to be more 'medical' in younger children, and more 'psychosocial' in older children and adolescents. Multidisciplinary clinics represent the gold standard of care, involving collaboration with multiple subspecialists in paediatric/adolescent rehabilitation, neurosurgery, urology, orthopaedics, general paediatrics and internal medicine once transitioned to adult care.

Major disabilities

PARALYSIS

Associated problems include immobility, dependence versus independence, joint contractures, anaesthetic skin risks and pressure necrosis of soft tissues. Barriers to mobility as well as behavioural problems and some degree of cognitive impairment.

Management involves a team approach:

1. Physiotherapy (e.g. ambulation training, wheelchair mobility).
2. Occupational therapy (e.g. functional training, ADLs).
3. Clinical motion analysis: Paediatric Gait Analysis Laboratory (see CP section).
4. Positioning orthoses (e.g. ankle–knee orthoses [AKO], hip-positioning brace).
5. Orthopaedic surgical procedures (e.g. tendon releases or transfers, surgery for dislocated hips). Surgery can be performed on many areas during the same operation.
6. Mobility aids (e.g. crutches, reciprocating gait orthoses (usually younger patients with higher lesions [lower thoracic]), hip–knee–ankle–foot orthoses (HKAFOs [for lesions at lower thoracic level, or L1–L2, adds to ability to be ambulatory]), walkerette, parapodium, wheelchairs).
7. Education regarding risks to skin integrity (e.g. tight clothes, temperature of bath water, sunburn, overtight tying of booties in babies or even hospital identification labels on ankles, ill-fitting orthoses, standing on hot sand at the beach). Aggressive management of pressure necrosis.

SPHINCTER DISTURBANCE

Associated problems include the social disability of incontinence and its medical implications (e.g. infection, renal impairment, hypertension).

BLADDER AND RENAL FUNCTION

Bladder management depends on the type of dysfunction (e.g. dribbling urine; dribbling with increased abdominal pressure, such as during crying or movement; urinary retention). Investigations may clarify this. On occasion, particularly in adolescents, a worsening of bladder control may be the first indication of a problem such as tethered cord, syringomyelia or a failing shunt.

Anticholinergic agents (e.g. oral oxybutynin) may increase bladder storage capacity, and alpha-adrenergic drugs may increase bladder outlet resistance. The combination of these, plus intermittent catheterisation, can prevent residual urine retention and increase continence. Self-catheterisation is encouraged when the child is old enough. Many units' management involves starting all babies on intermittent catheterisation as soon as possible, usually within the first 2 weeks of life. Indicators of high-pressure systems include urinary tract infection, hydronephrosis, vesicoureteric reflux and incomplete emptying; these all mean that intermittent catheterisation should be initiated—if it has not been as yet. Parents are trained in catheterisation, using an appropriately sized catheter with lubricant, starting at a frequency of 3–4 times daily. Generally, a French size 8 catheter is used until the age of 8 years, then size 10 until 10 years, then size 12 until 12 years, then size 14 after that. Other forms of management include BTX-A injection into the detrusor muscle, and intravesical oxybutynin.

Those children who cannot store any urine can be managed by incontinence clothing (pads and pants). Boys can use a penile appliance from about 8 years of age. An artificial sphincter may be considered in this group, although this is very rarely done now because of high complication rates.

If catheterisation is at all difficult, then a Mitrofanoff procedure can be done (the appendix, used as a conduit to the abdominal wall, is fashioned and catheterisation is performed via this stoma). This is useful as children get older and need to be more independent, especially for those with tight adductors or fine motor difficulties who cannot catheterise themselves.

Urinary tract infections (UTIs) need a full course of antibiotics for the acute infection. However, a positive urine culture in the absence of significant symptoms probably reflects urinary tract colonisation rather than infection per se. It is prudent to only treat for a UTI with antibiotics if the child is unwell; otherwise, antibiotic resistance would increase. Only give prophylactic antibiotics in the neonatal period when there is hydronephrosis or vesico-ureteric reflux (VUR). Urine specimens (MSUs) should be obtained to check for infection, when parents suspect (urine odour, child unwell). Surgery may be required for several urinary problems: augmentation cystoplasty if the bladder is small and hypertonic, bladder neck reconstruction or artificial external urinary sphincter. Surgery for VUR may be needed if recurrent UTIs occur despite treatment, and if there is renal scarring or persistent hydronephrosis. Urolithiasis can occur secondary to immobilisation.

Renal review by nephrologist or urologist, with ultrasound or renal scan, and nuclear or radiographic cystogram, are required yearly.

Chronic kidney disease (CKD) can occur in about 5–10% of patients, and the medical management is along standard lines, including peritoneal dialysis and renal transplantation (RTx). It should be noted that, in peritoneal dialysis, an indwelling catheter in the peritoneal cavity with an elevated risk of peritonitis is a consideration in patients with ventriculoperitoneal shunts who are prone to develop shunt infections. An ileal conduit is usually required for transplant as the neurogenic bladder is the cause of the renal failure.

CKD-mineral bone disorder (renal osteodystrophy) in this population is of interest: children with MMC are at increased risk of fracturing their paraplegic lower limbs, even with normal renal function, so that with renal impairment, bone mineralisation is compromised further by metabolic acidosis, secondary hyperparathyroidism and impaired hydroxylation of vitamin D. This can be treated with dietary restriction of phosphate, administration of phosphate binders and 1-OH-vitamin D. The correction of metabolic acidosis is particularly important, as MMC patients may have urinary conduits, bladder augmentation or urinary reservoirs, each of which can cause hyperchloraemic acidosis requiring alkali therapy. For more details on CKD, dialysis and RTx, see Chapter 12, Nephrology.

BOWEL

Bowel management principles include managing constipation with a range of laxatives. Movicol (comprising macrogol, NaCl, KCl and sodium bicarbonate) has proved very useful in some children who have major problems with constipation and faecal impaction. A low-fibre rather than a high-fibre diet is recommended. Rectal emptying by suppositories or enemas may be necessary (when the child reaches the usual age of toilet training). In children with problematic faecal incontinence and constipation, some SB teams recommend regular colonic enemas with hand-warm tap water or commercially prepared normal saline 0.9% solution, given at home from once a day to twice a week. This approach has been reported in one series as permitting the use of nappies/diapers to decrease from 90% to 40%, and allowing both faecal continence and high satisfaction with the procedure in two-thirds of patients. Another approach is a transanal irrigation system (e.g. Peristeen). If none of the above are successful, then consideration should be given to the MACE procedure, emptying the colon of stool using fluid (e.g. glycerine and normal saline) infused through a non-latex catheter inserted into a stoma in the proximal colon; this is done every 2 days to wash out the colon. Glycerine-based irrigants are preferred as they are effective in 95% of cases, and are associated with faster evacuation (averaging around 45 minutes) than other irrigants.

HYDROCEPHALUS

This is seen in 90% of all children with MMC, and is treated with a ventricular shunt. The caudal hindbrain anomaly of the Arnold–Chiari II malformation is present in almost all patients. Associated problems include an increased chance of intellectual impairment, and shunt complications such as infection, obstruction (underdrainage), low-pressure syndrome (overdrainage) or seizures. An average of two shunt changes are needed in the first 10 years. Management includes appropriate schooling for intellectual impairment, and education regarding complications of shunts and their presentation. (There is another procedure that has been used as an alternative to shunt placement: endoscopic third ventriculostomy [ETV], which has a success rate of up to 72%; this is mentioned for completion.)

Underdrainage can be due to blockage of the shunt tubing, the shunt breaking or parts becoming disconnected. Classic presentation includes headache (worse on waking, before rising in the morning), nausea, vomiting, dizziness, listlessness, lethargy, poor feeding, insidious deterioration in behaviour (e.g. irritable or disruptive) or intellectual functioning (worsening school performance), and onset of, or worsening of, fitting. In addition, shunt malfunction can present as a change in motor performance (e.g. decreased muscle strength, loss of previously acquired motor skills, increase in spasticity in upper or lower limbs), alteration in gait, change in bladder or bowel habit, change in lower cranial nerve function, back pain, worsening scoliosis and worsening of lower limb orthopaedic deformities. Very rarely, the sole indicator of shunt malfunction is papilloedema, so it is worth checking the fundi every time a doctor is seen.

Overdrainage has a somewhat similar presentation: headache (worsened by getting up from lying down), dizziness and fainting. If rapid, a subdural haemorrhage can result, with symptoms varying from headache to those of a stroke. If gradual, 'slit ventricle' syndrome can occur, and can cause high pressure to reappear, but with small ventricles on scanning). Various symptoms in a patient with a shunt may be attributed to the shunt unless a definite alternative diagnosis is apparent.

Infection of shunts is almost always due to bacteria getting into the cerebrospinal fluid (CSF) or shunt at the time of operation; hence it is most common within first 3 days of shunt placement. On occasion, infection can present as shunt blockage within weeks or months of operation. An infected shunt must be removed and replaced with a new clean shunt. Progress is being made in developing shunts that are resistant to bacterial infection.

In any child with a shunt, if there is any deterioration in neurological, orthopaedic or urological function, it should be assumed to be due to shunt dysfunction until proved otherwise. Generally, a cranial CT scan is performed in the first instance to exclude blockage.

Other useful investigations with shunt problems may include cerebrospinal fluid analysis, plain X-rays (head, chest, abdomen) to demonstrate shunt position and to check for disconnection, cranial CT or MRI scans, and radioisotope studies (e.g. computerised clearance study for clearance over 24 hours, or direct injection of isotope into the shunt to check shunt patency).

THE ARNOLD–CHIARI II MALFORMATION, SYRINGOMYELIA AND SCOLIOSIS

The *Arnold–Chiari II malformation* comprises downward displacement of the cerebellar tonsils and vermis through the foramen magnum, elongation and kinking of the medulla, caudal displacement of the cervical spinal cord and medulla, and obliteration of the cisterna magna. Descent of the hindbrain through the foramen magnum can cause compression of the brainstem and lead to dysfunction of the cerebellum, medullary respiratory centre and cranial nerves IX and X, and to hydrocephalus. It also incorporates other brain malformations (e.g. callosal dysgenesis, abnormalities of neuronal migration and brain sulcation) that may be associated with learning disabilities experienced by some children with spina bifida. It causes symptoms sufficient to require surgical treatment in about 15–35% of patients.

Symptoms can include: swallowing difficulties (due to lower cranial nerve or brainstem dysfunction), choking on foods (especially liquids), nasal regurgitation or gastro-oesophageal reflux when drinking or vomiting, repeated aspiration pneumonia episodes, dysarthria, OSA, cyanosis, stridor (inspiratory), hoarse or high-pitched cry, oculomotor dysfunction, weakness or spasticity of upper limbs, neck pain, headache, scoliosis, dizziness, clumsiness or poor coordination (the last three being cerebellar symptoms).

Surgical treatment involves decompression of the medulla and upper cervical cord, then insertion of a dural patch graft (duraplasty) to increase the size of the dural sac. Cervical laminectomy is performed below the lowest level of the cerebellar tonsils. In response to surgical decompression, brainstem abnormalities improve in 50%, and upper limb weakness, cerebellar function and pain improve in 80% of cases.

Syringomyelia is a cavity which communicates with the central canal of the spinal cord; hydromyelia is dilatation of the central canal; the term 'syringohydromyelia' encompasses the two, as differentiating between them is challenging. Syringohydromyelia can develop secondary to the Chiari malformation, causing abnormal cerebrospinal fluid dynamics. Apart from the bulbar symptoms, many of the problems described above can be attributed to syringohydromyelia. Syrinxes can be of varying sizes and range along the spinal cord. They can reach holocord dimensions, meaning that they have just a thin rim of spinal cord around the fluid-filled syrinx. Syringohydromyelia is significantly associated with scoliosis, and lower limb weakness and deformities. MRI can show the size and range of syrinxes. The size of the syrinx does not seem to correlate with the degree of associated scoliosis; it seems that the presence of syringohydromyelia is sufficient to cause scoliosis. Syrinxes can be seen on MRI in around 80% of patients with MMC, but are symptomatic in only 2–5%. Usual presenting features are upper limb weakness, back pain, scoliosis and spasticity or motor loss in the lower limbs. Extension of syringohydromyelia can affect lower cranial nerves and brainstem function. Symptoms from syringohydromyelia can be due to associated hydrocephalus or shunt malfunction, and resolve when this underlying cause is corrected. The posterior decompression of the foramen magnum and upper cervical spine to decompress the Chiari malformation often reduces the size of the syringohydromyelia. A shunt from syrinx to peritoneal cavity can relieve the problem.

Scoliosis in MMC patients can be caused by congenital malformations of the spine, but more often scoliosis is acquired due to intraspinal abnormalities, such as syringohydromyelia, tethered cord or shunt failure. When hydrocephalus with syringohydromyelia is drained, there are improvements in scoliosis if the Cobb angle is small (measuring less than 30°). Around 50% of children with MMC have scoliosis, the higher the lesion the more likely the scoliosis: thoracic rate 90%, mid-lumbar 40%, low lumbar 10%. Acquired scoliosis is due to spinal muscle weakness. It increases with age. Bracing does not work and could lead to more pressure sores. Larger curves (> 30°) require formal surgical interventions. Associated problems of scoliosis can include: impairment of balance (changed centre of gravity); decreased total lung capacity, with an increased risk of infection and cor pulmonale; impairment of height; need for surgery (e.g. Harrington rods) and consequent prolonged hospitalisation. The surgical goals are stopping the progressive development of curving, and correcting pelvic obliquity, for improved sitting and fewer pressure sores. Spinal fusion, the usual definitive treatment, is reserved for children who have completed the majority of their growth. The fusion is often left short of the pelvis, as fusing the spine to the pelvis has led to some ambulatory patients losing their ability to walk, as they can no longer maintain balance.

There are now growing constructs (e.g. vertically expanding prosthetic titanium rib systems, growing rods) which enable still-growing younger children with more severe curves to achieve spinal stabilisation without any disadvantage to the final height of their trunk. Many units have found that when patients with subtle signs of neurological deterioration are closely followed, aggressively investigated, and dealt with by revising shunts for hydrocephalus or decompressing the Chiari malformation, then there is a marked decrease in patients who have scoliosis in their clinics at follow-up.

THE TETHERED CORD

This is present in virtually all children with MMC (seen on MRI dorsally in the area of the previous defect), because of the nature of the closure of the MMC, but only causes problems requiring surgical intervention in around one-third, who manifest symptoms or signs of tethering generally during growth spurts, as in adolescence. These include gait changes (especially crouched gait), back (at site of defect) or lower limb pain, worsening of motor function (decreased muscle strength or increased tone), change in sensory level, change in bladder or bowel habit, altered gait, or progressive orthopaedic deformities of the spine or lower limbs, particularly foot deformities (e.g. unilateral equinus deformity). Imaging includes MRI to confirm tethering and define the regional anatomy, and to identify any associated lesions (syringohydromyelia, lipomas) that could produce similar symptomatology or signs. Surgical untethering involves reopening the original repair wound, dissecting the scarred part of the cord from the dura and checking for any other areas of tethering (e.g. thickened filum terminale). The surgical outcome is very good: 72% of patients have improvement of preoperative motor impairments, 25% cause stabilisation of motor impairment, although 3% can worsen. Tethered cord can recur.

NEUROLOGICAL DISEASE PROGRESSION IN ADOLESCENCE

Because of their rapid growth, adolescents are particularly prone to neurological deterioration from the above conditions, including tethered cord, syringohydromyelia or Chiari malformation, or a failed ventricular-peritoneal (VP) shunt. Hence, if there is any deterioration, even subtle, in any aspect of the patient's wellbeing, such as progression in their scoliosis (which should always prompt exclusion of intraspinal anomalies), a recent change in a club foot, new levels or locations of weakness, new pressure sores on the foot, sacrum or pelvis, then these four areas must be given first priority as differential diagnoses: remember (in anatomically descending order): Scoliosis Causes: Shunt: Chiari, Syrinx, Cord (tethered) (SC, SC, SC).

Other significant disabilities (the six Ss)

SLEEP-DISORDERED BREATHING (SDB)

Around 20% of patients with MMC have sleep-disordered breathing (SDB), from simple snoring to OSA. Consequences of SDB include fragmented sleep, developmental delay, behaviour problems (often ADHD-like), learning problems, headaches, bed wetting, poor growth and cor pulmonale from the repetitive hypoxic episodes. A concerning statistic is an 8–9% incidence of sudden death during sleep in these patients. All patients with the Chiari malformation or with lesions above T10 should have formal sleep studies (for management, see the long case on OSA in Chapter 15, The respiratory system).

SPINE (SCOLIOSIS, KYPHOSIS)/SKELETON (HIPS, KNEES, ANKLES)/FRACTURES, BONE HEALTH

Scoliosis is discussed on the previous page. Kyphosis increases the risk for needing multiple shunt revisions. The natural history of sagittal plane kyphosis is progression at about 8° per year, leading to intolerance of sitting and loss of independent use of the hands while sitting. Associated skin instability and breakdown can occur. Kyphosis has a serious negative impact on self-esteem. Some centres operate at age 2–5 years. Surgical correction techniques have included excision of apical vertebrae, stabilised with instrumentation, and multiple lordosing intervertebral osteotomies (decancellation kyphectomy). Hip problems including subluxation, dislocation and contractures are all due to muscle imbalance. A counterintuitive observation in MMC is that unilateral or bilateral dislocated hip in an ambulant patient does not affect gait symmetry, and with unilateral dislocation, does not affect walking speed; in MMC the dislocated hip is essentially pain free, and the focus is not on relocating the hip(s), but on maintaining range of movement, which may mean contracture release. Knee flexion and extension contractures can both be seen, flexion in those with higher lesions with weak quadriceps muscles, due to prolonged sitting with knees flexed, and extension in those with mid-lumbar lesions due to unopposed quadriceps activity. Foot and ankle deformities are usual in MMC, such as congenital clubfoot (presents in 50%), and vertical talus; unbalanced forces secondary to muscle weakness lead to these deformities. A foot with a calcaneus deformity (very dorsiflexed) is due to unopposed tibialis anterior activity in MMC at L4–L5. Should a progressive foot deformity become apparent (e.g. evolving pes cavus), then a syrinx or tethered cord should be considered. Between 11 and 30% of children with MMC experience fractures, due to reduced bone mineral density secondary to decreased ambulation and to muscle weakness; fractures may be pain free in MMC, and are identified by warmth and swelling. Bisphosphonates are not standard treatment but can be considered for children with MMC who have already had a fracture.

SKIN

With loss of sensation below the waist, pressure ulcers are among the main reasons for hospital admission. Pressure sores can be graded from Stage 1 (intact skin) to Stage 4 (full-thickness skin loss). Any skin breakdown should be taken very seriously. Care in protecting the skin during simple ADLs can avoid prolonged hospitalisation. Burns can occur easily with normal activities (e.g. during a bath, resting against the hot tap).

Anaesthetic areas of skin can also lead to missing significant pathology that would normally present with pain (e.g. significant infections or orthopaedic injuries that are not felt, and only noticed by swelling or redness). Poorly fitting callipers, crutches or wheelchairs can cause substantial skin breakdown before it is noticed. All of these areas become more of a problem with increasing independence and self-care. In treating pressure areas, avoid film dressings, as these, in combination with the excessive sweating often seen in these children, worsen skin breakdown. The majority of commercially available wound dressings are adequate for pressure ulcers. Management also requires comprises pressure relief.

SENSES: VISION (SQUINT) AND HEARING

Squint can be associated with hydrocephalus and can lead to amblyopia if missed. Referral to an ophthalmologist is necessary. Hearing should be assessed routinely.

SIZE

These patients have a small stature, with short lower limbs, and are obese for their height. Some of these issues are related to HP axis disruption, which is caused by hydrocephalus. Recently endocrine aspects have been studied in MMC, such as leptin secretion, GH deficiency and precocious puberty. Leptin, from adipose tissue, regulates satiety. Leptin dysfunction leads to obesity and delayed puberty; treatment with leptin causes weight reduction and continuation of puberty. It has been reported that GH-deficient children with MMC have abnormal nocturnal leptin secretion. Precocious puberty is associated with precocious puberty; perinatal raised intracranial pressure in patients with MMC leads to early and precocious puberty. Between 30 and 70% of children with MMC have GH deficiency. Recombinant human growth hormone (rhGH) is appropriate for some children with MMC and small stature, particularly if they have CKD. Treatment with GH has been shown not only to improve height, but also to improve BMI and muscle strength, ambulation, and in a proportion of adults, to stop progression of scoliosis.

SEIZURES

Epilepsy occurs in 15–20% of children with MMC and should be managed with careful consideration to possible pregnancy in female patients and to the issue of fit-free periods before applying for a driver's licence.

Other problems
SOCIAL ISSUES

These can be the most important issues, particularly in older children. Problems include low self-esteem, with a propensity to depression. Those who are not socially continent have lower self-esteem. Other issues include ongoing dependence on parents, leading to living at home indefinitely, seeking partners who will 'care' for them (parent substitute), unrealistic expectations about marriage and employment prospects. One way to boost self-esteem is to encourage children to participate in decision-making (e.g. type of crutches, what kind of bracing, colour of wheelchair), and to include them in discussions about incontinence care and surgical interventions, if old enough. In terms of helping them to become more self-sufficient in society, their attention should be focused on the long-term picture, so that realistic educational and employment goals can be set.

Adolescence brings its own set of stresses. Those with MMC tend to be around 2 to 5 years behind typical adolescents, in the areas of self-care and autonomy. In these children, areas of concern include appearance and presentability. Problems such as pressure sores, obesity, leaking of urine and progression of scoliosis become paramount. Other problems include denial of disability, difficulty establishing identity, independence, friendships with the opposite sex and appropriate sexual functioning.

Adolescence brings its own set of stresses. Those with MMC tend to be around 2 to 5 years behind typical adolescents, in the areas of self-care and autonomy. In these children, areas of concern include appearance and presentability. Problems such as pressure sores, obesity, leaking of urine and progression of scoliosis become paramount. Other problems include denial of disability, difficulty establishing identity, independence, friendships with the opposite sex and appropriate sexual functioning.

When patients reach adulthood, the attendance rate at multidisciplinary clinics drops by around 50%, lack of motivation being but one possible cause. Secondary effects may include neglect of skin care or of adequate catheterisation techniques. Apathy due to having the disorder per se, as well as secondary depression, are not uncommon in adults, and the use of antidepressants may be warranted. Suicidal ideation is not uncommon, and anxiety issues often arise. The local doctor is usually best placed to assess for these sorts of problems.

TRANSITION TO ADULT CARE

The positive aspects of transition include patients wanting to be treated 'like an adult'. Parents, however, do not appreciate disconnecting lifelong relationships with their paediatric doctors, and being able to exert less control around medical issues. Transition discussions about timing should be during periods of relative wellness, not when the child is in hospital for a current clinical problem. The negative aspect of transition, as above, is the poor follow-up rate once adulthood is reached. This is a serious issue; many patients whose multidisciplinary SB clinics they attended either ceased or became inaccessible were lost to medical follow-up, and this led to significant morbidities including nephrectomy and amputation. A smooth coordinated transition to adult care is extremely important. The greatest barrier to such smooth transition is finding access to adult subspecialists with an interest in special needs patients. Some units refer to specialists involved in managing adult patients with spinal cord injury.

SEX EDUCATION

Sex education is an area of great importance. Because of years of incontinence, and catheterisation by helpers, modesty may not have been encouraged. This population is at risk of sexual abuse, and there is at least one paper that quotes 25% incidence (on self-report). Group discussions regarding sexuality in disabled people may be very beneficial. Group outings may improve socialisation skills, and encourage appropriate friendships.

YOUNG WOMEN WITH MMC

Females with MMC have normal fertility. Almost all females with lesions below L3 have vulval sensation and most can experience orgasm. Contraception must be discussed with any adolescent female patient. Folate supplementation must be stressed as vitally important. Pap smears and mammograms must not be overlooked. Pregnant women with SB require management by 'high-risk' experienced obstetricians. In labour, some patients may not feel contractions so need to depend on other signs of labour (e.g. rupture of membranes). An adolescent or adult female with MMC has an increased risk (1 in 20) with each pregnancy of producing a child with MMC. Antenatal screening should be discussed.

The problems of caring for a child with MMC when the parent is also disabled are indeed considerable. Most young adults with MMC wish to have children of their own.

YOUNG MEN WITH MMC

Many males with MMC have the ability to achieve erections (around 70%), ejaculation (dripping ejaculation in around 50%), orgasm (around 20%), and many are infertile.

There is a procedure **to max**imise sensation sexuality and quality of life (**TOMAX**); this is a microneurorraphy which attaches the ilioinguinal nerve to the dorsal nerve and increases sensation to the glans penis postoperatively, and improves quality of life. This attempts to restore the penile sensory impulses (normally these travel via two dorsal nerves and pudendal nerve to S2–S4 sacral roots, which is interrupted in MMC). This procedure is underused, presumably from lack of awareness of it among physicians.

LATEX ALLERGY

Children with MMC are 500 times more likely to develop latex allergy than the general population. Latex is a substance derived from the sap of *Hevea brasiliensis*, the functional unit being the rubber particle—a spherical drop of polyisoprene. There is a clinical and immunochemical cross-reactivity between latex and avocado, banana, kiwi, papaya and chestnut.

Exposure to latex antigen can occur by skin, mucosal or parenteral routes. Latex gloves are dusted in cornflour powder, which is a potent carrier of latex antigen. Exposure to latex occurs with surgical procedures, rectal disimpaction and bladder catheterisation. Up to 50% of SB patients may have latex-specific IgE. Children with a history of adverse reactions to latex should have serum RAST (radioallergosorbent test) or enzyme-linked immunosorbent assay to look for latex-specific IgE. The parents, carers and school, medical and allied health professionals involved with the child must be able to identify latex allergy reactions and respond appropriately if an allergic reaction does occur (e.g. availability of adrenaline if there has been a previous severe or anaphylactic reaction). The (obvious) treatment for the condition is avoidance of latex and the foods that cross-react with it. Operating in a latex-free environment is the usual practice in many paediatric institutions. Sexually active males and partners of sexually active females need to have access to latex-free condoms.

GENETIC ISSUES

The mother of a child with a NTD has triple the risk for another NTD-affected pregnancy with each subsequent pregnancy. The recurrence rate for a mother of a child with an NTD is between 1 in 100 and 1 in 200. The risk for a first-degree relative (e.g. sibling, child, parent) having a fetus with a NTD is between 1 in 30 and 1 in 140, and the risk for a second degree relative (e.g. half-sibling, grandchild, grandparent) is between 1 in 90 and 1 in 220. Antenatal screening involves detailed ultrasound at 16 weeks (95% accurate in experienced hands) and amniocentesis to measure alpha fetoprotein and acetylcholinesterase, which are elevated with an open MMC lesion. The accuracy of ultrasound together with amniocentesis clearly should exceed 95%. If a fetus is affected, options available for expectant mothers to consider include termination or expectant management, in most countries; in specialised centres in the US, a third option of in-utero repair of the MMC at 18–25 weeks' gestation may be available.

PROGNOSIS

Around 80% of children with MMC have IQs in the normal range. Among those with normal intelligence, 60% have some form of learning disability, particularly problems with mathematics, sequencing of information, problem-solving, language, and visual perception. Neuropsychological profiling can identify particular phenotypes and help to improve functioning. Unfortunately the difficulties with mathematics, executive function and language are not delays, but rather persist into adulthood. Problems with attention, of ADHD proportions, are often seen. Approximately 70% of surviving children walk well enough to function in the community. Social continence (free of urinary incontinence in social situations) is achieved in 85% of school-aged children. Of adult patients, 80% are independent in the community, 30% attend or finish tertiary education, and around one-third are employed.

LONG CASE: Neurofibromatous type 1 (NF1)

Background

Neurofibromatous type 1 (NF1, MIM#162200) is an autosomal dominant disorder, due to mutations in the NF1 gene, which is in the long arm of chromosome 17 at 17q11.2, and affects 1 in 3500 people. These mutations can be whole-gene deletions (in 4–5%) or partial gene deletions, insertions, amino acid substitutions, stop mutations, nonsense or missense mutations, splicing mutations (in 30%), nucleotide changes or intragenic copy number changes. There are well over 1000 pathogenic variants in NF1, many being specific to certain families. Around 50% of people with NF1 have a de novo mutation.

The NF1 gene is around 350 kilobases in size, and has 61 exons, and codes for *neurofibromin 1* (OMIM*613113), a 327-kD protein containing 2839 amino acids; it is a cytoplasmic protein found in neurons, oligodendrocytes, Schwann cells and leukocytes. The NF1 gene has a very high mutation rate.

Neurofibromin 1 regulates a number of different intracellular processes, including assembly of the cytoskeleton, activating *ras* GTPase (guanosine triphosphate-ase), which controls cellular proliferation (this suppresses tumour formation; *ras* was the first identified proto-oncogene, standing for *retrovirus-associated* DNA *sequences*), and regulating adenylate cyclase activity, and intracellular cyclic AMP generation. The *ras*-neurofibromin signal transduction pathway is a target for medical therapies.

Neurofibromin 1 is found throughout the nervous system, functioning as a tumour suppressor. Loss of neurofibromin 1 (by somatic mutation) leads to increased risk of development of tumours, both benign and malignant. Hence a loss of neurofibromin occurs in NF1-associated tumours, but many features are not accounted for by the interaction between neurofibromin and *ras*. The cells most affected by NF1 mutations are derived from the neural crest.

NF1 shows marked clinical variability. Clear genotypic-phenotypic correlations are few. Whole NF1 gene microdeletion (which also affects some adjacent genes) correlates with dysmorphic facial features, accompanied by more significant cognitive impairments, earlier-appearing and very numerous cutaneous neurofibromas, and overgrowth (somatic) with large hands and feet.

At the other end of the scale, there is a form of NF1 where there are the usual pigmentary findings but no cutaneous or plexiform neurofibromas or other severe complications; this is due to a three-base pair in-frame deletion of exon 17 (NF Consortium numbering; exon 22 for NCBI numbering).

Age-related presentation

In NF1, one can anticipate the emergence of different features at different ages. At any age, developmental delay/learning issues can occur, and plexiform neuromas can make an appearance. Diffuse plexiform neuromas affecting the head and neck typically occur before 1 year of age, and those affecting other parts of the body occur before adolescence.

From birth until 8, optic pathway tumours can occur. From 2 years onwards, hypertension can occur. With respect to skin findings, from birth to 2 years: café-au-lait macules (CALM); from 3 to 5 years: intertriginous freckling (axillae, groins); from 5 years onward, development of neurofibromas. Lisch nodules are expected to appear between 5 and 10 years.

Bony anomalies (long bone bowing [tibial pseudoarthrosis], and sphenoid wing dysplasia [SWD]) are congenital and usually noticed within the first 2 years. Rapidly progressive dysplastic scoliosis typically occurs between 6 and 10, whereas milder forms similar to idiopathic scoliosis occur during adolescence. Malignant peripheral nerve sheath tumours (MPNSTs) can occur from adolescence onward. Adults get progression of dermal neurofibromas.

Diagnosis

For a diagnosis of NF1, there are National Institutes of Health (NIH) criteria which must be met. These are two or more of: 1. six or more café-au-lait macules > 5 mm greatest diameter in prepubertal children, and > 15 mm diameter in postpubertal people; 2. two or more neurofibromas of any type, or one plexiform neuroma; 3. freckling in the axillary or inguinal region; 4. optic glioma; 5. two or more Lisch nodules (iris hamartomas); 6. distinctive osseous lesions such as sphenoid dysplasia or tibial pseudoarthrosis; and 7. a first-degree relative with the NF1.

These criteria apply extremely well to adults, and also to children 4 years and over. In younger children, however, unless they have an affected first-degree relative, only a proportion of children who do have NF1 meet the NIH criteria; at age one this is only around half these children meeting the criteria, but virtually all of these same children meet criteria by 8 years old.

Molecular genetic diagnosis is infrequently indicated: in cases where NF1 is suspected but does not fulfil criteria (e.g. developing an optic glioma, with no other features); in cases of at-risk relatives in families with spinal NF1, or with NF1 c.2970–2972 del AAT mutation, which may not meet criteria for NF1 in childhood. If molecular testing for NF1 is undertaken, there is a multi-step mutation detection protocol which finds > 95% of NF1 pathogenic variants in those fulfilling the clinical NIH criteria.

DIAGNOSTIC CRITERIA FOR NF1

Mnemonic **FIBROMA**

Fibromatous tumours (plexiform neuromas)	occur in 30–50%
Iris hamartomas (Lisch nodules) > 2	occur in 90%
Bone lesions: tibial pseudoarthrosis; SWD	occur in 2%; 1%
Relative (first degree) with NF1	occur in 50%
Optic pathway glioma (OPG)	occur in 15–30%
Macules (CALM): 6 > 5 mm pre-, > 15 mm postpuberty	occurs in > 99%
Axillary and inguinal freckling	occurs in > 90%

SKIN MANIFESTATIONS: CAFÉ-AU-LAIT MACULES, FRECKLING, NEUROFIBROMAS

Almost all patients with NF1 have *CAL macules*, and over 90% have intertriginous freckling with more freckling occurring in sun-exposed areas. CAL spots are typically 1–3 cm diameter, flat and seen more readily with a Wood's light; they do not occur on palms or soles. Adults with NF1 almost invariably have many benign skin *neurofibromas*; more neurofibromas develop throughout life; they can increase substantially and rapidly during pregnancy. Around 50% of NF1 patients develop *plexiform neuromas*, although these are frequently internal, hidden from clinical suspicion. They can cause significant disfigurement and can impinge on vital structures (such as the airway). Non-diagnostic skin findings can include *nevus anemicus* which is pale but does not redden when rubbed, and *juvenile xanthogranuloma* which are orange papules which tend to be in groups.

VISION

The most well-known features involving the eyes are *optic pathway gliomas (OPGs)* and *Lisch nodules*. OPGs are benign, pilocytic astrocytomas, but can be serious, especially in children under 7 years; they can cause loss of visual acuity, abnormal colour vision, visual field cuts, strabismus, proptosis or even hypothalamic dysfunction. *Lisch nodules* (hamartomas of the iris) cause no problems at all. Pulsatile proptosis can occur in patients with SWD which causes a bony defect behind the eyeball, and allows the temporal lobe to herniate into the orbit, causing the visible (brain) pulsatility. Non-diagnostic eye lesions can include *neovascular glaucoma* and *retinal vasoproliferative tumours*.

NEUROLOGICAL SYSTEM, LEARNING ISSUES AND BEHAVIOURAL PROBLEMS

Most children with NF1 have normal IQs. However, the majority (50–75%) have some memory or specific learning problems, ADHD symptomatology and difficulties at school. Around 30% have ASD features. Intellectual impairment is seen in 6–7%, which is about double that of the typical population. Particularly common are attentional issues, visual spatial problems and social competence difficulties. Low self-esteem is common. Poor interpretation of social cues is another well-recognised issue in NF1.

Children with NF1 have difficulties with running, hopping, skateboarding or riding a bike, as well as problems writing or drawing (holding a pencil is more challenging) or independently getting dressed. Seizures occur more in NF1 patients, especially focal seizures which can represent an underlying tumour or stroke.

Sleeping difficulties, and headaches (including migraine), are more common in NF1 patients than in the general populace. Rarer causes for headache in NF1 can include intracranial aneurysms, in addition to the more well-known intracranial tumours (e.g. brainstem glioma, cerebellar glioma). Diffuse polyneuropathy can occur with multiple nerve root tumours, and malignant transformation can occur, with the development of MPNSTs; around 10% of NF1 patients develop these. MPNSTs occur more often in those with whole-gene deletion, or with subcutaneous neurofibromas, or with a number of plexiform neuromas. Plexiform neuromas can be painful, as can be malignant transformation to a MPNST, so an alteration in pain warrants further evaluation.

MUSCULOSKELETAL

There are two forms of scoliosis seen in NF1. *Dystrophic scoliosis* is the less common form, which occurs earlier and can progress rapidly; it occurs under the age of 10 (often 6–8 years old), involves a shorter segment (usually 4–6 spinal segments), distorts the vertebral bodies, describes a more acute angle and is more common in girls. There can be an associated underlying plexiform neurofibroma. *Non-dystrophic scoliosis* is similar to idiopathic scoliosis, is mild and rarely needs any treatment.

Bone involvement can include the congenital diagnostic criterion: long bone dysplasia (such as tibial pseudoarthrosis [so-called as the bowing makes it almost appear as if there is a joint present]), which is an inherent anomaly of the bone itself; and SWD, which is associated with adjacent plexiform neuromas, and can present with asymmetry of orbits, or pulsating exophthalmos, or more commonly, strabismus. Vertebral dysplasia can occur in association with plexiform neuroma and/or dural ectasia.

NF1 is associated with decreased mineral bone density; contributing factors include increased bone resorption and vitamin D deficiency. In adults aged in their 40s, 50% have osteopenia and almost 20% have osteoporosis. There is an increased risk of fractures in NF1.

HYPERTENSION AND VASCULOPATHY

Hypertension occurs in around 2% of children with NF1. The differential diagnostic list is broad: coarctation of the aorta; renal artery stenosis; other renovascular causes;

and neuroendocrine derived tumours which produce vasoactive chemicals, such as phaeochromocytoma, ganglioneuroma or neuroblastoma. The management of hypertension depends on the cause.

NF1 vasculopathy involves larger vessels and can lead to abnormal cerebrovasculature, with narrowing of major arteries (internal carotid, middle cerebral, anterior cerebral). Moyamoya telangiectatic vessels develop around the narrowed segments. NF1 patients also have anatomical variants of the cerebral vessels more often than the general population. Coronary artery disease is also more common in NF1 patients.

CARDIAC

Pulmonary valve stenosis is the heart defect seen most often in NF1 (occurs in 2%); it is also a feature of three particular subgroups of NF1: those with whole-gene deletions; those with NF1-Noonan syndrome (see below); and those with Watson syndrome (see overleaf). Left heart obstructive lesions, such as coarctation of the aorta (where the narrowing can be long and fusiform), and aortic valve stenosis, occur with increased frequency in NF1. Those with whole-gene deletions can get several other types of congenital heart disease (pulmonary valve stenosis is just the most common), or hypertrophic cardiomyopathy. Intracardiac neurofibromas occur on occasion.

GROWTH

Children with NF1 often have head circumference above average and height below average. Whole-gene deletion NF1 demonstrate a quite different pattern, with overgrowth of all parameters, particularly height, especially between 2 and 6 years of age. Although both precocious puberty (especially with chiasmal tumours, and these children are taller) and delayed puberty (mechanism unclear) are well described in NF1, most children have normal puberty.

TUMOURS

The most common tumours are: benign neurofibromas (Schwann cell tumours) which can affect any nerve; optic gliomas (benign; females with NF1 are more likely to need treatment for these); and brain tumours (such as brainstem gliomas and cerebellar gliomas). Gliomas of the brainstem and cerebellum are less aggressive in NF1 patients. In patients with gliomas treated by radiotherapy, second tumours can arise in the radiation treatment field, such as non-optic gliomas, and MPNST.

MPNSTs are the most common malignancies associated with NF1, being encountered in around of 10% NF1 patients. The following list includes a selected number of tumours associated with NF1.

The list of tumours in NF1 can be expressed as an alphabetic run: **LMNOP + DR G**:

Leukaemia (juvenile chronic myelogenous leukaemia, myelodysplastic syndromes)
Meningioma/**M**alignant peripheral nerve sheath tumours (MPNSTs)
Neurofibromas (dermal, diffuse plexiform, deep nodular plexiform)/
  Neurofibrosarcoma/**N**euroblastoma
Optic pathway glioma (OPG)
Phaeochromocytoma/**P**ilocytic astrocytoma/**P**arathyroid adenoma/**P**ancreatic
  somatostatinoma
+
Duodenal carcinoid/**D**uodenal somatostatinoma
Rhabdomyosarcoma/**R**etinal vasoproliferative tumours
Gliomas (hypothalamic-optochiasmatic, brainstem, cerebellar, second tumours after
  XRT of first tumours)/**G**astrointestinal stromal tumours (GIST)

GASTROINTESTINAL FEATURES

GISTs tend to occur in the proximal small intestine, present with bowel obstruction or gastrointestinal bleeding. One study has identified an importance cooccurrence between GIST and phaeochromocytoma, leading to the suggestion that any child undergoing any surgical procedure to assess for GIST should be assessed for phaeochromocytoma first.

CORRELATIONS BETWEEN MUTANT ALLELES AND CLINICAL PHENOTYPES

Genotype-phenotype correlations so far described (as of 2016) include:

1. Large or complete gene deletions lead to severe disease, including cognitive involvement, cardiovascular disease, occurrence of benign and malignant tumours, dysmorphic features and somatic overgrowth including large hands and feet.
2. Mutations in the upper (proximal) third of the NF1 gene are associated with OPGs.
3. Constitutional missense or splicing mutations are associated with spinal NF1.
4. Truncating mutations are associated with solid malignancies and 'elephantiasis'.
5. Non-truncating mutations are associated with cardiac defects such as pulmonary stenosis.
6. p.Arg 1809 missense mutation correlates with 'Noonan-like' dysmorphic features, no skin manifestations and pulmonary stenosis.
7. A specific 3-base-pairs in-frame deletion of exon 17 (c.2970–2972 delAAT) which leads to typical pigmentary findings of NF1 but no neurofibromas.

Dual diagnoses and specific phenotypes

Some 12% of children with NF1 also have features of Noonan syndrome. The *NF1-Noonan phenotype* includes pulmonary stenosis, webbing of the neck, low-set ears, hypertelorism and downslanting palpebral fissures. It has a number of causes, including two dominant mutations occurring together in the one family; in most patients with NF1-Noonan syndrome, there are constitutional mutations of the NF1 gene as in point 6 above. The PTPN11 gene, which is found in 50% of Noonan syndrome patients, has also been reported in this phenotype. Both NF1 and Noonan syndrome involve mutations in genes encoding for proteins concerned with *ras* signalling; this shared pathway may be the reason for the phenotypic overlap.

Segmental NF1 refers to a condition where NF1 is limited to one part of the body, where neither parent is affected by NF1.

Watson syndrome (WTSN) (MIM 193520) is due to mutation in the NF1 gene; features include pulmonary valve stenosis, CAL spots, Lisch nodules, decreased cognition, short stature and macrocephaly; a third of affected children have sufficient criteria to diagnose NF1. Patients with WTSN do not have any neurofibromas.

History

Ask about the following.

PRESENTING COMPLAINT

Reason for current admission.

CURRENT SYMPTOMS

1. Cognitive abilities, or present developmental status (e.g. intellectual impairment), schooling details.
2. Learning issues at school (e.g. visual-spatial-perceptual skills, reading disability, executive functioning skills, any neuropsychometric testing by guidance officer), any help needed, attitudes of class teacher, fellow students.

3. Behavioural issues (e.g. ADHD, ASD symptomatology and any relevant medications such as stimulants), professionals involved in management (psychologist, psychiatrist, paediatrician, therapists).
4. Vision (e.g. decreased visual acuity, decreased field of view, prominence of eyes, agitation, known optic glioma progress with MRI results, frequency of ophthalmic/ MRI evaluations).
5. Speech, hearing, communication problems, professionals involved.
6. Growth and puberty (e.g. large head, short stature, tall stature, precocious puberty [tall stature plus precocious puberty suggesting optic chiasmal glioma], delayed puberty, disproportionate growth of extremities with plexiform neurofibromas). In those with complete deletion of the NF1 locus, there can be overgrowth between ages of 2 and 6.
7. Tumours (e.g. neurofibromas, which are benign Schwann cell tumours); when appeared, how presented, current known tumours, any changes in size or any pain (plexiform neurofibromas commonly associated with pain), previous treatment (e.g. radiotherapy, chemotherapy, what agents used [risk of second tumour higher if treated with alkylating agents in NF1 patients], current treatment regime).
8. Musculoskeletal problems: any bone issues (e.g. SWD with pulsatile proptosis; vertebral dysplasia; pseudoarthrosis [bowing] of tibia, fibula; osteoporosis), and management thereof, or any spinal problems (e.g. scoliosis, either the dysplastic type [which may need fusion] or the non-dysplastic type [may need bracing]) and management thereof; muscle strength (often reduced).
9. Hypertension (can be 'essential', or from typical 'NF1 vasculopathy' [which can include coarctation of aorta, renal artery stenosis], renovascular causes or vasoactive compound-producing tumours such as phaeochromocytoma or ganglioneuroma), anti-hypertensive therapy, monitoring BP; symptoms of headache, palpitations, abdominal pain, gastrointestinal symptoms.
10. Vasculopathy (can cause hypertension [above], involvement major arteries of brain or heart, cerebrovascular accidents, moyamoya, aneurysms).
11. Cardiac issues (e.g. pulmonary valve stenosis, other congenital heart lesions, hypertrophic cardiomyopathy [especially with whole-gene deletions], pulmonary hypertension, intracardiac neurofibromas).
12. Neurological symptoms: headache, focal neurological symptoms of CNS tumours, seizures, paraesthesiae (from multiple nerve root tumours causing diffuse polyneuropathy).
13. Skin: neurocutaneous markers; any effect of cosmetic appearance, any treatment, changes in any skin lesions.
14. Second autosomal dominant diseases (e.g. Noonan, multiple endocrine neoplasia type 2).

PAST HISTORY
1. Initial diagnosis: what age informed diagnosis of NF1.
2. Time period between being informed of NF1 diagnosis and development of symptoms.
3. What investigations undertaken to confirm diagnosis.
4. Evolution of symptoms referrable to neurodevelopmental, cognitive, behavioural concerns, communication, vision, hearing and speech, and professionals involved in any of these.
5. Evolution of symptoms referrable to any tumours, musculoskeletal concerns (scoliosis, hemihyperplasia), hypertension, vasculopathy, cardiac issues, any neurological

symptoms, skin concerns or recognition of second autosomal dominant disease (e.g. Noonan).
6. Number of hospitalisations and indications for these.
7. Development of complications (e.g. learning issues at school, ADHD and/or ASD symptomatology) and their management.
8. Previous medications tried (stimulants, anti-hypertensives), laser therapy (for smaller neurofibromas), surgical procedures (e.g. tumour resection).
9. Immunisations, allergies.

CURRENT MANAGEMENT

Present treatment in hospital, usual treatment at home (including physiotherapy, occupational therapy, speech therapy, exercise, medications taken), future treatment plans (e.g. surgical procedures), usual follow-up (by whom, where, how often), unproven (not really 'alternative') therapies tried (e.g. naturopathy).

SOCIAL HISTORY

1. Impact on child (e.g. delays or regression in development, difficulties at school, limitations on lifestyle, body image, self-esteem, peer reactions).
2. Impact on family (e.g. parental coping, difficulties between mother and father, effect on siblings, financial considerations, transport, hospitalisations, private health insurance).
3. Benefits received.
4. Social supports (e.g. social worker), early intervention services for children with disabilities (e.g. via the Australian Government's Department of Social Services at https://dss.gov.au, Better Start at www.betterstart.net.au).

FAMILY HISTORY

A three-generation family history is worth taking; can mention gene testing in discussion if NF1 suspected but not able to be diagnosed clinically in family members.

UNDERSTANDING OF DISEASE

Check understanding by the child, by the family (e.g. parents, siblings, grandparents) and by teachers. Ask about the degree of previous education about NF1 (e.g. in hospital, by local paediatrician), and contingency plans (e.g. sudden change in vision). At the completion of the history, think about what particular problems this family is experiencing at the moment, from the viewpoints of the child, the parents and the attending physicians. These three perspectives may be quite different.

Examination

See separate short case on NF1 in this chapter.

Management

SKIN: DISCRETE NEUROFIBROMAS AND PLEXIFORM NEUROFIBROMAS

The most concerning aspect of the disease for many patients is the disfigurement associated with neurofibromas. Plexiform neuromas can become very large, and can impinge on vital structures; however, many are hidden internally and unsuspected until found with MRI surveillance. Treatment for neurofibroma is surgical removal, or treatment with laser or electrocautery. *Radio **frequency** therapy* has been used with some success for facial diffuse plexiform neurofibromas, and for CAL macules. However, *radio**therapy*** is *contraindicated* for plexiform neurofibromas as it leads to development of second tumours in the radiation field, and can induce MPNSTs.

There is no specific medical therapy yet available for these skin lesions, but there is much research into various therapies which have included imatinib (which targets a 'c-KIT receptor', involved in mast cells infiltrating Schwann cells in developing plexiform neurofibromas), and PEGylated interferon.

Transformation into MPNSTs is one of the key concerns when symptoms develop such as new or different pain in a plexiform neurofibroma, development of new neurological signs, or when a previously quiescent plexiform neurofibroma starts to grow; these presentations are evaluated by MRI and PET scans. Complete surgical excision is the treatment for MPNSTs.

VISION AND NEUROLOGICAL SEQUELAE

Children with NF1 and under the age of 7 years are most at risk from symptomatic OPGs. Fifteen per cent of NF1 patients get OPGs. Treatment can comprise: chemotherapy with vincristine and cisplatinum; and surgery to debulk large chiasmal gliomas, manage proptosis or provide cosmetic palliation in a blind eye.

LEARNING AND BEHAVIOURAL ISSUES

There is no standard learning disability profile with NF1. Each child is unique, and no preschool neurodevelopmental assessments and school neuropsychological testing are important for educational purposes to identify areas requiring support for that particular child with NF1.

Difficulties with executive planning, problem-solving and speech intelligibility are well recognised. All the behavioural issues that can occur in typical children without NF1 also occur in NF1, and the same medications are used for children with ADHD, ASD, anxiety and depression. There are no NF1-specific medications as yet for learning or behavioural issues.

Self-esteem issues, however, are very much a particular concern in NF1 due to the many and varied physical signs which lead to teenagers with NF1 being more vulnerable than their typical peers, especially with concomitant learning problems. The child and family should be prepared for this by discussion with their paediatrician.

MUSCULOSKELETAL ISSUES

The treatment for dystrophic scoliosis involves surgery, as it does not respond to bracing. There are several potential complications depending on the degree of kyphosis, with risk of distal nerve damage and poor union; correction is rarely complete, and treatment goals must be discussed thoroughly pre-surgery. The surgery usually involves fusion, anterior and posterior.

The management of tibial pseudoarthrosis is very complicated, and a topic of much current research. It requires orthopaedic surgeons with experience in NF1; early recognition of bowing allows early bracing to prevent fractures occurring. Once fractures have occurred, the focus is on stability and adequate blood supply, and there are several orthopaedic procedures that can be used. However, if stable union cannot be maintained, there can be selective limited procedures, including below-knee amputations, ankle-saving procedures, amputation of the foot and replacement with prosthesis. There is no standard consensus approach to this problem as yet. Multiple operations are the usual course, with significantly long recuperation periods.

Osteoporosis in NF1 does not have a standard approach as yet. Trials with calcium and vitamin D have not shown benefit. Bisphosphonates are being studied.

HYPERTENSION, VASCULOPATHY AND CARDIAC ISSUES

The management of hypertension depends on the cause; essential hypertension is treated the same as in non-NF1 children; weight reduction if obese, salt restriction, correct recognised underlying problems (such as OSA) plus medications.

The drugs used are the same as used in adults: 1. blockers of the renin-angiotensin-aldosterone system (*ACE inhibitors*, and *sartans* [which inhibit the AT1 receptor of angiotensin II; also called *AT1 receptor antagonists*]); 2. beta blockers; 3. calcium channel blockers; and 4. diuretics. ACE inhibitors, sartans and beta blockers all disable the renin-angiotensin-aldosterone system, and they reduce vascular resistance. Calcium channel blockers directly vasodilate. Diuretics lower blood volume and increase natriuresis. In renovascular causes of hypertension, ACE inhibitors and sartans are preferred.

RECOMMENDED SURVEILLANCE

Children with NF1 should be assessed annually, concentrating on development and school progress, growth and pubertal development, cardiovascular examination, including BP (looking for phaeochromocytoma, renal artery stenosis) and auscultation for congenital heart disease (e.g. pulmonary valve stenosis), visual assessment (including acuity, fields and fundoscopy, plus colour vision testing), and examination of spine and skin. Other assessments should be determined by symptomatology.

MRI of the relevant organ/system is as follows: orbits (for poor vision, proptosis or precocious puberty); painful plexiform neurofibromas (to exclude MPNST); brain (for changing seizures, behavioural change or head circumference enlarging); abdomen (if hypertension, for phaeochromocytoma). If the BP is elevated, include 24-hour urinary excretion of catecholamines and their metabolites.

GENETIC COUNSELLING

This is recommended for all NF1 patients before they conceive. Prenatal diagnosis is available by direct mutation testing on fetal DNA derived from chorionic villous biopsy or amniocentesis. It is infrequent that prenatal testing is pursued, as there is no way to accurately predict severity of disease, although there are a number of genotype-phenotype correlations recently described (see the section on background information). Preimplantation genetic diagnosis is available, where single cells from 3-day-old embryos are tested for the NF1 mutation and those which do not carry it are implanted.

LONG CASE: Sturge-Weber syndrome (SWS)

Sturge-Weber syndrome (SWS), also called encephalotrigeminal angiomatosis, is an uncommon phakomatosis, characteristically comprising facial capillary malformations (termed 'port-wine stains' [PWSs] or 'port-wine birthmarks' [PWBs]) in the distribution of the trigeminal nerve, with ipsilateral leptomeningeal [pial] angiomas involving particularly the occipital and parietal lobes leading to calcification and laminar cortical necrosis. The resultant clinical picture can include hemiparesis, epilepsy, developmental delay and glaucoma. If there is an inpatient with this condition during an examination week, it is highly likely they will be asked to participate as either a long- or short-case patient.

Background

SWS (OMIM#185300) is due to a somatic mosaic mutation in the guanine nucleotide-binding protein, Q polypeptide (GNAQ) gene (OMIM#600998), the cytogenetic location of which is on the long arm of chromosome 9 at 9q21.2, and affects 1 in 50 000 people. Unlike NF1 and TSC, in SWS there is, as yet, no evidence of heredity. The recurrent somatic mutation identified is called c.548G>A (p.R183Q), a single-nucleotide variant in the GNAQ gene, which is a gain of function mutation, associated with increased gene expression of fibronectin in SWS port-wine-derived fibroblasts.

This mutation also causes capillary malformations, congenital (CMC) (OMIM#163000), also known as non-syndromic PWSs. The prevailing theory is that SWS represents an earlier occurring mutation in progenitor cells, which can then differentiate into various cell types, causing the range of phenotypic features, whereas PWSs could result when the mutation occurs later, and thus affect only vascular endothelial cells.

PWSs are the most common vascular malformations, seen in 0.3% of live births. The risk of having SWS, in the presence of some form of facial vascular lesion, is 8%. The overall frequency of SWS is around 1 in 20 000 to 1 in 50 000. PWSs affecting the complete ophthalmic division of the fifth cranial nerve (V1) are strongly associated with cerebral involvement and glaucoma (about 80% correlation) whereas if only a portion of V1 is involved the coexistence of neurological or ocular involvement is much lower, around 25%.

The GNAQ gene is around 315 kilobases in size, and codes for *guanine nucleotide-binding protein G(q) subunit alpha*, a 42-kD protein containing 359 amino acids; it is situated at the nuclear membrane.

GNAQ subunit alpha is involved in signalling between G protein-coupled receptors (GPCRs), including endothelin-1, angiotensin II receptor type 1, alpha-1-adrenergic receptors, vasopressin receptors type 1A and type 1B, serotonin and glutamate receptors, and effectors downstream, all of which are recognised as being important in vascular function in cardiovascular disease.

The mutation in GNAQ in SWS is the same as the mutation in melanocytes in adults which leads to uveal melanoma; in this condition there are already trials of therapies which could be applicable in the management of SWS. Also, the mutation in GNAQ has been shown to hyperactivate ERK-phosphorylation, and ERK inhibitors are available. Hence, targeted treatments may be available for SWS in the near future.

In SWS, there has been a failure of regression of the normal vascular plexus (the primitive cephalic venous plexus) that develops around the cephalic aspect of the neural tube between 6 and 9 weeks' gestation. With normal development, the primitive vascular system splits into three divisions: an external portion that supplies the scalp and facial skin; a middle portion that supplies the meninges; and an inner portion that supplies the brain. Where the plexus normally regresses, this does not occur in SWS so residual embryonic blood vessels form angiomas that exert their effect on the face, ipsilateral eye and leptomeninges.

A number of pathological processes can occur which cause the effects on the adjacent brain tissue, including (mnemonic **HIT VIVAS**) **H**ypoxia, **I**schaemia, **T**hrombosis, **V**enous occlusion, **I**nfarction, **V**ascular steal phenomena, **A**trophy and **S**eizures.

Although the actual leptomeningeal angiomas (LAs) are, technically and anatomically, *static* lesions, clinically this condition can progress and deteriorate. This seems related to seizure activity, and in addition a vascular steal phenomenon surrounding the angioma, leading to cortical ischaemia. Seizure activity and recurrent vascular events (transient hemiparesis) worsen the steal phenomenon, calcification and gliosis ensue, leading to the observed worse neurological outcomes, including more focal cerebral atrophy, when seizures have earlier onset.

Classification

SWS can be divided into three 'types', based on presence or absence of the facial PWS and the SWS CNS pathology, using the Roach scale:

1. Type I is also termed 'complete', and refers to the presence of both facial and leptomeningeal vascular malformations/angiomas, and the patients may well have glaucoma.
2. Type II ('incomplete') refers to facial PWS alone (no cerebral involvement), and the patient may have glaucoma.
3. Type III ('incomplete') refers to just the leptomeningeal vascular malformations/angiomas, with no PWS and usually no glaucoma either, and this is rare. Type III is a diagnostic consideration in presentations with intracranial unilateral calcification, complicated migraine, and seizures.

Skin manifestations

PWSs are vascular malformations comprising ectatic capillaries and postcapillary venules in the dermis ranging from 30–300 μm in diameter. A hallmark of SWS occurring in 96% of SWS patients, they occur in the distribution of the trigeminal (V) nerve, typically in the ophthalmic distribution (V1) and maxillary distribution (V2), but can occur beyond these confines with extra-cranial PWSs and soft-tissue overgrowth. Over 50% of SWS patients have PWSs in extra-cranial locations.

Seizures

Epilepsy occurs in 75–90% of patients with SWS, the onset can be anytime from birth until 23 years with a median at 6 months of age. If there is bilateral involvement, the incidence is higher than unilateral (93% versus 72%) and earlier than unilateral (median onset 4 months in bilateral disease, versus 8.5 months). Even in bilateral disease, one hemisphere predominates.

Three-quarters of children with SWS have seizures within their first year of life, 86% by 2 years and 95% by five. Up to one-third of those experiencing seizures present initially in the context of a febrile illness. The earlier that seizures commence, the more likely the seizures will be more frequent, and the more likely there will be developmental delays and a need for special education. According to the Sturge-Weber Foundation, 50% of SWS children get full seizure control, while 39% achieve partial control, with AEDs.

Seizures are associated with the vascular malformation/angioma affecting the leptomeninges found, usually, in the posterior occipital lobe. In some patients the angioma is more anterior, and this seems to correlate with a later seizure onset. There can be cortical dysgenesis in some children with SWS which may increase the propensity to fitting.

Most seizures are focal, with motor activity on the side contralateral to the angioma, but they can readily generalise. Various seizure types can be seen, including infantile spasms (which can be asymmetric), and generalised tonic–clonic seizures (GTCS) can present at the onset. Myoclonic-astatic epilepsy can occur, and gets worse on carbamazepine or oxcarbazepine. There can be a 'clustering' pattern where a number of seizures occur in succession, which is then followed by a lengthy duration of being seizure free; up to 40% of children with SWS experience this pattern at some stage; however, this does not mean a poorer prognosis. Gelastic seizures can occur, where the child seems to have uncontrollable laughter or crying as the manifestation of the fit.

Status epilepticus can be accompanied or followed by extended periods of hemiparetic weakness or new visual field cuts; these can last for variable periods of time, but are transient; they can last hours, days, weeks, even months, and are called 'stroke-like episodes'. These episodes can also occur with non-epileptic episodes of ischaemia.

Predictably, several prognostic factors portending poor outcomes relate to seizure activity, including seizures refractory to medical therapy, focal seizures which generalise, increasing seizure activity, and longer duration postictal deficits.

Focal neurology

There are permanent and transient types of focal neurological problems. Permanent hemiparesis occurs in a third of SWS patients. Ipsilateral cortical atrophy typically causes contralateral hemiparesis and contralateral hemianopia. These can present initially with early hand preference indicating hemiparesis, and head turning indicating visual field cuts. Hemiparesis is due to ischaemia, associated with venous occlusion and thrombosis. Temporary or transient episodes are termed 'stroke-like' episodes, and occur in 70% of SWS patients. These can occur in the context of seizures, increasing in severity with recurrence of seizures, or with migrainous headaches, inferring a vascular basis. There can be thromboses on a recurrent basis, or completed strokes. Permanent neurological defects are more common in adults, in keeping with the unfortunately progressive nature of SWS pathology. Increased severity of hemiparesis has been linked to earlier onset of seizures.

Younger children are particularly at risk of stroke-like episodes following on from minor head trauma, so activities likely to involve this should be avoided.

Some cases of hydrocephalus are described, attributable to impaired CSF resorption associated with inadequate venous drainage.

Vision

The more concerning ocular aspects of SWS are secondary to raised intraocular pressure. Ophthalmological signs can include conjunctival, episcleral and eyelid (particularly upper lid) vascular malformations/angiomas, diffuse choroidal vascular malformations/angiomas (in 40–50% of patients), tortuous retinal vessels can occur, with arteriovenous malformations.

Glaucoma occurs in 30–70% of SWS patients. It is usually ipsilateral to the PWS. It can occasionally be contralateral to the PWS. If there are bilateral PWSs, there is a 45% chance of bilateral glaucoma. Almost two-thirds of cases present as congenital glaucoma; there may be photophobia (neonate refusing to open their eyes; when the eyes are opened [in a dark room], there is corneal opacity/clouding or haziness due to corneal oedema) and buphthalmos ('ox eye', which refers to an enlarged globe with an abnormally enlarged cornea—in a short case, measure the [increased] corneal diameter—due to raised pressure especially seen in neonates, whereas presentations later in childhood tend not to involve eye enlargement).

Glaucoma presents earlier (under 2 years) when the tissues involved in the vascular malformation are those responsible for formation of the anterior chamber angle; if the vascular tissues involved are conjunctival and episcleral, then presentation with glaucoma is delayed until after 5 years of age. This corresponds with the noted second peak of glaucoma diagnosis at 5–9 years, when 15–23% of patients develop it.

There is a third peak after the age of 20 (when 20% of patients are affected). Glaucoma can present with frequent tearing (epiphora), almost constant blinking (blepharospasm) and blurred vision. The risk of glaucoma is lifelong in SWS; it can develop at any time.

Other ocular manifestations of SWS can include iris heterochromia (different-coloured eyes [irides]), colobomata of iris, amblyopia, myopia, anisometropia, visual field cuts, retinal degenerative changes, retinal detachment and blindness.

Cognitive, learning, behavioural and psychosocial aspects

Over 80% of children with SWS have some cognitive impairment, and eventually around 50% of patients may be diagnosed as having intellectual impairment. The patients most severely affected tend to be those with bilateral disease, those with intractable seizures, those with early seizure onset, and multiple seizure types, and those with a greater degree of cerebral atrophy. In cases with bilateral disease, there is an increased risk of autistic features if there is bilateral temporal lobe involvement, and increase risk of motor and developmental delays if both frontal lobes are involved. Behavioural and emotional problems are very common, including ADHD symptomatology, ASD (see Chapter 5, Behavioural and development paediatrics), oppositional defiant disorder (ODD) and depression (which is more common in those patients with normal intelligence, and is related to the extensiveness of their facial PWS). Social skills are problematic, especially for those with difficult-to-control seizures and more severe cognitive issues.

Headache

Migraine headaches are common in SWS and are attributable to the vascular disease component: the propensity to getting migraine in SWS is thought to be due to a greater vasogenic leakage of neuropeptides into the subarachnoid space as there are simply more vessels from which to leak. These 'symptomatic migraines' occur in around 30% of patients, including in patients under 10 years, and neurological manifestations (deficits) occur in about 60% of these patients.

Headaches in general (not specifying migraine) occur in 60–80% of SWS patients. Headaches are frequent in patients who experience stroke-like episodes. With a median onset at 8 years of age in a subgroup of SWS patients with seizures and headaches, headaches, at this age, are often considered of greater concern than seizures. Adult patients describe the following during migrainous headaches: sensation of facial pulsation, their facial PWSs becoming more discoloured, nausea, vomiting, dizziness and dysarthria.

Hemiplegic migraines are well documented in SWS, and can be prolonged, lasting days. During the episodes, imaging shows delayed hyperperfusion, hypermetabolism and more marked enhancement of the leptomeningeal vascular malformation, all of which can disappear after the episode is ended clinically.

Body asymmetry and overlap with other syndromes linked to Weber

All SWS patients have other skin lesions than the defining facial PWSs, and 96% of SWS patients have some degree of body asymmetry. Children with classic SWS may have other, extra-cranial, vascular malformations and overgrowth, including hemihyperplasia. There can be overlap with two other syndromes which also have 'Weber' in their names. *Klippel-Trénaunay-Weber* syndrome (KTW) (OMIM%149000) includes a triad of vascular malformations, abnormal lymphatics and hemihyperplasia; venous malformations in KTW are slow flowing. *Parkes Weber* syndrome (PKWS) (MIM#608355) includes micro-arteriovenous fistulas (AVFs) associated with skeletal and soft-tissue overgrowth; the AVFs in PKWS are fast flowing, and involved limbs are **p**inker and **w**armer than in KTW (recall **P**arkes **W**eber = **P**ink **W**armer → **p**erfused **w**ell [as *arterial*—venous, and fast flowing, rather than just venous and slow flowing like KTW]). In addition to the overlap with KTW and PKWS, there is soft-tissue hypertrophy in almost a quarter of SWS patients, and around 7% of children with SWS have scoliosis.

Other anomalies: endocrine; ears, nose and throat (ENT); OSA

Central hypothyroidism is described in 2.4% of children with SWS, but has been associated with treatment of SWS children with oxcarbazepine. Thyroid function testing should be performed in patients if they are receiving oxcarbazepine. Growth hormone deficiency is 18 times more common in SWS than in the general population; this suggests hypothalamic–pituitary axis dysfunction.

Mnemonic for features of SWS is **STURGE**:

Seizures/**S**urgical resections for refractory epilepsy (callosotomy, lesionectomy, hemispherectomy)/**S**troke, **S**troke-like episodes/**S**tructural leptomeningeal involvement/**S**trabismus/**S**coliosis/**S**poradic/**S**omatic mutation

Trigeminal nerve distribution (V1, V2)/**T**rabeculectomy requirement for glaucoma

Uveal tract: choroidal vascular malformation/**U**nderactive thyroid/**U**nderproduction pituitary GH/**U**neven growth (body asymmetry)

Regional defects—hemiparesis, hemianopia/**R**estricted vision: field cuts (homonymous hemianopia)

Glaucoma/**G**oniotomy requirement/**G**lobal delay/**G**ene = **G**NAQ/**G**rowth hormone deficiency

Encephalotrigeminal angiomatosis (alternate name for SWS)/**E**ye enlargement/**E**ye pressure increased/**E**ducational opportunities limited (intellectual impairment)

History

Ask about the following.

PRESENTING COMPLAINT

Reason for current admission.

CURRENT SYMPTOMS

1. Skin. Extent of skin involvement, social stigma noted, any cosmetic treatment (e.g. pulsed dye laser [PDL] photocoagulation).
2. Seizures. For each type of seizure, ask: age of onset; any prodromal symptoms (e.g. irritability, pallor); precipitating factors (seizure triggers); aura; initial cry or scream; initial localising signs (e.g. twitching of hand of hemiplegic side); description of all aspects of the seizure itself (e.g. eyes rolling back, cyanosis, tonus, clonus, incontinence); duration of seizure (range [e.g. between 2 and 20 minutes], usual time [e.g. 2 minutes], any episodes of status epilepticus [over 5 minutes]); frequency of seizures (range and 'usual'); time of occurrence (waking, going to sleep); date and time of last seizure; postictal events (e.g. sleeping, residual paralysis); usual treatment; recent/future planned surgical procedures for fitting (e.g. focal cortical resection, hemispherectomy); emergency plan for status epilepticus.
3. Focal neurology, *permanent*. Hemiparesis and hemianopia, ask: age first noted, extent of impairment, interference with ADLs (e.g. bathing, cleaning teeth, combing hair, dressing, writing and other hand usage, toileting, menses), muscle strength (often weak), imaging.
4. Focal neurology, *transient*: 'Stroke-like episodes', frequency, duration, pattern, whether worsening, management.
5. Vision. Glaucoma: age noted, any procedures (e.g. trabeculectomy, goniotomy); other ocular problems (e.g. diffuse choroidal haemangioma [DCH]), any procedures (e.g. radiotherapy for DCH).
6. Cognitive abilities, or present developmental status (e.g. intellectual impairment), schooling details.
7. Learning issues at school (e.g. executive functioning skills, any neuropsychometric testing by guidance officer), any help needed, attitudes of class teacher, fellow students.
8. Behavioural issues (e.g. ADHD, symptomatology and any relevant medications such as stimulants), professionals involved in management (psychologist, psychiatrist, paediatrician, therapists).

9. Headache. Symptomatic migraines: description of headache (aura, associated increased discolouration of PWS, nausea or vomiting, dizziness, sensation of facial pulsation, dysarthria), any treatment acute or preventative, known precipitants.
10. Body asymmetry. Any spinal problems (e.g. scoliosis; any treatment [fusion or bracing]), any hemihyperplasia or soft-tissue hyperplasia, any management thereof.

PAST HISTORY

1. Initial diagnosis: what age informed not just PWS.
2. Time period between being informed of SWS diagnosis and development of symptoms.
3. What investigations undertaken to confirm diagnosis.
4. Evolution of seizures, evolution of focal neurology, evolution/regression of development.
5. Number of hospitalisations and indications for these.
6. Development of complications (e.g. learning issues at school, ADHD symptomatology, central hypothyroidism, scoliosis) and their management.
7. Previous medications tried (AEDs, stimulants, medications for migraine, medications for glaucoma), surgical procedures (e.g. for seizures, for glaucoma, for scoliosis), dermatological procedures (PDL).
8. Immunisations, allergies.

CURRENT MANAGEMENT

Present treatment in hospital, usual treatment at home (including physiotherapy, occupational therapy, speech therapy, exercise, medications taken [including eye drops for glaucoma]), future treatment plans (e.g. surgical procedures), usual follow-up (by whom, where, how often), unproven (not really 'alternative') therapies tried (e.g. naturopathy).

SOCIAL HISTORY

1. Impact on child (e.g. delays or regression in development, difficulties at school, limitations on lifestyle, body image, self-esteem, peer reactions).
2. Impact on family (e.g. parental coping, difficulties between mother and father, effect on siblings, financial considerations, transport, hospitalisations, private health insurance).
3. Benefits received.
4. Social supports (e.g. social worker, the US-based Sturge-Weber Foundation at www.sturge-weber.org, Sturge Weber UK at www.sturgeweber.org.uk), early intervention services for children with disabilities (e.g. Australian Government's Department of Social Services at https://dss.gov.au, Better Start at www.betterstart.net.au).

UNDERSTANDING OF DISEASE

By the child, by the family (e.g. parents, siblings, grandparents) and by teachers. Ask about the degree of previous education about SWS (e.g. in hospital, by local paediatrician), and contingency plans (e.g. what to do if the following occur: bleeding from PWS, status epilepticus, transient stroke-like episodes, severe migraine). At the completion of the history, think about what particular problems this family is experiencing at the moment, from the viewpoints of the child, the parents and the attending physicians. These three perspectives may be quite different.

Examination

See separate short case on SWS in this chapter.

Management

SKIN MANIFESTATIONS

At the time of writing (2017), the gold standard of treatment for PWSs remains pulsed dye laser (PDL), but a small number of patients have lesions which are refractory to this, so there are many other treatments being explored including immune therapy and angiogenesis inhibitors.

SEIZURES

Intractable seizures occur in around 30–50%; management for these seizures can involve neurosurgical procedures such as lesionectomy, corpus callosotomy and hemispherectomy. After hemispherectomy, around 80% of patients have no further seizures, and somewhat surprisingly, the effects on motor abilities may not be severe. In children with bilateral disease, but with fitting coming mainly from one side, surgery is also an option. All parents should have an emergency action plan for seizures.

FOCAL NEUROLOGY

The recommended neuroimaging modalities include: MRI, with T1 weighted imaging with gadolinium, with susceptibility-weighted imaging (SWI); post-contrast fluid-attenuated inversion recovery (FLAIR) imaging and high-resolution blood oxygen level dependent (BOLD) magnetic resonance venography; functional MRI (may show abnormal occipital activation); fluorodeoxyglucose (FDG) PET may show disturbed glucose metabolism; SPECT may show disturbed cerebral perfusion.

Electroencephalogram (EEG) is typically asymmetric, with decreased voltage and background slowing. EEG can help differentiate causes of acute paroxysmal events, identifying whether these are seizures rather than stroke-like episodes or migraine. Quantitative EEG (qEEG) can be used in babies with PWSs to differentiate between those with SWS cerebral findings and those without; asymmetry in qEEG gives an indication of the degree of neurological impairment.

Because the pathology of deterioration in SWS is largely vascular, due to ischaemia, the use of aspirin to decrease platelet aggregation has shown a decrease in the frequency of completed strokes, and in some studies, a decrease in seizure frequency. Immunisation against varicella is recommended before aspirin is commenced to lessen the small risk of Reye's syndrome.

VISION

The management of glaucoma is complex. Topical anti-glaucoma eyedrops are required. Operative treatment may include fashioning openings in the normal drainage system (goniotomy, trabeculotomy), draining intraocular fluid via a new opening in the anterior chamber (trabeculectomy) or using external glaucoma drainage devices (e.g. the Ahmed glaucoma valve [AGV] or the Molteno glaucoma tube implant). Surgical procedures for glaucoma involve risks of low intraocular pressure (hypotony), choroidal bleeding and retinal detachment. Aqueous production can be decreased by diode laser or cryotherapy to the ciliary processes. Cataracts can occur after repeated intraocular procedures.

COGNITIVE, LEARNING AND BEHAVIOURAL ASPECTS

Psychosocial support is exceedingly important. Supportive agencies should be utilised. Educational support should be available from government-run education departments for those fulfilling criteria for intellectual impairment, motor impairment or ASD. Preschool neurodevelopmental assessments and school neuropsychological testing are important for educational purposes to identify areas requiring support for that particular child with SWS.

All the behavioural issues that can occur in typical children without SWS also occur in SWS, and the same medications are used for children with ADHD, ASD, anxiety and depression. There are no SWS-specific medications as yet for learning or behavioural issues or for seizures or stroke-like episodes. Self-esteem issues are very important in SWS due to the aesthetic effects of large PWSs and body asymmetry issues, which in addition to the cognitive impairments, hemiparesis and recurrent seizures lead to teenagers with SWS being much more vulnerable than their typical peers, especially with concomitant learning problems; the child and family should be prepared for this by discussion with their paediatrician.

HEADACHE

The treatment for migraine in SWS follows the usual treatment for typical children without such a diagnosis, with avoidance of any known triggers (e.g. oranges, cheese, chocolate). Although internet surveys indicate around 20% of SWS patients have used triptans, there are very serious potential adverse vascular effects, which suggests they may not be an appropriate choice; more research is needed before it can be known whether they could be effective, safe or detrimental in children with SWS.

BODY ASYMMETRY AND OVERLAP WITH OTHER SYNDROMES LINKED TO WEBER

All SWS patients have other skin lesions than the defining facial PWSs, and 96% of SWS patients have some degree of body asymmetry. Involvement of a dermatologist with an interest, and experience, in SWS is vital, as is involvement of an orthopaedic surgeon with an interest, and experience, in SWS and/or KTW and/or PKWS. Children with classic SWS may have other, extra-cranial, vascular malformations which may be amenable to laser therapy.

OTHER ANOMALIES: ENDOCRINE; EARS, NOSE AND THROAT; OSA

Growth and thyroid function must be monitored, especially in SWS children taking oxcarbazepine. Confirmation of growth hormone deficiency may lead to growth hormone replacement. ENT consultation should be sought in children with recurrent ear infections and for those with OSA.

CURRENT RESEARCH

Current (2017) research trials include the use of mTOR inhibitors for treatment of PWBs and of refractive seizures in SWS, and the use of cannabidiols to manage GNAQ hyperactivation.

LONG CASE: Tuberous sclerosis complex (TSC)

Background
BASIC DEFECT

Tuberous sclerosis complex (TSC), a neurocutaneous multi-system disorder associated with low-grade tumours, is an autosomal dominant disorder and is due to mutation in either the TSC1 gene or the TSC2 gene. **TSC1** is on the long arm of chromosome 9 at **9q34.13**, and codes for the protein *hamartin* that forms a complex with the protein *tuberin* which is coded for by **TSC2** and is on the short arm of chromosome 16, at **16p13.3**. The hamartin-tuberin heterodimer complex regulates cell proliferation.

Hamartin and tuberin regulate the AKT signal transduction pathway, other signalling pathways and other cell cycle pathways. TSC has an overall incidence of 1 in 5000 to 1 in 10 000 live births.

The TSC1 gene (MIM*605284) is around 50 kilobases in size, has 23 exons and codes for hamartin, a 130-kD protein containing 1163 amino acids; the TSC2 gene (MIM*191092) is around 45 kilobases in size, has 42 exons and codes for tuberin, a 200-kD protein containing 1807 amino acids.

TSC1 mutations can be small deletions and insertions (in 52.5%), nonsense mutations (34%), splicing mutations (8%), missense mutations (4.5%), or large deletions and rearrangements (1%). Almost all TSC1 mutations lead to truncation of the hamartin protein; there are over 460 known TSC1 mutations. Hamartin stabilises the hamartin-tuberin complex.

TSC2 mutations can be small deletions and insertions (in 29%), missense mutations (28.4%), nonsense mutations (22%), splicing mutations (12.8–15%), or large deletions and rearrangements (7.8%). Around 70% of mutations cause loss or truncation of the tuberin protein while the other 30% cause changes in one or a few amino acids in tuberin; there are over 1230 known TSC2 mutations. Tuberin is a regulator of small G-proteins (guanine nucleotide-binding proteins), RHEB (ras homolog enriched in brain) (MIM*601293) and mTOR (mechanistic target of rapamycin complex 1) (MIM*601231), and affects protein translation and cell growth and proliferation; also, it has GTPase-activating protein functions for small G-proteins, Rap1a and Rab5.

TSC genes essentially act as tumour suppressor genes. TSC proteins function in negative regulation of the mTOR pathway. The mTOR pathway is an intricate component in tumour cell proliferation, energy metabolism, development of the cerebral cortex and control of growth. Treatments involving mTOR inhibitors have revolutionised management of TSC in the last decade, as outlined below.

The first mTOR inhibitor was rapamycin (sirolimus). Derivatives of sirolimus ('rapalogs'), such as everolimus, have their effects by binding with FKBP12 followed by interaction with the FKBP12-rapamycin-binding domain of mTORC1, which blocks the serine-threonine activity of mTORC1 and stops mRNA translation. This effects restoration of the mTORC1 inhibition normally effected by TSC1/TSC2 complex, which do not work in TSC. Reversal of a number of features of TSC can be achieved by inhibiting mTOR at the cellular level. Rapamycin can reduce the volume of TSC-related tumours in the brain (subependymal giant cell astrocytomas [SEGAs]) and the kidney (angiomyolipomas), and can improve pulmonary function tests in lymphangioleiomyomatosis (LAM).

Diagnosis

There was a diagnostic criteria update in 2012 which incorporated genetic testing. Molecular testing for the genes discussed above leads to a positive result for a mutation in 75–90% of patients diagnosed by previous clinical criteria from the 1998 consensus. There is a significant minority (10–25%) of patients with TSC who do not have a demonstrable mutation identified, termed 'no mutation identified' (NMI) as yet, so a negative genetic testing result does not exclude TSC. It is likely mosaicism and the limitations of technology that account for these NMIs. There are now, therefore, two forms of diagnostic criteria:

1. *Genetic diagnostic criteria*: finding TSC1 or TSC2 pathogenic mutations in DNA from normal tissue.

2. *Clinical diagnostic criteria*: two major features, or one major feature and at least two minor features.

There are 11 major features:

- **Skin** (4). **SHAU**: **S**hagreen patch, **H**ypomelanotic macules (> 3, at least 5 mm diameter), **A**ngiofibromas (> 3) or fibrous cephalic plaque, **U**ngual fibromas (> 2).
- **Brain/eye** (4). **S**ub**e**pendymal **g**iant cell **a**strocytoma (**SEGA**), subependymal nodules (SEN), cortical dysplasias, multiple retinal hamartomas.
- **Others** (3). Heart, lung, kidney: cardiac rhabdomyoma, **l**ymph**a**ngioleio**m**yomatosis (LAM), angiomyolipomas (> 2) (of kidney).

There are six minor features:

- 'Confetti' hypomelanotic skin lesions, dental enamel pits (> 3), intraoral fibromas (> 2), retinal achromic patch, multiple renal cysts, non-renal hamartomas.

MNEMONICS FOR DIAGNOSTIC CRITERIA

Major features (mnemonic **ASH CLUE**; old term for hypomelanotic macules: 'ash leaf' macules):

Ash leaf (hypomelanotic) macules (> 3, > 5 mm)/**A**ngiofibroma/**A**ngiomyolipoma
Subependymal nodules (SEN)/**S**ubependymal giant cell astrocytoma (SEGA)/
Shagreen patches
Heart: rhabdomyoma, **H**amartomas (multiple retinal)
Cortical dysplasia
Lymphangioleiomyomatosis
Ungal fibromas
Establish genetic diagnosis: identifying TSC1/TSC2 pathogenic mutations sufficient

Minor features (mnemonic **MIND achromia**)

Multiple renal cysts
Intraoral fibromas (> 2)
Non-renal hamartomas
Dental enamel pits (> 3)
achromia: retina (achromic patch), skin ('confetti' hypomelanotic skin lesions)

AGE-RELATED MANIFESTATIONS

Age-related presentation can be represented approximately by three groups. There are four consistent aspects that occur across all ages (mnemonic **HEFS**):

Hypopigmented macules
Epilepsy
Facial angiofibromas
SEN

Age under 1 year (mnemonic **CHEFS**):

Cardiac rhabdomyoma
Hypomelanotic macules
Epilepsy
Facial angiofibroma
SEN

Age 5–15 (mnemonic **RHEFS**):

Renal angiomyolipoma
Hypopigmented macules
Epilepsy
Facial angiofibroma
SEN

Age 25–60 (mnemonic **LU-RHEFS**):

Liver hamartoma
Ungual hamartoma
RHEFS

DERMATOLOGICAL AND DENTAL

Classic skin findings in TSC include *four major features*:
1. ***Hypomelanotic macules*** (> 3, at least 5 mm in diameter) are seen in 90% children with TSC; usually they appear at birth. These are best seen with a Wood's light; hypomelanosis of the hair (poliosis) is considered of the same significance as skin macules.
2. ***Facial angiofibromas*** occur in 75%, usually appearing between 2 and 5 years. *Fibrous cephalic plaque* usually appear on the forehead, though they can be on the face or scalp. They occur in 25% of children with TSC.
3. ***Ungual fibromas*** (> 2) appear later, in adolescence or adulthood, with frequency of about 20%.
4. ***Shagreen patches*** appear in the first decade, appearing over the lower back in the lumbosacral area, as plaques 2–6 cm in diameter, with an 'orange-peel appearance' seen in 50% children with TSC. They are also called 'fibrous collagenoma'.

Skin and dental/oral minor findings include three minor features: 1. *'confetti' hypomelanotic skin lesions*, 1–3 mm in diameter, scattered over arms and legs; 2. *dental enamel pits* (> 3) which occur in all adults with TSC; and 3. *intraoral fibromas* (gingival fibromas are found in 20–50% people with TSC and are more common in adults; fibromas can be found also on the tongue, and buccal or labial mucosa).

OPHTHALMOLOGIC

Typical eye findings in TSC include one major feature, ***multiple retinal hamartomas***, which have similar histology to tubers in the brain (see below), and are found in 30–50% of TSC patients, but usually cause no problem with vision. A minor ocular feature is the *retinal achromic patch*, an area of hypopigmentation found in 39% TSC patients.

CNS: CEREBRAL STRUCTURE, TUMOURS, TUBERS AND TERMINOLOGY

Classic CNS findings include three major features:
1. ***Subependymal nodules (SEN).***
2. ***Subependymal giant cell astrocytoma (SEGA).***
3. ***Cortical dysplasia.***

SEN and SEGA have similar histology, and are fairly specific to TSC, arise during childhood or adolescence, and occur in 80% of TSC patients. *SEN* are benign, arising along the ependymal lining of the third ventricle and the lateral ventricles. *SEGAs* arise from SEN, occurring in 5–15% of patients with TSC, and can block the foramen of Munro, where they classically occur, causing hydrocephalus.

Newer terminology uses a different term for SEGAs: 'subependymal giant cell tumours' (SGCTs) (but they are called SEGAs in the diagnostic criteria update from 2012) based on their mixed glioneuronal lineage. *Cortical dysplasia*, found in 90% in TSC, involves failure of normal neuronal migration; areas of focal cortical dysplasia are termed cortical 'tubers' and give TSC its name; however, this term is being replaced with 'glioneuronal hamartomas'. 'White matter heterotopia' is another term used for dysplastic and demyelinated white matter. Cerebral white matter radial migration lines are believed to indicate dysmyelination, with disordered migration, and have similar pathology to 'tubers'. The most recent 2012 criteria require multiple areas of cortical dysplasia to count as one major feature.

EPILEPSY

This affects 80–90% of TSC patients overall, with 60% of patients affected in their first year, but it is *not* a diagnostic criterion/feature. Three-quarters of TSC patients have epileptiform findings on routine EEG (in 35–70% of TSC children). Types of seizures include infantile spasms, simple partial, complex partial and secondary generalised. There is a higher risk of epilepsy in patients with cortical glioneuronal hamartomas with low central signal on FLAIR MRI.

INTELLECTUAL IMPAIRMENT

This affects 45–65% of TSC patients. Essentially all TSC children with learning problems have had seizures, typically infantile spasms, generally before one year of age. Around 55% of TSC patients have normal IQ scores. 30% have profound impairment (IQ < 21). 15% have moderate to severe impairment. Intellectual impairment is *not* a diagnostic criterion.

BEHAVIOURAL AND NEUROPSYCHIATRIC ISSUES

There are a wide variety of TSC-associated neuropsychiatric disorders (TAND). Autistic spectrum disorder is common in TSC. ADHD symptomatology, anxiety and depression are all well described in TSC. Behavioural problems occur in 40–90% of children with TSC, some studies linking these to being more common in children with lower IQ and more frequent seizures. These are *not* diagnostic criteria. TAND-like presentations can occur, particularly with sudden changes in behaviour or activity level, due to CNS problems (e.g. SEGA, epilepsy), or renal failure (uraemic encephalopathy). TAND presentations must always be taken very seriously in TSC.

CARDIOVASCULAR

Cardiac rhabdomyomas are benign and ***major features***; they are found in 50% TSC patients; they tend not to cause serious issues; they tend to occur in the ventricular and septal walls, and can cause ventricular outflow tract obstruction, or impair valve functioning; highly specific for TSC; they tend to be multiple; can appear in fetus, but regress after birth; there can be associated rhythm disturbances in 20% of TSC patients with rhabdomyoma (atrial and/or ventricular arrhythmias), as well as Wolff–Parkinson–White syndrome; cardiac failure can occur rarely. Rhabdomyomas tend to regress spontaneously.

PULMONARY

Lymphangioleiomyomatosis (LAM) (MIM#606690) involves smooth muscle infiltrating the lung interstitium; it predominantly affects females, and is a ***major feature***; it is found in 30–40% of female TSC patients (and up to 80% females by age 40), but only in 12% of males with TSC; it becomes symptomatic in females by their third to fourth decade, with shortness of breath on exertion, and pneumothoraxes; it is very rare for males with TSC to become symptomatic; LAM is found in 30% of patients with TSC2 mutations.

RENAL

Angiomyolipomas (> 2) are seen in 80% TSC patients, most commonly in the kidney (occasionally in liver or other organs), and are ***major features***. Multiple renal cysts are a minor feature; seen in patients with TSC1 or TSC2 or those with a contiguous gene deletion syndrome (PKDTS, MIM#600273) affecting both the TSC2 and PKD1 (polycystic kidney disease) genes, which are neighbours, and both transcribed on chromosome 16p13.3, but in opposite directions. PKDTS causes a very severe renal phenotype. TSC2 mutations are associated with higher incidence and greater severity of renal angiomyolipomas and cysts. Renal disease follows severe intellectual impairment as a major cause of early mortality. Other non-diagnostic renal manifestations include renal cell carcinoma.

ENDOCRINE, GASTROINTESTINAL AND SKELETAL SYSTEMS

'Non-renal hamartomas' can occur in any of these system, and are minor features; uncommon, they have been described in: the adrenals, thyroid, pituitary, pancreas and gonads; the liver and rectum; bone.

History
Ask about the following.

PRESENTING COMPLAINT
Reason for current admission.

CURRENT SYMPTOMS

1. Seizures; infantile (epileptic) spasms are the most common seizure type at diagnosis, but various types can occur; for each type of seizure, ask: age of onset, any prodromal symptoms (e.g. irritability, pallor), precipitating factors (seizure triggers), aura, initial cry or scream, initial localising signs (e.g. twitching of hand of hemiplegic side), description of all aspects of seizure itself (e.g. eyes rolling back, cyanosis, tonus, clonus, incontinence), duration of seizure (range [e.g. between 2 and 20 minutes], usual time [e.g. 2 minutes], any episodes of status epilepticus [over 5 minutes]), frequency of seizures (range and 'usual'), time of occurrence (waking, going to sleep), date and time of last seizure, postictal events (e.g. sleeping, residual paralysis), usual treatment, recent/future planned surgical procedures for fitting (e.g. focal cortical resection, hemispherectomy), emergency plan for status epilepticus.
2. Cognitive abilities, or present developmental status (e.g. intellectual impairment), schooling details.
3. Learning issues at school (e.g. executive functioning skills, any neuropsychometric testing by guidance officer), any help needed, attitudes of class teacher, fellow students.
4. Behavioural issues (e.g. ADHD, ASD, anxiety, or depression symptomatology, and any relevant medications such as stimulants), professionals involved in management (psychologist, psychiatrist, paediatrician, therapists).
5. Cardiovascular disease; rhabdomyoma: structural obstructive or arrhythmic symptoms: shortness of breath, cyanosis, palpitations, chest pain, fainting.

Associated vascular symptoms attributable to coarctation of aorta, or renal artery stenosis (hypertension, headache), or thoraco-abdominal aneurysm.

6. Pulmonary disease; lymphangioleiomyomatosis (LAM) respiratory symptoms: dyspnoea on exertion, cough, haemoptysis, pneumothorax, oxygen requirement, mTOR inhibitor (sirolimus), future plans for lung transplantation.

7. Renal disease: hypertension (secondary to renal artery stenosis, polycystic kidney disease, renal cell carcinoma, large angiomyofibromas causing chronic kidney disease [CKD]), level of BP, anti-hypertensive therapy, monitoring BP; symptoms of headache; monitoring for angiomyofibroma, treatment with an mTOR inhibitor, awareness of potential need for surgical/embolic/ablative treatments in event of ruptured aneurysm within an angiomyolipoma, presenting as retroperitoneal haemorrhage with severe abdominal pain, vomiting and shock.

8. Surveillance history: how often having MRIs, HRCTs, USs and similar investigations.

PAST HISTORY

1. Initial diagnosis: what age informed diagnosis of TSC.
2. Time period between being informed of TSC diagnosis and development of symptoms.
3. What investigations undertaken to confirm diagnosis.
4. Evolution of seizures, evolution/regression of development.
5. Number of hospitalisations and indications for these.
6. Development of complications (e.g. learning issues at school, ADHD and/or ASD symptomatology) and their management.
7. Previous medications tried (AEDs, stimulants), surgical procedures (e.g. for seizures).
8. Immunisations, allergies.

CURRENT MANAGEMENT

Present treatment in hospital, usual treatment at home (including physiotherapy, occupational therapy, speech therapy, exercise, medications taken), future treatment plans (e.g. surgical procedures), usual follow-up (by whom, where, how often), unproven (not really 'alternative') therapies tried (e.g. naturopathy).

SOCIAL HISTORY

1. Impact on child (e.g. delays or regression in development, difficulties at school, limitations on lifestyle, body image, self-esteem, peer reactions).
2. Impact on family (e.g. parental coping, difficulties between mother and father, effect on siblings, financial considerations, transport, hospitalisations, private health insurance).
3. Benefits received.
4. Social supports (e.g. social worker, Tuberous Sclerosis Support via www.agsa -geneticsupport.org.au, early intervention services for children with disabilities (e.g. via https://dss.gov.au, via www.betterstart.net.au).

FAMILY HISTORY

A three-generation family history is worth taking; can mention gene testing in discussion if TSC suspected but not able to be diagnosed clinically in family members.

UNDERSTANDING OF DISEASE

By the child, by the family (e.g. parents, siblings, grandparents) and by teachers. Ask about the degree of previous education about TSC (e.g. in hospital, by local paediatrician), and contingency plans (e.g. status epilepticus). At the completion of the history, think about what particular problems this family is experiencing at the moment, from the viewpoints of the child, the parents and the attending physicians. These three perspectives may be quite different.

Examination

See separate short case on TSC in this chapter.

Management

EPILEPSY

Seizures in TSC (which occur in 85% of patients) are often refractory to treatment. TSC-associated epilepsy typically presents in the first 12 months of life as infantile spasms or as focal seizures, initially, and over half these children have multiple seizure types. The genetic make-up can influence this: those with TSC2 mutations have earlier seizures, more tubers and lower cognitive outcomes than those with TSC1 mutations. In general, the earlier the fits, the greater risk of neurodevelopmental and intellectual deficits. As the mechanism of tumour growth has been dissected, and the importance of mTOR pathways have become clear, mTOR inhibitors such as everolimus have shown significant success in the management of TSC-associated epilepsy, and particularly in the management of SEGAs. Everolimus can decrease SEGA tumour size by over 30%, in three out of four patients, and can decrease seizure activity in those same patients by over 50.

Recommended treatments for infantile spasms: first line: vigabatrin. Vigabatrin is dramatically effective in IS in TSC: 95% of children with IS due to TSC respond to vigabatrin, many more than in IS due to other conditions. There is improved long-term intellectual outcome if IS is treated earlier with vigabatrin. It is not known why vigabatrin is so effective in TSC.

Second line treatment: **h**ormone (ACTH) if **h**ypsarrhythmia on EEG, but topiramate if no hypsarrhythmia. Third line treatment: ketogenic diet, other AEDs; other: tailored surgical resection for focal area of dysplasia.

Recommended treatments for focal seizures: first line; vigabatrin under 1 year of age, GABAergic-inhibiting AEDs (topiramate or carbamazepine) over 1 year of age; second line: tailored surgical resection; third line: other AEDs for focal seizures, ketogenic diet, vagus nerve stimulation; other: for Lennox-Gastaut syndrome, recommended agent is rufinamide, which is unrelated to other AEDs, its exact mechanism of action unclear, although likely related to modulation of sodium channel activity; for atonic seizures (drop attacks) and tonic seizures, recommended agent is, again, rufinamide, also vagus nerve stimulation can be useful.

Surgery is generally limited to focal stereotypical seizures with a solitary EEG focus, in patients with fitting refractory to two AEDs; it is also considered if there is a single focus thought to be responsible for infantile spasms or bilateral seizures, or if there is a predominant seizure type which is most problematic in a child with other seizure types, where invasive recording can be very useful to assist in obtaining good surgical results.

In TSC, prophylactic therapy with AEDs can be justified if there are ictal EEG discharges without clinical evidence of fitting in children under 24 months, as early diagnosis and treatment may diminish the adverse effects of early onset seizures. EEG monitoring is recommended monthly for the first 6 months of life, then every 6 to 8 weeks (until 24 months of age). EEG also should be obtained if there are any sudden changes in behaviour or sleeping patterns, as this could be an epileptiform event rather than TAND.

Known SEGA with symptoms, either clearly referrable to ventricular enlargement, or alterations in usual neurological findings, or TAND, requires neurosurgical resection, which may include ventriculoperitoneal shunting; (*symptomatic SEGAs => surgery +/– shunt*). SEGA without symptoms, but growing and/or causing ventricular enlargement, requires either treatment with an mTOR inhibitor like everolimus, or resection.

Everolimus has US Food and Drug Administration approval for treatment of TSC patients with SEGA who are not surgical resection candidates. Dosage for everolimus is based on surface area, commencing at 4.5 mg/metre squared/day, then rounded to the nearest tablet size.

Side effects of everolimus can include hyperlipidaemia with elevated cholesterol and triglycerides (which may obviate a low-fat, low cholesterol diet, but is rarely a reason to stop the drug), transaminitis and leucopenia; thus testing with FBC, LFTs, fasting lipids, plus urea and electrolytes, is advised, prior to commencing everolimus. Therapeutic drug monitoring is important, starting 2 weeks after starting the drug. Mouth (aphthous) ulcers can occur in up to a third of patients receiving mTOR inhibitors.

Everolimus can reduce substantially the size of SEGA tumours, even reversing hydrocephalus and midline shifts in some cases. Interactions with AEDs are important to consider: drugs which induce the cytochrome P450 enzyme system, such as oxcarbazepine, can decrease everolimus levels; therefore, drugs like topiramate or levetiracetam are better choices if the child is receiving everolimus but seizures still require a new AED.

Sudden changes in behaviour should trigger rapid assessment to exclude SEGA as cause. MRI of the brain should be obtained every 1–3 years up to the age of 25, to screen for development of SEGA. It has been recommended that TAND be screened for yearly, but more comprehensively at several developmental ages: infancy (0–3 years), preschool (3–6 years), primary school (6–9 years), adolescence (12–16 years) and early adulthood (18–25 years). There are many trials currently evaluating everolimus therapy for neurocognitive problems and autism in TSC.

RENAL MANIFESTATIONS

MRI of the abdomen should be obtained every 1 to 3 years; angiomyolipomas are usually lipid-rich on MRI, appearing bright with T2-weighted images, but do not take up gadolinium (this differentiates them from the rarer renal cell carcinoma which are lipid-poor, take up gadolinium and grow more rapidly). The importance of angiomyolipomas is their potential to: 1. bleed, as larger angiomyolipomas (especially over 3–4 cm squared) have fragile vasculature and can lead to life-threatening retroperitoneal haemorrhage; 2. damage normal kidney tissue; 3. decrease renal function; or 4. compress other viscera.

Treatment for symptomatic angiomyolipomas which present with acute haemorrhage comprises embolisation by an interventional radiologist, and then corticosteroids; primary treatment for asymptomatic angiomyolipomas (larger than 3 cm^2) comprises an mTOR inhibitor such as everolimus; for those above 6 cm^2 in size, selective embolisation or resection, but avoiding nephrectomy. Around 40% of angiomyolipomas respond to mTOR inhibitor therapy. Renal function (including calculated GFR) and BP should be checked at least yearly.

PULMONARY MANIFESTATIONS

LAM predominantly affects young women. Complications include pneumothoraxes and chylous lung effusion. High-resolution CT (HRCT) scanning can diagnose LAM readily. Pulmonary function testing may demonstrate decreased forced expiratory volume in 1 second (FEV1) early in the clinical course of LAM. On occasion, early symptoms of LAM can be misdiagnosed as asthma. Surveillance recommendations include: if asymptomatic, 5–10 yearly HRCT; if symptomatic or known lung cysts, then 2–3 yearly HRCT and annual pulmonary function testing. Therapy with mTOR inhibitors (everolimus) can be used for moderate, severe or rapidly progressive LAM. Lung transplantation is another option if not precluded by comorbid TSC aspects, also remembering that anti-rejection drugs may lower seizure threshold and AEDs may impact negatively on anti-rejection drugs.

DERMATOLOGICAL, DENTAL, CARDIOLOGICAL AND OPHTHALMOLOGICAL MANIFESTATIONS

None of these are likely to be problematic, and there are minimal agreed approaches. Skin lesions have been treated successfully with surgical excision, laser therapy and topical mTOR inhibitors. Dental enamel defects rarely cause symptoms. Oral fibromas can be excised. Bony jaw lesions can be excised or undergo curettage. Cardiac rhabdomyomas regress, but warrant 1–3 yearly echocardiography until then, and regular ECGs at 3–5 year intervals to monitor for conduction defects. Annual eye evaluation is recommended, especially if the patient is receiving vigabatrin which can cause field cuts.

GENOTYPE—PHENOTYPE CORRELATIONS

Children with TSC2 mutations, as a group, have more severe phenotypic features, with an earlier age of seizure onset, a higher rate of intellectual impairment, and more tubers. However, within the group with TSC2 mutations, there are specific genotypes associated with less severe disease. A missense mutation of the central area of TSC2 (exons 23–33) leads to a lower risk of infantile spasms. The R905Q mutation leads to skin lesions and seizures which are very responsive to AEDs. The G1556S mutation leads to a mild phenotype with minimal cerebral effects. However, the same mutation can be associated with quite different phenotypes, from mild to severe.

SHORT CASE: Developmental assessment

Entire books have been written describing the approach to evaluating a child's development. This section is not meant to be a detailed description, but merely a guide to the general areas that should be covered, and a suggested overall plan.

All candidates will be familiar with at least one type of developmental assessment system, and should continue using one with which they are comfortable (e.g. the Denver Developmental Screening Test).

Candidates often fear the lead-in, 'Would you please perform a developmental assessment', simply because there is an associated mythology of difficulty, which is unwarranted. Once you know the first 18 months of development 'backwards', including the times of appearance and incorporation of all the primitive reflexes, then you should be fairly well equipped to interpret your findings, as this tends to be the age range that is more popular as an examination subject.

The problem with this case is not one of interpretation but of inappropriate actions, such as distracting an infant with a noise-making stimulus when testing vision, or not undressing the patient when assessing gross motor milestones. This section addresses those issues.

Begin by introducing yourself to the parent and patient. Inspect for the following:
1. Growth parameters; for example, failure to thrive, associated with syndromal or chromosomal anomalies. Undernutrition or chronic illnesses can be associated with developmental delay, as may be small or large head size.

2. Evidence of any dysmorphic features (various syndromal diagnoses).
3. Appearance of the 'ex-premature' infant (beware the 'ex-premmie' whose age is not corrected for prematurity).
4. Obvious neurological abnormalities (including 'floppy infant' posturing, hemiplegic posturing and involuntary movements).

The next step depends on the age of the child. A child small enough to be comfortably sat on his or her mother's knee should be positioned there for assessment of vision, hearing, language, personal–social interaction and fine motor control.

It is unwise to remove a child from his or her mother to perform a gross motor assessment first. Often, candidates seem too keen to do exactly that. It does not help rapport with the child, mother or examiner. If a child is older, then he or she may prefer to be examined sitting on a chair.

Always test vision before hearing. Fixing and following, and an approximation of visual acuity (e.g. the ability to pick up a 'hundred and thousand' for infants, or the ability to read in older children), are important. Testing of visual fields is not required. Testing each eye separately is desirable, but can be difficult to achieve without upsetting an infant.

Testing hearing, with the infant on the mother's lap, requires initial distraction with a non-noisemaking (i.e. purely visual) stimulus, directly in front of the child. This is then hidden, at which time the noise-maker (e.g. bell) is brought towards the ear from behind (out of range of visual fields) by an assistant (e.g. the chief examiner). On a signal given by yourself, the assistant makes a sound (e.g. rings the bell) at a certain distance from the ear (this varies for different ages), testing each ear in turn and noting whether the child's facial expression, or activity (in babies), changes, and if the head turns towards the stimulus, localising the sound (in older children). If the conditions are not optimal for testing hearing (e.g. fractious toddler), say so. If there is an equivocal result, it is reasonable to suggest a formal audiological assessment.

The fine motor assessment can then be performed. If the child is severely visually impaired, this makes assessment very difficult, and explains the logic of always testing vision first. Ensure that you have appropriate objects in your case to test fine motor functions, such as 'hundreds and thousands', raisins (testing pincer grip), 2.5 cm blocks (for stacking), different-sized beads and threads (threading a bead is a good test of coordination), a biro with a top (putting the top on a biro is another good test of coordination and fine motor development), and a plastic knife, fork and spoon set.

Throughout the testing described above, assessment of personal–social interaction and language can be performed. Do not forget to comment on any vocalising the child does, or on interactions with you (e.g. smiling, waving, laughing), as these may give very valuable information, which can be overlooked if it is not actively considered as part of a developmental assessment.

Finally, perform a gross motor assessment. In an infant, or severely impaired patient, this comprises the '180° examination', and in an older child, a gait examination.

The '180° examination' aptly describes the sequence of manoeuvres examined, as follows. Note that the gross motor assessment should be performed on a firm surface, so if the examining couch is not firm, a sheet or blanket can be spread on the floor (the examiners must be aware that you realise the need for a firm surface).

First, with the child lying supine, note the posture (e.g. adopting abnormal asymmetric tonic neck reflex [ATNR] positioning) and movement (e.g. choreoathetoid movements with cerebral palsy [CP], paucity of movement with some neuromuscular diseases).

Next, draw the child into the sitting position, by traction on the arms, noting the degree of head control/lag (e.g. marked head lag with spinal muscular atrophy).

With the child in the sitting position, note the amount of head and trunk control, and ability to sit, supported and unsupported.

Next, hold the child up to check weight bearing. This helps detect lower limb scissoring (as in CP), lower limb hypotonia and weakness (e.g. neuromuscular disorders causing the 'floppy infant' syndrome), and inappropriately 'advanced' weight bearing (in CP).

Then, hold the child in ventral suspension and describe the posture of the head, trunk and limbs. This position can demonstrate hypotonia well: if very severe, the infant describes a 'C' shape over the examiner's hand. The converse can occur with CP, where an exaggerated extensor posture may be adopted.

Finally, lay the child prone. Make sure that the hands are placed to either side of the infant's shoulders, with the palms apposed to the bed and elbows flexed, to optimise the ability to extend the upper limbs. Note the ability of the child to raise the head and trunk when placed prone.

The primitive reflexes may be checked separately after the 180° examination, or may be incorporated into the sequence (e.g. assessing the sucking, rooting, ATNR and neck-righting reflexes when supine, the grasp reflex when pulling the child to sit, the placing and stepping reflexes when held standing to check weight bearing, the Landau and Galant reflexes when held in ventral suspension), depending on personal preference. Whichever is chosen, leave the Moro and parachute reflexes until last, as they may upset the child.

If you are checking the primitive reflexes separately, the following is a suggested order, with the usual times of appearance and incorporation, or disappearance, of the reflexes. The elicitation of the lesser-known reflexes is detailed:

1. *Sucking* and *rooting* (birth to 4 months, when awake, and to 6 months when sleeping).
2. *Palmar grasp* (birth to 3 months).
3. *Placing, stepping* (both from birth to 6 weeks).
4. *Landau reflex*, a two-stage reflex. With the child supported prone (with your hand under the abdomen), the child should (normally) extend head, trunk and hips. This is the first, and more important, stage. Next, flex the head and neck; normally the response is flexion of trunk and hips, but this is less constant than the first stage (first stage from 4 months, plus second stage from 9 months; gone by 2 years).
5. *ATNR*. With the child supine, the head is rotated to one side. A 'fencing' posture develops, with extension of the ipsilateral upper and lower limb (i.e. the side towards which the head is turned) and flexion of the opposite side (2–6 months). Persistence beyond 6 months is indicative of upper motor neurone problems, especially CP. Maintaining the ATNR posture throughout the time that the head is held turned, such that the child cannot 'break' from that position, is similarly significant.
6. *Neck-righting reflex*. Rotation of the trunk to conform with the position of the head when the head is rotated to one side (6 months to 2 years).
7. *Moro reflex* (birth to 4 months). As with most primitive reflexes, persistence beyond the usual time of disappearance is pathological. Make a point of focusing not only on the limb movements but also the facial response, for asymmetry (e.g. in hemiplegic CP).
8. *Parachute reflex*. With the infant held in the prone position, move him or her rapidly, face downwards, towards the floor. The normal reaction is to extend both upper limbs as if to break the fall (appears between 6 and 12 months, usually at 9 months, and persists; its absence beyond 12 months is abnormal). Asymmetry occurs with hemiplegia.

Remember that primitive reflexes do not actually 'disappear', but become incorporated and kept under control by the CNS. The only primitive reflex which is never incorporated is the parachute reflex. Primitive reflexes which have 'disappeared' and then 'reappear' do so in the context of cerebral damage (such as the well-known glabellar tap in Parkinson's disease).

As the examination is proceeding, it is useful to comment on each finding as it is elicited, making sure that the examiners see that you know the significance of each sign found. Terms such as 'age appropriate' may be useful when normal findings occur.

A succinct summary at the completion of the examination should attempt to give a developmental age to each of the areas assessed, and state whether any delay detected is global, or whether there is a scatter of abilities (e.g. gross and fine motor delay only in Werdnig–Hoffmann disease, visual and gross motor impairment in an ex-premature baby, global delay in a child with congenital rubella or severe CP).

SHORT CASE: Eye examination—general

This is not an infrequent case. The number of possible pathologies is clearly enormous, but the candidate should be able to perform a comprehensive eye examination as outlined, and should be familiar with important paediatric eye conditions that can appear in examinations; a selected few are outlined below.

Background information: some important eye conditions
LIDS
Ptosis (short for blepharoptosis)
The muscle involved in elevation of the lid is the levator palpebrae superioris, supplied by the third cranial nerve. Congenital causes of ptosis are the most common. Acquired causes include myopathies and third cranial nerve palsy (and Horner's syndrome causes a partial ptosis). Mechanical problems such as orbital cellulitis or haemangioma may also cause ptosis. Bilateral ptosis should prompt examination for a neuromuscular cause.

IRIS
Aniridia
This is actually hypoplasia, not absence, of the iris; the root of the iris is present. Associated developmental anomalies of the eye include cataract, glaucoma and corneal opacification. There are at least two types of aniridia, one autosomal dominant, the other sporadic and associated with Wilms' tumour and genitourinary anomalies (deletion of chromosome 11).

LENS
Cataract
This opacity of the lens has a wide differential diagnosis, although in 50% of cases no cause is detected. Groups of causes include hereditary (e.g. autosomal dominant), chromosomal disorders (e.g. Down syndrome), other malformation syndromes (e.g. Noonan syndrome), congenital TORCH infections, metabolic disorders (e.g. diabetes mellitus, galactosaemia) and drugs (e.g. steroids). It is important to examine the child to detect these underlying problems.

Ectopia lentis
This displacement of the lens may be inherited as the sole anomaly, or may be associated with systemic conditions, such as Marfan syndrome (where it usually displaces superiorly;

mnemonic Mar*fan*—remember [ceiling] *fans are up* above) and homocystinuria (where it mostly displaces inferiorly; remember this as the opposite to Marfan).

RETINA
Colobomata
This defect, or lack of some portion, of tissue can involve any part of the eye. The most important types are chorioretinal and isolated optic nerve colobomata.

Optic nerve hypoplasia
This can be an isolated anomaly, or be associated with other eye anomalies (microphthalmos, aniridia) and neurological problems such as encephalocele. It is associated with absence of the corpus callosum.

Retinopathy of prematurity (ROP)
This can only occur before the retina is vascularised. As the peripheral retina is the region that is vascularised last in the eye of the baby, it is the most commonly involved area. ROP affects around 80% of babies under 1 kg and almost 10% of these will have their vision threatened. Among those between 1 and 1.5 kg, 50% are affected with ROP, and 2% of these will have their vision threatened. The stage, location and extent of ROP are the standard three aspects that determine management.

There are five stages of ROP:

Stage 1. Flat white demarcation line between avascular and vascularised retina.
Stage 2. Ridge due to arteriovenous shunting (demarcation line raised into vitreous).
Stage 3. Extraretinal fibrovascular proliferation (new vessels elevated into vitreous).
Stage 4A. Partial retinal detachment, macula attached (visual prognosis still hopeful).
Stage 4B. Partial retinal detachment, macula detached (visual prognosis poor).
Stage 5. Complete retinal detachment.

'Plus' is added to each stage if there are dilated and tortuous vessels in the posterior retina. This indicates a worse prognosis and more progressive disease.

Three zones are described:

Zone I. A circle centred on the optic nerve, the radius being double the distance from the optic nerve to fovea; disease here is the most dangerous.
Zone II. The edge of Zone I to the ora serrata (nasal side), to the anatomic equator (temporal side).
Zone III. The peripheral crescent on the temporal side.

The extent is described relative to the circumferential distribution, in clock hours, with the entire eye comprising 12 clock hours, divided into single clock hours of 30°.

If the disease is Stage 3 in 5–8 adjacent clock hours with plus disease in Zone II, treatment with cryotherapy is warranted; this is the threshold level. The small (less than 1000 g) sick baby who goes from crisis to crisis is at greatest risk.

SQUINT (STRABISMUS)
Certain terms should be known by the candidate:
- *Pseudostrabismus*: false appearance of squint (often due to epicanthal folds).
- *Orthophoria*: perfect condition of ocular balance.
- *Heterophoria*: latent tendency to squint (e.g. when tired).

- *Heterotropia*: permanent tendency to squint.
- *Non-paralytic squint*: not due to a problem with any extraocular muscles or the cranial nerves supplying them.
- *Paralytic squint*: due to a problem with extraocular muscles or cranial nerves.
- *Esotropia*: convergent squint.
- *Exotropia*: divergent squint.

Squint can be divided into non-paralytic and paralytic types.

NON-PARALYTIC

1. Convergent (i.e. esotropia). Types include infantile and accommodative. Accommodative squint typically presents around age 18 months to 2 years.
2. Divergent (i.e. exotropia). Types include intermittent and constant.

PARALYTIC

1. Third nerve palsy (frequently congenital; divergent squint, plus downward deviation of eye and ptosis).
2. Fourth nerve palsy (congenital or acquired from head trauma; accompanying head tilt towards opposite shoulder to eliminate a vertical deviation).
3. Sixth nerve palsy (frequently acquired from head trauma; convergent squint).

Procedure

The paediatric eye examination is best done with the child sitting on the side of the bed, in a chair or on the parent's lap, depending on the child's age. After introducing yourself, stand back and look at the overall appearance of the child, particularly for dysmorphic features (various malformation syndromes have eye involvement), facial features of the 'ex-premmie' (associated ROP) and growth parameters (e.g. may be small and microcephalic, with intrauterine infection). Also note any head tilt (e.g. with fourth cranial nerve palsy). After brief comments on general appearance, direct your attention to the eyes.

Irrespective of the child's age, eye examination is always started by inspection for external abnormalities. Commence by looking from in front, from the side and from above to detect any proptosis. Next, focus successively on each of the anatomical structures of the eye to detect any abnormalities (i.e. look at the eyebrows, eyelids, cornea, iris, sclera and conjunctivae). This systematic approach should prevent important signs being overlooked. If the child wears glasses, examine these also.

After inspection, proceed with testing of visual acuity in each eye. Response to a face is the best way of trying to assess whether or not an infant can see. Note whether the infant can fix and follow by moving your face in front of him or her. After a face, the next best target is a large bright object (e.g. red ball of wool). See if the child is fixing and following. If he or she can see a large object, then proceed to test with smaller objects down to the pinhead size of a 'hundred and thousand' cake decoration. If there is no response to your face, use a torch to check response to a bright light. In older children, Sheridan–Gardner Test Charts (preschool age) or the Snellen Test Charts (school age) can be used. If these tests suggest a problem with acuity, then comment on the need for formal testing.

Testing of the visual fields can then be performed. Again, the technique is age dependent. In infants, use a red ball of wool brought from behind the child's head: head turning indicates when it enters the visual field. In older children, a direct confrontation can be used, first with both eyes and then with each eye separately. The classic 'red hat pin' technique can be used with adolescents. (See Figure 13.3.)

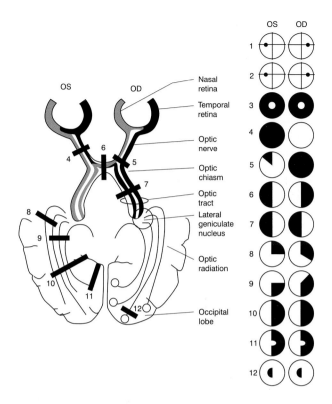

Figure 13.3 **Visual pathways (left side of diagram) and representative lesions resulting in visual field loss (right side of diagram). (1, 2 and 3 are represented only on the right side of the diagram.)**

Redrawn from; D. P. Edward, L. M. Kaufman, Pediatric Clinics of North America, Volume 50 (2003), pp. 16 to 17, Figure 14. (1) Normal visual field showing normal blind spot. (2) Bilateral macular lesion (exp. congenital toxoplasmosis) with central scotoma both eyes (OU). (3) Tunnel visual fields OU as seen in advanced glaucoma. (4) Optic nerve lesion in the left eye (OS), resulting in ipsilateral unilateral loss of vision. (5) Junction lesion in the right eye (OD) damaging optic nerve OD and decussating inferonasal retinal fibres OS that project into contralateral optic nerve (Wilbrand's knee), resulting in loss of vision OD and superotemporal wedge scotoma OS. (6) Optic chiasm lesion resulting in bitemporal hemianopsia. (7) Optic tract lesion on right, resulting in left homonymous hemianopsia. (8) Optic radiation fibres from the ipsilateral inferotemporal retina and contralateral inferonasal retina course laterally from the lateral geniculate nucleus into the parietal lobe. Lesions of these fibres on the left side result in bilateral incongruous right superior quadrantanopsia. (9) Optic radiation fibres from the ipsilateral supero temporal retina and contralateral superonasal retina course directly posterior from the lateral geniculate nucleus into the parietal lobe. Lesions of these fibres on the left side result in bilateral incongruous right inferior quadrantanopsia. (10) A complete left optic radiation lesion resulting in right homonymous hemianopsia. (11) Lesion of the ventral aspect of the left occipital cortex, resulting in right homonymous hemianopsia with macular sparing. (12) Lesion of the dorsal aspect of the right occipital cortex, resulting in left homonymous central scotoma. (Illustrations by Adrienne J. Boutwell and Lisa J. Birmingham D University of Illinois Board of Trustees 2002.)

Extraocular movements can then be tested (see the short case on motor cranial nerves in this chapter). It is probably easier to hold the child's head still with one hand, and have the child follow an interesting target (e.g. a small bright puppet) held by the other hand, than to keep asking the child to stop moving the head. Both eyes can be tested together, and the child should be asked, at each position of gaze, to indicate any diplopia: 'Say how many you see' or 'Say if you see two'.

The evaluation of eye movements in the newborn infant can be difficult. One way to overcome this is to pick the baby up and move him or her in various directions, watching the eye movements produced because of the vestibular ocular reflex (when the child is rotated, eyes move in the opposite direction, and nystagmus occurs; when rotation is ceased, after-nystagmus occurs). Thus, moving the child up and down, side to side and backwards and forwards will permit evaluation of the main directions of eye movement.

At this stage, in older children, depending on the clinical findings so far, it may be appropriate to check for lid lag (if there is a suggestion of thyrotoxicosis) and fatiguability on upward gaze (to screen for myasthenia gravis, particularly if there is bilateral ptosis or myopathic facies).

Near and far cover tests should be performed, with an interesting toy as the fixation target. If the child becomes upset when one eye is covered, this suggests poor vision in the uncovered eye (although this should have been detected when assessing visual acuity). Also, shine a torch into the eyes from a distance to detect a squint (although this will not detect microstrabismus).

Testing the pupillary light reflexes and fundoscopy are usually best left until the end, because of the cooperation required and time constraints. When assessing the pupils, note whether they are of normal size (or have been dilated for the examination) and if there is any asymmetry in size, and then check the light reflex (with a pen-torch; remember to place a hand between the eyes as a barrier to prevent any light reaching the opposite side to the one being tested; also watch for the Marcus Gunn phenomenon). Check the accommodation reflex.

Ophthalmoscopy is then performed. First, look for the red reflex. Then the anterior aspects of the eye should be examined, the cornea, the lens and finally retinoscopy. Remember that one of the 'golden eye rules' is 'never give an opinion through an undilated pupil'. However, the examiners may expect an opinion (the pupils may already be dilated; if not, it may be appropriate to comment that dilating the pupils would be helpful).

Finally, for completeness, offer to test the corneal reflex (do not just go ahead and do it, as children tend to find this very distressing), palpate for evidence of raised intraocular pressure (glaucoma) and then auscultate over each closed eyelid with the bell of the stethoscope (with the child holding his or her breath while you auscultate, if possible) for bruits.

At the completion of the examination, the examiners may ask whether there is anything else you would like to assess. This will depend on the most obvious finding, as in the following examples:

1. *Finding: papilloedema.* The next steps could include a neurological examination for signs of raised intracranial pressure, measuring the BP to detect hypertension and checking for asterixis from hypercapnia.
2. *Finding: retinopathy consistent with diabetes.* The next steps may include an endocrine assessment and urinalysis.
3. *Finding: nystagmus.* The next steps would include a full neurological examination; for example, for cerebellar signs, if there is horizontal nystagmus. See separate short case on nystagmus.

VISUAL ACUITY

At birth, all normal children can see, but normal 'adult' acuity takes a few years to develop. Expected acuity is as follows:

1. At birth, normal visual acuity is approximately 3/60.
2. By 6 months, normal visual acuity is 6/30.
3. By 18 months, it is 6/9.
4. By 2 years, it is 6/6.

STAGES OF VISUAL DEVELOPMENT (IN RELATION TO CLINICALLY APPLICABLE TESTING)

- Neonates turn their head towards a diffuse light source.
- By 6 weeks of age, babies follow a face or large, coloured (especially red) object (which should be silent, so that turning to sound is not misinterpreted). Also by this age the 'blink to menace' response is present.
- By 3 months, the eyes converge for finger-play.
- By 4 months, the infant follows objects through 180°, turning the head.
- By 5 months, infants reach for a toy within their visual field and are able to regard a small raisin on a table.
- By 6 months, they move the eyes together in all directions. A squint at this stage is abnormal. This is the earliest age at which the Stycar graded balls test can be used to test the vision.
- By 9 months, they are able to pick up a raisin (raking grasp), look for fallen toys and play peek-a-boo.
- By 12 months, babies are able to pick up a raisin with neat pincer grasp. At this stage, it is possible to test with rolling balls as small as 3 mm at a distance of 3 m. Also, the Stycar mounted balls test for ability to fixate and peripheral vision can be used. In the examination setting, a ball of red wool can be used for peripheral vision testing, bringing it from behind the child and watching the head turn towards the ball when it enters the child's visual field.

Between 1 and 2 years, the allure of rolling balls has diminished, and it is difficult to hold the child's attention, but if this is possible, the rolling and mounted ball tests remain useful. From 2 years, miniature toy-matching tests can be used. Remember that by the age of 2 years, acuity should be 6/6. For preschool children (31/2 to 51/2 years old), the Sheridan–Gardner test or the E test can be used. The former is a better test, as children are less likely to become confused because laterality is not involved. For school-aged children, the Snellen Test Charts can be used, or the E test if the child cannot recognise the Snellen Chart letters.

SHORT CASE: Eye examination—nystagmus

This is presented as a separate short case as it is complicated, but worth further consideration. Two 'mantras' are worth mentioning first:

1. '*Unilateral nystagmus is due to a tumour until proved otherwise*', or said another way, never make a diagnosis of spasmus nutans syndrome without a normal MRI of the brain and eyes.

   Unilateral → MRI

2. '*Look out for nystagmus in internuclear ophthalmoplegia*'. When a child with internuclear ophthalmoplegia (INO) looks to one side, there is a failure of adduction in the affected eye, while the contralateral eye abducts (hence, 'looking out'), and develops nystagmus. So this is another cause of apparent 'unilateral' nystagmus, although the unilaterality may alternate. Internuclear ophthalmoplegia indicates significant brainstem pathology affecting the medial longitudinal fasciculus (MLF). If the child with left-sided INO (with left MLF pathology) looks to the right, the left (affected side) eye fails to adduct, while the right eye can abduct (look out) to the right, but develops nystagmus.

   Look out for nystagmus → *abducting eye* gets nystagmus

Nystagmus can be defined as oscillations of the eyes which are rhythmic, involuntary, periodic and to-and-fro, and may have components described as 'pendular' (where the bilateral oscillations are of the same velocity in both directions) and/or components described as 'jerk' (where the eye movement in one direction is clearly faster than that in the opposite direction); children with congenital nystagmus usually have a combination of pendular and jerk waveforms, and these vary with direction of gaze and the age of the patient. In cases of jerk nystagmus, it is described by the direction of the fast movement, although this is the corrective movement; it is the slow movement which represents the pathology. Further descriptive subdivisions address whether both sides or just one side are involved, the form the nystagmus takes (horizontal, vertical or rotary, in the various fields of gaze), whether the movements are conjugate or dysconjugate, and whether there is a null point (where the oscillations are minimised or absent). Vertical nystagmus is rare in paediatric patients. Horizontal conjugate nystagmus in children is most commonly due to anticonvulsant medication, but for children with a negative drug history, cerebellar disease is the most common cause.

Nystagmus is typically divided into two groups: congenital and acquired causes. Most congenital causes are related to visual conditions, whereas acquired causes are more likely due to vestibular or cerebellar pathology, or medications. Afferent nystagmus, from congenital causes of impaired vision, is usually not seen until 2 or 3 months of age. Causes include congenital cataracts, high refractive errors, congenital optic atrophy and oculo-cutaneous albinism; these should be able to be identified by fundoscopy. Children whose vision is severely impaired before their second birthday almost invariably develop nystagmus, whereas children whose vision is severely impaired after they have turned 6 years of age do not; between these ages it is variable.

Congenital nystagmus is bilateral, conjugate and horizontal, typically having a null point at 10–30° for the primary position; waveforms vary (jerk, pendular or combination of both), and increase with fixation or lateral gaze. The direction remains horizontal and uniplanar, with vertical gaze; this occurs only in three conditions: congenital nystagmus, labyrinthine disease (peripheral vestibular nystagmus), and periodic alternating nystagmus (which is horizontal jerk nystagmus which intermittently changes direction, and can occur with cervicomedullary junction anomalies, such as Arnold–Chiari malformations). Patients with congenital nystagmus typically do not have abnormal visual sensory apparatus;

that is, there is no afferent nystagmus, and the wobbling movements are responsible for visual problems. There may be a head tilt to maintain the null point.

Examination procedure

Introduce yourself to patient and parent. Note whether the child looks well or unwell, note growth parameters, any dysmorphic features (many syndromes can include nystagmus, such as Bardet–Biedl, Crouzon, Down, Noonan) or features suggesting oculo-cutaneous albinism (white hair). Note the child's posture; see if there is any head tilt, as this may represent a null point for when the child is looking forwards. It is worth spending a few minutes watching the nystagmus movements in each of the nine main eye positions.

If the movement is **bilateral and roving**, the cause is most likely *visual*, so testing visual acuity is the first priority.

If the movement is **horizontal**, the cause may be *cerebellar, vestibular or visual*; it is still appropriate to check acuity first, and if this is not impaired, then it is prudent to move onto a full neurological assessment, which could focus on aspects of cerebellar examination, as well as examining for ear pathology which may indicate a vestibular cause.

In children under 2, the neurological testing could commence with the motor components of the developmental assessment followed by formal neurological examination (starting with lower limbs, then upper limbs, then motor cranial nerves); in children over 2, it can be commenced with a gait examination, then lower limbs, upper limbs and finally motor cranial nerves.

Testing hearing should be mentioned and/or performed if the ears are examined. Performing Weber's and Rinne's testing should be offered if relevant and age appropriate, although these may be notoriously inaccurate in children.

Vestibular nystagmus is usually horizontal or horizontal-rotary jerk nystagmus which is maximal in intensity when gaze is directed towards the fast phase.

In peripheral (end organ) vestibular pathology, jerk nystagmus in all fields of gaze is pointed permanently in the same direction, maximal in direction of the fast component and disappears with fixation. Peripheral vestibular nystagmus typically is associated with vertigo and can be caused by any inner ear pathology.

In central (nuclear) vestibular pathology, jerk nystagmus can change direction with change in gaze direction, and does not disappear with fixation. Central vestibular pathway pathologies include acoustic neuroma and intrinsic brainstem disease.

If the movement is **vertical**, this can indicate a *visual cause or a brainstem problem*, so again, visual acuity is tested first, and then a neurological examination should follow. If the movement is unilateral, or predominantly unilateral, the possibilities include a tumour, such as a chiasmal glioma, third ventricular tumour and some neurodegenerative diagnoses, so that concern should be voiced, and then proceed to complete an eye examination. Other causes of monocular nystagmus include monocular loss of vision, which is typically vertical, and *spasmus nutans*, which occurs in infants (4 months to 3 years) and comprises a triad of head nodding (first sign), nystagmus and head tilt.

Other notable forms of nystagmus include *dissociated nystagmus*, of which an example is internuclear ophthalmoplegia causing nystagmus of the abducting eye. There are various other forms of dissociated nystagmus where one eye seems independent of the other eye completely, such that one eye could be oscillating in a vertical direction, but the other could be moving in a horizontal direction, or there can be varying amplitudes between the two sides; this can occur with posterior fossa tumours or demyelinating conditions.

Downbeat nystagmus is a form that represents brainstem pathology, such as craniocervical junction disorders (e.g. Arnold–Chiari malformation). *Upbeat nystagmus* is a form that also represents intrinsic brainstem disease. *See-saw nystagmus* describes where one eye oscillates upwards as the other side oscillates downwards; this can occur with a parasellar mass such as a craniopharyngioma, with septo-optic dysplasia or with oculo-cutaneous albinism. Patients with large parasellar masses as the cause, can have accompanying bitemporal hemianopia.

Mnemonic for **infantile nystagmus syndrome** (also called congenital motor nystagmus) is **INFANTILE**:

Idiopathic
Nutans (spasmus nutans syndrome [SNS])
Fusion maldevelopment nystagmus syndrome (also called latent nystagmus)/**F**oveal hypoplasia
Albinism
Nerve (Optic) hypoplasia (bilateral)
Transilluminate iris (to confirm albinism)
Iris absence (aniridia)
LEber's congenital amaurosis 1 (LCA1) or other retinal dystrophy/**LE**ns opacity (cataract)

Mnemonic for *unilateral nystagmus* is **CHIASM**. Importance is excluding tumours of:

Chiasmatic glioma
Hypothalamic glioma
Internuclear ophthalmoplegia (indicates brainstem disease)
Amblyopia/**A**bsent vision on one side (complete blindness—unilateral)
Spasmus nutans syndrome (SNS)
Maldevelopment fusion nystagmus (also called latent nystagmus)

The other condition worth mentioning is the opsoclonus myoclonus syndrome (OMS), as this is a diagnosis that can be confused with nystagmus initially. If the lead-in is: 'This is Harry aged 2; his mother has noticed his eyes wobbling recently. Would you like to examine him from this perspective?', then OMS is in the differential diagnosis. OMS is a rare paraneoplastic condition, associated with neuroblastoma in 50% of cases, and comprises opsoclonus, which describes fast, repetitive eye movements in both horizontal and vertical directions also called 'dancing eyes', myoclonic jerks ('dancing feet'), plus ataxia, hypotonia and irritability. If this is the presentation, focusing on the abdominal examination and the BP may give the diagnosis.

SHORT CASE: Eye examination—proptosis and exophthalmos

The Greek word *proptosis* means a 'falling forwards', so the medical definition is a forward protrusion of the globe/eyeball with respect to the orbit. Radiologically, it is measured relative to the interzygomatic line, which is drawn at the most anterior aspects of the zygomatic arches, as seen on a CT scan. The term 'exophthalmos' derives from two Greek words—*ex* meaning 'out' or 'away from' and *ophthalmos* meaning eye—and is generally defined as an abnormal protrusion of the globe/eyeball.

Many use the terms 'proptosis' and 'exophthalmos' interchangeably, some use 'exophthalmos' purely in reference to endocrine diagnoses (such as thyroid eye disease [TED]), some use it to specify an increase of volume of orbital contents as the aetiology of the protusion forwards, and some use it to quantitate the degree of protrusion, meaning *severe* proptosis (in adults this means the eye protrudes more than 18 mm from the lateral orbital margin). In the examination format, the stem is likely to include 'prominent eye(s)'. Devices that measure the exact protrusion of the eye from the orbit have included 'exophthalmometers' and 'proptometers'; the former term is employed more often.

Irrespective of the terminology, the cause of protrusion of the globe in the majority of cases is an increased mass of tissue behind the globe, pushing it anteriorly, within the limited-volume confines of the bony orbit. An exception to this is the group of craniofacial syndromes, where the problem is due to a shallow orbit. Many authorities use the term 'proptosis' for non-endocrine-related protrusion of the globe and 'exophthalmos' as endocrine-related, as occurs in TED.

The most common cause of proptosis in *adults*, unilateral or bilateral, is TED, but TED is rare in paediatrics (despite thyroid disease, in general, not being uncommon).

Unilateral proptosis in children is more likely to be due to infectious causes, such as orbital cellulitis (from acute ethmoiditis), but can be caused by an intra-orbital and/or retro-orbital tumour (e.g. dermoid cyst, glioma of optic nerve, haemangioma, retinoblastoma, rhabdomyosarcoma or metastatic disease) or other forms of infiltrate.

Bilateral proptosis in children can be due to **TED**, more serious conditions such as **neuroblastoma** or **leukaemia**, or the syndromic group of **craniofacial conditions** which include craniosynostoses, such as Apert and Crouzon syndromes.

The following differential diagnosis for *proptosis* is arranged into the mnemonic **STARING CHILD**:

Sarcoma (metastatic Ewing's)/**S**arcoma (granulocytic [AML])/**S**arcoidosis
Thyroid eye disease (also called thyroid orbitopathy, thyroid-associated orbitopathy, Graves' orbitopathy, thyroid ophthalmopathy)/**T**hrombosis of cavernous sinus
Arachnoid cyst/**A**LL/**A**bscess
Rhabdomyosarcoma (orbital)/**R**etinoblastoma
Infection: orbital cellulitis/**I**nfiltrate: histiocytosis X
Neuroblastoma (metastatic)/**N**eurofibroma (orbital)
Glioma (optic nerve/chiasm)/**G**laucoma (includes in Sturge-Weber syndrome [SWS])
Chiasmal glioma/**C**raniosynostosis syndromes (Crouzon, Apert)
Haemangioma (orbital)/**H**istiocytosis X/**H**aemorrhage (orbital; e.g. trauma)
Inflammation: pseudotumour, paranasal sinuses (ethmoid, maxillary)
Lymphangioma (orbital)/**L**ymphoma (orbital)/**L**acrimal gland tumour
Dermoid cyst (orbital)/**D**istance in adult: protrusion of over 18 mm from the lateral rim of the orbit to corneal apex measured by exophthalmometer termed exophthalmos

There is a subgroup within proptosis, with a pulsatile quality; if there is a child with pulsatile proptosis, the differential is narrower. There are five causes worth knowing.

Pulsatile proptosis causes are the 5 **A**s:

Absent wing of sphenoid bone in NF1
Aortic incompetence
Arteriovenous malformation (carotid-cavernous sinus fistula)
Arachnoid cyst (intra-diploic in middle cranial fossa, expands bone, deforms posterolateral wall of orbit)
Accident (trauma): orbital roof fracture

Thyroid eye disease (TED)

TED is not common in paediatrics. Bilateral disease is more common in Graves' disease with hyperthyroidism. Unilateral disease is more common in ophthalmic Graves' disease. Some aspects of TED are due to the sympathetic/adrenergic potentiation caused by thyroid hormone excess itself: lid lag, lid retraction, infrequent blinking and widened palpebral fissures; other aspects are due to autoimmune-mediated inflammatory pathology affecting tissues within the orbit, particularly fat and extraocular muscles, with cellular infiltrates including lymphocytes, plasma cells and mast cells, and chemical changes including deposition of glycosaminoglycans and increased water content: proptosis, oedema (periorbital tissues, conjunctivae [chemosis]), increased orbital pressure, ophthalmoplegia and diplopia.

Lid retraction, which is due to spasm of the *levator palpebrae superioris* causing upper lid elevation, makes the sclera visible **above the iris**, between the margin of the upper lid and the cornea (if gaze forwards while head is vertical), giving a staring appearance. **Exophthalmos** leads to the sclera being visible **below the iris**, between the margin of the lower lid and the cornea.

Other autoimmune-mediated components of TED include:

1. Ophthalmoplegia (affecting gaze up and out first); can present with early morning transient diplopia in the direction of, and related to oedema of, the affected muscles accumulating overnight while asleep; so get *problems looking up and out when up and about*; more permanent tethering of the muscles can occur, especially of the inferior rectus, which can cause downward deviation of the globe.
2. Periorbital swelling affecting upper lids more than lower.
3. Conjunctival changes include inflammation, chemosis (oedema) and injection of the sclera laterally, over the insertion of the lateral rectus muscle.
4. Congestive ophthalmopathy.

The mnemonic for TED is **CHEMOSIS**:

Chemosis (conjunctival oedema)/**C**ornea: ulceration/**C**olour vision loss
Hyperthyroid signs: lid lag, lid retraction, infrequent blinking, wide palpebral fissure
Exophthalmos/**E**levated lid (lid retraction)
Muscles (extraocular) affected/**M**orning (transient) diplopia
Optic nerve compression if severe/**O**ptic atrophy (late)
Spasm of lids (blepharospasm) impersonates ptosis/**S**welling: periorbital
Impaired visual fields/**I**nflammation of conjunctivae
Sight threatened

An alternate mnemonic for TED is **EXOPHT**:

Elevated lid (lid retraction)
Xtra-ocular muscles (EOMs) movements impaired: ophthalmoplegia
Optic nerve compression can cause visual failure/**O**ptic atrophy (late)
Proptosis
Hyperthyroid signs: lid lag, lid retraction, infrequent blinking, wide palpebral fissure
Tethering of EOMs/**T**ransient (morning) diplopia

Examination procedure

Introduce yourself to the patient and parent. Note whether the child looks well or unwell (orbital cellulitis is the most common cause of proptosis in children). Note growth parameters, any dysmorphic features (many syndromes can include proptosis, such as Apert, Crouzon) or features suggesting hyperthyroidism (goitre, hyperactivity, tremor).

It is useful to ask for the vital signs at this point. In particular, has this child had a fever which would direct you to infectious or oncological causes, rather than endocrine or skeletal or neurocutaneous. The pulse rate may be elevated with an infectious cause or with hyperthyroidism. The BP could be elevated with underlying NF1, or neuroblastoma; pulse pressure could be elevated in hyperthyroidism or in aortic incompetence (which can cause pulsatile proptosis); the respiratory rate could be elevated with an infectious cause. After brief comments on general appearance and interpreting vital signs, focus on the eyes.

The best position for examination is with the child sitting on the side of the bed, in a chair or on the parent's lap, depending on the child's age. Inspect the eyes from in front, from the side and particularly from above as this is the best way to clinically detect proptosis. Describe the degree of proptosis in each eye, note whether both eyes are involved, whether there is asymmetry of involvement and whether there is visible pulsation. Note any accompanying external abnormalities. Focus successively on the anatomical structures of the eye to detect abnormalities (i.e. look at eyebrows, eyelids, cornea, iris, sclera and conjunctivae) that may indicate thyroid eye disease. If the child wears glasses examine these also.

After inspection, test visual acuity in each eye, then visual fields, then extraocular movements (see short cases in this chapter: Eye examination—general and Motor cranial nerves). Check for lid lag (hyperthyroid), near and far cover test, check for strabismus by shining a torch into the eyes from a distance, then test pupillary reflexes and offer fundoscopy. Finally, to complete the eye examination component, palpate for evidence of pulsatility (e.g. absent sphenoid in NF1 or AV fistula), and for evidence of raised intraocular pressure (TED or glaucoma).

By this stage, you should have an impression of whether there is bilateral proptosis (making TED or some of the craniosynostoses more likely) or unilateral proptosis. If unilateral does the child look unwell, or have an IV cannula in situ (orbital cellulitis or abscess), or show signs of current chemotherapy (e.g. alopecia) or haematological disease (pallor or bruising from ALL).

Look at the skin for any evidence of any neurocutaneous syndromes (e.g. NF1 or SWS) or haemangiomas.

If the proptosis is bilateral, mention TED as a possible cause and check for thyroid status; examine the neck for goitre, the cardiovascular system including heart rate for tachycardia, BP for wide pulse pressure and auscultation for any flow murmurs.

Look for tremor by having the child hold out their hands and place a sheet of paper on the dorsum of either hand to detect the fine tremor found in hyperthyroidism, and check the reflexes for briskness (but do not expect to find any of these classic signs in a euthyroid, appropriately treated child with Graves ophthalmopathy, who has come in just for the examination).

After checking the eyes and looking for thyroid signs, move on to a haematological examination, as other well-described causes of bilateral disease include leukaemia and neuroblastoma; incorporate examining for lymph nodes, bony tenderness and abdominal examination looking for hepatosplenomegaly (e.g. ALL, lymphoma) or adrenal masses (neuroblastoma).

The focus on the remainder of the examination depends on what has been discovered up until this point. If the diagnosis appears to be a craniofacial syndrome, look for features that could differentiate Apert from Crouzon syndrome, for example. If the diagnosis appears to be NF1, then looking for other features of NF1 would be appropriate (see short case on NF1 in this chapter).

This completes the examination. Give a differential diagnosis and suggest appropriate imaging (MRI, CT) and other investigations you would perform.

For completion, there are some conditions which can impersonate proptosis but there is no true protrusion of the globe. There are three well-described proptosis impersonators:
- Enophthalmos of contralateral eye.
- Microphthalmia of contralateral eye.
- Macrophthalmia of involved eye.

SHORT CASE: Motor cranial nerves

This is one of the most common neurological examinations requested. The introductions are variable (e.g. 'This child has had droopy eyelids since birth', or 'This boy has had facial weakness for several years'), but the specific instruction of 'Examine the motor cranial nerves' usually accompanies this type of lead-in. A smoothly performed motor cranial nerve examination can be comfortably achieved within 5 minutes. This is quite different from 'Cranial nerves', as the additional examination components of the vision, eyes, hearing and other sensory modalities are quite time-consuming.

A suggested approach follows for children of preschool age or older. For younger children, improvisation involving the use of interesting-looking toys and play is necessary.

First, introduce yourself to the patient and parent. Shake hands with both (although this is not a reliable test to detect myotonic dystrophy, it is worth doing, as it is polite and as myotonic dystrophy can be a differential diagnosis for motor cranial nerve pathology; if myotonic dystrophy is suspected, get the patient/parent to make a fist and then fully open the hand, spreading the fingers, as quickly as possible). Inspect the face carefully and scan the limbs, for any obvious signs such as ptosis, facial asymmetry or hemiplegic posturing.

Before checking the extraocular eye movements, the visual acuity needs to be quickly checked, to confirm that the child can see to follow an object (e.g. a finger puppet). Explain what you are doing as you proceed.

To test the extraocular movements, ask the child to follow your finger or other small object. Ask the child how many fingers (or objects) can be seen, in each of nine positions (right and left lateral gaze, up and down in central, right and left lateral positions, and straight ahead, i.e. central).

The findings sought include lack of movement, diplopia and nystagmus. If abnormalities are demonstrated, then each eye should be tested separately.

Third nerve lesions, when complete, cause ptosis, a 'down and out' position of the involved eye, and paralysis of most eye movements, sparing only lateral rectus and superior oblique function. They also cause a dilated pupil and lack of direct and consensual pupillary light response, but pupil light reactions do not need to be tested in a motor examination. (There are three types of third nerve dysfunction: 1. complete; 2. affecting only the parasympathetic fibres, which encircle the inner motor nerve [these are compressed with raised intracranial pressure, and can lead to, solely, a 'blown', dilated pupil, but no ptosis]; and 3. affecting only the motor component, so no dilated pupil.) Fourth nerve lesions cause diplopia on looking down and in. Sixth nerve lesions cause lack of lateral movement, with diplopia most marked on looking towards the affected side.

Next, examine the fifth nerve. You may ask the child the following, demonstrating each move as you proceed. 'Open your mouth': the jaw will deviate towards the weak side with a unilateral fifth nerve lesion, pushed by the normal pterygoid. 'Now keep it open; don't let me close it': this tests the pterygoids. 'Clench your teeth tight': feel the muscle bulk on each side. Then with your hand against the lateral aspect of the chin, 'Move your chin towards my hand', on each side. This tests each pterygoid in turn. Finally check the jaw jerk: 'Open your mouth a little; I'm just going to tap on your chin'. The jerk will be increased in pseudobulbar palsy.

The muscles of facial expression are then tested. 'Look up and raise your eyebrows': this tests the frontalis and is particularly useful in differentiating upper motor neurone lesions (upper facial muscles are preserved due to bilateral innervation) from lower motor neurone lesions, where the upper facial muscles are affected. 'Screw your eyes up tight': compare the two sides, noting any asymmetry between the degree the eyelashes are buried on either side. This may detect an obvious Bell's phenomenon, where there is rolling upwards of the eyeball when attempting to shut the eyes forcefully, as eye closure may not be possible in lower motor neuron lesions. Then try to open each eye: 'Keep them shut; stop me opening them'. This tests the orbicularis oculi muscles. 'Now show me your teeth' allows assessment of any asymmetry of the nasolabial grooves. The mouth will be drawn towards the normal side if there is a unilateral lesion of either upper or lower motor neuron type. 'Puff out your cheeks; keep them like that': demonstrate this and then tap with your finger over each cheek to detect ease of air expulsion on the affected side.

The ninth, tenth and twelfth nerves are then tested. 'Open your mouth wide': look (with a torch) at the uvula for any deviation to either side. 'Now say aaah': watch movement of the soft palate. With unilateral lesions of the tenth nerve the uvula is drawn towards the normal side. Inspect the tongue for fasciculations (tongue not protruding). Then say 'Poke out your tongue' and note any deviation. With a unilateral lesion, the normal side pushes the tongue towards the affected (weaker) side. Also check that the tongue can be equally well protruded towards each side. (For some reason, children love poking their tongues out at nervous examination candidates.) Get the child to speak (e.g. 'Which school do you go to?') to check for any evidence of hoarseness (unilateral recurrent laryngeal nerve lesion), and to cough to check for the 'bovine' cough of bilateral recurrent laryngeal nerve lesions: these are very rare in paediatric patients but are easy to test, for completeness.

The eleventh cranial nerve supplies the sternocleidomastoid and trapezius muscles. With your hand against the lateral aspect of the child's face say, 'Turn your head towards my hand', or if that is not understood, choose something for the child to inspect over his or her shoulder and say 'Look over there'. When this movement is performed, inspect and palpate the bulk of the sternomastoid, then repeat the process for the other side. Ask the child to 'shrug your shoulders' (demonstrate this), and then to repeat this against resistance (your hands). Note the bulk of the trapezius muscles.

At the completion of the examination, summarise your findings and give a differential diagnosis. The remainder of the examination should be directed towards confirming any suspected diagnosis, which may entail examination of the gait, lower limbs, upper limbs or neuromuscular assessment.

SHORT CASE: Neurological assessment of the upper limbs

This is a fairly common short case, and like most cases in neurology it necessitates careful inspection before laying of hands on the patient. Perhaps because most candidates are quite comfortable with a standard neurological examination procedure, they may be eager to test power, tone and reflexes before careful inspection.

For adequate exposure, the child should be completely undressed down to the waist. Watching the child remove the pullover or shirt may provide valuable clues to the underlying problem.

Introduce yourself to the parent and child, and shake hands with the child (this may detect the inability to release your hand, which indicates myotonic dystrophy).

Inspection

Initial inspection is best done with the child standing, and then sitting in a chair or on the edge of the bed, directly facing the candidate.

Stand back and look at the child. Inspection should not be confined to the upper limbs; it should also include rapid scanning of the face, neck, lower limbs and skin, for clues to the underlying pathology (see Table 13.3 for details).

Next, focus on the upper limbs. Note their resting posture (e.g. hemiplegia). Look for: muscle wasting of arms, forearms or small muscles of the hands (marked wasting being more likely due to lower motor unit pathology); fasciculations (which indicate lower motor unit degeneration, such as anterior horn cell disease, when in the presence of other signs of motor pathology); involuntary movements (e.g. chorea, tremor); contractures; scars (inspect thoroughly for these); growth arrest (compare size of thumb nail beds); and trophic changes, neurocutaneous stigmata (e.g. neurofibromata). When looking at the hands, also note any 'classic' signs of brachial plexus lesions: 'true claw hand' due to a lower (Klumpke's) lesion (C8, T1); or the 'waiter's tip' position of an upper (Erb) lesion (C5, 6).

Also note any 'classic' signs of peripheral nerve lesions: wrist drop due to radial nerve palsy, 'monkey hand' due to median nerve palsy and 'ulnar claw hand' due to ulnar nerve palsy.

After inspecting the upper limbs, quickly look at the neck for scars (e.g. removal of tumour) and the back, for scars of spinal surgery (e.g. spina bifida repair) or evidence of scoliosis (various neuromuscular causes such as anterior horn cell disorders, neuropathies, myopathies).

Have the child hold both upper limbs straight out in front, and ask her or him to close the eyes. Drifting of either arm may be due to loss of proprioception (posterior column disease), cerebellar hypotonia or weakness from pyramidal tract pathology.

PALPATION

Feel the muscle bulk in each muscle compartment and, if possible, have the child contract the muscles while they are being palpated, for a more accurate assessment. Also note any muscle tenderness (e.g. dermatomyositis). Feel for any hypertrophied peripheral nerves, such as the ulnar nerve at the elbow (e.g. Charcot-Marie-Tooth disease).

TONE

Assess the tone at the wrists and elbows. When moving the joints, ensure that the rhythm and rate at which this is done is irregular and not predicted, and resisted, by the child. Passive pronation and supination of the forearms is probably the easiest way of assessing tone accurately. Note whether there is spasticity, rigidity or hypotonia.

POWER

All candidates should be familiar with the grading of muscle power out of 5 (National Health and Medical Research Council Scale, see Table 13.2) and with the various motor root values and sensory dermatomes of the upper limb. While assessing power, note whether any weakness found is symmetrical or asymmetrical, is predominantly proximal or distal, and involves a particular muscle group, motor nerve root or the distribution of a particular peripheral nerve, or is in an 'upper motor neuron pattern', with weakness of abduction of the shoulder and extension of elbow and wrist.

Check the strength of the following:
1. Shoulder abduction (C5, 6): 'Hold your arms up like this (demonstrate abduction at shoulders with elbows flexed). Stop me pushing them down'.
2. Shoulder adduction (C6, 7, 8): 'Hold your arms up like this again. Stop me lifting them up'.
3. Elbow flexion (C5, 6): 'Pull my hands towards you'.
4. Elbow extension (C7, 8): 'Push me away'.
5. Wrist flexion (C6, 7): 'Hold your hands like this (demonstrate full flexion at wrists). Keep them like that; don't let me straighten them'.
6. Wrist extension (C6, 7): 'Hold your hands like this [demonstrate full extension at wrists]. Keep them like that; don't let me straighten them'.
7. Hand grip (C8, T1): 'Squeeze my finger as tight as you can. Don't let go'.
8. Finger abduction (C8, T1): 'Spread your fingers apart like this [demonstrate]. Stop me pushing them together'.

The following points may aid remembering motor root values:
1. The highest level is shoulder abduction (C4, 5).
2. Extensors (of elbow, wrist, fingers) are all supplied by C7 (**ext**ension from s**eve**n).
3. Wrist flexion and extension have the same motor roots (C6, 7).
4. The lowest level is grip and small muscles of the hand (T1) (**T**1 for in**t**rinsic muscles, '**T**1 for **T**rinsics').
5. Myotome nerve root nursery rhyme: 'Five, six, pick up sticks; seven, eight, lay them straight'.

If there is a suggestion of a myopathic problem, at the end of assessing power ask the child to make a fist and then open the hand as quickly as possible, to assess for myotonia. If this is positive, go on to tap over the thenar eminence for percussion myotonia.

REFLEXES

Check the reflexes. Remember to check with reinforcement, if there is no response on initial testing. Biceps and brachioradialis jerks both correspond to C5, 6. Triceps jerk corresponds to C7, 8 (so remember 5, 6, 7, 8).

COORDINATION

Check the finger–nose test: with the eyes open to assess for signs of cerebellar disease such as intention tremor, clumsy, jerking movements (dyssynergia) and overshooting the target (dysmetria); with eyes closed to assess for defective proprioception. In younger children, who cannot cooperate with the finger–nose test, putting a pen into a pen-top held out by the candidate may yield similar information. Also, threading a bead is a valuable test of coordination in young children. Check for dysdiadochokinesis.

SENSATION

Accurate testing of sensation is difficult in most children; it is also quite time-consuming and is impractical in younger children. It may thus be appropriate in some cases to comment on the lack of reliability of testing in children and omit sensation. The following description is for older, cooperative children.

It may be wise to commence with testing for proprioception (posterior columns), as this is not time-consuming and is fairly easy to do. Move the distal phalanx of the index finger (held from the sides) up and down, after demonstrating the procedure with the child's eyes open. Next, test vibration (also posterior columns) using a 128 Hz tuning fork, with the child's eyes closed. Start distally (over the head of the ulna). Move proximally (over elbow) if there is lack of distal sensation. The best way to check is to ask the child to tell you when the 'buzzing' has stopped, and then to stop the fork vibrating. Then, proceed with checking light touch, in dermatomal distribution, with a wisp of cottonwool; this can be very difficult in younger children. Finally, check for pain sensation (spinothalamic tracts) using a new blunt pin. This is left until last, so as not to frighten the child. Ask the child to close the eyes and say whether the pin is sharp or dull. As with testing of light touch, test in dermatomal distribution.

The easiest way to remember the segmental cutaneous supply of the upper limb is as follows: numerically, start at the shoulder (C4) and proceed down the radial aspect of the limb (C5 arm, C6 forearm), reaching the tips of the fingers (C7) and then continuing up the ulnar aspect of the limb (C8 forearm, T1 elbow), until you reach the axilla (T2). It is useful to practise this 'counting' technique on your own upper limbs.

FUNCTION

Finally, if it seems relevant to the findings noted (e.g. spasticity, sensory deficits), it may be appropriate to perform a functional appraisal, although this is not part of the 'standard' neurological examination. (This is really 'the icing on the cake', and omitting it would not be detrimental.) Ask the child to perform (or mime) some ADLs, such as writing (if old enough), using a knife, fork, spoon, cup, comb and toothbrush, and undoing buttons or turning on a tap.

Summary

When summarising your findings, it may be useful to give a general description of the type of lesion (e.g. lower motor unit disorder) and then a more specific diagnosis (e.g. anterior horn cell disease), followed by a differential diagnosis of this.

It may be appropriate to request permission to examine other areas to confirm your impression of the most likely diagnosis. This may include, commonly, examination of motor cranial nerves and gait if a myopathy is suspected, or gait and lower limbs if a peripheral neuropathy is suspected, or further assessment of cerebellar function if a cerebellar lesion is likely.

If the suspected diagnosis is inheritable, also make a point of looking at the parents (e.g. in patients with Charcot-Marie-Tooth disease or myotonic dystrophy).

If the examiners ask which investigations would be useful, do not make the error of asking to see the electromyogram and nerve conduction studies, because if given actual copies of these, you must then be able to interpret them. It is more prudent to ask for the results of these studies (as interpreted by an expert).

Table 13.3
Additional information: possible useful signs on inspection, neurological assessment of upper limbs
HEAD AND NECK
Horner's syndrome (look for neck pathology, check for chest expansion on that side—diaphragm)
Myopathic facies (think of myopathies, myotonic dystrophy, myasthenia gravis)
Facial nerve palsy (look for upper motor neurone signs, hemiplegia)
Short neck (think of the Klippel–Feil anomaly; look for signs of spasticity, findings of syringomyelia)
LOWER LIMBS
Posture
Muscle wasting (e.g. peroneal atrophy of CMT)
Involuntary movements
Growth arrest
Foot deformities (e.g. pes cavus)
SKIN
Stigmata of neurofibromatosis type 1 (NF1) (e.g. café-au-lait patches, axillary freckling, neurofibromata)
Stigmata of tuberous sclerosis (e.g. hypopigmented lesions)
GRADING OF POWER (NATIONAL HEALTH AND MEDICAL RESEARCH COUNCIL SCALE)
0 Complete paralysis
1 Flicker of contraction
2 Movement possible if gravity removed
3 Movement possible against gravity, but not against resistance
4 Movement possible against gravity and some resistance
5 Normal power

CMT = Charcot-Marie-Tooth disease; NF1 = neurofibromatosis, type 1.

SHORT CASE: Gait

This is one of the most commonly encountered cases. A smooth and complete approach is mandatory. It can be the introduction to evaluating most pathological processes that affect the nervous system, and is an intricate component of many other cases outlined in this chapter on neurology (e.g. seizures, large head, scoliosis). But 'gait' does not necessarily mean a neurological diagnosis. A gait examination also may be the lead-in to a primary orthopaedic or rheumatological problem, or even haematological problems such as haemophilia (presenting with a limp due to hip haemarthrosis or intrapsoas haemorrhage).

The 'stem' you are given may give a clue on how to proceed. Helpful stems could include: 'This 4-year-old boy has trouble climbing stairs. Could you please assess his gait?', which may lead you towards muscle pathology such as Duchenne muscular dystrophy (DMD), and ensure you do not forget Gowers' sign; or 'This girl was born at 23 weeks' gestation and has some difficulties with walking. Could you please assess her gait?' would lead you towards complications of extreme prematurity, and ensure careful assessment for spastic diplegia.

Begin by introducing yourself to the parent and patient, getting an impression of the child's cognition, and any problems with speech or eye contact. Also gain an impression of whether the parents have any gait/neurological problems themselves. Stand back, quickly scan the room for orthoses (e.g. ankle–foot orthoses [AFOs]), other aids, and scan the child for signs of neurological disorders, such as a large head, obvious eye signs (e.g. squint, ptosis or nystagmus), abnormal posturing (e.g. hemiplegic), abnormal movements (e.g. tremor, fasciculations) and asymmetry (e.g. growth arrest with hemiplegia, rib asymmetry with scoliosis). Inspect the limbs very carefully. Note the muscle bulk (look systematically at buttocks, thighs and calves for any wasting, or any enlargement of calves [calf pseudohypertrophy in DMD]), contractures and any deformities of the feet (e.g. talipes, pes cavus). Look for skin signs such as neurocutaneous stigmata or scars of procedures (e.g. tendon releases, ventriculoperitoneal shunts). Then, with the child's lower limbs adequately exposed (watch how the child undresses), you may proceed with the following steps in this suggested order:

1. *Normal gait.* This is the initial screening procedure. Note any characteristic pattern of the gait; for example, circumduction with hemiplegia, scissors (+/− crouching) gait with spastic diplegia, wide-based with cerebellar pathway dysfunction, waddling with proximal myopathies (pelvic girdle weakness, giving bilateral Trendelenburg gait), steppage gait with foot drop (paralysed ankle and foot dorsiflexors), unilateral Trendelenburg gait with unilateral dislocated hip, antalgic gait (limp from painful limb pathology) with orthopaedic problems. If no obvious recognisable pattern is seen, then look at each component of the gait in turn, focusing on the pelvis, hips, knees and feet, or in the reverse order, and simply describe what you see.

2. *Heel–toe walking.* This tests for cerebellar pathway problems. If the child is over 2 years, and quite unable to walk steadily, this may be due to pathology in the cerebellar vermis, but it may also be due to weakness or sensory deficits. Do not over-interpret this sign by itself. It is useful to get the child, after walking tandem in a straight line, to turn around quickly ('as fast as you can') and walk back the other way. If the child stumbles with the quick turn, this can be the *first* sign of vermal pathology. The author has seen a number of patients with cerebellar tumours, where this 'quick turn' was the 'key' sign to suspect the diagnosis.

3. *Walking on heels.* This tests for strength of dorsiflexion (L5) or contractures of the calf muscles. It is often difficult to do this in a large number of conditions (e.g. CP, anterior horn cell disease, peripheral neuropathies, DMD). This is a useful test in the school-aged child, but not necessarily younger. (By 2.5 years, 60% of children can walk on their heels; by 4 years, most children can walk on their heels, by 5 years almost all children can walk on their heels.)

4. *Walking on toes.* This tests for strength of plantar flexion (S1). It is usually possible for children with CP or DMD to do this well, but children with lesions affecting S1 (e.g. low lumbar myelomeningocele [MMC], peripheral neuropathies, anterior horn cell disease) may find it impossible. (By 2 years, 90% of children can walk on their tip-toes.)

5. *Walking on outsides of feet.* This is the Fog test. Maintaining the position of marked inversion brings out signs of subtle hemiplegia, with the mildly hemiplegic child adopting either a frank hemiplegic posture, or demonstrating a notable asymmetry in arm and leg positioning. Walking on the insides of the feet (marked eversion), often called the 'reverse Fog', has similar significance. It is important not to over-interpret the sometimes bizarre bilateral postures that children adopt when performing this part of the gait routine. It is the finding of asymmetry that is important.

6. *Running.* This also accentuates findings such as hemiplegia and proximal weakness (in the latter, a child may seem to be miming a run in slow motion). Only ask the child to run if there is adequate room to do so and if the child is over 2 years old. (By 18 months, 80% of children can run; by 2 years, 97% of children can run.)

7. *Standing on each foot.* By inspecting from behind and noting the position of the pelvis, by iliac crest position, this allows detection of any proximal instability and positive Trendelenburg's sign. This test is useful in children over 3 years old. (By 2.5 years, about 50% of children can stand on one foot for over 6 seconds; by 3 years, 95% of children can manage this.)

8. *Hopping on each foot.* This assesses for unilateral weakness and for balance, in school-aged children, especially over 7. (By 3.5 years, 50% children can hop for 3 metres. By 5 years, 92% of children can hop this distance. By 7 years almost all children can manage this.)

9. *Standing with feet together.* With eyes open, this tests for truncal (cerebellar) ataxia. With eyes closed, this checks for Romberg's sign (falling due to dorsal column pathology, and removal of visual input). The Romberg test, standing with feet together, is often combined with holding the upper limbs extended out in front of the child, with fingers extended, looking for parietal (proprioceptive) drift when eyes are closed, which occurs with contralateral parietal lesions, where the arm may drift away from the previous position, moving down (or up) because of unawareness of its position without visual reinforcement (a form of hemineglect).

10. *Bending forwards and touching toes.* This is to screen for scoliosis, which can occur with numerous neuromuscular disorders. The back should be inspected carefully for midline scars (e.g. MMC repair), hairy patches or lipomas. Scoliosis can be cause or effect of neurological disorders. The degree of scoliosis may reflect the severity of lower motor neuron (LMN) disorders such as the spinal muscular atrophies (SMAs), myopathies, DMD or upper motor neuron (UMN) disorders such as CP.

11. *Squatting and then rising from the squatting position.* Maintaining a squatting position tests more peripheral strength. This may be difficult in cases with peripheral neuropathy. Arising from the squatting position tests for proximal weakness. (By 12 months, 95% of children can squat.)

12. *Lying on the floor and then rising from this position.* This is called Gowers' manoeuvre, to elicit Gowers' sign, which occurs with proximal weakness, classically associated with DMD; where children essentially roll over, from supine to prone, before getting themselves into a position where they climb up their own legs to get upright. (See the sequential photographs in the long-case section on DMD in this chapter.) If a child over 2 years old does not sit bolt upright quickly, this suggests some proximal weakness. Do not routinely ask every child to perform this manoeuvre, as it is inappropriate except where one is specifically looking for proximal weakness, and there is no other pathology which would make it difficult or uncomfortable for them to get themselves off the floor.

After the manoeuvres just outlined, probably the safest next step is to examine the lower limbs, as over-interpretation of certain signs may lead the candidate off on an inappropriate tangent (e.g. unsteadiness due to weakness could be misinterpreted as being ataxia due to a cerebellar problem, and may cause the candidate next to check for nystagmus and dysdiadochokinesis, rather than to methodically examine the lower limbs).

Common findings include hemiplegia, spastic diplegia and muscle disorders.

If the findings suggest hemiplegia, proceed as per the hemiplegia short case and work out the level of pathology: cortical (accompanying visual field cuts or neglect, various agnosias); internal capsule (pyramidal tract motor fibres); and assess chronicity (hemiatrophy).

If the findings suggest spastic diplegia, after completing neurological assessment, proceed as per ex-premmie examination (as per chronic lung disease [CLD] long-case examination section); look for ex-premmie head shape, VP shunt from hydrocephalus secondary to intracranial haemorrhage (ICH), visual impairment from retinopathy of prematurity (ROP), chest wall deformity from CLD, and abdominal scars from surgery for necrotising enterocolitis (NEC).

If findings suggest a muscle problem, proceed as per the neuromuscular short case. Look for muscle biopsy scars, cardiac complications (DMD in boys, Pompe in infants), respiratory complications (tachypnoea, chest deformity, paradoxical breathing), complications of treatment, such as steroid side effects (Cushingoid, see long case on DMD in this chapter), and MedicAlert bracelets warning about steroid dependence (DMD) or anaesthetic hyperthermia (DMD, Limb Girdle dystrophy [LGD], myotonic dystrophy [MD], central core disease, multiminicore disease).

If the findings suggest ataxia, proceed as per the ataxia short case, including a full cerebellar examination (see the short case on cerebellar function in this chapter).

If the findings suggest a neuromuscular junction problem, proceed with a motor cranial nerve examination looking for ptosis, checking external ocular movements and facial muscle strength. Fatiguability can be mentioned, but is not expected to be demonstrated within the time constraints of a short case.

After the standard lower limb examination, you will probably have enough information to tell the examiners your thoughts about the probable pathology, and then to proceed to examine whatever else is relevant (this is most often the upper limbs).

Two real cases follow (each with a 'hidden' abnormal sign, and neither on YouTube).

The author's FRACP gait examination short case had a more general introduction of: 'This 6-year-old boy has had increasing trouble with walking lately. Could you please assess his gait?' On initial inspection, the boy had a large head, and a small scar on the abdomen (he was already in shorts with shirt off and shoes and socks off). He had normal facial expression and no dysmorphic features. Looking around the room, there were no mobility aids. His mother was present. His gait showed some asymmetry with mild left-sided hemiplegic posturing, but a wide base. On specific gait manoeuvres, he was unsteady on tandem gait and he could not stand on his toes nor could he walk on his heels. The Fog test exaggerated his hemiplegic posturing. Running caused circumduction of the hemiplegic side. He could not squat down and he could not maintain his balance. Gowers' sign was not attempted as he did not present with proximal weakness. Lower limb examination showed bilateral pes cavus, peripheral weakness and absent reflexes at ankles. Upper limb examination showed some bilateral grip weakness, with increased reflexes at the biceps and triceps on the left side. Examination of his head revealed an enlarged head, with a VP shunt. There were thus three pathologies: shunted hydrocephalus; a hemiplegia; and some form of peripheral LMN weakness. The next step was to clarify the LMN pathology, which seemed to be a peripheral neuropathy. The next step was to examine … the mother. She had on a long dress which covered her lower legs and ankles. She lifted her hem to reveal pes cavus, and peroneal muscular wasting, the 'inverted champagne bottle' appearance of Charcot-Marie-Tooth (CMT). So having a system is important.

Another real case, for the MRCP examination, had the introduction: 'This 8-year-old girl has put on some weight recently and has trouble walking. Could you please examine her gait?' It was winter, in London, and this girl was dressed in a heavy coat, a woolly hat, a turtle-neck sweater and jeans. Her centiles were requested. Her weight centiles showed a progression from 50th to 95th and back to 50th over a period of the past 12 months; her height centiles showed progression from 50th to 25th and back towards 50th over the same period, the sudden weight gain coinciding with the sudden cessation of increase in height. She removed the hat and coat and jeans. She walked with a waddling gait, consistent with marked proximal weakness. The examiners then asked what should be examined next. At this stage the findings pointed to two pathologies. The growth charts suggested some pathology that causes weight gain and cessation of height gain, which could be a number of endocrinopathies, such as hypopituitarism, hypothyroidism or Cushing's syndrome. The gait suggested proximal muscle weakness. The one condition which could have caused both was Cushing's syndrome. But this girl had no suggestion of Cushingoid features. And remember this girl had on a turtle-neck sweater. Why? This was asked to be removed, as the next step, revealing a goitre. This suggested acquired hypothyroidism as a cause for the growth parameter changes, but did not necessarily explain the gait. Then the examiners asked to assess one more sign and then synthesise a differential. The sign chosen was the pulse rate. If it was slow, then treatment had somehow been suboptimal; if it was fast, then this suggested hyperthyroidism, iatrogenic or otherwise. But the pulse was normal. This suggested this girl was euthyroid; she had *treated* hypothyroidism. The reason for the myopathy? Previous *over*treatment. This girl had taken an overly high dose of thyroxine for a period of time, immediately after the diagnosis of hypothyroidism was made, until the waddling gait presented and thyroid function tests showed a very high blood level of thyroxine. Residual muscle weakness had yet to have resolved.

There are many easy-to-access gait abnormalities shown in videos on YouTube. A suggested video playlist is: www.youtube.com/playlist?list=PLD74972DCFB2D58C8 which gives demonstrations of 14 gait patterns.

SHORT CASE: Neurological assessment of the lower limbs

This is one of the most common neurological short cases. It is best started with examination of the gait (see the short case on gait in this chapter), unless the examiners direct otherwise or the child is too young or too disabled to walk. The child's lower limbs should be adequately exposed, ideally undressed down to the underpants in younger children, with socks and shoes removed; some older children can become embarrassed, and most adolescents prefer to maintain their modesty. The candidate should demonstrate to the examiners their sensitivity to the patient's modesty.

Note that examination of the back is essential in assessing the lower limbs.

Inspection

Initial inspection is done with the child standing (before full gait examination). More thorough inspection may be done when the child is on the bed, after the full range of gait manoeuvres.

Stand back and look at the child. Inspection should not be confined to the lower limbs. It should include rapid scanning of the face, neck, upper limbs and skin, for clues to underlying pathology (for details, see the short case on neurological assessment of the upper limbs in this chapter). The back must be checked at some point, and this is most easily done when incorporated into the gait examination. Also note any peripheral signs, such as nearby crutches, splints, orthoses or a wheelchair.

Focus on the lower limbs themselves. Note the resting posture (e.g. diplegia). Look for: muscle wasting of thighs, calves or feet (marked wasting being more likely due to lower motor unit pathology); fasciculations (which indicate LMN degeneration, such as anterior horn cell disease, when in the presence of other signs of motor pathology); involuntary movements (e.g. myoclonus, chorea); contractures; scars (inspect thoroughly, including looking at posterior aspects of ankles and knees); growth arrest (compare size of great toe nail beds; may measure leg lengths); trophic changes; and neurocutaneous stigmata (e.g. café-au-lait macules).

When looking at the feet, also note whether there is pes cavus, which reflects neuromuscular disease. This finding should prompt consideration of lower spinal lesions, spinocerebellar degenerations or peripheral neuropathies. Two 'classic' examination cases that may present like this are Charcot-Marie-Tooth (CMT) disease and Friedreich ataxia.

Palpation

Feel the muscle bulk in each muscle compartment, and if possible, have the child contract the muscles while they are also being palpated, for a more accurate assessment. Also note any muscle tenderness (e.g. dermatomyositis). Feel for any hypertrophied peripheral nerves, such as the lateral popliteal at the knee (e.g. CMT).

Tone

Assess the tone at the knees and ankles. When moving the joints, ensure that the rhythm and rate at which this is done is irregular and not predicted, and resisted, by the child. Note whether tone is normal, increased (as in UMN or extrapyramidal lesions) or decreased (as in LMN or cerebellar lesions). Check for clonus at the knee and ankle. For the knee, place your hand on the lower quadriceps, and then push the patella down (towards the foot) briskly. For the ankle, position the limb with the knee bent and the hip externally rotated, then briskly dorsiflex the ankle. Sustained rhythmic contractions at either knee or ankle indicate UMN pathology. Note that up to 10 beats of ankle clonus may be present in the newborn, but this usually disappears by 2 months.

Power

All candidates should be familiar with the grading of muscle power out of 5 (see Table 13.2), and with the various motor root values and sensory dermatomes of the lower limb.

When assessing power, note whether any weakness found is symmetrical or asymmetrical, is predominantly proximal or distal, involves a particular muscle group, motor nerve root, or distribution of a particular peripheral nerve, or has an UMN pattern (i.e. weakness of flexion at hip, knee and ankle).

Check the strength of the following:

1. Hip flexion (L1, 2, 3): 'Lift your leg straight up. Don't let me push it down' (by your hand placed above the knee).
2. Hip extension (L5, S1, 2): 'Keep your leg on the bed. Stop me lifting it up'.
3. Knee flexion (L5, S1): 'Bend your knee. Pull your foot in towards your bottom. Stop me straightening it'.
4. Knee extension (L3, 4): 'Straighten your leg. Stop me bending it'.
5. Ankle plantar flexion (S1): 'Push down. Push my hand away'.
6. Ankle dorsiflexion (L4, 5): 'Pull your foot back like this (demonstrate with wrist extension). Stop me pushing it down'.

Remember the myotomes by the rhyme: 'One, two buckle my shoe' (S1 ankle plantar flexion, to get foot positioned to buckle shoe) and 'Three, four, kick the door' (L3, 4 knee extension, required to execute kick).

Reflexes

Check the reflexes. Remember to check with reinforcement (e.g. clenching teeth, or interlocking fingers in a 'monkey grip' and [almost] pulling apart hard just before the tendon hammer strikes the tendon) if there is no response on initial testing. Ankle jerk corresponds to S1, 2 and knee jerk corresponds to L3, 4 (so remember 1, 2, 3, 4).

Look for the crossed adductor reflex (adduction at the contralateral hip when the knee jerk is elicited) and other spread of reflexes (elicitable moving distally down the anterior aspect of the tibia) when checking the knee jerks. These indicate an UMN lesion in children older than 8 months. Check the plantar response. An extensor (Babinski's) response is normal under the age of 18 months, but after that time it reflects an UMN lesion.

Coordination

These manoeuvres are to detect cerebellar dysfunction. Check the heel–shin test: have the child slide his heel down his shin on each side, to check whether he can smoothly and accurately follow the line of the tibia. Next, check the toe–finger test (as with the finger–nose test): have the child lift his big toe to touch your finger, to detect intention tremor and past-pointing. Finally, test whether the child can tap the foot rapidly against your hand.

Sensation

Sensation is examined as for the upper limbs (see the short case on upper limbs in this chapter). When testing proprioception, the big toe is used rather than the index finger. When testing vibration, the points for placing the tuning fork are the ankle (medial malleolus), the knee (tibial tuberosity or patella) and the pelvis (anterior superior iliac spine). Sensation for light touch and pain (pin prick) is tested in dermatomal distribution.

The easiest way to remember the segmental cutaneous supply of the lower limb is as follows. Numerically start at the groin (L1) and proceed down the anterior aspect of the limb: L2 supplies upper thigh, and L3 the knee. It becomes a little complicated below the knee: L4 supplies the medial aspect of the leg; L5 supplies the lateral aspect of the leg and continues down on to the medial aspect of the foot. (Mnemonic: L5 is the lowest lumbar, lateral and long enough to reach the big toe.) S1 supplies the sole. S2 supplies the central posterior aspect of the leg and thigh.

Summary

When summarising your findings, it may be useful to give a general description of the type of lesion (e.g. LMN disorder) and then a more specific diagnosis (e.g. peripheral neuropathy), followed by a differential diagnosis of this.

It may be appropriate to request permission to examine other areas to confirm your impression of the most likely diagnosis. This may include, commonly, examination of the upper limbs and motor cranial nerves, or further examination of cerebellar function. If the suspected diagnosis is inheritable, also make a point of looking at the parents (e.g. in patients with CMT or myotonic dystrophy). See the short case on the upper limbs in this chapter for comments on investigations.

SHORT CASE: Cerebellar function

Occasionally, the examiners may give a very directed lead-in such as, 'This boy has a problem with his coordination. Would you assess his cerebellar function please?' If this is the introduction, then the following approach is useful.

First, make general observations, such as noting any nystagmus or tremor. Then ask the patient his name and age. With an older child, ask him to say 'sizzling sausage', which is more discerning in detecting cerebellar dysarthria. Next, examine the eyes for horizontal nystagmus (maximal if looking towards the side of the lesion). Have the child extend the upper limbs and note any drift or static tremor (due to hypotonia). Then check the finger–nose test for intention tremor and past-pointing. Test for dysdiadochokinesis by having the child rapidly pronate and supinate the hand. In older children, it is also worth checking for 'rebound', where the child lifts his arms up very quickly from the side and then suddenly stops this movement. Cerebellar hypotonia may prevent the child from being able to stop the arms. Next, test for truncal ataxia by having the child sit up from lying down, with the arms folded. When the child is sitting up, test for pendular knee jerks (these only occur in severe cases).

Have the patient walk normally, then heel–toe. Get the child to walk heel–toe in one direction, and then ask the child to turn around as quickly as possible and walk in the opposite direction; if there is any truncal ataxia, this manoeuvre will bring out staggering at the point of turning rapidly around, and cause trouble maintaining balance. Also, have the child walk around a chair in both directions, as this will bring out staggering towards the affected side.

Then, return the patient to the bed and examine the lower limbs for hypotonia, check the heel–shin test and the toe–finger test (the lower limb equivalent of the finger–nose test), and also have the child tap each foot rapidly against a firm surface (e.g. a clipboard).

This examination should take no more than 5 minutes, after which time a summary of the positive findings can be given and then the examination can be directed towards eliciting the cause. It may be worthwhile asking the examiners whether the child is taking anticonvulsants, if no obvious cause is discernible.

SHORT CASE: Large head

The most important things to remember in this case:
1. Always measure the head yourself, until a constant result around the largest diameter is obtained (usually three times is enough).
2. Always measure the parents' heads (in a similar fashion).
3. Always request the progressive percentiles of the child (parents' charts unavailable).
4. Always examine the back, to avoid missing spinal dysraphism.
5. Always examine the lower limbs before the upper limbs, as the lower limbs are first affected in hydrocephalus, because the tracts supplying them run closer to the ventricles.
6. Always examine the eye movements, in particular the upward gaze (for Parinaud syndrome, from raised intracranial pressure [ICP] compressing the mesencephalic tectum/superior colliculus) and lateral rectus function (for raised ICP compressing the sixth nerve).

Background information

To interpret the abnormal, you need to know the normal. There is a sex difference, and charts of head circumferences are readily available in all hospitals.

It is easy to remember the following average figures:
- 35 cm at birth.
- 47 cm (another 12 cm) at 12 months.
- 49 cm (another 2 cm) at 2 years.
- 50 cm at 3 years.
- 52 cm at 6 years.
- 53 cm at 10 years.
- 56 cm as adult.

In the examination, do not rely on remembering this. Always check the charts.

Correct interpretation of the percentile charts is mandatory. Measurements crossing percentile lines usually indicate significant pathology, except in the case of the benign condition, familial large head, where the 98th percentile line may be crossed (at, say, 12 months) and continue to deviate from the percentile curve, before it stabilises after 2 years of age.

The pattern of head growth on the percentile chart can give an indication of the type of hydrocephalus a child may have. Acquired hydrocephalus (e.g. from bacterial meningitis) will show normal growth until the time of the meningitis insult, and then will show deviation. Congenital problems (e.g. aqueduct stenosis) show much earlier deviation from the norm.

A large head can result from large bones, a large brain, large ventricles or a large bleed. This is outlined below with examples of each group.

Large bones, better referred to as 'bony disorders':
1. Achondroplasia.
2. Rickets.
3. Osteogenesis imperfecta (OI).
4. Chronic haemolytic anaemias.
   Large brain (increased brain substance), *generalised* megalencephaly:
1. Sotos syndrome (cerebral gigantism): SOTOS1 (MIM#117550); SOTOS2 (MIM#614753).
2. Weaver syndrome (MIM#277590).
3. Neurocutaneous syndromes (see individual long and short cases for NF1, TSC, SWS):
   a. Neurofibromatosis type 1 (NF1; MIM#162200).
   b. Tuberous sclerosis complex (TSC1; MIM#191100; TSC2; MIM#613254).
   c. Klippel-Trénaunay-Weber syndrome (KTW; MIM%149000).
   d. Sturge-Weber syndrome (SWS; MIM#185300).
4. Inherited metabolic disorders: lipidoses, mucopolysaccharidoses, leucodystrophies.
   Large brain (increased brain substance), *localised* enlargement:
1. Cerebral tumours (e.g. gliomas [astrocytoma, ependymoma], medulloblastoma).
2. Cerebral abscess.
   Large ventricles/subarachnoid spaces, due to excessive CSF; that is, hydrocephalus:
1. Obstructive ('non-communicating'): aqueduct stenosis, posterior fossa tumours.
2. Failure of CSF absorption ('communicating'): meningeal adhesions post-meningitis.
3. Overproduction of CSF (also 'communicating'): choroid plexus papilloma.
   Large bleed: subdural haematoma (uni/bilateral): accidental/non-accidental injury (NAI).

The following approach should detect the above groups. As the approach to the infant and older child is slightly different, both are discussed.

Examination

INFANT

Introduce yourself to the parents and child. Note the child's level of alertness, movement and any obvious features of syndromal diagnoses or neurocutaneous disorders. Look at the head for signs suggestive of hydrocephalus (e.g. 'sun-setting' of the eyes, and prominent scalp veins).

Measure the head circumference yourself, and then measure the head circumference of each parent. Request the percentile charts and comment on the findings. Inspect the shape of the head: this is best done with the child sitting up on the mother's lap. In this position, other important signs may be readily apparent, such as any titubation of head or trunk, or truncal ataxia from Dandy-Walker syndrome (DWS; MIM#%220200). The shape of the head should be assessed from all angles, and is best described in terms of 'anteroposterior diameter', 'biparietal diameter', 'frontal bossing' and 'occipital prominence'. Inspect the back for evidence of a repaired spina bifida lesion at this point, in case it is overlooked later.

Palpate the head for suture separation, fontanelle patency (posterior fontanelle normally closes by 4 months, anterior fontanelle closes by 18 months) and pressure, which must be checked in a sitting position, as a false impression of bulging may be obtained when the infant is prone or supine. Palpate carefully for shunts (there may be more than one, so be thorough) and, if present, trace shunt tubing, and inspect the abdomen for scars. Abdominal scars would indicate a ventriculoperitoneal shunt but remember shunts can also be drained to the pleural and rarely pericardial spaces.

While palpating, interact with the child, watching eye movements and responsiveness. Do not do anything never done before, such as attempting percussion of the head, or transillumination (the proper equipment for this is unlikely to be available).

Auscultate for evidence of an arteriovenous malformation (AVM) involving the great vein of Galen. Listen over both temporal fossae, both eyeballs and both retroauricular regions.

Next, a full eye examination should be performed. When eye movements are being examined, do not forget that frontal bossing, if severe, can itself be a visual barrier, and may give a false impression of an upward-gaze palsy.

Examination of the back is essential; children with spina bifida are frequent cases.

Following this, lower and upper limbs should be examined for motor and cerebellar signs. Testing sensation may be omitted in view of time restrictions, unless very relevant (e.g. sensory level in spina bifida).

A developmental assessment (gross motor, fine motor, personal–social and hearing) may then be performed. Abdominal examination is performed if a storage disorder is suspected.

A suggested order of approach is outlined in Fig. 13.4. A more comprehensive listing of possible findings, for reference, is given in Table 13.4.

1. Introduce self
Interact with child, gain impression of
    development

2. General observations
Alertness
Dysmorphic features
Skeletal anomalies
Growth parameters
Movement
Skin

3. Head
Inspect
Measure
Percentiles
Shape
Look at back at this point
Palpate
Auscultate

4. Eyes
Inspect
  • Visual acuity
  • Visual fields
  • External ocular movements
  • Pupils
  • Fundi

5. Back
Inspect
  • Midline scar (spina bifida)
  • Scoliosis (associated spina bifida,
    NF1)

6. Lower limbs
Full examination of motor system
  • Upper motor neurone signs
    (hydrocephalus, intracranial
    tumour)
  • Lower motor neurone signs (spina
    bifida, leukodystrophies)
  • Cerebellar signs (D-W)

7. Upper limbs
Full motor examination (as with lower
    limbs)

8. Developmental assessment
Gross motor
Fine motor
Hearing

9. Abdomen
Hepatosplenomegaly (MPS)

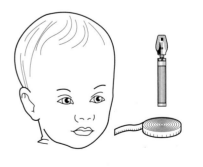

D-W = Dandy-Walker syndrome; MPS = mucopolysaccaridoses; NF1 = neurofibromatosis, type 1.

Figure 13.4 **Large head—infants**

Table 13.4
Additional information: possible physical findings in the child with a large head
GENERAL OBSERVATIONS
Dysmorphic features (e.g. Sotos, mucopolysaccharidoses)
Skeletal anomalies (e.g. achondroplasia, OI)
Parameters • Height: tall (e.g. Sotos); short (e.g. achondroplasia) • Weight: failing to thrive (e.g. Tay–Sachs, subdural from NAI, congenital toxoplasmosis)
Movement • Quality (e.g. hypotonia, poor head control in Tay–Sachs) • Symmetry (e.g. hemiplegia from subdural haematoma) • Upper limb versus lower limb (e.g. spina bifida)
Skin • Neurocutaneous stigmata (e.g. TS, NF1, SWS, KTW) • Bruising (NAI)
HEAD
Initial inspection • Size, shape (see below) • Signs of hydrocephalus (scalp vein prominence, shiny skin, sun-setting eyes) • Eye signs, e.g. squint (see below)
Size
Measure head circumference: patient; parents
Request progressive percentiles
Shape *(Describe with infant supine initially; then sit child up)* • Frontal prominence (obstructive hydrocephalus) • Parietal prominence (subdural fluid, porencephalic cyst) • Occipital prominence (D-W) • Small posterior fossa (aqueduct stenosis)
(Look at the back at this point, for spina bifida)
Palpate
(With child sitting up; interact with child and observe responsiveness, eye movements) • Craniotabes (rickets) • Split sutures (hydrocephalus) • Bulging fontanelle (hydrocephalus) • Absent fontanelle pulsation (hydrocephalus) • Shunts—trace shunt tubing, look for chest (VA) and abdomen (VP) scars
Auscultate
Bruit (AV malformation of great vein of Galen, causing increased CSF)
EYES
Ptosis (third nerve palsy)
Nystagmus (brainstem tumour)
Squint (sixth, third nerve palsies)

Table 13.4 (continued)
Proptosis (NF1 with orbital wall defect or optic nerve tumour)
Corneal clouding (MPS)
Visual acuity (impaired) • Retinal causes (e.g. optic atrophy, retinal haemorrhage) • Optic pathway causes (e.g. intracerebral glioma, optic nerve glioma; both can occur in NF1)
Visual fields: field defect (e.g. porencephalic cyst, intracerebral tumour)
External ocular movements • Third nerve palsy (e.g. raised ICP) • Sixth nerve palsy (e.g. raised ICP) • Upward gaze palsy (e.g. pinealoma)
Pupils • Enlarged (third nerve palsy) • Unreactive to light (Parinaud's syndrome from dilated third ventricle)
Lens: cataracts (congenital toxoplasmosis)
Fundi • Papilloedema (raised ICP with closed fontanelle) • Optic atrophy (long-standing raised ICP) • Retinal haemorrhage (NAI) • Astrocytic hamartoma (TS) • Chorioretinitis (congenital toxoplasmosis) • Macular degeneration (lipidoses)
Developmental assessment
Gross motor: delayed (e.g. hydrocephalus, inherited metabolic diseases)
Fine motor: delayed (e.g. inherited metabolic diseases, neurocutaneous disorders)
Hearing: impaired (e.g. post-meningitis, MPS)

AV = arteriovenous; CSF = cerebrospinal fluid; D-W = Dandy-Walker syndrome; ICP = intracranial pressure; KTW = Klippel-Trénauney-Weber syndrome; MPS = mucopolysaccharidoses; NF1 = neurofibromatosis type 1; NAI = non-accidental injury; OI = osteogenesis imperfecta; SWS = Sturge-Weber syndrome; TS = tuberous sclerosis; VA = ventriculoatrial; VP = ventriculoperitoneal.

OLDER CHILD

The approach to the older child is fairly similar to the examination of the infant. Again, begin with general observations and a full examination of the head and eyes, in a similar fashion to the examination for the infant. Perform a full gait assessment, look for scoliosis, examine the lower and then the upper limbs. Next, test the hearing and then the abdomen.

SHORT CASE: Small head

A less common case than the large head, it requires a similar well-structured approach. There are several important points that must be remembered:

1. Always measure the head circumference of the patient, and of the parents and siblings, yourself (three times), and assess the percentile charts (including those of height and weight) before proceeding further.
2. Differentiate between true microcephaly (inferring microencephaly) and craniosynostosis.
3. Always include examination of vision and hearing in the assessment.

Background information

To interpret the abnormal, you must be able to remember the normal. Average head circumference measurements at various ages are given in the section on the large head case. Correct interpretation of the head circumference percentile charts is mandatory. Measurements crossing percentile lines usually indicate significant pathology. The other growth parameters, height and weight, are very important, because they give valuable indications as to the underlying aetiology. Percentile charts should be appropriate for the child's ethnic origin.

There are essentially three patterns of percentile findings:

1. Head circumference, height and weight all at the same percentile. Possibilities here include various syndromal diagnoses, endocrine causes such as hypopituitarism, and constitutional growth delay.
2. Head circumference small, but weight and height percentiles are even lower (i.e. relative sparing of the head). Possibilities here include various chronic illnesses, undernutrition and maternal neglect.
3. Head circumference small, height and weight at significantly higher percentiles and may be within the normal range. Possibilities include all the causes of microencephaly (see below) and craniosynostosis.

It is the latter group that is most commonly represented in the short-case setting.

A small head can result from 'small bones'—that is, premature fusion of one or more sutures (craniosynostosis)—or from a small brain (microencephaly). These are discussed below.

CRANIOSYNOSTOSIS

This is labelled according to which sutures are involved. If there is premature fusion of one or two sutures, there is no restriction of growth of the brain. However, if there is fusion of multiple sutures, this can prevent normal brain growth and lead to raised intracranial pressure and significant neurological impairments.

Table 13.5 gives a list of the sutures involved, the names given for premature closure of that suture, and the resultant head shape.

MICROENCEPHALY

Causes of microencephaly include primary defects in brain development, either of prenatal onset (e.g. chromosomal anomalies such as the trisomies; malformations such as holoprosencephaly, lissencephaly and other syndromes; hereditary conditions such as autosomal recessive or autosomal dominant microcephaly) or postnatal onset (e.g. malformation syndromes including Aicardi, Angelman's, Fanconi and Rubinstein-Taybi).

Table 13.5		
Sutures involved in craniosynostosis		
SUTURE	**NAME FOR PREMATURE CLOSURE**	**RESULTANT HEAD SHAPE**
Sagittal	Scaphocephaly (also called dolichocephaly)	Elongated in the anteroposterior diameter, or boat-shaped, with decreased transverse diameter
Coronal	Brachycephaly	Widened in the transverse (biparietal) diameter, with high vault; decreased anteroposterior diameter
Single suture: unilateral coronal or lambdoid suture (or both), i.e. asymmetric craniosynostosis	Plagiocephaly	A 'skewed' shape
Metopic	Trigonocephaly	Midforehead ridging, with pointed, narrow appearance to forehead, and hypotelorism
Fusion of four or more sutures	Oxycephaly (also called turricephaly or acrocephaly)	A high, narrow, 'towershaped' skull; can cause significant neurological sequelae

Secondary (acquired) abnormalities may similarly be of prenatal onset (e.g. intrauterine TORCH infection, fetal alcohol spectrum disorder [FASD], maternal phenylketonuria [PKU]) or postnatal onset (e.g. perinatal asphyxia with resultant hypoxic encephalopathy, infections such as perinatally acquired herpes simplex encephalitis, or bacterial meningitis, head injury, undernutrition, inherited metabolic disease such as PKU, or endocrine anomalies such as hypothyroidism and hypopituitarism). Note: TORCH refers to **t**oxoplasmosis, **o**thers (includes syphilis, *Listeria monocytogenes,* HIV and Zika virus), **r**ubella, **c**ytomegalovirus (CMV) and **h**erpes, both simplex (HSV) and varicella zoster (HVZ).

Examination

Introduce yourself to the parents and patient. Note the sizes of the parents' heads and whether they appear to have normal intelligence. Note the child's alertness. Scan for any dysmorphic features and note the presence of spectacles or hearing aids (e.g. intrauterine TORCH infection).

Look at the child's posture, as well as quality and symmetry of movement (voluntary and involuntary). Also inspect the skin for neurocutaneous stigmata.

Measure the head circumference yourself, and then measure the head circumference of the parents. Request the height and weight of the child and the percentile charts. Comment on the findings. If the birth parameters are not given and a prenatal onset seems likely from the later percentile readings, request these. If prenatal onset is confirmed, this will direct the remainder of the examination towards disorders such as intrauterine infection and chromosomal anomalies.

Note the child's overall growth; in particular, whether the child looks generally small (e.g. syndromal diagnoses, constitutional growth delay) or whether just the head is small (e.g. autosomal recessive microcephaly).

Request the percentile charts to confirm your impression. Note whether the head circumference lies at a lower, an equal or a higher percentile than the other parameters (weight and height). This is a very important step (see above).

Examine the head for any scars (e.g. surgical repair of craniosynostosis, closure of encephalocele, decompressive craniotomy for severe head trauma) and visible ridging along suture lines (the metopic being seen most readily).

Next, focus on the shape of the head, assessing it from all angles. This is best done with the child sitting on the parent's lap. Head shape is best described in terms of 'anteroposterior diameter' and 'biparietal diameter'. Possible findings include the 'tower' skull of oxycephaly, or the sloping forehead and flat occiput of autosomal recessive microcephaly.

Palpate the head for ridging along suture lines and any deformities of skull contour (craniosynostosis) or bony defects (repaired encephalocele). A feature of congenital Zika virus infection is craniofacial disproportion (i.e. the cranial vault looks markedly too small for the size of the face).

Check the fontanelles. The posterior fontanelle closes by 4 months, and the anterior fontanelle by 18 months. A large anterior fontanelle occurs with the trisomies, congenital rubella and congenital hypothyroidism.

Table 13.6

A comprehensive list of possible findings on examination for small head

GENERAL OBSERVATIONS
Alertness
Dysmorphic features (e.g. de Lange, Rubenstein–Taybi)
Wearing glasses (e.g. TORCH, CP, neurodegenerative disease)
Wearing hearing aid (e.g. TORCH, CP, Cockayne, neuroaxonal dystrophy)
Skeletal anomalies (e.g. rhizomelia with RCDP)
Posture • Hemiplegic (e.g. CP, Cockayne) • Quadriplegic (e.g. CP, neurodegenerative disorders) • Decorticate (e.g. Krabbe disease)
Voluntary movements • Quality (e.g. poor head control with CP, neurodegenerative disorders) • Symmetry (e.g. hemiplegia due to CP, Cockayne, HIV-1)
Involuntary movements (beware CP or neurodegenerative disease) • Choreoathetosis (e.g. CP, PKU, Pelizaeus–Merzbacher) • Myoclonus (e.g. CP, PKU, infantile ceroid lipofuscinosis, Alpers, Aicardi, incontinentia pigmenti) • Tremor (e.g. PKU, HIV-1-related encephalopathy)
Skin • Neurocutaneous stigmata (whorled splashes of brown pigmentation in incontinentia pigmenti)
PARAMETERS
Head circumference: measure patient and parents
Request progressive percentiles
Height: short stature • Same percentile as head (syndromal diagnoses, constitutional delay, endocrine disorders) • Higher percentile than head (TORCH, Seckel, Cockayne, any severe encephalopathy in infancy) • Lower percentile than head (causes of failure to thrive, chronic illness)
Disproportionate (RCDP)
Weight (failing to thrive): comparing weight and head percentiles, causes as outlined for height comparison above

Table 13.6 (continued)

HEAD

Size (as above)

Shape (describe with child sitting up)
- Elongated AP diameter (sagittal synostosis)
- Wide with high vault (coronal synostosis)
- Asymmetric (e.g. unilateral lambdoid synostosis)
- Narrow forehead, midforehead ridge (metopic synostosis)
- Tower shaped (multiple synostosis)
- Sloping forehead (autosomal recessive microcephaly)

Palpate (with child sitting up; interact with child and observe responsiveness, eye movements)
- Ridging along sutures (craniosynostosis)
- Wide fontanelle (e.g. trisomies, congenital rubella)

EYES

Dysmorphic features
- Microphthalmos (e.g. TORCH)
- Hypotelorism (holoprosencephaly)
- Upward slant (e.g. Down syndrome)
- Downward slant (e.g. trisomy 9)
- Epicanthic folds (e.g. trisomies)

Squint (e.g. TORCH, CP)

Nystagmus (e.g. TORCH, any cause of severe visual impairment, such as neurodegenerative disorders)

Corneal opacity (e.g. Cockayne, congenital rubella, herpes)

Glaucoma (e.g. congenital rubella)

Visual acuity (impaired)
- Retinal causes (see below)
- Optic pathway causes (e.g. CP)

Visual fields: field defect (e.g. hemiplegic CP)

Eye movements: restricted upward gaze (HIV-1)

Pupils
- Anisocoria (e.g. congenital varicella)
- Unreactive to light (retinal or optic path causes of visual loss)

Lens: cataracts (e.g. TORCH, incontinentia pigmenti)

Fundi
- Chorioretinitis (TORCH)
- Pigmentary degeneration (neurodegenerative disorders, e.g. ceroid lipofuscinosis, incontinentia pigmenti), Cockayne, TORCH)
- Optic atrophy (e.g. disorders with pigmentary degeneration, TORCH, Krabbe)
- Papillitis (e.g. incontinentia pigmenti)

NOSE

Saddle shape (congenital syphilis)

Prominent (Cockayne, Seckel)

Midline groove (holoprosencephaly, hypopituitarism)

Continued

Table 13.6 (continued)
FACE
Dysmorphism assessment of facies (syndromes)
HEARING
Hearing impairment (e.g. TORCH, Cockayne, neuroaxonal dystrophy)
NECK
Goitre (hypothyroidism)
BACK
Scoliosis (e.g. CP, neurodegenerative disorders)
CHEST
Full praecordial assessment for congenital heart defects (congenital rubella, trisomies, other syndromes)
ABDOMEN
Hepatosplenomegaly (e.g. TORCH)
Dysmorphic features (e.g. umbilical, genital or anal anomalies in various syndromes)
LIMBS
Dysmorphism assessment   • Hands (e.g. simian crease: Down syndrome)   • Joints (e.g. contractures: COFS)   • Proximal shortening (e.g. RCDP)
GAIT, LOWER AND UPPER LIMBS (OLDER CHILD)
Full assessment (excluding sensory) for: • Upper motor neurone signs (CP, TORCH, neurodegenerative disorders)   • Lower motor neurone signs (neuropathies with some neurodegenerative disorders, e.g. Krabbe)   • Cerebellar signs (CP, some neurodegenerative disorders, e.g. Pelizaeus–Merzbacher)
Gross and fine motor development (infants)
Full assessment for developmental delay (CP) or regression (neurodegenerative disorders)
Full lower and upper limb assessments (as above)

COFS = cerebro-oculo-facial skeletal syndrome; CP = cerebral palsy; PKU = phenylketonuria, RCDP = rhizomelic chondro-dysplasia punctata; TORCH = toxoplasmosis, others (includes syphilis, *Listeria monocytogenes* and HIV), rubella, cytomegalovirus and herpes (both simplex and varicella-zoster).

By this stage, it should be clear whether you are dealing with craniosynostosis or microencephaly. If it is the latter, then proceed as outlined below. If it is craniosynostosis, proceed as outlined later in this section.

Note any dysmorphic facial features (various syndromal diagnoses) as you proceed. Inspect the eyes for dysmorphic features. Perform a full eye examination (the relevant findings are given in the comprehensive list in Table 13.6). In particular, check the visual acuity (impairment from various pathologies, including TORCH or trisomies), the lens for cataracts (e.g. TORCH and trisomies) and the fundi for chorioretinitis (TORCH).

After examining the eyes, check the hearing (impairment with various pathologies, e.g. TORCH, kernicterus). Assess the face for dysmorphic features, then examine the neck for goitre (hypothyroidism). Next, assess the praecordium for congenital heart defects (e.g. congenital rubella), the abdomen for hepatosplenomegaly (e.g. TORCH) and the genitalia for size (e.g. micropenis with hypopituitarism) and structure (e.g. cryptorchidism and/or hypospadias in various syndromal diagnoses).

Finally, assess the limbs, looking for dysmorphism such as joint contractures with cerebro-oculo-facial-skeletal syndrome (COFS; caused by at least four genes, *ERCC1, ERRC2, ERRC5, ERRC6*), cicatricial skin lesions and limb deformity with congenital varicella, or rhizomelia (proximal shortening) with rhizomelic chondrodysplasia punctata (RCDP; a peroxisomopathy causing hypertelorism, micrognathia, contractures and intellectual impairment).

Next, assess the gross and fine motor development. In an infant, perform the standard '180° examination' (see the short case on the floppy infant in this chapter). In an older child, a gait examination can be performed, followed by a neurological assessment of the lower and then the upper limbs, concentrating on the motor system.

At the completion of your examination, summarise the findings and give a differential diagnosis. You may then comment on investigations that you would find helpful. These will depend on your findings; the following may be of use.

Investigations

IMAGING

1. MRI for cerebral malformations, evidence of perinatal asphyxia or intrauterine infection.
2. CT scan with 3D reconstruction can define craniosynostosis and also detect calcifications seen in congenital infections.

BLOOD TESTS

1. Serological tests for intrauterine TORCH infections.
2. High-resolution karyotype (e.g. trisomy syndromes).
3. Chromosome Microarray (CMA).
4. Neonatal screening tests for PKU, congenital hypothyroidism, other IEMs.
5. Metabolic studies (for specific IEMs where clinically appropriate).

URINE

For metabolic screen, and to detect CMV excretion with congenital CMV.

CSF

To detect intrauterine or perinatal TORCH infections.

Examination procedure for craniosynostosis

Once craniosynostosis has been found, the examination is directed towards finding associated abnormalities and complications. In particular, abnormalities of the eyes and of the neurodevelopmental examination are sought.

Examine the eyes fully for signs such as proptosis (may occur with brachycephaly or with oxycephaly), hypotelorism (with trigonocephaly; may be associated with holoprosencephaly), colobomata (may occur with trigonocephaly), strabismus (especially sixth nerve palsy), and retinal findings of papilloedema or optic atrophy (with raised intracranial pressure). Next, check the hearing, as oxycephaly can be associated with auditory and vestibular impairments due to a narrowed internal auditory canal.

Then, assess the child from a neurodevelopmental perspective. Vision and hearing having been assessed already, proceed with evaluation of personal–social and language abilities, and gross and fine motor functions. Follow this with a full examination of the lower and upper limbs for long-tract signs, including assessment of balance and cerebellar function, in view of the possibility of vestibular dysfunction, as mentioned previously.

Generally, scaphocephaly is associated with a normal intellectual and neurological examination, as is plagiocephaly. Brachycephaly may be associated with neurological abnormalities, especially eye signs, and oxycephaly may well be complicated by raised intracranial pressure and significant neurological sequelae. Trigonocephaly can be associated with intellectual impairment and midline defects such as cleft palate, so the palates of children with trigonocephaly should be examined using a torch and spatula. In cases with plagiocephaly, check for congenital torticollis as the cause of the asymmetric head shape, rather than craniosynostosis.

SHORT CASE: Seizures

Children with seizures may occasionally be encountered in the examination as short-case subjects. The introduction may direct the candidate to examine for the aetiology of the seizures. Less frequently, the introduction may be directed towards finding more acute problems resulting in the current seizure activity.

A differential diagnosis mnemonic for seizures (especially afebrile) is **HEADSPACE**:

Hypo-glycaemia, calcaemia, magnesemia, natremia/**H**ypertension/**H**aemorrhage/**H**ead injury
Encephalopathies/**E**ncephalitis
AV malformation/**A**neurysm
Developmental syndromes (e.g. NF1, TSC, SWS)/**D**rugs
Stroke—ischaemic or haemorrhagic/**S**hunt (VP shunt)/**S**OL/**S**torage disorders
Prolonged QT interval/**P**oisons (toxins)
Abscess + other CNS infections: meningitis/intrauterine TORCH infections
Cerebral palsy/**C**ancer (primary/secondary brain tumours)/**C**losed head injury (occult)
Epilepsy

Recurrent seizures

Introduce yourself to the parents and patient. Look for diagnostic skin rashes (neurocutaneous syndromes). Look for asymmetry (stand child with hands and feet together), as occurs in long-standing hemiplegia (relative growth arrest of affected side).

Check/request the BP. Hypertension may be causative, or a coincidental finding in a disease that causes seizures by another mechanism (e.g. NF1). Trousseau's sign, for hypocalcaemia, can be mentioned here but is best left until the end of examination.

The head and neck are examined (Fig. 13.5). Start with the head (e.g. microcephaly with CP, syndromes; macrocephaly with hydrocephalus, intracranial tumours). Examine the eyes fully (e.g. findings in raised ICP and in CP). Check hearing (e.g. impaired with CP, congenital rubella) and examine the lower motor cranial nerves.

Long-tract signs are screened for by gait examination, then by abbreviated lower and upper limb examinations (omit sensation testing to save time).

Any significant intracranial pathology may be identified by this stage.

Next, examination of the abdomen may be performed to detect any hepatosplenomegaly due to neurometabolic disorders.

Finally, request the temperature chart and the urinalysis.

Figure 13.5 outlines this approach. Table 13.7 gives a more comprehensive listing of possible physical signs, for reference only.

Recent acute seizure

If the lead-in is 'This child has just had a seizure. Would you please examine him?', the approach is somewhat different. This is similar to the real-life situation of seeing a child in the accident and emergency department who has just had a seizure (irrespective of a past history of recurrent seizures).

The examination should assess for the following:

1. Acute infections precipitating seizures (e.g. meningitis, encephalitis).
2. Evidence of recent trauma to the head (examine the head for bruising, fractures).
3. Hypertension (as in acute post-streptococcal glomerulonephritis).
4. Hypocalcaemia (Chvostek's and Trousseau's signs).
5. Long-tract signs (assess gait, lower and upper limbs).

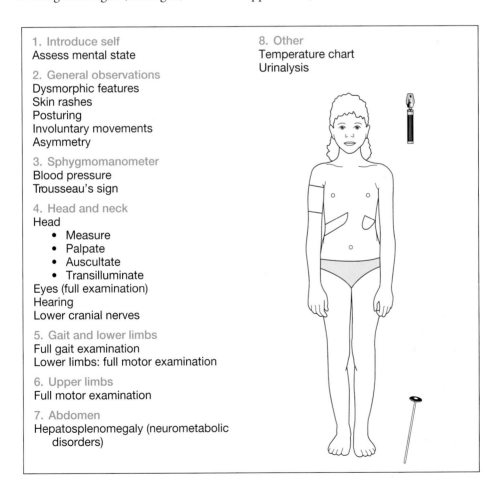

1. Introduce self
Assess mental state

2. General observations
Dysmorphic features
Skin rashes
Posturing
Involuntary movements
Asymmetry

3. Sphygmomanometer
Blood pressure
Trousseau's sign

4. Head and neck
Head
  • Measure
  • Palpate
  • Auscultate
  • Transilluminate
Eyes (full examination)
Hearing
Lower cranial nerves

5. Gait and lower limbs
Full gait examination
Lower limbs: full motor examination

6. Upper limbs
Full motor examination

7. Abdomen
Hepatosplenomegaly (neurometabolic
    disorders)

8. Other
Temperature chart
Urinalysis

Figure 13.5 **Recurrent seizures**

Table 13.7

Additional information: a more comprehensive listing of possible physical findings in children with recurrent seizurest

GENERAL OBSERVATIONS
Dysmorphic features (e.g. Angelman, trisomy 13)
Skin rashes • Facial port wine vascular malformation (SWS) • Facial naevus sebaceous (linear sebaceous naevus sequence) • Forehead fibrous plaque (TS) • 'Adenoma sebaceum' (facial fibroangiomatous lesions) (TS) • Facial butterfly rash (SLE) • Hypopigmented macules (TS) • Pigmented flecks and whorls (incontinentia pigmenti) • Café-au-lait spots (NF1) • Vascular malformations (KTW) • Axillary freckling (NF1)
'Neurometabolic' facies • Coarse features (e.g. generalised gangliosidosis) • Doll-like (Tay–Sachs)
Spastic posturing (e.g. CP)
Involuntary movements (e.g. CP)
Asymmetry (hands and feet together) • Facial (Parry–Romberg, Proteus) • Limbs (hemiplegia, KTW, NF1, Proteus)
SPHYGMOMANOMETER
Elevated blood pressure (as cause, or coincidental: e.g. NF1)
Trousseau's sign (hypocalcaemia)
HEAD
Size • Small (e.g. TORCH, CP, syndromes) • Large (e.g. IC tumour, hydrocephalus)
Shape • Flat occiput (e.g. Angelman) • Prominent forehead (e.g. generalised gangliosidosis)
Scars (craniotomy for intracerebral haemorrhage, tumour; encephalocoele repair; bolt for ICP monitoring)
Scalp veins prominent (hydrocephalus)
Palpation • Shunts (hydrocephalus) • Sutures: separated (hydrocephalus) • Skull bony defect (e.g. surgical removal, trisomy 13, encephalocoele) • Fontanelles: delayed closure (e.g. trisomy 13)
Percussion: 'cracked pot' sign (hydrocephalus)
Auscultation: bruit (arteriovenous malformation)
Transillumination • Unilateral illumination (porencephalic cyst, subdural fluid) • Bilateral illumination (hydrocephalus)
HAIR
Lightly pigmented, broken, sparse, texture like steel wool (Menkes)

Table 13.7 (continued)
EYES
Inspection • Ptosis (e.g. linear sebaceous naevus, head injury with third nerve palsy) • Squint (e.g. CP, raised ICP, congenital rubella) • Nystagmus (e.g. Aicardi, congenital rubella or herpes) • Corneal enlargement (SWS) • Iris: Lisch nodules (NF1)
Function • Visual acuity: impaired (e.g. CP, Aicardi) • Visual fields: field defects (e.g. IC tumour, haemorrhage, cyst) • Visual neglect (e.g. parietal lobe tumour or haemorrhage)
External ocular movements • Upward gaze palsy (pineal tumour) • Lateral gaze palsy (e.g. IC tumour, haemorrhage) • Sixth cranial nerve palsy (e.g. IC tumour causing raised ICP)
Pupil: dilated (third nerve palsy from IC tumour or trauma)
Ophthalmoscopy
Lens: cataracts (e.g. congenital rubella)
Retinae • Papilloedema (IC tumour causing raised ICP) • Optic atrophy (e.g. raised ICP) • Haemorrhage (NAI) • Chorioretinitis (e.g. congenital toxoplasmosis) • Circular 'holes' (Aicardi) • Cherry red spot (Tay–Sachs)
HEARING
Impaired (e.g. CP, congenital CMV, or rubella, kernicterus)
LOWER MOTOR CRANIAL NERVES
Examination of the fifth, seventh, ninth, eleventh and twelfth nerves for signs of IC pathology (e.g. hemiplegic CP, tumour)
Chvostek's sign (hypocalcaemia)
ABDOMEN
Injection sites (T1DM with recurrent hypoglycaemia)
Hepatosplenomegaly (neurodegenerative disorders, e.g. Niemann–Pick type C, Gaucher type II, generalised gangliosidosis)
OTHER
Temperature chart (precipitating fever)
Urinalysis • Glucose (T1DM) • Protein (renal disease) • Blood (precipitating UTI, CKD) • Nitrites (precipitating UTI) • Specific gravity (high with SIADH, low with CKD)
Cardiovascular examination: if evidence of long-tract signs, for underlying cyanotic congenital heart disease
Hyperventilation to induce absence seizures can be mentioned (use pinwheel)

CP = cerebral palsy; CKD = chronic kidney disease; IC = intracranial; ICP = intracranial pressure; KTW = Klippel-Trénauney-Weber syndrome; NF1 = neurofibromatosis type 1; SIADH = syndrome of inappropriate antidiuretic hormone secretion; SLE = systemic lupus erythematosus; SWS = Sturge-Weber syndrome; T1DM = type 1 diabetes mellitus; TS = tuberous sclerosis; UTI = urinary tract infection.

SHORT CASE: Facial weakness

The lead-in may request examination of the face, or may be directed specifically; for example, 'This child has had droopy eyelids since birth. Please examine the motor cranial nerves', or 'This child has facial weakness. Would you please assess?' Generally, the best approach to this case involves examining the motor cranial nerves (see short case in this chapter), and then, depending on those findings, go on to examine other areas of the nervous system. The weakness may be bilateral, as in the case of myopathic diseases or neuromuscular junction disorders, or unilateral as in Bell's palsy (lower motor neuron [LMN]) or as part of hemiplegia (usually upper motor neurone [UMN]).

There are three main groups of facial findings:

1. Ptosis and/or ophthalmoplegia with bilateral facial involvement. The differential diagnosis here includes Möbius syndrome (also spelt Moebius; MIM%157900), myasthenia gravis (MG), infant botulism and myotonic dystrophy (DM1; MIM#160900 and DM2; MIM#602668).
2. No ptosis with bilateral facial involvement. Possibilities include facioscapulohumeral dystrophy (FSHD1, MIM#158900; FSHD2, MIM#158901), bilateral LMN VII palsy with Guillain-Barré syndrome (GBS), and CP, which can cause bilateral UMN VII palsy.
3. Unilateral involvement. Unilateral facial weakness can be due to a unilateral LMN VII palsy, a unilateral UMN VII palsy or asymmetric crying facies (not really weakness, but hypoplasia of the depressor anguli oris muscle).

As with several neurological cases, examination of the mother or father is an essential part of the assessment (e.g. for myotonic dystrophy [DM], or FSHD). At certain points, depending on findings, the examination may be redirected towards other aspects of the nervous system.

Introduce yourself to the parents and patient. Engage the child briefly in conversation, note any dysphasia (associated hemiplegia) or dysarthria (DM), and gain an impression of mentation (decreased in DM, some causes of hemiplegia). Looking at the parents for 'myopathic facies'; if this is present, examine the parents after examining the child.

With the child undressed above the waist, inspect for 'myopathic facies' and ptosis including whether there is unilateral or bilateral involvement in the weakness. Look carefully for and ophthalmoplegia and diplopia (MG, sixth nerve palsy can be seen in Möbius syndrome). Visually scan the neck, trunk and upper limbs for wasting (e.g. FSHD), hemiplegic posturing, limb anomalies or hypoplastic fingers (Möbius syndrome).

If there is bilateral facial involvement, and ptosis is demonstrated, examine the motor cranial nerves. If there is any abnormality of the external ocular movements, have the child look up for at least 30 seconds to elicit evidence of MG. Next examine the upper limbs, starting at the hands, looking for myotonia; percuss the thenar eminence. If this demonstrates myotonia, continue as outlined below for further signs and complications of DM. If there is no suggestion of myotonia, go on to examine for tone, power and reflexes, for evidence of neuropathy (e.g. Kearns-Sayre Syndrome [KSS, MIM#530000]; a mitochondrial cytopathy).

If there is bilateral involvement and no ptosis, examine the motor cranial nerves. If the facies appear myopathic, examine for myopathy (particularly FSHD). Describe the muscle bulk, look for winging of the scapula and check the tone, power and reflexes of the upper limbs. Then check the gait, including having the child squat and rise from lying on the floor determining whether Gowers' manoeuvre is employed to do so. If the face is not myopathic (i.e. has bilateral LMN or UMN VII palsy), check the head circumference (CP) and the remaining cranial nerves, followed by the gait (GBS, CP).

If there is unilateral LMN involvement, examine the eighth cranial nerve (acoustic neuroma) and the ears (for vesicles in Ramsay–Hunt syndrome), followed by gait (brainstem glioma), and request the BP (hypertension as cause). If there is unilateral UMN involvement, examine the visual fields and gait (for hemiplegia).

If myotonia is suspected, examine for percussion myotonia at the thenar eminence and the deltoid. Have the child make a fist and then open the hand as fast as possible. After confirming myotonia, look for other associations (in older children), such as lens opacities, retinitis pigmentosa and choroid colobomata, and cardiomyopathy and conduction defects. After this, perform a functional assessment to assess the degree of impairment on the ADLs.

SHORT CASE: Floppy infant

This can be a difficult case if not well practised. The introduction/written stem, which gives the candidate 2 minutes to plan an approach, is commonly a variation on 'Caitlin is a 6-month-old girl whose mother feels she is floppy. Would you please assess her?' Other possibilities include combinations of 'apnoea and feeding difficulties', 'feeding and respiratory difficulties', 'has trouble holding her head up' and 'is unable to sit supported'. Careful initial inspection in the latter situations should allow the approach outlined here to be followed as with the more obvious lead-in of 'floppy infant'.

In daily practice, infants can be floppy for a wide variety of reasons, including prematurity (under 28 weeks), acute illness (e.g. sepsis), chronic conditions (e.g. malnutrition), endocrinopathies (e.g. hypothyroidism), connective tissue disorders (e.g. Marfan syndrome), and many and varied neurological and genetic causes. In the examination format, candidates are more likely to encounter a neurological, genetic or, infrequently, a connective tissue cause.

Hypotonia can be due to central or peripheral nervous system disorders. Central disorders include pathology at the levels of the cerebral cortex, cerebellum or brainstem, all of these being above the level of the anterior horn cell; therefore, these are termed 'upper motor neurone' (UMN) disorders. Children affected by these may be hypotonic but they are not weak, hence the colloquial term 'floppy strong' applies to them; an older term is 'non-paralytic hypotonia'.

Disorders from the anterior horn cell to the muscle cell are termed 'lower motor neurone' (LMN) disorders. Children affected by these disorders are weaker than typical children and the term 'floppy weak' applies; an older term is 'paralytic hypotonia'.

The causes of being 'floppy weak' can be divided into pathologies at the anterior horn cell, motor nerve, neuromuscular junction (NMJ) and muscle. It is worth knowing at least two aetiologies at each level.

Disorders that may be encountered in the exam include the following:

1. **'Hypotonic' cerebral palsy** is the single most common central (nervous system) cause of hypotonia. *Central causes* of hypotonia account for 60–80% of cases of floppy infants. They include: hypoxic ischaemic encephalopathy (HIE, in around 20%); genetic/chromosomal syndromes (in around 30%; includes: Down [and other trisomies]; Prader–Willi syndrome [P–WS]; 1p36 deletion syndrome; 22q13 deletion syndrome [Phelan-McDermid]; 22q11.2 deletion syndrome [DiGeorge/velocardiofacial; 'CATCH-22']; Williams; Wolf-Hirschhorn; Sotos; Smith-Magenis; Kabuki; cri-du-chat, achondroplasia); brain malformations (in around 15%); intracranial haemorrhage; congenital infection (TORCH); metabolic conditions (congenital disorders of glycosylation, Smith-Lemli-Opitz and other inborn errors of metabolism [IEMs], Zellweger and other peroxisomal disorders); and maternal drugs.

2. **Type 1 spinal muscular atrophy (SMA1; MIM#253300)**, also called Werdnig–Hoffmann disease, is the most common and severe form of spinal muscular atrophy (SMA). SMA describes a number of genetic disorders which lead to degeneration of anterior horn cells of the spinal cord, and lower motor (bulbar) nuclei in the brainstem.

   SMA1 presents during the neonatal period with progressive proximal weakness; features include: alert facies; normal external ocular muscles and facial expression; preserved social interaction; tongue atrophy and fasciculations; postural tremor of fingers; absent deep tendon reflexes (DTRs); and paradoxical, 'see-saw' breathing pattern (chest indrawing with inspiration secondary to intercostal weakness but sparing of diaphragm; also spares facial expression muscles and pelvic sphincters).

   SMA is related to homozygous deletions or point mutations in the survival motor neuron 1 (*SMN1*) gene situated at 5q13.2. SMN protein is involved in mRNA production within motor neurons. Around 95–98% of patients with SMA have homozygous deletion of exon 7 (lack of exon 7 in both copies of *SMN1*); the remaining 2–5% are compound heterozygotes for deletion of *SMN1* exon 7 and an intragenic mutation which inactivates SMN1.

   Variations in SMN protein production and phenotype expression are due to a second SMN gene, *SMN2*, which is adjacent to *SMN1* and only varies from its composition by five base pairs. Some patients have more than one copy of *SMN2* (range is 0–5 copies). The more SMN2 protein produced, the better (milder) the phenotype; if the child with SMA has three or more copies of *SMN2*, the phenotype is milder.

   The investigation to diagnose SMA1 is targeted mutational analysis of the *SMN1* gene. SMA1 accounts for around 2% of floppy infants. Other pathologies that target the anterior horn cell include poliovirus and enterovirus 71(EV71).

3. **Dejerine-Sottas syndrome** (DSS; MIM#145900; genetic heterogeneity: can be caused by mutations in: *MPZ, PMP22, PRX, EGR2, GJB1*), also called Charcot-Marie-Tooth type 3 (CMT3); this is a demyelinating peripheral neuropathy that has its onset in infancy (unlike CMT1 and CMT2 which present in older children; CMT describes a spectrum of genetic disorders causing peripheral neuropathy).

   There is another condition with significant clinical overlap: CMT4E (also called severe congenital hypomyelinating neuropathy, CHN; MIM#605253; genes: *MPZ, EGR2*). Both present with hypotonia, distal muscle weakness and areflexia; may develop scoliosis, pes cavus.

4. **Neonatal myasthenia gravis (MG)** can be due to transient acquired neonatal myasthenia (in 10–15% of children born to mothers with MG, due to passive placental transfer of antibodies against the acetylcholine receptor [AChR] protein) or due to congenital myasthenic syndromes (CMS), which can be caused by a number of genes, some which code for proteins which are found in the neuromuscular junction, including for subunits of the AChR (genes: *CHRNA1, CHRNB1, CHRND, CHRNE*). Babies with CMS may require ventilation from birth, and may have arthrogryposis, ptosis, generalised weakness or episodic apnoea. Diagnosed by response to IV or SC edrophonium chloride. Babies with the transitory form may develop symptoms from within hours of birth to 3 days of age and may need respiratory support, but resolve after an average of 18 days. Other pathologies that target the NMJ: magnesium toxicity, aminoglycoside toxicity, infant botulism (*Clostridium botulinum*).

5. **Congenital myopathies** are divided into subgroups based on the histopathological appearance of the muscle biopsy, including: nemaline bodies, which are accumulations

of protein (nemaline myopathy [NEM1: gene *TPM3*; MIM#609284; NEM2: gene *NEB*; MIM#256030]); and cores lacking mitochondrial oxidative activity (central core disease [CCD; gene *RYR1*; MIM#117000] and multiminicore disease [MMD; gene *RYR1*; MIM#255320]).

Myopathies can present with ophthalmoplegia, facial weakness and bulbar weakness, which helps differentiate them from anterior horn cell disorders and peripheral neuropathies. Reduced muscle bulk with preservation of deep tendon reflexes is a clue.

6. **Congenital myotonic dystrophy (DM1; MIM#160900)**, an autosomal dominant disorder, is caused by a mutation in the dystrophica myotonia protein kinase gene (*DMPK*) comprising a trinucleotide (CTG) repeat expansion; normal people have 5 to 37 repeats of CTG; a repeat length beyond 50 copies of CTG is pathogenic; patients with classic DM1 have 100–1000 repeats, babies with the congenital onset DM1 inherit the mutated gene from their affected mother, and have an amplified CTG repeat of over 2000 repeats by maternal transmission; this repeat expands in successive generations. Features can include requirement for ventilation from birth (due to inadequate intercostal muscles and diaphragm), weak cry, poor suck, facial diplegia, tented upper lip, high arched palate, open mouth, thin cheeks, wasting of temporal muscles, weakness of proximal muscles and myotonia; there also may be arthrogryposis, dislocated hips and club feet. Reflexes usually are absent.

7. **Congenital muscular dystrophies (CMD)** are a group of inherited muscle disorders, genetically heterogeneous. The major subtypes comprise: laminin alpha-2 (merosin) deficiency (MDC1A); collagen VI-deficient CMD; LMN-related CMD (L-CMD); *SEPN1*-related CMD; and the dystroglycanopathies. Infants present with progressive weakness, joint contractures, spinal rigidity, respiratory compromise and cognitive impairment.

8. **Prader–Willi syndrome (P–WS; MIM#176270)** is a contiguous gene syndrome caused by deletion of paternal copies of *SNRPN* and *NDN* within 15q11–q13. This is a cause of central hypotonia. An old mnemonic was **H3O**, meaning **H**ypotonia, **H**ypomentia, **H**ypogonadism (hypogonadotropic) and **O**besity. Also, hands and feet are small. Onset of obesity between 6 months and 6 years. Growth deceleration in adolescence. Dysmorphic facies: almond-shaped eyes, upslanting palpebral fissures, squint, thin upper lip and small mouth with down-turning corners. Skeletal features can include scoliosis and kyphosis. Mild to moderate intellectual impairment is usual.

The examination should first elicit whether the infant is 'floppy weak' or 'floppy strong'. Infants who are floppy and weak usually have disorders involving the LMN. The pathology can be at the level of anterior horn cell, peripheral nerve, NMJ or muscle. Infants who are floppy and strong usually have central neurological (UMN) causes, or non-neurological causes, such as connective tissue disorders (e.g. Marfan syndrome).

Remember to look at the mother's face for evidence of myotonic dystrophy. If this is suspected, the parent can be asked to make a fist and then open the hand quickly; this will detect myotonia more easily than a handshake. Look for evidence of MG in the mother.

Commence inspection by noting any dysmorphic features, and describe the infant's alertness, posture, movements, head size, facial features, any interventions such as nasogastric tube, oxygen catheter, tracheostomy or gastrostomy, and any tachypnoea paradoxical breathing, use of accessory muscles, and note the cry. The suggested procedure is outlined in Figure 13.6. A comprehensive listing of findings sought is given in Table 13.8 (see also Fig. 13.7).

1. Introduce self
Look at parents' faces (myotonic
    dystrophy, myasthenia gravis)

2. General observation
Dysmorphic features
Head size
Facial features
Posture
Movement
Previous intervention
Respiratory difficulties

3. Manoeuvres: the 180°
    examination
a. Observe infant in supine position
To describe: posture, movement
b. Pull to sit
To detect: degree of head control/lag
c. Sitting
To describe:
  - Degree of head control
  - Degree of trunk control
  - Ability to sit unsupported
d. Attempted weight bearing
To detect:
  - Lower limb hypotonia/weakness
  - Lower limb scissoring (CP)
  - 'Advanced' weight bearing (CP)
e. Ventral suspension
To describe:
  - Posture of head, trunk and limbs
    (degree of hypotonia; infants with
    CP may have extensor posture)
f. Place infant prone and observe
To describe:
  - Degree of head control
  - Ability to lift head/trunk

4. Limbs
Inspect (small hands and feet in P–WS)
Palpate
Tone
Power
Reflexes

5. Primitive reflexes
Test for:
  - Suck
  - Grasp
  - Stepping

  - Placing
  - ATNR
  - Moro reflex

6. Head
Head
  - Inspect
  - Palpate
  - Auscultate
  - Transilluminate
Eyes
  - Full examination for evidence of
    intrauterine infection, CP,
    retinopathy of prematurity
Hearing
  - Test with bell and rattle for
    deafness from kernicterus,
    intrauterine infection, CP

7. Abdomen
Examine for hepatosplenomegaly due to
    intrauterine infection MPS (central),
    glycogen and lipid storage
    myopathies (peripheral)
Genitalia (hypoplastic in PWS)

8. Chest
Examine praecordium for cardiac
    enlargement and dysfunction due to
    glycogenoses types 2 or 3, or for
    congenital heart disease due to
    congenital rubella

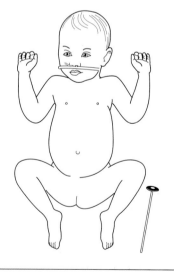

CP = cerebral palsy; MPS = mucopolysaccharidoses; P–WS = Prader–Willi syndrome; ATNR = asymmetric
tonic neck reflex.

Figure 13.6 **Floppy infant**

Table 13.8
Additional information: possible findings on floppy infant examination
GENERAL OBSERVATION
Dysmorphic features (e.g. Down, PWS, MPS, lipidoses)
Head size • Microcephaly (e.g. CP) • Macrocephaly (e.g. associated myelomeningocele, congenital toxoplasmosis)
Facial features • 'Ex-premmie' appearance (prematurity per se, CP) • Alert (e.g. SMA) • Expressionless (e.g. some congenital myopathies, MD, MG) • Ptosis (as above) • Ophthalmoplegia (as above) • Nasogastric tube (e.g. hypotonic CP, some congenital myopathies, MD, MG) • Oxygen catheter (e.g. hypotonic CP, SMA, some congenital myopathies, MD, MG) • 'Fish' (triangular) mouth (e.g. congenital myopathies or MD) • Tongue fasciculation (SMA)
Posture • 'Frog-leg' lower limb posture (e.g. especially SMA, congenital myopathies) • Fisted hands (CP) • Arthrogryposis (e.g. congenital muscular dystrophy, MD)
Main areas affected • Face (congenital myopathies, MD or MG) • Lower limb (myelomeningocele) • Proximal limb (e.g. SMA) • Distal limb (congenital MD)
Normal movement (e.g. connective tissue disorders)
Fasciculations (e.g. SMA)
Previous intervention • Tracheostomy/scar (e.g. infant botulism) • Gastrostomy/scar (e.g. hypotonic CP, congenital MD)
Respiratory difficulties
Upper airway noises (e.g. CP) • Tachypnoea (e.g. aspiration with SMA, CP, congenital MD, Pompe) • Paradoxical breathing , bell-shaped chest, splayed lower ribs (e.g. SMA)
LIMBS
Inspection • Decreased muscle bulk (e.g. SMA, undernutrition) • Fasciculation (e.g. SMA) • Muscle biopsy site
Palpate • Confirm hypotonia • Contractures (causes of arthrogryposis) • Joint hypermobility (connective tissue disorders)
Power • Weak (e.g. SMA, congenital MD, muscular dystrophy or myopathies) • Normal (e.g hypotonic CP, other central causes, connective tissue disorders)
Reflexes • Absent (e.g. SMA) • Decreased (e.g. neuropathies or, later, myopathies) • Normal (e.g. connective tissue disorders) • Increased (CP)

CP = cerebral palsy; MD = myotonic dystrophy; MG = myasthenia gravis; MPS = mucopolysaccharidoses; P–WS = Prader–Willi syndrome; SMA = spinal muscular atrophy.

A. SUPINE
To describe
Posture
Movement

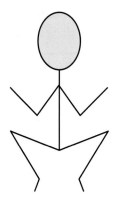

B. PULL TO SIT
To detect
Degree of head
control/lag

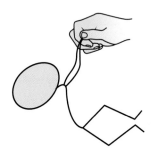

C. SITTING
To describe
Degree of head control
Degree of trunk control
Ability to sit
unsupported

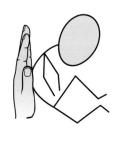

D. ATTEMPTED WEIGHT-BEARING
To detect
Lower limb
hypotonia/weakness
Lower limb scissoring
(CP)
'Advanced' weight-bearing (CP)

E. VENTRAL SUSPENSION
To describe
Posture of head, trunk
and limbs (degree of
hypotonia; infants with
CP may have extensor
posture)

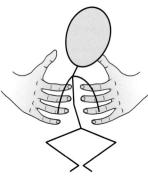

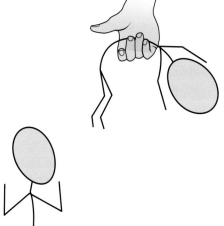

F. PRONE
To describe
Degree of head control
Ability to lift head/trunk

Figure 13.7 **Floppy infant—manoeuvres**

When describing posture, use appropriate terminology; comment on the joint positioning in terms of 'external rotation at hips' and 'flexion at knees'. 'Frog leg' posture is a well-recognised term, but should be supplemented with these more accurate terms.

Assessment of movement should focus on whether the baby can move against gravity, any difference between proximal and distal movement, and upper limbs versus lower limbs. SMA type 1 may be associated with some degree of sparing of the hands and feet (e.g. finger and toe movement only), as well as the face. Lumbar myelomeningocele (MMC) affects the lower limbs. Some congenital myopathies affect all limbs and face.

Describe any lack of movement with appropriate terms, such as 'paucity of movement'.

Inspection of the face can give many clues to the diagnosis. Infants with Werdnig–Hoffmann disease have alert, bright faces, respond appropriately to surroundings and are visually interactive, whereas those with NMJ or muscular disorders may have ptosis, ophthalmoplegia, facial diplegia, a tented mouth and an expressionless 'myopathic facies'. Infants with central disorders may have a depressed level of consciousness, may not fix or follow, and may appear lethargic and not interactive. Babies with facial weakness (NMJ or myopathies) cannot keep their eyelids closed when any attempt is made to open their lids.

Always check for tongue fasciculation, which is seen in SMA1. The presence of a nasogastric tube or gastrostomy suggests a feeding or swallowing problem, which may occur in several conditions, including SMA, some myopathies, and intracranial ischaemia or haemorrhage.

An oxygen catheter in situ implies respiratory difficulties. Respiratory distress may be due to aspiration with SMA, CP or congenital MD, or diaphragmatic 'see-saw' breathing in SMA. A tracheostomy scar indicates previous intensive treatment for conditions that may improve with time, such as infant botulism, congenital MD or an intracranial catastrophe.

Next, the manoeuvres comprising the '180° examination' may be performed to quantify the degree of hypotonicity. During these manoeuvres, signs such as scissoring with CP, or a posterior midline scar with MMC may be noted.

When assessing the infant's ability to raise his/her head and trunk when placed prone, the infant's hands should be placed to either side of the shoulders (with the palms apposed to the bed and elbows flexed) to optimise the infant's ability to extend the upper limbs. If the child is positioned with the hands beneath the trunk, or with arms extended, an accurate assessment will not be possible.

Following the manoeuvres, the limbs are examined; examine the lower limbs first. Confirm hypotonia, check joint mobility, note any contractures and joint dislocations (especially at the hips). The strength should then be assessed. Note whether the child can raise their limbs fully against gravity and sustain them in that position. The strength of a withdrawal response can be easily tested (tickle the feet).

At this point, indicate to the examiners whether the child is 'floppy weak' (i.e. peripheral) or 'floppy strong' (i.e. central) group. This directs the remainder of the examination. More common causes of a floppy weak infant are SMA1, congenital DM1 and congenital myopathies. More common causes of a floppy strong infant are hypotonic cerebral palsy and Down syndrome.

Tendon reflexes are helpful. If reflexes are very brisk, LMN pathology is unlikely. Reflexes are always absent in SMA1. Reflexes may be absent in severe congenital myopathies and congenital DM due to inadequate muscle bulk to generate a movement.

If the cause appears peripheral, give a differential diagnosis at this stage. If a myopathy seems most likely, go on to examine the abdomen for hepatomegaly and the praecordium for cardiomegaly, for myopathy due to glycogenoses types 2 or 3. If a hereditary neuropathy seems most likely, request permission to examine the mother (e.g. for pes cavus). If a neuromuscular junction problem is likely, request permission to examine the mother for MG.

At the completion of the examination, request the reports on electromyography, nerve conduction velocity and muscle biopsy. Do not request the actual test, as if this is supplied, interpretation is expected! Be prepared to tell the examiners the usual findings of the disease you suspect.

If the cause appears central, go on to check the primitive reflexes, which may provide evidence of CP. Then examine the head, eyes and hearing for evidence of intrauterine infection, and complications of prematurity that can lead to CP. Finally, check the abdomen for hepatosplenomegaly (TORCH) and praecordium (for congenital heart disease due to congenital rubella). At the completion of the examination, request relevant investigations (see below).

Despite the fact that a number of diagnoses have been stressed, the important point is the method of examination. The candidate should aim to give an overall picture of the child, then categorisation and, lastly, actual diagnosis.

Relevant investigations that may be appropriate:

- *Central hypotonia*:
  - High-resolution karyotype.
  - Chromosomal microarray (CMA).
  - Thyroid function tests.
  - Vitamin B_{12}.
  - Lactate.
  - Amino acids.
  - Ammonia.
  - Very long chain fatty acids (VLCFAs; elevated in peroxisomal disorders).
  - Fluorescent in-situ hybridisation (FISH) test for P-WS.
  - For intrauterine infection, TORCH serology.
  - MRI brain and spine.
  - For inborn errors of metabolism, urine metabolic screen.
- *Peripheral hypotonia*:
  - For SMA1: targeted mutational analysis of *SMN1* gene.
  - For DM1: test for size of CTG repeats in *DMPK* gene.
  - For DSS/CMT: nerve conduction studies (differentiates forms: demyelinating/axonal/intermediate/pure motor).
  - For myopathies: EMG, muscle biopsy (also for mitochondrial, metabolic, storage) including electron microscopy and histochemistry.
  - For congenital muscular dystrophies: test for CK.
  - For dystrophinopathy: CK; MLPA for dystrophin.
  - For Pompe disease (acid maltase deficiency, AMD): acid maltase (acid alpha-glucosidase) blood spot; CK; liver function tests (aspartate aminotransferase [AST], lactic dehydrogenase [LDH] elevated); EMG; ECG (short PR interval, tall broad QRS); muscle biopsy (vacuoles stain for glycogen).
  - For LMN: 'neuromuscular gene panel' which can detect over 400 genetic causes.
  - If neuromuscular panel negative: whole exome sequencing (WES).
  - If WES negative: whole genome sequencing.

Connective tissue diagnoses, presenting as a floppy strong infant, can include joint hypermobility (which is defined in older children using the Beighton score), and a number of heritable disorders of connective tissue including Marfan syndrome, various forms of Ehlers-Danlos syndrome (the six main groups of which share a triad of joint hypermobility, skin hyperextensibility and tissue fragility) and Loeys–Dietz syndrome (LDS).

LDS comprises a triad of progressive aortic aneurysmal disease, hypertelorism, and bifid uvula or cleft palate; a Marfanoid habitus, craniosynostosis and micrognathia can also occur. LDS is associated with congenital heart disease: atrial septal defect (ASD), patent ductus arteriosus (PDA), bicuspid aortic valve (BAV) and mitral valve prolapse (MVP). Orthopaedic findings in LDS include congenital dislocated hips, talipes equinovarus, pectus excavatum and scoliosis. There are five groups of LDS described, due to four mutated genes: *TGFBR1*, *TGFBR2*, *SMAD3*, *TGFB2* (both LDS2 and LDS4 are due to *TGFBR2* mutations). Clinically, LDS acts like an overlap between Marfan and Ehlers-Danlos syndromes. The importance of recognising this condition is the associated generalised arterial tortuosity and risk of arterial rupture. Osteogenesis imperfecta (OI), caused mainly by mutations in genes that code for type 1 procollagen (*COL1A1*, *COL1A2*), can also present with joint hypermobility.

SHORT CASE: Hemiplegia

Children with hemiplegia are usually included in the short-case section under the introduction of 'Examine the gait'. The task is not just to identify the hemiplegia, but to ascertain the level of the problem and the aetiology. The examination can assess these factors sequentially as outlined here. The overall plan is as follows:
- Demonstrate the physical signs of hemiplegia in the lower and upper limbs.
- Demonstrate the level by assessing, as a minimum, the seventh cranial nerve (lower motor neuron involvement implies pathology in the region of the pons; upper motor neuron involvement implies a lesion above the pons) and the visual fields (involvement implies site of lesion at internal capsule or above), and look for parietal lobe signs (cortical lesion).
- Look for the cause.

The causes can be divided into two groups: arterial ischaemic stroke (AIS), and haemorrhagic stroke.

Causes of *AIS* include: cerebral arteriopathies (responsible for 50–80%), cardiac causes (acquired or congenital), sickle cell anaemia (SCA), thrombophilia and infections.

A mnemonic for *AIS* is **SCA**:

Sickle cell anaemia/**S**epsis
Cardiac causes/**C**lotting tendency (thrombophilia)
Arteriopathies

Causes of *haemorrhagic* stroke include: cerebral vascular abnormalities (responsible for 40–90%; including AVM, cavernous malformations, aneurysm), bleeding disorders, brain tumour and hypertension.

A mnemonic for *haemorrhagic* stroke is **CHAT**:

Cerebral vascular abnormalities/**C**oagulopathies
Hypertension/**H**aemophilia
AVM/**A**neurysm
Tumour (cerebral)/**T**hrombocytopaenia

The causes can also be grouped as systems.

Cardiovascular causes

1. Hypertension.
2. Cyanotic congenital heart disease (CHD): before 2 years of age, usually cerebral thrombosis; after 2, cerebral abscess.
3. Subacute bacterial endocarditis (SBE).
4. Cerebral arteriovenous malformations (AVM).
5. Cerebral vaso-occlusive disease; for example, moyamoya disease.
6. Sturge-Weber syndrome (SWS): cerebral vessel anomalies.

Traumatic causes

1. Non-accidental injury (NAI).
2. Brain trauma; for example, motor vehicle accidents (MVA).
3. Intraoral trauma.

Infective causes

1. Herpes simplex encephalitis (HSE).
2. Bacterial meningitis.
3. Cerebral abscess.

Systemic disorders

1. Systemic lupus erythematosus (SLE).
2. Sickle cell anaemia (SCA).
3. Homocystinuria.
4. Neurofibromatosis type 1 (NF1).
5. Acute leukaemia, non-lymphocytic (ANLL) or lymphocytic (ALL).

Examination

In practice, there is a significant percentage of children with acute hemiplegia in which the cause is not yet known. A suggested approach is as follows.

GENERAL OBSERVATIONS

Introduce yourself to the child and parent. Ask the child simple things, such as name, age and school. Note any dysphasia (dominant hemisphere) and note any obvious intellectual impairment (secondary to meningitis, HSE, NAI, MVA, homocystinuria).

Have the child adequately exposed, being sensitive to their modesty. Note the posture and describe it carefully. Note any asymmetry of the limbs (growth arrest). Assess the growth parameters. If tall or Marfanoid habitus, think of homocystinuria. Comment on whether the child is well or unwell, as she or he may be recovering from recent insults (e.g. encephalitis) or may be in distress from acute problems (SBE, CHD with cardiac failure). Check whether the child is cyanosed (CHD).

Examine the skin for the following:

1. Bruising/purpura (NAI, ANLL, ALL).
2. Pallor (SCA, ANLL, ALL).
3. Neurocutaneous stigmata (SWS, NF1).
4. Cigarette or electric heater burns (NAI).

GAIT (OLDER CHILD) OR GROSS MOTOR ASSESSMENT (INFANT)

Now, after thorough inspection, take the child through a full gait examination (for details, see the gait short-case approach in this chapter). In subtle cases of hemiplegia, manoeuvres such as the Fog test and 'reverse Fog' test may reveal the problem. Remember to check for sensory neglect when the child is standing up (when testing for Romberg's sign).

In infants too young to walk, where the introduction will obviously not be 'gait' but perhaps 'not using one side' or '6 months old and prefers the left hand', a gross motor developmental assessment replaces the gait manoeuvres. Instead of the Fog test, use the 'cover' test, where the child's face is covered with a cloth, and each handheld in turn to see if the cloth can be removed equally well using either one. Also check the primitive reflexes for signs such as asymmetric Moro or parachute reflexes.

LOWER LIMBS

Check tone, power and reflexes. Remember to test for clonus at both ankle and knee, crossed adductor response (abnormal after 9 months of age) and spread of reflexes. In view of time constraints, it is reasonable to omit sensory testing, or postpone it until later, if the examiners agree when you suggest this.

ABDOMINAL REFLEXES

For a complete assessment of pyramidal tract function, these should be included. They correspond to spinal segments T7–T12.

UPPER LIMBS

As with lower limbs, just test tone, power and reflexes, and omit or postpone sensory testing.

HEAD

Inspect and describe facial features; there may be obvious facial asymmetry (e g. seventh cranial nerve lesion). In this case, it is best to examine the motor cranial nerves, starting with the twelfth nerve and working up. Check for tongue deviation (twelfth), asymmetry of shoulder shrugging (eleventh), asymmetry of palate elevation (ninth), eyebrow raising, tight closing of eyes, showing teeth and puffing out cheeks (all seventh) and external eye movements (third, fourth and sixth; note that the third cranial nerve nucleus is in the midbrain, and the fourth is in the pons). At completion of motor cranial nerves, check the visual fields for field defects and for parietal visual neglect. A field defect implies a lesion at or above the internal capsule.

Now examine the higher centres for parietal lobe signs.

In older children, test for receptive dysphasia, agraphia ('write your name for me'), astereognosis (e.g. unable to recognise key in hand), ideomotor apraxia (e.g. 'show me how you brush your teeth') and left/right confusion. These occur when the dominant side is involved. Also test for constructional apraxia (e.g. ask the child to draw a clock), which occurs when the non-dominant side is involved, and finally examine for sensory extinction, which can occur with either side involved.

In younger children, the 'higher centres' part of the examination is more general, and works best if simple things are asked first, such as name, address age, sex ('Are you a boy or a girl'), and naming parts of the body (e.g. pointing at nose, eyes, ears, arm and asking 'What's this?'). If the child is unable to succeed at the latter, point to something such as your watch, ask 'Is this a dog? A cat? A watch?' and note the responses.

Note that if there is no involvement of any cranial nerves or higher centres, then a spinal cord lesion is possible, and warrants a sensory examination being performed, as well as assessment of the spine itself.

By this stage the level will have been ascertained, and the cause can be sought. An approach is set out overleaf.

Inspect and palpate the head for the 'S' signs:
1. **S**ize: head circumference may be increased with subdural haematoma, or intracranial tumour.
2. **S**cars (e.g. craniotomy for repair of AVM, evacuation of subdural haematoma).
3. **S**utures and fontanelles (widened sutures, full fontanelle with raised intracranial pressure: e.g. with intracranial tumour, hydrocephalus).
4. **S**hunts (e.g. hydrocephalus, chronic subdural collection).

Auscultate the skull for bruits (AVM). Inspect conjunctivae for pallor (SCA). Examine the retinae for retinal haemorrhage (NAI), papilloedema (raised intracranial pressure). Inspect the oral cavity for haemorrhage from oral trauma.

CARDIOVASCULAR

Perform a full cardiovascular examination, looking for clubbing (cyanotic CHD), hypertension, central cyanosis (CHD), murmurs (CHD, SLE), carotid pulsation (decreased in arteritis), carotid bruits, hepatomegaly (SCA, ALL) and splenomegaly (SCA).

SPINE

This is an essential part of the examination if there is no involvement of any cranial nerves or higher centres. If this is the case, the above head and cardiovascular assessments should be postponed.

Inspect for scoliosis (e.g. NF1, spinal tumour) and scars (e.g. excised spinal tumour). Palpate for tenderness and masses. Auscultate for arteriovenous malformations or vascular tumours.

URINALYSIS

This is for blood (e.g. post-streptococcal glomerulonephritis with hypertension, SCA) and protein (chronic kidney disease with hypertension).

SHORT CASE: Intellectual impairment

The approach outlined here may be useful in assessing the aetiology for clinical problems such as developmental delay or developmental regression in the long- or short-case setting (the technique for performing a developmental assessment is discussed in a separate short case). It is imperative to differentiate between static and progressive causes of intellectual impairment. The examination procedure outlined here is quite comprehensive, covering multiple aetiologies of both groups of causes. Several neurodegenerative conditions (progressive causes) are mentioned. The examiners will not expect detailed knowledge of the individual conditions; they are simply mentioned for completeness, and of course many are relevant only in certain age groups or with certain dysmorphic or other salient clinical features.

You should still be able to assess in general terms for neurodegenerative conditions: remember that those predominantly affecting grey matter may present with dementia and seizures, while those affecting white matter tend to have problems of spasticity, cortical deafness and blindness.

Examination

Introduce yourself to the patient and parents. Note the age and sex of the child, to allow age and sex-appropriate neurodegenerative conditions to be borne in mind. Examples include: males with X-linked conditions such as fragile X, Menkes, adrenoleucodystrophy

(ALD) and Hunter syndromes; infants with conditions such as tuberous sclerosis complex (TSC) and epileptic spasms; older children with disorders such as subacute sclerosing panencephalitis (SSPE), and Wilson disease (WD).

Stand back and scan for obvious dysmorphic features (e.g. Down syndrome, mucopolysaccharidoses), neurocutaneous stigmata (e.g. cutaneous findings of TSC, ataxia-telangiectasia [AT], Sturge-Weber syndrome [SWS], incontinentia pigmenti [IP]) and other skin abnormalities, such as thick skin with the mucopolysaccharidoses (MPSs). Note any abnormal posturing, such as spastic quadriparesis with CP, late stages of white matter degenerations; hypotonic posturing in infants with atonic CP, Down syndrome and various degenerative conditions (see short case on the floppy infant in this chapter).

Note any involuntary movements, such as extrapyramidal movements (CP, WD), static tremor (WD), intention tremor (WD, Friedreich), myoclonic jerks (SSPE) or seizure activity (CP, TSC, peroxisomal disorders [e.g. Zellweger], degenerative grey matter disorders [gangliosidoses], some white matter diseases such as ALD).

Note the growth parameters, particularly the head circumference. This may be large with several inherited neurodegenerative disorders (Gaucher, mucopolysaccharidoses [MPSs]), or with hydrocephalus or chronic subdural effusion. Head circumference may be small with several syndromal diagnoses (Cornelia de Lange, Seckel), intrauterine infections (TORCH) or autosomal recessive microcephaly. Measure the head circumference yourself, and request progressive percentile measurements. Height is infrequently a useful guide, as most of the disorders can be associated with short stature (genetic disorders, hypothyroidism, fetal alcohol spectrum disorder [FASD], TORCH). Marked obesity can indicate Prader–Willi syndrome (P–WS), hypothyroidism or pseudohypoparathyroidism. Request the progressive percentiles of these parameters.

The systematic examination can be commenced at the head. After measuring it, inspect carefully for scars and shunts, and palpate for fontanelle and suture patency in infants, shunts or bony defects (e.g. repaired encephalocele). Transillumination may be worth mentioning (for hydrocephalus, hydranencephaly, subdural effusion or porencephaly), so that the examiners know you have thought of it, although most candidates are probably not armed with an appropriate torch. Feel the hair in male infants (in Menkes kinky hair syndrome, it feels like steel wool). Assess the face from a dysmorphic perspective. Note the size and position of the ears, and then make a detailed evaluation of the eyes, looking at external features (e.g. epicanthic folds [Down], corneal clouding [MPSs, congenital rubella]), function (e.g. blindness, squint) and ophthalmological findings (e.g. cataracts, optic atrophy, cherry red spot [gangliosidosis]). Assess the nose, mouth, chin, neck and hairline for dysmorphic findings. Also examine the neck for goitre (hypothyroidism).

Next, a neurological assessment can be performed. Depending on the ability of the patient, this may be commenced with a full gait examination, including checking the back for scoliosis (e.g. CP, Friedreich ataxia [FRDA], AT), kyphosis (MPSs) and gibbus (GM1 gangliosidosis), or with a gross motor developmental assessment.

Assess whether the patient has muscle weakness. This includes a comment on any facial myopathy and muscle bulk. In the cooperative child, ask them to rise from the floor assessing for Gowers' manoeuvre. Certain congenital muscular dystrophies, myotonic dystrophy and DMD are associated intellectual disability.

This is then followed by examination of the lower and upper limbs, both for dysmorphic features and neurologically, especially for tone (e.g. hypertonia with CP, PKU, Gaucher; hypotonia with hypotonic CP, Down, PWS) and reflexes (e.g. hyperreflexia with CP; hyporeflexia with metachromatatic leucodystrophy [MLD] which causes peripheral neuropathy).

The abdomen can then be examined for hepatosplenomegaly (intrauterine TORCH infection, Gaucher, Niemann-Pick, Hurler, GSDs) and the genitalia for dysmorphic features (various malformation syndromes) or large testes in the postpubertal male (fragile X).

Next, the chest is examined for dysmorphic features and the praecordium for any evidence of cardiomegaly (e.g. MPSs) or congenital valvular heart disease (e.g. 22q11.2 deletion [CATCH-22], Down, Noonan, other malformation syndromes).

After this, the hearing should be tested (e.g. impairment with intrauterine CMV, kernicterus, MPSs).

With completion of this assessment for aetiology, the examiners may request an opinion regarding the level of impairment. If so, go on to perform a developmental assessment (see the short case on this in this chapter). This will give an approximation only of the true intelligence quotient.

The examiners will expect you to be familiar with the definitions of the various levels of intellectual disability:

- IQ below 20: profound.
- IQ 20–34: severe.
- IQ 35–50: moderate.
- IQ 50–70: mild.

The examination procedure outlined here is thus primarily a neurological evaluation, but also incorporates a dysmorphology assessment, as numerous malformation syndromes are associated with intellectual impairment (Down syndrome, fragile X syndrome). Also sought are associated findings of both syndromal and neurodegenerative diagnoses.

Note that prior knowledge is assumed regarding which conditions are degenerative and which are not, as with many physical signs, static and progressive causes are listed side by side.

The diseases listed in parentheses are scant examples only of most of the physical signs enumerated. Comprehensive lists of causes of each of these diagnostically helpful signs can be found in the standard textbooks of neurology. For reasons of space, many of the names of diseases are abbreviated, such that Down syndrome is listed as 'Down' and Wilson disease as 'Wilson'.

At the completion of your examination, summarise your findings, give a brief differential diagnosis and then discuss which investigations would be relevant to this particular child; these obviously depend on the physical signs found.

This is clearly an enormous topic, but an attempt is given below to list, broadly, groups of investigations that may be useful.

Minimum investigations

All children with intellectual impairment should have the following investigations.

BLOOD

1. Microarray (array-based CGH).
2. High-resolution karyotype (at least at the 650 band of resolution) (e.g. Down).
3. Fragile X testing (DNA analysis of promoter region FraX).
4. TORCH serology in infants.
5. Thyroid function tests: TSH, T4 and T3.
6. Creatine phosphokinase (CK) in boys (Duchenne muscular dystrophy).
7. Vitamin B_{12} (especially in vegan/vegetarian families).

IMAGING

Cranial CT or MRI scanning is often useful, both to exclude space-occupying lesions such as intracranial tumours, hydrocephalus and chronic subdural effusion, and to diagnose degenerative conditions such as the leucodystrophies (hypodensity of white matter) and grey matter disorders.

NEUROPSYCHOLOGICAL ASSESSMENT

A formal neuropsychological assessment by a psychologist will also be appropriate. The following is a brief selection of some of the psychometric tests in common use for general aptitude (intelligence).

1. Bayley Scales of Infant Development: age range 2–49 months.
2. Stanford–Binet Intelligence Scale: age range 2–23 years.
3. Wechsler Preschool & Primary Scale of Intelligence-Revised (WPPSI-R): age 3–7.25 years.
4. Wechsler Intelligence Scale for Children–IV (WISC-IV): age range 6–16 years, 11 months.
5. McCarthy Scales of Children's Abilities: age range 2.5–8.5 years.
6. Vineland Adaptive Behaviour Scale–II: neonates to adults.

Further investigations

Further tests are determined by the clinical picture. The following is a more comprehensive listing of groups of investigations that may be relevant.

BLOOD

1. If clinically indicated, there are a number of conditions (contiguous gene deletion syndromes) which can be elucidated on FISH testing, including: CATCH-22 (catch FISH), cri-du-chat (cats like FISH), some double-barrel names (in ascending chromosome number order: Wolf-Hirschhorn Syndrome [WHS, MIM#194190; mnemonic: **W**arrior **H**elmet **S**eizures] caused by hemizygous deletion at 4p16.3; Williams–Beuren Syndrome [WBS, MIM#194050] caused by deletion at 7q11.23; Prader–Willi [P–WS, MIM#176270]/Angelman's [AS, MIM#105830]; both P-WS and AS can be caused by mutations at 15q11.2–q13; P-WS caused by deletion of *Paternal* copies of SNRPN and NDN genes at 15q11–q13; AS [MIM#105830] caused [in 70% cases] by de novo *maternal* deletions [so remember **P**rader from **P**ater, and **A**ngelman's from **A**ngelic **M**ater]; Miller–Dieker lissencephaly syndrome [MDLS, MIM#247200]; deletion involving genes PAFAH1B1 and YWHAE at 17p13.3; Smith-Magenis syndrome [SMS, MIM#182290]; deletion, or RAI1 mutation, at 17p11.2).
2. Metabolic conditions presenting with intellectual disabilities are fairly rare and routine testing gives very low yield; the following are only ordered if there are clear pointers to these diagnoses: plasma amino acids (aminoacidopathies); plasma 7-dehydro-cholesterol reductase deficiency (7-DHC) (Smith-Lemli-Opitz Syndrome, SLOS, MIM#270400); lactate and pyruvate (mitochondrial disorders); ammonia (urea cycle disorders); uric acid (Lesch–Nyhan in boys); caeruloplasmin (Wilson); measles serology (SSPE), very long chain fatty acids (peroxisomal disorders). Lead testing is also useful in children with risk factors.
3. White cell lysosomal enzymes, to diagnose lysosomal storage diseases (LSDs):
   a. Sphingolipidoses (e.g. Gaucher, Niemann-Pick, MLD).
   b. Mucopolysaccharidoses (e.g. Hurler, Hunter).
   c. Mucolipidoses (Types I, II, III and IV).
   d. Oligosaccharidoses (e.g. mannosidosis, fucosidosis).

URINE
1. Organic acids (organic acidurias).
2. Mucopolysaccharides and oligosaccharides (mucopolysaccharidoses).

CSF
1. Protein (elevated in MLD).
2. Glucose + paired serum sample (ratio CSF:serum glucose < 0.4 in GLUT1-DS).
3. Gamma globulin (elevated in SSPE).
4. Measles antibody titre (SSPE).

TISSUE BIOPSY AND ELECTRON MICROSCOPY

Muscle, nerve, brain, rectal tissue, bone marrow, skin, liver or leucocyte may be required, depending on the disease suspected.

ELECTROPHYSIOLOGICAL STUDIES
1. Visual evoked response/potential (VER/P) and electroretinography (ERG). VER tests the function of the optic nerve pathways (i.e. white matter), while ERG evaluates the retina (i.e. grey matter). They are useful in differentiating grey from white matter disorders (e.g. some LSDs), and in diagnosing cortical blindness.
2. Brainstem evoked response audiometry (BERA) evaluates electrical activity in the cochlea and the auditory pathways in the brain, to detect hearing loss.
3. Nerve conduction studies and electromyelography (e.g. some LSDs).
4. EEG is not part of the routine investigation of intellectual impairment (only useful in context of fitting/suspected epileptic syndrome, if suspect SSPE; can be helpful also for some LSDs).

OTHER

In children with dysmorphic features, a computerised searching system may be very useful in pinpointing a syndromal diagnosis. Molecular genetic analysis is available in many diseases presenting with intellectual impairment.

SHORT CASE: Involuntary movements

This is a somewhat infrequent case. The approach outlined here covers the following four types of involuntary movement: chorea, athetosis, dystonia and tremor. Hemiballismus, tics, myoclonus and seizure activity are mentioned briefly.

Background information

The following are brief descriptions only of the types of involuntary movements—comprehensive descriptions are in all standard neurology texts.

- *Chorea.* This describes irregular rapid movements involving any muscle group, especially distal. Causes include CP, Sydenham chorea, Wilson disease (WD), systemic lupus erythematosus (SLE), moyamoya disease and degenerative conditions such as AT, Huntington disease (HD), Lesch–Nyhan syndrome (LNS) and phenylketonuria (PKU). Chorea is due to pathology affecting the corpus striatum.
- *Athetosis.* This describes slow writhing movements of proximal extremities. It can accompany chorea, as in dyskinetic CP, WD, LNS and AT. Athetosis is due to pathology affecting the outer region of the putamen.
- *Dystonia.* This comprises sustained abnormal posturing, which may be brought on rapidly in 'dystonic spasms'. Causes include drugs (tardive dystonia), degenerative disorders such as WD, HD and posthemiplegic.

- *Tremor.* There are three basic types:
  1. *Static tremor*: present at rest, disappears with action. Causes include WD, HD and Parkinson diseases.
  2. *Postural tremor* is most notable when the arms are outstretched in front of the body, but can occur through a range of movement. Causes include thyrotoxicosis, phaeochromocytoma, familial tremor, physiological tremor and WD.
  3. *Intention tremor* is marked at end points of movement, but is not present during the course of movement. Causes include many disorders affecting the cerebellar hemispheres and pathways, including WD. Note that asterixis, or 'flapping tremor', is not actually a tremor, and should be differentiated from this. Causes include liver failure and hypercapnia.
- *Hemiballismus.* This is unilateral random gross rotatory movements of the proximal portion of a limb. Exceptionally rare in paediatrics, it is due to pathology in the sub-thalamic region on the side opposite to the affected side.
- *Tics.* These are brief, separate, defined movements, usually involving the head and face, that can be voluntarily suppressed. Causes include benign childhood tics, and the Gilles de la Tourette syndrome.
- *Myoclonus.* This is sudden, disorganised, irregular contraction of a muscle or muscle group (distinguished from fasciculations, which cannot cause movement of a complete muscle group). Causes include seizure disorders (e.g. infantile spasms, benign juvenile myoclonic epilepsy), degenerative conditions (neurocutaneous syndromes, WD), structural brain anomalies (Aicardi syndrome, porencephaly), cerebrovascular accidents, anoxic brain injury, infections (SSPE) and metabolic disorders (aminoacidopathies).

It is clear from surveying the aetiologies of the various disorders, above, that WD and CP can cause choreoathetosis, tremors, dystonia or myoclonus, so the examination needs to evaluate thoroughly for these two conditions, irrespective of the type of movement disorder.

It is often difficult to differentiate between the types of movement; for example, between hemiballismus and chorea. It does not matter if the candidate is unable to decide. What is important is to describe what is seen accurately and to have an approximate idea of the likely region of the pathology (e.g. basal ganglia). For this reason, the outline given below is essentially similar, whether the problem is chorea, athetosis, dystonia or tremor.

Remember that movement disorders can coexist: for example, dystonic spasms can be accompanied by tremor and myoclonus. If myoclonus or seizure activity seems most likely, indicate this to the examiners, and then proceed as outlined in the case on recurrent seizures, as myoclonus may be associated with primary seizure disorders, as well as with degenerative or other disorders that can be associated with seizures (as noted above). Any accompanying change in consciousness should help decide if the myoclonus is seizure related.

Examination

Begin by introducing yourself to the patient and parent. Try to gain an impression of whether there is any intellectual impairment (e.g. CP, HD, PKU) or hearing impairment (e.g. kernicterus) and note the speech (e.g. cerebellar dysarthria, palilalia with Parkinson disease).

Stand back and inspect for evidence of stigmata of chronic liver disease (WD), telangiectasia (AT), facial butterfly erythema (SLE), fair complexion with blond hair (PKU), mask facies (Parkinson), prominent eyes (thyrotoxicosis), evidence of self-mutilation (LNS) or spastic posturing (CP).

Make a point of looking at the parents (HD). Describe the quality and distribution of the movements: whether they are unilateral or bilateral; involve face, arms, trunk, or legs; are fast or slow, regular or irregular, distal or proximal.

A series of manoeuvres can then be performed to establish more clearly which sort of movement is occurring.

Have the child shake hands with you and then squeeze your finger. This is to detect a 'milkmaid grip', which occurs with chorea. Then ask the child to hold out his or her hands, first with palms up, and then with palms down. This may detect static tremor or chorea. Ask the child to hold the arms outstretched to either side of the body. Then have the child try to put both index fingers to either side of the nose, as close as possible to the nose without touching. This is a sensitive test for several involuntary movements, including intention tremor. Finally, have the child hold his or her wrists back in extension to exclude asterixis.

Have the child hold both arms up above the head. Look for the development of pronation (pronator sign) with chorea. If there is any suggestion of intention tremor, check for dysdiadochokinesis. Check the upper limb tone (decreased with chorea, increased with CP), power and reflexes. A rapid functional assessment (e.g. write name, drink from a cup) may be performed at this stage to assess the degree of incapacity caused by the movement.

By this stage it may be clear whether the problem is (most probably) chorea or tremor. This will allow much of the following to be omitted, as it will not be relevant.

If the type of movement is not yet clear, a full gait examination can be performed, looking for evidence of CP, cerebellar disease, and WD or HD. Take note of heel–toe walking (cerebellar disorders), squatting (thyrotoxicosis), and also have the child walk, turn quickly, stop and recommence walking (Parkinson). This can be followed by a neurological lower limb evaluation for tone, power, reflexes and cerebellar function.

The head may then be examined. Measure the head circumference (decreased with CP). Inspect the face for malar flush (SLE). Look at the eyes for lid retraction or proptosis (thyrotoxicosis), telangiectasia (AT), Kayser-Fleischer rings (WD), nystagmus (cerebellar disease, AT) and oculomotor dyspraxia (AT). Test the extraocular movements, looking for nystagmus, and check for lid lag (thyrotoxicosis). Check the ears for telangiectasia (AT); test the hearing (kernicterus, CP), and if it is abnormal perform Rinne's and Weber's tests. Have the child poke out the tongue, to detect a 'Jack-in-the-box' tongue, which may occur with chorea. Check the neck for goitre (thyrotoxicosis).

Next, the cardiovascular system can be examined for evidence of rheumatic heart disease (Sydenham chorea). Check the pulse for abnormal wave form (e.g. aortic incompetence) and tachycardia (thyrotoxicosis). Request or take the BP (for phaeochromocytoma as the cause of tremor). Palpate and auscultate the praecordium for valvular disease.

Examine the abdomen for prominent abdominal wall veins, hepatosplenomegaly or ascites (WD) and look for peripheral signs of chronic liver disease. If tremor is the problem, also look for abdominal wall needle marks (diabetic hypoglycaemia as the cause of tremor) and palpate for the adrenal glands (but check with the examiners that there is no contraindication to deep palpation, as palpating a phaeochromocytoma can cause an acute hypertensive crisis).

At the completion of the case, summarise your findings, present a differential diagnosis and discuss which investigations would be in order.

SHORT CASE: Neurofibromatosis type 1 (NF1)

As children with NF1 often appear in both the long- and the short-case sections of the examination, it is worth having a systematic approach to examining for the myriad complications of this condition.

The short-case approach to NF1 should include assessment of the growth parameters, eyes, BP and spine in particular, just as should occur with each review of any patient with NF1 in the outpatient clinic setting.

Begin by introducing yourself to the patient and parents. Ask the child her or his age, school and grade: you may gain an impression of any significant intellectual impairment.

General observation should commence with growth parameters: patients with NF1 often have macrocephaly and short stature. Macrocephaly in this context usually reflects a large brain, but may also be due to an intracranial tumour mass or hydrocephalus secondary to aqueductal stenosis or to a tumour, such as astrocytoma, causing obstruction to CSF flow. Measure the head circumference, height and lower segment (LS) yourself. Calculate the US:LS ratio (may be decreased with scoliosis) and request progressive percentile charts for head circumference, height and weight. The weight can decrease rapidly, with diencephalic syndrome from chiasmal glioma compromising the hypothalamic function.

Inspect the skin for café-au-lait macules (CALMs): count them (and measure their maximal diameter with a tape measure if there is any doubt about fulfilling the diagnostic criteria). Make a show of looking for axillary and inguinal freckling. Look also for neurofibromas, and note any associated scratch marks (due to excessive pruritis: neurofibromas have a high mast cell content).

It is worth knowing at what age certain skin manifestations appear:

1. CALMs are usually present at birth; they are obvious by the end of the first year of life.
2. Axillary freckling develops in mid-childhood.
3. Peripheral neurofibromas usually appear at the onset of puberty.

    Next, perform a Tanner pubertal staging (can be precocity or delay).

Request the BP. Hypertension in NF1 may be due to a number of causes: renal artery stenosis, phaeochromocytoma, coarctation of the aorta, or noradrenaline-producing neurofibromas (usually paraspinal, of autonomic ganglia).

A series of manoeuvres can then be performed to assess for scoliosis and other skeletal anomalies. First, look at the child's back in the standing position. Have the child bend forwards and touch their toes: look at the back from all angles for kyphoscoliosis or scars (e.g. posterior fusion and insertion of metal rod). Describe in detail any abnormality found (e.g. scoliosis: site, convexity to which side, associated scapular and iliac crest positions-for details, see the short case on scoliosis in this chapter). Then, inspect the chest from the front and side for pectus excavatum. Have the child stand with the legs together and hands together with arms extended, and inspect the entire body for asymmetry (e.g. hemihypertrophy or segmental hypertrophy due to plexiform neurofibromas). Focus on the lower limbs for any evidence of tibial bowing (usually congenital, directed anterolaterally, at the lower third of tibia; secondary to bony dysplasia), genu varum or valgum, or pes cavus (secondary to spinal cord involvement: e.g. compression by neurofibromas, untreated kyphoscoliosis or vertebral collapse from erosions associated with neurofibromas).

Next examine the head. Look for scars (resection of intracranial tumour, shunt insertion for hydrocephalus). Feel for suture separation, shunts and their tubing, or bony defects (especially occipital, associated with cerebellar hypoplasia). Note any facial asymmetry, or disfigurement due to soft-tissue masses (especially in the periorbital area). Note that large plexiform neuromas of the head and neck are almost always obvious by 12 months of age and do not develop after this time.

A full eye examination can then be performed, looking in particular for proptosis, which may be non-pulsating due to neurofibromatous tissue within the orbit (e.g. optic glioma), or pulsating (transmitted brain pulsation) when associated with a congenital bony defect (sphenoid wing dysplasia) of the posterior orbital wall, ptosis (plexiform neuroma can cause 'S-shaped' lid) and Lisch nodules (small, light brown, dome-shaped iris hamartomas, seen in 90% of patients by 5 years of age by slit lamp examination). Make the examiners aware that they are only very occasionally visible to the naked eye. Assess visual acuity and external ocular movements. Presenting signs of optic nerve or chiasmal gliomas can include diminished visual acuity or strabismus.

Hearing should be tested, as impairment may be treatable. However, if this is done at this stage, it may give the examiners the impression that the candidate does not appreciate the difference between NF1 and NF2. Acoustic neuromas are particularly unusual in NF1. The author would defer checking the hearing at this stage, and perform it at the end of the examination.

In the child over 2 years of age, a gait examination can be performed next (in those under 2, a neurodevelopmental assessment is more appropriate at this point), followed by a full neurological assessment of the lower limbs. Look for long-tract signs reflecting cerebral involvement (e.g. tumours, cerebrovascular accidents due to hypertension or berry aneurysm rupture) or spinal cord involvement (e.g. spinal neurofibroma). Also examine for cerebellar signs (e.g. cerebellar astrocytoma, asymmetrical cerebellar hypoplasia).

Next, a thorough neurological examination of the upper limbs can be performed, again looking for evidence of long-tract and cerebellar involvement (e.g. neurofibromas arising from cervical or brachial plexuses; intracranial tumour or haemorrhage). If time permits, a higher functions assessment may be performed (mild intellectual impairment occurs in up to one-third of NF1 patients).

The abdomen can next be examined, particularly for large visceral neurofibromas (may be evident in the loin) and renal artery stenosis.

At the completion of your examination, summarise your findings and outline the investigations you would perform.

SHORT CASE: Sturge-Weber syndrome (SWS)

Commence in the usual fashion by introducing yourself to the patient and parents. Note the growth parameters, particularly the size of the head. Look for any asymmetry (growth arrest with hemiplegia; facial hemihyperplasia from angiomatosis, sometimes just an enlarged ear ipsilateral to the port-wine stain [PWS] vascular malformation), any hemiplegic posturing and any current seizure activity (as these children may have very frequent seizures). Inspect the skin thoroughly and describe the distribution of the PWS; remember it may extend onto the neck, back or chest, so make sure to gain adequate exposure. Some children have more widespread PWSs such as on their extremities, which can overlap with Klippel-Trénaunay-Weber (KTW) syndrome (MIM%149000; cytogenetic location 8q22.3), or with Parkes Weber syndrome (PKWS) (MIM#608355; cytogenetic location 5q14.3).

There may be hemihyperplasia due to either KTW or PKWS. If the child has had some laser therapy for the PWS, there may be multiple small (7–10 mm) circular discs of normal looking skin within the PWS.

Next, measure the head circumference yourself, and request progressive centiles. Look at the eyes carefully for any evidence of glaucoma, which can lead to buphthalmos ('ox eye') with enlargement of cornea or entire eye, due to raised intraocular pressure; look for corneal clouding, tearing or tortuous vessels on the conjunctivae or sclera on the affected side; also, there may be heterochromia of the irides, and superficial haemangiomatous changes on the eyelid (actually venous dilatation only) ipsilateral to the PWS. If there are bilateral PWSs, check both eyes carefully for glaucoma, as above, as 45% of bilateral PWSs have bilateral glaucoma.

Look for any evidence of strabismus, which can occur secondary to optic nerve damage from glaucoma. Check the visual fields carefully for evidence of homonymous hemianopia.

Offer fundoscopy, while commenting that one should not give an opinion through an undilated pupil (i.e. if they haven't just been dilated for the exam, which is unlikely but not impossible). Fundoscopy could identify a tomato-ketchup coloured fundus (ipsilateral to the PWS), and diffuse choroidal haemangiomas (DCHs).

Using a torch, look at the mouth for evidence of angiomatosis on buccal mucosa, palate, tongue, gums or lips; look for evidence of unilateral hypertrophy (e.g. of tongue).

Next, perform a neurodevelopmental assessment if the child is 2 or under, or a standard gait examination if the child is 3 or over.

In infants, particularly note hand preference by offering toys; the cover test is useful (a cloth is placed over the face [after asking parental permission to do this] and each hand in turn gently restrained, to see if the child is capable of using either hand to remove the cloth); developing hand preference under 12 months may indicate underlying hemiplegia. In infants, assessment of fine motor skills (as is the case when testing vision and hearing) is best tested with the child sitting in the parent's lap.

After evaluating fine motor, gross motor, language and personal–social skills, go on to assess long tracts, and finally the primitive reflexes. In older children, after the gait examination, assess the long tracts fully (but omit sensation in view of time constraints).

Before finishing, mention checking the femoral pulses, as coarctation has an increased incidence in patients with SWS. Finally, request urinalysis and stool analysis for blood, as angiomatosis can affect mucous membranes of viscera.

SHORT CASE: Tuberous sclerosis complex (TSC)

The TSC short case focuses on demonstrating skin manifestations, and a full neurodevelopmental assessment including fundoscopy. It could be introduced by: requesting direct inspection of any of the major skin features; mentioning the combination of fitting and skin findings; or the diagnosis could be given and the candidate can demonstrate their knowledge of the condition. As with other cases, introduce yourself to the patient and parents and try to gain an impression of any significant intellectual impairment, lack of verbal communication (autistic features can be seen) or behavioural problems such as hyperactivity (ADHD \-type behaviours can be seen).

Note the growth parameters, in particular the head circumference (for macrocephaly due to hydrocephalus, secondary to ventricular obstruction from subependymal nodules [SEN], or subependymal giant cell astrocytoma [SEGA]). Note whether the child looks well or unwell, and note the vital signs. Cardiorespiratory problems (see overleaf) can manifest as tachypnoea, and/or tachycardia. Request the BP and urinalysis. Renal complications can cause hypertension and haematuria; these include renal failure secondary to multiple renal cysts or renal tumours (angiomyolipomas), or, less commonly, compression of the ureters or renal pelvis. Mention you will examine the abdomen after scanning the skin.

Carefully examine the skin for hypomelanotic macules (classic lesions are 'ash leaf' shaped), smaller hypomelanotic 'confetti' or 'white freckles'. Comment on the need to re-examine with a Wood's light, a long-wave ultraviolet light source, for a more accurate appraisal. Hypomelanotic macules appear at birth or early infancy. Note any depigmentation of hair, eyebrows, eyelashes (the term for hypopigmented hair is 'poliosis') or iris. Look for any fibrous plaque on the forehead or any facial angiofibromas (previously given the misnomer 'adenoma sebaceum'), which are small flesh-coloured papules which affect the cheeks and chin but tend to spare the upper lip; these tend to occur between the ages of 2 and 5 years.

Next, in older children and adolescents, look at the fingers and toes for ungual fibromas. Next, in older children, look for shagreen patches, which are leathery or 'orange peel' yellowish plaques on the trunk predominantly in the lumbo-sacral region. (Note that café-au-lait macules are *not* increased in prevalence in TSC patients; they are *not* a sign of TSC.) After the skin examination, check in the mouth for fibromas in the gums around the teeth, and on the lips, or the tongue, and check for pitting of teeth, which is due to focal areas of enamel hypoplasia.

Next, perform a neurodevelopmental assessment, commencing with examination of the head (measure the circumference yourself), then the eyes. Mention at this point that you would like to examine the fundi (although the mantra 'never give an opinion through an undilated pupil' comes to mind); this could be deferred until the end of the examination, but it should not be forgotten. Vision and hearing should be checked as part of the developmental assessment in younger children, to interpret personal–social, language, fine and gross motor abilities.

Eye findings on fundoscopy include multiple retinal hamartomas, and retinal achromic (hypopigmented) patches, although neither of these tend to affect vision per se. Hearing is usually normal. Next, check for long-tract signs starting with the lower limbs and working up. In older children, a standard gait examination can be performed followed by lower limb, and then upper limb examination. Abnormal focal neurological signs are rare in TSC, but complications such as hydrocephalus and giant cell astrocytoma can be detected.

After this, concentrate on other manifestations of TSC, namely detection of lesions involving chest (heart for rhabdomyomas, which when intracardiac can cause outflow tract obstructive lesions or valve lesions, or when intramural cardiac failure or arrhythmias; and lungs for lymphangioleiomyomatosis [LAM], which can cause subjective dyspnoea or objective tachypnoea) and abdomen (for nephromegaly from angiomyolipomas or multiple cysts, in particular, plus for hepatomegaly or splenomegaly from angiomyolipomas of these organs).

It is worth knowing the ages of appearance of the various skin manifestations, as a separate list: hypomelanotic macules can be seen at birth; angiofibromas are rare before 2, usually appear after 4, but may not occur until puberty; gingival fibromas appear between 4 and 10 years; and shagreen patches and ungual fibromas appear around the time of puberty.

SHORT CASE: Neuromuscular assessment

The request to perform a neuromuscular assessment does not mean that the problem is neuromuscular disease. A common error is to assume that there is neuromuscular pathology, even when the patient has an obvious problem such as hemiplegia or spastic paraparesis. The candidate should first form an opinion as to whether the problem is neuromuscular. Having determined that it is, another common problem in differential diagnosis is to fail to think of major levels of lesion (anterior horn cell, peripheral nerve, neuromuscular junction and muscle fibre).

There are several possible introductions: for example, 'This boy has increasing difficulty climbing stairs', or 'This girl has been having trouble with increasing tiredness and weakness'. Essentially, a neuromuscular assessment is a modified neurological examination. Specific manoeuvres are included that aim at eliciting relevant signs of various neuromuscular disorders. The procedure outlined below describes several of these.

Start with general observations. Enquire whether the child can stand for you. Then, focus your attention systematically on the following:

1. Posture (e.g. as in DMD; see the long case in this chapter).
2. The face: for myopathic facies, ptosis, presence of nasogastric tube or oxygen catheter, tongue fasciculations (spinal muscular atrophy [SMA]).
3. The neck: for tracheostomy tube, or scars from a previous tracheostomy, goitre (hyperthyroidism can cause myopathy), muscle bulk (for facioscapulohumeral dystrophy), contractures (Emery-Dreifuss muscular dystrophy [EDMD]). Weakness of neck flexors is a good pointer to DMD.
4. Upper limbs: for horizontal axillary skin folds (DMD), proximal muscle wasting (most myopathies), distal muscle wasting (myotonic dystrophy [DM], neuropathies), fasciculations (SMA), scars (tendon releases or transfers), contractures.
5. The back: for scoliosis, kyphosis, lordosis.
6. Lower limbs: for proximal or distal wasting, fasciculations, scars (tendon releases or transfers), contractures, foot deformity such as pes cavus.

Remember to glance at the parents for any evidence of myopathic facies, peroneal atrophy or pes cavus.

After this, ask whether the child can walk for you. Have the child go through a full gait examination (i.e. walking normally, walking on toes, walking on heels, walking heel to toe, running, hopping, jumping, using stairs, stepping up on to a chair or stool, squatting and rising, lying on floor and rising, performing push-ups). This may give very valuable clues to help differentiate between neuropathy and myopathy.

Next, ask the child to hold up both arms above the head, to test for proximal upper limb weakness. Have the child make a fist and then quickly open the hand (easier to assess than a handshake) and finally percuss the thenar eminence (these manoeuvres involving the hands are to detect myotonic dystrophy). If positive, go on to tap the deltoid muscle with a tendon hammer, for myotonia, and ask the mother to make a fist and then open her hand quickly and percuss over her thenar eminence as well.

Next, ask the child to look upwards at the roof (unless there is already ptosis) for a full 30 seconds (screening for myasthenia gravis).

Following these screening tests, perform a standard neurological examination of the lower limbs and upper limbs (including palpating for hypertrophied lateral popliteal, ulnar and greater auricular nerves), followed by the motor cranial nerves. By this stage, the type of problem should be apparent and will allow guidance as to what else should be examined.

If a myopathic process is most likely, then at the end of the neurological examination, it may be wise to examine the cardiorespiratory system next (cardiac muscle can be involved in DMD, Pompe disease [in infants]; conduction defects can occur in DM, EDMD and mitochondrial cytopathies), and then the abdomen (for storage diseases).

SHORT CASE: Scoliosis

Candidates may seldom consider this case, and as such it can prove difficult. The first thing to determine is the classification of the scoliosis: whether it is postural, compensatory or fixed (structural). Most often, it will be the latter group, which can itself be conveniently subdivided into three major groups of causes:

1. Idiopathic (congenital and later onset).
2. Paralytic (i.e. neuromuscular causes).
3. Bony or ligamentous (e.g. connective tissue disorders).

Thus, the examination focuses firstly on manoeuvres to assess classification.

Once classified as fixed, the numerous causes of this are sought. Inspection will give valuable clues to several groups, such as skeletal dysplasias, neurocutaneous stigmata and malformation syndromes. A thorough neurological evaluation is essential, as there are potential causes at most levels of the neuraxis. Examples include CP, spinocerebellar degenerations (Friedreich ataxia [FRDA]), anterior horn cell disease (Kugelberg-Welander disease), peripheral neuropathies (Charcot-Marie-Tooth disease [CMT]), myopathies (mitochondrial cytopathies), muscular dystrophies (DMD) and myotonic disorders (e.g. myotonic dystrophy [DM]). Finally, the child should be evaluated for complications of the scoliosis itself, such as cardiorespiratory compromise.

Begin by introducing yourself to the patient and parents. Try to gain an impression of the child's intelligence (impairment with Coffin–Lowry syndrome [CLS], homocystinuria). The child should be undressed down to the underwear. Inspect for any dysmorphic features (Turner, Noonan, CLS) or other obvious signs of underlying disease (disproportionate short stature, limb bowing, Marfanoid habitus, neurocutaneous stigmata). Note the growth parameters, in particular height. Short stature may be due to the scoliosis per se or an underlying problem (e.g. skeletal dysplasias, metabolic bone diseases, neurofibromatosis type 1 (NF1), Turner or Noonan syndromes). Tall stature may be due to Marfan syndrome or homocystinuria. Macrocephaly may occur with NF1 or hydrocephalus. For completeness, the height, arm span and lower segment can be measured by the candidate, the upper segment:lower segment (US:LS) ratio calculated, and the degree of trunk shortening (or limb shortening in skeletal dysplasias) quantified. Inspect thoroughly for neurocutaneous stigmata such as café-au-lait macules and axillary freckling with NF1, which can cause scoliosis by several mechanisms including muscle imbalance, hemihypertrophy, hemivertebrae and 'dumbbell' tumour. Other rarer neurocutaneous syndromes that may lead to scoliosis include incontinentia pigmenti and hypomelanosis of Ito.

Next, focus on the back itself; look for thoracotomy scars (e.g. from repair of associated abnormalities such as congenital diaphragmatic hernia or CHD) or posterior midline scars (myelomeningocele [MMC] repair), hairy patches or lipomas. Describe in detail the following features (mnemonic: all starting with 'S'):

Scoliosis (site and convexity to which side)
Shoulders and hands (higher on side to which primary curve convex)
Scapulae (prominence on which side)
Skin (loin) crease symmetry
Superior iliac spine position
Spare ribs (rib cage rotation posteriorly or anteriorly)
Space between arms and body (asymmetry)

Look for any limb bowing (e.g. rickets). Inspect for evidence of neuromuscular problems, such as pes cavus (CMT, FRDA), 'champagne bottle legs' (CMT) or prominent calf muscles (DMD).

Note whether the occiput aligns directly over the buttock crease. To be more accurate, a 'plumb-line' can be dropped from the occiput to ascertain whether there is failure of alignment.

Following this initial inspection with the child standing, there are three manoeuvres to assess the degree of correctability of the curve.

1. Have the child bend forwards and touch the toes. Reassess the curve, look at the rib hump, and describe these. This manoeuvre can confirm a fixed scoliosis or exclude a postural scoliosis.
2. Sit the child down on a chair and re-evaluate the curve. Sitting will eliminate any contribution of unequal leg length to the curvature.
3. Applying upward traction on the proximal upper limbs (lifting under the axillae) should straighten any mobile component of the curve.

Next, palpate and percuss over the spine for tenderness from metabolic disorders (e.g. rickets), inflammatory disorders (e.g. chronic tuberculosis) or tumour, and then auscultate over the apex of the curve (for vascular tumour such as haemangioma as underlying cause).

Now examine the back movements. Forward flexion should cause a measurable increase of 10 cm between C7 and S1 in postpubertal patients, and fingers should be able to reach the toes (with knees extended). Extension to 30° is normal, with lateral flexion to 35°, and rotation (sitting, which anchors the buttocks) to 45°.

The next part of the examination assesses for neuromuscular causes or consequences of the scoliosis. Perform a standard gait examination, followed by a lower limb examination. Measure the actual lower limb lengths (anterior superior iliac spine to medial malleolus), inspect for scars, muscle wasting, contractures and foot deformities (e.g. pes cavus), and then test power, tone and reflexes, cerebellar function, and sensation (can omit the latter, as it is time-consuming). Then, percuss the bladder (for neurogenic storing bladder) and offer to test the anal wink.

It is important not to overlook evidence of weakness of intrinsic muscles of the feet, decreased ankle jerks and evidence of bladder involvement, as these may be the only clues to tethering of the spinal cord.

Examination of the upper limbs, again for neurological causes, is followed by evaluation of the head for macrocephaly (NF1, hydrocephalus), the eyes for evidence of NF1 (Lisch nodules of iris, strabismus from optic glioma, proptosis), or FRDA (nystagmus), Marfan syndrome (upwardly dislocated lenses) or osteogenesis imperfecta (blue sclerae).

After the neurological assessment, examine the chest for cardiorespiratory complications. Examine the heart for evidence of cor pulmonale, a complication of scoliosis per se, and for heart disease associated with possible underlying aetiologies (e.g. CHD associated with congenital thoracic scoliosis, mitral valve prolapse in Marfan syndrome, pulmonary valve stenosis with NF1). Do not forget to take the BP (may be elevated in NF1, Marfan syndrome, MMC or with congenital renal anomalies in association with thoracolumbar scoliosis). Finally, check the chest expansion and request a peak flow reading, to give some indication as to whether restrictive lung disease is present.

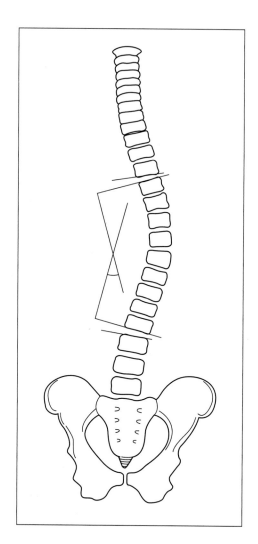

Figure 13.8 **Assessing the Cobb angle**

Figure 13.8 shows how to assess the Cobb angle. First, find the upper and lower vertebrae of the curve by erecting tangents to the vertebral bodies and identifying where the disc spaces first become widened on the concavity of the curve. Next, draw perpendiculars from the tangents at the top of the upper vertebra and the bottom of the lower vertebra, and measure the angle between them. Note that if the tangents of the upper and lower vertebrae are extrapolated, they intersect at a point that is the centre of a circle of which the curve is an arc. This method can be repeated for each of multiple curves.

SHORT CASE: Spina bifida (SB)/Myelomeningocele (MMC)

A comprehensive short-case approach to spina bifida is very useful in both long- and short-case contexts. It is one of the few cases where it can be better to start at the bottom and work up. It is important to have a good knowledge of sensory dermatomes, and to know the motor root values, of the entire body (not just the lower limbs).

The general plan for this case is as follows:

1. Demonstrate the level of the lesion.
2. Functional assessment.
3. Look for associated abnormalities/complications.

This case may be introduced in several ways: for example, 'This boy has spina bifida. Would you please assess him/his function above the level of the lesion?' Other introductions (e.g. big head, scoliosis, talipes) may have spina bifida as the underlying diagnosis. When the diagnosis is reached, the candidate may then proceed with assessment of function (e.g. ability to walk) and disease complications (e.g. hydronephrosis, hydrocephalus).

Thorough inspection is crucial in this case, particularly when the patient is an infant. Much can be gleaned from simply taking one minute to stand back and look. In particular, the child's posture and spontaneous movement is valuable in indicating the level of the lesion before the back is inspected directly.

A few points worth noting are outlined below—the positions described refer to those seen with the child supine:

1. Hip flexion corresponds to L1 and L2, so is affected in high lesions.
2. Lesions above L1 cause total paraplegia, as hip flexion is absent. Thus, in thoracic lesions, the lower limbs are flaccid, in a 'frog leg' position of external rotation, with some degree of passive abduction and flexion at the hips, and the knees slightly flexed, the ankles plantar flexed.
3. Lesions in the high lumbar zone cause the child to lie in a position of flexion and adduction at the hips.
4. Lesions with L3 preserved allow an infant to exhibit some kicking movements when upset, with some knee flexion and extension.
5. Lesions in the low lumbar zone result in a position of hip flexion and adduction, good knee flexion and extension, and ankle dorsiflexion, due to unopposed action of the tibialis anterior (L5).
6. Hip extension corresponds to L5, S1 and S2, and so is affected in all but the lower sacral lesions.
7. Lesions at S3 or below completely spare lower limb sensory and motor function, but cause paralysis of bladder and anal sphincters, and 'saddle anaesthesia'.

The examination procedure given here covers children of any age, and is thus quite detailed. It should, of course, be modified to suit the individual patient. If it were followed as it stands, it would appear too rigid and reflect rote learning, which is not the idea of this book—nor will it meet with approval from the examiners.

The introduction, and the child's age and degree of cooperation, will determine the best order to perform the examination. If the lead-in is a functional assessment above the level of the lesion, do not start by describing the foot deformities.

Examination

Begin by introducing yourself to patient and parents. The child should be undressed down to nappies or underpants. Interact with the child: if old enough, ask name, age and school to gain an impression of their development. In infants, note the degree of alertness, the pitch of the cry, which is high-pitched with raised intracranial pressure in cases with the Arnold–Chiari malformation (ACM) and resultant hydrocephalus. The presence of a nasogastric tube, stridor or apnoea and, in older children, a hoarse voice may all occur with lower cranial nerve palsies due to brainstem compression with severe ACM. Note the respiratory rate: tachypnoea may be a sign of aspiration pneumonia (due to lower cranial nerve palsies) or of cardiac failure (due to hypertension, or cor pulmonale in patients with severe kyphoscoliosis).

Stand back and inspect carefully the child's posture and spontaneous movement. the posture in detail, focusing on each joint systematically (e.g. 'flexed at hips, hyperextended at the knee') and noting any deformities (e.g. talipes equinovarus). Note the muscle bulk, comparing lower limbs with upper limbs. Observe the child's movements, again lower limbs versus upper. If the child's movements seem unsteady, this may be due to weakness in higher lesions, or severe ACM which may cause ataxia. Do not hurry your description of posture and movement.

Next, inspect the head, noting its size (hydrocephalus from ACM) and any obvious shunts. Look at the eyes for squint or nystagmus (either can occur with ACM). Scan the abdomen for any scars (ventriculoperitoneal shunt). Note the child's growth parameters: the head may well be enlarged due to hydrocephalus, so measure it yourself. Request the other growth parameters. The height is usually decreased, due to a short trunk (associated kyphoscoliosis) and short lower limbs (decreased growth and contractures). The weight for the actual height implies obesity, but should be compared to the arm span instead, to give a more accurate indication of true obesity. Generally, these children are not obese for their arm span.

Next, focus your attention on the back. Note the site of the lesion, the size of the repair scar and look for any kyphosis, scoliosis or scars (fixation rods for kyphoscoliosis).

Then, the examination proceeds well if started at the lower limbs. A thorough neurological examination is necessary. In an infant with no spontaneous lower limb movement, a pinprick stimulus may still result in a flexion withdrawal of the legs. This is a spinal reflex due to elements of the spinal cord, distal to the clinical level of the lesion, that are preserved. The fact that the child makes no facial or emotional response from which to infer a painful sensation should prevent misinterpretation of this response.

Examination of the abdomen may then be performed, followed by the head and the upper limbs. Next, take the BP and examine the chest. After this, you may perform a functional assessment in older children, looking at the ADLs, such as reading, writing, using a knife, fork, spoon, comb, toothbrush, and the ability to attend to personal hygiene (i.e. toileting, insertion of tampons). In younger children, perform a developmental assessment (see the short case on this in this chapter). Several of the findings sought are listed in Figure 13.9 and Table 13.9.

1. Introduce self

Interact with child, gain impression of development

2. General inspection

Alertness

Cry (high-pitched with ACM)

Nasogastric tube (severe ACM)

Respiratory distress

Hoarse voice (severe ACM)

Posture
- Deformity (e.g. TEV, dislocated hips)

Muscle bulk
- Lower versus upper limb

Movement
- Lower versus upper limb
- Ataxia (with ACM)

Head
- Size
- Shunts
- Eye signs

Skin

3. Back

Lesion
- Site: closure scar (describe)
- Spinal deformity: scoliosis, kyphosis

Scars (e.g. fixation rod)

4. Lower limbs

Inspect

Palpate

Tone

Power

Reflexes

Joint movement

Sensation

5. Abdomen and pressure areas

Inspect
- Scars (e.g. VP shunt)
- Distension (lax muscles)
- Ileal conduit
- Patulous anus
- Dribbling of urine
- Tanner staging (precocity)
- Pressure sores

Palpate
- Kidneys (hydronephrosis)

Percuss
- Bladder (urinary retention)

Check
- Abdominal reflexes

- Anal wink
- Anal tone

Urinalysis
- To detect CRF, shunt nephritis, UTI

6. Head

Inspect
- Size
- Shape (e.g. frontal prominence with ACM)
- Signs of hydrocephalus (scalp vein prominence, shiny skin, sun-setting eyes, shunt scars)

Measure head circumference

Request progressive percentiles

Palpate (sitting up)
- Fontanelles
- Sutures
- Shunt, trace tubing

7. Eyes

Inspect
- Nystagmus (severe ACM)
- Squint (e.g. with ACM)

Visual acuity

External ocular movements
- Sixth nerve palsy (raised ICP)
- Impaired upward gaze (Parinaud's syndrome with hydrocephalus)

Fundi
- Papilloedema (raised ICP)
- Optic atrophy (long-standing raised ICP)

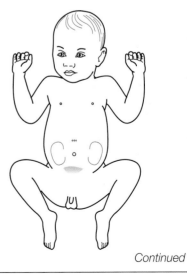

Continued

Figure 13.9 **Spina bifida**

8. Hearing and bulbar function
Assess hearing
Check lower cranial nerves (nine, ten, eleven, twelve)
Suck and swallow
Gag reflex (if cannot swallow)
Tongue atrophy

9. Upper limbs
Full examination, for signs of syringomyelia

10. Blood pressure
Hypertension (CRF)

11. Chest
Full examination of praecordium and lung fields for signs of cardiac failure due to:
• Hypertension (CRF)
• Cor pulmonale (kyphoscoliosis)

12. Functional/developmental assessment
Assess ADL in older children
Perform developmental assessment in infants

ACM = Arnold–Chiari malformation; ADL = activities of daily living; CRF = chronic renal failure; ICP = intracranial pressure; TEV = talipes equinovarus; UTI = urinary tract infection; VP = ventriculoperitoneal.

Figure 13.9, continued

Table 13.9

Additional information: details of possible findings on spina bifida examination

GENERAL INSPECTION
Respiratory signs • Stridor (severe ACM) • Apnoea (severe ACM) • Tachypnoea (aspiration pneumonia, cardiac failure)
Skin • Pressure sores • Scars (e.g. of VP shunts, tendon releases)
Growth parameters • Head circumference: increased (hydrocephalus) • Height: usually decreased • Arm span (use instead of height): may be normal for age • Weight: obese for height, not for arm span
LOWER LIMBS
Inspection • Muscle bulk, wasting • Joint deformity (e.g. dislocated hips, talipes) • Contractures • Scars (e.g. tendon releases, transfers or osteotomies) • Spontaneous movement
Palpation: muscle bulk (each muscle compartment)
Check tone, power, reflexes (including with reinforcement)
Joint movement • Hip (e.g. fixed flexion deformity; check for dislocation last) • Knee (e.g. fixed hyperextension) • Ankle (e.g. fixed dorsiflexion)
Check hips for dislocation
Sensation: demonstrate the sensory level (may use a new pin in infants; full examination in older children)

ACM = Arnold–Chiari malformation; VP = ventriculoperitoneal.

SHORT CASE: Ataxia

The word ataxia derives from *ataktos*, a Greek word meaning 'lack of order'; it has been defined variously as: a failure of coordination of the muscles; irregularity of muscle action; difficulty with walking/gait; problem with movement orientation because of abnormal agonist–antagonist muscle coordination; or motor incoordination most notable when walking or sitting. There is a spectrum of unsteadiness in walking, from 'clumsy' otherwise normal children to those with profound ataxias. The latter group includes many hereditary-degenerative forms, the most well described being named after Friedreich, who differentiated 'his' condition from ataxia due to syphilis (syphilitic locomotor ataxia). As the children in short case exams seldom fit into a neat category, but are generally presented with 'This boy has trouble walking' or 'This girl has developed unsteadiness in her walking; please examine her', then this short case approach covers the spectrum of unsteadiness. Some use another term 'pseudoataxia' for unsteadiness that is not cerebellar in origin.

In simple terms, ataxia, in exam situations, is usually due to cerebellar disease or proprioceptive disorders. Friedreich ataxia combines the two main pathologies (cerebellar dyssynergia and loss of proprioception/posterior column sensation) such that patients with this condition may be seen in examinations despite its rarity. Some children with significant weakness can have marked unsteadiness that some would call ataxia, others pseudoataxia; irrespective of the name, these children can present in the exam, with the same lead-in/stem as ataxias due to cerebellar problems or proprioceptive disorders. So for each child, think of the three groups: cerebellar disease; proprioceptive problems; and weakness.

Ataxia can be divided into three groups: acute; recurrent (also called episodic or intermittent); and chronic/progressive.

Acute ataxia (meaning evolution of symptoms within 3 days) has a few common causes which account for 80% of children with this: 1. intoxications; 2. infectious causes (varicella); and 3. post-infectious causes (Guillain-Barré syndrome).

Recurrent ataxia can be due to mitochondrial disorders or other metabolic disorders (aminoacidurias [e.g. Hartnup disease], organic acidaemias [e.g. Maple Syrup Urine Disease (MSUD)], or lysosomal storage diseases [e.g. Niemann-Pick type C]).

Progressive ataxia has a wide differential including hereditary ataxias, metabolic disorders, brain tumours, and neurodegenerative conditions such as leucodystrophies (adrenoleucodystrophy, metachromatic, Pelizaeus–Merzbacher disease).

Acute ataxia usually has a benign cause, recurrent and progressive ataxia generally indicates more serious pathology.

The following mnemonics related to ataxia include one for all groups of causes (FLAMING SPINNER, see overleaf); the other mnemonics are for some of the classic exam cases.

Causes of ataxia are acute, episodic and progressive (**FLAMING SPINNER**):

FRDA (Friedreich ataxia) (MIM#229300)
Labyrinthitis (vertigo causing ataxia)/**L**ysosomal storage diseases
AT (ataxia-telangiectasia) (MIM#208900)/**A**betalipoproteinaemia (MIM#200100)/**A**rgininosuccinic aciduria (MIM#207900)
Medulloblastoma/**M**etabolic: **M**SUD (maple syrup urine disease) (MIM#248600)/**M**LD (metachromatic leucodystrophy, also called arylsulfatase A [ARSA] deficiency) (MIM#250100)/**M**etal disease: Wilson disease (MIM#277900)/**M**igraine: basilar artery/**M**itochondrial disorders (Kearns-Sayre [MIM#530000], MERRF (*m*yoclonic *e*pilepsy with *r*agged *r*ed *f*ibres) [MIM#545000], NARP (*n*europathy, *a*taxia and *r*etinitis *p*igmentosa) [MIM#551500])/**M**ultiple sclerosis/**M**yxoedema (hypothyroidism)
Infection (e.g. cerebellitis, meningitis, mastoiditis)/**I**EMs (Inborn errors of metabolism e.g. OTC [*o*rnithine *t*rans*c*arbamylase deficiency] [MIM#311250])
Neuroblastoma (occult)
GBS (Guillain-Barré syndrome)/**G**enetic (hereditary) ataxias (many)

SCAs (spinocerebellar ataxias, autosomal dominant)/**S**CARs (spinocerebellar ataxias, autosomal recessive)/**S**PAX (spinocerebellar ataxias with prominent spasticity)/**S**upratentorial tumours
Post-infectious cerebellitis/**P**osterior fossa tumours/**P**aroxysmal vertigo/**P**ellagra (niacin deficiency; can cause the four Ds: dermatitis (photosensitive), diarrhoea, dementia and death)/**P**ellagra-like dermatosis (Hartnup disorder [HND]) (MIM#234500)/**P**yruvate **C**arboxylase deficiency (MIM#266150)/**P**sychogenic (not real ataxia, but impersonating this)
Intoxication/**I**ngestion (drugs)/**I**nner ear pathology (e.g. labyrinthitis)
Nutritional deficiencies: deficiencies of vitamin B_1 (thiamine), B_3 (niacin/nicotinic acid), B_6 (pyridoxine), B_{12} (cobalamin), E
Neurodegenerative disorders
Ependymoma/**E**A (episodic ataxias)
Refsum disease (MIM#266500)/**R**ett syndrome (MIM#312750)

Ataxia-telangiectasia (AT) (**ATAXIA CASE**):

ATM (ataxia-telangiectasia mutated) gene codes for serine-protein kinase ATM; only known cause/**A**ge: **a**taxia/cerebellar dysfunction (onset 1–4 years) **an**tedates telangiectasia/Ig**A** (Immunoglobulin **A**) decreased
Telangiectasia of exposed areas (bulbar conjunctivae, nose [bridge], ears, neck, antecubital fossa): age 3 to 10 years/**T**en years of age often require wheelchair/**T**runcal ataxia/**T**one decreased/**T**hree out of ten develop malignancy (usually [85%] leukaemia or lymphoma)
Apraxia of eye movement (cannot follow object across field; vertical and horizontal saccadic movements affected) and nystagmus
X-ray of chest (CXR) for sinopulmonary infection (increased susceptibility)
Immune deficiency (cell mediated immunity decreased)/**I**onising radiation sensitivity
Absent reflexes

Choreoathetosis/Cancer risk 40–100 times normal; especially ALL, AML, lymphoma, brain tumours, adenocarcinoma of stomach, basal cell carcinoma, ovarian dysgerminoma

Alpha feto-protein (AFP) increased/Ageing appears premature (grey hair)

Speech slurred (dysarthria)/Susceptibility to sinobronchopulmonary infections and serious neoplasia (as above)

Elevated carcinoembryonic antigen/Endocrine: insulin resistant diabetes/Elasticity skin lost/Eleven = chromosome locus (11q22.3)

Friedreich ataxia (FRDA) (**FRIEDREICHS**):

FXN gene (at 9q13) codes for frataxin, a mitochondrial protein; only known cause/Five–fifteen age group/Feet: pes cavus

Reduced sense of vibration, position/Romberg test positive/Recessive

Impaired sense of vision

Eyes: optic atrophy/nystagmus

Dysarthria/Deafness

Reflexes in lower limb absent, but …

Extensor plantar/Equinovarus feet (plantar flexors, inverters affected)

Insulin requirement (T1DM)/Iron misdistribution in mitochondria allows oxidative damage, decreased ATP production

Cardiac disease; hypertrophic non-obstructive cardiomyopathy

Hyperglycaemia (diabetes in up to 30%)

Spastic lower limbs (pyramidal weakness)/Scoliosis

Mitochondrial disorders (**MITOCHONDRIALS**):

Myopathy (proximal)/Myoclonus/Migraine

Inheritance recessive

Tubular (renal) defects

Optic atrophy

Cataract/Chorea

Heart: cardiomyopathy/pre-excitation syndromes

Ophthalmoplegia

Neuropathy/Neurogenic weakness/Neurologic: encephalopathy

Deafness (sensorineural)/Diabetes/Dementia

Retinopathy (pigmentary)

Increased lactate: blood (fasting > 3.0 mmol/L); CSF > 1.5 mmol/L

Ataxia

Lid: ptosis

Seizure/Stroke-like episodes/Spasticity

Examination procedure

Start by introducing yourself to the parent and the child. Note the child's level of consciousness, alertness (medications [toxins] or encephalopathies—e.g. acute disseminated encephalomyelitis [ADEM] can alter these), quality of movement (e.g. choreoathetosis with AT) and any obvious asymmetry, such as head tilt (ataxia plus head tilt equals posterior fossa tumour until proved otherwise), or scoliosis (can occur in ataxic cerebral palsy or in FRDA), or asymmetrical ataxia (which can mean brain tumour, stroke or demyelinating disease). If the child is sitting or lying down when first seen, look around for any nearby peripheral aides such as a wheelchair. If the child's feet are uncovered, note any pes cavus (FRDA).

Stand back and look for any rash, such as telangiectasia over the eyes and ears and bridge of nose in AT, or resolving varicella (acute cerebellitis, post-infectious cerebellar ataxia); pellagra-like rash, with hyperpigmented crusted and fissured well-defined plaques on sun-exposed areas of the face, dorsum of hands and legs (Hartnup disease; 'pellagrous glove and boot'); urticaria (Kawasaki) or purpura (Henoch–Schönlein); or (rarely) ichthyosis with Refsum disease. Ask the child a few age-appropriate questions (e.g. their age, school, grade, teacher's name, favourite subjects, and in older children, specifically ask their full name, current location and day of the week), to get an impression of their orientation in time, place and person (for intoxications or encephalopathies) and the quality of their speech (e.g. slurring with AT).

If the child is sitting or lying down initially, ask the child, parent or examiners whether the child can walk. If the child can walk, then perform a gait examination. Focus on heel–toe (tandem) walking in particular to check cerebellar vermis function. Ask the child to walk across the room and back normally, then ask them to walk heel–toe 'like on a tight rope', and explain you would like them to turn around as quickly as they can, and then walk back to you, when you say so. Watch for truncal ataxia as the child walks across the room, then get the child to quickly turn; if the child then staggers, this is the earliest marker of truncal ataxia and vermal disease. This means cerebellar pathology, which can be hereditary, metabolic or a tumour, such as a medulloblastoma.

The rest of the gait examination should be completed, particularly looking for a positive Romberg's test for proprioceptive loss. Romberg's test comprises asking the child to stand with their feet together, then ask the child to close their eyes. Make sure you have your arms in a position to catch the child should their test be positive. If closing the eyes makes the child stagger or sway, then this is a positive test, as closing the eyes removes the ability of the child to maintain balance with visual and vestibular input despite their proprioceptive disorder. During the other components of the gait examination, note any weakness, particularly when the child squats and gets up, and also on checking for Gower's sign, to check for weakness as a cause of, or contributor to, the ataxia. Also note any scoliosis during the gait examination, which can occur with any of the more progressive neurodegenerative disorders, or with FRDA, Rett disorder or ataxic cerebral palsy. When the child is walking on their heel and on their toes, any pes cavus should be seen easily (FRDA).

See the short case on gait and also the short case on cerebellar function both in this chapter. The remainder of the examination is a standard neurological examination, focused on cerebellar and proprioceptive functions in particular.

Next, examine the lower limbs, again focusing on cerebellar and proprioceptive function, and muscle strength; see the short case on lower limbs in this chapter. Then, examine the upper limbs as per the upper limb short case; in addition, take particular note of the muscle bulk in the hands (for peripheral neuropathy), and take the pulse for any arrhythmia (embolic cause of cerebellar stroke, mitochondrial disease with pre-excitation, cardiomyopathy with mitochondrial disease or FRDA).

Following examination of the lower and then upper limbs, there are two possible approaches; the head and neck can be examined next, followed by motor then sensory cranial nerves, or alternatively, the neurological focus can continue, deferring the head and neck examination until this is completed, so that the motor cranial nerves are examined next (see short case in this chapter; make a point of mentioning to the examiners you will look at the fundi after the motor cranial nerves).

During the motor cranial nerve examination, thoroughly check the third, fourth and sixth nerve function, and look for nystagmus (many hereditary ataxias) or opsoclonus (neuroblastoma), followed by examination of the sensory nerves, checking the hearing (acute middle and inner ear pathology, FRDA, Refsum). Check the eyes carefully for visual acuity, visual fields and then ask to examine the fundi (for evidence of papilloedema, retinitis or optic atrophy).

Whichever order is chosen, the other findings sought on head and neck examination include checking the head circumference (for hydrocephalus, such as from aqueduct stenosis or tumours), looking for scars of shunts or other neurosurgery, feeling the head for shunts, reservoirs. Feel the hair (abnormal in argininosuccinic acid, and in AT), look at the eyes (bulbar conjunctivae) nose and ears, for telangiectasia (AT). Next check the ears, nose, throat and mastoids for infection (labyrinthitis) and, if relevant, perform the Dix-Hallpike manoeuvre (only suggest this if you really think the patient could have benign paroxysmal vertigo). Then check for any other site of infection (for infectious or post-infectious ataxia causes), including checking for signs of meningitis if the child is febrile.

A full cardiorespiratory examination is appropriate. The BP is checked for hypertension (neuroblastoma, or hypertension as cause of stroke). The heart is examined for murmurs or arrhythmias (embolic stroke). The chest is examined for two reasons: first to check for involvement in any neurological process that can affect respiratory reserve, as with GBS (get the child to count out loud; how far can they count?), and second to check for signs of chest infection, such as *Mycoplasma* which may present with crackles and wheezes.

The abdomen can then be examined for hepatosplenomegaly (EBV) or any masses (neuroblastoma).

At the completion of your examination, present a relevant differential diagnosis, and suggest the investigations most appropriate to confirm your diagnosis. This is a vast area. Suggesting brain (+/– spinal cord) imaging, and gene tests are often appropriate.

Reference

Bushby, K. et al. (2010). Diagnosis and management of Duchenne muscular dystrophy, part 1; diagnosis, and pharmacological and psychosocial management. *The Lancet Neurology*, 9(1), 77–93.

Chapter 14

Oncology

LONG CASE: Oncology

The last few years have seen significant advances in paediatric oncology, including a more detailed understanding of the genetic basis of cancer, the development of disease-specific therapies and investigations, the increasing role of immunotherapeutic approaches and an expansion of disease classifications.

One such change has been the development of cancer-specific drugs, the prototype being imatinib. This drug targets the inappropriately activated tyrosine kinase generated by a fusion gene created through the Philadelphia chromosome translocation (t(9;22) (q34;q11)). The use of imatinib has revolutionised the treatment of both Philadelphia chromosome positive chronic myeloid leukaemia (CML) and acute lymphoblastic leukaemia (ALL). In both forms of leukaemia, the role of bone marrow transplantation has been refined and reduced.

There have been significant advances in the use of monoclonal antibodies (mAbs) with the development and release for clinical use of mAbs that can target specific malignancies. In addition, mAbs have now been developed that recruit and amplify endogenous immune response to target cancers. In addition, mAbs have been developed which are conjugated to specific cytotoxic drugs and delivered directly to cancer cells (e.g. anti-CD33 gemtuzumab ozogamicin for acute myeloid leukaemia [AML], anti-CD30 brentuximab vedotin for Hodgkin disease). mAbs can also be linked to radioactive molecules to deliver local targeted radiotherapy (e.g. 90Y-Ibritumomab, which is a modified anti-CD20 antibody for non-Hodgkin lymphoma).

In recent years, there has been significant success in using antigen-specific T-cells which have genetically modified chimeric antigen receptors (CAR-T-cells) to target specific malignancies. Results in treating patients with relapsed and refractory acute lymphoblastic leukaemia have been promising and this has led to an expanded effort to develop this treatment modality for other forms of leukaemia and solid tumours. Another significant immunotherapy advance has been the development of bispecific T-cell engager antibodies (BsAbs), which have dual binding specificities targeting through direct attachment both a specific tumour antigen on the cancer cell as well as a specific immune effector T-cell which is then activated to destroy the malignant cell.

Blinatumomab is a BsAb which can direct CD3+ T-cells against CD19+ acute lymphoblastic leukaemia (ALL) cells.

Other advances have led to the recognition that prognosis and relapse risk for patients can be better defined by use of molecular biology techniques to detect cancer-specific genetic changes, which are used to monitor the kinetics of disease response by monitoring minimal residual disease (MRD) burden during therapy, particularly during the early phases. Stratifying patients into risk-adapted treatments based on disease response as measured by MRD techniques utilising flow cytometry or polymerase chain reaction is now routine and regarded as standard of care.

There is now a better understanding of the interacting abnormal genetic mechanisms that are responsible at a molecular level for the pathogenesis of neoplasms.

The role of haematopoietic stem cell transplantation (HSCT) continues to evolve and be refined. The indications for HSCT will change as frontline therapies improve. Currently, HSCT plays a significant role in haematological malignancies, including various subgroups of patients with ALL, AML and myelodysplasia.

Of great importance is the role of medical practitioners to provide long-term sensitive surveillance and follow-up. A web-based comprehensive set of guidelines for management of such survivors, the Children's Oncology Group's *Long-term Follow-up Guidelines for Survivors of Childhood, Adolescent, and Young Adult Cancers*, can be found at www.survivorshipguidelines.org. Such initiatives have expanded the literature significantly and are very useful to many candidates.

In the UK, the National Cancer Survivorship Initiative (NCSI) has developed a survivorship framework and care pathways.

In Australia and New Zealand, all major paediatric centres are members of the US-based Children's Oncology Group (COG), a consortium of childhood cancer centres that promotes clinical and laboratory research trials in paediatric oncology.

The general principles of care are similar for patients with haematological malignancies, solid tumours or brain tumours.

The dramatic advances in cancer genomics have provided the platform on which a new era of precision therapeutics has evolved in the field of oncology. This shift in approach is based on extensive and individual analysis of each patient's cancer to identify and define the principal causative (so-called 'driver') mutations and other molecular abnormalities that determine the properties and behaviour of individual cancers such as growth kinetics, drug resistance, response to therapy, resistance to apoptosis, metastasis, angiogenesis and ability to evade recognition and surveillance by the immune system.

The information from this molecular profiling, together with data relevant and specific to each patient, is used as the basis for developing targeted approaches to the prevention, diagnosis and treatment of disease. Therapies are based on therapeutically exploiting these molecular abnormalities rather than relying on the histological classification of the cancer to define treatment regimens. This approach has shown significant potential and success in driving the development of new drug targets as well as diagnostic tests, enabling delivery of tailored treatments to patients.

In addition, extending these strategies and techniques to genomic molecular profiling of constitutional DNA from individuals provides additional information such as personalised risk profiles for specific diseases such as cancer and risk of toxicities from therapy. The information can be used to identify those patients with an underlying genetic predisposition to cancer and to quantify the extent of an individual's risk of specific cancers. This in turn enables healthcare providers to implement evidence-based strategies (such as lifestyle modifications) to minimise or prevent cancers, as well as institute appropriate surveillance programs. This approach in oncology is broadly referred to as precision medicine.

The oncology long case provides an opportunity for a general paediatrician to display competence in assessing and managing a child with cancer, and his or her family, both within multiple contexts: the domestic situation, schooling requirements, wider social relationships and within the medical framework. The medical needs reflect the multilayered levels of care required for the patient and delivered by the general practitioner, the general paediatrician, the paediatric oncologist and other consultants whose help may be required from time to time.

The general paediatrician (the candidate) should be able to demonstrate that he or she can competently handle the medical aspects of a child with cancer as well as the complex professional interrelationships that are involved in coordinating care. The candidate should also be familiar with any recent advances that could affect the management of the patient, which requires a close relationship with the treating oncologist.

An approach to any oncology long case can potentially fit into the following scheme.

History: an overview

At the outset of the interview, it is important to identify clearly the primary and secondary diagnoses, as well as important historical landmarks such as the date of diagnosis, the date of completion of therapy, the history of relapse, or major secondary events such as significant sequelae of therapy (e.g. endocrinopathies or second tumours). Spend your time wisely and carefully in the interview. Limit yourself to about 1–3 minutes to synthesise an overview of the child's condition and focus on gathering data relevant to the presentation. Parents of oncology patients have frequently had sustained and prolonged medical contact, and could fill hours recounting 'what the doctor said'. This approach is very time consuming and often unhelpful.

BEFORE DIAGNOSIS

1. Initial symptoms (with particular reference to the usual non-specific nature of oncology symptoms). A notable difference from adult presentation is the paucity of these symptoms. Unlike adults with cancer, it is very unusual for a child to present with weight loss, haemoptysis or haematemesis and melaena. Symptoms that may present in children include a mass, and the 8 Ps:

   Pyrexia, Pain, Pallor, Purpura, Persistent squint, Personality change, Posterior fossa symptoms, and do not forget the Pretenders (i.e. ALL or neuroblastoma impersonating arthritis, or mediastinal lymph nodes impersonating asthma).

2. Symptom duration (may give a guide to disease 'tempo'). For example, patients with B-cell lymphoma may present as extremely ill, with a history of illness spanning a few days, compared to a patient with a brain tumour or other solid tumour, who may have experienced symptoms for many months.

3. Parental guilt about acts of commission or omission that may have contributed to their child developing cancer.

4. An enquiry about the parent's feelings towards the diagnosis is often revealing. Most parents are initially very angry, an anger that may be self-directed and related to guilt, or directed at doctors or others who they perceive as having failed in their duty to provide an early diagnosis; although, at the time, the non-specific symptoms may not have suggested malignancy as a likely possibility.

Factors 3 and 4 (above) will impact on the family's approach to their sick child and possibly bias the relationships that they establish subsequently with people entrusted with the care of their children, particularly as the care and follow-up of a child with cancer nowadays can be expected to span in excess of 10 years for long-term survivors (over 80% of cases) whom we expect will survive.

POST-DIAGNOSIS PHASE

Important aspects in the history include an appreciation of the parents' understanding of the details and significance of the diagnosis, or even whether the family is aware of the precise diagnosis. The candidate should enquire about the level of knowledge of treatment-related details that the family has acquired in the interval from diagnosis. The examinee should determine the family's understanding of the prognosis, which falls into two broad categories: what they have been told by their doctor, and what they believe. The level of parental awareness and understanding of the condition is important, as this affects the parents' level of care for the child and compliance with medication requirements and appointments. It also influences whether they strive to maintain a near-normal lifestyle for the child, or withdraw him or her from social interaction in anticipation of early death, perceived needs of additional protection and suchlike.

The candidate should enquire about the impact of the diagnosis on siblings, the marital relationship, the financial situation for the family and job stresses. Parents may respond inappropriately in the post-diagnosis phase, by selling their house to relocate closer to the hospital, resigning from stable employment or moving away from familiar and supportive communities, because they believe they are acting in the best interests of the child.

CURRENT STATUS OF THE PATIENT

The details of the therapy received in the specific treatment protocol for that patient should be sought. The details should be general. Is most medication oral, IV or IM? Is there a central line? How many visits have been made to the hospital for treatment? Can the local doctor or local hospital give any chemotherapy? No candidate will be expected to be familiar with all protocols. Be sure to ask about complementary therapies.

Enquire about problems such as infections (especially pulmonary), marrow suppression and complications arising from this (such as febrile neutropenic episodes, anaemia and thrombocytopenia), compliance with oral chemotherapy and *Pneumocystis* prophylaxis with cotrimoxazole (or a similar drug), and any other side effects from therapy, including nausea, vomiting and rashes. Then concentrate on the current status, particularly the immediate (rather than late) effects of treatment and their consequences, such as: lethargy and easy fatigability from anaemia; nausea, vomiting and anorexia, resulting in weight loss; alopecia; limitation of activities (e.g. swimming) because of the presence of central lines; or ostomies involving the gastrointestinal or genitourinary tracts.

OTHER

The impact on daily activity of amputation of a lower extremity for bone tumour should be explored (and secondary consequences such as kyphoscoliosis sought during physical examination). Growth and development should be explored with the families. Social issues and schooling can then be discussed in the light of the foregoing information.

Finally, details of late effects of treatment and underlying illness should be sought.

Any family history of conditions associated with a predisposition to malignancy should be noted (e.g. immunodeficiencies, neurofibromatosis type 1).

From the above, the candidate should be able to formulate a comprehensive problem list, picking up items from each of the sections, prioritising these and being ready to discuss them.

Examination

See the short-case section in this chapter on late effects of oncology treatment.

Management plan

The following is an outline of the major issues that the general paediatrician may need to address, divided into general and specific problem areas.

DISCUSSION POINTS

1. Relapse of primary disease.
2. Growth and development, including specific late effects.
3. Development of second tumour.
4. Social issues.
5. Schooling.
6. Infection.
7. Immunisation.
8. Issues of ongoing chemotherapy (crisis intervention for bone marrow suppression).
9. Supportive care.
10. Haematopoietic stem cell transplantation (HSCT).
11. Therapeutic modifications: risk-adapted therapy.
12. The dying child.

RELAPSE OF PRIMARY DISEASE

Note that patients who relapse are unlikely to be selected for an examination. However, this does not diminish the importance of properly assessing the issues regarding relapse.

In seeking symptoms from the parents or patient, the candidate ought to enquire whether any new symptoms resemble those present before the diagnosis, and determine the level of anxiety that these new symptoms are causing.

Progressive symptoms such as weight loss, unexplained anorexia, nausea, fever or the appearance of lymphadenopathy, organomegaly, excessive bruising, bleeding, gum oozing, knotty palpable masses or painful bony masses all warrant further investigation.

GROWTH AND DEVELOPMENT

Irradiation is the single most important factor in determining long-term growth and development. The candidate should know which structures were within the treatment portal, and the total dose used. Patients treated with craniospinal irradiation will be at the combined risk of hypopituitarism and relative shortening of the vertebral column. In addition, even if the pituitary is spared, the thyroid gland may well receive sufficient radiotherapy to result in biochemical hypothyroidism that requires intervention (because if it is untreated, the risk of thyroid cancer is enhanced). Any irradiated area may demonstrate relative soft-tissue atrophy.

In the past, cranial radiotherapy was used for central nervous system (CNS) prophylaxis in a majority of patients with ALL. Modern treatment regimens now restrict the use of cranial radiation to 10% or less of patients with ALL. Up to 50% of children treated for acute leukaemia with cranial radiotherapy can have decreased growth hormone secretion. Loss of final height can also be influenced by early (rarely precocious) onset of puberty or (too) early institution of testosterone therapy for hypogonadism in boys. The management usually comprises growth hormone, delaying treatment with testosterone.

If there has been a bone marrow transplant, the eyes should be checked by a paediatric ophthalmologist regularly (say, 12–24 monthly) for cataracts from total body irradiation (or from steroids). Hearing may be impaired by drugs such as cisplatin or aminoglycosides, and requires regular review and audiological assessment.

Ideally, a formal psychological assessment should be carried out before any cranial irradiation. After treatment, psychological assessment may be repeated on a regular basis, in conjunction with neurological examination, MRI scanning and assessment of school performance, to monitor neuropsychological outcome and provide early rehabilitative intervention if needed. The spectrum of CNS damage varies from decreased performance at school, to frank leukoencephalopathy, spasticity and significant intellectual impairment. Intravenous methotrexate may result in leukoencephalopathy in children with ALL, especially after irradiation. Pubertal development may be early (rarely precocious); however, delayed puberty is more common, with high gonadotropin levels from end-organ gonadal damage.

Cardiac toxicity

The use of anthracycline-containing chemotherapy plus mediastinal irradiation in treating leukaemia and lymphoma can lead to cardiotoxicity; subclinical myocardial dysfunction occurs in 18–57% of long-term survivors of childhood cancer. Cancer survivors are more likely than their (control) siblings to have heart failure, myocardial infarction, atherosclerosis, pericardial disease or valvular disease, and require coronary angiography. Cardiac abnormalities tend to worsen over time. Periodic assessment of left ventricular ejection fraction (LVEF) should be done, using echocardiography or radionuclide ventriculography (RVG).

Children with Down syndrome treated for AML with anthracyclines have an especially high risk of developing cardiomyopathy.

Treatment for asymptomatic left ventricular dysfunction, or symptomatic heart failure comprises ACE inhibitors as first-line agents. Cardiac transplantation may be needed, in those with higher lifetime cumulative doses of doxorubicin or daunorubicin.

Fertility preservation

One important issue to address in adolescent patients is future reproductive potential. In boys with tumours such as Hodgkin's disease, sperm storage should be considered before irradiation and chemotherapy. In girls, ovarian tissue storage is now available.

In both sexes, cranial irradiation can cause hypogonadotropic hypogonadism. In girls, chemotherapy, particularly alkylating agents, can cause hypergonadotrophic hypogonadism. Management may include oocyte cryopreservation, pubertal induction and female hormone replacement therapy. In boys, chemotherapy, especially alkylating agents, and gonadal radiotherapy or total body irradiation (TBI) can cause azoospermia and hypergonadotrophic hypogonadism. Management may include semen analysis and cryopreservation, pubertal induction and testosterone supplementation.

Bone health and low bone mineral density (BMD)

Childhood survivors of cancer are more likely to develop low bone mineral density (BMD) if they: had malignant bone disease, or were exposed to chemotherapeutic agents which affect bone metabolism such as methotrexate, or corticosteroids; had growth hormone or sex hormone deficiency secondary to their treatment; or had poor nutrition or a sedentary lifestyle.

To determine BMD, dual-energy X-ray absorptiometry (DXA) is used, using normative Z scores based on age, height and Tanner pubertal staging. Treatment may involve calcium and vitamin D supplements, sex hormone or GH replacement, and weight bearing exercises.

Metabolic syndrome and obesity

The risk factors for developing metabolic syndrome (hypertension, dyslipidaemia and visceral adiposity) are cranial, abdominal or TBI; this increases the risk of developing type II diabetes mellitus and atherosclerosis. The prevalence of obesity in childhood cancer survivors is around 40%; obesity occurs more often in: those exposed to dexamethasone, or cranial irradiation; female sex; younger age; in particular, survivors of ALL, brain tumours and HSCT have the highest rate of obesity.

Thyroid dysfunction

This can be central (secondary) or primary. Central hypothyroidism is caused by the hypothalamic–pituitary (HP) axis being exposed to radiation to the HP axis (> 30 to 40 Gy), or surgery affecting the HP area. Primary hypothyroidism is caused by a direct effect on the gland by radiation (including I-131) or by drug therapy with tyrosine kinase inhibitors. Screening involves annual measurement of TSH and T4, or more frequently if periods of rapid growth.

Cognitive/psychosocial effects

Cranial irradiation can induce cognitive decline; the younger the age and the higher the dose, the greater the deficit. All survivors are at increased risk for psychosocial problems, learning difficulties and may need additional educational support.

DEVELOPMENT OF SECOND TUMOUR

The risk of developing a second malignancy may approach 15–20% at 20 years in long-term survivors of childhood cancer, and appears to be related to the original diagnosis and treatment modalities. In ALL, children who have received cranial irradiation when under 6 years of age are susceptible to brain tumours, and children who have had extensive treatment with epipodophyllotoxins (teniposide and etoposide) are at greater risk of developing AML.

SOCIAL ISSUES

Some long-time survivors have trouble adjusting to the stress of normal life. This can be assessed by simple interview and psychometric testing. Potential problems include diminished school performance, behavioural problems, impaired attainment of social skills, ongoing anxiety regarding relapse and the financial burden of the child's treatment on the family. These areas should be explored so that appropriate intervention can be made.

SCHOOLING

Survivors of ALL in particular are at risk of school-related problems, including repeating grades and a need for special education. This may relate to neurological damage from CNS prophylactic therapy. Assessment of school performance allows evaluation of problems with memory, concentration and attention span: all well-recognised sequelae. The amount of schooling that a child missed during treatment should be noted. Has the trend of school absence continued after therapy was completed? If so, determine the reasons. Is it excessive concern about infections such as varicella or measles (exposures to which are not relevant more than 6 months from the end of treatment)? The school situation must always be explored at follow-up.

INFECTION

The child on chemotherapy

Common childhood infections occur in children receiving therapy for cancer just as in normal children, and many can be managed in the usual way, provided that the child does not appear toxic, there is an identifiable localised infection, the neutrophil count is greater than $1.0 \times 10^9/L$ and regular follow-up is provided. Often chemotherapy may be continued, after consultation, through the course of mild infections, be they bacterial or viral. If a child is unwell at home, with a fever and rhinorrhoea, the parents should be advised to contact the paediatrician. If the temperature is above a previously agreed level (e.g. 38°C), then the child should be seen either in hospital.

All children on therapy who are febrile need prompt assessment, and in most cases antibiotics should be started early (without waiting for result of blood count). Blood cultures should be collected before antibiotics.

If the neutrophil count is low (below $0.5 \times 10^9/L$), the child should be admitted to hospital. The management of febrile neutropenia should include broad-spectrum parenteral antibiotic therapy (e.g. ceftriaxone, tobramycin, teicoplanin). Antibiotics ideally should be commenced within 1–2 hours of the child reaching the emergency room. It is inappropriate to wait for the results of the blood count before starting therapy with antibiotics, especially if there is any delay in processing the sample in the laboratory. In such circumstances, antibiotics should be started. If the count is normal, there is less cause for concern. Remember, however, that many patients have central venous access devices in place, which can be the cause of serious infections despite normal neutrophil numbers. *Always* remind the family that fevers occurring within 6–8 hours of flushing a central line may be due to the introduction of bacteria into the patient from an infected central venous line. For more details, see below.

Granulocyte colony stimulating factor (G-CSF) can decrease hospitalisation duration for prolonged febrile neutropenia after intensive remission induction chemotherapy. G-CSF can be started 24 hours after cytotoxics and is given subcutaneously daily for 10 days. G-CSF may be ceased when the neutrophil count is greater than $1.0 \times 10^9/L$, and beyond the nadir. A long-lasting form of G-CSF, Peg-G-CSF, is administered as a single dose 24 hours after completing the chemotherapy course.

Exposure to certain viruses requires specific intervention. In the case of varicella contacts, varicella zoster immune globulin should be given within 96 hours of exposure, and is more efficacious the earlier it is given. With measles contacts, standard immunoglobulin is recommended. In patients who are at risk of significant infection with herpes simplex virus (HSV), valaciclovir can be used (this has a longer half-life than aciclovir). Ganciclovir is often used for CMV prophylaxis in the setting of stem cell transplantation.

For prophylaxis against oral candidiasis, oral nystatin or amphotericin B lozenges can be given. In patients with prolonged neutropenia and/or lymphopenia, fluconazole may be used (covers *Candida* but not *Aspergillus*) or itraconazole (covers aspergillosis, e.g. posttransplant). Cotrimoxazole is recommended as prophylaxis against *Pneumocystis carinii*, particularly in patients with prolonged lymphopenia (lymphocytes less than $1.0 \times 10^9/L$ or CD4 count below 400). In patients where cotrimoxazole causes neutropenia, or there are unacceptable side effects, pentamidine may be considered.

Mouth care is important in children with mouth ulceration or mucositis, or in those at risk of these if they are neutropenic ($< 1.0 \times 10^9/L$). Chlorhexidine mouthwash may be useful, as it is bactericidal.

The child off chemotherapy

For the first 3–6 months after completion of chemotherapy, there is a continued susceptibility to infection, although this is quite small. This risk is much greater for patients who continue to receive immunosuppressive therapy; for example, post-BMT for chronic graft-versus-host disease (GVHD). Children with chronic GVHD are immunosuppressed, as they are generally receiving steroids and anti-T-cell medications (cyclosporine or mycophenolate). They are often relatively neutropenic. Patients with active GVHD should not attend school. It is advisable for the schoolteacher to notify the parents, within the first 6 months of ceasing chemotherapy, of any outbreaks of chickenpox or measles in the class.

IMMUNISATION

Susceptibility to live vaccines is maximal during chemotherapy and for the first 6 months after chemotherapy. Thus, avoidance of live vaccines is recommended, with the exception of live varicella vaccine, which can be given safely during the maintenance therapy for ALL (but not during the early intensive phases—the first 6 months of treatment). This, however, is *not* routine practice in Australia. Killed virus vaccines (e.g. Salk vaccine) can be given.

Some authorities avoid administering live measles and mumps vaccine to siblings, as there is a small risk of transmission. Others consider this risk minimal and the vaccine safe. Influenza vaccine is safe and may have a place in patients with chronic chest symptoms.

Hepatitis B recombinant vaccine is safe, but as these patients are immunosuppressed, adding a further booster dose is recommended. Titres may be checked 12 months later to assess efficacy. There are now recommendations regarding immunisation in two distinct groups: those who receive standard therapy and those who require stem cell therapy.

Immunisation with standard dose chemotherapy

There is a decrease in the concentrations of vaccine–antigen-specific antibodies after completing chemotherapy. During chemotherapy, children are immunosuppressed and so cannot have live vaccines such as measles, mumps and rubella (MMR). Non-live vaccines can still be given according to the routine immunisation schedule. After completion of chemotherapy, it is wise to re-immunise children, following the routine immunisation schedule of the child's country of residence, starting 3–6 months after the cessation of treatment. Immune function recovery can occur as early as 3 months post-treatment.

Immunisation with HSCT

HSCT recipients are significantly immunosuppressed for months after transplantation. Immune reconstitution occurs faster with autologous than with allogeneic transplantation. They have extensive alterations in their immune function and are especially susceptible to infection with polysaccharide-encapsulated organisms.

For autologous HSCT, the immunosuppression is mainly due to pretransplant treatment. For allogeneic HSCT, the immunosuppression is due to a combination of pretransplant conditioning, GVHD and immunosuppressive therapy following HSCT.

B-lymphocyte reconstitution occurs 3–6 months after transplant, and immunoglobulin isotypes start normalising 6 months after transplant, but there is an IgG subclass imbalance, with low IgG2 levels for 18 months or more after transplant. T-lymphocyte reconstitution starts at 1–2 months, peaks at 3–6 months and reaches normal levels by 1–2 years after transplant. It is important that these children receive the full immunisation schedule of their country of residence, usually 18 months after cessation of therapy, and this should include immunisation against *Streptococcus pneumoniae* with the seven-valent pneumococcal conjugate vaccine 7vPCV and the 23-valent-pneumococcal polysaccharide vaccine 23vPPV, and against *Neisseria meningitidis* with the meningococcal C conjugate vaccines MenCCV and the tetravalent meningococcal polysaccharide vaccines 4vMenPV. The current version of *The Australian Immunisation Handbook* outlines the schedule post-HSCT.

ISSUES RELATED TO ONGOING CHEMOTHERAPY

For oncology patients receiving chemotherapy, there are misconceptions about how best to 'protect' children. This advice is standard in paediatric oncology centres.

1. Check that relatives are well before visits.
2. Patients can swim in swimming pools (even with central lines, but they require prompt cleaning after the swim). Swimming policy varies between units—generally advise against swimming if there is an external central line.
3. Children can go shopping in supermarkets and attend group gatherings (e.g. church, birthday parties).
4. Prophylactic cotrimoxazole is essential.

Crisis intervention

The candidate should be familiar with medical practices in his or her own teaching hospital's oncology unit. For example, prophylactic platelet transfusions for severe thrombocytopenia (platelet count below 10×10^9/L) is not standard practice in all units.

It would be uncommon for a candidate to be asked about any theoretical oncological emergencies, as they could have applied to the long case patient acutely. However, it is worth candidates being cognisant of local procedures to deal with some of the more common acute issues such as: tumour lysis syndrome (may require hyperhydration, blocking uric acid production and correcting electrolytes); spinal cord compression (dexamethasone, imaging, neurosurgery); seizures (ABC, O_2, IV midazolam, IV phenytoin as second line); acute abdomen (beware typhlitis [necrotising colitis, localised to caecum and ascending colon] in severe neutropenia); perianal cellulitis/abscess (antibiotics against *Pseudomonas* plus anaerobes plus G-CSF if neutropenia); and anaphylaxis (adrenaline, then H_1-antagonist, H_2-antagonist, steroid). Anaphylaxis occurs not infrequently, to **a**sparaginase, **a**ntibiotics, **A**TGAM, **a**mphotericin, **a**mifostine (the cytoprotective adjuvant) and biologics.

Drug toxicities

The paediatrician must be aware of the various side effects of the many drugs used in the treatment of the malignancy, and be cognisant of a confusing complaint (e.g. ataxia in a child with leukaemia) being possibly due to drug toxicity (e.g. vincristine neuropathy) rather than necessarily meaning CNS relapse.

Thrombocytopenia is one of the more common drug side effects. If the platelet count is below 20×10^9/L, spontaneous bleeding can occur. If the platelet count is below 50×10^9/L, minor trauma can result in bleeding.

If there is no overt bleeding, then simple precautions suffice, such as avoiding injurious activities or invasive procedures (unless essential, which may require them to be covered by platelet transfusion), body-contact sports, strenuous exercise or hard-bristled toothbrushes. Note that severe headaches may indicate CNS haemorrhage. Avoidance of drugs such as aspirin or antihistamines (which can interfere with normal platelet function) is important.

Febrile neutropenic episodes

Neutropenia means a neutrophil count of below 1.0×10^9/L, but most infections occur with a level below 0.5×10^9/L, and most of those are below 0.2×10^9/L. Clinically, the problem can be very difficult to assess, as there are no classic signs or symptoms. Particular areas on which to focus include the skin, mucous membranes (ulceration, candida, herpes), chest, central-line site and perianal region (ischiorectal abscesses can be very subtle).

Management usually includes admission to hospital, culture of the potential sites outlined, blood cultures and administration of broad-spectrum parenteral antibiotic therapy. Most units withhold chemotherapy until the child is afebrile for more than a day and the neutrophil count has returned to above $1.0 \times 10^9/L$.

Pulmonary infections

These are among the most common form of severe infection seen in oncology patients, and there are many possible pathogens. The neutrophil count plus the chest X-ray may be useful guides in management. Note that in the presence of neutropenia, pulmonary markings may not be prominent, despite significant infection. Approximately 50% of bacterial infections are due to gram-positive bacteria and the remainder are due to gram-negative organisms: thus, broad-spectrum antibiotic therapy cover is advisable. Opportunistic infections can occur, such as *Pneumocystis carinii* (although most patients are on cotrimoxazole prophylaxis for this), opportunistic viruses (e.g. cytomegalovirus), fungi, *Mycobacterium* or *Mycoplasma*. Note that radiological findings may be due to non-infectious causes (e.g. leukaemic infiltration or toxicity from chemotherapy or radiotherapy).

Central venous access devices

These may be central lines or totally implantable venous access devices, such as portacath and Infuse-A-Port. These devices are routinely used in most conditions encountered in oncology. They require regular heparin flushes to avoid clots forming, and may on occasion become infected, particularly with *Staphylococcus* species.

SUPPORTIVE CARE

Mouth care

Mouth care is important in children with mouth ulceration or mucositis, or in those at risk of these if they are neutropenic ($< 1.0 \times 10^9/L$). Chlorhexidine mouthwash is useful, as it is bactericidal. In very young patients, chlorhexidine gel is appropriate, and before meals xylocaine viscous is useful.

Antiemetics

All chemotherapy protocols include the use of 5-HT_3 antagonists such as ondansetron, as vomiting occurs predictably after many specific chemotherapeutic agents. Ondansetron can be given intravenously or orally, the latter being significantly cheaper and available in the form of wafers or syrup. If ondansetron is not enough, metoclopramide or dexamethasone provide additional antiemetic effect.

Many of the drugs used in solid tumour protocols are very emetogenic. These include Adriamycin, carboplatin, cisplatin, cyclophosphamide (CPA) and ifosfamide. Ondansetron is usually given before, during and after each chemotherapy infusion.

HAEMATOPOIETIC STEM CELL TRANSPLANTATION (HSCT)

In allogeneic HSCT, healthy haematopoietic stem cells are harvested from a separate donor, related or unrelated, though clearly human leukocyte antigen (HLA) matched cells would be ideal, and used to replace the patient's abnormal cells; in autologous HSCT, the patient is his or her own donor, where healthy haematopoietic stem cells are harvested, stored and reinfused after cytoreduction.

Allogeneic donors for SCT in children can be of several types: these include cells from bone marrow, umbilical cord blood, mobilised peripheral blood, unmanipulated or T-cell depleted, or CD34 or CD133 selected grafts. (The use of T-cell depletion and high-dose infusions of CD34+ cells can reduce the rate of severe GVHD, and can improve the rate of engraftment.) The selection of donors depends on underlying diagnosis, risk for relapse, availability, age of patient (younger preferred), size of patient, cytomegalovirus (CMV) status (negative preferred), sex of donor (male preferred; female donors, especially those with high parity, have association with a higher rate of GVHD); but the most important consideration is high-resolution HLA matching; identification of an HLA donor at the DNA level is prioritised. Matching at 10 out of 10 alleles would be ideal; a low mortality rate is reported in SCT in children 7 out of 10 or 8 out of 10 HLA allele-matched unrelated donors with the use of antithymocyte globulin. Even the availability of a matched sibling, or a 10 out of 10 allele-matched unrelated donor, does not prevent transplant-related complications including GVHD.

Autologous HSCT can be used in the treatment of neuroblastoma, AML and Hodgkin's and non-Hodgkin's lymphoma. Allogeneic HSCT can be used in the treatment of ALL, AML, CML and Hodgkin's and non-Hodgkin's lymphoma.

Allogeneic stem cell transplantation: selected haematological malignancies

- *Acute lymphoblastic leukaemia*: certain patients who relapse after initial treatment, plus subgroups of patients with high-risk features of relapse, will proceed to an allogeneic SCT; in the latter, this can occur while in the first remission. SCT may be the only curative therapy for the former. Relapsed ALL is the fourth-commonest malignant disease in childhood (with a higher incidence than many newly diagnosed paediatric tumours). Outcomes for SCT are best when performed during first or second complete remission.
- *Acute myeloid leukaemia*: the best therapy during first remission is controversial; SCT is preferred for patients with less favourable prognoses, such as those with complex karyotypes (e.g. −5, del(5q), −7, 3q abnormalities) or hyperleucocytosis. Allogeneic SCT during the second remission is associated with better outcome after relapse.
- *High-grade myelodysplastic syndrome*: allogeneic SCT is the treatment of choice.
- *Therapy-related myelodysplastic (MDS) syndrome and AML*: these are clonal malignant disorders occurring after exposure to cytotoxic agents. They tend to be more aggressive than the de novo disorders, and SCT may be the only curative therapy available.
- *Chronic myeloid leukaemia (CML)*: allogeneic transplantation from a matched related family donor is the only curative approach.

HSCT: bone marrow transplantation (BMTx)

In the weeks leading up to bone marrow transplantation (BMTx), especially in late autumn/early winter, isolating the children is a good idea, because if they get RSV, parainfluenza, adenovirus or influenza, this will delay the BMTx.

Candidates should know that pretransplant preparative regimens usually combine very high-dose cytotoxic agents and immunosuppressive agents (e.g. CPA, melphalan, cytosine arabinoside [ara C], etoposide, thiotepa, busulfan, fludarabine) with various doses (e.g. 12 grey to 15.75 grey before allogeneic transplantation for leukaemia) of fractionated total body irradiation (TBI). Non-TBI-based regimens usually use busulfan or CPA, with or without melphalan, etoposide, thiotepa and fludarabine. The preparative regimen should have sufficient cytotoxic anti-leukaemic effect combined with adequate immunosuppression to ensure engraftment.

After BMTx/HSCT

All recipients of allogeneic marrow are at risk of GVHD post-engraftment. Agents used to prevent this occurring include methotrexate (MTX), cyclosporine (CSA), prednisolone, tacrolimus and mycophenolate mofetil. The main target organs of acute GVHD are the skin (maculopapular rash), liver (cholestatic jaundice) and gut (anorexia/diarrhoea).

Acute GVHD may require treatment with prednisolone, antithymocyte globulin, tacrolimus, psoralen plus ultraviolet light (PUVA).

In the first 6 months after transplant, the child should not attend school, and social contacts should be limited (especially with GVHD). There are no firm recommendations regarding the use of live viral vaccines for these patients. If the child is well, and has no GVHD, then after 12 months live viral vaccines are safe.

Late effects post-BMTx/HSCT

Chronic GVHD appears around 80 days post-BMTx. The main target organs are the skin (epidermal atrophy, focal dermal fibrosis, scleroderma, loss of hair and nails), liver (cholestatic jaundice), eyes (keratoconjunctivitis sicca) and mouth (erythema, lichenoid lesions of buccal mucosa). Less often, the lungs, gut and neuromuscular system may be involved. If GVHD is extensive, treatment may involve the use of prednisolone with CPA, prednisolone with tacrolimus, azathioprine or PUVA.

Other effects related to the BMTx process include graft rejection and immunological dysfunction (short-lasting, donor-derived T- and B-lymphocyte immunity [TBI]; reimmunisation of patients should occur 12 months post-BMTx).

Complications of the preparative regimen include lung disease (both restrictive and obstructive defects can occur long term), development of second malignancies (at 15 years, around 6% if no TBI, but 20% if received TBI), endocrine dysfunction (growth hormone deficiency, gonadal dysfunction, hypothyroidism) and neuropsychological problems.

Alternative transplantations: umbilical cord blood transplantation (UCBT) and haploidentical transplantation

Umbilical cord blood (UCB) is an alternative source for transplantable stem and progenitor cells. Cord blood can be collected from the placenta via the umbilical vein after the baby is delivered. GVHD occurs at lower rates than matched-sibling BMTx. Cord blood is available at short notice. Disadvantages include the potential for unknowing transmission of genetic diseases (e.g. immune deficiency and storage diseases), and the limitation of volume and cell content of what is collected (i.e. the finite number of stem cells in the cord blood unit). UCBT may be very useful for those without a matched donor for BMTx. Predictors of success after UCBT include the number of cells in the UCB graft, and the degree of HLA disparity; a cell dose of 3×10^7 per kg have a much higher survival rate.

Haploidentical transplantation with T-cell depletion using CD 34+ positive selection from mobilised peripheral stem cells can be successful, without GVHD, with outcomes comparable to matched unrelated donor transplantation.

With the addition of matched or partially matched UCB and haploidentical donors to the pool of available donors, most children with high-risk haematological malignancies should be able to have a donor found for them, and then have an allogeneic transplantation if the risk–benefit ratio is favourable.

THERAPEUTIC MODIFICATIONS: RISK-ADAPTED THERAPY

As the number of survivors has increased, so there has been heightened awareness of the potential consequences of treatment. This has led to modifications to therapy to enhance the quality of life for survivors. The following brief summary outlines risk-adapted therapies aimed at diminishing complications, the latter grouped according to the organ system involved.

Cardiopulmonary

Decreased dose of radiation; improved shielding of heart and lungs; decreased doses of anthracyclines (cardiotoxic) and bleomycin (pulmonary toxicity); newer anthracyclines with decreased cardiotoxicity; the use of cardioprotective agents (dexrazoxane); routine monitoring (e.g. echocardiography, pulmonary function tests).

Endocrine

Lower doses and volumes of radiotherapy; routine oophoropexy during pelvic radiotherapy; reducing doses of alkylating agents in patients with good prognoses; routine testing for deficiencies of various hormones (e.g. growth hormone, oestrogen, thyroid hormone) and replacement thereof; ovarian tissue and sperm storage.

Genitourinary

The use of mesna, a uroprotectant drug that binds to toxic metabolites in the urine, after CPA or ifosfamide, and decreases haemorrhagic cystitis; new analogues with less renal toxicity (e.g. carboplatin compared with cisplatin); routine monitoring (e.g. blood testing for electrolytes, including phosphorus, and magnesium).

Neurological

Elimination of intrathecal and intravenous methotrexate after cranial irradiation has decreased leukoencephalopathy; delaying therapeutic radiation until older (aiming for over 3 years) by utilising systemic chemotherapy; routine monitoring of neuropsychological status.

Second malignancy

Decreased exposure to alkylating agents, plus limiting volume of radiation in Hodgkin's lymphoma; greatly diminished use of epipodophyllotoxins in leukaemia; increased education of survivors about potential of late effects of their specific therapy.

THE DYING CHILD

There are many issues that need to be addressed in a child for whom no further beneficial therapy is possible. Most children nowadays die at home. Palliative treatment involves issues of control of pain, nutrition and appreciation of the psychosocial dynamics of the family. These children may show an inability to cope by features such as denial of their illness, withdrawal or unwarranted anger.

The family's mourning can include, again, denial, anger and depression, and very often seeking further opinions or considering alternative forms of therapy. These processes should be understood and accepted by the paediatrician. For the child who dies in hospital, the major objective is ensuring maximum comfort. This can be aided by surrounding the child with familiar possessions from home and having no restriction on visitors. Invariably, other children on the ward become aware of the change in the management of these patients, and frank discussion should be encouraged, as well as permitting interaction with the dying child.

The death of the child invariably is associated with confusion and shock, irrespective of the degree of expectation and preparation. Prior discussions regarding issues of postmortem examination and, if the child dies at home, transport of the body to the hospital, are usually beneficial to the family. The role of the paediatrician extends beyond the death of the child to helping the family cope with caring for siblings, discussing unresolved issues and intervening, by appropriate referral, where an abnormal grief reaction is apparent, such as acting out by siblings, or severe depression and contemplation of suicide in the parents. As the most severe grief may occur some months after the child's death, follow-up should be for many months rather than weeks.

SHORT CASE

SHORT CASE: Late effects of oncology treatment

Late effects of oncology treatment plus common signs of disease relapse (in particular, acute leukaemia) are outlined in Table 14.1. This is incomplete, of course, due to the

Table 14.1
Late effects of oncology treatment
GENERAL OBSERVATIONS
Introduce yourself: ask name, age, school; assess intelligence (is child alert, conversant?) (leukoencephalopathy secondary to treatment [XRT, MTX]; subnormal IQ with intracranial tumours); note hearing aids, glasses, glass eye, deformities, amputations, prostheses
Parameters • Height (short stature: growth hormone deficiency, panhypopituitarism [cranial XRT, MTX], hypothyroidism [thyroid XRT or MIBG], steroid therapy, skeletal changes from spinal XRT) • Upper segment:lower segment (US:LS) ratio (skeletal changes from radiation of spine) • Weight + BMI • Head circumference • Percentile charts, noting trend since treatment, look at growth velocity
Tanner staging (delay: alkylating agents, radiation to gonads, cisplatin, carboplatin)
Cushingoid features (steroid therapy)
Tachypnoea, cyanosis or cough (radiation- or chemotherapy-induced pneumonitis, or pulmonary infection)
Skin • Pallor: anaemia from marrow suppression (most agents), or bone marrow relapse of leukaemia (or development of secondary leukaemia) • Bruises: thrombocytopenia from marrow suppression (most agents) or (rare) coagulopathy from L-asparaginase, or bone marrow relapse of leukaemia • Dermatitis (MTX, 6-MP, 6-TG) • Hyperpigmentation (chronic GVHD from BMT) • Desquamation (bleomycin) • Jaundice (MTX, 6-MP, 6-TG, bleomycin, radiation to liver) • Pigmented naevi (increased by most agents)
MANOEUVRES
Stand with hands and feet together (asymmetry from XRT to limbs or hemihypertrophy with Wilms' tumour—do not confuse the two)
Gait: full examination for evidence of neuropathy (VCR), spasticity (leukoencephalopathy), cerebellar ataxia (L-asparaginase), antalgic limp (marrow relapse of leukaemia) or proximal myopathy (steroids); also may detect evidence of cerebral tumour (second malignancy)
Romberg's test (neuropathy from VCR)

Table 14.1 (continued)

BACK

Effects on bony skeleton (XRT, steroids, GVHD, MTX, BMT, endocrinopathy; poor mineral density, growth anomalies, avascular necrosis); effects on paraspinal soft tissues (XRT, steroids, GVHD; muscle weakness, hypoplasia, impaired mobility)

Inspect; look for scars, any vertebral masses (secondary malignancy)

Bend forwards and touch toes (to assess for scoliosis or kyphosis from spinal irradiation, particularly if unilateral)

Palpate for tenderness (steroids; rickets from ifosfamide)

UPPER LIMBS

Effects on bony skeleton (XRT, steroids, GVHD, MTX, BMT, endocrinopathy; poor mineral density, growth anomalies, avascular necrosis; effects especially on large joints); effects on soft tissues (XRT, steroids, GVHD; muscle weakness, hypoplasia, impaired mobility)

Inspect; look for scars (previous diagnostic or curative surgery)

Asymmetry (limb radiation, hemihypertrophy)

Contractures (limb XRT, chronic GVHD)

Peripheral stigmata of chronic liver disease (MTX, 6-MP, radiation to abdomen)

Palmar crease pallor (marrow suppression)

Pulse (bradycardia; untreated hypothyroidism from XRT to thyroid, or busulfan, BMT, MIBG)

Neurological examination
Peripheral neuropathy (vinca alkaloids, usually reversible; test reflexes and sensation to document this)
Functional assessment if:
- any asymmetry or contractures suggestive of radiation to limb, or
- scars from resection of tumour with potential neurological or vascular complications, or
- amputation—examine function with prosthesis; check how well fits, any loosening or infection

Blood pressure (elevated from steroids, bleomycin, MTX nephrotoxicity, radiation nephritis, renal damage from GVHD; low from adrenal insufficiency from XRT to adrenal area, BMT, metabolic syndrome)

HEAD AND NECK

Alopecia (*reversible*: ADR, bleomycin, CPA, daunorubicin, VCR; *irreversible*: post-BMTx; busulfan; cranial XRT + anthracycline given close together)

Scars (previous diagnostic, curative or debulking surgery)

Midfacial hypoplasia, small nose, chin (XRT to head and neck → altered growth bone/soft tissue)

Eyes (XRT, busulfan, steroids, GVHD)
- Aniridia (association with Wilms' tumour, not a late effect)
- Conjunctival pallor (marrow suppression, various agents)
- Scleral icterus (bleomycin, MTX, 6-MP, 6-TG, radiation to liver)
- External ocular movements for evidence of cranial nerve palsy (CNS relapse of leukaemia, VCR neuropathy)
- Cataracts (corticosteroids, radiation to eyes)
- Papilloedema (CNS relapse of leukaemia)

Ears
Hearing impairment/hearing aid (XRT, cisplatin, carboplatin, antibiotics)

Mouth
- Dry (salivary gland dysfunction from XRT)
- Mucositis (MTX, 6-MP, 6-TG, actinomycin D)

Temporomandibular joint: note interdental distance (normally should be able to fit three fingers lined up vertically, between lower and upper teeth); limited range of movement (XRT)

Continued

Table 14.1 (continued)
Teeth (XRT, BMT; tooth/root agenesis, root thinning/shortening, enamel dysplasia) • Microdontia; poor enamel and root formation (radiation to head) • Dental caries (most agents)
Thyroid: look and palpate for nodules (thyroid carcinoma from craniospinal XRT)
CHEST
Scars (previous diagnostic, curative or debulking surgery)
Praecordial assessment for cardiomegaly (cardiomyopathy) from anthracyclines (the 'rubicins') or radiation (mediastinal XRT), pericarditis (reversible—from mediastinal XRT), evidence of congestive cardiac failure (from cardiomyopathy), abnormal rhythms
Full respiratory examination for tachypnoea, cough or crackles due to interstitial pneumonitis or pulmonary fibrosis (bleomycin, busulfan, MTX, CPA, XRT, GVHD), pulmonary infection (opportunistic viruses, bacteria/fungi if still on chemotherapy)
Assess bony tenderness at sternum, clavicles, spine (marrow relapse: leukaemia, secondary leukaemia)
ABDOMEN
Scars (previous diagnostic, curative or debulking surgery)
Prominent veins (chronic liver disease from MTX, 6-MP or XRT to abdomen)
Hepatomegaly (MTX, 6-MP or relapse of leukaemia or lymphoma)
Splenomegaly (relapse of leukaemia or lymphoma)
Genitals: Tanner staging (delay from alkylating agents or gonadal XRT); ambiguous genitalia with Denys–Drash syndrome (association with Wilms', not a late effect)
Testicular enlargement (relapse of leukaemia)
Undescended testes (association with Wilms', not a late effect)
LOWER LIMBS
Effects on bony skeleton (XRT, steroids, GVHD, MTX, BMT, endocrinopathy; poor mineral density, growth anomalies, avascular necrosis; effects on large joints); effects on soft tissues (XRT, steroids, GVHD; muscle weakness, hypoplasia, impaired mobility)
Asymmetry (limb radiation, hemihypertrophy)
Contractures (limb XRT, chronic GVHD from BMT)
Ankle oedema (from cardiac, liver or renal disease; see above)
Bony (tibial) tenderness (marrow relapse of leukaemia)
Neurological examination • Peripheral neuropathy (vinca alkaloids; usually reversible; test ankle and knee jerks and sensation to document this) • Delayed relaxation of ankle jerks (hypothyroidism from thyroid radiation, busulfan, BMT) Functional assessment if: • any asymmetry or contractures suggestive of radiation to limb, or • scars from resection of tumour with potential neurological or vascular complications, or • amputation: examine function with prosthesis; check how well it fits, any loosening, or infection
OTHER
Temperature chart: fever with intercurrent infection (myelosuppression with various agents) or (rare) radiation pneumonitis
Urinalysis • Blood (CPA-induced cystitis) • Proteinuria (radiation nephritis) • Glucose (corticosteroids)

ADR = Adriamycin; BMT = bone marrow transplantation; CNS = central nervous system; CPA = cyclophosphamide; GVHD = graft-versus-host disease; MIBG = radioactive iodine metaidobenzylguanidine; MTX = methotrexate; 6-MP = 6-mercaptopurine; 6-TG = 6-thioguanine; VCR = vincristine; XRT = radiotherapy.

nature of the wide range of tumours and their individual modes of relapse. Some of the findings mentioned will be relevant only to children still on chemotherapy. This approach may be found useful in assessing children in follow-up clinics. Several of the findings can only be ascertained fully by involving other specialised areas, such as neuropsychology and audiology. Neurocognitive dysfunction is the area that worries survivors of cancer and their parents the most. Survivors of (especially) ALL and CNS tumours, head and neck tumours requiring radiation therapy and patients treated with HSCT are most at risk. Cranial radiotherapy is the main risk factor for adverse neurocognitive outcome. In ALL patients, exposure to chemotherapy alone will still be associated with neurocognitive decline in two-thirds of patients. These children tend to have problems with executive function, memory, attention and concentration, processing speed and visual perceptual skills, which translates to inattention in class, inconsistent academic performance, not finishing homework, incomplete assignments, careless errors, and trouble with planning and organisation, with specific problems in the areas of mathematics, reading and spelling. It is usually in the later years of school that these sorts of problems become apparent, when rote learning is replaced with reasoning, and organisational skills and time management skills become of paramount importance. Simple educational accommodations may help (sitting at the front of the class, being allowed extra time to complete exams).

These features cannot be assessed in a short-case setting, but the examiners will appreciate the candidate mentioning the importance of these areas, after the physical examination is complete.

Chapter 15

The Respiratory System

LONG CASES

LONG CASE: Asthma

Recent advances in management have included: improved understanding of the importance of genetic and environmental interactions; the emerging approach of conceptualising asthma as a condition of varied phenotypes, with specific management approaches; improved understanding of the underlying pathophysiology of asthma; and clinical trials of a range of new treatment approaches. Risk factors for developing asthma are better understood.

It has become clear that inhaled corticosteroid (ICS) and long-acting beta-agonist (LABA) combination therapy is not appropriate to prescribe as first-line preventer therapy in children with asthma. Inappropriate use of ICS–LABA is associated with risks: 1. lack of efficacy, with a 2009 Cochrane review concluding little additional benefit (mainly improvements in spirometry) of LABAs over ICS alone; 2. adverse effects consisting of loss of effectiveness of short-acting beta-agonist (SABA) reliever medication and loss of effective prevention of exercise-induced asthma; and 3. a specific Arg[16] beta 2 receptor genotype, (homozygous for arginine at codon 16), found in 15% of asthmatic children, has been found to be associated with tachyphylaxis and higher susceptibility to exacerbations in asthmatic children receiving LABAs regularly—this genotype would put children taking LABAs at risk of SABAs not working efficiently when needed during acute wheezing episodes.

The *Australian Asthma Handbook* (AAH) recommends LABAs not be prescribed to children under 5 years, as does the Global Initiative for Asthma (GINA) guideline. A review of deaths from childhood asthma, 2004–2013 in New South Wales, noted 15 of the 20 children who died had been prescribed ICS–LABA combination therapy.

A proof-of-concept study in 2013 addressed personalised medicine based on genotype in these children with homozygosity for the susceptible Arg[16] genotype, using montelukast, instead of LABAs, as a 'tailored therapy'. Montelukast is known to have a range of side effects. They are commonly minor, such as pharyngitis, but more significant side effects such as sleep and behaviour disturbances and even neuropsychiatric symptoms have been documented. In line with this, some have proposed personalising treatment in adults, based on physiological and clinical features combined with biomarkers which predict clinical reactions to specific drugs. In keeping with this approach of treating based on phenotype, patients with a clinical phenotype characterised by atopy and reversible airway obstruction, for example, could use the biomarker of serum IgE to select omalizumab.

Although several genes have been reported to be associated with various asthma phenotypes, no single gene has emerged as responsible for asthma susceptibility. Other risk factors which increase the development of asthma include: positive family history; urbanisation; high-income lifestyle; sedentary lifestyle; high body mass index; 'stress'; low birth weight; prematurity; caesarean delivery; rhinitis; atopic sensitisation; ingestion of fast food, salt or trans-fatty acids; medications (paracetamol, antibiotics, beta agonists); or infection with rhinovirus, respiratory syncytial virus or pertussis.

Risk factors for life-threatening asthma may include persistent asthma, atopy, food allergies, history of anaphylaxis, low socioeconomic status and psychosocial difficulties.

In children who have died from asthma, risk factors have included suboptimal asthma control, attending hospital in the year before death, lack of written asthma action plan (AAP) or lack of adherence to an AAP. Poor asthma control is most often due to misdiagnosis, lack of adherence to medication and poor inhaler technique. The AAH notes that up to 90% of asthmatics have suboptimal/poor inhaler technique. Education can fix this.

There is an increasing number of medications targeting interleukin pathways; anti-interleukin antibodies include T-helper-2 (Th2)-directed monoclonal antibodies trialled in severe asthma in adults (e.g. benralizumab, dupilumab, lebrikizumab, mepolizumab [recently approved], reslizumab, tralokinumab and QGE031 [which has 50 times the affinity for IgE than omalizumab, the first approved humanised antibody for asthma treatment; see later this chapter]).

The long-case management aims remain: control of cough and wheeze, enabling the child to participate in normal daily activities, and educating both child and parents to manage asthma within the family's lifestyle. One should not underestimate an asthma long case, as important issues could be omitted such as: the child's technique of using aerosols, spacers and peak flow meters; what treatment is taken during holiday trips to remote areas in a severe asthmatic with previous life-threatening episodes; whether the adolescent is actually taking his or her recommended inhaled steroids twice daily (or at all); or whether he or she smokes actively.

History

PRESENTING COMPLAINT

Reason for current admission.

SYMPTOMS

Dyspnoea, wheeze, cough, tightness in the chest, exercise tolerance (last in races?), nocturnal symptoms (cough, wheeze, wakening), morning symptoms (tightness, wheeze), use of bronchodilators, viral upper respiratory tract infections, cyanosis, syncope. Provide a detailed expansion of important or specific symptoms; for example, for cough, note duration, nature (e.g. productive/loose), frequency, timing (day/night), effects (vomiting, awakening, family disruption), sputum (amount, colour, blood), associated symptoms (fever, wheeze, shortness of breath, symptoms of allergic rhinitis, upper airway obstructive symptoms such as snoring and obstructive sleep apnoea), responsiveness to beta-2 agonists/ antibiotics, any lessened effect of beta-2 agonists after starting LABAs.

PATTERN OF EPISODES

Frequency of attacks (infrequent [less than every 4–6 weeks] or frequent [more than every 4–6 weeks], episodic, chronic), control (severity; e.g. how often needing bronchodilators or oral steroids at home—once patients are taking preventers, it is preferable to talk about asthma 'control' rather than 'severity'), time of year (perennial, seasonal), diurnal variation, geographical variation.

PRECIPITANTS

Usual triggers: viral upper respiratory tract infection (URTI), environmental tobacco smoke, indoor wood fires, bushfires, household aerosols, gas heaters, weather, pollution, temperature change, humidity, cold dry air, exercise, allergic precipitants (animals [e.g. birds, furry animals such as cats], cockroaches, pollen, house dust mite, moulds, thunderstorms [airborne pollens, moulds]), food (e.g. Chinese food with MSG, pickled onions, juices, bee products [e.g. royal jelly], cold drinks), emotion, laughter, drugs (aspirin, other non-steroidal anti-inflammatory drugs [NSAIDs], beta blockers), echinacea, inhalants, perfumes, aerosols.

TYPICAL ACUTE EXACERBATION

Initial symptoms, precipitants, tempo of progression, rate of recovery, how child handles the illness, usual outcome, treatment required.

SOCIAL HISTORY

Disease impact: on child (school missed, limitation of activities, effect on development, education, behaviour, peer interaction); on family (financial issues such as costs of nebuliser, peak flow meters, oxygen cylinders, frequent hospitalisation, private health insurance; disruption of family routine); on siblings (changed holiday plans to allow nebulisation or hospital access for emergencies); personal or family smoking history; social supports (e.g. Asthma Foundation, local parent groups).

PAST HISTORY

Age at onset, diagnosis, the number of hospitalisations, treatment required, changes in clinical course, previous investigations, past complications (e.g. pneumothorax, intensive care admissions), any other clinical history that may suggest this is not just asthma (e.g. past history of severe respiratory illness in early life, developmental disability suggesting aspiration, history to suggest structural airway problem, productive cough as the main symptom), other atopic features and treatment of those (potential impact of treatment of allergic rhinitis on improving asthma control).

FAMILY HISTORY

Asthma, 'wheezy bronchitis', hay fever, allergies, eczema.

MANAGEMENT

Present treatment in hospital, usual treatment at home (inhaler/spacer; technique used), school, before exercise, previous medications tried, side effects (e.g. steroids), physical activity (e.g. swimming), holiday camps, compliance, alternative therapies tried, allergen avoidance, immunotherapy, dietary manipulation (appropriate or not), use of MedicAlert or Emergency ID bracelet, home monitoring with peak flow meter, crisis plan. Get the child to demonstrate his/her inhaler/spacer technique.

UNDERSTANDING OF DISEASE

By child and by parents. Ask about the degree of previous education (by doctors, by reading, by attending lectures). Ask whether they know the differences between preventers and relievers.

Examination

GENERAL IMPRESSION

Note any facial features suggesting Cushing syndrome (flushed cheeks, moon face) or atopy (swollen, discoloured eyelids; transverse nasal crease from 'allergic salute'). Check percentiles (decreased weight and height from disease or its treatment), Tanner staging (delayed puberty), sick or well, tachypnoea at rest, and use of accessory muscles. Note the skin (e.g. dry skin, atopic eczema at elbows, knees). Note any clubbing (e.g. obliterative bronchiolitis with bronchiectasis mimicking asthma). If cough is a current symptom, ask older patients if they can produce sputum, as it may indicate a complicating factor such as chronic bronchitis or bronchiectasis.

VITAL SIGNS

Pulse (rate, palpable paradox), blood pressure (side effects of steroids or beta-2 agonists), temperature (precipitating viral URTI).

RESPIRATORY EXAMINATION

1. Hands: tremor (beta-2 agonists).
2. Chest: deformity, increased anteroposterior diameter, Harrison's sulcus, expansion, tracheal position, apex position, palpable pulmonary valve closure, right-ventricular overactivity, percussion, auscultation.
3. ENT: ears—serous otitis media; nose—allergic rhinitis; pale, swollen, nasal mucosa, visible inferior turbinates, green/clear discharge; throat—tonsillar size, redness or exudate. Cervical nodes: lymphadenopathy.

GENERAL EXAMINATION

Steroid side effects (e.g. proximal muscle weakness, dermopathy, cataracts), accurate Tanner staging, and the remaining systems involved in the child with multiple problems.

Signs of life-threatening asthma

Candidates may be asked these in hypothetical scenarios. A mnemonic based on **S** and **C** is:

Silent child (can't speak)
Silent chest (poor air entry)
Cyanosis (or oxygen saturation < 90%)
Consciousness altered (due to hypoxia)
Collapse (exhausted)
Cardiac arrhythmia or **C**ardiac rate **s**low (pre-arrest)
Slow breathing (pre-arrest)

Diagnosis and investigations

Generally a clinical diagnosis; on occasion, some investigations may be warranted.

PEAK EXPIRATORY FLOW RATE (PEFR) MEASUREMENTS AND SPIROMETRY

PEFR monitoring is unreliable in children under 7 years and is easily manipulated by older children and adolescents. It adds little to noting symptoms and use of bronchodilators in those with severe asthma. Spirometry in those over 5 years can be measured, as this gives a more reliable and sensitive measure of airways obstruction. Symptom-based asthma action plans have been shown to be just as effective as those using symptoms plus PEFR monitoring.

CHEST X-RAY

This is only helpful if there is doubt about the diagnosis. Inspiratory and expiratory films may exclude an inhaled foreign body or other structural lesions. In acute asthma, the only indications are suspected pneumothorax or first-ever presentation (to exclude other diagnoses).

OTHER INVESTIGATIONS

Provocation inhalation challenge testing (mannitol, hypertonic saline, exercise challenge) may be useful to confirm airway hyperresponsiveness in cases with diagnostic difficulty, recurrent cough or recurrent breathlessness or exercise-induced dyspnoea. Exercise testing may also be useful to elucidate the cause of exercise-induced dyspnoea.

Tests to exclude other diagnoses that may present with cough or wheeze are as follows: 1. to exclude *cystic fibrosis* (CF)—sweat test, CF genotype; 2. to exclude *alpha-1-antitrypsin deficiency*—alpha$_1$-antitrypsin phenotype; 3. to exclude *infection*—sputum microscopy and culture, nasopharyngeal aspirate for viral pathogens; 4. to exclude *immune deficiency* states—full blood count, T-cell subsets, immunoglobulins, including IgG subclasses, vaccine antibody responses, complement levels, HIV testing; 5. to exclude *structural airway disease*—bronchoscopy, endobronchial ultrasound, CT 3D reconstruction, which may detect congenital tracheomalacia or bronchomalacia, especially if wheeze and hyperinflation commenced early in life, and are unresponsive to anti-asthma treatment; 6. to exclude *parenchymal pathology* such as bronchiectasis or congenital structural lung lesions—high-resolution CT (HRCT) scan of thorax; 7. to exclude *mediastinal or vascular lesions* (e.g. vascular ring)—helical CT scan or MRI with vascular reconstruction; 8. to exclude *occult cardiovascular disease*—electrocardiogram.

Treatment

ACUTE

1. *Position.* Sit child up, for ease of chest expansion and diaphragmatic excursion.
2. *Oxygen.* All children with acute severe asthma are hypoxic. Always check pulse oximetry. The aim is maximum inspired oxygen; keep the SaO$_2$ above 90%.
3. *Beta-2 agonists* (e.g. salbutamol). Nebulised for severe, life-threatening asthma; for mild and moderate asthma, pressurised metered dose inhaler (pMDI) with spacer. For very severe asthma, continuous nebulised therapy (dose 0.3 mg/kg per hour; prevents rebound bronchospasm); for moderately severe cases, either intermittent nebulised therapy (dose 0.15 mg/kg per dose [to maximum of 5 mg]) or 6–12 puffs of pMDI (100 μg per actuation) via spacer, every 20 minutes, initially. If nebulised therapy is needed, the optimum volume of drug in the 'acorn' of the nebuliser is 4 mL, with the driving oxygen rate being 8 L/min; can give with ipratropium bromide (see below).
4. *Anticholinergics.* Ipratropium bromide augments the actions of beta-2 agonists. The inhalation solution concentration is 250 μg/mL, and unit dose vials come as 250 μg/mL, the dose being 0.25–1 mL every 4–8 hours, or 4–8 puffs pMDI (20 μg per actuation) via spacer; it can be given (with salbutamol) every 20 minutes for three doses initially, then continued at 4–6 hour intervals.
5. *Corticosteroids (CS)* (oral prednisolone, IV hydrocortisone or methylprednisolone). Used in all moderate to severe episodes; decreases morbidity. A 3-day course usually suffices, using prednisolone 2 mg/kg as an initial dose, and then 1 mg/kg for further daily doses. The treatment for any longer duration should be slowly weaned, the main reason to wean is to prevent rebound in those with more persistent asthma; it is now accepted that oral steroids can be given for up to 2 weeks without the need

to wean to avoid adrenal suppression. Studies have failed to show any additional benefit of oral steroids in preschool children with mild to moderate viral-induced wheezing.

6. *Intravenous magnesium sulfate.* An initial bolus of magnesium sulfate 50%: 0.1 mL/kg (50 mg/kg) over 20 minutes, then an infusion of 0.06 mL/kg per hour (30 mg/kg) with serum drug level goal 1.5–2.5 mmol/L. Magnesium sulfate has been shown to be effective and safe in acute severe asthma in children. It is worth considering in a child with refractory asthma, with impending respiratory failure.

7. Other medications
   a. *Intravenous beta-2 agonists.* If nebulised therapy is not working, when inspiratory flow rates are very low, or the need for high-flow oxygen precludes nebuliser. An initial salbutamol bolus is followed by an infusion, incrementally increased until there is a good response. Toxicities: hypokalaemia, tachyarrhythmias, metabolic acidosis.
   b. *Theophylline preparations.* These are used less, due to concerns regarding efficacy and toxicity. There is a narrow therapeutic/toxic margin. Toxicities include vomiting, arrhythmias and, in cases of inadvertent overdosage, intractable seizures. IV aminophylline still has a use in the child not responding to other treatments in the paediatric intensive care setting.
   c. *Intravenous adrenaline.* 'Back to the wall' treatments include IV adrenaline ('God's own inotrope') and *isoprenaline*.
   d. Non-conventional therapies in acute severe asthma include helium–oxygen, general anaesthesia with halothane or ether, extracorporeal membrane oxygenation (ECMO) or even bronchial lavage.

8. *Non-invasive positive pressure ventilation (NIPPV), also called bilevel positive airway pressure (BiPAP).* Safer than intubation and mechanical ventilation, BiPAP is a combination of inspiratory positive airway pressure (IPAP) and expiratory positive airway pressure (EPAP, also called CPAP or PEEP). The IPAP component augments inspiratory effort, decreases work of breathing and increases tidal volume; the EPAP component decreases resistance to air flow, inflates the lungs, decreases the work of the respiratory muscles and recruits the expiratory muscles. This can reverse deterioration such that children will request it once they have experienced it. Bronchodilators can be nebulised through the circuit. BiPAP has two levels of support, a higher level during inspiration and a lower level during expiration.

9. *Intubation and mechanical ventilation.* A last resort. Indications are respiratory arrest, extreme fatigue or relentless hypercapnia. A treacherous path, with morbidity risks including barotrauma, gas trapping (compromised cardiac function), dysrhythmias, atelectasis and nosocomial pneumonia. Strategies to minimise these include: initial rapid sequence induction, oral intubation; sedation and paralysis; permissive hypercapnia; minimal positive end expiratory pressure (PEEP); prolonged expiratory time; low rate; and limitation of peak inspiratory pressure (PIP).

PREVENTATIVE

1. Modification/avoidance of precipitants

The use of beta-2 agonist or cromolyn before exercise, initiating regular inhaled therapy at home at the onset of viral URTIs. Avoid cigarette smoke (active and passive) and known allergens. House dust mite is a problem, with a Cochrane review concluding that none of the methods of house dust mite avoidance have proven clinical benefits for the patient.

2. Inhaled corticosteroids (ICS): fluticasone propionate (FP), budesonide (BUD), hydrofluoroalkane-beclomethasone dipropionate (HFA-BDP), ciclesonide (CIC), mometasone (MOM)

ICS are the mainstay of treatment in persistent asthma. FP, BUD and BDP are used in most countries; the newest ICS are CIC and MOM. CIC has been available in Australia since 2008; MOM is available in the UK and the US. Concerns regarding side effects centre around hypothalamic–pituitary–adrenal (HPA) axis suppression and effects on linear growth. To evaluate the risks, the equivalent corticosteroid dosing must be appreciated, as follows, from least to most potent: BUD 200 microgram = BPD-HFA 100 microgram = FP 100 microgram = CIC 80 microgram. The most appropriate dosage is the lowest that gives symptom control.

Suggested initial doses are 400 µg/day for BUD, 200 µg/day for FP or HFA-BPD, or 160 µg/day for CIC, then back titrate the dose to the lowest dose that maintains control. If these doses are insufficient, then step-up medication options include increasing the ICS, adding a leukotriene antagonist (especially for those with exercise-induced symptoms), or adding a LABA (being aware of all the risk factors associated with LABA use, and only for those 6 years or over).

ICS side effects are minimal in doses below 200 µg of FP or equivalent daily in children over 5, for periods of at least 24 months. If doses of 200 µg or above are used, side effects may include short-term growth suppression (at 400 µg, a decrease in linear growth of 1.5 cm per year; reversible) and adrenal suppression. Approximately 36 µg/kg per day of BUD will cause some HPA axis suppression.

Clinical adrenal suppression has been described in children receiving over 400 µg (FP equivalent) ICS daily, presenting with hypoglycaemia. Most cases of adrenal crisis have been associated with high doses of fluticasone. At higher doses, add-on agents (such as leukotriene modifiers [LTMs]) should be used.

Once the dosage exceeds 400–500 µg (FP equivalent) daily, side effects increase but the clinical effect does not: it plateaus (flat dose–response curve). ICS given as pMDI should always be given through a spacing device (increases the amount delivered to airways and decreases oral candidiasis from pharyngeal deposition from the aerosol).

After taking ICS, children should rinse the mouth and spit (can do when cleaning teeth); this decreases topical side effects such as oral candidiasis, but not systemic absorption as this is due to pulmonary deposition. ICS potential side effects include decreased bone mineralisation and cataracts.

Ciclesonide is taken as a prodrug, des-ciclesonide, which is converted to the active drug mainly by the lungs; it has high topical potency, very low systemic bioavailability and minimal systemic levels. It is given as once daily dosing. Mometasone has similar potency to FP (double that of BUD), and also can be given once daily.

3. Cromones: sodium cromoglycate, nedocromil sodium

These are effective in 70% of asthmatic children; and useful as first-line preventers, for exercise-induced asthma, as steroid-sparers or for asthmatic cough (nedocromil is particularly useful here). They are now not commonly used because of problems with clogging of inhalers (as the CFC-free formulation is stickier than the original) and because of the advent of montelukast as a daily oral non-steroidal alternative.

4. Leukotriene modifiers (LTMs)

There are two classes: 1. leukotriene receptor antagonists (LTRAs) (e.g. montelukast, zafirlukast); and 2. 5-lipoxygenase inhibitors (e.g. zileuton).

The main indications for LTRAs are mild persistent asthma or frequent intermittent asthma; the more frequently prescribed LTRA, montelukast sodium, is a specific inhibitor of the cysteinyl leukotriene CysLT1 receptor, and is used as an alternative to cromones or low-dose inhaled corticosteroids. LTMs can improve FEV_1 by 10–20%, with the greatest improvement within first 4 weeks of starting treatment. Given orally, once or twice daily, LTRAs are as effective as cromones or around 300 μg of beclomethasone (BEC). They are particularly useful in aspirin-induced asthma. Montelukast may protect against viral-induced wheeze in children with intermittent asthma, either as continuous treatment or as acute brief courses responding to respiratory tract infections.

There is evidence of efficacy of LTRAs as protection against exercise-induced bronchoconstriction, where it could be an alternative to SABAs; single-dose montelukast can be taken the night before, or at least 2 hours before, exercise. LTRAs can be used as steroid-sparers, and for prevention of exercise-induced bronchoconstriction, where they are superior to LABA. Well tolerated, montelukast is a chewable tablet, available in a 4 mg size (for ages 2–5) or a 5 mg size (for ages 6–15); the maximum effect is 12 hours after the dose is given. Specific side effects described include raised liver enzymes with higher than recommended dosage (zileuton), and 'unmasking' of eosinophilic vasculitis (Churg–Strauss disease) suppressed by steroids, becoming evident as steroids withdrawn. Recently, concerns have been raised about behavioural issues and depression with use of montelukast.

LTRAs have been approved by the PBAC for children 6–14 years as an add-on therapy for children with ongoing activity-related symptoms. LTRAs are second-line agents in mild asthma (if inhaled therapy is not viable) and can be given with a low-dose ICS in moderate persistent asthma. There is little evidence to support the use of LTRAs in children with moderate to severe asthma; these children are better treated with ICS therapy. Another potential role of montelukast is in coexisting allergic rhinitis, where it reduces symptoms of sneezing, itching and nasal congestion, although it may not be effective in controlling throat itch or tear secretions; intranasal corticosteroids remain the most effective pharmacological therapy for allergic rhinitis in children.

5. Long-acting beta-2 agonists (LABAs): salmeterol xinafoate, eformoterol fumarate dihydrate

These are *not recommended* for children *under 5 years* of age, at all, and even in combination with ICS, *ICS–LABA should **not** be used as first-line prevention*. LABAs are mentioned here, as inappropriate prescribing of them is widespread, despite the amount of information of concern about their use. In 2010, the American FDA concluded a review of the use of LABAs and recommended that: the use of LABAs for asthma be *contraindicated* in patients of all ages without concomitant use of an asthma-controller medication such as an ICS. It is well recognised that there is a potential for increased exacerbations and loss of SABA effectiveness if using LABAs, even in patients using LABA with ICS. Also, LABA use can be associated with loss of exercise bronchoprotection. Although not preventers, LABAs have been prescribed most often in combination medications with ICS, and as such make up a large percentage of the medications taken for 'prevention'. These are symptom relievers, providing bronchodilation for up to 12 hours.

Eformoterol has an onset of action similar to that of salbutamol, and faster than that of salmeterol: it is not used for acute asthma; it has been used for symptomatic poorly controlled asthma, especially nocturnal waking. Eformoterol was initially promoted as protective against exercise-induced asthma for up to 9 hours, but tachyphylaxis does occur. No child should receive LABAs without ICS. For breakthrough symptoms, or as a prophylaxis against exercise-induced asthma, SABAs are preferred. Montelukast is superior to LABAs in terms of protection against exercise-induced bronchoconstriction.

6. Combination therapies

As above, these are mentioned for completeness.

ICS + LABAs: fluticasone propionate (FP) + salmeterol xinafoate (SX); budesonide (BUD) + eformoterol fumarate dihydrate (EFD)

In Australia, these are available as follows:

- FP dose/SX dose (μg)—Accuhaler (powder for inhalation): 100/50, 250/50, 500/50. SX dose fixed (50); FP dose varies. FP dose/SX dose (μg): pMDI 50/25, 125/25, 250/25; SX dose fixed (25); FP dose varies.
- BUD dose/EFD dose (μg)—100/6, 200/6, 400/12 (not recommended under 18). These combination medications should not be used as first-line prevention in children.

7. Theophylline

This has anti-inflammatory effects and is used in low doses as add-on treatment, which significantly reduces the concerns over side effects. There is still evidence for efficacy in low doses.

8. Omalizumab

This is a murine recombinant monoclonal humanised antibody that blocks IgE (and skin allergy tests in atopic patients), which suppresses early- and late-phase allergic responses (EPR and LPR) and sputum eosinophilia. It is given as a subcutaneous injection, 2- to 4-weekly, for an extended period. It is known to be effective in the treatment of allergic rhinitis, and is being assessed for therapy and prevention of anaphylaxis, food allergy and atopic dermatitis.

In asthma, it improves symptoms and reduces the need for ICS. It can be considered in children requiring unacceptably high doses of ICS or oral CS, or those with CS-induced side effects. A disadvantage is its expense, and the dose being based on IgE levels makes it impractical in patients with very high IgEs.

9. Other treatments

Tiotropium is a long-acting anticholinergic drug, and has been widely used for chronic obstructive pulmonary disease (COPD). It may be given once daily via a soft mist Respimat inhaler (dosage: two inhalations of 2.5 μg), or as a dry powder via a HandiHaler device (dosage: 18 μg per inhalation). There is evidence supporting its use in asthma in adults. The main side effect is dry mouth.

There have been anecdotal reports in the use of anti-inflammatory drugs (AIDs) and immunomodulator approaches. It has been noted that asthma symptoms in children with cancer are less with chemotherapy. *Methotrexate* and *intravenous gamma globulin* have been used in very problematic asthmatics.

SMOKING

Cigarette smoke has emerged as having adverse effects at multiple levels, not just through maternal smoking in pregnancy, but with a separate and additional risk of paternal smoking, plus childhood smoking increasing adolescent asthma. The effects of exposure to tobacco smoke, the most important environmental factor that can adversely affect the asthmatic population, are largely determined by whether children have a particular glutathione-S-transferase (GSTM1) genotype.

Adverse effects (increased risk of development of asthma and wheezing) after in utero exposure to tobacco products are determined largely by the GSTM1 null genotype being present. An increased prevalence of asthma related phenotypes does not occur in children exposed in utero to tobacco smoke who possess the GSTM1+ genotype.

DELIVERY METHODS

The child must have an age-appropriate mode of drug delivery. Most anti-asthma drugs can be given by pMDI + spacing devices ± mask; pMDI + spacing devices ('spacers') have replaced nebulisers in all but life-threatening asthma. The breathable fraction of an aerosol represents that part which is deposited in the small airways and alveoli, corresponding to particle sizes (termed the 'mass median aerodynamic diameter' [MMAD]) of between 0.5 and 5 µm.

SPACERS

The delivery of inhaled medications is ideally via spacer. Spacers can be used at all ages. Small-volume (150 mL) spacers with face masks (e.g. AeroChamber, Breath-A-Tech) are useful in young infants and children up to 4 years. Large-volume (750 mL) devices (e.g. Volumatic, Nebuhaler) are ideal for those over 4. They are very useful and effective in acute severe asthma if no nebuliser is available; can give 6–12 puffs pMDI via spacer, on the way to hospital. Three important points in the daily use (not rescue use) of a spacer are as follows:

1. Load with one puff pMDI at a time.
2. Allow 30 seconds (timed) for inhalation of drug from the loaded spacer.
3. Do not clean the spacer more than once a month, unless the valve 'clogs up', as cleaning or actively drying with a cloth or paper can cause electrostatic charge on the inside of the spacer, to which the minimally charged medication particles of the pMDI 'stick'.

It is worth cleaning the spacer after a URTI or LRTI. In short, 'one puff, 30 seconds; don't clean it until you have to'. When cleaning is needed, use detergent and leave to air dry.

NEBULISER THERAPY

This remains the treatment of choice in life-threatening severe asthma. There are still parents who prefer their child under the age of 2 years to have nebuliser therapy, as they find it more effective, or because their child struggles with spacers, or because they do not wish to wake a sleeping child who needs treatment. Less than 10% of the dose in the nebuliser reaches the lungs. The particle MMAD usually is 1 to 5 µm.

DRY POWDER INHALERS (DPIs)

These devices may use capsules in an Aerolizer (eformoterol) or be breath-activated such as the Accuhaler (salmeterol, salmeterol plus fluticasone, fluticasone) or the Turbuhaler (terbutaline sulfate, budesonide plus eformoterol, budesonide, eformoterol). These are useful from 8 years of age, but only 10–20% reaches the lungs.

An inspiratory flow of at least 30 L/min is needed to disperse the medication adequately to reach the lungs. The particles generated have MMADs ranging from 1 to 2 µm.

PRESSURISED METERED DOSE INHALERS (pMDIs)

These devices are the most widely used, releasing their drug at speeds of 30 m/sec, as particles with MMADs of 2 to 4 µm. Standard pMDIs (salbutamol, ipratropium bromide, beclomethasone, ciclesonide, fluticasone propionate, sodium cromoglycate, nedocromil sodium, salmeterol plus fluticasone, budesonide plus eformoterol) can be used alone in children over 8 years, but only 10–20% reaches the lungs. Standard pMDIs should always be used with spacers, as this can triple the amount of drug delivered. Breath-activated pMDIs including the Autohaler (salbutamol, beclomethasone) can automatically administer the dose on commencement of inspiration.

The development of pMDIs with hydrofluoroalkane (HFA) propellants, introduced in accordance with the Montreal Protocol to protect the ozone layer, have led to smaller size of aerosol droplets with smaller MMADs and improve the deposition to the lung of the drugs. The minimum inspiratory flow rate needed to use a standard pMDI without a spacer is 20 L/min.

Optimum management for the child

The Australian National Asthma Campaign set out a six-point plan in 2006 as follows: 1. assess asthma severity; 2. achieve best lung function; 3. maintain best lung function—avoid trigger factors; 4. maintain best lung function with optimal medication; 5. develop an action plan; and 6. educate and review regularly. This plan still holds, but has been updated and expanded. In keeping with these principles, note the following:

1. Every child should have a written asthma treatment program, fully explained, and an appropriate crisis management plan.
2. Every child requires regular monitoring of his or her disease and its treatment, plus the complications of each, including growth (failure of linear growth can be due to undertreatment, or to overtreatment with steroids). Other treatment complications should be sought: tremor; hyperactivity (SABAs, LABAs); Cushingoid features (ICS, oral steroids); nausea, vomiting (theophylline).
3. Every child should be assessed for any inadequacy in current treatment, suggested by the following:
   a. Frequent waking to use inhaled bronchodilators.
   b. The need for inhaled treatment immediately upon awakening.
   c. Evidence of bronchospasm during physical activity, and limitation of activity.
   d. Using more than one pMDI per month.
   e. Conversely, using less than one pMDI per 3 months (non-compliance), particularly preventative therapy.
   f. Using SABAs more than three times a week for relief of symptoms.
   g. Time off school/work.

COMMON MANAGEMENT ISSUES

In the long case, the medical therapy may well be adequate, and the 'big opening' for discussion may be social and psychological issues related to asthma. The following headings include many of the more common problems encountered.

IS CONTROL OPTIMAL AT HOME?

The child should be able to participate in all ordinary daily activities. The symptoms outlined above should be sought, and the treatment considered with respect to the child's age and ability. Maintaining physical fitness with exercise (e.g. swimming) and the treatment of exercise-induced asthma are very important. Allergen avoidance and removal from exposure to cigarette smoke also should be addressed, if relevant.

ARE THERE ANY UPPER AIRWAY ISSUES?

Allergic rhinitis can contribute to poor asthma control, and treating this can improve control. Ask about symptoms such as runny nose, blocked nose, sneezing, itchy eyes, runny eyes, throat clearing, hoarse voice, mouth breathing, halitosis, pain/pressure over sinuses, loss of sense of smell, coughing after first lying down at night, headaches, poor sleep or snoring. Management may include allergen avoidance and pharmacological treatment. For continuous treatment, intranasal corticosteroid (INCS) is the treatment of choice. Intranasal mometasone, fluticasone, budesonide and triamcinolone do not have a significant effect on the hypothalamic–pituitary–adrenal (HPA) axis. Treating the coexisting allergic rhinitis can improve asthma control significantly. Obstructive sleep apnoea (OSA), from whatever cause, including allergic rhinitis, can contribute to poor asthma control and successful treatment of this may aid in asthma control. See the long-case approach to OSA in this chapter.

IS THE CRISIS PLAN APPROPRIATE?

Is a nebuliser, or spacer, available for emergencies? How far away is the local doctor (is there a nebuliser there)? Where is the nearest ambulance station? Where is the nearest hospital? Has this child's asthma received appropriate priority triage in the past (both for ambulance and the department of emergency medicine at the nearest hospital)? The candidate should stress the importance of ensuring appropriate triaging of this child with severe asthma. Does the disease severity warrant home oxygen, subcutaneous terbutaline or adrenaline? Do the parents know when to 'bail out' nebulising at home, and bring the child to the hospital? Parents should know to seek medical aid if they are worried by their child having a bad attack, if the child needs beta-2 agonists 2-hourly, if wheezing is not settling and continuing for over 24 hours, if symptoms worsen quickly or there is little relief from beta-2 agonists.

IS THERE ADEQUATE EDUCATION OF THOSE INVOLVED?

This includes education of the child, parents and teachers:
1. *The child.* Should know to take beta-2 agonist before exercise.
2. *The parents.* Need to understand the treatment and know when to initiate more frequent treatment; how to monitor the child. Do they understand that the child should not avoid sport at school? Are they aware of the prognosis?
3. *The teachers/school.* Is a pMDI with spacer available to the child at all times? Do teachers appreciate the need for treatment? Do sports instructors inappropriately exclude the child from games?

WHAT IS THE MAIN WORRY OF THE PARENTS?

Uncertainty regarding the nature and outcome of asthma, effects on schooling and home management of acute exacerbations are common causes for parental anxiety. Sometimes their fears are based on hearing about a severely affected patient, and then incorrectly extrapolating this to their child. The management of these parents is through education. However, in other children the approach is quite different. The risk of dying can be the major concern (and a realistic one) of the mother of a 10- to 14-year-old steroid-dependent asthmatic, who is exactly the sort of patient you may encounter in the examination. This issue should be addressed. In children with life-threatening asthma, the crisis plan must be clear, with consideration given to home oxygen, parenteral treatment, wearing an identification bracelet with medical details and moving closer to the hospital.

IS THERE A PROBLEM WITH ADHERENCE TO TREATMENT?

Adherence to treatment in adolescence is often a problem, and there may also be parental concern about long-term corticosteroid usage, which can lead to non-adherence on their behalf. The added risk of smoking induced by peer pressure or of medication avoidance is not an uncommon management problem. Another compliance issue is the parents' almost invariable inability to stop smoking or, in many cases, even smoke away from the child, despite constant requests. This has been documented by testing the urine of the child for cotinine (a metabolite, and anagram, of nicotine) levels before and after education about smoking. The other point to explore is the responsibility of care—whether it belongs predominantly to the patient or parent—as this is a key issue in adolescence.

IS THERE AN INAPPROPRIATE AMOUNT OF SCHOOL BEING MISSED?

If long periods of school are being missed, the reason may not just be hospitalisation, and this area should be explored. There can be parent–child interdependence, or school avoidance, related to asthma. Parents not infrequently fear that school may aggravate the disease (related to exposure to viral illnesses, or assuming that rest at home is somehow beneficial). Treatment is planned around normal schooling.

IS THIS SEVERE REFRACTORY ASTHMA OR DIFFICULT ASTHMA?

Severe refractory asthma refers to severe asthma where alternative diagnoses have been definitively excluded, triggers are appropriately identified and compliance with treatment is good. Difficult asthma, however, refers to asthma that is still uncontrolled because of poor adherence to treatment, aggravating factors (commonly smoking), and comorbidities (such as obesity, OSA). Parents who smoke should be encouraged to quit at each medical interaction. The family's general practitioner is best placed to follow the National Smoking Cessation Guidelines for Health Professionals, and can prescribe nicotine replacement therapy. Convincing parents to quit for their children, or even for financial reasons, is challenging. Telling smoking fathers of asthmatic children about the well-recognised effect of smoking causing permanent erectile dysfunction (impotence being a marker of vasculopathy that predates coronary artery disease), can be persuasive. Telling smoking mothers about the well-recognised effect of smoking causing premature aging of the face can be persuasive also.

ARE SOCIAL SUPPORTS SUFFICIENT?

The family needs to be aware of the many supportive groups and services available (e.g. the Asthma Foundation), where to get printed information regarding asthma and the benefits and financial assistance to which they may be entitled, and should have access to a social worker to assist in these areas. Whether the family is coping, with the current supports, needs to be explored.

IS THIS A CASE FOR PSYCHOLOGICAL ASSESSMENT AND FAMILY THERAPY?

There is evidence that family therapy can be very beneficial in the management of asthma, particularly asthma control, in selected cases, where there are problems within the family that may be causing the child stress, which in turn makes the asthma worse. It is well recognised that psychosocial and emotional factors have a significant impact on asthma. A Cochrane review in 2005 described two studies that evaluated family therapy being used in addition to standard asthma therapy, and found evidence of family therapy reducing asthma symptoms.

USEFUL WEBSITES

- All candidates should read the *Australian Asthma Handbook*, which comprises national guidelines for asthma management; the National Asthma Council Australia website is excellent. For links to key articles/studies/videos see www.nationalasthma.org.au and www.nationalasthma.org.au/health-professionals/australian-asthma-handbook.

- A Quick Reference guide pdf can be found at: www.asthmahandbook.org.au/uploads/555143d72c3e3.pdf
- Asthma resources for parents can be found at: www.asthmaaustralia.org.au

LONG CASE: NICU graduate—Chronic lung disease/bronchopulmonary dysplasia (CLD/BPD)

Chronic lung disease (CLD)/bronchopulmonary dysplasia (BPD) in the neonatal intensive care unit (NICU) graduate is defined as an oxygen requirement beyond 36 weeks' post-conceptual age. The term 'CLD' is used interchangeably with the term describing the pathology of the condition, 'bronchopulmonary dysplasia' (BPD).

Currently (2017) neonates born at 23–26 weeks' gestation have a significantly improved rate of survival; this is 8–10 weeks more premature than the original babies with BPD. Lung injury mechanisms have altered. BPD as initially described (which will be termed 'old') occurred in moderately premature babies treated with pressure-limited time-cycled ventilators and a high oxygen concentration for significant time intervals. Since the late 1980s, with ubiquitous use of antenatal steroids, use of surfactant and the advent of gentler, non-invasive ventilating strategies ('gentilation'), a 'new' BPD has emerged.

The new BPD is not often seen in infants over 1500 g, but it still occurs, and may be becoming more frequent, in extremely premature babies, so a large number of children with BPD are available for long-case participation. Many have had postnatal steroid therapy for prevention and/or treatment of BPD. There is clear evidence that the risks of steroid therapy used postnatally in babies with BPD outweigh the possible benefits. 'Early' dexamethasone (before day 8) increases risks of cerebral palsy (CP), neurosensory disabilities, hypertrophic cardiomyopathy and gastrointestinal perforation; it is unclear whether 'late' dexamethasone has similar harms to these latterly described. It is well recognised that late dexamethasone can cause hypertension, hyperglycaemia and may increase retinopathy of prematurity (ROP).

Decreased dexamethasone use between 1997 and 2006 was associated with increased BPD incidence in babies born at 23–28 weeks' gestation. However, as the use of dexamethasone reduces the risk of BPD, despite the significant adverse effects profile, some authorities still recommend consideration of dexamethasone use, depending on the likelihood of developing BPD: **if the risk of BPD is above 60%, dexamethasone decreases the rate of death or CP**, but **if the risk of BPD is 33%, then dexamethasone significantly increases the rate of death or CP**.

Recent progress has been made in the understanding and management of BPD. In studies by the NeOProM collaboration (SUPPORT, BOOST and COT), evaluating oxygen saturation (SpO_2) targeting and effects on various outcomes including BPD and ROP, it has become apparent that **in babies of under 28 weeks' gestation, the SpO_2 target must be higher than 85–89%, as levels lower than this leads to increased mortality; the suggestion now is for targeting SpO_2 of 90–95%**. It has been hypothesised that hypoxaemic episodes could make these infants more susceptible to later death from causes such as BPD, pulmonary hypertension, necrotising enterocolitis or sepsis.

Of the many strategies aimed specifically at reducing the incidence of BPD, there are only two pharmacological therapies which have sufficient high-quality evidence to support use in extremely preterm babies, to prevent BPD: caffeine and parenteral vitamin A.

Caffeine is a methylxanthine. It decreases CNS effects of adenosine. It stimulates breathing by enhancing carbon dioxide sensitivity, increasing diaphragmatic activity and increasing minute ventilation. The Caffeine for Apnea of Prematurity (CAP) trial showed that caffeine decreased the risk of BPD.

If caffeine is started before day 3 of life, additional benefits are conferred, especially in babies without severe respiratory distress. Caffeine also improves neurodevelopmental outcomes at 18–21 months. Caffeine also decreases requirement for treatment for patent ductus arteriosus (PDA) (drug or surgical), and it decreases ROP.

Vitamin A includes a number of fat-soluble compounds including retinol and beta-carotene (provitamin). Vitamin A is involved in forming photosensitive visual pigment in the retina, growth of epithelial cells in the respiratory system, and in immune regulation. Vitamin A deficiency was found to contribute to development of BPD. In 1999, a large randomised controlled trial showed reduced BPD in extremely low birth weight babies treated with IM vitamin A for 4 weeks. Disadvantages include cost and need for intramuscular administration. An international study of oral vitamin A supplementation in extremely premature babies is planned.

In babies less than 1000 g, up to 30% develop BPD. It is not known how much of BPD is iatrogenic and how much is unpreventable. Pulmonary immaturity (yet to develop protectants: surfactants; antioxidants; proteinase inhibitors) is the number one risk factor for BPD; other risk factors include prolonged mechanical ventilation, high oxygen concentration, maternal factors (smoking, illicit drugs, malnutrition, infection), neonatal sepsis, fetal growth restriction, PDA, Caucasian race, male gender and family history of asthma. Some have termed BPD a 'neo-iatro-epidemic'.

'New' BPD occurs in the context of multi-hit insults to the developmentally immature lung (especially under 26 weeks' gestation), positioned between canalicular and saccular phases of lung growth (at 23–30 weeks). There is the intrinsic problem of developmental arrest of alveologenesis and vasculogenesis, with dysregulated angiogenesis, resulting in large simplified alveoli and dysmorphic lung vasculature, in addition to a premature anti-oxidant system, surfactant deficiency and a very compliant chest wall; these intrinsic qualities increase susceptibility to the noxious effects of extrinsic problems. These extrinsic problems include mechanical ventilation and ventilator-induced lung injury which include, especially, *volutrauma* (from overdistension), and also *atelectotrauma* (from insufficient tidal volume), *biotrauma* (from infection, inflammation), *rheotrauma* (from inappropriate airway flow) and *barotrauma* (from pressure, although this is of much less importance than volutrauma); these forms of trauma (mnemonic: **Bio BRAVo** for **Bio**trauma, **B**arotrauma, **R**heotrauma, **A**telectotrauma, **V**olutrauma) alter the integrated morphogenic program of pulmonary development. Other inhibitors of alveolarisation and lung growth include: oxygen toxicity; intrauterine, lung and systemic infections; and cytokine exposure. BPD is still the most prevalent sequel of preterm birth. Requirement for supplemental oxygen at 36 weeks' postmenstrual age (PMA) is the commonest accepted definition of BPD at present (2017).

More very premature babies are surviving, and more survivors will develop BPD. Premmie survivors with 'new' BPD, compared to survivors without BPD, have higher rates of neurological problems, including: 1. CP; 2. specific movement disorders; 3. poor fine and gross motor skills; 4. impairments in hearing, vision and visuospatial perception; 5. delayed development of speech and language (receptive and expressive); 6. lower cognitive abilities; 7. attentional impairments; 8. memory and learning problems; 9. difficulty with executive skills; and 10. behavioural problems.

Premmies are at increased risk of neurodevelopmental impairment, but BPD is an independent additional risk factor. Some aspects of this could be attributed to postnatal steroids, some to recurrent desaturation/hypoxia and some to poor growth. BPD is associated with global developmental impairment, the severity of which correlates with that of the BPD.

Around 50% of BPD survivors are re-hospitalised in the first 2 years of life. Rates of bronchial hyperresponsiveness are higher in BPD survivors than in ex-premmies of similar size and age without BPD until they enter school age. BPD survivors have more respiratory tract infections in childhood, and BPD survivors at 18 years have worse lung-function variables reflecting airflow than non-BPD ex-premmies.

BPD mostly occurs in infants under 30 weeks' gestation, with birth weights < 1500 g. BPD is a multi-system disorder; associated conditions include pulmonary hypertension, neurodevelopmental delay, hearing impairments and ROP. Survivors of BPD, at any age, have lower spirometry values reflecting airflow; the mean FEV_1 values in BPD survivors approximate the lower limit of the normal range of controls. However, these data do not reflect those with 'new' BPD.

Unfortunately, almost 30% of people born prematurely smoke as young adults, which causes a steeper age-related decline in lung function. BPD is no longer a disease of childhood, as BPD survivors may have obstructive lung disease that persists into adulthood. Lung abnormalities that may persist into adulthood include airway obstruction, airway hyperreactivity, bronchiectasis and emphysema.

The single most significant predictor of CLD developing is low gestational age. Complications of CLD may include pulmonary hypertension (if oxygenation not maintained), recurrent hospitalisation with lower respiratory infections such as RSV, and bronchial hyperreactivity. The lungs of a baby with CLD have low compliance, with increased work of breathing.

History

PRESENTING COMPLAINT

Reason for current admission: commonly a deterioration associated with an intercurrent viral illness, or related to other complications of prematurity.

PAST HISTORY

1. Pregnancy, gestation, delivery, birth weight, Apgar scores, reason for premature delivery.
2. Initial resuscitation required, when intubated, underlying respiratory diagnosis (e.g. hyaline membrane disease, meconium aspiration), duration of ventilation, continuous positive airways pressure (CPAP), oxygen requirement.
3. Complications of ventilation (e.g. air leaks, subglottic stenosis, tracheal stenosis, tube blockage), apnoeic episodes, associated problems (e.g. PDA, intraventricular haemorrhage [IVH], periventricular leukomalacia [PVL], ROP).
4. Drugs/treatments used (e.g. salbutamol, ipratropium bromide, theophylline, corticosteroids, diuretics, RSV intravenous immune globulin [RSV Ig], palivizumab).
5. Monitoring since extubation, discharge details (e.g. age, weight, treatment).
6. Hospitalisation details (frequency, duration, usual treatment).
7. Outpatient clinics attended (where, how often, usual tests: e.g. chest X-ray, pulse oximetry).
8. Any recent change in symptoms or management.

CURRENT STATUS

1. Symptoms:
   a. Respiratory-specific; for example, tachypnoea, poor feeding, poor weight gain, fatigue, wheeze, cough, fever, cyanosis, apnoea, respiratory noises, plus symptoms related to O_2 use (epistaxis, nasal problems: discharge, obstruction).
   b. Non-respiratory-specific for conditions that the child is at risk of: gastro-oesophageal reflux (GOR), vomiting, feeding difficulties, aspiration.

2. Home management; for example, nasal oxygen, nebulised bronchodilators, oral theophylline, diuretic (e.g. frusemide), antibiotics.
3. Status of other systems where ex-premmies have increased risk of dysfunction; for example, ears, eyes, development, renal, cardiac, gut from necrotising entero-colitis (NEC).

SOCIAL HISTORY

Disease impact on family, financial consideration (e.g. nebuliser, oxygen cylinders, oxygen 'concentrator'—actually a blender), social supports, understanding of disease, expectations for future, access to paediatrician, hospital, any exposure to tobacco smoke.

IMMUNISATION

Routine (what age given). Specific (RSV Ig; palivizumab).

Examination

Table 15.1 gives an approach to the cardiorespiratory examination (specifically) of the NICU graduate. It does not include looking for other complications of prematurity (e.g. IVH), but does include toxicities relating to ventilation and oxygen.

Table 15.1
An approach to the cardiorespiratory examination of the NICU graduate
GENERAL OBSERVATIONS
Parameters • Weight • Height • Head circumference • Percentiles
Sick or well, pallor, cyanosis, alertness, movement
Nutritional status: visual scan for muscle bulk, fat
Respiratory • Distress (tachypnoea, tracheal tug, intercostal, subcostal recession) • Audible wheeze • Stridor (subglottic stenosis, vocal cord damage from intubation) • Cough • Cyanosis • Oxygen cannula
CHEST
Inspection
Breathing pattern
Respiratory rate
Chest deformity • Pectus carinatum • Increased anteroposterior diameter (hyperinflation) • Rib rosary (vitamin D deficiency)

Table 15.1 (continued)
Scars • Previous tracheostomy • Intercostal catheters • Repair of patent ductus
Palpation • Tracheal position • Apex position • Palpable pulmonary valve closure • Right-ventricular overactivity
Percussion can be deferred until after auscultation, as it may cause crying in younger infants
Auscultation
Lungs • 'Air entry' • Breath sounds • Vocal resonance • Crackles • Wheezes
Heart • Loudness of second heart sound (pulmonary hypertension) • Murmur of PDA
Percussion • For hyperinflation, consolidation
After the above, palpate the liver for ptosis (hyperinflation) and percuss for liver span (hepatomegaly from congestive cardiac failure [CCF])
UPPER LIMBS
Hands: scars of previous intravenous cannulae
Nails • Clubbing • Cyanosis
Pulse • Rate • Paradoxus • Hyperdynamic (PDA) • Pulsus alternans (CCF)
Blood pressure: hypertension (renovascular hypertension due to umbilical catheter, corticosteroid use or renal dysfunction)
HEAD
Eyes • Nystagmus (ROP) • Visual acuity (ROP) • Fundi: ROP (and grading of this)
Nose: deformity due to prolonged intubation
LOWER LIMBS
Palpate for ankle oedema (CCF)
OTHER
Temperature chart (infection)

CCF = congestive cardiac failure; PDA = patent ductus arteriosus; ROP = retinopathy of prematurity.

Management

Adequate oxygenation (and nutrition discussed below) is the most important factor for growth and development. Home oxygen is usually administered via nasal prongs. Low-flow oxygen (less than 2 L/min) can be provided via various different-sized cylinders. All families must be supplied with cylinders: size E, which are small and portable, and size C, which are larger and to be kept at home.

Oxygen is needed if the child's PO_2 in air is below 60 torrs. The aim is for the oxygen saturation (SpO_2) to be between 90% and 95% in the awake and asleep phases. Aiming for higher levels may worsen lung disease, and does not necessarily improve long-term growth or development. Oxygen administration is associated with increased weight gain, decreased pulmonary hypertension, decreased SIDS-like events, and decreased morbidity and mortality. Home oxygen therapy avoids prolonged and expensive hospitalisation.

At discharge from NICU, the average requirement for BPD is low-flow nasal oxygen at 250–1000 mL/min. The median duration of oxygen requirement is 6–10 months. Weaning should occur very slowly, over about 12 weeks, guided by regular saturation monitoring. An intercurrent acute respiratory tract infection may require reinstitution of oxygen.

Increased oxygen is needed during increased activity, feeding and sleeping (rapid eye movement sleep is associated with increased activity and irregular breathing, and carries a risk of hypoxia), so that monitoring of these times indicates when the child is able to cope in air. Oxygen is discontinued first when awake, then eventually when asleep. These children may be admitted to hospital overnight, for oximetry off oxygen while asleep. If the saturation level is consistently below 95%, oxygen therapy is still required; if it stays at or above 97%, then oxygen can probably be discontinued. Alternatively, as an outpatient, a period of oximetry for one hour when awake demonstrating saturations consistently above 97% indicates that supplemental oxygen is no longer required. Once oxygen is discontinued, weight gain is watched closely over the ensuing few weeks to ensure that adequate growth is occurring. As above, note variation of acceptability of minimum SpO_2.

GROWTH AND DEVELOPMENT

Children with BPD are at high risk of associated neurodevelopmental and growth problems. Much of the child's energy expenditure is related to the work of breathing, and this contributes to failure to thrive unless nutritional supplementation to 120–150% of usual requirements is achieved. Motor delay is not uncommon (e.g. poor muscle bulk, general debility) and, if not associated with intellectual impairment, may improve with time. Developmental assessment (intellect, vision, hearing) is regularly performed to enable appropriate intervention.

NUTRITION

As mentioned above, adequate nutrition is of paramount importance. Tachypnoeic infants do not feed well, the time they take for a breastfeed or bottle being proportional to the severity of their BPD. As these children may need to avoid fluid overload, the quality of feed should be altered, not the quantity. Usual requirements are around 140–180 kilocalories (kcal) per kg per day, but the real test is whether the child grows, and these figures are guides only. Calorie supplementation may be achieved by increasing the caloric content of infant milk formulae to 24–32 kcal per 30 mL. Added calories may comprise increased measures of milk powder (extra scoops), glucose polymers, vegetable oil or medium-chain triglyceride oil. In breastfed infants, small-volume high-calorie supplements can be given. Calorie wastage must be avoided; this occurs when too many calories are given.

Reasons for 'difficult feeding' include oral aversion, volume or acid reflux, aspiration (especially when neurodevelopmental problems are present) and dysphagia. Another problem is the lack of oral intake early (while in NICU), with poor tolerance to and lack of interest in feeds, which may persist. Some children require feeding at night via gastrostomy (often with fundoplication), particularly infants with GOR. Nasogastric tube feeding is generally avoided (it can aggravate reflux and cause increased nasal problems), but is sometimes necessary. Provision of adequate vitamins and minerals (especially iron, folate and fluoride) is important. Supplemental oxygen can improve nutrition.

OBSTRUCTIVE AIRWAYS DISEASE AND BRONCHODILATORS

These patients have obstructive lung disease, but variable airway hyperactivity, and lack uniformity in their response to drugs. Many have hypertrophied lung smooth muscle and respond to bronchodilators (even when preterm) earlier than true 'asthmatics'.

Combinations of inhaled beta-2 agonists, ipratropium bromide and inhaled corticosteroids are widely used, with variable success. Most units try these medications for at least some weeks to ascertain efficacy. Despite the common usage, there is inadequate long-term data to recommend the use of any beta-agonist, or ipratropium bromide, in BPD.

FLUID BALANCE AND DIURETICS

These infants tend to accumulate interstitial lung fluid; fluid overload should be avoided. Fluid intake of up to 180 mL/kg per day are usually well tolerated. Diuretics may need to be used (especially in children with some degree of cor pulmonale). Diuretics may act as pulmonary vasodilators. Initially, frusemide with potassium supplementation is used for short periods. For longer-term use, hydrochlorothiazide and spironolactone may be used (fewer side effects than frusemide). Serum urea and electrolytes should be monitored to avoid side effects (hypokalaemia, hyponatraemia, metabolic alkalosis). Prolonged frusemide therapy (over 2 weeks) can cause renal calcification, detectable on ultrasound. Diuretics improve lung mechanics and oxygenation in the short term only; no long-term benefits have been demonstrated.

IMMUNISATION AND RSV IMMUNE PROPHYLAXIS

Routine immunisation is particularly important in these children. Often allowed to lag behind because of their prolonged stay in the NICU, immunisation should be given at the appropriate chronological age, uncorrected for prematurity. Some units use RSV Ig. Prophylaxis with IV or IM RSV Ig (which is very expensive) significantly decreases the incidence of RSV infection and subsequent hospitalisation by about 50%. It can be given on an individual needs basis on discharge from hospital, and then monthly during the peak RSV season.

The other preparation used for immune prophylaxis is palivizumab, a humanised RSV monoclonal antibody given intramuscularly. Infants with a gestational age below 28 weeks can benefit from prophylaxis up to 12 months of age, whereas infants with a gestational age of 29–32 weeks may benefit up to 6 months of age. Treatment is for children under 2 years of age who are still having oxygen, and is used in the anticipated RSV season for 4–6 months of the year.

AVOIDANCE OF TOBACCO SMOKE

Smoking in the house is forbidden if a baby is receiving oxygen, because of the fire hazard. However, exposure to smoke still occurs. Exposure to smoking increases pulmonary inflammation, worsens lung function, increases the risk of developing respiratory tract infections and increases the risk of cot death. Parents should be encouraged to stop smoking, but this is rarely successful, and this is a difficult issue. At the very least, parents should be encouraged to smoke outside of the house, well away from any verandah/patio or front or back doors, wearing some sort of jacket or shirt, and a hat, to decrease the deposition of tobacco smoke on the parents' own clothes, hair and skin, and then take off the hat and jacket, leaving them on a hook outside the house, and then wash their hands and face (and ideally clean their teeth) before going near the child.

SOCIAL ISSUES

The degree of psychosocial difficulty depends to some extent on the associated problems that the child has. If there is severe neurological impairment, there is a parental separation rate approaching 50%. There tend to be three phases after the initial discharge of the child from hospital: first, a 'euphoric' phase, which may last about 6 weeks; then a period of despair and exhaustion, lasting from around 6 weeks to 6 months post-discharge; and finally, the stage of acceptance. Another common problem is the 'vulnerable child syndrome', a parent–infant behaviour disorder that may include problems with feeding, difficulty separating from the mother, overindulgence and overprotection, leading to the child 'running the household'. This may be prevented by spending more time with the parents, educating them in potential problem areas that are well recognised, by normalising the management of the baby, and by normal and appropriate discipline.

ASSOCIATED APNOEA AND BRADYCARDIA

Children with BPD appear to be at higher risk of apnoea and sudden death than other infants. Some units provide monitors for the first few months after discharge home. Sleep laboratory studies may show unrecognised bradycardia/apnoea and may guide therapy (e.g. caffeine), but are not useful in prognosis. Adequate oxygenation by low-flow oxygen is the most important aspect to prevent unrecognised hypoxia and bradycardia.

OTHER PROBLEMS

Excluding the numerous other complications of prematurity, the other common problem that these children experience is that of intercurrent viral illnesses, which can become complicated by bacterial superinfection, which is life-threatening. Early institution of antibiotic therapy for respiratory infections is recommended. If these children become acutely unwell, with respiratory distress, the parents should have the child checked, preferably by a doctor familiar with them, or at the nearest hospital. They should be told to resist wanting to 'turn up the oxygen', or recommence it if discontinued previously.

PROGNOSIS

Most problems with BPD occur in the first year of life. Long term, most children with BPD have minimal functional abnormalities, mainly due to the increase in the number of alveoli that occurs from birth (20 million saccules at term; air/tissue interface 2.8 m^2), producing new alveoli up to 8 years old (300 million alveoli; air/tissue interface 32 m^2).

LONG CASE: Cystic fibrosis (CF)

This is a common long case and it is expected to be handled well. Cystic fibrosis (CF) is becoming an adult disease with, currently, some 50% of CF patients in Australia being adults. Survival continues to increase, with overall mean survival in Australia at the time of writing (2017) at around 42 to 50 years (males older, females younger). The median age of survival in Canada in 2013 was 50.9, compared to 31.9 in 1990. This improved survival is largely the result of standard care, intervening earlier and aggressively treating every respiratory exacerbation, optimised by the ability to eradicate *Pseudomonas* (in 1998, 44% of children were infected with *Pseudomonas*, versus 12% in 2007), the optimal use of mucolytics (dornase alpha, hypertonic saline 7%), utilising the anti-inflammatory effects of azithromycin, and recognition of the utility of improvements in infection control to prevent person-to-person transmission of organisms.

The most exciting recent advance in CF management has been the development of cystic fibrosis transmembrane conductance regulator (*CFTR*) modulators. In 2015 a landmark study by Wainwright et al., published in the *New England Journal of Medicine*, showed that treatment with Lumacaftor and Ivacaftor, in combination, of patients with CF homozygous for *Phe508del-CFTR*, could decrease the rate of pulmonary exacerbations by one-third, decrease the need for hospitalisation and decrease the need for antibiotics.

CF is associated with airway infection from the first few months of life and a range of recognised pathogens have been identified from bronchoalveolar lavage (BAL) samples in very young children, most commonly including: *Staphylococcus aureus*; *Pseudomonas aeruginosa*; *Haemophilus influenzae*, *E. coli* and *Streptococcus pneumonia*. These organisms continue to be found in respiratory samples in older patients along with a range of organisms such as *Burkholderia cepacia* complex, *Achromobacter xylosoxidans*, *Stenotrophomonas maltophilia*, *Klebsiella* species, *Enterobacter* fungal species and non-tuberculous mycobacteria.

Discussion in the long case could well centre around aspects other than lung disease, as longer survival has led to more patients developing complications such as cystic fibrosis-related diabetes (CFRD), CF liver disease, adverse effects of medications including drug allergies, complications of venous access, mental health issues and musculoskeletal disorders.

Genetics

CF is inherited as an autosomal recessive condition. CF is caused by mutations in the cystic fibrosis transmembrane conductance regulator gene (CFTR); the locus is on the long arm of chromosome 7 (7q31.2), and the protein is called CFTR. Over 2000 different mutations in the CFTR gene are known to date (2016); almost all are point mutations or small (1–84 base pair) deletions although not all of them have functional consequences with approximately 250 variants having evidence for disease-causing effects. The CFTR gene comprises 27 coding exons spanning over 250 kb on the long arm of chromosome 7. CFTR is a cyclic-AMP-regulated chloride (and bicarbonate) channel on the apical surface of epithelial cells. CFTR is the only ATP binding cassette (ABC) transporter that acts as an ion channel. The deficiency of CFTR function leads to abnormal regulation of chloride channels, and reduction in anion permeability, and decides the phenotype of the epithelial cells. Lack of CFTR (the main epithelial ion regulator) causes decreased ion conductance with ionic dysregulation. Dehydration of both mucus and the airway surface liquid may occur and result in disturbance of mucociliary clearance and an increased risk of airway infection and inflammation associated with progressive lung disease. The most common mutation worldwide is the *Phe508del-CFTR*, where there is deletion of phenylalanine at the 508th amino acid within the CFTR protein; this accounts for 30–80% of mutant alleles, depending on the ethnic group.

CFTR mutations have been categorised into six classes; however, many mutations may have features of different classes. For example, *Phe508del-CFTR* is regarded as a Class II mutation but it also has reduced gating and features of Class III and it is less stable so has features of Class VI (see below).

- Class I mutations result in no functional CFTR protein production, and are associated with nonsense, frameshift or splice junction mutations (e.g. *Gly542X*: 2.5% of cases).
- Class II mutations are associated with *protein trafficking defects* and almost no CFTR protein expression at the epithelial cell surface, and are associated with missense mutations and amino-acid deletions (e.g. *Phe508del*: 70% of cases in Australia).
- Class III mutations are gating mutations with defective regulation of CFTR and while CFTR is present at the apical surface of epithelial cells, it functions very poorly (e.g. *Gly551Asp*: 4% of cases worldwide and around 6% in Australia).
- Class IV mutations are associated with *altered conductance of the CFTR chloride channel* (e.g. *Arg117His*: 3% of patients with CF).
- Class V mutations are associated with reduced quantity of normal CFTR protein due to *aberrant splicing of CFTR* (e.g. *Ala455Glu*).
- Class VI mutations are associated with *decreased stability of normal CFTR*, (e.g. *120del23* or *4326delTC*).

Different mutations are more common in different countries. It is not necessary to be homozygous for the same mutation to have CF. The most common defects can be detected within hours by polymerase chain reaction (PCR). Gene mutations are weakly correlated with clinical severity: genotype/phenotype correlations are strongest for pancreatic insufficiency (PI), with patients homozygous for the *Phe508del* mutation being almost always pancreatic insufficient (99%).

Classes I, II and *III* mutations are severe mutations as they lead to no functional CFTR protein at the epithelial cell surface and patients with two severe mutations are more likely to have PI and more severe disease.

Classes IV, V and *VI* mutations are partial function mutations with reduced CFTR function. Patients with these mutations are more likely to be pancreatic sufficient and have milder disease.

The gene frequency varies across different populations but in Caucasian populations is 1 in 25, giving an incidence of around 1 in 2500. In contrast, incidence in African-Americans is 1 in 15 000 and in some Asian populations approximates 1 in 31 000.

History
PRESENTING COMPLAINT

Reason for a current admission: often a combination of loss of weight, appetite and energy, and an increase in cough, sputum and school/work missed and a fall in lung function or concern regarding infection status and a plan for eradication treatment of a particular organism.

CURRENT STATUS

Respiratory disease

1. Symptoms: pulmonary exacerbations (intermittent worsening of usual respiratory symptoms), URTI symptoms, impaired exercise tolerance (important but relatively uncommon in children); cough frequency, severity (cough syncope extremely rare), nocturnal or exercise-induced wheeze or asthma, recent change in pattern; sputum volume, colour, blood and any recent change in these; fatigue, dyspnoea, wheeze, response to bronchodilators, peak flow pattern (limited value); need for home oxygen; chest pain; chronic sinusitis; glue ears; nasal polyps (nasal polyps produce symptoms of rhinorrhoea, nasal blockage, snoring and even occasionally have protruded from the nose).
2. Infective agents: acquisition of chronic infection with *Pseudomonas* aeruginosa is an important prognostic factor, with early chronic infection (under 5–6 years) of *Pseudomonas aeruginosa* especially mucoid phenotype being associated with increased morbidity and mortality, especially in females. Also, *Burkholderia cepacia complex* acquisition is important.
3. Past complications; for example, pneumothorax, moderate-to-large haemoptyses, allergic bronchopulmonary aspergillosis (ABPA).
4. Investigations; for example, sputum culture, chest X-ray, pulmonary function tests, overnight oximetry.
5. Home management; for example, exercise, airway clearance (frequency, type and by whom), device used (positive expiratory pressure [PEP] mask, flutter, vest and so on); nebulised antibiotics, saline, bronchodilators or dornase alpha; pMDIs (bronchodilators, ICS); oral antibiotic including use of oral azithromycin for anti-inflammatory modulation and reduction in pulmonary exacerbations or corticosteroids; venous port access for parenteral antibiotics.
6. Future therapy plans: use of antibiotics, oral or nebulised; corticosteroids; consideration of lung transplant, gene therapy, experimental therapies.

Gastrointestinal disease

1. Symptoms; for example, growth, weight loss, appetite, dietary history, stool pattern (oily, pale, bulky or offensive, blood, melaena), passing wind and burping (may not be popular, but can have an impact on kids at school), abdominal pain, vomiting, haematemesis, heartburn.
2. Past complications; for example, meconium ileus early surgical and especially important to document removal of bowel and risk of short gut, meconium ileus equivalent later (which is termed 'DIOS' [distal intestinal obstruction syndrome]), rectal prolapse, CF liver disease, portal hypertension, GOR disease, fibrosing colonopathy, gastrostomy.
3. Investigations; for example, faecal elastase (not affected by use of enzymes), liver function tests, hepatobiliary ultrasonography or rarely abdominal CT scan or Tc-99m scintigraphy.
4. Home management; for example, pancreatic enzymes, vitamins, salt tablets.
5. Future plans; for example, endoscopy, gastrostomy, sclerotherapy, liver transplantation.

Other systems

Symptoms, past complications including episodes of dehydration (which is a significant problem in warmer climates, and which increases the risk of pneumonia and DIOS), investigations, home management and future plans regarding diabetes mellitus, growth failure, pubertal delay and arthropathy.

PAST HISTORY OF CF

Initial symptoms, investigations and management prior to diagnosis, diagnosis (when, where, how), subsequent investigations and management, progress of the disease, hospitalisation details (frequency, duration, usual treatment), complications of the disease and treatment, outpatient clinics attended (where, how often, routine tests performed), any recent change in symptoms or management.

Immunisations (especially pneumococcal, influenza vaccines).

Venous access is a serious issue, especially as aggressive treatment now starts earlier. The complications of totally implantable venous access devices can be serious.

Allergy may be an important issue, with some children requiring desensitisation.

SOCIAL HISTORY

Disease impact on patient

Treatment regime, disruption of going to hospital, recurrent/permanent loss of: normal social life, being part of peer group, being part of family, freedom, independence, normal childhood, trust, self-esteem (impaired growth, development, may have short stature, delayed puberty, gastrostomy button, intravenous access ports, offensive flatus, cough, requirement for treatment [pancreatic enzymes, vitamins, bronchodilators], decreased ability for physical activity, stamina). By around 8–12 years, aware of differences from normal peer group, and shame and embarrassment can become very prominent. There is the question of 'Why me?' Other issues: seeing friends or relatives with CF deteriorating in hospital, requests for transfer to adult care, compliance (reluctant to take medications in front of peers), schooling (attendance, performance, teacher awareness of disease and its treatment, peer interactions), employment prospects, limitation of activities of daily living (including sport), depression (inevitability of death), consideration of marriage, and prevention (smoking).

Fertility must be discussed: What has been said and to whom? Many units normally talk with boys around 14 years of age and discuss all health-related issues, including normal sexual function, reduced ejaculate, and choices for the future with micro-aspiration sperm and IVF techniques. Smoking must be discussed. Alcohol is another discussion area for the pancreatic-sufficient children, as they have an increased risk of pancreatitis.

Disease impact on parents

Restricted social life, marriage stability, maternal depression, denial, fears for the future, requirement to stop smoking, financial considerations (medical treatment, food, travel, petrol, parking fees, awareness of benefits available, modifications of holiday plans), problematic parenting (overprotective or too lenient), knowledge of terminal nature of CF, time constraints of treatment regime, most treatment is organised/carried out by the mother.

Disease impact on siblings

Sibling rivalry, hostility, isolation, alienation, resentment, guilt ('survivor guilt'), concern, worry, effect of family's financial burden, genetic counselling. There are camps for siblings (e.g. CF sibling camps). A useful website is www.siblingsaustralia.org.au.

Disease impact on family unit

Factors that impact on family adaptation include the severity of the disease, the illness course, the financial costs, the stability of the family and their support network. Frequent coping styles include optimism, relying on self, humour, realistic appraisal of circumstances and maintaining normal lifestyle.

Social supports

Social worker (their role: advocacy, liaison with school, organising referrals, evaluating child protection risks), Cystic Fibrosis Association, community nurse, extended family, close friends, CF 'social network', respite from managing child, financial support.

Coping

Who attends with the patient, who gives treatment, confidence with management, parents' main concerns, degree of understanding of the disease, expectations for the future, understanding of prognosis (by patient and parent).

Access

To local doctor, paediatrician, CF clinic sister, Cystic Fibrosis Association, hospital.

FAMILY HISTORY AND GENETIC ASPECTS

Other members with CF; whether other siblings screened, more children planned, prenatal diagnosis (and subsequent management for positive result) discussed; patient's fertility, female patient's contraception, pregnancy risk—have these been addressed?

IMMUNISATION

Routine, early measles immunisation, gamma globulin for measles contacts, requesting yearly influenza vaccine.

Examination

The approach given in Table 15.2 assesses patients with CF for disease progression, severity and the current status of the disease. It looks particularly at clubbing, flap, chest deformity, cor pulmonale, nutrition, puberty, diabetes, chronic liver disease and hypertrophic pulmonary osteoarthropathy. Two very important signs are the cough and the sputum, and these may give a better indication of the state of the lungs than any other finding on physical examination.

Table 15.2
Examination of the child with cystic fibrosis
GENERAL INSPECTION
Position patient: standing, with adequate exposure, for a complete examination, but sensitive to the patient's modesty—although ideal, the patient being fully undressed (as stated in previous editions) is neither practical nor sensitive in most patients, and should not be encouraged
Parameters • Weight • Height • Head circumference • Percentiles
Sick or well
Pubertal status (delay)

Continued

Table 15.2 (continued)

Vital signs
- Respiration
- Pulse
- Temperature
- Urinalysis (glucose)

Nutrition
- Muscle bulk (protein) (e.g. biceps, quadriceps)
- Subcutaneous fat (e.g. mid-arm, subscapular)
- Pallor (anaemia)

Peripheral stigmata of CLD

Oedema (hypoproteinaemia)

UPPER LIMBS

Nails
- Clubbing
- Cyanosis
- Leukonychia (CLD)

Fingers
- Fingertip prick marks (BSL testing)
- HPOA

Palms
- Erythema (CLD)
- Crease pallor (anaemia)

Pulse
- Paradoxus (severity of airway obstruction)
- Alternans (CCF)
- Bounding (hypercarbia)

Flap
- Hypercarbia
- Liver failure (rare)

Joints: arthropathy

Skin
- Bruising or petechiae (CLD, vitamin K deficiency)
- Spider naevi (CLD)
- Scratch marks (cholestasis)

Muscle: bulk (palpate, if not done already)

Axilla: hair, odour (Tanner staging)

HEAD

Eyes
- Conjunctival pallor
- Scleral icterus
- Retinal venous dilation (hypercarbia)

Ears
- Secretory otitis media
- Hearing (aminoglycosides)

Table 15.2 (continued)

Nose: nasal polyps

Mouth
- Angular cheilosis
- Central cyanosis (lips, tongue)
- State of teeth, dental hygiene
- Oral thrush

Face
- Cushingoid (systemic corticosteroids)
- Acne and facial hair (pubertal status)

CHEST

Inspection
- Chest deformity: pectus carinatum, increased AP diameter (hyperinflation), thoracic kyphosis
- Scars: previous pneumothorax, bilateral lung transplant, venous access port (e.g. Port-A-Cath, Hickman)
- Tanner stage of breast development
- Harrison's sulcus
- Chest expansion

Cough: moist, productive, request sputum

Perform peak flow measurement if meter available (limited usefulness)

Palpation: tracheal position, apex position, palpable pulmonary valve closure, right-ventricular overactivity

Percussion for hyperinflation, consolidation

Auscultation (note: may be normal even in moderately severe CF)
- Air entry
- Breath sounds
- Vocal resonance
- Adventitious sounds
- Crackles
- Wheezes
- Loudness of second heart sound (pulmonary hypertension)
- Gallop rhythm (cor pulmonale)

ABDOMEN

Inspection
- Distension (poor abdominal musculature with protein–calorie malnutrition, ascites with CLD)
- Scars (e.g. gastrostomy, previous meconium ileus, hepatobiliary surgery for common bile duct stenosis, fundoplication)
- Venous access port (e.g. Infuse-A-Port)
- Prominent abdominal wall veins (CLD)
- Needle marks (diabetes mellitus)
- Tanner stage of pubic hair
- Striae (corticosteroids)

Palpation
- Liver ptosed (chest hyperinflation); liver edge—is it firm, or is it bumpy (cirrhotic)?
- Hepatomegaly (fatty liver with malabsorption or corticosteroid use, CCF with cor pulmonale)
- Splenomegaly (portal hypertension)
- Faecal masses (DIOS can present as a right iliac fossa mass)
- Herniae

Assess for ascites (fluid thrill, shifting dullness)

Examine genitalia
- Tanner staging
- Hydrocoele

Inspect anus for rectal prolapse

Continued

Table 15.2 (continued)
LOWER LIMBS
Inspection • Toe clubbing • Bruising (vitamin K deficiency, CLD) • Joint swelling (arthropathy)
Palpation: ankle oedema (hypoproteinaemia)
Gait examination • Peripheral neuropathy (vitamin E deficiency) • Cerebellar ataxia (vitamin E deficiency) • Proximal muscle weakness (corticosteroids)
(Note that clinically evident vitamin deficiencies are very rare in CF, so signs of vitamin A and D deficiencies are extremely unlikely to be seen)

BSL = blood sugar level; CCF = congestive cardiac failure; CLD = chronic liver disease; HPOA = hypertrophic pulmonary osteoarthropathy.

Investigations

DIAGNOSTIC

Neonatal screening

Most infants with CF are detected in this way in Australia at present (2017), as neonatal screening is now universal across Australia and New Zealand. Each Australian state performs this slightly differently, although all check immunoreactive trypsin (IRT) on the neonatal screening blood test, followed by gene analysis on the top 1% IRTs. Blood immunoreactive trypsin (IRT) levels are measured in the Guthrie blood sample. IRT levels in CF are 2.5–7.5 times the normal range. Samples with IRT levels above the 99th centile have genetic testing and the number of mutations tested varies between the different states in Australia. Making the diagnosis early in life does have a significant positive impact on prognosis.

The critical aspect is accurate diagnosis; it needs to be confirmed. Sweat tests should be carried out only in centres that do at least 50 per year (so private pathology laboratories may not be appropriate for this test). The diagnosis is based on two CF-causing mutations plus a positive sweat test, or consistent clinical features, or one mutation plus a positive sweat test. It is possible to have two mutations, but a normal sweat test and no clinical manifestations (except possible male infertility). Also, there can be difficult scenarios with borderline sweat test results. Two mutations alone does not equal diagnosis unless they are two recognised severe mutations; children with borderline sweats are at risk of CF-related disease over time and still need to be followed closely.

Sweat testing

The Gibson–Cooke classic technique requires 100 mg of forearm sweat obtained by pilocarpine electrophoresis. Many centres are now using pilocarpine iontophoresis to collect sweat and smaller volumes of sweat may be collected using this technique. Most patients with CF have a sweat chloride > 60 mmol/L, which is diagnostic. However, a small proportion of patients have sweat chlorides below this level, usually between 50 and 60 mmol/L (the equivocal range), and some will have a value in the forties. Understanding the genetic mutations carried by the patient will be important and this may require either more extensive genetic testing or sequencing of the *CFTR* gene. False-negative sweat results can occur in children with oedema. False-positive results can occur in children with malnutrition (e.g. due to coeliac disease or emotional deprivation), immune deficiency (e.g. AIDS, hypogammaglobulinaemia), eczema, adrenal insufficiency and hypothyroidism.

Other

Pancreatic stimulation testing can diagnose CF in cases with normal or borderline sweat tests; it will always reveal abnormal ductal function in CF. At diagnosis, patients need a faecal sample to check for faecal elastase, to document the presence and severity, or absence, of steatorrhoea. Eighty-five per cent of CF patients have fat malabsorption with pancreatic insufficiency (PI). Serum vitamin levels are checked early, as vitamin levels may be low and can be easily corrected. Vitamin E deficiency that persists over several months in early life and is not corrected may be associated with a small loss of IQ, and with newborn screening in place there is an opportunity to ensure complete prevention of this complication of CF.

MONITORING OF DISEASE

Not many routine tests are done in CF:

1. At diagnosis infants are usually seen very frequently initially (every few days or weekly) and this can be extended as the child gets older and in a stable clinical situation. Routine clinic visits usually occur at least every 3 months: note weight, height nutritional status, respiratory cultures, lung function using spirometry and/ or other tests such as lung clearance index.
2. Documentation of disease progression at annual review. The following are usually done: sputum culture including culture for non-tuberculous mycobacteria in older patients or those taking azithromycin, chest X-ray (CXR), nutritional assessment, pulmonary function tests, liver function tests, full blood count, vitamin levels and work-up for ABPA with total IgE. An oral glucose tolerance test is routine annually from the age of 10 years but may be added earlier in younger patients with concern especially around nutritional status and growth or unexplained fall in respiratory status, and of course with any symptoms suggestive of diabetes. A high-resolution CT scan of the thorax in primary and secondary school can assess progress of bronchiectasis and in some centres is used more often.

OTHER INVESTIGATIONS AS INDICATED

1. Cardiac: electrocardiography, echocardiography (right-ventricular hypertrophy) usually only done when heading for transplant.
2. Gastrointestinal: serum protein and albumin, liver function tests, coagulation studies, abdominal X-ray (meconium ileus, equivalent or peritonitis), abdominal ultrasound (gallbladder, liver), pancreatic function tests.
3. CFRD should be screened for, with an oral glucose tolerance test (GTT) in children over 10 years. A fasting blood glucose is not particularly useful in this context, as it does not exclude diabetes and can be normal in patients with significant CFRD; a GTT is a better test. Urea and electrolytes may be used to assess salt loss, and dye studies in patients with venous access ports can be used for assessment of port function as needed.

Management

Aims of management include: 1. ensuring optimal growth and development; 2. delaying progress of pulmonary disease; 3. preventing/treating complications; 4. normal lifestyle; 5. patient and family education; and 6. recognition and treatment of psychological problems.

HOSPITALISATION

Parameters used in assessing the need for hospitalisation (usually patients are seen in clinic every 2–3 months) include decreasing weight (or poor appetite), diminished exercise tolerance or deteriorating lung-function test results, increased cough and sputum production. School holidays are usually chosen (if possible), as this interferes less with lifestyle, although the reality of hospital bed shortages often means that patients are admitted when a bed is available rather than when it is convenient to the child.

TREATMENT OF LUNG DISEASE

The focus of CF treatment over the next decade will include the prevention of lung disease.

Pseudomonas aeruginosa can be eradicated in 77% of those treated aggressively after a single treatment cycle. Early intervention is essential, before FEV_1 decline. Optimal use of proven medications to assist chest clearance (dornase alpha, inhaled hypertonic saline, mannitol), anti-inflammatory therapy (include the macrolide azithromycin) and careful infection control will continue to be very important. An Australian 10-year bronchoscopy and CT scans in CF study (completed in December 2009) has shown that at 5 years, structural lung disease is almost universal, although nutritional status and lung function are mostly normal. Two-thirds of children have gas trapping on CT by 12 months of age, and 40% have bronchiectasis by age 4. The median age of acquisition of a first isolate of *Pseudomonas aeruginosa* is 26 months, early acquisition being a known risk factor for bronchiectasis.

CF MICROBIOLOGY: 'OLD' ESTABLISHED AND 'NEW' EMERGING PATHOGENS

The microbiology of lung pathogens dictates the usual treatment plans. Initially, the main organisms encountered are *Staphylococcus aureus, Streptococcus pneumoniae, Haemophilus influenzae, P. aeruginosa* non-mucoid (probably the cause of at least 30% of exacerbations in children under 2 years of age) and mucoid strains of *P. aeruginosa* (in > 50% of adult CF patients). *B. cepacia complex* infections may be associated with rapidly progressive lung disease. Approximately one-third of CF patients have precipitating antibodies to *Aspergillus fumigatus*, and two-thirds have positive skin tests for this. Infection control issues are important. Cross-infection must be minimised, avoiding the risk of transmission of viral and bacterial pathogens.

The above pathogens have been recognised for decades in the CF population, and could be termed 'old' organisms.

There are now emerging newer pathogens:

- *MRSA (methicillin-resistant Staphylococcus aureus).* This can be associated with a rapid decline in lung function and chronic infection with this pathogen is now recognised as associated with both increased morbidity and mortality. This can be eradicated and different regimens are used in different clinics.
- *Stenotrophomonas maltophilia.* This is an aerobic gram-negative organism, aquatic and previously classified in the genus *Pseudomonas.*
- *Achromobacter xylosoxidans.* This is an aerobic gram-negative bacillus. *Atypical non-tuberculous mycobacteria.* These can colonise, or actively infect. Should look for signs of disease before treating; can repeat sputum cultures, and perform CXR or CT scan of lung fields.
- *Fungi: Aspergillus.* Around 30% CF patients may culture this fungus in sputum samples and patients exposed to inhaled antibiotics have a greater risk of positive cultures with this fungus. Should look for signs of disease features of ABPA (see below), such as wheezing, positive IgE, positive skin test, and CXR consistent with ABPA.
- *Fungi: Scedosporium apiospermum.* Poor sensitivity to antifungal drugs. Similar to *Aspergillus*, it is the second commonest filamentous fungus in CF patients (after *Aspergillus*). It is a saprophyte, obtaining nutrition by assimilating decaying organic matter. Its presence may prevent transplant.

ANTIBIOTICS

The following is a general guide. Intermittent oral antibiotics can be used for exacerbations of disease with minimal respiratory symptoms. Ciprofloxacin, plus nebulised antibiotics such as tobramycin or colistin, may be used in patients with chronic *P. aeruginosa* infection. Continuous oral antibiotics may be appropriate with persistent sputum production or deteriorating lung function. The standard of care for patients with chronic *Pseudomonas aeruginosa* infection includes inhaled antibiotic therapy which is usually cycled 1 month on, 1 month off, and in patients with deterioration in the month off alternating tobramycin/colistin month by month is sometimes used. Intravenous (IV) therapy is reserved for a sick child or deterioration in clinical status, or specifically for eradication-type therapy, if that is required. Occasionally, regular admissions are booked for children with severe lung disease.

1. *Sputum cultures.* These reflect lung flora in CF (but only in children who can produce sputum easily). Induced sputum is now routine in many centres; it is well tolerated and is successful in 60–80% of patients. Oropharyngeal cultures have poor sensitivity and positive prediction (around 55%), and better specificity and negative prediction (around 85%). Frequent cultures are required to detect early infection, and in very young children who are unable to manage induced sputum oropharyngeal cultures are usually performed and sampled four times per year; this is associated with better health outcomes likely related to earlier pick up of infection with *Pseudomonas aeruginosa* which may be eradicated if detected early.

2. *Choice of antibiotic.* For hospital treatment, this usually includes two IV antibiotics to reduce the chance of the development of antibiotic resistance and also to ensure better coverage of a range of potential organisms and to eradicate/or substantially reduce airway load of organisms. The standard treatments usually include an antipseudomonal penicillin (e.g. ticarcillin with clavulanate, or piperacillin with tazobactam or a cephalosporin such as ceftazidime) and an aminoglycoside (e.g. tobramycin).

3. *Dose of antibiotic.* Abnormal metabolism, and rapid excretion, of antibiotics occurs. Higher doses of antibiotics are usually needed compared with the non-CF population, especially aminoglycosides (e.g. tobramycin, gentamicin), and aminoglycoside use requires therapeutic drug monitoring. As patients get older, the aminoglycoside dose may need to be wound back. Aminoglycosides are usually given as single daily doses.

4. *Route of antibiotic*:
   a. *Intravenous (IV).* Issues include the problem of venous access: peripheral lines (standard and 'long') versus implantable devices, or venous access 'ports' (Infuse-A-Port, Port-A-Cath). Complications of 'ports' or central venous lines can include thrombosis, infection, haemorrhage, embolism, loss of venous access and needle phobia.
   b. *Inhaled.* Many units use nebulised antibiotics (e.g. colistin, ticarcillin, tobramycin) at home in some children. Their use is associated with a dramatic decrease in hospital admissions. Disadvantages include allergy, resistance, expense, bronchoconstriction (infrequent) and time required for nebulisation (compliance problem). It is important to have the appropriate nebuliser device for the drug. There are three types of nebuliser; ultrasonic, jet (including breath-assisted open vent and breath-actuated types) and a range of newer 'vibrating mesh' nebulisers.

      There are many different types on the market, some only available when the patient is taking a particular antibiotic (e.g. the I-neb with Promixin [colistimethate], where it only operates where there is a microchip/disc programmed to the drug

Promixin; other discs are available to allow nebulisation of other medications, such as hypertonic saline, salbutamol, rh-DNase and tobramycin). Improved technology has shortened the period of time and inconvenience of nebulising significantly.

c. *Oral.* For mild-to-moderate exacerbation of lung disease (outpatient management), directed against the most likely (non-pseudomonal) flora. Cotrimoxazole or amoxycillin with clavulanic acid can be used. If no improvement occurs with the first choice, change antibiotics based on sputum sensitivities. Some centres give oral flucloxacillin prophylactically in the first year.

Ciprofloxacin, an oral antipseudomonal quinolone, can be used in older children for a short period, usually 2–3 weeks. However, resistance can develop quickly.

Most exacerbations of chest disease are probably due to viral infections but if symptomatic, respiratory cultures need to be collected and antibiotic cover is required to reduce the risk of a more prolonged bronchitic exacerbation.

Some patients, especially with chronic infection with *P. aeruginosa*, take regular azithromycin, which may be associated with a reduced rate of pulmonary exacerbations requiring IV therapy, thought to be related to anti-inflammatory properties. It can be used as an adjunct treatment, particularly with the aim of reducing the number of days of IV antibiotic use required. It has a long intracellular half-life and can be given three times a week.

Some older drugs have been given newer formulations: aztreonam lysinate inhaled has become available overseas although is not currently funded in Australia (uses an eFlow rapid nebuliser); tobramycin has become available as dry powder capsules; ciprofloxacin solution has become available, and once-daily inhaled amikacin is being developed.

ERADICATION OF *PSEUDOMONAS AERUGINOSA*

P. aeruginosa produces alginate biofilms, which protect it from antibiotics and neutrophils. Having *P. aeruginosa* by 2 years of age is highly correlated with later bronchiectasis. Standard therapy is now 1 month of inhaled tobramycin for inhalation, although many centres will admit children who have respiratory symptoms for 2 weeks of intravenous antibiotics prior to the month of tobramycin for inhalation. Recurrent infections are often treated more aggressively and patients may be admitted for 2 weeks' IV antibiotics followed by oral ciprofloxacin and nebulised colistin or nebulised tobramycin for 1–2 or even 3 months.

CHEST PHYSIOTHERAPY: AIRWAY CLEARANCE TECHNIQUES

Parents and patients are educated in home physiotherapy from the time of initial diagnosis. 'Classical' physiotherapy comprises postural drainage, percussion and vibration, and requires the assistance of a partner. It is usually performed for 10–20 minutes, once or twice a day. It is most useful in children with chronic sputum production, but its value is uncertain in older children with 'dry' chests. It remains useful in acute exacerbations of disease.

Other methods encourage independence and may be used in combination with the above. Positive expiratory pressure (PEP) treatment is commonly used even in very young children. The resistance of the mask is variable and requires expert physiotherapists and inhaled hypertonic saline may be used during this treatment as well. There are many other forms of airway clearance now being used and the techniques chosen will vary according to clinical status, developmental stage and determination of the optimal treatment for airway clearance for each individual child. The important factor is that the child has regular multidisciplinary review including from specialist respiratory physiotherapists.

Forced expiratory technique can be taught from 8–9 years. Exercise should be encouraged from a very young age and especially encouraged to continue in the teenage years.

NEBULISED TREATMENT

Bronchodilators, saline, hypertonic saline and mucolytics may be used, and are best given before chest physiotherapy. Antibiotics, cromolyn or corticosteroids, when used, are best given immediately after physiotherapy. Hypertonic (7%) saline (HS) can be useful acutely in hospital, in patients with significant symptoms, given twice daily. However, HS has not been shown to reduce exacerbations in children with normal lung function (whereas dornase alpha has; see below).

BRONCHODILATOR TREATMENT

Increased bronchial reactivity is found in 40–75% of patients with CF. Standard anti-asthma treatment may be used, including inhaled (nebulised or pMDI) beta-2 agonists (e.g. salbutamol). Note that the condition of some patients can deteriorate following bronchodilators, with a loss of airway wall tone, and dynamic airway compression.

HYDRATOR TREATMENT

Hydrators are osmotic agents which increase surface liquid in airways which are dehydrated in CF. Hypertonic (7%) saline can decrease pulmonary exacerbations and enhance lung function, and is used in patients with moderate to severe lung disease. Mannitol also is used as a hydrator and improves lung function; this also is available as a dry powder inhaler (DPI). Both hypertonic saline and mannitol can have irritant effects, so are given after pre-treatment with bronchodilators.

DISEASE-MODIFYING THERAPY: CFTR MODULATORS

1. Read-through compounds for Class I mutations. Class I mutations lead to no CFTR due to premature stop codons (e.g. *Gly542X*). Corrective therapy for this enables synthesis, by read-through of stop codons by ribosomes; compounds which can do this are being developed. It is recognised that aminoglycoside antibiotics including gentamicin and tobramycin have some effect; however, they are not indicated for this purpose and have side effects that preclude their use at this stage for CFTR modulator therapy.
2. Correctors for Class II mutations. Class II mutations lead to no CFTR trafficking (e.g. Phe508del). *Lumacaftor*, the most successful 'corrector' so far, is designed to fix the trafficking defect; by itself, it only decreased sweat chloride levels and had no effect on lung function, but in combination with the potentiator ivacaftor (see overleaf) there was a significant positive effect.
3. Potentiators for Class III or IV mutations. *Ivacaftor* was the first modulator drug used. A selective CFTR potentiator, it increases the function of the faulty CFTR in patients with the Class III mutation *Gly551Asp* (which is present in around 4% of CF patients) at the apical surface of the cell, restoring channel activity. It has been approved by the FDA in the US for several other Class III mutations which comprise around 5% of all CF patients. Other potentiators which can activate chloride conductance, and bypass the gating defect of Class III mutations, include *genistein*, an isoflavone angiogenesis inhibitor and phytoestrogen, and other flavonoids.
4. Antisense oligonucleotides (AONs), correctors and potentiators comprise the approach for Class V mutations (e.g. *3849+10kbC→T*), aimed at correcting the splicing defect. AONs or antisense RNA can bind to pre-mRNA, regulating gene splicing.

5. Phe508del-CFTR stabilisers can be used for Class VI mutations (e.g. *4326delTC*); these include activators of Rac1 signalling, such as hepatocyte growth factor (HGF), which anchor CFTR to the cell surface.

ANTI-INFLAMMATORY TREATMENT

Long-term use of oral corticosteroids (OCS) and of ibuprofen has been shown to slow the progress of CF. Azithromycin is used for its anti-inflammatory effects. Studies on inhaled corticosteroids (ICS) are somewhat contradictory; a retrospective analysis of 2978 patients with CF receiving inhaled steroids suggested there may be a lessening in the rate of lung-function decline, whereas a Cochrane Review of 506 adults and children suggested that inhaled steroids do not improve lung function and, furthermore, that high-dose fluticasone might slow growth in children. Asthma should be managed appropriately.

MUCOLYTIC TREATMENT: DORNASE ALFA (RECOMBINANT HUMAN DEOXYRIBONUCLEASE 1) (PULMOZYME)

Dornase alfa (rhDNase 1) is an enzyme that cleaves extracellular DNA and decreases the viscoelasticity of purulent lung secretions. It is used in children with chronic suppurative disease or obstructive disease. The lung function changes seen acutely with use of dornase do not indicate long-term potential benefit in reducing exacerbations. A small number of patients may get worse or show no change, and a third will show a marked improvement in lung function. In most cases, the response can be judged within 2 weeks of starting treatment. It is given once daily through an approved nebuliser (not ultrasonic; preferably with a mouthpiece).

UNPROVEN (NOT REALLY 'ALTERNATIVE') THERAPIES

These are frequently used, often cost large amounts of money and can be dangerous. Occasionally, unscrupulous operators have tried to sell household bleach as something that kills germs and can be nebulised. There was a fad for nebulising tea tree oil as well. Silver is used by many, and can cause severe discolouration of the skin and anaemia. It is always worth asking about alternative therapies.

ALLERGIC BRONCHOPULMONARY ASPERGILLOSIS (ABPA)

This is difficult to diagnose in CF, as the features of ABPA (CXR findings, increased serum immunoglobulins) occur in CF, except for IgE. A high IgE level is suggestive of ABPA if other features are present. ABPA can occur in progressive stages: acute stage (upper- and middle-lobe infiltrates, eosinophilia, IgE level very high, prednisolone responsiveness); remission (after 6 months; normal CXR, no prednisolone); recurrent exacerbation stage (recurrence of infiltrates, eosinophilia, IgE elevated, prednisolone responsiveness, if steroid resistant respond to omalizumab); steroid-dependent asthma stage (chronic obstructive airways disease, responds to prednisolone or inhaled steroids, or omalizumab); fibrotic stage (diffuse airway disease, with obstruction and fibrosis, variable CXR, poor response to steroids; this phase can be terminal). Treatment is stage dependent. Agents used may include: prednisolone; methylprednisolone pulses; antifungal agents (the '-conazoles'—itraconazole, voriconazole or posaconazole); anti-IgE agent (omalizumab); granulocyte colony-stimulating factor (G-CSF); granulocyte–macrophage colony-stimulating factor (GM-CSF); interferon; tumour necrosis factor (TNF); and therapeutic bronchoscopy/surgery. For acute stage, management often includes steroids and antifungal agents for 6 months. Progress may be monitored by IgE levels. ICS may ease the asthma symptoms.

HAEMOPTYSIS

This is a common complication of moderate to severe lung disease. No specific treatment is needed for minor haemoptysis; treat the infection and reassure the child. Any haemoptysis over 15–20 mL probably warrants hospital admission, and may need oxygen, vitamin K or transfusion with larger bleeds. Massive haemoptysis (over 300 mL blood loss in 24 hours, with falling haematocrit and hypotension) can occur from bronchial collateral vessels (usually upper lobe). Treatment includes upright position, stopping chest physiotherapy, arranging cross-match, treating with intravenous antibiotics, vitamin K and reassurance. More severe cases may require more emergent treatments such as bronchial artery embolisation or, with respiratory failure, intubation with balloon tamponade and emergency lobectomy. For frequent life-threatening haemoptyses, lung transplantation may be needed.

PNEUMOTHORAX

Pneumothorax is a complication of severe lung disease. Generally, the more severely affected lung collapses. It is a poor prognostic indicator (75% die within 3 years), and recurrence is common.

Acute management involves oxygen—a conservative approach if possible, but each case should be treated on its merits. The prospect for future lung transplantation is adversely affected by more aggressive intervention, such as tube thoracostomy (can scar the pleura and may also cause bronchopleural fistula), chemical pleural sclerosis or surgical pleural abrasion. Needle aspiration may bring symptomatic relief.

COR PULMONALE OR RIGHT-HEART FAILURE

This is a poor prognostic indicator (median survival is 6 months). Treat hypoxia with home nocturnal oxygen. Diuretics may be needed. Treat any infection. BiPAP can be used in patients with respiratory failure to maintain them and avoid heart failure. Cor pulmonale can resolve with lung transplantation (discussed next).

LUNG TRANSPLANTATION

CF is the most common indication for paediatric lung transplant. CF does not re-occur in transplanted lungs. Bilateral sequential single-lung transplantation is now the operation of choice, the sole option for long-term survival of terminal patients. The mainstem bronchus and pulmonary artery are connected by end-to-end anastomoses; the two pulmonary veins from each lung are harvested intact with a patch of the left atrium of the donor, and then each left atrial patch is sewn to the recipient's left atrium. This is performed using cardiopulmonary bypass. Living-donor lobar transplantation (LDLT) is another option, which is rarely performed because of technical and ethical complexities: it requires two donors, each undergoing a lower lobectomy to provide a right and left lower lobe to serve as right and left lungs for the recipient; for adolescents taller than 152 cm, the donors need to be tall enough to provide adequate lung tissue.

The main indications are: life expectancy less than 2 years (usually corresponds to FEV_1 below 30% of predicted), quality of life impaired (oxygen dependent at home, doing nothing) or frequent life-threatening haemoptysis (initial attempted control will be by bronchial artery embolisation). Other indications for referral to a transplant unit include hypercapnic respiratory failure, exacerbation of lung disease sufficient for ICU care, increased frequency of pulmonary exacerbations requiring antibiotic therapy, and recurrent or refractory pneumothorax.

The ideal clinical status includes no major systemic disease (and preferably no surgical procedure to the chest), optimal nutrition (between 70 and 130% of ideal body weight), not on a ventilator and on no more than a low-dose steroid (5 mg or less of prednisolone per day), adequate psychological status, adequate social supports and no major psychiatric illnesses.

There are virtually no contraindications to transplantation. Advice from local tertiary centre transplantation centres should be sought for each case considered. There are, however, areas for discussion in cases with: progressive neuromuscular disease; previous malignancy in the last 2 years; pleural space disease; active infection with *Aspergillus*, *Mycobacterium* or multiply resistant bacteria, such as some strains of *B. cepacia*; high-dose steroids; gross malnutrition; and some psychosocial areas (non-compliance with recommended treatment, major psychoaffective disorders). Donor–recipient matching is based on ABO blood group incompatibility, CMV antibody status and the size of the thoracic cage. Immunosuppressive regimes may include a calcineurin phosphatase inhibitor (e.g. tacrolimus), a purine synthesis inhibitor (e.g. mycophenolate mofetil) and prednisolone.

Complications fall into three groups.

1. *Immediate phase* (first few days posttransplant). Subgroups include the following:
   a. Hyperacute rejection (due to prior exposure to foreign tissue antigens, complement-mediated vascular injury and thrombosis that can lead to loss of the graft; rare).
   b. Early graft dysfunction due to ischaemic injury during harvesting and reimplanting the lungs; occurs in 13–35%; manifests as pulmonary oedema (non-cardiogenic), with decreased lung compliance and poor oxygenation; managed supportively (ventilation, extracorporeal membrane oxygenation [ECMO], nitric oxide).
   c. Surgical complications (airway and vascular anastomoses can break down; bleeding from vascular anastomoses or chest cavity can be persistent; vocal cord and hemidiaphragm paresis or paralysis can occur, but usually resolve in a few months; early re-operation needed in around 10% of cases).
   d. Infection of pulmonary allograft, secondary to poor mucus clearance (impaired ciliary function), poor cough (pain), impaired diaphragm function (phrenic nerve injury), low IgG (from cardiopulmonary bypass) and immune suppression.
2. *Early phase* (first few weeks posttransplant). Subgroups include the following:
   a. Acute rejection (common; may present with dyspnoea, fever, hypoxia, abnormal CXR with perihilar infiltrates or effusions, or obstructive-pattern spirometry); diagnosed on bronchoscopy, bronchoalveolar lavage, transbronchial biopsy; treated with high-dose IV methylprednisolone; if persists, treated with a mono- or polyclonal T-cell antibody preparation (e.g. antithymocyte globulin [ATG]).
   b. Infection: CMV—treat with valganciclovir; bacterial lower respiratory tract infection—treat with IV antibiotics.
   c. Side effects of surgery (narrowing at suture line of airway anastomosis): treated with bronchoscopic balloon dilatation; distal intestinal obstruction syndrome (DIOS; see p. 40); arrhythmias, usually atrial, from interference with integrity of muscle along suture lines, where donor atrial patches with pulmonary veins are attached (see previous section on lung transplantation).
   d. Side effects from medication (triple immunosuppression with calcineurin phosphatase inhibitor [e.g. tacrolimus], a purine synthesis inhibitor [e.g. mycophenolate mofetil] and prednisolone; for discussion of these drugs, see other sections on organ transplantation—e.g. renal, liver, heart).
   e. Seizures (can be due to tacrolimus or cyclosporine, secondary to cerebral vasoconstriction).

f. Hypertension (in 36% of cases at 1 year, 71% at 5 years; may be due to tacrolimus or cyclosporine, or steroids): treat with calcium channel blockers or angiotensin-converting enzyme (ACE) inhibitors.

g. Diabetes mellitus (occurs in 20% at 1 year, 28% at 5 years) can be precipitated by steroids or tacrolimus.

h. Renal dysfunction (hypomagnesaemia, renal tubular acidosis, chronic renal insufficiency; more common in re-transplantation).

3. *Late phase* (months posttransplant). Subgroups include the following:

a. Bronchiolitis obliterans (OB) (the main reason that lung transplantation is not as successful as solid organ transplantation); treatment difficult—tried treatments include ATG, cyclophosphamide, methotrexate, total lymphoid irradiation; better management of rejection has led to improved rates of OB.

b. Malignancy (most often posttransplant lymphoproliferative disorder (PTLD); in 6.5% at 1 year, 8.2% at 5 years): treatment—reduced immunosuppression plus CD20 antibodies.

c. Renal failure (due to calcineurin inhibitors and other nephrotoxic drugs [e.g. aminoglycosides]; occurs in 7.7% at 1 year, 26% at 5 years).

Posttransplant, any acute respiratory illness or acute febrile illness should be investigated and treated aggressively. One needs to be aware that many medications (anticonvulsants, macrolides, antifungals) can interact with the main immunosuppressive agents used (tacrolimus, cyclosporine); MIMS or a similar reference should be checked each time a new medication is contemplated.

The drug levels of antirejection therapy such as cyclosporine must be closely monitored, as inadequate pancreatic enzyme supplementation and erratic absorption of medication can decrease the levels, allowing rejection to occur. If there are many episodes of graft rejection within 2 months of lung transplantation, there is a high frequency of PTLD.

Females may require transplantation earlier than males, as they have a shorter median survival than males. Overall, the survival rate posttransplant approaches 90% at 1 year, 70% at 5 years and 50% at 10 years. For those surviving 10 years, their age at transplant predicts ongoing survival, being less favourable if the transplant occurred under 18 years of age. Three significant factors for poor outcome are repeat transplant, mechanical ventilation at transplant and co-existent congenital heart disease. The three main causes of death are early graft dysfunction (most deaths in the first 30 days posttransplant), infection (first year posttransplant) and bronchiolitis obliterans (beyond the first year posttransplant, for cadaveric transplant recipients; rare in LDLT). Preoperatively, a 2-week assessment in hospital in necessary. The usual age has been around 17–19 years. The rate-limiting factor for this treatment is the scarcity of donor organs. To overcome this, as well as LDLT, reduction surgery and xenograft transplantation from genetically engineered porcine donors have been developed. Concurrent heart and lung transplants have been performed in patients with severe CF lung disease and significant associated cor pulmonale. A study reported in 2007, based on a retrospective cohort study of 514 children with CF on a transplant waiting list, of whom 248 had lung transplants, estimated that only five patients would clearly have improved survival from lung transplantation, inferring that lung transplantation was not necessarily associated with an improved survival in children. Some 50% of lung-transplanted patients have obstructive lung disease in 4 years. Patients can have re-transplants.

END-OF-LIFE CARE

Limited organ availability means that some patients die waiting for a transplant. End-of-life discussions can be held too close to the time the patient dies. 'End-of-life' refers to the period of time when the patient's clinical state is deteriorating relentlessly, and death is likely within a limited time frame (usually 2 years); at this juncture, consideration is given to transplantation and palliative care. A discussion regarding potential transplantation, and its requisite assessments/work-up, allows an opportunity to bring up end-of-life issues at that point, rather than postponing consideration of palliative care and end-of-life issues.

INVASIVE RESPIRATORY SUPPORT

The most appropriate indications for such support are acute reversible conditions such as pneumothorax-precipitating respiratory failure (while waiting for the lung to reinflate after initiating drainage), massive haemoptysis (while awaiting bronchial artery embolisation) or postoperatively, after major surgery.

NON-INVASIVE POSITIVE PRESSURE VENTILATION (NPPV)

NPPV has been reported as being effective in treating impending respiratory failure (in the context of upper abdominal surgery or severe acute pulmonary exacerbation) and avoiding intubation. NPPV also has been reported as improving airway clearance and gas exchange during sleep in patients with CF, and improving respiratory muscle performance and decreased oxygen desaturation episodes during chest physiotherapy.

IMMUNISATION

As well as routine vaccination, many paediatric respiratory units actively encourage influenza vaccination, particularly for very young patients and for those with severe lung disease. Illnesses resembling influenza may be treated with antiviral agents; for example, oseltamivir oral preparation makes it suitable for children from 12 months of age. *Pseudomonas* vaccines are being trialled.

BURKHOLDERIA CEPACIA INFECTION

This can be associated with rapid decline in lung function, and increased mortality. It is now recognised that this organism can survive in respiratory droplets on environmental surfaces for prolonged periods, such as in CF clinics. Person-to-person spread occurs. Patients with *B. cepacia* infection are usually seen separately in outpatient clinics and are nursed in isolation as inpatients. The organism is found in the environment and sporadic infections are seen. It is important to strain type *B. cepacia* and to ensure that there is no person-to-person spread; vigilance is required with all aspects of care, including healthcare professionals' hand washing, equipment use and cleaning in pulmonary function laboratories.

SINONASAL DISEASE

Most children with CF have sinonasal disease, but it is underreported. On CT scan, 92–100% of CF patients have chronic rhinosinusitis, the average age of onset being 5–14 years. Nasal polyps are seen in 18% of children under 6 years old, and eventually seen in 30–50% of adolescent CF patients, versus 0.1% of non-CF/normal children; of these in CF patients, only around 60% are symptomatic.

The history for sinonasal disease may include nasal obstruction, mouth breathing, cough, nasal discharge, post-nasal drip, headache, facial pain, facial pressure, hyposmia, anosmia, poor sleep, snoring, limited activity, hoarseness and halitosis. Examination findings may include congested turbinates, post-pharyngeal oedema, nasal polyps, medialisation of the lateral nasal wall and craniofacial distortion. Nasal polyps can be managed medically, with oral antibiotics, nasal toilet with normal saline irrigation, irrigation with tobramycin or nasal inhalation of Pulmozyme.

Only in exceptional circumstances will surgical treatment of polyps go ahead, when refractory to any other treatment, because of the attendant risks of anaesthetising a patient with CF (these patients can get severe mucus plugging of their airways during anaesthesia, especially when intubated), the possible complications (especially injury to surrounding structures: CSF leak, meningitis, medial rectus damage, optic nerve damage, blindness, cerebral injury, orbital bleeding) and because surgical treatment is not a cure, but a symptomatic treatment only, and up to three quarters can need surgical revision within 2 years. The usual surgery performed is endoscopic sinus surgery comprising polypectomy, wide middle meatal antrostomies, anterior and posterior ethmoidectomies, and removal of polypoid disease in the frontal recess. Postoperatively: saline, steroids, antibiotics and clinic follow-up for division of synechiae (between inferior turbinates and septum).

Treatment of gastrointestinal disease
PANCREATIC INSUFFICIENCY (PI)

The degree of PI is determined by the specific nature of the CF mutation. Certain mutant alleles are associated with PI or pancreatic sufficiency (PS). Fat absorption improves from about 60% without therapy, to 85–90% with pancreatic enzyme replacement therapy (PERT). Dosage regimens have been revised since recognition of the association between high-strength PERT (over 6000 units of lipase per kg) and the development of fibrosing colonopathy.

PERT doses should be derived from a ratio of lipase units per gram of dietary fat ingested; an upper limit of 10 000 units of lipase per kg per day has been suggested. Usual dose ranges from 2000–2500 units of lipase per kg per meal (more details below).

Pancreatic enzyme supplements contain lipase, amylase and proteases. Most units use enteric-coated microspheres. Three preparations are available in Australia: Cotazym-S (capsules contain 10 000 units of lipase), Creon (capsules can contain 5000, 10 000 or 25 000 units of lipase) and Panzytrat 25000 (capsules contain 25 000 units of lipase). The amounts of protease and amylase also vary between preparations. Adjusting PERT to the fat content of foods ingested can lead to increased absorption of fat, despite no change to the total capsule number. PERT guidelines for infants suggest 500–1000 units of lipase per gram of dietary fat, starting with a minimum dose (2500 units of lipase per 120 mL formula/breast feed), increasing the dose according to weight gain and bowel signs. For children, the guidelines suggest 500–4000 units of lipase per gram of dietary fat. For the average child, whose requirement is around 5000 units of lipase per 3–4 g of fat, this is roughly one 5000-lipase-unit capsule per kg body weight per day. Adjustment should be in concert with medical staff, not independently. For younger children, the contents of the capsules should be mixed with acidic fruit gel or yoghurt, not chewed, and the oral cavity should be cleared with a finger after the feed to remove residual microspheres, as enzymes work for up to 30 minutes after ingestion. Older children and adults should swallow the capsules whole just before or during eating. PERT should be given with all foods and fluids that contain fat. The aim is for normal growth and normal stools.

Some patients appear refractory to PERT (i.e. stool fat output persistently above 25% of fat intake), related in some to duodenal acidity. Treatment for these patients may include gastric acid suppression with antacids, H_2-receptor blockers (e.g. ranitidine), proton pump inhibitors (e.g. omeprazole) or prostaglandin analogues (e.g. misoprostol) to aid fat digestion. An alternative pancreatic enzyme preparation may be tried, as dissolution profiles may vary, or preparations may be given at the start of the meal, for earlier onset.

NUTRITION

A high-energy diet is recommended. CF patients require approximately 120% of normal energy requirements because of increased energy use (due to the effort of breathing, and infection), decreased protein synthesis with acute exacerbations of chest disease, nutrient loss with malabsorption, anorexia and raised basal metabolic rate. Less than optimal nutrition may lead to poor growth, impaired respiratory function and decreased exercise tolerance.

Diet should be liberal, with a high intake of a variety of foods, rich in fat (extra margarine, butter, ice-cream, cream), sugar (unless diabetic), salt, milk products, protein foods, cereals and bread. Breastfeeding is desirable for babies with CF; soy milks are not recommended.

In advanced lung disease, with loss of weight and anorexia, despite optimal oral intake, long-term supplementation of nutrition may be appropriate by invasive means (e.g. nasogastric tube or gastrostomy). Caloric supplementation may result in improvement in growth and wellbeing. Nutritional and respiratory status influence each other; if one should deteriorate, so will the other.

VITAMINS

Patients are at risk of deficiencies of fat-soluble vitamins A, D, E and K, especially at diagnosis. Children under age 2 can take a liquid preparation such as Penta-vite liquid multivitamins (which, curiously, contains seven vitamins: vitamin A, thiamine [B1], riboflavin [B2], nicotinamide [B3], pyridoxine [B6], vitamin C and cholecalciferol [vitamin D3] 0.45–0.9 mL daily), plus a vitamin E (alpha tocopherol) preparation such as Micelle E 0.2 mL daily, and vitamin K (phytomenadione) 2.5 mg daily. An alternative is VitABDECK 1–2 mL daily. Preschoolers take Penta-vite chewable tablets, plus Micelle E 0.4 mL daily, and vitamin K 5 mg twice weekly. Again, an alternative is VitABDECK two capsules daily; additional Micelle E or vitamin K may be needed. School-age children can take vitamin A 5000 units daily, vitamin E 100 units daily, and vitamin K, 10 mg twice a week. The aforementioned are the recommendations of the Cystic Fibrosis Standards of Care, Australia, 2008. Recommendations vary on vitamin supplementation in other units in other countries.

SALT

Many units use oral rehydration solutions (e.g. Glucolyte or Gastrolyte) as a source of salt, as fluid, as well as salt, is useful, particularly in younger children. Guidelines for recommended amounts of salt are as follows:
1. Under 6 months: 0.5 g/day (1 g/day in hot weather).
2. 6–12 months: 1 g/day (1.5 g/day in hot weather).
3. 1–5 years: 2 g/day (3 g/day in hot weather).
4. Over 5 years: 3 g/day (4 g/day in hot weather).

Salt replacement may be needed several times a day in hotter weather. Parents can add salt to food, and offer their children salty snack foods. In infants, salt can be given as oral rehydration solutions, or as pinches of salt added to the bottle. As children get older, they may switch to salt tablets with added drinks. The fluid component is important to reduce DIOS.

OTHER GASTROINTESTINAL PROBLEMS

The spectrum of gastrointestinal involvement is as follows:
1. Pancreas: insufficiency (see the previous page); pancreatitis (in patients with PS).
2. Liver: focal biliary cirrhosis, multilobular biliary cirrhosis (complications include portal hypertension, liver failure), intrahepatic stones and sludge.
3. Gallbladder: non-functioning, stones.

4. Common bile duct: stones, stricture, rarely carcinoma.
5. Oesophagus: GOR (increased abdominal pressure from coughing and wheezing, depressed diaphragm from hyperinflation), oesophagitis, oesophageal varices (from portal hypertension; beta blockers can reduce portal venous pressure, and risk of bleeding with varices in CF, but 1 in 5 get bronchospasm).
6. Stomach: portal gastropathy (congested stomach, with purpura in stomach, from portal hypertension).
7. Duodenum: ulcer.
8. Small intestine: meconium ileus (with or without the associated complications of volvulus, atresia, perforation), meconium ileus equivalent (DIOS), intussusception.
9. Large intestine: rectal prolapse, constipation with acquired megacolon, meconium plug, fibrosing colonopathy.
10. Gastrointestinal malignancy: occurs more frequently in CF, although the overall risk of cancer anywhere is no different to that for the general population.

MECONIUM ILEUS

Meconium ileus (MI) occurs in association with PI almost exclusively. Management may include careful monitoring of fluid status and conservative enema (e.g. Urografin and Tween 80 isotonic mixture) if uncomplicated. In some patients with MI refractory to Urografin enemas, T-tube ileostomy with installation of N-acetylcysteine or Gastrografin has been tried with success as an alternative to surgical decompression. Operative management is needed if complicated (includes meconium peritonitis from in utero perforation, gangrene, volvulus and atresia), or if more conservative means fail. Usually, the Bishop–Koop procedure is used.

MECONIUM ILEUS EQUIVALENT—DISTAL INTESTINAL OBSTRUCTION SYNDROME (DIOS)

DIOS is due to abnormally viscid mucofaeculent material in the terminal ileum and right colon, presenting with attacks of bowel obstruction with pain and vomiting, but with normal stool frequency and consistency initially. Predisposing risk factors include PI, suboptimal PERT, meconium ileus and dehydration. DIOS is common in both PI and PS patients. Classic DIOS will cause bilious vomiting and fluid levels on erect abdominal X-ray. If obstruction becomes complete, management may include nasogastric decompression, intravenous hydration and enemas. In incomplete obstruction, paraffin oil, stool softeners, osmotic laxatives such as poly ethylene glycol, a low-residue diet, enemas or a colonic electrolyte lavage formulation (GoLYTELY) flush, by nasogastric tube, may be used. Once an episode has resolved, review PERT; consider a high-fibre diet and laxatives. If the problem persists, consider stimulant laxatives, or even oral N-acetylcysteine or Gastrografin (sodium meglumine diatrizoate). It often presents as a mass in the right iliac fossa and may be asymptomatic. Acute episodes may be confused with appendicitis or appendix mass. Management needs CF team involvement and careful multidisciplinary assessment. Prevention needs to be focused on improving fluid and salt intake.

RECTAL PROLAPSE

This usually occurs in the first few years of life; spontaneous resolution by age 5 years is usual. It is associated with inadequate control of steatorrhoea, and may resolve with adequate PERT. Conservative management is with manual reduction, stool softeners (mineral oil or lactulose) and improved nutrition. Not infrequently, patients learn to self-reduce the prolapse with pelvic floor muscles, and do not need manual pressure on the prolapsed rectum. If prolapse is persistent, it may require general anaesthesia and pararectal triple saline injection, but this is very rare.

CF-ASSOCIATED LIVER DISEASE (CFLD): LIVER AND BILIARY TRACT DISEASE

CFLD is an indolent process. Focal biliary cirrhosis occurs secondary to inspissated bile. Cirrhosis is the third leading cause of mortality in CF patients. CFLD occurs in around 15% of the CF population, cholelithiasis in 12%, cirrhosis in 10%, portal hypertension in 2–5% and clinically significant disease in 1–2%. The average age of presentation is around 10 years, with the peak incidence at 16–20 years. Once cirrhosis has developed, the duration of survival is 4–5 years.

In the liver, only intrahepatic biliary epithelial cells express CFTR chloride channels, affecting water and solute movement through chloride secretion and thence bile flow. In CF, bile fibrosis leads to biliary cirrhosis, which in turn leads to multilobular cirrhosis. CFLD is more common with PI. Management of cholestasis may include giving ursodeoxycholic acid (URSO), which mimics endogenous bile acid production. Investigations include LFTs and liver ultrasound, which can diagnose cirrhosis (nuclear scans such as HIDA have been abandoned, having been neither sensitive nor specific enough for precise diagnosis).

The gold standard for diagnosis remains liver biopsy. CFLD has two major effects: *portal hypertension* (leading to varices and hypersplenism) and *end-stage liver disease* (ESLD). Splenic enlargement can squash the stomach and splint the diaphragm, and can cause abdominal pain via the splenic capsule being stretched or via small peripheral splenic infarcts. Management of portal hypertension may include sclerotherapy, variceal bonding, endoscopic variceal ligation, portosystemic shunting or transjugular intrahepatic portosystemic shunt placement. If progressive, irreversible hepatic insufficiency develops and liver transplantation (LTx) is the treatment of choice; LTx is a relevant management option in around 5% of CF patients. Long-term survival after LTx in CF is comparable to LTx performed for other indications (see LTx in the Chronic liver disease case in Chapter 8, Gastroenterology). Lung function can also improve after LTx. Distal common bile duct stricture, recurrent pain or biliary tree obstruction can be managed with surgical intervention: cholecystojejunostomy if the gallbladder is functioning, or choledochojejunostomy for non-visualised gallbladder, or microgallbladder. Annual screening with LFTs and ultrasound is worthwhile.

SMALL BOWEL BACTERIAL OVERGROWTH (SBBOG)

Normally the small intestine is relatively sterile, compared to the colon, where around 95% of bacteria reside. SBBOG is when the bacterial load in the jejunum is $> 10^5$ per millilitre. SBBOG can occur due to several mechanisms in CF such that, theoretically, almost all patients should have it. Mechanisms include decreased gastric acidity to sterilise ingested bacteria, decreased intestinal flushing by decreased secretion volume, abnormally viscid mucus and gut dysmotility, less secretory IgA, and impaired access of 'defensins' trapped in intestinal crypts.

Complications from SBBOG include competition for nutrients, inflammation from enterotoxic metabolites, deconjugated/inactive bile acids, malabsorption, bloating, nausea and weight loss. The treatment involves flushing out with Gastrografin or GoLYTELY via percutaneous endoscopic gastrostomy (PEG), and the use of motility agents and antibiotics (e.g. macrolides, norfloxacin, ciprofloxacin), and usually needs to be repeated.

PROTRACTED NAUSEA

When lung disease is stable, and not the cause, there is a wide range of pathologies for this not uncommon complaint. There are over a dozen common causes (mnemonic **FASTING**):

Fat maldigestion

Abdominal pain (functional; this is probably intestinal hypervigilance, where minor sensations become major)

Small bowel bacterial overgrowth/**S**plenic enlargement (portal hypertension)/**S**inusitis

Treatment: prescribed drug side effects; over-the-counter drug side effects

Inflammatory bowel disease, IBD (especially Crohn disease, which is 12 times more common in CF)/**I**ncreased intracranial pressure (ICP)

Non-prescribable (alternative/complementary) treatments

Gastrointestinal tract causes (5 **G**s): **G**astro-oesophageal reflux, **G**astritis, **G**astroparesis (diabetic), **G**allstones, **G**iardia—to sort out which is the case, investigations can involve endoscopy and imaging; treatment may involve treating CFRD, PERT tailoring and medications (depending on the likeliest diagnosis, the possibilities include high-dose proton pump inhibitors, metronidazole, domperidone, ondansetron or even antidepressants)

ABDOMINAL PAIN

This can be a diagnostic and management problem, not dissimilar, in scope, to protracted nausea as above. Constipation is a common cause. Other causes are many (mnemonic **GUARDING**):

Gastro-oesophageal reflux/oesophagitis

Underdosing PERT

Appendicitis

Renal stones/**R**espiratory disease related: lower-lobe pneumonia, muscle strain (rectus)

DIOS/**D**uodenal ulcer

Inflamed pancreas (pancreatitis)/**I**BD/**I**ntussusception

Non-organic/functional (e.g. grief reaction with death of friend with CF; recognising own mortality with deteriorating health—may be unrelated to CF)

Gallbladder/biliary related: cholelithiasis, common bile duct stricture, cholecystitis

The treatment for constipation comprises paraffin oil (in those over 2 years) or lactulose. DIOS management is discussed above.

LOSS OF WEIGHT

Causes can include non-compliance with one or more aspects of therapy, inadequate caloric intake, inadequate PERT, chest infection, CFRD, or co-existent conditions such as celiac disease or inflammatory bowel disease. Other causes overlap with the causes of protracted nausea and of abdominal pain, as above. Loss of weight should always prompt review by the paediatric team.

FIBROSING COLONOPATHY

This is an iatrogenic complication of the treatment of CF. The risk is greatest in children under 12 or with a history of DIOS. Colonic strictures/stenoses, frequently long segment, occur from submucosal thickening by fibrous connective tissue, leading to intraluminal narrowing related to high-dose PERT. Patients may present with abdominal pain, diarrhoea and haematochezia, before strictures form. It seems likely that a methacrylic acid co-polymer in the enteric coatings of some PERT preparations is the putative agent. Since particular PERTs have been withdrawn from the market, it is reported less. Management in the past has included colectomy.

CYSTIC FIBROSIS-RELATED DIABETES (CFRD)

CFRD is the most common comorbidity in CF, seen more often due to the increasing life span of CF patients: it occurs in 9% of 5–9 year olds, 26% of 10–20 year olds and 50% of patients by 30. CFRD can be a fluctuating diagnostic state; CFRD can occur with or without fasting hyperglycaemia; the usual CFRD developmental path begins with early, variable intermittent postprandial hyperglycaemia, followed by impaired glucose tolerance, then diabetes without fasting hyperglycaemia (plasma glucose < 7 mmol/L fasting, but 2-hour glucose level > 11.1 mmol/L), followed by diabetes with fasting hyperglycaemia. CFRD increases the mortality rate in CF sixfold, and the prediabetic state is associated with increased morbidity. CFRD is treated with insulin, not oral hypoglycaemic agents.

CFRD tends to develop insidiously. Clues may include delayed puberty, failure to gain weight/decreased growth velocity, unexplained deterioration in lung function, or the more obvious presentation of polyuria and polydipsia. Microvascular complications occur, but are rare before 10 years' duration with CFRD; they include microalbuminuria (14%), retinopathy (16%), gastropathy (50%) and neuropathy (55%). CFRD is linked to the common Phe508del mutation.

The pathology is fibrosis and fatty infiltration of the pancreas, which disrupts the islet architecture, causing insulin deficiency (which can be severe but not absolute); this process also can cause impaired glucagon secretion. Insulin resistance occurs because of decreased peripheral glucose uptake and inadequate insulin suppression of hepatic glucose production.

Several aspects to CFRD are quite different to both type 1 and type 2 diabetes. Calorie restriction is contraindicated, as a high-calorie high-fat diet is indicated in CF. Diabetic ketoacidosis (DKA) is rare, due to persistence of endogenous insulin production and impaired glucagon response. CFRD can first present when insulin resistance is increased (e.g. during immunosuppression posttransplant with tacrolimus usage, with steroid treatment, with increased calories from nasogastric overnight feeds). It is more severe with co-existent liver disease. HbA1c is unreliable in CFRD.

The insulin regime in CFRD is managed along standard lines used for type 1 diabetes, but particular difficulties can occur with concomitant corticosteroid usage and dietary requirements. Overnight feeding may require isophane and regular insulins to cover. Basal insulin requirements can increase fourfold with acute illness, but they also drop rapidly once the intercurrent acute illness is resolved. For further discussion on insulin, see the long and short cases on diabetes in Chapter 7, Endocrinology.

Treatment of other complications

CYSTIC FIBROSIS-RELATED BONE DISEASE (CFR-BD)

Musculoskeletal complications are increasingly recognised with longer life span. The best predictors of bone health are nutritional status and severity of lung disease in early adolescence:

- Hypertrophic pulmonary osteoarthropathy (HPOA) is the most common disorder (it occurs in 2–7% patients with CF). It is characterised by digital clubbing, and long-bone and joint pain (especially wrists, knees and ankles), worsened by pulmonary exacerbations. The aetiology remains unclear. Bone scan can detect HPOA early. Management includes optimising pulmonary care and aggressive treatment of exacerbations. NSAIDs may relieve discomfort.

- Kyphosis with an angle over 40° occurs in over 75% of adult female CF patients, and around one-third of adult male patients. Both HPOA and kyphosis are associated with deteriorating lung function, and are seen as markers of a poor prognosis.
- Low bone mass is common, despite supplementation with vitamin D, calcium and PERT. Bone mineral density decreases and fracture risk increases with increasing age. Osteoporosis and crush fractures can lead to significant back problems. Rib fractures are also reported. Severe bone loss occurs in transplant patients.
- CF episodic arthritis usually presents with recurrent (non-destructive) mono-articular involvement or a symmetrical polyarthritis. It can be managed by standard therapy (NSAIDs or aspirin). Glucocorticoids may be required, orally or intra-articularly. It has been observed that antibiotic therapy for lung disease can improve joint symptoms. Eruptions resembling erythema nodosum may occur in association with it.
- Rheumatoid arthritis has been reported, and treated along standard lines.
- Ciprofloxacin-induced arthralgia is treated by stopping the drug.

GROWTH AND RECOMBINANT HUMAN GROWTH HORMONE (rhGH)

Poor linear growth and inadequate weight gain are very common, and adults with CF have lower than average final adult heights. Poor weight gain and worsening of clinical state are well known. It has been hypothesised that improved linear growth can allow greater lung mass, leading to improved lung function. Many studies of rhGH in children with CF have shown significant improvement in height velocity, weight velocity, bone accumulation, forced vital capacity and exercise tolerance.

ADOLESCENCE AND FERTILITY

Females with CF are mildly subfertile (related to suboptimal body weight, thick cervical mucus, low body fat and associated oestrogen deficiency). Many pregnancies are successful, although pregnancy can be associated with risk of cardiorespiratory failure and fetal loss; however, the only contraindication is cor pulmonale. Tolerance of pregnancy depends on the severity of lung disease, and is better tolerated in those with milder disease and in those with a certain ideal body weight before conception. Risk factors for a poorer outcome of pregnancy include $FEV_1 < 50\%$ predicted, undernutrition and CFRD.

The choice of contraception can be difficult and should be individualised. Barrier methods such as condoms are very effective. Liver disease is a contraindication to the use of the combined oral contraceptive pill. Implanon (etonogestrel) implants and 3-monthly Depo-Provera (medroxyprogesterone acetate) have been used for contraception, although some units avoid Depo-Provera due to concerns about adverse effects on bone health in the long term. Oral contraceptives have been avoided in adolescent females, because frequent use of different antibiotic therapies may affect drug levels and effectiveness, and patients may have liver disease, but oral contraception remains the commonest form used in adult women with CF. The hormone levels of the OCPill are not affected by concomitant ingestion of ampicillin, ciprofloxacin, clarithromycin, doxycycline or roxithromycin. Oral contraceptives are also used for medical/hormonal purposes, such as acne or painful menses.

With increased survival, many CF patients request genetic counselling and fertility assessment. Genetic screening of partners detects around 90% of carriers. Females with CF can overcome difficulties with conception by in vitro fertilisation techniques.

Males with CF usually have congenital bilateral absence of the vas deferens (CBAVD), but the resultant infertility can be managed by having spermatozoa retrieved by direct aspiration from the head of the epididymis, then intracytoplasmic sperm injection (ICSI) into an oocyte obtained by egg harvesting.

DRUG ALLERGIES

In adult CF clinics, some 35% of patients with CF eventually will have an allergy to more than one class of anti-*Pseudomonas* antibiotic, and 1 in 8 will have allergy to two or more beta lactam-containing antibiotics. This is due to cumulative exposure.

Common management issues

WHAT SHOULD THE PATIENT KNOW ABOUT THE ILLNESS?

Most patients are diagnosed through neonatal screening, so that the parents receive education about the condition. As children get older, simple explanations are required to explain why they require physiotherapy and medications.

Fertility should be discussed at around age 13–17 years, explaining infertility to boys and implications of pregnancy to girls. With acceleration in the ease of information retrieval, most children and parents will have obtained much information from the internet and will be asking challenging questions regarding these issues earlier than in the past.

HOW MUCH SHOULD SCHOOL/PEERS BE TOLD?

School should be told about the diagnosis, the need for exceptions to school rules (e.g. running late for class due to treatment at home, running to toilet, being exempt from sport) when necessary, and the need for free access to bronchodilator therapy. Schoolfriends can be given information when they ask, keeping answers simple, but there is little point in trying to keep the diagnosis secret. It is important that the school is aware that if there is more than one patient with CF in the school, the children should not be in the same class, to avoid prolonged contact and risk of transmission of organisms from patient to patient. It is of key importance that children and parents have a positive attitude to prognosis and ensure adequate education. The majority of children born with CF today will live to adult life, will need to work and may have a family of their own.

WHEN SHOULD THE PATIENT TAKE RESPONSIBILITY FOR SELF-CARE?

Children can generally manage to swallow their pancreatic enzymes by age 5. Adolescents often start to have some time alone with the doctor during consultations by around age 14 and achieve total self-care by the end of adolescence.

WHEN SHOULD THE PATIENT TRANSFER TO ADULT CARE?

The appropriate time is more dependent on maturity and physical health than age. Some units feel the year after leaving school is the appropriate time, with prior introduction to the adult physician. A common problem with transfer is decreased compliance (factors include loyalty, rapport with new doctors, physiotherapists, change in treatment, clinic environment, drug costs and loss of parental supervision). Positive reasons for transfer include recognition of transition to adulthood and patient preference (but a problem can be disease stability at the time). Negative reasons include crowding of paediatric outpatient clinics and disinclination of paediatricians to manage adult problems. Most young people are happy to transfer care when they finish school or if they take on adult responsibilities and behaviours earlier. Many units make the transition to adult care after completion of grade 12. Most patients are happy with this and, although most parents are worried, the doctors and therapists usually have no concerns.

IS MODIFICATION OF CURRENT MEDICAL TREATMENTS WARRANTED?

Alternate daily oral steroids may impact negatively on growth and bone density, and increase the risk of diabetes, although previously reported positive effects have included increased growth and appetite, decreased infection and increased wellbeing in some patients. Home intravenous antibiotics using venous access ports had appeared promising, and seemed as effective as hospital antibiotics, but many studies subsequently showed home IV treatment may require a longer time on therapy, compared to hospital care, to achieve the same end points. Many units reserve this for patients who are very well motivated and have a lot of support. Home oxygen is useful for later-stage 'restless' nights and morning headache with significant oxygen desaturation overnight: this needs assessment (e.g. overnight oxygen saturation monitoring, echocardiography to detect cor pulmonale).

IS LUNG TRANSPLANTATION AN OPTION FOR THIS PATIENT?

This is an area to be evaluated in any terminal patient with CF. Bilateral sequential single-lung transplantation is the sole option for long-term survival of such patients. See the discussion in the section on the treatment of lung disease.

If there is a second major organ failure, a second organ transplant may be appropriate (for co-existent liver failure, liver–lung transplantation; for co-existent heart failure, heart–lung transplantation). In the past, heart–lung transplant had been considered for cor pulmonale associated with pulmonary hypertension; however, it is now recognised that the right-sided heart dysfunction of cor pulmonale resolves after lung transplantation.

IS THE FAMILY COPING AT PRESENT?

There may be a need for increased financial and social support. Depending on the state of the child's illness, there may be a need for grief counselling. This is useful at any of the more stressful times in the parents' lives, including the initial diagnosis, the next hospital admission, the death of someone else's child, crisis times (e.g. increased hospitalisation, start of school), antenatal diagnosis and termination of pregnancy, and transfer to adult hospital. Grief reactions can include shock, denial, sadness (e.g. loss of expected healthy child/life span), anger ('Why me?') that may be directed at health workers, relief (symptoms have a name), guilt (they transmitted the disease), resentment, anxiety (fear for the future) and somatic problems (e.g. headaches).

ARE THE PARENTS PLANNING MORE CHILDREN?

Discussion must include prenatal diagnosis and the ethical problem of what to do should the result be positive. The education of the parents in the genetic considerations should be explored to prevent misunderstanding (e.g. 'The next three will be all right because the risk is 1 in 4').

Prognosis

Life expectancy is increasing. Mean age of survival in Australia is 42–50 years in 2016. Over 90% of mortality is due to lung disease. Poor prognostic factors include:

- Female sex (teenage and young adult age period).
- Pancreatic insufficiency.
- Complications, including CFRD or CFLD, or ABPA.
- Abnormal CXR 12 months after diagnosis.
- Age of acquisition of chronic pulmonary infection with *P. aeruginosa* and, in particular, mucoid *P. aeruginosa* under 6 years.
- Lung infection with *B. cepacia*.
- Fall-off in growth curves.
- Recurrent haemoptysis.
- Pneumothorax.
- Onset of cor pulmonale.
- Cigarette smoke exposure.
- Poor socioeconomic status.
- Non-CF-clinic care.

LONG CASE: Obstructive sleep apnoea (OSA)

Background information

OSA is at the severe end of the obstructive sleep-disordered breathing (SDB) spectrum, and is the hypoventilation disorder most likely to be encountered in the examination context. With an estimated incidence of 2%, OSA can occur in children of any age, the peak ages being between 2 and 8 years.

In a long-case format, the patient may well have one of the several underlying conditions, such as craniofacial anomalies, neuromuscular disorders or significant obesity. In addition to disruption of normal breathing and sleep architecture, episodes of partial or complete airway obstruction during sleep may lead to significant neurocognitive, cardiovascular or metabolic morbidities. The pathophysiology is complex (a disorder of anatomy and neuromuscular control of the upper airway), involving increased upper airway resistance (most commonly associated with lymphoid tissue [adenotonsillar] hypertrophy, or mandibular/maxillary narrowing or retropositioning), decreased neuromuscular activation, altered ventilatory control, changed arousal thresholds and other abnormalities of sleep architecture. There is typically repetitive collapse of the pharyngeal airway, intermittent hypercarbic hypoxia (IHH) and recurrent transient arousal; IHH and sleep fragmentation impair sleep restoration. Neurocognitive and behavioural morbidities (learning deficits, inattention and hyperactivity) can be attributed to sleep fragmentation and intermittent hypoxia.

The main two determinants of upper airway patency during sleep are, firstly, the anatomical structure/size of the bony and soft tissues of the airway and, secondly, the tone of the upper airway/pharyngeal dilator muscles (genioglossus is the best studied). Accordingly, the anatomy is affected by:

- Various craniofacial syndromes that cause midfacial hypoplasia (Apert, Crouzon, Pfeiffer, Treacher Collins).
- Macroglossia (Beckwith-Wiedemann).
- Relative macroglossia/small pharynx (Down).
- Glossoptosis (Pierre Robin sequence).
- Short cranial base (achondroplasia; which also causes midface hypoplasia, reduced size of foramen magnum [with potential for cervicomedullary compression] and hydrocephalus).

Other conditions causing anatomical impingement on the airway calibre include those that:

- Decrease the bony cross-section of the lower face, such as sickle cell anaemia (SCA), via bone marrow hyperplasia, and juvenile idiopathic arthritis (JIA), via micrognathia from temporomandibular joint (TMJ) involvement.
- Increase airway soft tissue (adenotonsillar hypertrophy, obesity [parapharyngeal fat deposits], mucopolysaccharidoses [MPSs], airway papillomatosis).
- Cause collapsible upper airway tissues (Marfan; important to pick OSA because its presence may increase the risk of aortic root dilatation; other contributors to OSA in Marfan syndrome are crowded teeth, high-arched palate and narrowed jaw).
- Cause laryngeal/tracheal narrowing (laryngomalacia, subglottic stenosis).

Various neurological conditions affect the muscle tone, whether upper motor neurone (cerebral palsy) or lower motor neurone (spinal muscular atrophy [SMA], myasthenia gravis, various myopathies).

Some causes of OSA (including genes) are as follows (mnemonic **COMPACTED BREATHING**):

Crouzon syndrome (FGFR 2 & 3)/**C**ervical fusion (Klippel–Feil syndrome)
Obesity/**O**verbite (and other dental anomalies)
Marfan syndrome (FBN 1)/**M**oebius sequence/**M**yelomeningocele
Pfeiffer syndrome (FGFR 1,2)/**P**rader–Willi (deletion at 15q11-q13)/**P**aralysed vocal cord
Adenotonsillar hypertrophy/**A**pert syndrome (FGFR 2)/**A**chondroplasia (FGFR 3)
CP/**C**HARGE (choanal stenosis/atresia; CHD7)/**C**hotzen (Saethre-Chotzen; TWIST)
Tracheal/subglottic stenosis/**T**racheomalacia/laryngomalacia
Extra tissue (fatty infiltration upper airway structures, storage disorders, airway papillomatosis, cystic hygroma [lymphatic malformation], nasal polyps in CF)
Down syndrome (normal-size tongue, small pharynx causing relative macroglossia)

Burns to head and neck/**B**eckwith-Wiedemann (11p15.5) (macroglossia)
Rhinitis (allergic)/**R**obin sequence (hypoplasia of mandibular area before 9 weeks in utero causes glossoptosis)/**R**epaired cleft lip/palate/pharyngeal flap
Endocrine disease: hypothyroidism/hypopituitarism (both cause decreased muscle tone)
Arthritis (JIA; TMJ involvement causing micrognathia)/**A**rnold–Chiari malformation (ACM) type II (including in spina bifida)
Treacher Collins syndrome (TCOF 1)
Haematological: SCA/**H**allermann–Streiff syndrome (malar hypoplasia, micrognathia with hypoplastic rami and anterior displacement of TMJ, high narrow palate)
Inborn errors of metabolism: mucopolysaccharidoses (MPSs)
Neuromuscular weakness (SMA, myasthenia gravis, myopathies)
Goldenhar syndrome (hemifacial microsomia: 1st and 2nd branchial arch syndrome [14q32])

Diagnosis of OSA

Polysomnography (PSG) is a multichannel recording of physiological parameters during sleep. It is the gold standard for diagnosis of OSA, but criteria for the paediatric population are inconsistent. The parameters recorded on PSG are (mnemonic **SLEEPING OVER**):

Submental EMG
Limb movements via EMG
EEG–AASM recommended
Eye movement
Position of body
Intensity of respiratory effort
Nasal airflow

Grade snoring (frequency and/or volume)
Oxygen saturation (detects brief drops in SpO_2 by lowering averaging time to 2 seconds)
Video recording
End-tidal CO_2 signal (reduced in hypopnea; absent in apnoea)
Rhythm ECG

Polysomnographic criteria for diagnosis of OSA in children: the apnoea hypoxic index (AHI), equal to the average number of apnoeas and hypopnoeas per hour of sleep: greater than one is abnormal (whereas in adults the number cut-off is five) and consistent with the diagnosis of OSA. A minimum oxygen saturation less than 92% is also considered abnormal.

Less time-consuming and cumbersome 'abbreviated tests' have been disappointing, as they lack sensitivity. Nocturnal pulse oximetry has a high positive predictive value (over 96%) and a high specificity (over 97%), but a low negative predictive value (under 50%) and a low sensitivity (under 50%). Hence this test is of no utility if it is negative.

HISTORY

Despite many studies demonstrating a lack of reliability of history in assessing OSA, it is prudent to take a thorough detailed history, focusing on the three most useful diagnostic symptoms (the 3 Ss): 1. Snoring (especially the majority of nights; breathing pauses/observed apnoeas); 2. Snorting (the mechanism of breaking obstructive events, and increased work of breathing); and 3. Sleep disturbance (movement to find a better position for stable sleep). The history can be divided into night-time/sleep symptoms and daytime/awake symptoms, and varies somewhat depending on the age of the patient. No particular combination of symptoms and signs can differentiate OSA from primary snoring. Parental impressions of sleep problems do not correlate with sleep study findings (as shown in a study where 57% of 56 children aged 4–63 months with Down syndrome had OSA proved on polysomnography). Similarly, a normal score on an OSA-18 disease-specific quality-of-life questionnaire (OSA-18) does not exclude OSA in children.

PRESENTING COMPLAINT
Reason for current admission.

SYMPTOMS

Night-time/sleep: snoring: duration (how long aware of snoring); frequency (every night, most nights); intensity (loud enough to be heard outside of bedroom); when noticed more (second half of night, as OSA worse during rapid eye movement [REM] sleep, associated with relative hypotonia of upper airways and diminished respiratory drive); whether documented (tape recording, video recording); quality of breathing (pauses in breathing: duration, frequency [how many per hour], associated inspiratory noises at end of pause); mouth breathing; increased work of breathing (use of accessory muscles of respiration, tracheal tug, intercostal recession, sternal recession, subcostal recession); additional noises (snorting, gasping, choking); associated symptoms including unusual/abnormal sleeping position, hyperextended neck, restlessness, restless legs syndrome (RLS, leg discomfort, motor restlessness, worse at night), period limb movements disorder (PLMD, repetitive flexion of hips, knees, ankles; a PSG diagnosis), sweating, bruxism/teeth grinding, secondary nocturnal enuresis.

In infants, also ask about disturbed sleep with recurrent episodes of crying, whether there is an established day/night cycle, any poor sucking/feeding, any ambulance calls for apparently life-threatening events.

In toddlers, ask about whether 'niggly' or 'grouchy', crying spells, night terrors and witnessed apnoeas.

In preschoolers, ask about drooling during sleep, confusional arousals, night terrors, sleepwalking, whether hard to wake up, need for napping and poor eating.

In school-aged children, ask about sleep-talking, insomnia, daytime fatigue, aggression, shyness, depression, low self-esteem, delayed puberty, dental problems (e.g. overcrowded teeth, malocclusion, severe enough to see a dentist/orthodontist). The increase in partial arousal parasomnias (sleepwalking, night terrors) is due to compensatory increase in slow-wave sleep in response to sleep fragmentation.

Daytime/awake: symptoms on waking include headache, thirst, jaw pain (from bruxism), stiff neck (from neck hyperextension), mouth breathing, dry mouth, hyponasal speech, nasal 'congestion', rhinorrhoea (allergic rhinitis), difficulty swallowing (tonsillar hypertrophy), hearing problems, poor appetite, excessive daytime sleepiness (usually the predominant symptom), taking naps, disruptive behaviour (easily frustrated, agitated, irritable, aggressive, moody, emotionally labile, impulsive, increased activity), ADHD-like symptoms (poor attention span, academic problems, may have been diagnosed as ADHD, may be taking stimulants), oppositional behaviour, conduct problems, increased somatic complaints (internalised; *sleepiness is associated with attention loss; poor executive abilities reflect hypoxaemia to frontal lobe*), neurocognitive difficulties (learning problems, poor school performance, any psychometric testing, IQ score), cardiovascular symptoms (hypertension noted by local doctor or paediatrician—*hypoxia and microarousals most likely lead to stimulation of the sympathetic nervous system and elevated blood pressure*), growth aspects (obesity as a cause, including from hypothyroidism; failure to thrive/asthenia, secondary to increased energy expenditure with increased work of breathing), precipitants of more severe OSA (intercurrent URTIs with tonsillar enlargement, exposure to cigarette smoking [doubles frequency of URTIs], allergic rhinitis).

SOCIAL HISTORY

Disease impact on child (effect on development, education, behaviour); on family (effect of snoring on other family members [if snoring in most/all members of family, presentation may be late, as thought 'normal'], responsibility for home CPAP, financial issues; CPAP driver, private health insurance); on siblings (especially if share a room).

PAST HISTORY

Age at onset, diagnosis, where and when made, investigations undertaken (e.g. formal sleep study), number of hospitalisations, treatment required (e.g. adenotonsillectomy), complications of OSA (e.g. pulmonary hypertension) or its treatment (e.g. post-adenotonsillectomy complications: nasopharyngeal stenosis, pulmonary oedema), investigation, diagnosis and treatment of underlying condition (e.g. details of craniofacial syndromes/neuromuscular disorders). Any co-existent obesity hypoventilation syndrome.

FAMILY HISTORY

OSA, underlying inheritable diagnoses (e.g. craniofacial syndromes), atopic or allergic history, who at home smokes. Ask about any family history of sudden infant death syndrome (SIDS) or apparently life-threatening events (ALTEs), in addition to the family history of OSA, as there has been a report of OSA in infants being associated with a multiple family history of SIDS, ALTE or OSA. The family history of sleep apnoea is a risk factor for sleep apnoea in children.

ALLERGIES

Allergic rhinitis (can contribute to/cause OSA, by nasal obstruction).

MANAGEMENT

Present treatment in hospital, usual treatment at home (e.g. CPAP, BiPAP).

UNDERSTANDING OF DISEASE

By child and by parents. Ask about the degree of previous education (by doctors, by reading).

Examination

The following has been set out as a short-case approach for the lead-in of OSA, essentially as a combination of three approaches: the 'dysmorphic child' plus a full respiratory with an abbreviated neurological examination. If no dysmorphic features are immediately apparent, then respiratory and gait examinations usually will detect the cause, or give sufficient clues to lead to the next system. In the long case, the diagnosis will be known and so direct the examination to all findings relevant to that condition.

GENERAL IMPRESSION

Note any dysmorphic facial features suggesting any of the craniofacial syndromes or other syndromes/conditions listed within the background information. Note whether there are 'allergic facies', with 'allergic shiners' (swollen discoloured eyelids; transverse nasal crease from allergic salute or 'adenoidal facies'). Inspect the head shape, measure the head circumference (HC; many with craniofacial syndromes, and those with some neurological disorders, will have decreased HC and abnormal skull shapes, whereas those with hydrocephalus [e.g. Arnold–Chiari type II] or thicker bones [sickle cell anaemia, mucopolysaccharidoses] will have increased HC).

Note the morphology of the eyes (microphthalmia in Hallermann–Streiff, proptosis in Crouzon and Pfeiffer, hypertelorism in Apert, Crouzon, Pfeiffer and Saethre-Chotzen, iris coloboma in CHARGE), ears (displaced and malformed in Goldenhar and Treacher Collins) and jaw. Look for midface hypoplasia (Apert, Crouzon, Pfeiffer and Saethre-Chotzen). Note any facial asymmetry (Beckwith and Goldenhar). Check size of jaw from the side (micrognathia with Robin sequence, TMJ involvement in JIA and Hallermann–Streiff). Look for any neck swelling (goitre from hypothyroidism, cystic hygroma). Check percentiles (increased weight as a cause, or decreased weight as a consequence, increased height [Marfan], decreased height [various syndromes]), Tanner staging (delayed puberty), sick or well, stridor, tachypnoea at rest, tracheal tug and use of accessory muscles. Note the skin (e.g. atopic eczema, coarse features [MPSs, hypothyroidism], acanthosis nigricans [obesity]).

RESPIRATORY AND CARDIOVASCULAR EXAMINATIONS

Examine the ears (dysmorphic with Treacher Collins and Goldenhar) and nose (inspect nasal mucosa [pale and swollen, with visible inferior turbinates, and green/clear discharge with allergic rhinitis], look for nasal polyps, then check whether both nasal airways are patent by getting child to breathe through the nose onto the cold metal of the stethoscope; there will be condensation from expired air if the nostrils are patent, if the metal is cold enough) and throat (size of tonsils, size of tongue). Note that there is *no reliable relation* between the size of the tonsils and the presence or degree of OSA.

Examine the chest for: asymmetry (left chest prominence with chronic increased right-ventricular activity, Beckwith-Wiedemann), deformity (Marfan), expansion, tracheal position, apex position, palpable pulmonary valve closure, right-ventricular overactivity, percussion and auscultation. Examine the cardiovascular system, noting any signs of pulmonary hypertension (single S2, P2 loud, ejection click, early diastolic murmur of pulmonary incompetence, systolic murmur of tricuspid incompetence) or cor pulmonale (signs of right-sided failure: hepatomegaly, ankle oedema).

NEUROLOGICAL EXAMINATION

The neurological system is most quickly assessed by starting with the gait and working up, through the lower limbs, upper limbs and then the motor cranial nerves, with sensory cranial nerves last, as they are the most time-consuming and less likely to be relevant in the examination of most children with OSA.

In the long-case scenario, examine every system thoroughly. In the short case, target relevant systems. If there are dysmorphic features, then examine as per the short case in the genetics chapter. If there are coarse features suggesting a storage disease (e.g. MPS), examine the abdomen for hepatosplenomegaly. If there is hypotonia, determine whether it has a neurological cause, or a connective tissue cause; perform a neurological examination to ascertain the level of hypotonia (upper motor neurone, or lower motor neurone; if the latter, whether anterior horn cell, peripheral nerve, neuromuscular junction or muscle); perform manoeuvres to test for hypermobile joints as in Marfan syndrome (see short case on tall stature in Chapter 7, Endocrinology, and the discussion in long-case section of Chapter 6, Cardiology).

Management

Treatments for OSA with known efficacy include the following.

SURGICAL PROCEDURES

1. *Adenotonsillectomy* (tonsillectomy and adenoidectomy, Ts & As) remains the key treatment for OSA, and leads to significant improvement in most children with OSA, with regard to breathing, sleeping and quality of life. Reports have been somewhat contradictory as to whether there may be improvements in concentration, school performance, cognitive or developmental progress. Adenotonsillectomy has been reported as reducing the need for CPAP in morbidly obese children with OSA. Adenotonsillectomy with the addition of uvulopharyngopalatoplasty (UPPP) has been used in some units for patients with Down syndrome or cerebral palsy (CP), but other units warn against UPPP, as there is a success rate of only around 50%, and complications can include velopharyngeal incompetence.

    • Adenotonsillectomy is not without some risks. There are a number of antecedent risk factors that predict requirement for paediatric ICU care postoperatively. These include: age under 2 years, craniofacial anomalies (especially midface hypoplasia and retrognathia), failure to thrive, or just thin-body habitus, hypotonia, cor pulmonale, marked obesity, previous upper airway trauma, severe OSA on PSG, concomitant UPPP and a history of prematurity. In each of these cases, as postoperative upper airway compromise is not too infrequent, here nasal mask CPAP can be useful.

    • Complications of adenotonsillectomy include anaesthesia-related complications, bleeding (immediate or delayed), upper airway obstruction, nasopharyngeal stenosis, pulmonary oedema, pain (local, odynophagia, otalgia), infection, nausea and vomiting, velopharyngeal insufficiency and hypersomnolence. The mortality rate is around 1 in 4000 to 1 in 27 000; morbidity is around 5–10% overall, but the morbidity rate in patients with OSA is 18–34%. Adenotonsillectomy has an overall efficacy of around 75% in improving or normalising respiratory pattern during sleep.

2. Other surgical therapies: for patients with life-threatening OSA (usually patients with craniofacial syndromes), then the following could be needed: mandibular distraction, maxillomandibular advancement, plus or minus tracheostomy (see overleaf). Procedures to relieve nasal obstruction include inferior turbinate reduction, septoplasty, nasal valve surgery and rapid maxillary expansion. Procedures to relieve retroglossal obstruction include tongue reduction, genioglossus advancement and hyoid myotomy.

3. *Tracheostomy* is another surgical treatment that is available for selected patients with life-threatening OSA, particularly those with craniofacial anomalies (e.g. Pierre Robin sequence, CHARGE, Treacher Collins and Beckwith-Wiedemann syndromes), craniofacial and laryngeal tumours, or bilateral vocal cord paralysis.

MEDICAL THERAPIES

1. Intranasal corticosteroids are effective in decreasing OSA in children with moderate to severe adenoidal hypertrophy (associated with some decrease in adenoid size), those with allergic rhinitis and those with residual postoperative OSA following adenotonsillectomy.
2. Leukotriene antagonists; the combination of intranasal corticosteroids and oral montelukast is effective in resolving mild residual OSA after adenotonsillectomy.
3. Weight loss is recommended as supplementary therapy for obese children.

MECHANICAL VENTILATORY SUPPORT

Non-invasive mask ventilatory support; for example, nasal mask continuous positive airways pressure (*nasal CPAP*) or nasal mask bilevel positive airway pressure (*BiPAP*) are both considered efficacious in paediatric OSA, but there is a high drop-out rate. CPAP provides positive pressure to the airway lumen and reduces airway collapsibility. CPAP can be titrated during PSG to ascertain optimal pressures. A snug-fitting mask is particularly important. BiPAP provides a back-up rate and gives some ventilatory assistance, which is particularly useful for patients with OSA who also have sleep-related hypoventilation due to neuromuscular disease or obesity.

Long-term CPAP or BiPAP can lead to midface hypoplasia, so maxillomandibular growth has to be monitored carefully. CPAP can be indicated where Ts & As have not relieved OSA completely, or where adenotonsillectomy is not indicated or contraindicated, and before surgery in children with severe OSA.

Other therapies, which have been tried but are not used often in children, include oral appliances (such as tongue retainers and mandibular advancing devices) and supplemental oxygen therapy, which eradicates the desaturation episodes, but has no effect on the obstructive component and can worsen hypoventilation.

SHORT CASES

SHORT CASE: The respiratory system

This is a common case, expected to be performed well. On occasion, the patient may have a chronic rare condition such as hypoplastic lung, congenital lobar emphysema or Kartagener's syndrome (primary ciliary dyskinesia), but more common problems include CF and CLD. Specific approaches for the latter two cases are given in the long-case section. The approaches for 'stridor' and for a 'chest' examination are described after this section.

'Examine the respiratory system' implies something different from 'Examine the chest'. The former includes the hands (starting with the nails for clubbing), chest wall, praecordium, lungs, ears, nose, throat and regional lymph nodes. The latter includes chest wall (starting with this, not the hands), heart and lungs, as the primary focus of the examination, only then followed by more peripheral signs. The key is to do exactly what the examiners ask, and not interpret their instructions inappropriately.

Commence the examination of the respiratory system by introducing yourself. Note the child's voice, which may be hoarse (e.g. in laryngotracheobronchitis). Stand back and give a general description of the child, in particular noting the growth parameters (e.g. failure to thrive with CF, BPD), nutritional status (e.g. poor fat stores in CF) and any dysmorphic features (e.g. Pierre Robin facies, with micrognathia).

At this point, the child's chest should be fully exposed, except in the case of an infant, where more subtle manoeuvring may be necessary to avoid upsetting the patient.

Note whether the child looks well or unwell, cyanosed or acyanotic, and describe any notable respiratory noises, such as stridor or wheeze, any cough and the nature of the cry in infants. Note the degree of respiratory distress (e.g. tracheal tug, intercostal, substernal and subcostal recession) and count the respiratory rate. Describe any IV lines (look at what is in the fluid being given; e.g. salbutamol, aminophylline, hydrocortisone or antibiotics), oxygen being administered (at what rate), and any nebuliser or spacer at the end of the bed.

Note any monitoring devices present, such as pulse oximetry or transcutaneous monitoring devices, and their readings. Also note any useful signs on the cot or bed. Describe any chest deformity, asymmetry, any scars and any venous access devices, and ask the child to cough. Request inspection of sputum if there is a moist, productive cough in an older child, and no sputum cup to be seen in the vicinity of the bed.

Commence the general systematic examination of the child with the hands. Then examine the head, followed by the chest, abdomen, ears, nose, palate, throat and regional lymph nodes, and the lower limbs, and request the temperature chart.

Only ask for the PEFR if it would be relevant (making sure you know the appropriate expected values for that patient). Depending on the prior findings, further examination of the fundi, skin and neurological system may be required. The various findings sought are listed in Figure 15.1, and a comprehensive listing of possible signs on initial inspection is given in Table 15.3.

Table 15.3
Additional information: details of findings on respiratory examination
INSPECTION
Dysmorphic features • Robin sequence • Down syndrome • Apert syndrome • Cleft lip sequence
Nutritional status • Muscle bulk • Subcutaneous fat
Intervention • Intravenous line • Oxygen mask or catheter • Spacer +/− mask, or nebuliser at end of bed • Nasogastric tube
Monitoring devices • Pulse oximeter • Cardiorespiratory monitor

Continued

Table 15.3 (continued)
Colour
Respiratory rate
Respiratory noises: stridor, wheeze, cough, cry
Respiratory distress, degree of: • Tracheal tug • Sternal recession • Intercostal, subcostal, substernal or supraclavicular retraction
Chest deformity: barrel chest, Harrison's sulcus, pectus carinatum or excavatum, rib flaring, scoliosis, kyphosis
Asymmetry (e.g. hypoplastic lung, congenital lobar emphysema)
Scars (e.g. multiple intercostal drain tubes, lobectomy, associated congenital heart defects)
Venous access devices (e.g. for antibiotics, in CF patients)
Cough (ask older child to do this and request inspection of any sputum collected)
UPPER LIMBS
Nails: clubbing (suppurative lung disease, pulmonary fibrosis, co-existent cyanotic heart disease)
Fingertips: prick marks (BSL testing in CF patients with diabetes)
Palms: crease pallor (anaemia)
Dorsum of hand: scars of previous multiple IVs (NICU graduate)
Joints: swollen (HPOA; very rare)
Pulse • Tachycardia (hypoxia, fever, treatment with beta-2 agonists) • Pulsus paradoxus (e.g. in severe asthma)
Asterixis: CO_2 retention
OTHER
Lower limbs • Toenail clubbing • Ankle oedema (right-ventricular failure)
Temperature chart
Peak flow meter readings in older children
Fundi: retinal venous dilatation (CO_2 retention)
Skin: eczema (e.g. with asthma)
Neurological system for predisposing causes of respiratory distress (e.g. bulbar palsy [aspiration]), spinal muscular atrophy (diaphragmatic breathing)

BSL = blood sugar level; CF = cystic fibrosis; HPOA = hypertrophic pulmonary osteoarthropathy; NICU = neonatal intensive care unit.

After inspection, ask the child to take a deep breath in and observe the chest expansion for asymmetry. This tends to be more useful than actually palpating during deep inspiration. Next, palpate for the apex beat, parasternal heave, palpable pulmonary valve closure and tracheal position, before percussion. Tactile fremitus can be omitted, as it is unlikely to be helpful in most children.

1. Introduce self
Voice: hoarse (e.g. laryngitis)

2. General inspection
Position patient: standing, fully
    undressed; then sitting
Well or unwell
Parameters
- Height
- Weight
- Head circumference
Dysmorphic features
Nutritional status
Intervention (e.g. IV line, oxygen mask,
    nasogastric tube)
Monitoring devices
Colour
Respiratory rate
Respiratory noises
Respiratory distress
Chest deformity
Asymmetry
Scars
Venous access devices
Cough

3. Upper limbs
Nails
Palms
Joints
Pulse
Asterixis

4. Head
Face
- Dysmorphic
- 'Ex-premmie' (BPD)
- Cushingoid (treatment with
    corticosteroids)
Mouth
- Cyanosis
- Cleft lip
- Tongue: cyanosis

5. Chest
Reinspect (for anything missed on
    general inspection)
Palpate
- Apex beat (displacement)
- Parasternal area (RV heave)
- Pulmonary area (palpable
    pulmonary valve closure)
- Trachea (displacement)
Chest expansion (symmetry in older
    children; inspection better in
    younger children)

Percuss
Auscultate
- Lungs
- Praecordium, for evidence of
    pulmonary hypertension, cor
    pulmonale

6. Abdomen
Liver
- Ptosis (hyperinflated chest)
- Enlarged (right heart failure)
Spleen
- Enlarged (portal hypertension in
    CF)

7. ENT and lymph nodes
Ears: otitis media, acute or chronic
    serous
Nose: polyps (CF)
Mouth: cleft palate
Throat: tonsillitis
Lymph nodes
- Occipital, postauricular (from in
    front)

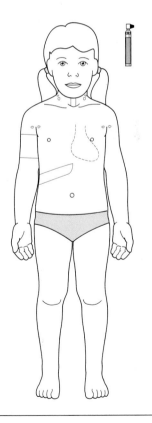

BPD = bronchopulmonary dysplasia; CF = cystic fibrosis; RV = right ventricle.

Figure 15.1 **The respiratory system**

Percussion must be performed well; have consultants check your technique while practising cases. Ensure that percussion is performed symmetrically. The apices are best percussed from behind. When percussing the axillae, it is easier with the child's hands on his or her head. Next, auscultate in the standard manner, again symmetrically. Vocal resonance can usually be omitted. If any rhonchi are noted, it is worth asking the examiners when the last dose of bronchodilator was given.

Consultants differ in their approach to examining the chest. Some prefer to examine the anterior chest wall completely, and then the posterior aspect of the chest completely. Others prefer percussion of front and back, then auscultation in a similar manner. There is no right or wrong way to do it: the important thing is to stick to one method with which you are comfortable; do not change it on exam day.

At the completion of the physical examination, the CXR can be requested; logical and succinct interpretation is expected (see the section on reading CXRs at the end of this chapter).

SHORT CASE: The chest

With this introduction, the examiners want you to start with the chest, not the hands. After general inspection, looking for the various findings sought in a cardiac or respiratory short case, with the child's chest fully exposed, perform a thorough examination of the lungs (as in a respiratory case) and the heart (as thoroughly as in a cardiac short case), as well as the bony structures (sternum, ribs, clavicles, spine), for findings such as scoliosis. Only when every component of the chest per se has been assessed should the systematic examination move peripherally, the direction this takes depending on the findings noted.

SHORT CASE: Stridor

This is a variation of the respiratory examination. The patients seen are usually infants, often with congenital stridor. There is a wide differential diagnosis.

After introducing yourself, stand back and give a general description of the child. Note if he or she appears well or unwell, note the growth parameters, and look for any dysmorphic/syndromal features (e.g. Opitz syndrome, with hypertelorism, cleft lips, protruding ears and laryngeal cleft), or the features of the 'ex-premmie' NICU graduate (prolonged intubation, resultant subglottic stenosis).

Scan the child for any evidence of capillary haemangiomata, particularly in the 'beard' distribution of the face and neck (associated subglottic haemangioma).

Note the infant's colour, posture (e.g. hyperextended neck with supralaryngeal problems, hypertonic spastic posturing in infants with cerebral palsy and pseudobulbar palsy), activity (paucity of movement with some neurological causes) and the degree of respiratory distress. Note the respiratory rate, tracheal tug and degree of chest recession (sternal, intercostal, substernal, subcostal or supraclavicular). Also note the following:

1. Whether the child is receiving any supports, such as nasogastric feeding (which implies at least one patent choanal opening), intravenous fluids, oxygen.
2. Whether the child has been receiving supports (which are temporarily unnecessary), such as bronchodilator therapy (an MDI, spacer or mask), or an oropharyngeal airway, on the bedside cupboard, or whether there is perinasal linear skin reddening, suggesting recent removal of tape securing a nasogastric tube or high-flow nasal oxygen.
3. Whether the child is being monitored; for example, with pulse oximetry.

Observe whether the child is a nose or mouth breather (mouth breathing inferring nasal obstruction; e.g. due to choanal stenosis), and if there is any drooling (suggesting supralaryngeal obstruction) or pooling of secretions (neurological causes).

Listen to the child's breathing to determine in which phase of respiration the noise occurs. Note that fixed obstructive lesions causing significant cross-sectional area reduction of the airway (anywhere) can cause inspiratory and expiratory (biphasic) stridor, irrespective of whether the lesion is extrathoracic (above the clavicles) or intrathoracic (below the clavicles).

Purely inspiratory stridor suggests a non-fixed obstruction, usually above the clavicles/extrathoracic, such as a laryngeal or supralaryngeal obstruction. Inspiratory and expiratory (biphasic) stridor may infer a non-fixed lesion with tracheal involvement. Expiratory noises alone are more likely non-fixed and below the clavicles (tracheal). Laryngeal problems may change the character of the voice (e.g. a hoarse voice with unilateral vocal cord paralysis, or with laryngitis) or the cry (e.g. weak with vocal cord problems; note that bilateral vocal cord palsy is more often associated with a normal cry and normal voice). Crying itself worsens the stridor in laryngomalacia or subglottic haemangioma. Note the relative timing of inspiration and expiration: in laryngeal disorders, inspiration is prolonged; while in bronchial obstruction, expiration is prolonged.

If the mother changes the infant's position when the child is distressed, note any change in the stridor with the crying and with the repositioning.

The child's head posturing must be noted, as it may give a clue to the level of the problem. Laryngeal or supralaryngeal narrowing tends to make a child hyperextend the neck (classic example: epiglottitis) to increase the upper airway diameter.

Inspect the nose, noting whether it permits passage of a nasogastric tube and whether there is any movement of mucus with respiration, inferring patent nostrils. Inspect the mouth for any scars from repaired cleft lip, glossoptosis or micrognathia (syndromal diagnoses) and, when the child opens the mouth, note any obvious cleft palate.

Inspect the neck for any asymmetry (e.g. lymphatic malformation ['cystic hygroma'], neoplasm). Inspect the chest for scars (e.g. previous tracheostomy, previous multiple intercostal drain tubes in the NICU graduate), deformity (e.g. pectus excavatum, Harrison's sulci), increased anteroposterior diameter (e.g. in co-existent CLD in the NICU graduate) and degree of chest recession.

Before the child is too distressed, if you suspect nasal obstruction, the 'metal condensation test' can be performed in a few seconds. Simply hold the metal arm of your stethoscope under the infant's nostrils, and as the metal is (usually) cold, any nasal breathing will result in moisture condensing on the metal, confirming nostril and choanal patency.

Some aspects of the examination of the mouth are unpleasant and are best deferred until the end of the examination, but must not be omitted (see overleaf).

Palpate the neck for any masses (e.g. lymphatic malformation [cystic hygroma]). If any masses are present, examine these in the standard manner for any lump (i.e. size, shape, consistency, pulsatility, attachments, fluctuation, transillumination, auscultation, regional lymph nodes). At this stage, if there is a neck mass, turn the child's head to either side, then flex and extend the neck to assess if this worsens or alleviates the stridor.

Palpate the trachea to detect any deviation. Also palpate the apex beat (deviation), any parasternal heave or palpable pulmonary valve closure (pulmonary hypertension and cor pulmonale), and then percuss across the upper chest to detect any retrosternal mass compressing the airway. Auscultate the lungs (to confirm the timing of the stridor, and detect associated respiratory disease; e.g. CLD) and the heart, for loud second sound and any evidence of right-heart failure or co-existent heart disease (as in some syndromal diagnoses). Now, with auscultation completed, move the infant into a supine and then a prone position, to detect any change in the stridor: in laryngomalacia, the stridor diminishes when prone.

At this point, it may be worthwhile looking carefully at the skin for any 'strawberry' haemangiomata that may have passed unnoticed.

Now come the least pleasant aspects of the examination:

1. Inspect the oral cavity, using a spatula and torch, looking for cleft palate and any obvious swellings or tumours (e.g. retropharyngeal or tonsillar).
2. Test the gag reflex and the suck (for bulbar dysfunction in neurological causes).
3. Palpate the tongue all the way back to detect any mucus retention, cyst or other obstructive lesion.
4. If the condensation test suggests complete obstruction, it is now time to request a feeding tube and pass this down each nostril. Only do this at the very end of the examination, as it always upsets the child.

If a syndrome seems likely, look for other dysmorphic features.

If there is a suggestion of a neurological aetiology, perform a gross motor assessment, followed by testing the long tracts, and then the motor cranial nerves (starting from cranial nerve XII and progressing upwards to III).

Always request the temperature chart at the completion of your examination (e.g. for retropharyngeal abscess).

Give a brief, logical differential diagnosis, and after this request a posteroanterior (P-A) CXR and a lateral airways film.

SHORT CASE: Chest X-rays

Accurate interpretation is expected. Note the date of the X-ray and the name, to check that it is the correct film. Then note which side is labelled 'right' to avoid missing dextrocardia (although it should have been noted clinically), particularly in the child with clubbing and purulent sputum, who has Kartagener's syndrome (immotile cilia/primary ciliary dyskinesia) and not CF. Note whether the film is well centred. This is the time to quickly scan the bony structures, as rotated films will show asymmetry of clavicles on the P-A view. Check the chest symmetry and note any scoliosis or rib crowding. Check that the film is well penetrated, and has been taken during a full inspiration. Expiratory films are notoriously difficult to interpret and may be quite misleading. Note the centring of the trachea and the cardiac shadow, checking for any deviation.

Assess the cardiac size: the cardiac diameter is normally 50% or less of the cardiothoracic diameter (except in neonates, where it can be 60%) (see Fig. 15.2).

The heart may be enlarged due to pathology related to the lungs, such as cor pulmonale. The cardiac contour is then inspected, looking for evidence of the following:

1. Loss of right-heart border definition, which indicates right middle-lobe involvement.
2. Loss of apex definition, which indicates lingula involvement.
3. Increased opacification behind the heart, usually in a 'sail' or triangular shape, indicating left lower-lobe involvement.
4. A prominent pulmonary artery shadow, which can indicate pulmonary hypertension (PHT).
5. A prominent right-atrial shadow, which can occur with PHT.
6. A prominent right-ventricular region, which can occur with PHT (see Fig. 15.3).

Focus on the lung fields. Note any asymmetry in the lucency of the lungs (e.g. in congenital lobar emphysema), any hyperinflation (as in asthma, with 'flattened' diaphragm shadows and increased lucency).

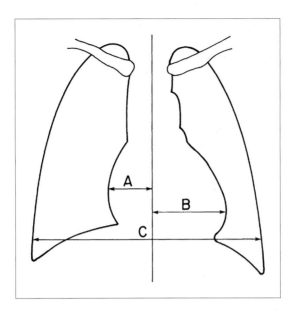

Figure 15.2 **Chest roentgenography. Diagram showing how to measure the cardiothoracic (CT) ratio from the posteroanterior view of a CXR film. The CT ratio is obtained by dividing the largest horizontal diameter of the heart (A–B) by the longest internal diameter of the chest (C).**

Source: Park, M.K. (2007). *Pediatric Cardiology for Practitioners* (5th ed.). Philadelphia: Elsevier. Figure 4.1, p. 66.

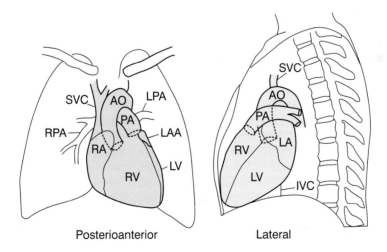

Figure 15.3 **Posteroanterior and lateral projections of a normal cardiac silhouette. Note that in the lateral projection, the right ventricle (RV) is contiguous with the lower third of the sternum and that the left ventricle (LV) normally crosses the posterior margin of the inferior vena cava (IVC) above the diaphragm. AO, aorta; LA, left atrium; LAA, left atrial appendage; LPA, left pulmonary artery; PA, pulmonary artery; RA, right atrium; RPA, right pulmonary artery; SVC, superior vena cava.**

Source: Redrawn from Park, M.K. (2007). *Pediatric Cardiology for Practitioners* (5th ed.). Philadelphia: Elsevier. Figure 4.2, p. 66.

Focus on the diaphragm shadows, looking for the following:

1. Loss of the line of the left hemidiaphragm suggests left lower-lobe involvement.
2. Loss of the line of the right hemidiaphragm suggests right lower-lobe involvement.
3. Loss of a clear costophrenic angle suggests pleural effusion (remember to examine the apices for a pleural cap).
4. The right hemidiaphragm is normally higher than the left, due to the liver; if the lungs are hyperinflated, the hemidiaphragms may be at almost the same level.

Note any focal areas of increased opacification, and any generalised increase in opacification in perihilar or peripheral areas. If it is unclear on assessing the P-A film which region of the lung is involved (as is particularly the case in consolidation affecting the 'midzone' of the lung fields), request a lateral film.

In assessing the lateral film, first note the bony structures. Note the degree of opacification of the vertebrae: normally the upper vertebrae are quite opaque, due to the overlying shoulder region, and as one progresses down the spine, the vertebral bodies appear increasingly lucent, because of the lack of overlying soft tissues in that region. Thus, if there is increased opacification of the lower vertebral area, there may be consolidation, or other process, involving the posterior segments of the affected lobe. Also note any kyphosis (rare) or rib abnormalities. Check the tracheal position followed by assessing the positions of the hemidiaphragms. Now inspect the lung fields; they are normally obscured in the postero-superior aspect (by the shoulders) and in the anteroinferior aspect (by the heart). Look for the interlobar fissures, which may delineate a collapsed or consolidated area.

Reference

Wainwright, C.E. et al. (2015). Lumacaftor-Ivacaftor in patients with cystic fibrosis homozygous for Phe508delCFTR. *New England Journal of Medicine*, 373, 220–231.

Chapter 16

Rheumatology

LONG CASE: Juvenile idiopathic arthritis (JIA)

Biological disease-modifying anti-rheumatic drugs (bDMARDs, or 'biologics') have enabled the management of JIA to evolve remarkably in the last decade. Trials of these agents in JIA have taken place through international collaborative efforts. Mirroring major advances in the understanding and the evidence base of JIA management, the escalation of chemotherapeutic agent usage and the evolution of biological therapies have transformed the outcome goals sought in JIA, where the expectation now is to be able to *switch off* inflammation, not just control it. Early aggressive treatment that induces remission rapidly is the aim. There are now effective therapies available for the following:

- Systemic JIA (sJIA). These include interleukin-1 blockers anakinra and canakinumab, and the interleukin-6 blocker tocilizumab.
- Polyarticular JIA (pJIA). These include the tumour necrosis factor (alpha) (TNF) inhibitor etanercept, and abatacept, a humanised selective T-cell co-stimulatory modulator, and the monoclonal antibodies adalimumab and infliximab.
- Enthesitis-related arthritis (ERA). These include the TNF inhibitors etanercept, adalimumab and infliximab.

Methotrexate remains the key conventional disease-modifying anti-rheumatic drug (DMARD), and intra-articular corticosteroid injections (IACI) the recommended initial therapy for oligoarticular JIA (oJIA).

By convention, disability, remission, structural damage and death have been the main outcome measures in arthritis. In JIA, extra-articular comorbidities such as uveitis have also been measured as the disease outcome. There is no single measure that could represent all outcomes in JIA. Health-related quality of life (HRQOL) may be studied using various tools that have been developed to measure single outcomes, or a combination of these outcomes. These include the Childhood Health Assessment Questionnaire (CHAQ), the Child Health Questionnaire (CHQ) and the Pediatric Quality of Life Inventory Generic Core Scales (PedsQL). Measurement of change may be undertaken by using internationally agreed-upon core set variables, often in the context of response to treatment. These variables include: physician global assessment of disease activity; parent/patient assessment of overall wellbeing; the disability index (CHAQ score); the number of joints with active arthritis; the number of joints with a limited range of movement; and a measurement of inflammation, such as the erythrocyte sedimentation rate (ESR) or C-reactive protein (CRP). Recently devised definitions of clinical remission, on and off medication and minimal disease activity will assist in comparing and contrasting different treatment regimens. The American College of Rheumatology (ACR) has developed criteria that quantify improvement in at least three of six core variables, as a percentage of improvement, so the ACR Pediatric 30 criteria define an improvement of > 30% in at least three of six core variables, the ACR Pedi50 criteria define an improvement of > 50%, the ACR Pedi70 of > 70% and the ACR Pedi90 of > 90%, respectively.

The definition of a 'flare-up' in the disease has been based on these same criteria, with > 40% worsening of two of six components, with no more than one component improving by 30%.

Children with JIA are often used as long-case subjects, as their care is multifaceted and often difficult. The candidate should be well versed in the range of available drugs and newer biological agents employed, their important adverse effects, the role of physical and supportive therapies, the associated disorders and the long-term outcomes.

Current classification of JIA

OLIGOARTHRITIS (FOUR OR FEWER JOINTS INVOLVED WITHIN THE FIRST 6 MONTHS); oJIA

The most common form of JIA, oligoarthritis is defined as arthritis affecting one to four joints during the first 6 months after onset of the disease. Accounting for approximately 45% of all JIA, this form predominantly occurs in females aged between 12 months and 5 years (peak 3 years). This group is at risk (up to 30%) of chronic uveitis, which is almost always asymptomatic, although it can occasionally result in photophobia, red eyes and visual changes. The untreated uveitis can result in complications such as band keratopathy, cataract and glaucoma. This is the leading cause of blindness in children in developed countries. As such, all children in this group require regular slit-lamp examination, every 3–4 months, by an ophthalmologist. Antinuclear antibody (ANA) positivity (which occurs in about 50% of this group) is associated with the occurrence of uveitis in this group. The knees are most commonly affected, although the ankles (including the subtalar joints), wrists and elbows may also be involved. Hip involvement as the presenting joint is very rare. Erosive disease does occur particularly in the extended oligo form.

The presence of some historical or laboratory features may exclude the diagnosis of oligoarthritis. These include several conditions which meet diagnostic criteria for other forms of JIA: 1. a positive family history of psoriasis; or 2. a positive family history of spondyloarthropathy in a first-degree relative; or 3. a positive rheumatoid factor; or 4. positive HLA B27 in male over 6 years; or 5. a diagnosis of SJIA. A favourable outcome is dependent on appropriate and timely management, which may include intra-articular steroid injection, physiotherapy and exercise, all aimed at restoring the pre-morbid joint status. While NSAIDs may be used to treat symptoms and enable more intensive physical activity, DMARDs may be used to maintain the joint and prevent recurrence of inflammation. In this way, joint complications such as asymmetrical growth, subluxation or ankylosis can be avoided.

PERSISTENT OLIGOARTHRITIS

Persistent oligoarthritis is defined as affecting no more than four joints during the course of the disease. Provided that treatment has been implemented, the arthritis prognosis in this group is relatively better than other subtypes of JIA. The associated uveitis has a better prognosis when discovered by screening than by symptomatic referral.

EXTENDED OLIGOARTHRITIS

Extended oligoarthritis is defined as arthritis affecting one to four joints during the first 6 months of the disease, and a cumulative total of five joints or more after the first 6 months of the disease. Specific exclusions are as outlined on the previous page. Methotrexate (MTX) is the agent of choice for maintenance of arthritis in this group. This subtype of JIA can be quite severe and can continue into adult life.

POLYARTHRITIS RF-NEGATIVE (pJIA)

'Polyarthritis RF-negative' is defined as arthritis affecting five or more joints during the first 6 months after onset of the disease. This accounts for around 25% of JIA with female predominance, at any age. There is arthritis involving both the large and small joints of the upper and lower limbs, as well as the cervical spine and temporomandibular joints, and it may be symmetrical or asymmetrical. Uveitis may occur in approximately 10% and requires screening. ANA may be positive in over 25%. It can remit in late childhood, although continuation into adult life may also be seen. NSAIDs may be used to treat symptoms, while methotrexate is the agent of choice for maintenance of disease. Some patients may need higher doses of MTX, and as absorption of oral MTX may be variable and subject to first-pass metabolism by liver, parenteral administration may be required. Subcutaneous MTX is as effective as intramuscular MTX, but less painful and more likely to be adhered to.

POLYARTHRITIS RF-POSITIVE (pJIA)

Polyarthritis RF-positive is defined as arthritis affecting five or more joints during the first 6 months of the disease, associated with positive rheumatoid factor tests on at least two occasions 3 months apart. This accounts for around 5–10% of JIA with female predominance and late childhood/teenage onset. Resembles adult rheumatoid arthritis, with a *symmetrical* polyarthritis affecting the upper (e.g. metacarpophalangeal joints most common) and lower limbs. Other features include subcutaneous nodules and early erosive changes radiologically. Untreated, it often follows a progressive course, with eventual joint destruction. Unremitting severe disease and poor functional outcome occur in over 50%. This group responds to the same drugs as for adult rheumatoid arthritis.

SYSTEMIC JIA (sJIA)

1. Early onset (1–4 years; peak at 2), but can occur throughout childhood, equal sex incidence, up to 10% of JIA.
2. Systemic symptoms: fever (typically single or double quotidian pattern with high spikes daily, occurring at similar times every day); rash (evanescent, coming and going with fever spikes; discrete salmon pink macules 2–10 mm, usually around upper trunk and axillae; show Koebner phenomenon; rarely pruritic; not purpuric); polyarticular arthritis (can be late feature).
3. Other features: lymphadenopathy, hepatosplenomegaly, serositis (pericarditis, pleuritis), and inflammatory ascites, haematological changes (anaemia, leucocytosis, macrophage activation syndrome).
4. An occasional feature is myocarditis.
5. Systemic features can precede arthritis by months. Natural evolution: systemic features followed by polyarthritis; this remains while systemic features regress.
6. Rheumatoid factor (RF) negative and usually ANA negative.
7. Approximately 50% remit in 2–3 years.
8. Untreated, joint destruction occurs in most cases.

9. Systemic arthritis is the only type of JIA without a specific age, gender or HLA association.

10. Most mortality from JIA is in this subgroup. Deaths can be due to infection secondary to immunosuppression, myocardial involvement or macrophage activation syndrome (MAS). MAS is a rare complication of systemic arthritis, involving increased activation of histiophagocytosis. Triggers include preceding viral illness (e.g. EBV) and additional medications (particularly NSAIDs, sulfasalazine and etanercept). Clinical findings include lymphadenopathy, hepatosplenomegaly, purpura, mucosal bleeding and multiple organ failure. Investigations may show pancytopenia, prolonged prothrombin time and partial thromboplastin time, elevated fibrin degradation products, hyperferritinaemia, hypertriglyceridaemia and low ESR. Treatment involves pulse methylprednisolone and cyclosporine A, or dexamethasone and etoposide. Increasingly, biologic medications such as anakinra are being used as second-line agents.

11. Uveitis is rare, although ophthalmological surveillance is necessary to detect cataracts or glaucoma as complications of steroid treatment.

The ILAR classification lists three criteria that are *definite*: 1. documented quotidian fever for at least 2 weeks, of which at least on three consecutive days a quotidian pattern has been recorded; 2. evanescent, non-fixed erythematous rash; and 3. arthritis. There are also criteria for *probable* systemic disease, in the absence of arthritis—criteria 1 and 2, together with any two of: generalised lymph node enlargement; hepatomegaly or splenomegaly; or serositis.

ENTHESITIS-RELATED ARTHRITIS (ERA)

Approximately 15% of all JIA, this predominantly occurs in males in pre-teenage years, with lower limb involvement, especially the hips and sacroiliac joints. Many show features common to spondyloarthropathies (e.g. enthesitis, decreased lumbar flexion). Involvement of the spine is uncommon in childhood. Rarely buttock pain occurs, reflecting sacroiliitis.

Imaging the sacroiliac (SI) joints with magnetic resonance imaging (MRI) scan is more sensitive than plain radiographs, and will detect inflammatory changes before cartilage and bone destruction occurs. Bone scan may be useful if there are positive findings; however, a negative result does not rule out sacroiliitis. Uveitis in this subtype may occur in 25% of cases, and usually presents as an acute red eye with pain and photophobia. (This is quite different to the chronic asymptomatic uveitis that occurs in oligoarthritis or extended oligoarthritis.) HLA-B27 antigen is positive in 80%; ANA- and RF-negative.

ERA is defined by: 1. arthritis and enthesitis; or 2. arthritis or enthesitis, with at least two of the following: sacroiliac joint tenderness, inflammatory spinal pain, HLA-B27 positive, a family history (first- or second-degree relatives—at least one of 1. acute anterior uveitis; 2. spondyloarthropathy confirmed by a rheumatologist; or 3. inflammatory bowel disease) or acute anterior uveitis.

Specific exclusions are a positive rheumatoid factor or a positive family history of psoriasis in a first-degree relative. Treatment, just as for other subtypes, must be targeted at obliteration of active synovitis or enthesitis. This may require intra-articular or peri-entheseal long-acting corticosteroid injection (e.g. triamcinolone), as well as commencement of sulfasalazine (SSZ) for maintenance and prevention of recurrence of inflammation. Methotrexate is normally used if SSZ does not achieve this, although other cytotoxics (e.g. azathioprine) may also be useful. TNF inhibitors have been successful and are used when earlier steps have failed. NSAIDs may be useful to treat symptoms, but they do not change structural outcomes such as erosive disease. Prolonged use of NSAIDs may have long-term health consequences (renal or cardiovascular) and should be avoided.

ERA includes patients previously known as 'juvenile ankylosing spondylitis'. This terminology has been now updated, however, and is best avoided. The diagnosis of IBD-related arthritis does not come under JIA, as in the presence of a specific diagnosis arthritis can no longer be regarded as 'idiopathic'. Extra-articular manifestations of ERA, in addition to anterior uveitis, include aortitis, aortic incompetence, muscle weakness and fever (usually low grade).

PSORIATIC JIA (psJIA)

psJIA has a female predominance and tends to occur in mid-childhood. The arthritis is frequently *asymmetrical* and may have oligoarticular onset, although a polyarticular course is commonly present. Dactylitis (sausage digits) is seen in younger patients and DIP joint involvement is common. The inflammation may involve tendon sheaths, and in its severe form cause 'arthritis mutilans', a very destructive arthropathy. There is often a family history of psoriasis. Fingernail pitting, onycholysis or other nail dystrophic changes may be seen. About half of the patients have the rash of psoriasis before the arthritis, while in the others the rash may present much later, or never at all. Few cases may develop both symptoms simultaneously. Uveitis can occur, and is seen in about 10%. (Both ANA and HLA-B27 antigen may be present.)

Treatment of the psoriatic arthritis subtype is along similar lines as for other JIA subtypes, utilising intra-articular steroid injections for rapid control of acute inflammation, and DMARDs for maintenance of the disease and prevention of relapse. Both methotrexate and steroids may not be as efficacious in the treatment of psJIA, and the use of TNF inhibitor may be indicated to prevent irreversible joint damage, or to reverse erosive changes.

UNDIFFERENTIATED ARTHRITIS

This group includes patients with arthritis whose presentation does not fulfil the criteria of any other specific groups. An example is systemic arthritis in the presence of positive RF.

Presentation of a long case with JIA

The child with JIA may have a very long and complicated history. Clarity of presentation to the examiners is essential. Long cases with JIA particularly lend themselves to pictorial display. This method can be used for recording the history and allows the examiners to appreciate clearly the progress of the illness. If the candidate wishes to try this technique, it should be practised on trial cases before the exam. Figure 16.1 demonstrates an example: a 15-year-old girl with difficult-to-control polyarthritis RF-positive JIA. The diagram shows progress over a 5-year period, with arthritis activity and drugs used. Investigation results can be shown on the same diagram.

History

The history given here includes questions regarding possible differential diagnoses, which would be relevant only in a newly presenting patient. Differentials are given after their symptoms, in parentheses. Ask about the following.

PRESENTING COMPLAINT

Reason for current admission.

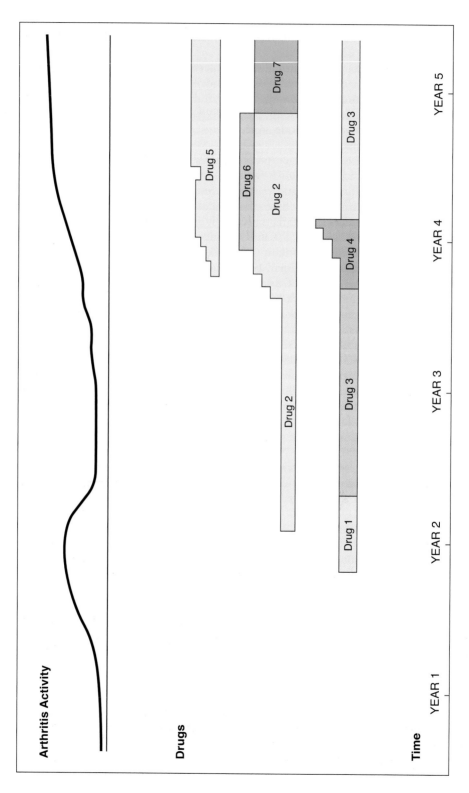

Figure 16.1 The 5-year history of a 15-year-old girl with difficult-to-control polyarthritis RF-positive JIA

CURRENT SYMPTOMS

1. General health; for example, constitutional symptoms (fever, pallor, weight loss), exercise tolerance, quality of sleep.
2. Joint symptoms; for example, early morning stiffness, nocturnal discomfort/night waking, pain, tenderness, swelling, limitation of movement, problem joints (e.g. knees, hands), splints and orthoses used.
3. Level of functioning with activities of daily living (ADLs); for example, eating or pain on mastication, poor dental hygiene (limited jaw opening reflecting temporomandibular joint [TMJ] involvement), dressing, writing, walking, aids required (e.g. dressing sticks, adaptive utensils, wheelchair, computer), home modifications required (e.g. ramps, bathroom fittings), ability to attend/manage school, limitations of sporting and social activities, depression.
4. Skin rashes; for example, salmon rash of systemic JIA, malar flush (SLE), heliotrope of eyelids (dermatomyositis), psoriasis, rheumatoid nodules.
5. Chest symptoms; for example, pain from pleuritis, pericarditis.
6. Bowel symptoms; for example, diarrhoea with inflammatory bowel disease (IBD).
7. Eye problems; for example, uveitis, cataract, glaucoma.
8. Neurological symptoms; for example, seizures, drowsiness (JIA or SLE), personality change or headache with SLE.
9. Growth concerns; for example, short stature, delayed puberty, requirement for growth hormone, self-image effects.
10. Nutritional issues; for example, anorexia from drug side effects (e.g. methotrexate), cachexia, persistent high inflammatory state, mechanical issues (TMJ involvement), bone mineral density (BMD) measurements (increased fracture risk with osteopenia [low bone mass for age, BMD between 1 and 2.5 standard deviations below the mean for age and sex] or osteoporosis [BMD more than 2.5 standard deviations below the mean for age and sex]), whether taking calcium or vitamin D supplements, muscle mass measurements.
11. Jaw involvement; for example, micrognathia, effect on self-image.
12. Drug/agent side effects; for example, steroid effects (poor height gain, obesity, myopathy), NSAIDs (GIT upset), methotrexate (leukopenia, hepatotoxicity), bDMARDs (increased number of infections).

PAST HISTORY

Initial diagnosis (when, where, presenting symptoms, initial investigations), apparent triggers (e.g. immunisations, precedent illness), number of hospitalisations, sequence of joint involvement, development of complications and their management.

MANAGEMENT

Present treatment in hospital, usual treatment at home and school (including occupational and physiotherapy, exercises, sports, drugs), previous treatments used (including effects, and why stopped), side effects, monitoring of levels, compliance, use of identification bracelet, alternative therapies tried (e.g. naturopathy), elimination diets.

SOCIAL HISTORY

1. Disease impact on child; for example, school absenteeism, limitation of ADLs, self-image.
2. Impact on parents; for example, financial considerations such as the cost of home modifications, splints, wheelchairs, transport, frequent hospitalisations, drugs.
3. Impact on siblings; for example, resentment from not getting enough attention/time from parents.

4. Benefits received; for example, Child Disability Assistance Payment, Health Care Card.
5. Social supports; for example, Arthritis Australia; internet resources used by parents.

FAMILY HISTORY

Arthritis, autoimmune conditions, inflammatory bowel disease, psoriasis, enthesitis, uveitis.

At the completion of presenting the history, the examiners should have a clear impression of the following:
1. The patient's current functioning (e.g. ADLs).
2. The patient's current (and past) treatment modalities, such as physiotherapy, drugs and alternative therapies tried (e.g. naturopathic).
3. The social situation (e.g. the child's expectations for the future, the geographical situation relative to the treating hospital).

Examination

See the short case on joints in this chapter. This gives an approach to the lead-in 'Please examine this child's joints', so that it covers not only signs found in JIA, but also signs indicating other diseases, such as SLE. These latter features are not usually relevant in the JIA long case, unless a diagnostic dilemma exists.

Diagnosis

Although it is the most common chronic inflammatory arthropathy in children, JIA remains a clinical diagnosis of exclusion. Some of the diseases to be excluded have been enumerated already. The diagnosis has been made categorically in patients used as long-case subjects. However, the candidate may be asked which investigations would have been appropriate when the child was initially seen. Thus, a differential diagnosis is worth considering, even in established cases, if only for possible discussion purposes.

Investigations

In terms of differential diagnoses, there are too many to allow a brief but worthwhile list to be given. However, arthritis in the context of infections (e.g. EBV), neoplastic disease (leukaemia) or other connective tissue diseases (SLE, mixed connective tissue disease [MCTD]) should be considered. The most appropriate investigations obviously depend on the clinical situation.

A mnemonic of selected differential diagnoses is **VIRAL JOINT**:

Viral (Parvo, EBV)/**V**asculitides (Henoch–Schönlein, Kawasaki)
Infective (bacterial: septic joint, osteomyelitis, discitis, sacroiliitis, Lyme)
Reactive (post-streptococcal, rheumatic fever, Reiter, serum sickness)
Autoimmune (SLE, dermatomyositis, systemic sclerosis, MCTD, psoriasis, Behçet's)
Leukaemia (ALL, AML)

JIA + other inflammatory disorders (inflammatory bowel disease, sarcoidosis)
Osteo: benign (osteoid osteoma/osteoblastoma)/malignant (osteosarcoma/Ewing)
Immunodeficiency (common variable immunodeficiency)
Neoplasia (neuroblastoma, rhabdomyosarcoma)
Trauma

The following investigations may be helpful in JIA.

BLOOD TESTS
Haematology

1. Full blood examination may reveal normochromic normocytic anaemia, neutrophil leucocytosis or thrombocytosis. Anaemia, and low-normal platelet count ± leucopenia may suggest the presence of leukaemia.
2. ESR/CRP: often raised; but may be normal. May be useful for ongoing disease monitoring.

Serology

1. IgM rheumatoid factor (RF): 10% seropositive. Higher IgM RF titres carry a worse prognosis as regards permanent disability, and a greater likelihood of systemic features. The presence of CCP antibodies may add specificity to a positive RF test. Very high RF titres (> 1000) may suggest SLE or MCTD to be the primary diagnosis.
2. Antinuclear antibody (ANA): positive in 50%, and mainly in oligoarthritis and extended oligoarthritis subtypes. While the titre of ANA does not correlate with disease severity, by convention values ≥ 80 are regarded as positive. Very high ANA titres (> 1000) may suggest that SLE or MCTD is present.

Immunology

1. Immunoglobulins: all immunoglobulin types may be elevated as a hypergamma-globulinaemia response. The presence of specific Ig deficiency can cause arthritis, although this precludes diagnosis of JIA.
2. Complement: C3 and C4 may be elevated as a part of an inflammatory response, and a low C2 may occasionally be found (associated C2 complement deficiency), although deficiency in early complements may suggest diagnosis of SLE.

HLA typing

1. B27; for example, enthesitis-related arthritis especially in males 6 years and above, psoriatic arthritis, arthritis associated with IBD.
2. DR4 (polyarthritis: RF-positive).

IMAGING
Plain radiography

Plain radiographs are useful in excluding other differential diagnoses such as osteomyelitis, septic arthritis, trauma and malignancy. It is not necessary to X-ray the lumbosacral region in most children with JIA, as a negative study does not exclude the absence of sacroiliac joint involvement and the radiation dose is high. Common findings on plain X-rays include:
1. Soft-tissue swelling.
2. Joint-space narrowing (only in established untreated cases).
3. Periarticular osteoporosis.
   (The above three are the most common findings in RF-negative JIA.)
4. Joint erosions (development may lead to changed management), disappearing joint line, ankylosis/subluxation.
5. Leg-length discrepancy (accelerated maturation due to hyperaemia around the joint and low grade inflammation; also can have decreased bone growth due to growth plate destruction).

ORTHOPANTOMOGRAM (OPG)

This is used to screen for TMJ involvement (condylar resorption), although direct lateral views provide better detail.

ULTRASOUND

Ultrasound can be useful in:
1. Effusions (especially useful assessing hips, shoulders).
2. Synovitis/tenosynovitis (increased echogenicity with inflamed tissues).
3. Acute synovitis (assessing for increased vascularity on Doppler).
4. Guiding intra-articular therapy.

Magnetic resonance imaging (MRI)—enhanced with gadolinium (gadopentetate dimeglumine)

MRI is significantly more sensitive than a conventional X-ray, being useful in demonstrating anatomy, including soft tissue and cartilage, to assess:
1. Early joint damage.
2. Positive effects of treatment before they are clinically apparent.
3. The amount of inflamed synovium (when performed with gadolinium enhancement).
4. Long-term effects in difficult-to-monitor joints (cervical spine, TMJ, hips).

Management

The goals of JIA management are as follows:
1. Switch off inflammation, hence preventing permanent joint damage.
2. Provide analgesia.
3. Maintain joint function.
4. Prevent deformities.
5. Treat complications and extra-articular manifestations.
6. Ensure optimal nutrition.
7. Rehabilitation.
8. Ensure optimal psychosocial health.
9. Educate parents/patient regarding disease.

1. SWITCH OFF INFLAMMATION
Local corticosteroid injections

Long-acting steroid preparations (e.g. triamcinolone hexacetonide) injected intra-articularly are safe, effective and useful for any joint with significant persistent inflammation. With successful treatment of joint inflammation, symptomatic treatment (e.g. NSAID treatment) may no longer be needed. Joint injections can be performed as a day case, using nitrous oxide inhalation or under conscious sedation for older children (over 8), or under general anaesthesia for younger children, for difficult-to-access joints (e.g. fingers, hips) or when multiple joints are being injected.

Image intensification or ultrasound may be useful, particularly in the shoulders, hips and subtalar joints. For the TMJ, injection under CT or US guidance may be required, especially in patients with effusion or pannus evidenced on TMJ MRI. Paediatric rheumatologists are using intra-articular therapy much earlier in the treatment of JIA than previously, as there is evidence to show that this improves protection against erosions and will delay relapses. The positive effects of the steroid are noted usually within a few days, with effects usually lasting for several months. For those cases with recurrent synovitis, especially if a polyarticular course is present, simultaneous maintenance treatment (e.g. methotrexate) will be required.

Systemic corticosteroids

Pulse intravenous steroids may have a place when a rapid therapeutic effect of the systemic steroids is required, such as in pericardial or pleural effusion, or macrophage activation syndrome (MAS) in sJIA. MAS is a complication in sJIA, or any other connective tissue disease with persistently high inflammation, and if left untreated can cause multi-system failure and death. In addition to steroids, a maintenance agent, usually cyclosporine A, will be required. The treatment regimen consists of IV methylprednisolone (30 mg/kg [up to 1 g maximum dose] as an infusion given over 1–2 hours for three consecutive days). Repeating this schedule a week later may be associated with less recurrence.

Non-steroidal anti-inflammatory drugs (NSAIDs)

Non-steroidal anti-inflammatory drugs (NSAIDs) should not be a part of ongoing maintenance therapy as they do not modify the natural history of the condition. They can decrease pain and stiffness, as well as increase the range of movement. Analgesic response is rapid, although the anti-inflammatory effect may take longer to commence. The average time to achieve a therapeutic response is around 1 month. Nearly all patients who are going to respond to a particular NSAID will do so within 3 months. Common side effects include anorexia, abdominal pain and behavioural issues. More serious side effects include gastrointestinal ulceration (rarer in children than in adults; medications such as antacids or H_2 blockers may be required), bruising from abnormal coagulation and pseudoporphyria skin rashes on sun-exposed areas. NSAIDs are unpredictable, their effectiveness being largely idiosyncratic. Around 50% of JIA children respond to their first NSAID.

NSAIDs include naproxen, diclofenac (avoided if history of aspirin allergy, as cross-sensitivity with aspirin), ibuprofen, indomethacin (especially ERA or unresponsive sJIA), piroxicam, aspirin. With the past adverse publicity relating to salicylate usage and Reye's syndrome, aspirin is used rarely and is not recommended.

Conventional disease-modifying anti-rheumatic drugs (DMARDs)

Conventional DMARDs are those medications (other than biologics) that reduce the rate of adverse structural outcomes such as joint erosions. These include methotrexate (MTX), sulfasalazine (SSZ) and leflunomide. The use of a particular agent may depend on the JIA subtype.

DMARDs are continued until such time that the underlying disease activity is sufficiently low (remission), or if intolerance to them cannot be managed.

Methotrexate (MTX)

Methotrexate (MTX) is effective in all forms of JIA, although less so in the sJIA, psJIA and ERA subtypes. With over 30 years of experience in its use, low-dose, once-a-week MTX is safe and reliable. Folate supplementation decreases side effects. MTX is given at a dose of 10–15 mg per m^2 of surface area once a week, by an oral or parenteral (usually subcutaneous) route. Higher doses may be more effective, but this is at the expense of an unacceptable increase in toxicity; therefore, they are rarely used. The parenteral route of administration is associated with fewer side effects, although the need to train someone to administer the medication, as well as the need to eliminate the cytotoxic waste, make this more cumbersome. Side effects include appetite loss, nausea and oral ulcers (lessened by treating with folate), as well as raised liver enzymes. Less commonly, a low neutrophil or platelet count is seen, while agranulocytosis is a very rare complication. Regular blood tests (monthly or second monthly) are performed to detect any liver impairment or marrow involvement. Long-term studies of MTX in JIA have yet to be published. Theoretical risks of carcinogenesis, infertility or interstitial lung disease have not transpired with several years of treatment. MTX is a teratogen and contraception should be considered. It has been shown to slow and even stop the progression of bone destruction in adults with rheumatoid arthritis. MTX has allowed remission to be achieved early in many patients.

Sulfasalazine (SSZ)

This is only used in ERA; some rheumatologists use this before MTX. The effective moiety of the drug is 5-aminosalicylic acid. A trial of at least 3 months, and usually longer, is needed to judge efficacy. Side effects include hypersensitivity reactions, hepatotoxicity and bone marrow alterations.

Leflunomide (LEF)

This is not used frequently. It is a pyrimidine synthesis inhibitor of dihydroorotate dehydrogenase. It appears safe and effective, comparing favourably to MTX, both in efficacy and in having fewer side effects. Its side effects include diarrhoea, elevated liver enzyme levels and mucocutaneous abnormalities. Leflunomide may have teratogenic effects; and in patients of child-bearing age, effective contraception is required during and for up to 2 years after use, because of prolonged enterohepatic circulation ('washout' regimens are available to shorten this interval if needed).

Biological disease-modifying anti-rheumatic drugs (bDMARDs)

bDMARDs can block, selectively, pro-inflammatory cytokines and can decrease production of cytokine acting through B- or T-lymphocytes. These include: the tumour necrosis factor-alpha (TNF-α) inhibitors etanercept, infliximab and adalimumab; the IL-1 inhibitor anakinra; the IL-6 inhibitor tocilizumab; the anti-CD20 (plasma cell receptor) rituximab; and the T-cell proliferation inhibitor abatacept. With the exception of rituximab, these agents are to be used simultaneously with methotrexate.

This is to improve efficacy and minimise the possibility of developing drug antibodies in the patient, which will cause tachyphylaxis. All of these agents can cause immunosuppression, and live virus vaccines should be avoided in a patient on these medications for this reason. Varicella-susceptible children should be ideally immunised 3 months before starting these agents; however, the severity of the arthritis usually does not allow any delay in starting them. TNF inhibitors (TNFIs) can lead to reactivation of latent tuberculosis (TB), so before starting therapy with these agents, tuberculin (PPD) non-reactivity needs to be confirmed, and a screening chest X-ray is performed. If the results are positive, then treatment with isoniazid should commence a month before starting the TNF inhibitors, to avoid reactivation of latent tuberculosis. Biological agents are used in children with severe disease that is refractory to standard therapy. Most have been shown to reverse erosions and promote bone remodelling, although this is limited to the initial phases of erosive disease. They are occasionally associated with allergic reactions (infliximab), although their medium-term side effects commonly relate to a higher rate of upper respiratory tract infections (etanercept) and injection site reactions (anakinra, etanercept).

Long-term safety data for use of these agents are becoming more available, with 30 cases of neoplastic disease occurring in children who received TNFIs reported to the Food and Drug Administration (FDA) in the US, during the decade from 1998 to 2008. A further potential increased risk is that of fungal infection.

At the time of writing, there were only three PBS-funded biologics available for prescription by rheumatologists in Australia: for patients with JIA, the funded medications are etanercept and adalimumab for all types of JIA, and tocilizumab for sJIA and pJIA.

There are three available IL-1 antagonists: anakinra, which is PBS funded, rilonacept and canakinumab. Anakinra and canakinumab are used in sJIA. No IL-1 blockers are funded for JIA in Australia. However, anakinra and more recently canakinumab are used for sJIA.

There is an IL-6 antagonist, tocilizumab, which can be used in pJIA and sJIA, and a chimeric antibody against the CD20 receptor, rituximab, which has been used in sJIA.

Note that all the drugs ending in 'cept' are soluble re**cep**tor antagonists, acting as decoy receptors; all the drugs ending in 'mab' are **m**onoclonal **a**nti**b**odies; and the 'mabs' with an 'x' in them (infliximab and rituximab) are 'cross-bred', with murine components to the antibodies; the other 'mabs' are more fully humanised; drugs which involve inhibiting interleu*kin*s may have 'kin' in their name (ana*kin*ra [an IL-1 receptor antagonist], and cana*kin*umab [monoclonal antibody against IL-1 beta]).

TNFIs should not be used at the same time as other bDMARDs. It is acceptable to switch from one type of TNFI to another TNFI. TNFIs should not be started until at least 8 weeks after trying other types of bDMARDs, like abatacept, rituximab or tocilizumab.

RTX should not be used at the same time as other bDMARDs. Rituximab should not be started until at least 4 weeks after etanercept, or 8 weeks since TNFIs, abatacept or tocilizumab.

TNF Inhibitors (TNFI)

Adalimumab (ADA) (humanised monoclonal anti-TNF-α antibody)

ADA is given by subcutaneous (SC) injection every 2 weeks. It is used for JIA with a polyarticular course. It is especially efficacious when MTX is given concurrently. The half-life of adalimumab is 14 days. The onset of benefit is 2–4 weeks. It is effective in pJIA, ERA, psJIA and oligoarthritis.

Etanercept (ETN) (recombinant p75 soluble tumour necrosis factor receptor [sTNFR]: Fc fusion protein)

ETN was the first anticytokine therapy used in JIA. Now a well-established therapy for JIA, it is used for patients with a treatment-resistant (failed to respond to MTX) active polyarticular course (pJIA). It has a response rate of 77%, although it has been found to be less successful in treating sJIA. The dose in children/adolescents aged 4–17 is 0.4 mg/kg (max 25 mg) twice-weekly by SC injection.

Parents are trained in reconstituting the etanercept and administering the injection using the aseptic technique. Autoinjectors (as used for diabetics) can be useful. Injection site reactions are common, occurring in about 40%, although these resolve after a few injections. Other common adverse events include upper respiratory tract infections, rhinitis, headache, rash and gastrointestinal symptoms. It is contraindicated in sepsis.

In previous years, numerous case reports were published about patients in whom uveitis developed after commencement of etanercept treatment, or worsened if pre-existent. Stopping this treatment for 2 weeks (washout period) and commencement of infliximab or adalimumab controlled the uveitis in most cases.

When effective, etanercept causes significant reduction in disease activity within 2 weeks of commencement, with sustained benefit as long as treatment is continued. In JIA with a polyarticular course, it controls pain and swelling, improves laboratory parameters and slows radiographic progression of the disease. The drug is named to indicate that it intercepts TNF-α, a cytokine important in the pathogenesis of RA and JIA.

It is made up of two components: the extracellular ligand-binding domain of the 75-kD human receptor for TNF-α, and the constant portion of human immunoglobulin (IgG1): hence the term 'fusion protein'. There is a low serious adverse event rate. Up to 8 years' continuous therapy with ETN has demonstrated no cases of opportunistic infection or malignancies. Around one-third of patients achieve remission; however, the relapse rate after cessation of maintenance therapy is high. The half-life of etanercept is 3.5 days. The onset of benefit is 2 to 4 weeks. It is effective in pJIA, ERA, psJIA and oligo.

Infliximab (IFX) (chimeric monoclonal anti-TNF-α antibody)

IFX binds to soluble TNF-α and its precursor, neutralising their action. IFX may be as efficacious as ETN in treating JIA with a polyarticular course, although head-to-head studies have not been conducted. It is given intravenously (IFX is IV). A higher dose of infliximab, at a level of 6 mg/kg, has a better safety profile than the dose used in the initial studies (3 mg/kg); it is given at time 0, 2 and 6 weeks, then every 6–8 weeks. Its half-life is 3 weeks. The onset of benefit is 2–4 weeks. It is not commonly used in JIA.

IL antagonists

Anakinra (ANA) (recombinant IL-1 receptor antagonist)

This is useful in recalcitrant sJIA, where it has a response rate approaching 80%. It is given by SC injection daily. The half-life of anakinra is 6 hours. The onset of benefit is 4–12 weeks. It is used in sJIA, where it is highly effective, sometimes within days of commencement. It seems of particular benefit when started early in the course of the disease, when systemic aspects are far more prominent than articular aspects.

Tocilizumab (TCZ) (humanised anti-interleukin-6 [IL-6] receptor antibody)

TCZ almost completely blocks transmembrane signalling of IL-6. IL-6 is a key cytokine in the pathogenesis of systemic arthritis. It appears promising in the therapy of recalcitrant systemic arthritis, used at a dose of 8–12 mg/kg. It leads to significant improvement in disease activity indices, and a decrease in acute phase reactants.

Adverse reactions can include anaphylactoid reactions, bronchitis and gastrointestinal haemorrhage.

Cell-targeting agents

Abatacept (ABA; CTLA4-Ig)—T-cell targeting

ABA is a fusion protein made up of the extracellular domain of human CTLA4 (a second receptor for the B-cell activation antigen B7) and a fragment of the Fc portion of human IgG1 (hinge and CH2 and 3 domains), and binds human B7 (CD80/86, on antigen-presenting cells) more strongly than CD28 (on native T-cells). It targets T-cell activation, and inhibits T-cell proliferation. It has been used successfully in patients who fail to respond to TNF inhibitors. The half-life of abatacept is 13 days. The onset of benefit is 4–8 weeks. It is effective in pJIA, and in refractory oJIA.

Rituximab (RTX) (chimeric monoclonal antibody targeting cells with CD20 surface markers)—B-cell targeting

RTX depletes the B-cell population. It has been used in conjunction with MTX in patients who are resistant to TNF inhibitors. It is given intravenously, at day 1 and then at day 15, then 6-monthly. Its half-life is 21 days, its onset of benefit at 12 weeks. It is useful for sJIA and uveitis. The main adverse effects have included infusion reactions from minor to anaphylactic, interstitial lung disease and rarely progressive multifocal leukoencephalopathy.

In Australia, Medicare requirements for the funded supply of bDMARDs are that application must be made for an authority for specialised drug use, and that the patient must be under the care of a recognised paediatric rheumatology service. This is the case for ADA, ETN and TCZ—none of the other drugs are funded for JIA in Australia.

Side effects of bDMARDs, especially TNFIs, as noted in adults, can be remembered by the mnemonic **AMPLE HINTS** (all initial headings are noted in any TNFIs; other agents are specified):

Autoimmune-like syndromes (TNFIs)
Malignancy, especially lymphoma (TNFIs)
Pancytopaenia/neutropenia (TNFIs, TCZ)/pregnancy should be avoided (TNFIs, ANA, RTX, ABA, TCZ)
Liver transaminase elevation (TNFIs, TCZ)/Lipid elevation (TCZ)
Eczema and psoriasis (TNFIs, RTX)

Heart failure: can be worsened by IFX
Infections: if serious bacterial infection occurs, stop or do not start TNFIs, ANA, RTX, ABA or TCZ
Injection site/Infusion reaction: common; treat with antihistamine, steroids, slowed rate (TNFIs, ANA, RTX, ABA, TCZ)
Immunisation: immunise before treatment; no live-attenuated vaccine during treatment (TNFIs, ANA, RTX, ABA, TCZ)
Neurological syndromes: Guillain-Barre, optic neuritis
Tuberculosis: increased susceptibility to TB or reactivation of TB (TNFIs)
Surgical procedures: because of potential effects on wound healing, withhold drugs for specific times—ETN 4 weeks, ADA, IFX 8 weeks, RTX 4–8 weeks, TCZ 2 weeks prior

Monitoring disease activity

An essential component of controlling the inflammatory process is that of clinical and laboratory monitoring:
1. Clinical disease (e.g. fever, worsening joint count, worsening joint function).
2. Erythrocyte sedimentation rate.
3. MRI/X-ray showing disease progression.
4. Degree of anaemia.

Sequence of drugs/agents

The examiners may ask about your approach to the use of the drugs noted previously. In all subtypes of arthritis, active synovitis almost always needs treatment with intra-articular or systemic (IV or oral) steroids to achieve rapid remission. In polyarticular course and systemic arthritis, simultaneous commencement of MTX may be necessary:
1. For life-threatening systemic arthritis, pulse corticosteroids are the agents of choice. MTX is simultaneously started as a maintenance agent, which in time will allow reduction in the amount of oral systemic steroids used (hence the term 'steroid-sparing agent' used for MTX). If MTX is unsuccessful, and the disease severity is significant, commencement of biological agents may be indicated.
2. For non-life-threatening and non-systemic disease, try the following sequentially: in oligoarthritis, intra-articular corticosteroids with NSAIDs. Sometimes repetition of IAS may be required to achieve a therapeutic response. If the relapse rate is high, the addition of a DMARD (usually MTX) will be required.

The management algorithm for each type ends with biological agents, after (steroids and/or) MTX along the way.

2. PROVIDE ANALGESIA AND TREAT STIFFNESS

Pain

1. Assess severity, timing.
2. Analgesic (e.g. paracetamol).
3. Ice packs (e.g. pack of frozen peas wrapped in a moist towel) for acutely inflamed joints or hot packs (especially if there is associated stiffness) may be useful.

Morning stiffness

1. A warm bath/shower or hot packs may be helpful.
2. May be seen the morning after a particularly physical and busy day (e.g. school sport).
3. Treat with nocturnal, longer-acting, non-steroidal anti-inflammatory drugs (NSAIDs) (e.g. dispersible piroxicam, naproxen, indomethacin), or by taking a morning dose of shorter-acting types (e.g. ibuprofen).

3. MAINTAIN JOINT FUNCTION

1. Physiotherapy (including hydrotherapy) to maintain the joint range of movement (ROM) (e.g. stretching), muscle strength (exercise) and gait education. Particularly useful types of activity that help joint range and strength are walking, cycling and swimming, which need to be done at least 4–5 times during the week.
2. Attention to footwear (e.g. sports shoes with a supportive arch are comfortable and often appropriate) or wearing custom-made orthotics for leg-length discrepancy or deformities (e.g. genu valgus, from epiphyseal overgrowth; measure the intermalleolar distance to monitor this).
3. Even in the presence of acute synovitis, active physiotherapy is encouraged to minimise muscle wasting and to maintain joint ROM. Hydrotherapy may be particularly useful, as the warm water promotes better mobility, and the buoyancy reduces the required power to move the body.
4. Occupational therapy assistance for those with upper limb involvement, particularly for wrist and hand involvement. This assists with fine motor movement, and ADLs such as dressing, feeding and toileting, as well as for writing and for using a keyboard.

4. PREVENT DEFORMITIES

1. Splinting:
   a. Resting splints (for acutely inflamed joints) will promote loss of ROM and muscle wasting, and are discouraged.
   b. A corrective splint (to increase joint ROM; by serial splinting/casting, placing in optimal ROM or dynamic splinting) may be necessary at times to improve a severely deformed joint, or to prevent nocturnal ROM loss.
   c. Functional splinting (to protect joint during ADLs; e.g. ankle–foot orthoses, wrist cock-up splint).
2. Insoles and medial arch support (for hindfoot valgus).
3. Prone lying (for hip/knee contractures in particular).
4. Nocturnal traction (especially for hip pain).
5. A cervical collar (for torticollis, pain, occipito-atlanto dislocation and before general anaesthesia requiring intubation).
6. Surgical intervention may be needed where conservative treatment has failed to prevent deformity. Possible interventions include soft-tissue releases (e.g. for fixed flexion deformities at hips or knees), stapling (e.g. of medial femoral and

tibial epiphyses to correct valgus deformity), osteotomy and fusion/arthrodesis. Synovectomy (surgical or radioactive) may be occasionally needed for persistent pain and swelling (e.g. hips, knees). Total joint replacement may be offered to individuals with severely damaged joints who have an unacceptable level of pain or functional loss, although with modern treatment fewer and fewer patients will need this.

5. TREAT COMPLICATIONS

Eye involvement

All patients with JIA are at risk of uveitis, although the incidence and type of uveitis may vary between subtypes. The oligoarthritis subtype (including extended oligoarthritis, which happens to have the highest rate of positive ANA test), young age and female gender bear the highest risk for severe chronic anterior uveitis. The ERA or PsA subtypes are more commonly associated with acute anterior uveitis (painful red eye), although chronic anterior uveitis may also occur. In addition, patients who have received long-standing systemic/topical steroid treatment are at risk of steroid effects (cataracts and glaucoma).

1. Chronic uveitis: all patients need regular uveitis screening by a trained ophthalmologist; 3–4 monthly for those at higher risk; 6–12 monthly if risk is lower.
2. Active uveitis is usually treated with steroid eye drops and mydriatics.
3. MTX has a therapeutic effect on uveitis.
4. The anti-TNF agents infliximab and adalimumab are efficacious in controlling uveitis. Etanercept has occasionally been held responsible for exacerbation or evolvement of uveitis.

Infection

Treat with appropriate antibiotics and general supportive measures. Immunosuppressants will need to be withheld if active infection is present, and live vaccinations (e.g. MMR, chicken pox) are to be avoided.

Amyloidosis

Fortunately, with modern aggressive treatment this complication has become extremely rare. It may present with hepatosplenomegaly, abdominal pain, diarrhoea or albuminuria, and is diagnosed by rectal or renal biopsy. Treatment is with chlorambucil. Children with severe systemic arthritis are more likely to have this complication: the overall incidence of amyloidosis in some studies in this subtype has been as high as 9%, but these rates are old and probably do not reflect current treatment cohorts.

6. ENSURE OPTIMAL NUTRITION

Nutritional status is paramount and must not be overlooked. Active disease or TMJ involvement, as well as side effects of drug therapy (e.g. NSAIDs, MTX), can lead to suboptimal intake, inadequate energy and muscle bulk, which can negatively impact on other aspects of treatment.

7. REHABILITATION

Occupational therapy

1. School: use of adaptive pencil holder, standing desks, ramps, decreasing inter-class distances, avoiding stairs, potential for use of laptops/tablets in place of writing.
2. Home: dressing sticks and hoops, large buttons, Velcro fasteners, adaptive utensils, handheld shower, use of computers, tape recorders (if writing difficult).

Physiotherapy

Exercise: active/passive (including isometric exercises) to improve joint ROM, and to strengthen muscles. Also aim to improve endurance.

Family support

Social worker, parent support groups, Health Care Card, Child Disability Assistance Payment, disabled parking authorisation.

8. ENSURE OPTIMAL PSYCHOSOCIAL HEALTH

1. Promote as much independence as possible.
2. Encourage the child to take responsibility for management, as appropriate for age.
3. Build self-esteem.
4. Help the child deal with peer-group problems (e.g. school liaison, addressing bullying).
5. Family psychosocial support, including siblings.

9. EDUCATE PARENTS AND PATIENT REGARDING DISEASE

1. Ensure adequate understanding by parents, patients and siblings of the disease, treatment, drug side effects, importance of compliance and prognosis.
2. Encourage contact with reputable consumer groups (e.g. Arthritis Australia) and suggest trustworthy websites.
3. Dispel myths and false beliefs (e.g. held by other, older family members) regarding JIA, drugs used and alternative therapies (unproven therapies that are popular [despite no data in existence to support their use], including glucosamine and hyaluronic acid).

Prognosis

It has been estimated that about one-third of patients with JIA will still have active disease as adults, which may well interfere with their ADLs and lifestyle. This prognosis depends on the type of JIA. RF-positive patients have the worst prognosis for ongoing disease activity: these are usually females with onset as teenagers.

If adequately treated, children with only a few joints involved do better than children with ongoing systemic disease or polyarthritis, although the risk of uveitis may be higher. If untreated, serious ocular damage occurs in 10–20%. In patients treated for systemic arthritis, 40–50% will go into remission; while up to one-third may develop destructive polyarthritis. The average duration of disease activity has been reported to be 6 years. In a follow-up study of JIA patients with disease duration over 10 years, around one-third had depression, related directly to disability and ongoing disease activity. Death from complications is extremely rare (less than 0.3% in North America).

LONG CASE: Juvenile idiopathic inflammatory myopathies (JIIMs)—juvenile dermatomyositis (JDM)

The IIMs of childhood are rare diseases, but are not uncommon in examination settings.

Background

Since 1975, the criteria of Bohan and Peter have been used widely. The five diagnostic criteria include:

1. Characteristic rashes. Two are pathognomonic: (a) *Gottron's papules*—scaly red papular areas over the knuckles (MP) and IP joints (papules can also overlay elbows, knees and malleoli); (b) *heliotrope rash*—a violaceous or purplish, somewhat oedematous, discolouration around the eyes, particularly over the eyelids (capillary telangiectasia), which may cross the nasal bridge and include the nasolabial folds. Other rashes encountered include scaly red rash on the sun-exposed areas; the face, neck and upper chest (V-sign), the shawl area (shawl sign) and over the extensor tendons, particularly of the hands (linear extensor erythema). Commonly there is an erythematous rash involving extensor surfaces (elbows, knees), which may be mistaken for psoriasis.

   The other criteria, of which three out of four are required, are as follows:

2. Symmetrical proximal muscle weakness (although in practice distal muscles, as well as the oropharynx are also involved).
3. Elevated muscle-derived enzymes (creatine kinase [CK], aldolase, lactate dehydrogenase [LDH] and transaminases [AST and ALT]).
4. Muscle histopathology confirming the typical pattern of myofibre atrophy and drop out necrosis with fibre regeneration, and chronic inflammatory infiltrate involving blood vessels.
5. Electromyography (EMG) changes of inflammatory myopathy (fasciculations at rest, bizarre high-frequency discharges). EMG interpretation is dependent on appropriate placing of the electrode in areas of inflammation. MRI is used to select the sample site (inflammatory muscle involvement causes non-uniform changes in muscle, abnormal increased signal on T2-weighted images and normal signal on T1).

   In 2006, Brown et al. reported an international consensus survey and suggested expanded criteria. Most rheumatologists reported finding the first two criteria to be essential, used by 100% of those surveyed, while the third criterion was used by 86.9%, but then, there were a number of suggested criteria considered to be as important as muscle biopsy and EMG, especially:

1. Typical findings for JDM on MRI and ultrasonography of muscle, as an alternative to, but in preference to, biopsy or EMG.
2. Capillaroscopy of nail folds (nail-fold telangiectasias, periungual erythema).
3. Calcinosis cutis (affecting elbows, knees, extremities; within 3 years of diagnosis).
4. Dysphonia (often coexisting with dysphagia).

   MRI has been used more often to detect skin, fascia and subcutaneous abnormalities, as well as muscle inflammation, which can be helpful in clarifying the extent of involvement in difficult cases, therefore aiding with devising a management plan. MRI is likely to replace the more painful, invasive tests of muscle biopsy and EMG, and become one of the official diagnostic criteria.

   JDM is an occlusive small-vessel vasculopathy, involving arterioles and capillaries. There can be very diffuse vasculitis (which may include nail-bed telangiectasia, digital ulceration, infarction of oral epithelium and gastrointestinal ulceration) and vasomotor instability. Other extramuscular manifestations including cardiac involvement and arthritis.

In 1997, Rider and Miller suggested a clinicopathological classification of the juvenile IIMs, listing 11 subsets in keeping with the myositis subsets recognised in adults.

The incidence of JDM is around 2–3 per million. The gender ratio varies around the world: in the UK and the US, girls are affected more often (up to twice as often), but in India and Japan, boys are affected more often. The mean age of onset varies also: it is around 7 years in the US and in the UK, but in the UK it has bimodal incidence, with one peak at age 2–6 and the other at age 12–13.

Susceptibility to developing JDM has been associated with several HLA alleles, including the class II major histocompatibility complex (MHC) allele HLA-DQA1*0501, which is found in 86–92% of patients, versus 28–46% of controls. Other alleles that are more common in JDM include HLA-B8, HLA-DRB1*0301 and HLA-DQA1*0301.

Tumour necrosis factor-alpha (TNF-α) is an immunomodulator and pro-inflammatory cytokine; TNF polymorphisms are associated with several rheumatic diseases, including JDM. Polymorphisms at the TNF-308 locus are associated with a longer disease course of over 36 months, and the development of calcification. The TNF-308 allele also is associated with an increase in concentration of thrombospondin-1, an anti-angiogenic factor that may predispose to increased vascular occlusion.

Maternal microchimerism (the persistence of maternal blood cells transferred by placenta) has been found in CD4 or CD8 peripheral blood cells and in skin lesions and muscle of children with JDM. It has been postulated that this could lead to a graft versus host reaction presenting as autoimmune disease. Maternally derived chimeric T-cells demonstrate a memory response to the child's lymphocytes.

There is no strong evidence to support the role of any environmental agent in the pathogenesis of JDM. Some immune responses have been elucidated: complement-mediated damage to vessels is a major mechanism, as is overexpression of adhesion molecules (e.g. intracellular adhesion molecule-1 [ICAM-1]; vascular cell adhesion molecule-1 [VCAM-1]), which belong to the immunoglobulin superfamily and recruit inflammatory cells. Increasing myositis-specific autoantibodies are being detected in patients with JIIM. These can be useful in predicting clinical manifestation and prognosis.

There is some evidence of involvement of type-1 interferons in JDM. Genes regulated by type-1 interferon mediate immunomodulation, upregulate MHC class I and support dendritic maturation; they also activate natural killer cells' cytotoxic effects, and promote activated T-cell survival. The degree of gene expression of the chemokine interferon-inducible protein 10 (IP-10) and the monocyte chemoattractant protein (MCP-1) correlates with activity of the disease. However, the mechanism by which this could lead to the pathogenesis of JDM is not known.

At diagnosis, all children have weakness and rash, and can be irritable. Anasarca (severe generalised tissue oedema) and skin ulceration are signs of severe disease and call for aggressive treatment. Most have muscle pain and fever, and 20–50% have dysphagia or hypernasality of voice, abdominal pain and/or arthritis. Soft-tissue calcification (calcinosis) is seen in 30–70% of patients eventually, in sites exposed to trauma (buttocks, knees, elbows) and seems to reflect the severity and duration of disease; it is relatively rare at diagnosis.

The mechanism of calcinosis is thought to be due to damaged muscles releasing mitochondrial calcium into matrix vesicles that promote mineralisation. Calcinosis is related to hydroxyapatite accumulation; it can occur as superficial lumps, plates along fascial planes or widespread exoskeleton distribution.

Calcification can resolve spontaneously, and drain a white exudate, leaving pitted scars. Abscess formation may be seen in the muscles and become infected with *Staphylococcus aureus*. Calcification can persist in fibrotic muscle in sheath-like forms, impairing function. Both the skin and the muscle manifestations may be precipitated or exacerbated by sun exposure.

Gastrointestinal involvement, through muscle weakness and/or vasculitis, can lead to impaired speech from soft palate involvement, decreased oesophageal motility with impaired swallowing, oesophageal reflux, aspiration pneumonia, ulceration, colonic perforation, haemorrhage, pneumatosis intestinalis and malabsorption.

Cardiopulmonary involvement can cause asymptomatic conduction abnormalities, myocarditis, dilated cardiomyopathy, widespread cardiac vasculopathy and pulmonary fibrosis. Respiratory muscle weakness can occur in around a third of patients.

Gastrointestinal and cardiorespiratory symptoms may evolve within 3 months of diagnosing JDM.

A candidate could be asked what investigations may have been ordered when the patient first presented. A list of the usual diagnostic work-up is useful, after stressing the importance of clinical examination and exclusion of mimics of JDM. Investigations commonly ordered include: blood for muscle enzymes, ESR, CRP and autoantibodies (antinuclear antibodies [ANA], anti-ds-DNA, extractable nuclear antibodies including anti-Sm, anti-RNP and anti Jo-1, myositis-specific antibodies); imaging (MRI of proximal muscles, chest X-ray); pulmonary function tests; ECG; and nail-fold capillaroscopy. Consider muscle biopsy.

Other manifestations include the following:

- Vasculitis involving the central nervous system (causing seizures and organic psychosis—even fatal brainstem infarction has been described).
- Ophthalmological complications include retinopathy (retinal exudates, 'cottonwool' spots, optic atrophy, visual impairment), glaucoma (from steroids) and cataracts (from steroids).
- Renal tract: renal failure secondary to myoglobinuria from muscle breakdown; ureteral (middle third) necrosis secondary to vasculopathy.
- Reproductive system: active disease can delay menarche, interrupt menses or adversely affect pregnancy outcomes.
- Raynaud's phenomenon.
- Lipodystrophy: this is a slowly progressive symmetrical loss of subcutaneous fatty tissue that typically involves the upper half of the body; mainly in females; it can be associated with acanthosis nigricans, hirsutism, hepatomegaly, hyperlipidaemia (especially hypertriglyceridaemia) and insulin-resistant diabetes mellitus; the pathophysiology is unknown.
- Juvenile polymyositis (JPM) is identical to JDM but without the skin rash. It is exceedingly rare.
- Amyopathic JDM is the rash without the muscle findings.

There are recognised subgroups based on the course of the disease: monocyclic (full recovery without relapse, recovering within 2 years on treatment; occurs in around 24–40%), whereas most patients (50–60%) have a chronic course, either chronic polycyclic (prolonged relapsing course), chronic continuous (persistent disease despite maintenance treatment) or ulcerative.

In recent years, a number of groups have collaborated internationally and produced accurate, reliable and validated outcome measurement tools. The three commonly used are the Childhood Health Assessment Questionnaire (CHAQ; initially developed to measure physical function in children with arthritis), Manual Muscle Testing (MMT; a score that assesses the muscle strength of seven proximal and five distal muscle groups, bilaterally; it predicts disease activity) and the Childhood Myositis Assessment Scale (CMAS; a 14-activity assessment of physical function, strength and endurance). These standardised tools allow comparisons between groups throughout the world.

History

At the completion of presenting the history, the examiners should have a clear impression of the patient's current functioning (e.g. ADLs), current (and past) treatment modalities (such as physiotherapy, drugs and alternative therapies [e.g. naturopathic] tried) and social situation (e.g. transport issues, distance from home to treating hospital).

Ask about the following.

PRESENTING COMPLAINT

Reason for current admission.

CURRENT SYMPTOMS

1. General health (e.g. fever, weight loss, nutritional status).
2. Musculoskeletal symptoms; for example, general pain or tenderness, asthenia, muscle weakness, cramps, joint symptoms (early morning stiffness or 'gelling' after inactivity, nocturnal discomfort, pain, tenderness, swelling, limitation of movement [contractures or calcinosis of tendon sheaths], problem joints), contractures and the requirement for serial casting.
3. Skin rashes; for example, heliotrope of eyelids, Gottron's papules (knuckles), photosensitive rashes, scarring and atrophy.
4. Calcinosis; for example, problem areas (e.g. buttocks, extensor surfaces).
5. Level of functioning with ADLs; for example, speech (tongue involvement), eating (chewing difficulties from involvement of muscles of mastication), swallowing (soft palate weakness, abnormal oesophageal motility), sitting (buttock soft-tissue calcification), walking, negotiating stairs, squatting, assistance devices (e.g. adaptive utensils, wheelchair, computer) and home modifications required (e.g. ramps, bathroom fittings).
6. Gastrointestinal tract (GIT) symptoms: oral, upper GIT and lower GIT (e.g. ulceration, perforation, haemorrhage, malabsorption).
7. Genitourinary symptoms; for example, discoloured urine (episodes of myoglobinuria), renal impairment, ureteral involvement and interference with menstruation.
8. Eye problems; for example, visual impairment, retinopathy, glaucoma and cataracts.
9. Neuropsychiatric symptoms; for example, mood swings and depression.
10. Drug side effects; for example, steroid effects (Cushing's syndrome, stunted linear growth, myopathy), cytotoxics (e.g. myelosuppression, opportunistic infection, hepatotoxicity [MTX], hypertension [CPA]) and IVIG (infusion-related toxicities, other IVIG complications such as aseptic meningitis, thromboembolism).
11. Other systems review; for example, cardiopulmonary symptoms, Raynaud's phenomenon.

PAST HISTORY

Initial diagnosis (when, where, presenting symptoms, initial investigations), possible triggers (e.g. infectious agents [parvovirus, enteroviruses, hepatitis B], excessive sun exposure), pattern of illness (monocyclic, chronic polycyclic, continuous), hospitalisations, the development of complications and their management.

MANAGEMENT

Current treatment in hospital, usual treatment at home (e.g. occupational therapy and physiotherapy, exercises, medications), previous treatments used (e.g. steroids, azathioprine, IVIG), responses to treatment, side effects, monitoring of effect, alternative therapies tried.

SOCIAL HISTORY

1. Disease impact on: (a) child (school absenteeism, limited ADLs, poor self-image); (b) parents (financial considerations: home modifications, wheelchairs, computers, transport, frequent hospitalisations, drugs); (c) siblings (rivalry).
2. Benefits received; for example, Child Disability Assistance Payment.
3. Social supports.

FAMILY HISTORY

Any connective tissue/autoimmune diseases (most common association is with type 1 diabetes mellitus and SLE).

Examination

The approach given in Table 16.1 could be used for a short case or clinic follow-up.

The following is the sequence suggested for the joint examination component of that approach (for detail, see the joints short case in this chapter). Inspect the distribution of joint involvement (symmetry); note swelling, loss of normal contours, angulation, deformity, redness and muscle wasting. Next, feel the joint and periarticular areas for tenderness, warmth, effusion, 'boggy' swelling (thickened synovium and fluid) and contractures.

Range of movement (ROM) is then examined, active movement first. Test passive movement to assess for any restriction (tenosynovitis, arthropathy) or tenderness. Describe ROM by qualifying statements (restricted, very restricted or absent), stating that formal measurement of joint ROM is carried out by a goniometer in the hands of a trained person.

A suggested order for a systematic examination of all the joints is as follows: hands (distal and proximal interphalangeal [DIP and PIP] and metacarpophalangeal [MCP] joints), wrists, elbows, shoulders, temporomandibular joints, cervical spine, lumbar spine, hips, knees, ankles, feet (i.e. hand to head, and head to toe). A good initial position is with the child sitting in a chair, or on the side of a bed, with the hands resting on the thighs.

The easiest places on the body to visualise capillaries are the nail folds (dermatoscope or auroscope may be needed) and along the teeth/gum line. This is where the underlying pathological lesion, capillary vasculopathy, can best be assessed. The findings of capillary branching/tortuosity and dilation, areas of haemorrhage and reduced number of capillaries (< 3 per mm) can all be seen with nail-fold capillaroscopy. Paediatric rheumatologists may use a stereomicroscope with microscopic oil to cut down on skin reflection, or simply a magnifying glass with water-soluble gel. Counting capillaries at the distal nail fold can predict disease activity, muscle strength and function, as well as skin activity.

Table 16.1
Examination for juvenile dermatomyositis (JDM)
INITIAL IMPRESSION
Well or unwell
Face • Cushingoid (steroids) • Heliotrope eyelid rash Malar rash with sparing of nasolabial folds • 'Chipmunk' facies (masseter atrophy)
Parameters • Height (short from steroids) • Weight (obese from steroids; thin from hypercatabolism or malabsorption)
Lipodystrophy (symmetrical loss of subcutaneous fatty tissue, mainly upper body; occasionally asymmetrical; usually in females; can be associated with acanthosis nigricans, hirsutism and clitoral hypertrophy)
SKIN
Photosensitive rashes (distribution of sun exposure)
Vasculitic rash
Subcutaneous calcification (buttocks, elbows, knees), scars/pits of old calcinosis
Atrophy
Hypertrichosis (cyclosporine); hirsutism (steroids)
UPPER LIMBS
Hands • Raynaud's phenomenon • Digital ulcers/scars
Nails: nail-fold capillary bed telangiectasia or periungual erythema
Palms • Anaemia (drug side effects, e.g. cytotoxics)
Knuckles • Gottron's papules
Elbows • JDM rash
Blood pressure • Elevated (e.g. steroids, nephropathy, cyclosporine); if elevated, make a point of requesting urinalysis now
Neuromuscular assessment • Palpate muscles (tenderness) • Range of movement of joints (active then passive); tone (contractures from sheathing of tendons) • Power • Reflexes
Joint assessment • All joints of upper limbs (as for the joints short case)
Functional assessment • Activities of daily living (e.g. writing, brushing teeth, combing hair, turning taps on or off, feeding self, carrying household objects)

Table 16.1 (continued)

HEAD AND NECK

Eyes
- Conjunctival pallor
- Visual acuity
- Glaucoma (steroids)
- Cataract (steroids)
- Retinopathy (retinal 'cottonwool' spots; optic atrophy)

Mouth
- Inflamed mucous membrane
- Gum hyperplasia (CSA)
- Dysphonia

CARDIORESPIRATORY

Auscultate
- Praecordium
- Lung fields

ABDOMEN

Tenderness (gastrointestinal haemorrhage/ulceration)

Buttock rash

GAIT, LOWER LIMBS AND BACK

Neuromuscular assessment
- Full gait examination

Squat
- Proximal weakness (JDM per se; steroids)

Test for truncal weakness: get the child to do a sit-up from a lying position on the bed, or resisted head lift off the bed (truncal weakness can take quite some time to return to normal, often lagging behind limb strength improvements)

Lower limbs (neurologically)
- Palpate muscles (tenderness)
- Range of movement of joints (active then passive); tone (contractures from sheathing of tendons)
- Power (Gower's sign)
- Reflexes

Back
- Palpate for tenderness (osteoporosis)
- Examine joints

Joint assessment
- All joints of lower limbs (as per joints short case)

Functional assessment
- Activities of daily living (e.g. sitting, getting out of chair, climbing stairs)

Continued

Table 16.1 (continued)		
OTHER		
Temperature chart • Fever (intercurrent illness, from steroids/cytotoxics)		
Urinalysis • Myoglobinuria • Proteinuria (nephropathy: JDM per se, or cytotoxics) • Haematuria (nephropathy: JDM per se, or cytotoxics)		
Stool analysis • Blood		

CSA = cyclosporine A.

Management

GOALS OF JDM MANAGEMENT

1. Control inflammation.
2. Restore muscle strength.
3. Maintain functional abilities.
4. Prevent and treat complications.
5. Minimise treatment side effects.
6. Educate the parents and patient regarding the disease.

FIRST-LINE TREATMENT

There is a paucity of randomised controlled trials for treatment choices in JDM. Corticosteroids (CS) are needed in relatively high doses to restore muscle power as quickly as possible, while commencement of a maintenance agent (e.g. MTX) will allow weaning the steroids later and helps with controlling the skin rash. Physiotherapy is started as early as possible, and other allied health professionals, such as a speech therapist, may be needed to assess the aspiration risk. The use of steroids has reduced the mortality in JDM from 40% to 3%, although with modern treatment this rate is probably even lower. It is likely that residual disability and the extent of calcinosis have been diminished by CS as well (although CS can occasionally cause muscle weakness, osteoporotic fractures and avascular necrosis, which can adversely affect disability). The oral prednisolone/prednisone dosage is usually 1–3 mg/kg per day, although doses larger than 1 mg/kg are associated with far greater side effects without much additional therapeutic benefit.

The aim of the treatment should be to start weaning the CS dose as soon as the patient's clinical condition allows, to minimise side effects. Oral CS are given as a morning dose to minimise their impact on growth, and alternate-day doses must be avoided to reduce the possibility of relapse. Intravenous methylprednisolone pulses (IVMP) are used if the overall disease severity is deemed high, or if there is incomplete response to oral CS. Aggressive induction of therapy, including the use of IVMP, seems to lead to less relapsing disease, residual weakness or calcinosis. IVMP also may be useful for treating serious complications such as myocarditis or dysphagia, as well as for treating the skin manifestations.

High-dose IVMP is a potent immunosuppressive agent. Meticulous attention is needed to detect any developing infection, with aggressive treatment of the same required. During the infusion, side effects may include flushing, headache, a metallic taste in the mouth and hyper/hypotension, requiring measurement of vital signs every 15 minutes.

Recently, there has been a trend to use IVMP at a dosage of 30 mg/kg/day for 3 to 5 days, then repeat this intermittently, subsequently. Many paediatric rheumatologists would give DMARDs, especially methotrexate, in combination with CS. Cyclosporine and IVIG are a popular combination in Europe, particularly for illness flares. Hydroxychloroquine is used for mild disease, and where cutaneous lesions predominate. Cyclophosphamide has been used for interstitial lung disease and in ulcerative cases. IVIG has been used for severe refractory disease and those with significant skin involvement.

The drugs used, other than steroids, may include (mnemonic **MB I CATCH MD**):

Methotrexate (MTX)
Biological disease-modifying anti-rheumatic drugs (bDMARDs)

Intravenous immunoglobulin (IVIG)

Cyclophosphamide (CPA)
Azathioprine (AZA)
Tacrolimus (TAC)
Cyclosporine (CSA)
Hydroxychloroquine (HCQ)

Mycophenolate mofetil (MMF)
Diltiazem (calcium channel blocker for calcinosis)

The use of any of these agents may be determined by the severity of disease and its complications, or the extent of vasculitis.

Methotrexate (MTX)

MTX inhibits dihydrofolate reductase, which is needed to make DNA and some amino acids, although its exact mechanism of action is not understood. Lower doses are used in rheumatology than in oncology. MTX was originally a second-line agent used with steroids for refractory disease, but recently there has been a shift towards earlier use of MTX as a steroid-sparing agent. Benefit is apparent within 6–8 weeks after the dosage is optimised (although it can take up to 12 weeks before a positive effect is seen).

The side effects include the following (mnemonic **MTX**):

Mucositis/**M**yelosuppression
Transaminase increase (i.e. hepatotoxicity)
X-rays warranted (*chest* X-ray for pneumonia [e.g. varicella pneumonia] or pneumonitis [exceedingly rare])/**X**tra folate recommended

Other opportunistic infections can occur; for example, cutaneous herpes zoster, herpes simplex, *Listeria monocytogenes* meningitis and tuberculosis. Varicella fulminans may complicate treatment of patients who have not been immunised or exposed in the past. Therefore, measurement of VZV antibody titres is recommended prior to commencement of CS or immunosuppressive therapy. In combination with CS, there is an increased risk of opportunistic infection. Unfortunately, not all patients will respond to the combination of steroids and MTX.

Biological disease-modifying anti-rheumatic drugs (bDMARDs)

Biological agents are being trialled increasingly in children with severe disease that is refractory to standard therapy. Rituximab, a depleter of CD20+ B-cells, has shown some positive results in open label trials and case reports, with between 70% and 83% of treatment-refractory patients improving. Patients with particular serological markers (anti-Jo-1, anti-Mi2 and anti-SRP antibodies) are more likely to respond. The main side effects are infusion reactions, increased rate of infections, and, rarely, progressive multifocal leukoencephalopathy.

Other bDMARDs being trialled include alemtuzumab (anti-CD52), eculizumab (anti-complement C3), tocilizumab (anti-interleukin-6), anakinra (anti-interleukin-1), secukinumab (anti-interleukin-17) and gevokizumab (anti-interleukin-1 beta).

One group of bDMARDs, tumour necrosis factor (TNF) inhibitors, (TNFIs), are ineffective; these include etanercept (ETN), infliximab (IFX) and adalimumab (ADA); these can worsen preexisting disease or can trigger disease. There is some evidence for etanercept, infliximab and adalimumab, although it is not conclusive.

Intravenous immunoglobulin (IVIG)

IVIG has multiple mechanisms of action. IVIG suppresses inducer T- and B-cells, induces suppressor T-cells, blocks the complement cascade, blocks Fc receptors on macrophages, enhances remyelination and downregulates inflammatory cytokines. A regimen of 2 days' consecutive treatment monthly leads to the peak effect after 3 months. Some units use this monthly treatment for up to a year.

The response to IVIG is comparable to that of pulse methylprednisolone and cyclosporine, although this is variable and depends on individual cases. Side effects include infusion-related toxicities (e.g. hypotension, fever), aseptic meningitis, and thromboembolic events caused by increased viscosity.

Azathioprine (AZA)

This is a purine analogue, metabolised to 6-mercaptopurine, which inhibits purine ribonucleotide synthesis. It can lead to complete or partial remission in up to 70% of patients when used as the second-line immunosuppressive. It has relatively fewer side effects than the other cytotoxics, although it may not be as efficacious. Measurement of thiopurine methyltransferase (TPMT) enzyme is required to assess the risk of leucopenia. Its onset peak effect is at 3–6 months after initiating treatment. It can cause gastrointestinal upset, and bone marrow suppression with leucopenia. In combination with CS, there is an increased risk of opportunistic infection.

Side effects (mnemonic **AZATHIOPS**):

Alimentary system effects (anorexia, nausea, vomiting, diarrhoea)
Zoster and other infections (especially opportunistic)
Aplastic anaemia (various forms of myelosuppression)/**A**lopecia
TPMT low means increased myelotoxicity
Haematological malignancy (AML, lymphoma)/**H**aemorrhage (low platelets)
Interstitial pneumonitis (rare)
Occlusive hepatic (hepatic veno-occlusive disease; rare)
PML (progressive multifocal leukoencephalopathy; rare)
Skin cancer/**S**teatorrhoea

Cyclophosphamide (CPA)

Pulse IV-CPA (0.5–1.0 g/m^2 monthly for 6–14 doses) has been used for severe disease with vasculitic predominance; for example, skin and gut ulceration and interstitial lung disease. It can also improve calcinosis cutis.

The side effects are as follows (mnemonic **CPA**):

Cystitis (haemorrhagic)
Pancytopenia
Alopecia/**A**ctivation of latent/opportunistic infections (e.g. herpes zoster, TB, PCP)

Tacrolimus (TAC)

A fungus-derived macrolide, TAC inhibits the activity of a calcium-regulated enzyme, calcineurin, required for transmitting activating signals from T-cell receptors. In adults, its use in DM enhances muscle strength and lung function. It has been used successfully in patients with interstitial lung disease, and patients with anti-synthetase or anti-SRP autoantibodies. Its side effects include nephrotoxicity, hypertension, hypomagnesaemia and tremor. Noteworthy side effects (mnemonic **TACROLIMUS**) include:

Tremor/**T**ingling (neurotoxicity)
Alimentary (diarrhoea, constipation, nausea, vomiting, anorexia)/**A**naemia
Cancer risk increased
Renal toxicity (includes irreversible vasculopathy, interstitial fibrosis, tubular damage)
Osteoporosis
Lymphoproliferative disease/**L**ow Phosphate
Increased: blood pressure, [K$^+$], (creatinine)
Magnesium low
Urea high
Sugar diabetes

Cyclosporine (CSA)

Like TAC above, CSA is a prodrug derived from fungi, binding to an intracellular protein 'cyclophilin', which inhibits activity of calcineurin. Noteworthy side effects (mnemonic **CSA**):

Compromised kidneys (nephrotoxicity includes irreversible vasculopathy, interstitial fibrosis, tubular damage)
Secondary malignancy potential (especially lymphoproliferative)
Anaemia/**A**ccelerated blood pressure (hypertension), hair growth (hypertrichosis) and gums (gingival hyperplasia)/**A**dditional myopathy (caused by CSA per se; this can contribute to osteoporosis)

There is little published evidence to support the use of CSA in JDM, though anecdotally some paediatric rheumatologists will quote it as being effective.

Hydroxychloroquine (HCQ)

This is an antimalarial drug and a DMARD. It inhibits the production of acute phase reactants, stabilises lysosomal membranes and inhibits the activity of collagenase and proteases which cause cartilage breakdown. Its half-life is 32–50 days. Side effects include renal and retinal toxicities (maculopathy) and gastrointestinal symptoms. Rarely, cardiomyopathy and neuromyotoxicity have been reported.

Mycophenolate mofetil (MMF)

This is an antimetabolite that interferes with purine metabolism in B- and T-lymphocytes. Patients who respond to MMF can tolerate lower steroid doses. It has similar toxicities to AZA. In a study in 50 children receiving MMF for 1 year, it significantly reduced the disease activity scores for muscle and skin involvement.

Diltiazem

This is a calcium blocker, and has been used to treat calcinosis cutis. It inhibits influx of extracellular calcium, during depolarisation, across muscle cell membranes, both of heart muscle and of vascular smooth muscle. This inhibits contraction of myocardial smooth muscle, leading to dilation of coronary and systemic arteries; this increases myocardial oxygenation. It is thought to reduce calcium influx in tissues affected by calcinosis and in macrophages.

PROGNOSTIC PREDICTORS

Some units use second-line agents in patients with factors known to portend a worse prognosis, including those with: 1. severe disease—vasculitis and anasarca, particularly with complications of calcification, ulceration, interstitial lung disease or significant dysphagia; 2. particular myositis-specific autoantibodies (MSAs), including anti-synthetase and anti-SRP autoantibodies; or 3. delayed treatment.

LIFE-THREATENING DISEASE (E.G. MYOCARDITIS, SEVERE DYSPHAGIA)

Treatments have included pulse methylprednisolone, oral CPA, pulse IV-CPA, plasmapheresis or combination therapies (e.g. MTX + AZA; IVIG + CSA, rituximab). Cell-based therapy may have a place. There are reports of patients with severe refractory disease entering prolonged remission after autologous stem cell transplantation, after immunoablation with fludarabine, CPA, anti-thymocyte globulin, and engraftment using a CD3/CD19-depleted graft.

EXTRAMUSCULAR DISEASE

Calcinosis cutis (CC)

This is more common where there has been a delay in starting treatment, and in polycyclic disease, local trauma and treatment with low CS doses. Calcinosis is dystrophic calcification with normal calcium and phosphorus levels. The calcium deposits (which contain calcium hydroxyapatite, osteopontin, osteonectin and bone sialoprotein) typically present as nodules over bony prominences, especially elbows and knees. In samples of these calcinosis nodules, IL-1, IL-6 and TNF-α are found. Bone resorption is increased in patients with connective tissue diseases and CC, and this can lead to calcium being deposited in soft tissues.

CC occurs in 20–40% of children with JDM. There are four subtypes: superficial calcium masses; deep calcium masses; linear deposits; and subcutaneous deposits around the torso.

All the treatments for CC listed here have little evidence for their efficacy, although there is common agreement that aggressive treatment of active disease will treat or reduce calcinosis. Thus, aggressive anti-inflammatory treatment for JDM (with IVMP, pulses, IVIG, CPA, MMF, bDMARDs) can improve CC in over 50% of patients. Otherwise, treatments specifically aimed at CC include: colchicine; surgical removal (some cases; usually not recommended as can be complicated by draining sinuses, ulceration, infection and recurrence); diltiazem (has been successful in around 50% of patients with JDM and CC, but can induce flares of myositis); aluminium hydroxide; oral, intralesional and intravenous magnesium sulfate and magnesium lactate; pamidronate (a bisphosphonate); and lithotripsy.

Some studies note benefits for diltiazem given with bisphosphonates, or aluminium hydroxide given with CS, respectively. Bisphosphonates (including etidronate, alendronate and especially pamidronate) decrease bone resorption and inhibit calcium turnover (inhibiting conversion of calcium phosphate into crystalline hydroxyapatite, and the nucleation of hydroxyapatite), and inhibit macrophage function, so can inhibit ectopic calcification. Other options, including haematopoietic stem cell transplantation, and the immunomodulator thalidomide (which inhibits TNF-α and IL-6 mRNA expression in peripheral blood mononuclear cells), have shown some promise in treating this complication.

Skin disease/protection from ultraviolet A and B light (UVA and UVB)

Sun protection using sunscreens, and sun avoidance (wide-brimmed hats, photoprotective clothing, avoiding sun during peak daylight hours), are paramount to help controlling disease and prevent relapse. Hydroxychloroquine as an adjunct to MTX or other cytotoxics may be useful. Antihistamines may be needed for associated pruritus. Other agents that can improve rashes include methylprednisolone, MTX, CSA, IVIG and dapsone.

Osteoporosis

This is multifactorial: 1. steroid use; 2. decreased muscle bulk and mobility; 3. deposition of resorbed bone calcium in calcinosis; 4. decreased GIT calcium absorption; and 5. production of cytokines that resorb bone (during active disease). With steroid therapy, if dietary intake is inadequate, supplementation with calcium and vitamin D is recommended.

REHABILITATION

A multidisciplinary approach is important to avoid significant morbidity and mortality. Physiotherapy, occupational therapy, speech therapy and dietetics intervention all will likely be necessary to: maintain muscle strength; avoid contractures with stretching; use splinting and assistive devices; cope with weak swallowing muscles; instruct on food consistency; optimise positioning of head, chin and tongue; and investigate dysphagia with videofluoroscopic swallow studies (VFSS). Exercise training is safe and worthwhile. Supervised twice-weekly aerobic and resistance exercise training improves muscle strength and function, bone mass, muscle mass and health-related quality of life within 12 weeks without any adverse effects on muscle enzyme levels.

There are a range of validated assessment scales: the Childhood Health Assessment Questionnaire (CHAQ) assesses physical function; the Childhood Myositis Assessment Scale (CMAS) assesses muscle strength, muscle endurance and functional capacity; the Disease Activity Scale (DAS) assesses muscle and skin involvement; and the Cutaneous Assessment Tool (CAT) assesses cutaneous findings in JDM.

PROGNOSIS

The mortality rate has been quoted as 3%, although this is probably lower with modern therapy and an aggressive approach. Morbidity is relatively high, especially from delay of treatment, or from medication side effects. Treatment should generally be continued for a couple of years for consolidation and maintenance, although in individual cases this may be shortened (monophasic disease in adolescents). A periungual capillary count of < 3 per mm is associated with relapse if treatment is withdrawn.

LONG CASE: Systemic lupus erythematosus (SLE)

SLE is a multi-system autoimmune disease that usually affects older children and adolescents, although rarely younger children (< 9 years old) can be affected. SLE is a complex condition which involves immune dysregulation of both the innate and adaptive immune system including production of autoantibodies and hypergammaglobulinaemia. SLE can arise spontaneously or in response to specific triggers, such as drug-induced SLE. SLE also can be caused by specific single gene abnormalities such as C1q deficiency. Compared to adults with SLE, there is a change (increase) in the frequency of several aspects of SLE in children (mnemonic **CHANGE**):

Chorea
Hepatosplenomegaly
Avascular
Necrosis
Glomerulonephritis
Exclusively paediatric problems: growth abnormalities, neonatal lupus

Paediatric SLE (pSLE) is a multifaceted chronic disease both in terms of the problem list and management, and would be an ideal long case.

Background information

The incidence of SLE with paediatric onset (under 19 years), is up to 19 per 100 000 in white females, and higher in African American (20–30 per 100 000) and Puerto Rican (16–36 per 100 000) females. It is nine times more common in females. It usually becomes apparent in the second or third decade. In Australia, it is more common in Indigenous Australians and people of South-East Asian or South Pacific heritage; also, it is more common worldwide in African Americans, Asians and Arabs.

There is a genetic component, with 30% concordance in monozygotic twins, an increased susceptibility to SLE with certain HLA haplotypes (HLA-DQ loci) and deficiency of early complement components (homozygous deficiency of C1q, C1r, C1s, C4, C2). These deficiencies remain strong susceptibility factors to SLE, but there are many more recently identified risk loci discovered by genome-wide association studies, including ITGAM, FCGR, PRDM1-ATG5 and TNFAIP3.

The development of lupus is related to defects in apoptotic clearance (apoptosis = programmed cell death). It is hypothesised that SLE could be due to failure to maintain self-tolerance, secondary to defective removal of apoptotic cells. A common feature of the autoantigens in SLE, particularly chromatin and the phospholipids, is that they are components of the surface blebs of apoptotic cells. Condensation and fragmentation of the nucleus, plus internucleosomal cleavage of chromatin, lead to the formation of apoptotic bodies and blebs. If there is disturbed removal of apoptotic cells, these could become antigenic targets for autoantibodies.

The Euro-lupus project (prospective cohort study of 1000 SLE patients followed from 1991) has noted approximately half of *all* SLE (not just pSLE) patients present with arthritis, around a third have malar rash, and just over a quarter present with active nephropathy. Having double-stranded DNA antibodies was predictive for haemolytic anaemia and nephritis, and having lupus anticoagulant was predictive for antiphospholipid syndrome.

Other non-genetic factors that may increase the likelihood of developing SLE include oestrogens (whereas androgens are protective), UV light (UVA2 and UVB), vitamin D deficiency, cigarette smoking, pesticides, phthalates and certain medications. There is a range of medications that are definitely associated (e.g. tumour necrosis factor inhibitors [TNFIs], procainamide, penicillamine, hydralazine), and several that are possibly associated (e.g. minocycline) with SLE.

History

PRESENTING COMPLAINT

Reason for current admission.

SYMPTOMS

This is essentially an extensive systems review. The three common organ systems involved in pSLE are the skin, and the musculoskeletal and renal systems. The most common clinical features include (in approximate descending order): *rash* (any type), *arthritis*, *fever*, *nephritis* (all of these are present in *over 50%* at presentation in pSLE), *lymphadenopathy*, *hepatosplenomegaly*, *malar rash* (specifically, these present in about *one-third* at presentation), neuropsychiatric disease, gastrointestinal disease, pulmonary disease and cardiovascular disease (these last four are uncommon in pSLE).

Constitutional symptoms such as fever, fatigue/malaise and weight loss are very common at presentation and with flares of disease:

1. General (anorexia, malaise, pallor, weight loss, fatigue).
2. Skin (malar rash, purpura), mucous membrane (palate ulcers, usually painless), hair loss or scalp ulceration.
3. Joints: symmetrical polyarthritis, usually non-erosive (Jaccoud's type of arthritis; reversible subluxation due to tenosynovitis) may present with morning stiffness, pain and swelling.
4. Cardiovascular (Raynaud's phenomenon, cardiac failure symptoms due to myocarditis, chest pain from serositis or, less likely, myocardial ischaemia).
5. Respiratory (recurrent chest infections, pleuritic chest pain, dyspnoea).
6. Renal (hypertension, oedema, haematuria).
7. Neuropsychiatric (headache, cerebrovascular disease, seizures, chorea, personality change, decreased school performance, depression, suicidal ideation, acute confusional state, anxiety, cognitive dysfunction, psychosis [occurs in 50% of patients with neuropsychiatric involvement]).
8. Abdominal pain (e.g. serositis, pancreatitis).
9. Menstrual abnormalities (due to SLE per se or steroids).
10. Endocrine (diabetes).
11. Drug effects (e.g. steroid effects: Cushing's syndrome, hypertension, poor height gain, myopathy, osteoporosis (± fracture or vertebral body collapse), avascular necrosis (AVN), especially hips and knees.

PAST HISTORY

Initial diagnosis (when, where, presenting symptoms, initial investigations), recognised aetiologies such as complement deficiencies, drug-induced disease (e.g. tumour necrosis factor inhibitors [TFNIs], hydralazine, alpha-methyldopa, penicillamine, isoniazid, chlorpromazine), number of hospitalisations, sequence of complication developments and their management.

MANAGEMENT

Present treatment in hospital, usual treatment at home, previous treatments tried, side effects, compliance, use of identification bracelet.

SOCIAL HISTORY

Disease impact on child (e.g. school absenteeism, limitation of ADLs, impact of disease manifestations and side effects of treatment, such as malar rash, hair loss from cyclophosphamide or weight gain from steroids). Impact on family (financial considerations, such as cost of frequent hospitalisation, private health insurance), impact on siblings (e.g. sibling rivalry), benefits received (e.g. Child Disability Allowance), social supports (e.g. Lupus Association).

UNDERSTANDING OF DISEASE

By child and by parents. Ask about the degree of previous education (e.g. in hospital, by local paediatrician) and contingency plans (e.g. who to contact first when the child is unwell).

Examination

The procedure outlined here would also be suitable for a short-case approach.

GENERAL OBSERVATIONS

1. Well or unwell.
2. Pallor (anaemia; various mechanisms).
3. Cushingoid features (steroid treatment).
4. Parameters: height (e.g. short due to steroids); weight (e.g. obese due to steroids).
5. Skin rashes.
6. Joint swelling, gait problems.
7. Peripheral oedema (renal disease).
8. Posturing (e.g. hemiplegic).
9. Involuntary movements (e.g. chorea, hemiballismus, tremor, parkinsonian-like movements).
10. Respiratory distress (e.g. pneumonitis, pulmonary oedema).
11. Impression of mental state (e.g. depressed, or difficulty concentrating, with neuropsychiatric involvement).
    In a short-case setting, request the following:
1. Temperature chart (fever, e.g. infection from leucopenia, steroids or cytotoxics).
2. Blood pressure (hypertension, from renal disease or steroids).
3. Urinalysis (blood, protein [renal disease]; glucose [steroids, or frank diabetes]).
    After this, the systems involved are screened sequentially.

SKIN, HAIR AND MUCOUS MEMBRANE

Thorough inspection of the skin for rashes (including malar rash over cheeks and nasal bridge, sparing nasolabial folds, photosensitive rash, vasculitic rash [may include ulceration, nodules and palpable purpura], discoid lesions, Raynaud's phenomenon, palmar/plantar erythema); digital ulcers; hair for alopecia, broken hairs; mucous membranes (oral and nasal) for hyperaemia and petechial rashes on the hard palate, ulcers (painless) or infection.

JOINTS AND BONES

Full joint screening examination (after enquiring if the child has pain anywhere; always get the patient to move his or her joints first [active range of movement] before passive investigation [the candidate moving the joints] and ask if any joints hurt; if this order is forgotten, the patient could be hurt). Particularly note wrists, hands, knees and feet, as these tend to be more commonly affected. Get the patient to walk normally (looking particularly for limp; avascular necrosis of the hips or knees can occur in around 10% of pSLE). Perform Trendelenburg's test to detect proximal weakness (with unilateral or bilateral hip disease, or proximal myopathy; both can occur due to steroids). Detailed examination of any involved joints is important (but be aware of time constraints).

NEUROLOGICAL AND EYES

Look for lateral localising signs, screening eye examination for common complications; for example, glaucoma or cataracts.

GAIT AND LOWER LIMBS

Full gait examination, to detect limp (e.g. from AVN of femoral head or knee due to steroids), hemiplegia, other focal deficits, cerebellar ataxia, peripheral neuropathy or proximal myopathy (steroids, SLE per se).

UPPER LIMBS AND/OR CEREBELLAR INVOLVEMENT

Arms held straight out in front of body (screen for chorea, tremor, monoplegic posturing). Finger–nose test (screen for cerebellar ataxia with eyes open, and for sensory neuropathy with eyes closed).

CRANIAL NERVES

Test motor cranial nerves (mononeuritis multiplex; trigeminal neuropathy, facial nerve palsy, extraocular muscle weakness). Look for nystagmus (cerebellar involvement). If the child has focal deficits, also check the visual fields (e.g. for hemianopia). Inspect for episcleritis. Ophthalmoscopy: check for cataracts (steroids); retinal cottonwool exudates, haemorrhages.

CARDIORESPIRATORY

Before palpating the chest, take the pulse (e.g. tachycardia or arrhythmia with myocarditis) and count the respiratory rate. Check the blood pressure (if you have not already requested this, in the short case) for narrow pulse pressure (myocarditis) or hypertension (renal involvement). Examine the praecordium (for cardiac manifestations; e.g. pericarditis, pericardial effusion, myocarditis). Examine the posterior aspect of the chest: percuss the lung fields for pleural effusion; percuss over the vertebrae for compression fractures (steroid side effect); auscultate the lung fields (e.g. for pleuritis, pneumonitis). Examine the lymph nodes (lymphadenopathy).

ABDOMEN

Inspect for scars (e.g. peritoneal dialysis, renal transplant, laparotomy for acute abdomen). Palpate for tenderness (serositis), hepatosplenomegaly (SLE per se) and inguinal lymphadenopathy (SLE per se). Percuss for shifting dullness if there is any peripheral oedema or pleural effusion.

Diagnosis

The Systemic Lupus International Collaborating Clinics (SLICC) published a classification system in 2012 designed to replace the 1997 American College of Rheumatology (ACR) criteria. The SLICC system has 11 clinical criteria and 6 immunological criteria, with a sensitivity and specificity of 94% and 92% respectively. Using the newer SLICC system, a child is said to have SLE if 4 or more of 11 selected criteria are present, with at least one clinical criterion *and* one immunological criterion, or lupus nephritis as the sole criterion in the presence of ANA or anti-dsDNA antibodies.

Each criterion has a specific definition (refer to Petri M et al., *Arthritis Rheum* 2012; 64:2677–86). The 11 *clinical* criteria are: acute cutaneous lupus (includes malar rash and photosensitivity); chronic cutaneous lupus (includes discoid rash); oral ulcers or nasal ulcers; non-scarring alopecia; synovitis (involving at least two joints); serositis; renal disorder (includes red cell casts); neurological disorder (includes seizures, neuropathies); haemolytic anaemia; leukopenia or lymphopenia; and thrombocytopenia. The six *immunological* criteria are: antinuclear antibody (above laboratory reference range); anti-double-stranded DNA antibody (above laboratory reference range); anti-Sm; antiphospholipid antibody positivity; low complement C3, low C4, low CH50; and direct Coomb's test in the absence of haemolytic anaemia.

Investigations

SLE is characterised by the production of autoantibodies directed against a wide range of proteins: histone, non-histone, RNA-binding, cytoplasmic and nuclear proteins. The following lists the antibodies and their approximate frequency in SLE (derived from adult data):

- *Antinuclear antibodies* (ANA): up to 100%.
- *Anti-U1 RNP antibodies* (an RNA-binding protein): 70–90%.
- *Anti-DNA antibodies*: 60–70%.
- *Anticardiolipin* (aCL) antibodies (*antiphospholipid* antibodies): 50%.
- *Anti-Sm antibodies* (another RNA-binding protein): 40–50%.
- *Anti-Ro antibodies*: 30–40%.
- *Lupus anticoagulant* (LAC) antibodies (*antiphospholipid* antibodies): 20%.
- *Anti-La antibodies*: 15–20%.
- *Antiribosomal antibodies*: 15%.

This list is given for completeness, and does not indicate clinical usefulness, which is covered by the SLICC system, and expanded below. The following investigations may be useful.

SIMPLE SCREENING TESTS

1. Haemoglobin (e.g. haemolytic anaemia; relative macrocytosis, or normocytic anaemia of chronic disease).
2. White cell count (e.g. leukopenia).
3. Platelet count (e.g. thrombocytopenia).
4. Antinuclear antibodies (ANA), directed against a number of autoantigens. This is one of the hallmarks of SLE, and an SLICC criterion. This is the best simple screening test. Be aware that persistently positive ANA in the absence of other objective evidence of rheumatic disease does not suggest a chronic rheumatic disease by itself. The vast majority of ANA-positive children do not have SLE. At least 10% of the normal paediatric population are positive for ANA.
5. Inflammatory markers: ESR is typically elevated in the presence of a normal CRP. If the latter is elevated, infections must be searched for meticulously.
6. Urea, creatinine, electrolytes (to assess renal function).
7. Urinalysis (for protein, blood or cellular casts).

MORE SPECIFIC TESTS FOR PSLE

Blood

1. *Double-stranded DNA (dsDNA)* antibodies (SLICC criterion; specific to SLE; correlates with more severe systemic involvement, e.g. renal disease); DNA–Farr (radioimmunoassay); DNA–Crithidia titre (immunofluorescence). DNA binding is also useful. dsDNA may be useful in disease monitoring; for example, renal or CNS disease.
2. Antibodies to extractable nuclear antigens (e.g. Ro [SSA], La [SSB], Sm, RNP). Antibodies to Ro and La are associated with neonatal lupus, and occur with increased frequency in children of mothers with SLE. Antibodies to Sm are very specific for patients with SLE: they are found in 40–50% of SLE patients.
3. *CH-50, C3, C4* (SLICC criterion; usually low values in active disease). C3 and C4 are useful in monitoring disease activity. Isolated deficiencies (e.g. C2) may be found.
4. *Coomb's (direct antibody) test* (e.g. positive with immune-mediated anaemias; SLICC criterion in absence of haemolytic anaemia).
5. Clotting profile (e.g. prolonged PTT with circulating lupus anticoagulant; paradoxically, a tendency for thrombotic events in vivo).
6. *Antiphospholipid antibodies* (aPL): includes anticardiolipin antibody (aCL) and lupus anticoagulant (LAC); SLICC criterion. Associated with recurrent thromboembolic events.
7. Liver function tests (raised enzymes in salicylate hepatotoxicity or active SLE).
8. Creatine phosphokinase (myositis).

Cerebrospinal fluid

No consistent cerebrospinal fluid (CSF) abnormalities are found with neurological sequelae of SLE, although pleocytosis, elevated protein level and low glucose level may occur. CSF examination helps to exclude haemorrhage and infection, but is not part of a standard assessment of a patient with SLE.

Imaging

1. Chest X-ray (e.g. pneumonitis, myocarditis).
2. Bone X-rays (e.g. vertebral collapse).
3. Neuroimaging (all but MRI scan are research tests so far):
   a. Cranial MRI scan (e.g. localised areas of vasculitis), MR angiogram, MR venogram.
   b. SPECT (single-photon emission computerised tomography) imaging (e.g. areas of hypoperfusion; often in parietal and cerebellar lobes).
   c. NMR (nuclear magnetic resonance) spectroscopy (e.g. areas with decreased ATP [adenosine triphosphate] levels).
   d. PET (positron emission tomography) scanning (areas of hypometabolism; often in temporal and parietal lobes).
   e. Conventional cerebral angiography is not usually performed. It is usually normal in patients with neurological or psychiatric manifestations of SLE (perhaps due to the small size of the vessels affected by lupus vasculopathy), although a positive result may suggest vasculitis or antiphospholipid syndrome.
4. Cardiac imaging: echocardiography—M-mode, two-dimensional, Doppler and/or transoesophageal (endocarditis vegetations, mural thrombi, other cardiac source for emboli).

Neurophysiological testing
1. EEG (abnormalities may occur in children with neurological sequelae of SLE, but are non-specific).
2. ECG (e.g. pericarditis, arrhythmias).

Urine

A 24-hour urine collection for creatinine clearance and protein.

Other

1. Renal biopsy is indicated if significant abnormality is detected in the urinalysis. Many children with SLE will have a renal biopsy. The vast majority of children with SLE have some form of renal disease. Various forms of glomerulonephritis (GN) can occur; for example, mesangial GN, focal and segmental proliferative GN, diffuse proliferative GN (DPGN), membranous GN and mixed patterns.
2. Pulmonary function testing (e.g. interstitial lung disease).
3. Neuropsychological assessment (for children with neurological involvement; there is some evidence that this may be the best test for CNS lupus).

Management

The treatment goals are as follows:
1. Control disease activity (prevent and suppress disease flaring) to restore health towards normal.
2. Prevent scarring of organs (e.g. kidneys, brain).
3. Minimise adverse drug side effects (e.g. Cushing's syndrome).

In general, systemic (oral or intravenous, or a combination) steroids are used for their quick onset of action to reduce disease activity. As with the treatment for JIA, a maintenance agent will be needed to allow reduction of the steroid dose as soon as possible. This could include methotrexate, azathioprine or mycophenolate mofetil. Hydroxychloroquine is used for its beneficial effect on skin rashes, and for long-term protection against cardiovascular events.

GENERAL MEASURES

The role of the general paediatrician (the candidate) is as a coordinator of overall care, in conjunction with a paediatric rheumatologist and other health professionals (e.g. a nephrologist). The candidate should ensure that the family is appropriately educated regarding SLE, and its complications and treatment (and its side effects), and that there are adequate contingency plans in case of intercurrent illnesses or flares in disease activity. An identification bracelet should be worn (indicating whether taking steroids), and general measures such as adequate exercise and a well-balanced diet should be encouraged.

Sun exposure should be minimised, as it can cause a systemic flare and worsen the skin component. Use sun-blocking agents with a high sun-protecting factor and protective clothing (long sleeves, wide-brimmed hat). Photosensitive rashes, especially annular erythema, are associated with anti-Ro and anti-La antibodies.

The child should receive the normal immunisations, unless receiving cytotoxics or high-dose steroids, when live viral vaccines are avoided. Sulphonamide drugs are best avoided, as children with SLE may have severe toxic reactions to them.

Preventative management for osteoporosis may include adequate exercise, a high calcium intake and adequate doses of vitamin D.

There may well be a number of social issues, including those specifically related to adolescence. A chronic disease conflicts with the desires for independence, peer acceptance and sexual activity, and SLE can have particularly obvious physical stigmata (e.g. malar rash). Problems to be addressed can thus include low self-esteem, poor self-image, lack of compliance and even suicidal ideation.

The issue of pregnancy while on cytotoxics needs to be discussed with the adolescent. Although the majority of female patients can probably tolerate an oral contraceptive pill, this should only be prescribed with caution, as the pill can induce SLE, and cause hypertension, thrombosis and chronic active hepatitis. For this, combined preparations with low-dose oestrogen, or progesterone only preparations, are preferable. In addition, barrier methods should be encouraged (a condom or diaphragm with spermicidal foam). The risks of pregnancy (which can be particularly hazardous if the patient is taking cytotoxics, or has renal disease) must be discussed with the adolescent girl. She should be aware of the following:

1. The occurrence of the 'postpartum backlash'; that is, relapse of the disease.
2. The SLE association with increased miscarriage, and neonatal lupus with congenital heart block (see later).
3. Pregnancy must be carefully planned (i.e. with blood pressure, renal disease and haematological indices under control) and is best timed when in remission, or stable for over 12 months.

Steroid usage can cause amenorrhoea, without interfering with ovulation, giving the patient a false sense of security. This may lead to unprotected intercourse and an unplanned pregnancy. Male adolescents receiving cytotoxics should be informed about the availability of sperm banks.

A key to managing an adolescent is allowing the patient to self-manage their disease as much as is practicable.

SPECIFIC MEASURES

There is some variation between different centres regarding optimal treatment, including whether to treat only clinical disease flares or to treat serological flares (e.g. rising anti-double-stranded DNA antibodies, falling complement; decreases in C4 preceding, and decreases in C3 coinciding with, disease flares), or a balance between these options. Treatment is individualised for each patient; in selected patients, serological measurements may be useful guides to timing of treatment courses.

A staging system has been developed, mirroring the example of the oncologists, by the Hospital for Special Surgery in the United States. There are 10 stages of increasing severity.

MAIN AGENTS USED

Corticosteroids (CS)

Most children with SLE will need steroids at some stage of their management, as most children have systemic disease. Severe systemic disease (e.g. renal involvement, haematological complications, pleuritis, pericarditis) requires steroids. Steroids will rapidly bring more minor problems (e.g. fever, arthritis and myositis) under control. Severe active disease is not likely to respond to oral steroids alone, and the use of IV methyl prednisolone (IVMP) may be indicated. Although this treatment is often well tolerated, its use must be carefully monitored, as occasional side effects may include hypertensive crises and fatal cardiac arrhythmias.

The side effects of steroids are well known and already alluded to in the section under JIA treatment. Children generally develop Cushingoid features if they take over 0.25 mg/kg prednisolone per day for over a month. A radioreceptor assay can measure steroid activity (plasma prednisolone equivalents). Catch-up growth after cessation of treatment may not be complete, as chronic disease may also compound growth failure. Children who have had more steroids are more likely to develop more significant sepsis.

Non-steroidal anti-inflammatory drugs (NSAIDs)

This class of medications may be used to control the symptoms of disease; for example, fever or arthralgia/joint stiffness. All NSAIDs can adversely affect the glomerular filtration rate (GFR), so caution or avoidance in renal disease is recommended.

Hydroxychloroquine (HCQ)

This may be useful for skin and joint involvement and fatigue, and also may be useful in nephritis. It is antithrombotic and decreases cholesterol concentration. Side effects include renal and retinal toxicities (maculopathy) and gastrointestinal symptoms. HCQ has immunomodulative effects mediated by toll-like receptor 9 (TLR9) without causing immunosuppression; it also increases lysosomal pH, and alters antigen. Rarely, cardiomyopathy and neuromyotoxicity have been reported.

Disease-modifying anti-rheumatic drugs (DMARDs)

Methotrexate (MTX), a folate antimetabolite which inhibits DNA synthesis, is effective as a steroid-sparing agent in musculoskeletal disease. Low-dose (10–20 mg per m^2), once-a-week MTX is safe; folate supplementation decreases side effects. It is given orally, although the parenteral route has more efficacy and is associated with less toxicity. Side effects include oral ulcers, gastrointestinal and bone marrow toxicities. Regular (1–2 monthly) blood tests are performed to detect any liver impairment or marrow involvement.

Other cytotoxics can be useful in children with uncontrolled progressive disease, or severe steroid side effects (e.g. significant growth failure), again based largely on anecdotal evidence. Agents used include oral azathioprine (AZA) or cyclophosphamide (CPA), and intravenous cyclophosphamide (IV-CPA) pulses.

Azathioprine (AZA) is a purine analogue which inhibits synthesis of xanthylic and adenylic acids, which then suppresses synthesis of DNA. It can be used as induction and maintenance therapy for lupus nephritis classes III and IV (see later in the case for details). It is used for systemic features of SLE and allows steroid sparing, decreasing steroid requirement.

Mycophenolate mofetil (MMF), which inhibits monophosphate dehydrogenase (blocking synthesis of guanosine nucleotides, decreasing proliferation of T- and B-lymphocytes), has been trialled head-to-head against oral cyclophosphamide and found to be as effective in treating nephritis with fewer side effects. MMF can be used both for induction and remission of nephritis, and for moderate to severe SLE.

IV-CPA pulses can have short-term effects including bone marrow suppression and significant hyperemesis (which can be minimised, either by giving frusemide 8–12 hours after the CPA dose, or by using ondansetron, the $5-HT_3$ receptor antagonist). Long-term effects of IV-CPA such as risks of infertility (around 17%) and neoplasia also need consideration.

Cyclosporine A (CSA) can be used for class V nephritis, as an alternative to AZA or MMF. A paediatric rheumatologist should decide if, when and which cytotoxics should be used, after careful discussion of the risk–benefit profile with the family.

Leflunomide (LEF) inhibits dihydroorotate dehydrogenase, which is essential for synthesis of pyrimidine and cellular protein kinases, and so blocks synthesis of DNA. Its side effects include diarrhoea, elevated liver enzymes and mucocutaneous abnormalities.

Tacrolimus (TAC) is a calcineurin inhibitor. It can be effective in treating lupus nephritis and also cutaneous lupus.

A major use for these agents is severe renal pSLE. These children may need prolonged treatment. The role of DMARDs in treating extrarenal disease is less clear.

Biological disease-modifying anti-rheumatic drugs (bDMARDs)

Patients who do not respond to conventional cytotoxic agents are increasingly being considered for bDMARDs. The most interest in SLE treatment has been in agents which block B-lymphocytes. Most of these are monoclonal antibodies (mAbs), either 'Umabs' or 'Imabs'. Some are cytokine re*cept*or blockers, or 'Cepts'. The following is brief list of those either established as effective, or those being trialled, in SLE.

- Rituximab is a B-cell depleter whose effect lasts up to 12 months; it is a chimeric monoclonal antibody to CD20; it leads to apoptosis induction. It is used rarely in JIA (see JIA long case in this chapter). Rituximab is established, as both ACR and EULAR (European League Against Rheumatism) guidelines mention it in context of active lupus nephritis where conventional therapies have been ineffective.
- T-cell targeting: **ART**; **A**batacept, **R**uplizumab, **T**oralizumab (T-cell function inhibitors). Abatacept is used in JIA; see JIA long case for details.
- **T**umour **N**ecrosis **F**actor **I**nhibitors (**TNFIs**): Etanercept, Infliximab. These are both used in JIA (see JIA long case for details of these drugs).

Intravenous immunoglobulin (IVIG)

IVIG can be useful in very refractory severe antiphospholipid syndrome, refractory to other treatment. It also has a place in active disease where DMARDs or bDMARDs cannot be used because of co-existent infection, or pregnancy.

Medications used for varying activity/severity of disease in SLE

- Mild (rash, arthralgia, fatigue): HCQ, NSAIDs.
- Moderate (arthritis, serositis, early renal, ulcers, rash): CS + MTX or AZA or MMF.
- Severe (non-renal; cerebritis, severe serositis, severe rash): initial: CS (IVMP) + MMF or RTX or CPA; maintenance: CS + MMF or AZA.
- Severe (renal; hypertension, oedema): initial: CS + IV-CPA or MMF or RTX; maintenance: CS or MMF or AZA.

APPROACH TO TREATMENT OF SPECIFIC SYSTEM INVOLVEMENT

Life-threatening systemic disease

Intravenous steroid pulses (IVSP), IV-CPA and plasmapheresis, are options.

Kidneys

Renal involvement in SLE is as follows (simplified schema of WHO classification):

- WHO class I: Normal light microscopy.
- WHO class II: Mesangial lupus nephritis (around 20% of cases).
- WHO class III: Focal proliferative glomerulonephritis (GN) (around 20% of cases).
- WHO class IV: Diffuse proliferative GN (just under 50% of cases).
- WHO class V: Membranous GN (around 10% of cases).
- WHO class VI: Sclerosed glomeruli.

Treatment is based on renal histology. Severe renal involvement requires intensive and prolonged treatment. Steroids (high-dose oral prednisone, or pulse IV doses of methylprednisolone [IVMP]) and DMARDs (conventional or biological [bDMARDs]) often are needed. Either CPA or MMF are appropriate induction agents for lupus nephritis, and MMF or AZA can maintain remission.

- WHO class II: low-dose steroids—short course, slow taper, excellent outcome. Some nephrologists use angiotensin-converting enzyme (ACE) inhibitors, or angiotensin receptor blocking agents (ARBs) alone, to decrease proteinuria.
- WHO class III and IV: high-dose steroids—slow taper, add second agent after biopsy to confirm histology. Second agent: MMF, AZA or CPA. MMF and AZA are safer, and MMF may be superior in African Americans. Class IV usually responds to steroids. For active SLE complicated by class IV, intravenous (IV-)CPA may be indicated. The Euro-lupus regimen comprises six pulses of IV-CPA every 2 weeks, at lower doses of CPA than other regimes, and a lower infection risk. Other effective regimens have included: six once-monthly CPA pulses as induction, and concomitant use of DMARDs for maintenance; monthly IV-CPA for 7 months, then IV-CPA every 3 months for the next 30 months. As the CPA-related toxicity is cumulative, there is a recent trend to use only six once-monthly CPA pulses as induction, and concomitant use of DMARDs for maintenance.

    With this treatment, many children have exhibited marked improvement in their overall wellbeing, including a decrease in infection, cerebritis, arthritis and emergency hospitalisation. If nephrotic syndrome occurs, AZA may be useful.

- WHO class V: may well respond to low-dose steroids. Some patients require prolonged steroids, then CSA, AZA or MMF. ACE inhibitors or ARBs are used as well to decrease proteinuria. Anticoagulation may be required, due to the risk of renal vein thrombosis, and possible pulmonary embolism.

Some children have histology that demonstrates more than one pathology type; for example, WHO classes II, III, IV and V. Treatment is directed against the most serious (proliferative) component.

Hydroxychloroquine therapy is associated with greater rates of renal response, less relapses and decreased development of renal damage.

Biological agents, such as rituximab (RTX, an anti-B-cell [CD20] antibody), have been effective in small studies, in severe treatment-resistant lupus nephritis; RTX has also been used successfully for severe haematological involvement.

Autologous stem cell transplantation has been successful in inducing remission in severe treatment-resistant cases.

Children with significant renal disease usually manifest haematuria and proteinuria within 6 months of initial diagnosis of their SLE. Progression to chronic renal failure (CRF) is associated with class IV, persistent hypertension lasting over 4 months, abnormal urinalysis, elevated creatinine and anaemia. If CRF and then end-stage renal disease (ESRD) supervene, dialysis may be needed while awaiting renal transplantation (RTx). Lupus can recur in transplants, but only rarely.

Children who receive RTx have a better prognosis than those on dialysis (see the section on RTx in Chapter 13, Nephrology). Those children with poor prognostic factors are treated aggressively, and those with ESRD have transplants as soon as possible.

Hypertension

Thiazide diuretics and beta blockers are the first line. If there is renal disease, especially with proteinuria, blockers of the renin-angiotensin-aldosterone system (RAAS), such as captopril (an ACE inhibitor), is first line. Avoid drugs that can cause SLE (e.g. hydralazine, methyldopa). Second-line agents include calcium channel blockers and minoxidil. If hypertension is uncontrolled, it can aggravate vasculitis and renal disease. Hypertension will be aggravated by steroid treatment.

Cardiovascular

The main cardiovascular system morbidity in pSLE is premature atherosclerosis. The most common cardiac manifestation is pericarditis with pericardial effusion. Other forms of involvement include endocarditis and myocarditis, which can be treated with steroids. Pericarditis can respond to NSAIDs alone. Valvular heart disease can occur, in association with aPL antibodies or with non-infective endocarditis. Libman–Sacks verrucous endocarditis can occur in acutely ill children with pSLE. The most commonly affected valves in order (left two, then right two) are as follows: mitral, aortic, pulmonary, tricuspid. There is an inflammatory infiltrate first, then the formation of nodules of fibrinoid necrosis of the supporting connective tissue of the valve. Treatment may involve high-dose steroids, DMARDs or surgery.

The main cardiovascular morbidity, however, is premature atherosclerosis. The main risk factor for this is ongoing chronic inflammation of pSLE itself. Steroids could theoretically make atherosclerosis worse.

Most children with SLE will develop significant dyslipidaemia, which increases their risk of atherosclerosis in later life. Antimalarials such as hydroxychloroquine have an advantage of lipid-lowering among their many effects. Input from dieticians and physiotherapists will help avoid high blood lipid levels and obesity, and will help optimise physical exercise. In North America, the Childhood Arthritis and Rheumatology Research Alliance (CARRA) has launched the Atherosclerosis Prevention in Pediatric Lupus Erythematosus (APPLE) prospective study, assessing the role of statins in the prevention of atherosclerosis—the largest prospective study ever undertaken in pSLE.

Pulmonary

For mild to moderate pulmonary disease oral steroids, plus antibiotics if infection is suspected. If severe pulmonary haemorrhage occurs, use pulse IV steroids and DMARDs. In severely ill patients, multiple antibiotics, high-dose steroids and positive pressure ventilation may be required. Children with pSLE should have opportunistic infections excluded (such as herpes, *Pneumocystis carinii*, legionella or fungal infections) before introducing DMARDs/bDMARDs.

Neuropsychiatric SLE (NP-SLE)/CNS lupus

The aetiology of NP-SLE is multifactorial, involving immune complexes, autoantibodies and cytokines; there are at least 11 known brain-specific antibodies and 9 systemic autoantibodies. The most common antibodies found in NP-SLE patients are anticardiolipin antibodies, which correlate with NP features such as chorea and intellectual impairment. It can be difficult to differentiate NP-SLE from antiphospholipid syndrome.

In 1999, the ACR divided NP-SLE into 19 separate conditions, including headache, psychosis, mood disorder/depression, cognitive dysfunction, cerebrovascular disease, seizures and movement disorders. An infrequent manifestation of NP-SLE is neuropathy (cranial [more common] and peripheral). As the area is complex, treatment decisions should involve a team including psychiatrists, psychologists, neurologists and rheumatologists. In general, high-dose steroids and DMARDs (AZA or CPA) are used. Psychotropic drugs, antidepressants and anticonvulsants may be needed as well. Analgesia can be ineffective in lupus headache.

The underlying cause for the headache must be sought and that cause treated (e.g. cerebral vein thrombosis [CVT], raised intracranial pressure from CNS infection or pseudotumour cerebri, active CNS vasculitis or systemic steroids). It may be difficult to determine whether behavioural problems are secondary to having a chronic illness or secondary to NP-SLE.

Aggressive treatment of NP-SLE is indicated, as this complication can be fatal. There have been no published NP-SLE treatment trials in paediatric populations. In adults, high-dose CPA with or without autologous haematopoietic stem cell transplantation has been used with success in severe life-threatening SLE with neuropsychiatric manifestations that are unresponsive to other treatment.

Joints

A combination of hydroxychloroquine and MTX is often used as maintenance treatment, while low-dose steroids and NSAIDs may be used to treat joint symptoms. Physiotherapy, including a personalised goal-oriented home exercise program (HEP), is essential to maintain joint function and aerobic fitness, as well as minimising bone loss.

Skin

Avoid sun exposure wherever possible. Adopt appropriate clothing and the use of sunscreen (with a sun protection factor of at least 30), topical steroids for discoid lesions, and oral agents (hydroxychloroquine, methotrexate, with or without low-dose steroids).

Raynaud's phenomenon is less common in paediatric than in adult SLE: management is by avoidance of cold exposure, appropriate clothing (e.g. insulated mittens [rather than gloves]; multiple layers of clothing; hats, hand and feet warmers) to keep extremities warm, low-dose aspirin (if there is no thrombocytopenia) and, if these are inadequate, oral nifedipine or low-dose steroids, or topical nitroglycerine paste. Severe digit-threatening disease can be treated with a prostacyclin infusion.

Other organ system involvement

As seen above, the most common organ systems involved in pSLE are the skin, and the musculoskeletal and renal systems. However, other systems can be involved, albeit less often than in adults.

Gastrointestinal, liver and spleen involvement

Lupus-associated vasculitis can manifest as an acute abdomen; abdominal pain can be due to peritoneal inflammation (serositis), pancreatitis, acute ischaemic enteritis, pseudo-obstruction or paralytic ileus; or the involvement of periappendiceal tissue can mimic appendicitis.

Vasculitis is the underlying cause in 60% of patients with SLE who develop an acute abdomen. Mesenteric vasculitis or thrombosis can inflame the bowel wall and present with cramping abdominal pain and diarrhoea. Lupus enteropathy may also present as malabsorption, or protein-losing enteropathy. Hepatomegaly occurs in around 40% of patients; up to a quarter have abnormal liver function tests; this can be due to fatty liver secondary to prolonged steroid use—if the liver function tests are significantly elevated, then lupoid hepatitis may need consideration. Splenomegaly occurs in around 30%, while functional asplenia is common and increases predisposition to infection.

Endocrine involvement

The organ most commonly involved is the thyroid; hypothyroidism or hyperthyroidism can occur, the former more often. Up to a third of pSLE patients have anti-thyroid antibodies, and a third of these develop overt hypothyroidism. Diabetes mellitus, induced by steroids, occurs in 5–10% of pSLE patients, and usually needs insulin.

Other endocrine complications include delayed puberty and irregular menstruation. Ovarian failure can occur as a complication of CPA, and is dose dependent; this is one reason why CPA is falling out of favour in this population, and is avoided wherever possible.

Antiphospholipid (aPL) antibodies

Antiphospholipid (aPL) antibodies are associated with an increased risk of thrombotic events (TE), chorea, epilepsy, migraine, livedo reticularis and avascular necrosis; the most commonly measured of these antibodies are anticardiolipin (aCL) antibodies (50%) and lupus anticoagulant (LAC) antibodies (25%). The risk of thrombosis is less in the paediatric population than in adults. In aPL-positive children, arterial and venous thromboses have been reported, including deep venous thrombosis (DVT), pulmonary embolism, superior vena cava thrombosis, ischaemic stroke, transverse myelitis, retinal artery occlusion and renal artery occlusion. Persistently positive LAC is associated with the highest risk of TE.

Neonatal lupus

Adolescent girls with pSLE contemplating having children need to be fully aware that babies of mothers with SLE can develop features of SLE. Transient features are entirely due to transplacental passage of maternal antibodies, as they resolve with clearance of the antibodies. Examples include thrombocytopenia, leukopenia, hepatosplenomegaly, myocarditis, pericarditis and the photosensitive discoid skin rash.

The other group is permanent features, their aetiology being only partially explained by transplacental antibody passage. Examples include congenital complete heart block (CCHB; associated with antibodies to SSA/Ro [particularly to the 52-kD Ro polypeptide rather than the 60-kD Ro] and SSB/La; these antibodies cross the placenta from 12 weeks' gestational age), endomyocardial fibroelastosis and other forms of structural heart disease. Fetuses with congestive cardiac failure, CCHB and pericardial effusions have been treated with some success by giving the mother dexamethasone.

Prognosis

Overall survival in pSLE (ESRD-free) approximates 95–100% at 5 years, 94% at 10 years, and 90% at 15 years. Mortality rates are connected to socioeconomic status and disease activity. The most common cause of death remains infection, usually associated with the use of steroids and DMARDs/bDMARDs. Other more common causes of mortality are cerebritis, pancreatitis, pulmonary haemorrhage, renal failure and myocardial infarction. The poorest prognosis is with class VI nephritis and severe CNS involvement. After the first 2 years of disease, new organs are much less likely to become involved, with the exception of the CNS.

SHORT CASE

SHORT CASE: Joints

This is not an infrequent case. The approach given here has three basic components:
1. Thorough general inspection.
2. Systematic examination of all joints.
3. Examination for extra-articular manifestations of JIA and other diseases affecting joints, plus detection of drug side effects.

Figure 16.2 outlines the findings sought on inspection, plus those sought on assessing for extra-articular manifestations and drug side effects. A suggested order for this is: skin, hands, blood pressure, hair, eyes, mouth, neck, chest, abdomen and lower limbs neurologically, plus temperature chart, urine and stool analysis.

Examination

The examination for each joint comprises inspection, palpation, movement (active first, as passive movements may cause distress and immediate loss of rapport with patient and examiners), measurement and finally assessment of functional ability.

A useful initial screen, on being introduced to the patient, is to ask him or her to walk a short distance (for antalgic gait), take off a jumper or shirt (for upper limb function) and then write her or his name for you (hand function).

Although, ideally, the child should be undressed down to underwear, there are many children who can become embarrassed, particularly those approaching adolescence. Showing sensitivity to the child's modesty will be well received by examiners and parents alike. If the child is younger and does not get embarrassed, then watching the child undress may yield valuable clues regarding involved joints. A good position for the examination is confrontation/mirroring (i.e. positioning yourself immediately opposite the child), so that you can demonstrate clearly what movements are required of the child, while using your own joints as reminders regarding normal range of movement.

The following is the sequence suggested for whichever joints are being examined. Inspect the distribution of joint involvement (symmetry) and note swelling, loss of normal contours, angulation, deformity, redness and muscle wasting. Next, feel the joint and periarticular areas for tenderness, warmth, effusion, 'boggy' swelling (thickened synovium and fluid), enthesitis and contractures.

The ROM is then examined, active movement first. Test passive movement, paying attention to the presence of soft-tissue restriction; for example, tenosynovitis or joint loss of ROM. Remember to watch the child's face to detect any discomfort. Any loss of ROM should be quantified by descriptive terms such as minimally, moderately or severely reduced (see the section on JIA). Finally, function (which correlates with strength) should be tested.

A suggested order for a systematic examination of all the joints is as follows: hands, wrists, elbows, shoulders, temporomandibular joints, cervical spine, lumbar spine, hips, knees, ankles, feet (i.e. hand to head, and head to toe). A good initial position is with the child sitting in a chair, or on the side of a bed, with the hands resting on the thighs.

1. Introduce self

2. General inspection

Well or unwell

Age and sex (e.g. JIA under 5 years usually female; JAS usually older male)

Cushingoid (steroids)

Obvious skin rash (e.g. SLE, psoriasis, HSP – see below)

Parameters
- Height (short from steroids)
- Weight (obese from steroids; thin from hypercatabolism)

3. Skin

Butterfly malar erythema (SLE)

Heliotrope eyelids (dermatomyositis)

Purpura (HSP, PAN)

Psoriasis

Vasculitic rash (e.g. SLE dermatomyositis, MCTD)

Maculopapular rash (systemic JIA)

Subcutaneous calcification (dermatomyositis)

Nodules (JIA, JRA)

Tight skin (scleroderma, MCTD)

Pigmentation and depigmentation (sclerodermal)

4. Upper limbs

Hands
- Raynaud's phenomenon (SLE, MCTD, scleroderma, PAN)

Nails
- Subungual haemorrhage (SLE)
- Pitting (psoriasis)
- Nail-bed telangiectasia (dermatomyositis)

Palms
- Anaemia (systemic JIA, SLE, drug side effects)
- Flexor tendon nodules (scleroderma)
- Flexor tenosynovitis (JIA)

Elbow region
- Epitrochlear nodes (systemic JIA, SLE, MCTD)
- Nodules over elbows (scleroderma)
- Rheumatoid nodules (JRA)

Blood pressure
- Elevated (e.g. HSP, steroids, PAN, SLE with nephropathy); if elevated, make a point of requesting urinalysis now

Axillae
- Lymphadenopathy (e.g. systemic JIA, SLE, Kawasaki's, MCTD)

5. Head and neck

Hair: alopecia (SLE)

Eyes: signs of seronegative JIA
- Iridocyclitis (usually need slit lamp to see)
- Band keratopathy
- Posterior synechiae (pupil shape change)
- Glaucoma

Eyes: signs of seropositive JIA
- Dry eyes (Sjögren's)
- Scleritis, episcleritis
- Scleromalacia perforans

Eyes: less specific signs
- Conjunctival pallor
- Cataract (JIA, steroids or chloroquine)

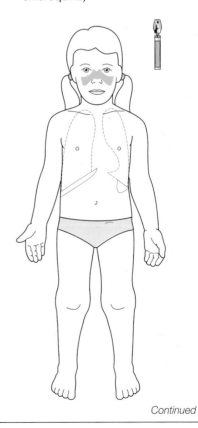

Continued

Figure 16.2 **Joint disease: extra-articular manifestations and drug side effects**

- Retinopathy (chloroquine)
Parotid: swelling (Sjögren's, MCTD)
Mouth
  - Inflamed mucous membrane (e.g. SLE, dermatomyositis)
  - Petechiae, purpura (e.g. SLE)
  - Ulcers (e.g. SLE, gold penicillamine)
Dysphonia (dermatomyositis)
Hoarseness (cricoarytenoid arthritis, laryngeal nodules with JRA)
Neck: lymphadenopathy (e.g. SLE, Kawasaki's, systemic JIA, MCTD)

6. Chest
Auscultate praecordium
  - Cardiomegaly (myocarditis with SLE or systemic JIA)
  - Pericarditis (SLE, systemic JIA)
  - Murmurs (SLE, SBE, rheumatic fever)
Auscultate lung fields
Pleuritis (systemic JIA, SLE)
Pleural effusion (SLE)

7. Abdomen
Tenderness (e.g. serositis with SLE, enteritis with IBD)

Hepatosplenomegaly (systemic JIA, SLE, MCTD)
Perianal disease (IBD)
Buttock rash (HSP)

8. Gait and lower limbs
Gait examination: screen for neurological signs (atlanto-axial subluxation with JIA; very uncommon)
Squat: proximal weakness (steroids, dermatomyositis, JA)
Lower limbs (neurologically)
  - Power (myopathy)
  - Reflexes (atlanto-axial subluxation)

9. Other
Temperature chart
  - Quotidian fever (systemic JIA)
Urinalysis
  - Proteinuria (penicillamine, amyloid, SLE, HSP, PAN, scleroderma)
  - Haematuria (SLE, HSP, PAN, naproxen)
Stool analysis
  - Blood (HSP, IBD, dermatomyositis)

HSP = Henoch–Schönlein purpura; IBD = inflammatory bowel disease; JAS = juvenile ankylosing spondylitis; JIA = juvenile idiopathic arthritis; JRA = juvenile rheumatoid arthritis (seropositive for IgM rheumatoid factor); MCTD = mixed connective tissue disease; PAN = polyarteritis nodosa; SBE = subacute bacterial endocarditis; SLE = systemic lupus erythematosus.

Figure 16.2, continued

SPECIFIC JOINTS

Note that the normal ROM at each joint is given in degrees, in parentheses.

Upper limbs
Hands and wrists

Look at the dorsum first: note any skin rash or muscle wasting. Methodically inspect the wrist, followed by the metacarpophalangeal (MCP) joints, proximal and distal interphalangeal (PIP and DIP) joints, and the nails. Then have the child turn the hands over and look at the palmar aspect in the same systematic fashion.

Look for palmar or periungual erythema or punctuate vasculitic rash of SLE. Check for Gottron's papules over PIP and MCP joints. Next, palpate each joint for tenderness and effusion.

Flex and extend the child's fingers while palpating over the flexor tendon sheaths (for tenosynovitis). Check ROM (active, then passive). Normal ROM values (in degrees) are as follows:

1. Wrist: flexion (80°), extension (70°), radial deviation (20°), ulnar deviation (30°).
2. MCP joints: flexion (90°), extension (30°).
3. PIP joints: flexion (100°).
4. DIP joints: flexion (90°), extension (10°).

Note that the thumb can flex to contact the tips of the other digits, and abduct from the index finger (50°).

Now, test the hands with respect to function. Simple tests include: grip strength; write with pencil; use knife, fork, spoon, cup; hold toothbrush; undo and do up buttons; turn key.

Elbows

Inspection (rheumatoid nodules, JDM rash) and palpation are followed by checking ROM:
1. Flexion (135°).
2. Extension (0–10°).
3. Supination (90°).
4. Pronation (90°).

Note that supination and pronation should be tested with the elbow flexed (if possible) at 90°; a pencil held in the closed hand (making a fist) can simplify assessment of the position.

Functionally, check if the child can turn an (imaginary) doorknob, comb hair, hang out the washing or answer a telephone.

Shoulders

After inspection and palpation, test ROM. It is usually easier to test younger children with play-like activities that produce the required movements that are to be tested. For example, you can tell the child:
1. 'Put your hands above your head' (demonstrate to the child): tests flexion (90°) and abduction (180°).
2. 'Give yourself a hug' (demonstrate): tests adduction (45°).
3. 'Scratch your back' (demonstrate): tests external rotation (45°).
4. 'Hide your hands behind your back' (demonstrate): tests internal rotation (55°) and extension (45°).

Functionally, several of the tests overlap with those for the elbows: comb hair, take off clothing, hang out washing, scratch near bottom (toileting function) and use a telephone.

JAW AND NECK

Look at the jaw (especially for acquired micrognathia) and teeth (for malocclusion), and feel for tenderness, crepitus or clicking over the temporomandibular joints (TMJs), with the child opening and closing the mouth. Note the interdental distance (inter-incisor distance) and show to the examiners (if relevant) that you are aware of the importance of measuring this to follow the progress of TMJ disease. A normal child should be able to fit the three middle fingers, lined up vertically, between the upper and lower teeth. Look for asymmetric opening, and absence of translation (anterior movement of the jaw at maximal opening) with the chin moving towards the affected side.

Next examine the cervical spine: inspect, palpate and check ROM:
1. Flexion: chin touches chest (45°).
2. Extension: head touches back (50°).
3. Rotation: turning chin to be in line with shoulder (80°).
4. Lateral flexion: ear to shoulder (40°).

THORACOLUMBAR SPINE

Inspect with the child standing, and then bending forwards (for scoliosis or kyphosis). Palpate for tenderness, over the spinous processes, the paraspinal and interspinous areas, and the sacroiliac joints. Check ROM.

1. Flexion: should be able to touch toes. Best assessed by Schöber's method.
2. Extension: arching back (30° at lumbar area).
3. Lateral bending (50° to each side)/flexion. This has equal contributions from the thoracic and lumbar spine.
4. Lateral rotation: most easily checked with child sitting (40° to each side). This is almost entirely thoracic.

To assess function, the child can be asked to pick an object up from the floor and to put on socks and shoes.

Schöber's test measuring lumbar spine flexion can be performed; in older children, more than 4 cm of movement should be measured. With the child standing upright, a mark (e.g. marker pen) is made 5 cm below the iliac crest, in the midline, and a second mark 10 cm above the iliac crest, in the midline. The child is then asked to bend forwards to touch their toes and the distance between the marks is measured. In adults, an increase in the distance between the two points of less than 5 cm indicates restriction of movement.

SACROILIAC JOINTS

Palpate for tenderness over the joint; additionally, press the pelvis from each side towards the midline to assess for pain (pelvic work test). Another manoeuvre is the **FABER** test, which comprises **F**lexing the hip to 90°, and **AB**ducting and **E**xternally **R**otating the hip (which is achieved by asking the child to put the foot of the affected side on the opposite knee), then simultaneously applying pressure to the medial aspect of the ipsilateral knee (push down the knee) and the contralateral anterior superior iliac spine (push down the opposite anterior superior iliac spine [ASIS]); this compresses the SI joint by applying pressure over the ASIS; if the child feels pain in the SI area, this indicates SI joint involvement/inflammation.

LOWER LIMBS

Examination can commence with watching the child walk (for antalgic gait), stand on each leg (for Trendelenburg's sign) and squat (for proximal weakness or instability). Beware of ankle tenderness, which can result in asymmetric placement of feet on squatting. Kneeling will stress the knee joints by testing them under partial weight bearing.

Hips

Inspect the resting position (e.g. external rotation with active synovitis) and muscle bulk. Palpate for tenderness. Measure the true leg length (ASIS to medial malleolus of ankle). With the child lying on the back, check ROM. Flexion (120°) can be checked first with active movement. Then perform Thomas' test for fixed flexion deformity.

Then test:

1. Internal rotation (35°).
2. External rotation (45°).
   (Both 1 and 2 are tested with hips at 90° flexion.)
3. Abduction (50°).
4. Adduction (30°).

Note that the pelvis should be stabilised (by one hand fixing the ASIS) when checking all these movements. Then, have the child turn over onto the abdomen and test extension (30°). Gait examination serves as a functional assessment.

Knees

Inspect, noting the quadriceps bulk. Feel for temperature and tenderness, and palpate entheses (at 10, 2 and 6 o'clock positions on the patella) and any synovial thickening or effusion. Test for the 'bulge sign' by 'milking' any joint fluid down the lateral aspect of the joint (look for a bulge medially) and then stroking upwards on the medial aspect, moving any fluid present into the suprapatellar bursa. Next, test for a patella tap. It may be appropriate to measure the muscle bulk of the thighs and calves if there appears to be a difference between the two sides: measure the circumference at a fixed distance (e.g. 5–10 cm) above the superior aspect of the patella, and at 10 cm below the tibial tuberosity. Also, if not already done, measure the leg length. 'True leg length' is measured from the ASIS to the medial malleolus of the ipsilateral leg.

Next, check the ROM: flexion (135°); extension (up to 10°).

Finally, check for knee stability. This should not be done if the knee is acutely inflamed, as the test will be painful and unnecessary. Test for anteroposterior movement with the knee joint flexed, with position fixed by sitting on the child's foot. Check for the 'Lachman sign' signifying damage to the cruciate ligaments (if there is movement when the leg is pulled forwards, the anterior cruciate is ruptured; if there is movement when the leg is pushed backwards, the posterior cruciate is ruptured). Also check for lateral mobility with the knee fully extended, for lesions of the medial or lateral ligament; normally, there is no lateral movement.

The McMurray sign is illustrated by applying external rotational movement on the knee while extending from 90° flexion and feeling for a click, or eliciting pain/apprehension in the joint, and signifies a meniscal tear.

Ankles and feet

Inspect for swelling, and loss of definition of the Achilles tendon (synovial thickening at the ankle joint). Palpate the ankle joint and entheses (Achilles insertion into calcaneus, metatarsal heads, plantar fascia insertion to calcaneus). Check the ROM.

1. Ankle: plantar flexion (50°); extension (dorsiflexion) (10–20°).
2. Subtalar joint: inversion (35–40°); eversion (15–20°).
3. Midtarsal (talonavicular and calcaneocuboid) joints: abduction (10°); adduction (20°). The midtarsal joint is tested by stabilising the calcaneus with one hand and moving the forefoot with the other.
4. First metatarsophalangeal (MTP) joint: plantar flexion (45°); extension (dorsiflexion) (70°). Note any crepitus or pain on moving the first metatarsal joint (may be selectively involved in spondyloarthropathies).

At the completion of the examination, summarise the positive findings, noting the number of joints involved, symmetry (symmetrical like juvenile rheumatoid arthritis, or asymmetrical like psoriatic arthritis), the activity of the disease (active with pain, redness), the functional severity (most important) and the differential diagnosis.

References

Brown, V.E., Pilkington, C.A., Feldman, B.M. & Davidson, J.E. (2006). An international consensus survey of the diagnostic criteria for juvenile dermatomyositis (JDM). *Rheumatology*, 45, 990–993.

Rider L.G. & Miller F.W. (1997). Classification and treatment of the juvenile idiopathic inflammatory myopathies. *Rheumatic Disease Clinics of North America*, 23, 619–655.

Suggested reading

The preparation for any examination, particularly the Fellowship Examination, requires the candidate to read widely. Reading allows the candidate to strengthen weaker areas and consolidate stronger ones. In recent years, the most popular source of information for local trainees/candidates has been UpToDate, an evidence-based resource available through the internet, computers and mobile devices. Another favourite is DynaMed, also an evidence-based reference tool that is available through the internet. The author finds both of these very useful.

The following list of non-internet-based sources of information is incomplete, but contains updated versions of textbooks that the author and his colleagues found useful in preparing for the Fellowship Examination. It is not expected that the prospective candidate will read all these tomes, but reference to at least some of them will be necessary.

The edition or year of publication of the medical texts is not listed, as the candidate should seek out the latest edition.

MEDICAL BOOKS

Barrett, K.E., Barman, S.M., Boitano, S. & Brooks, H. *Ganong's Review of Medical Physiology.* New York: McGraw-Hill.

Behrman, R.E., Kliegman, R.M. & Jenson, H.B. (eds). *Nelson Textbook of Pediatrics.* Philadelphia: WB Saunders.

Cohen, M. & Duffner, P. *Weiner & Levitt's Pediatric Neurology (House Officer series).* Baltimore: Williams & Wilkins.

Douglas, G., Nicol, F., Robertson, C. *Macleod's Clinical Examination.* Edinburgh: Churchill Livingstone.

Fauci, A.S., Braunwald, E., Kasper, D.L., Hauser, S.L., Longo, D.L., Jameson, J.L. & Loscalzo, J. *Harrison's Principles of Internal Medicine.* New York: McGraw-Hill.

Hall, J.E. *Guyton and Hall Textbook of Medical Physiology.* Philadelphia: WB Saunders.

Hardman, J., Limbard, L. & Gilman, A. *Goodman and Gilman's The Pharmacological Basis of Therapeutics.* New York: McGraw-Hill.

Illingworth, R.S. *The Development of the Infant and Young Child.* Edinburgh: Churchill Livingstone.

Jones, K.L. *Smith's Recognizable Patterns of Human Malformation.* Philadelphia: Elsevier Saunders.

Katzung, B. *Basic and Clinical Pharmacology.* New York: McGraw-Hill.

McIntosh, N., Helms, P., Smyth, R. & Logan, S. *Forfar & Arneil's Textbook of Pediatrics.* Edinburgh: Churchill Livingstone.

McMillan, J.A., Feigin, R.D., DeAngelis, C.D. & Jones, M.D. (eds). *Oski's Pediatrics: Principles and Practice.* Philadelphia: JB Lippincott.

Menkes, J.H. *Textbook of Child Neurology.* Philadelphia: Lea & Febiger.

Park, M.K. *Pediatric Cardiology for Practitioners.* Philadelphia: Mosby/Elsevier.

Rang, H., Dale, M. & Ritter, J. *Rang & Dale's Pharmacology.* Edinburgh: Churchill Livingstone.

Roberton, D.M. & South, M. (eds). *Practical Paediatrics.* Edinburgh: Churchill Livingstone.

Rudolph, C.D., Rudolph, A.M., Lister, G.E., First, L. & Gershon, A.A. *Rudolph's Pediatrics.* New York: McGraw-Hill.

Sondheimer, J.M., Levin, M.J., Deterding, R.R. & Hay, W.W. (eds). *Current Pediatric Diagnosis and Treatment.* New York: McGraw-Hill.

Stevenson, T., Wallace, H. & Thomson, A. *Clinical Paediatrics for Postgraduate Examinations.* Edinburgh: Churchill Livingstone.

Talley, N.J. & O'Connor, S. *Clinical Examination.* Sydney: Elsevier.

Taussig, L., Landau, L. & Le Soeuf, P. *Pediatric Respiratory Medicine.* St Louis: Mosby.

Thomson, A., Wallace, H. & Stevenson, T. *Short Cases for the MRCPCH.* Edinburgh: Churchill Livingstone.

Wilson, G.N. & Cooley, W.C. *Preventive Management of Children with Congenital Anomalies and Syndromes.* Cambridge: Cambridge University Press.

MEDICAL JOURNALS

Paediatric journals

Since candidates are expected to know of the advances in physiology, biochemistry and pharmacology applicable to paediatrics, studying the review articles, leading articles, annotations and editorial comments in appropriate medical journals is essential in the candidate's preparation for the Fellowship Examination. The following are recommended:

- *Archives of Disease in Childhood*
- *Journal of Paediatrics and Child Health*
- *Journal of Pediatrics*
- *Pediatrics*
- *The Pediatric Clinics of North America.*

Internal medicine journals

Internal medicine journals that are recommended are as follows:

- *Annals of Internal Medicine*
- *Australian and New Zealand Journal of Medicine*
- *Medicine International*
- *The American Journal of Medicine*
- *The British Medical Journal*
- *The Lancet*
- *The New England Journal of Medicine.*

Other paediatric journals

Other paediatric journals well worth looking at, especially in preparation for the clinical examination, are as follows:

- *Current Problems in Pediatrics*
- *Pediatric Annals*
- *Pediatrics in Review.*

Quick reference mnemonics

Chapter 5

Behavioural and developmental paediatrics

ANOREXIA NERVOSA

Indications for admission to hospital are as follows:
(Mnemonic **POLICE WT**, police weight)

Physiological instability; **P**ostural hypotension (drop in systolic pressure of over
20 mmHg, from lying to standing)/**P**urpuric rash
Obvious (over 5%) dehydration/**O**xygen saturation < 85% (exceedingly rare)
Loss of weight: 1. to the point of significant cardiovascular compromise, *or* 2. < 75%
expected body weight; *or* 3. rapid weight loss/**L**ow white cells (neutropenia)
Intractable vomiting
Cardiovascular compromise (hypotension [BP < 80/50], bradycardia [< 50 bpm],
postural tachycardia [> 20/min.], slow capillary return, cyanosed extremities)
Electrolyte abnormalities: hypokalaemia < 2.5 mmol/L, hyponatraemia <
130 mmol/L, hypophosphataemia < 0.5 mmol/L/**E**CG changes: prolonged QTc
interval > 450 msec (particularly with low potassium)

Worrying ideation (parasuicidal, depression, self-harming)/**W**eak muscles: squat
test—'Get down/squat on your haunches and stand up without using your
hands'—unable to get up without use of arms for leverage
Temperature low (hypothermia: < 35.5°C)

ADHD

**Conditions which increase the risk of sudden cardiac death and preclude prescription
of stimulants for ADHD are as follows:**
SCD has three main groups of causes: cardiomyopathies, primary electrical disease, and
congenital heart disease (especially cyanotic or repaired).
(Mnemonic **ABCD HELPs WPWMarfan**)

Arrhythmogenic right ventricular dysplasia
Brugada syndrome
Coronary artery anomalies
Dilated cardiomyopathy

Hypertrophic cardiomyopathy (HCM)
Ex-cardiac surgery (especially TGA, TOF, HLHS, AS, ASD, AV canal)
Long QT syndrome (LQTS)
Pulmonary hypertension/**P**rimary ventricular fibrillation or tachycardia

Wolff–**P**arkinson–**W**hite syndrome
Marfan's syndrome

ASD
DDx for ASD
(Mnemonic **TACT FREE MANNERS** [references lack of emotional reciprocity in ASD])

Tuberous sclerosis complex (TSC)
Angelman syndrome
CHARGE/**C**FC (cardiofaciocutaneous)/**C**ATCH-22 (22q11.2 deletion)/
   Channelopathies/**C**iliopathies (e.g. Joubert)/**C**ohen/**C**ornelia de lang/**C**ostello/
   Cowden/**C***NTNAP2* (at 7q35)
Trisomy 21/**T**imothy

Fragile X syndrome
Rett syndrome
Epilepsies: named: channelopathies, creatine deficiency, pyridoxine deficiency
Epilepsies: initialled: SYN1; SSADH (succinic semialdehyde dehydrogenase)
   deficiency; *CNTNAP2* (think: 'can't nap 2'; association of insomnia with autism);
   UBE*3A* duplication or triplication

Mitochondrial cytopathies/**M**etabolic disorders/**M**yotonic dystrophy
Autism spectrum disorders (OMIM) numbers: AUTS1, AUTS3–AUTS18; X-linked:
   AUTSX1–AUTSX6
NF1 (neurofibromatosis type 1)/**N**RXN1 (neurexin1) deletion
Noonan
Epilepsies: numbered: **1**q21.1 del, **7**q11.23 dup, **15**q11.1q13.3 del and dup,
   16p11.2 del, **17**q12 del, **18**q12.1, **22**q11.2 (CATCH-22)
Rubinstein–Taybi/**R**enpenning
SHANK3 mutations (Phelan-McDermid, 22q13.3 del)/**S**impson–Golabi–Behmel
   (both overgrowth syndromes)/**S**mith–Lemli–Opitz (SLOS)/**S**mith–Magenis
   (SMS)/**S**torage diseases (e.g. lysosomal storage diseases [LSDs])

ASD

Hypoactive brain regions in ASD
The brain regions known to be hypoactive in ASD in tasks where cognition and social
perception are used include the following.
(Mnemonic **FAST Pre-med**)

Fusiform gyrus
Amygdala
Superior temporal sulcus
Temporoparietal junction

Prefrontal cortex
medial aspect

Management of autism

Management can be divided into seven groups of headings.
(Mnemonic **SPECIAL**)

School-based special education (for children over 3 years)
Pharmacotherapeutic intervention
Education of, and support for, parents
Community supports
Intervention
Alternative treatments
Learning/**L**inks: useful websites

Differential diagnoses

(Mnemonic **PLACED**)

Pitt-Hopkins syndrome (PTHS): mutation in gene TCF4 on chromosome 18; developmental delay, intermittent hyperventilation and apnoea, but distinctive facial features including wide mouth)
Lennox-Gastaut syndrome (LGS)/**L**eucodystrophies
Autism spectrum disorder (ASD)/**A**ngelman (15q11-13 maternal deletion) syndrome/**A**taxias (spinocerebellar ataxia [multiple types], spastic ataxia)
Cerebral palsy (CP)
Encephalitis
Deletion (micro-deletion) syndromes, affecting chromosomes 12 to 22/**D**eafness/**D**isturbed vision

In children with suspected RTT, where there are no RTT-related pathogenic mutations of MECP2, FOXG1 or CDKL5, then investigations for the above differential diagnosis list may be performed if clinically appropriate, but if they are all unremarkable, then the diagnosis of RTT can still be made if the clinical criteria for RTT are fulfilled.

Extrapyramidal motor findings in RTT represent a **PROBLEM**

Proximal myoclonus
Rigidity
Oculogyric crises
Bruxism/**B**radykinesia
Lack of expression (hypomimia)
Excessive drooling
Muscle dystonia

RTT
Evolution of symptoms (stages)/current symptoms
(Mnemonic **DRUMBEATS**)

Delayed development (Stage I): milestones (e.g. age when first smiled, sat, spoke, crawled, stood, walked)

Regression of development (Stage II): loss of acquired skills (e.g. language, hand use), loss of interest in toys, loss of social interaction

Unapparent slow deterioration (Stage III): return of any abilities

Motor deterioration (late) (Stage IV): loss of ambulation, use of wheelchair, requirements for interventions (e.g. gastrostomy)

Breathing irregularities (almost always awake; rarely asleep; nocturnal central apnoea (rare): CPAP, BiPAP)/**B**ruxism/**B**lue hands and feet

Eye contact (decrease during regressive stage)/**E**ye pointing, or 'Rett's gaze' (developing during Stage III)/**E**pilepsy/**E**xpression (facial) and interpretation of others' expressions

Autism spectrum disorder—like symptomatology/**A**taxia/**A**praxia/**A**pnoeic episodes

Tone abnormalities: hypotonic (early), spasticity, rigidity (later)

Spinal deformities: **S**coliosis (double curve or single C curve), kyphosis/**S**tereotypies (mainly midline, hand stereotypies) including clapping, clasping behind back, grasping, held at sides, releasing, tapping, touching, washing, wringing/**S**leep phenomena (including screaming, laughing, occasionally central apnoea)

RTT
Rett syndrome features
(Mnemonic **RETTS MECP2 BASED**)

Regression: fine motor (loss purposeful hand movement); cognition; communication/**R**ecovery (partial) post-regression, then slow worsening

Epilepsy: in 90%; many seizure types, except absence; infantile spasms (severe) in separate cause from MECP2 gene: CDKL5 gene mutation

To and fro rocking and retropulsion/**T**witching/**T**rembling/**T**urning head

Twisting hands plus squeezing, wringing, clapping/**T**one: rigidity

Speech lost/**S**lowing (early) head growth/**S**tagnation of development/**S**low deterioration after partial recovery phase/**S**tereotypic movements (licking, grabbing)/**S**creaming/**S**tages; four described

Methyl-CpG binding protein 2 encoded by MECP2, on Xq28; mutations in 95–97% RTT/**M**alnutrition; nutrition supplements with gastrostomy/**M**yoclonic jerks

Eating: impaired (problems: chewing; swallowing; choking; regurgitation)

Cardiac: increased QTc, **C**oding regions MECP2 gene: 3; multiple mutations (e.g. truncations/missense proteins)/**C**-shaped scoliosis worsen rapidly

Parameters (growth): decreased head, then weight, then height percentiles/**P**ubertal changes in height and weight diminished/**P**erforation of stomach or bowel (from aerophagia, especially with fundoplication)

(over) 250 known MECP mutations can cause RTT

Bradykinesia/Breathing disorder: *awake*: hyperventilation; hypoventilation; apnoea/Broad-based gait/Bruxism/Bone density decreased/Back: scoliosis +/– kyphosis

Autonomic dysfunction (peripheral vasomotor anomalies; cold feet)/Aspiration/ Absence-like stopping (non-epileptic): staring, breath-holding, pupil dilation/ Apraxic/Ataxic gait/Absent walking (later)/Aberrant response to pain (delayed and diminished)/Aerophagia (swallowing air)

Sporadic mutations cause RTT/Sympathetic tone increased/Sleep architecture abnormal (waking disruptive, crying, laughing, screaming; shortened duration night)/ Scoliosis

Expression (facial) diminished (masking of facial expression = hypomimia)/ Extrapyramidal motor dysfunction: hands, gait/Eyes: oculogyric crises

Drooling/Dystonic and Dyskinetic tongue movements/Dysfunctional oropharynx/Dysmotile upper GIT/Dystonia/Deceleration of head growth +/–, weight +/– and height/Double-curved scoliosis thoracic + lumbar common

ADHD

Differential diagnosis of ADHD
(Mnemonic ACCURATE DIAGNOSIS HIGHLY DESIRABLE)

Autism spectrum disorder (ASD)/Anorexia nervosa (AN, overactive to lose weight)
Cerebral palsy (CP)/Cerebrovascular accident (CVA)/Cerebral tumour (frontal lobe)
Conduct disorder/Congenital heart disease (22q11, cyanotic, TAPVD, HLHS)
Urea cycle disorders
Reaction to social set-up (new partner/blended family)/Reactive attachment disorder
Acquired brain injury (ABI, especially frontal lobe damage, e.g. post-MVA), Abuse/ Attachment/Adjustment/Anxiety disorders/A duplicate of a hyperactive dad
Teratogens in utero (cocaine, heroin, methadone)/Tourette syndrome/Twins ('hype' each other when *together*)/Tuberous sclerosis complex (TSC)
Expressive language disorder/Encephalitis/meninitis sequelae

Deafness/Drugs (illicit)/Disrupted family (divorce)/Disruptive mood dysregulation
Intellectual impairment/Impaired: vision, hearing, speech, language, reading
Alcohol: fetal alcohol spectrum disorder (FASD)/Alcoholic parents
Global developmental delay (later termed intellectual impairment; various causes)
Neurocutaneous syndromes (e.g. NF1)/NICU graduate (ex-premmie, < 1500 g)
Obstructive sleep apnoea (OSA)/Oppositional defiant disorder (ODD)
Small for gestational age (SGA)/Smoking in pregnancy/Schizophrenia
Iron deficiency/Inborn errors of metabolism (e.g. phenylketonuria, PKU)
Syndromes: fragile X, Down, Williams, XXY, XYY, Sturge-Weber (SWS), Sotos

Hydrocephalus/Head injury/Haemorrhage (IVH/ICH in ex-premmie)
Intrauterine disorders: infections (TORCH)/teratogens (cocaine, heroin)
Graves' hyperthyroidism/Government benefits: faking ADHD to obtain (parent instructs child to trash paediatrician's office to prove he needs stimulants)
Hypothyroidism ('dreamy' inattention)/Hypoxic insult (drowning, strangulation)
Lead intoxication/Leukaemia survivor (cerebral irradiation)
Young/inexperienced parents (unrealistic beliefs; e.g. 12 month old referred!)

Depression/Drug acquisition (faking ADHD to get dexamphetamine, to make 'ice')
Epilepsy: childhood absence epilepsy (CAE, 'petit mal') or 'temporal lobe absences'
Sickness in family member (reaction to)/Substance use disorder/Stereotypies
Iatrogenic (phenobarbitone/beta-2-sympathomimetics/antihistamines/thyroxine)
Reaction to trauma (posttraumatic stress disorder)/Reaction to food/food additives
Attention seeking/Acting out/Absent dad: 'Acute Dad Deficiency'
Bright but bored (i.e. gifted and curious)/Bipolar disorder
Learning disorder (specific, SLD)/Language disorders/Lack of stable family
Environmental stressors at school or home (doing poorly in class; chaotic house)

AUTISM
Differential diagnosis of autism
(Mnemonic DIFFERENT CHILD)

Deafness (hearing loss alone, or combined with visual impairment [can cause poor
  eye contact, stereotypic head nodding, hand/finger flapping])/Disordered mood
  (bipolar or unipolar mood disorders)/Down syndrome
Intellectual impairment (any cause)
Fragile X syndrome
Fetal (intrauterine) TORCH infections/Fetal alcohol syndrome (FAS)
Expressive language disorder
Rett syndrome (females almost exclusively)
Elective mutism
Neurodegenerative conditions/Neurocutaneous conditions (other than tuberous
  sclerosis, which has the strongest association, ASD also has been associated with
  neurofibromatosis type 1 [NF1] and hypomelanosis of Ito)/Neglect (or abuse)
Tuberous sclerosis complex (TSC)

Cerebral palsy/Cerebral tumour/Childhood schizophrenia/Chromosomal syndromes
  (Smith-Lemli-Opitz, Smith–Magenis, Cohen, Joubert, Timothy, 15q and 16p
  duplication)
Hyperactivity with attention deficit disorder/'Happy puppet' (Angelman) syndrome
Inborn errors of metabolism (presenting with encephalopathy) (PKU)
Landau–Kleffner syndrome (acquired epileptic aphasia)/Lead intoxication
Disintegrative disorder

RTT
Alliterative mnemonic for important aspects of RTT examination: the Gs
Growth, Gait, Gaze, Gasping (irregular breathing patterns), Grasping (hand stereotypies),
Grinding (teeth), Gelastic episodes (laughter, unprovoked)
Introduction: Growth, Gait, Gaze, Gasping, Grasping, Grinding, Gelastic
Quality of movement and posture: Gait
Growth parameters, nutritional assessment, Tanner staging: Growth
Dysmorphology examination (head and neck): Grinding
Vision: Gaze and hearing
Speech: Gelastic
Cardiorespiratory system: Gasping, Gelastic
Full neurological examination: Gait, Gaze, Grasping
Developmental assessment: Gait, Gaze, Grasping

Chapter 6

Cardiology
CYANOTIC CONGENITAL HEART DISEASES
(Mnemonic 6 **T**s, 1 **P** and 1 **H**)

TGA: Listen: loud S2, no murmur. *CXR: egg on string*. ECG: may be normal

ToF: RV heave; *murmurs: RVOT, collaterals*. *CXR: boot*. ECG varies: T +ve V1, RVH

Tricuspid atresia: single S2, VSD murmur. *CXR: pulmonary oligaemia*. *ECG: LAD*

Tricuspid ectopia (Ebstein): TI murmur. *CXR: cardiomegaly*. *ECG: P waves > QRS*

Truncus: *truncal valve regurgitant murmur*. *CXR: pulmonary plethora*. ECG: LVH, RVH

TAPVD: loud S1, split S2, flow murmurs (RVOT, tricuspid). *CXR: snowman*; ECG: RAD

PA: (a) **PA-VSD**, continuous murmurs: CXR, ECG like ToF; variants + *PDA*, + *MAPCAs*. (vii) (b) **PA-IVS**, murmurs: PDA, TI. CXR: big RA, pulmonary oligaemia ECG: peaked P

HLHS: loud single S2. CXR: cardiomegaly, pulmonary plethora. ECG: RAD, RVH

MARFAN SYNDROME

Cardiology: features of Marfan syndrome
Clinical diagnosis of Marfan syndrome is based on major and minor criteria; there are four findings with major significance.
(Mnemonic the 17 **D**s)

Dilatation or **d**issection of *aorta* at level of sinuses of Valsalva

Displacement of *lens* (ectopia lentis); directed upward; cataract formation

Dural ectasia (lumbosacral)

Dolichostenomelia: disproportionately long extremities; decreased upper to lower segment ratio (US:LS < 0.85 for older children/adults) or arm span to height ratio > 1.05; other diagnostic skeletal features include the following:

Deformation of spine (scoliosis > 20°, or spondylolisthesis)

Deformation of sternum (pectus: excavatum or carinatum, requiring surgery)

Deep acetabulum with accelerated erosion (protrusio acetabulum)

Decreased elbow extension (< 170°) (in contradistinction to hypermobility of other joints)

Digit-related eponymous signs: 1. the thumb (Steinberg) sign, this being an extension of the whole distal phalanx of the thumb beyond the ulnar border of the hand when apposed across the palm (Fig. 6.31); and 2. the wrist (Walker–Murdoch) sign, this being overlapping of the distal phalanx of the thumb with the distal phalanx of the little finger when encircling the opposite wrist (Fig. 6.32)

Downward (medial) rotation of medial malleolus causing pes planus; four of these skeletal features are considered one major criterion

Distinctive facial features (**d**olichocephaly, **d**own-slanting palpebral fissures, **d**eeply set eyes [enophthalmos], **d**ecreased malar prominence [malar hypoplasia], **d**iminished jaw [retrognathia])

FEATURES OF MARFAN SYNDROME

The acronym **MARFANS** also can be used as an (alternative) aide-mémoire.

Mitral prolapse ± **M**itral regurgitation

Ascending aorta dilatation (involving sinuses of Valsalva)/dissection/**A**rched palate (high arched, with tooth crowding)/**A**cetabuli (protrusio acetabuli)

Regurgitation of aorta/mitral valve/**R**etinal detachment/**R**educed US:LS ratio

Fibrillin defective/**F**acial gestalt (dolichocephaly, down-slanting palpebral fissures, deeply set eyes [enophthalmos], decreased malar prominence [malar hypoplasia], diminished jaw [retrognathia])/**F**lat cheek bones/**F**lat cornea/**F**lexible joints (joint hypermobility)

Apical blebs (on CXR)/**A**ir leaks (spontaneous pneumothorax)/**A**rachnodactyly

Near-sightedness (myopia)/**N**eurological involvement related to dural ectasia; stretching of dural sac in the lumbosacral region/**N**erve entrapment: CSF leak from dural sac (causing postural hypotension and headache)

Scoliosis/**S**ternal deformation/**S**keletal dolichostenomelia/**S**acral dural ectasia

FEATURES OF NOONAN SYNDROME (NS)

The acronym **NOONANS** can be used as an aide-mémoire of the various features.

Neurodevelopmental problems: 25% learning disability, 10-15% special education, <30% mild intellectual impairment, 72% articulation problems, nonverbal abilities better than verbal, specific learning problems/**N**euromuscular: hypotonia (floppy strong); joint hyperextensibility/**N**eurosurgical: Arnold–Chiari type I

Obstructive heart lesions: RVOT (pulmonary valve); left-ventricular outflow tract (LVOT) (HCM)/**O**ther: ASD, VSD, ToF, coarctation of aorta, branch pulmonary artery stenosis

Ocular anomalies in up to 95%: strabismus, refractive errors, amblyopia, nystagmus; hypertelorism, epicanthic folds, droopy eyelids, vivid blue or blue–green irises

Neoplasia risk: juvenile myelomonocytic leukaemia (JMML); myeloproliferative disorders; Noonan-like/multiple giant-cell lesion syndrome (granulomas and joint and bone anomalies); hepatosplenomegaly (related to subclinical myelodysplasia)

Abnormal coagulation (33% have one or more defects)/**A**bnormal lymphatics: lymphoedema (hands/feet/scrotum/vulva), lymphangiectasia (lung, gut or testis)

Neck webbing, with low-set posteriorly rotated ears/**N**ipples widely set/**N**ephrological anomalies: duplex collecting systems, renal hypoplasia

Sternal deformity (superior carinatum, inferior excavatum)/**S**hort stature (GH responsive)/**S**econdary sexual characteristics: delayed puberty, cryptorchidism in males/**S**kin: pigmented naevi (25%), café-au-lait patches (10%), lentigines (3%)

COSTELLO SYNDOME: A RASOPATHY

(Mnemonic **COSTELlo**)

Cardiac (PS, HCM)

Ocular (epicanthic folds, hypertelorism)

Short stature

Tumours (papillomata, neuroblastoma, rhabdomyosarcoma)

Educational difficulties

Limb involvement (splayed fingers, ulnar deviation) (**lo**)

CARDIAC FINDINGS IN 22Q11.2 DELETION SYNDROME

Neural crest-associated conotruncal defects

This includes the following syndromes: DiGeorge (DGS), Velocardiofacial (VCFS), Shprintzen, Conotruncal Anomaly Face (CTAF), Caylor Cardiofacial, Autosomal dominant Opitz G/BBB). The 22q11.2-deletion-associated cardiac defects include 3 **TAP**s.

Truncus arteriosus, **T**etralogy of Fallot and **T**ricuspid atresia with d-malposition of the aorta (3 **T**s)

Aortic arch interruption, **A**trial septal defect and **A**berrant right subclavian artery (3 **A**s)

Pulmonary atresia and ventricular septal defect, **P**ulmonary valve absence and **P**atent ductus arteriosus (3 **P**s)

FEATURES OF 22Q11.2 DELETION SYNDROME

This includes the following syndromes: DiGeorge (DGS), Velocardiofacial (VCFS), Shprintzen, Conotruncal Anomaly Face (CTAF), Caylor Cardiofacial, Autosomal dominant Opitz G/BBB).

The acronym **CATCH-22** can expand to **CATCHING-22** to include more features.

Cardiac (3 TAPs; see above)/**C**orneal

Abnormal face/**A**utoimmune diseases

Thymic hypoplasia, T-cell deficiency

Cleft palate and palatal anomalies/**C**raniosynostosis and other skeletal anomalies/ **C**roup-like: laryngotrachealoesophageal anomalies

Hypoparathyroidism/**H**ypocalcaemia/**H**earing loss

Intellectual issues/**I**mpaired swallowing/feeding

Neurologic/**N**ephrologic/**N**eoplastic: '*blastomas*'

Growth hormone deficiency/**G**enitals/**G**astrointestinal/**G***P1BB* mutation can cause coexistent Bernard–Soulier syndrome (BSS)

WILLIAMS SYNDROME

(Mnemonic **WILLIAMS HYPERCALCAEMIA**)

Williams–Beuren Syndrome Critical Region (WBSCR); chromosome locus 7q11.2

Intelligence quotient (IQ) average 50–60/**I**mpaired vision: reduced stereopsis

Low tone (hypotonia)/**L**ow pitched or hoarse voice, vocal cord paralysis

Lax joints (joint hypermobility)/**L**oquacious, over-friendly, excessively empathic

Impaired feeding; tactile sensory defensiveness (difficulty with food textures); vomiting

ADHD symptomatology/**A**nxiety (somatisation can lead to abdominal pain)

Mitral valve prolapse (MVP)

Supravalvular aortic stenosis (SVAS)/**S**coliosis, kyphosis/**S**ternum: excavatum

HYpercalcaemia, **HY**percalciuria, **HY**pertension
Peripheral pulmonary arterial stenosis (PPW)/**P**uberty early (but not precocious)
Elastin arteriopathy (SVAS, PPS, aortic insufficiency, stenosis of mesenteric arteries)/**E**ndocrine: hypothyroidism; IDDM in adults/**E**lfin face (see below under A)
Renal anomalies (nephrocalcinosis, pelvic kidney)
Chronic otitis media (50%)/**C**haracteristic personality: over-friendly, people-orientated, empathic
Audiological: high-frequency sensorineural hearing loss, hyperacusis (in 90%)
Linear growth failure; postnatal growth rate 75% of normal/**L**oquacious personality
Cognitive: good verbal short-term memory, language; poor visuospatial construction
Appearance: broad brow, bitemporal narrowness, medial eyebrow flare, short palpebral fissures, epicanthic folds, blue stellate iris, short nose, full nasal tip, full cheeks, malar hypoplasia, long philtrum, full lips, wide mouth, small jaw, prominent earlobes
Eyes: hypotelorism, strabismus (50%), amblyopia, refractive errors (hyperopia in 50%)
Malocclusion, microdontia, enamel hypoplasia, widely spaced teeth, missing teeth
Intestinal problems: constipation, diverticulosis, coeliac disease
Abdominal pain: reflux oesophagitis; cholelithiasis; diverticulitis; ischaemic bowel

PRINCIPLES/ASPECTS OF MANAGING CONGESTIVE CARDIAC FAILURE (CCF)
(Mnemonic **ASPECTS**)

Afterload reduction: ACEIs, ARBs, brain natriuretic peptide (BNP), milrinone, nitrates
Sympathetic inhibition: beta blockers, BNP, digoxin
Preload reduction: BNP, diuretics
Enhanced contractility (inotropy): digoxin
Cardiac remodelling prevention: mineralocorticoid inhibitors (spironolactone)
Timely surgical repair of structural congenital heart disease
Systemic disease recognition and treatment (of pathology underlying CCF)

INDICATIONS FOR HEART TRANSPLANTATION
Heart transplant: life-saving: **CC**, **UU**, **RR**
CCF with symptomatic ventricular dysfunction secondary to myocardial disease or palliated CHD
Complex CHD with failed surgical correction
Unresectable tumours
Unresectable ventricular diverticula
Rhythm disturbances: life-threatening (arrhythmias), resistant to therapy
Retransplantation (graft vasculopathy, ventricular dysfunction)

Heart transplant: life-enhancing: **CC**, **FF**, **II**
CCF associated with pulmonary hypertension
Cardiomyopathy—restrictive, with poor survival overall
Fontan circulation with protein-losing enteropathy resistant to medical therapy
Fontan failing with decreased exercise tolerance, and declining quality of life
Inoperable AV valve or aortic regurgitation
Inoperable CHD with severe oxygen desaturation

Chapter 7

Endocrinology

CEREBRAL OEDEMA (CO) IN T1DM

There are three groups of criteria, described by Muir et al. (2004) to delineate CO:
Diagnostic criteria are **four** 2 **P**s and 2 **C**s.

Pain response abnormal: verbal or motor
Posture decorticate or decerebrate
Cranial nerve palsy (especially III, IV, VI)
Cheyne Stokes or other abnormal respiratory pattern

Major criteria are **three**
(Mnemonic 3 **C**s)

Consciousness level altered
Cardiac deceleration (drop by > 20 beats per minute)
Continence lost (age-inappropriate incontinence)

Minor criteria are **five**
(Mnemonic **HALVED**)

Headache
Age young (< 5)
Lethargy
Vomiting/**E**mesis
Diastolic pressure high (> 90 mmHg)

If a child has 1 diagnostic criterion, 2 major criteria, or 1 major and 2 minor criteria, then this gives 92% sensitivity, and 96% specificity for identifying CO soon enough to intervene.

Risk factors for CO are 10
(Mnemonic 10 **F**s)

Five years or under (especially under 2 years)
Fast insulin (insulin given as bolus)
Fast fluids/**F**looding with fluids (giving IV fluids [especially dangerous if hypotonic] too rapidly)
Failure to correct serum sodium (hyponatraemia developing with treatment, or failing to rise)
First serum sodium high (especially > 160 mmol/L)
First presentation of T1DM with DKA
First hour insulin (insulin given within first hour of treatment)
First arterial PCO_2: low
First serum urea: high
Flooding with bicarbonate (excessive administration)

HYPOPITUITARISM: PRESENTING BEYOND NEONATAL PERIOD
(Mnemonic **CRASH**)

Craniopharyngioma (and other intracranial tumours in hypothalamic/pituitary region)/**C**HARGE syndrome/**C**ombined pituitary hormone deficiency (CPHD)
Radiotherapy (cranial irradiation for CNS or non-CNS tumours, late effects of oncology treatment)
Acquired brain injury, including neonatal encephalopathy (can term **A**sphyxia purely for recall)
Septo-optic dysplasia (most common CNS structural cause)
Holoprosencephaly (failure of prosencephalon to divide adequately into two hemispheres)/**H**istiocytosis (Langerhans cell histiocytosis [LCH])

HOLOPROSENCEPHALY: FEATURES
(Mnemonic **HPE FUSED**)

Hypotonia/**H**ypothalamic dysfunction/**H**ead size: microcephaly common, macrocephaly uncommon (**H**ydrocephalus)
Pituitary deficiency: posterior or anterior pituitary hormones; central DI/**P**neumonia (aspiration)
Epilepsy (often hard to control)

Feeding difficulties (multiple causes, including poor tone, poor suck)
Uncoordinated oral-sensory function
Spina bifida can accompany/**S**leep disturbances
Eating slow/**E**sophageal reflux
Developmental delay

EXAMINATION FOR HYPOPITUITARISM
(Mnemonic **GREEN**)

GRowth (parameters, measurements)
Eye (acuity, fields)
Endocrine (Tanner stage, BP, pulse)
Neurological (gait, reflexes, disease-specific signs for underlying aetiology signs [e.g. SOD association, signs of raised ICP])

ENDOCRINOLOGY
The mnemonic **IS NICE** lists various headings/causes for aetiologies of short stature.

Idiopathic (constitutional delay in growth and puberty [maturational delay]; familial short stature)/**I**ntrauterine (SGA, TORCH, fetal alcohol syndrome [FAS])
Skeletal causes (dysplasias, OI)/**S**pinal defects (scoliosis, kyphosis)/**S**yndromes (Russell–Silver, Kallmann)/**S**epto-optic dysplasia (SOD)

Nutritional (e.g. malabsorption)/**N**urturing (4deprivation)
Iatrogenic (steroids, radiation)
Chronic diseases (CKD, congenital heart disease, CF, IBD)/**C**hromosomal (Turner, Down)/**C**raniopharyngioma (or other central tumour)
Endocrine (e.g. GH deficiency, GH insensitivity, hypopituitarism, hypothyroidism, Cushing's syndrome, T1DM, pseudohypoparathyroidism)

A mnemonic for PCOS, which includes most of the features of virilisation per se (plus common features of PCOS asterisked), is **HYPERANDROGENISM**.

Hirsutism (excessive growth in androgen-dependent sites; differentiate from hypertrichosis, which is excessive vellus or non-androgen responsive hair)
Y (chromosome, i.e. male) body habitus; remodelling of limb–shoulder girdle
Pubic hair towards umbilicus (male escutcheon)
Enlarged larynx (and elevated lipids: dyslipidaemia)
Reduced ovulation
Acanthosis (velvety hyperpigmentation: neck, axilla, under breasts, genitals)
Nigricans (*)
Deepening of the voice (vocal cord coarsening)
Reduced breast size
Obesity (*) in around 55% of patients with PCOS (and OSA increased [*])
Genital enlargement (clitoromegaly) (in sexually mature females, > 35 mm^2)
Enlarged striated muscle mass (masculine musculature)
Non-insulin-dependent diabetes mellitus (type 2 diabetes mellitus) (*)
Insulin level elevated; insulin resistance (*)
Skin; seborrhea, acne
Menstrual disturbance (oligo- or amenorrhoea)/**M**etabolic syndrome (*)

A differential diagnosis of the causes of premature and/or excessive development of pubic hair in girls (not just virilising conditions) follows.
(Mnemonic **PREMATOUR**)

Pituitary causes: true precocious puberty (see the short case on precocious puberty); gonadotrope neoplasia or hyperplasia/**P**olycystic ovary syndrome (PCOS)
Remote (ectopic) causes: chorionic-gonadotropin secreting tumours: hepatoblastoma; pineal dysgerminoma; retroperitoneal tumours
Exogenous: anabolic steroids; corticosteroids (Cushing's syndrome)
Metabolic: congenital adrenal hyperplasia: three forms: 21-OHD, 11-OHD, HSD3B
Adrenal causes: premature adrenarche, CAH (above), tumour (below), Cushing's syndrome
Tumour, virilising: adrenal—adrenocortical carcinoma, adenoma; ovary— arrhenoblastoma (usually benign); pineal—dysgerminoma; pituitary— gonadotrophin-releasing tumours
Ovarian causes: virilising tumour (arrhenoblastoma); PCOS
Unexplained (and unimportant pathology-wise): premature pubarche
Reductase (5-alpha-reductase) deficiency in an undervirilised XY child (can suddenly virilise at puberty, from previously phenotypically normal female)

Chapter 8
Gastroenterology
IBD

Medications used to *induce* remission
Induction of remission in CD **BEEN SAS**
Biologics, **EEN**, **S**teroids, **A**ntibiotics, **S**urgery
Induction of remission in UC **BASS**
Biologics, **A**minosalicylates, **S**teroids, **S**urgery

IBD

Medications used to *maintain* remission BIAS in CD and UC
Biologics, **I**mmunomodulators, **A**minosalicylates, **S**upplementary enteral nutrition in CD, **S**urgery in UC

TNF-α ANTIBODY INHIBITORS (TNFIs)
Side effects in *adults*
(Mnemonic **AMPLE HINTS**)

Autoimmune-like syndromes
Malignancy, especially lymphoma
Pancytopaenia/neutropenia (pregnancy should be avoided)
Liver transaminase elevation
Eczema and psoriasis

Heart failure: can be worsened by IFX
Infections: if serious bacterial infection occurs, stop, or do not start TNFIs/**I**njection site/**I**nfusion reaction: common; treat with antihistamine, steroids, slowed rate/**I**mmunisation: immunise before treatment; no live attenuated vaccine during treatment
Neurological syndromes: Guillain-Barré, optic neuritis; may be same frequency as normal population; if these occur, stop or do not start, TNFIs
Tuberculosis: increased susceptibility to TB or reactivation of TB
Surgical procedures: due to effects on wound healing, withhold drugs for 8 weeks prior)

CHRONIC LIVER DISEASE: METABOLIC CAUSES
(Mnemonic **WATCH**)

Wilson disease (WD)
Alpha-1-antitrypsin (AAT) deficiency
Tyrosinaemia type 1
Cystic fibrosis (CF)
Hereditary fructose intolerance (HFI)

COMPLICATIONS OF CIRRHOSIS
(Mnemonic **HEPATIC**)

Hypersplenism
Encephalopathy/**E**sophageal varices
Portal hypertension/**P**rotein calorie malnutrition
Ascites
Thrombosis of portal vein
Infection (spontaneous bacterial peritonitis)
Coagulopathy/**C**arcinoma (hepatocellular, many years later)

CAUSES OF HEPATOMEGALY
(Mnemonic for causes of hepatomegaly is **SHIRT**)

Structural
Extrahepatic biliary atresia (EHBA), choledochal cyst, paucity of bile interlobular ducts (PBID; Alagille syndrome) polycystic disease, congenital hepatic fibrosis

Storage/metabolic
Gaucher disease, Niemann–Pick syndrome, carnitine deficiency, MLs, T1DM, GSDs (1, 3, 4, 6), HFI, galactosaemia, Cushing's syndrome, MPSs, tyrosinaemia 1, UCDs, Wilson disease, CF, PCM, TPN, AAT deficiency

Haematological
Thalassaemia, sickle cell disease (chronic haemolysis and transfusion haemosiderosis), acute leukaemia, chronic myeloid leukaemia

Heart (congestive cardiac failure (CCF), constrictive pericarditis, obstructed IVC)

Infection
Viral (rubella, CMV, enteroviruses, Hepatitis A, B, C, D, E, EBV), bacterial (neonatal septicaemia, *E. coli* UTI, TB, syphilis), parasitic (hydatid, malaria, schistosomiasis, toxoplasmosis, visceral larva migrans)

Inflammatory (CAH, chronic persistent hepatitis, IBD associated liver disease)

Infiltrative (histiocytosis X, sarcoidosis)

Reticuloendothelial (non-Hodgkin lymphoma, Hodgkin disease)

Rheumatological (systemic-onset juvenile idiopathic arthritis (sJIA), SLE)

Tumour/hamartoma
Primary (hepatoblastoma, hepatocellular carcinoma), secondary (neuroblastoma, Wilms, gonadal tumours), vascular malformations/benign neoplasm (infantile haemangioendothelioma, cavernous haemangioma)

Trauma (hepatic haematoma)

CAUSES OF SPLENOMEGALY
(Mnemonic **CHIMPS**)

Cardiac
Subacute bacterial endocarditis (SBE)

Connective tissue disease
sJIA, SLE

Haematological
Chronic haemolytic anaemias: hereditary spherocytosis (HS), glucose-6-phosphate dehydrogenase (G6PD) deficiency, beta thalassaemia major

Infection
Viral: EBV, CMV; bacterial: SBE, typhoid; protozoal (malaria, toxoplasma)

Injury
Haematoma

Malignancy
Leukaemia, lymphoma

Portal hypertension
1. Extrahepatic: post-neonatal umbilical vessel catheterisation or sepsis
2. Hepatic: the various causes of cirrhosis, congenital hepatic fibrosis
3. Suprahepatic: Budd–Chiari syndrome

Storage diseases
Gaucher, Niemann–Pick

Splenic cyst or hamartoma

Chapter 9

Genetics and dysmorphology

TURNER SYNDROME COMPLICATIONS

(Mnemonic **TURNER ULLRICH'S**)

Thyroiditis and other autoimmune disease (juvenile idiopathic arthritis [JIA], coeliac disease)
Undermineralised bone
Root of aorta dilatation risks (BAV, aortic stenosis, aortic coarctation, hypertension)
Neck short, webbed/**N**ails hyperconvex/**N**ormal intelligence (but impairments in memory, maths, spatial perception, goal-setting, goal-attainment, attention span)
Endocrine deficiency (pubertal failure, short stature)/**E**ye findings (epicanthic folds, strabismus, ptosis, congenital glaucoma)/**E**ars (unusual shape, rotation)
Reproductive technology assistance (egg donor programs)

Ulcerative colitis/Crohn's disease
Left-sided heart problems/**L**inear growth deficiency
Lymphoedema/**L**ymphatic malformations (e.g. cystic hygroma)
Renal anomalies (hydronephrosis)
Infertility
Cancer risks (gonadoblastoma, neuroblastoma, colonic carcinoma)
Hearing loss/**H**ypertension/**H**epatic cirrhosis
Skeletal (DDH, Madelung)/**S**pine (scoliosis, kyphosis, lordosis)

ISOLATED HEMIHYPERPLASIA

(Mnemonic **HEMIS**)

Hemihyperplasia of spine, limbs, hands, feet
Embryonal tumours
Muscle hypertrophy in affected areas, **M**yelomeningocele
Intellectual impairment: seen in 20%
Spine involvement: **S**coliosis, myelomeningocele

BECKWITH-WIEDEMANN SYNDROME (BWS)

(Mnemonic **BECKWITH EMG**)
(Exomphalos-Macroglossia-Gigantism syndrome)

Blastomas (gonado-, hepato- and nephro-blastoma) (Wilms)/**B**lood count high in neonates (polycythaemia)/**B**one age advanced first 4 years
Eyes: prominent/**E**ar lobe: linear fissures, creases
Craniofacial anomalies/**C**apillary vascular malformation central forehead/**C**ardiac disorders: **C**ardiomegaly (isolated), **C**ardiomyopathy (focal), **C**ardiac hamartoma
Kidneys enlarged
Wilms tumour
Indentation posterior rim helix/**I**slet cells excess, **I**nsulin high (pancreatic hyperplasia)
Tumours: adrenal carcinoma, embryonal cancers, gonadoblastoma, hepatoblastoma,
Hepatomegaly/**H**ypoglycaemia (early infancy)

Exomphalos (also called omphalocele)
Macroglossia/**M**acrosomia/**M**uscle mass increased/**M**etaphyseal flaring/**M**alocclusion (**M**andibular: **M**axilla relative position: prognathism due to mandibular overgrowth, maxilla less prominent)/**M**etopic ridge/**M**icrocephaly (mild)
Gigantism/**G**enito-urinary: large ovaries, hyperplastic uterus, bicornate uterus, clitoromegaly, hypospadias, undescended testes

RUSSELL–SILVER SYNDROME
(Mnemonic **RUSSELL**)

Retrognathia/micrognathia/**R**enal: Wilms tumour, renal anomalies/**R**efractive errors
Uniparental (maternal) disomy of chromosome 7 in 10%/**U**rethral valves (posterior)
Small stature (prenatal onset)/**S**mall face/**S**mall fifth finger with clinodactyly
Skin: cafe au lait/**S**clera blue/**S**houlders: **S**prengel's deformity/**S**eminoma/**S**yndactyly
  second and third toes/**S**low development (delay)/**S**weating: excessive
Eleven, chromosome number (11p15.5)/**E**pigenetic alterations: DNA
  hypomethylation at H19/IGF2-imprinting control region/**E**sophageal reflux,
  Esophagitis/**E**ndocrine: fasting hypoglycaemia aged 10 months to 3 years
Linear growth decreased, growth hormone deficiency/**L**imb asymmetry
Large fontanelle/**L**iver: hepatocellular carcinoma

PROTEUS SYNDROME
(Mnemonic **PROTEUS HEAD VARIABLE**)

Ptosis, **P**alpebral fissure downslant, **P**ectus excavatum, **P**alate (cleft, submucous)
Renal: enlargement, hydronephrosis, cysts, haemangiomata
Ophthalmological: macrophthalmia; microphthalmia; nystagmus; strabismus;
  cataract/**O**pen mouth
Tumours: ovarian adenoma, parotid adenoma, yolk sac tumour of testis/**T**hyroid
  enlargement/**T**hymus enlargement
Elongation head and trunk
Uneven growth pattern: normal at birth, features appear over first year; progress
  throughout childhood; hamartomata growth completed by puberty; normal
  adolescent somatic growth, final height normal
Skin: thickened; café-au-lait macules/**S**ubcutaneous tumours (epidermal naevi,
  lipomas)

Hyperpigmentation (skin)/**H**eart: Hypertrophic cardiomyopathy (HOCM);
  conduction defects/**H**ead: enlarged; craniosynostosis/**H**yperostoses: skull, facial
  bones, jaw, external auditory canal, nasal bridge, alveolar ridges
Enlarged genitals (testes and penis)
Absent fat (regional)
Dolichocephaly/**D**epigmentation of skin/**D**ermoids (epibulbar)/**D**eep venous
  thrombosis (DVT)/**D**islocated hips/**D**igits: enlarged, clinodactyly

Vascular malformations: capillary, lymphatic, venous (esp. thorax, upper
  abdomen)/**V**ertebral dysplasia and enlargement (mega-spondylo-dysplasia)/**V**algus
  deformities of feet
Atrophy: muscles
Renal enlargement
Intellectual impairment in 20%
Angulation defects: knees
Back: scoliosis, kyphosis, spinal stenosis
Lipoma/**L**ipomatosis (abdominal and pelvic)/**L**ong face/**L**ung cysts
Epidermal naevi

Chapter 10

Haematology

MUSCULOSKELETAL TREATMENTS

Musculoskeletal bleeds benefit from:
(Mnemonic **RICES**)

Rest/immobilisation
Ice
Compression of the affected part
Elevation of the affected part
Splinting

SICKLE CELL ANAEMIA (SCA) CRISIS PRECIPITATORS

(Mnemonic **ACIDOSES**)

Acidosis
Cold
Infection
Dehydration
Oxygen lack
Stress
Elevated temperature
Sport (exercise)

VASO-OCCLUSIVE COMPLICATIONS OF SICKLE CELL DISEASE

(Mnemonic **SICKLE CELL**)

Sequestration (spleen and liver)
Infection
Cerebrovascular accidents (CVAs)
Kidney disease
Lung disease (ACS, pulmonary hypertension)
Eye disease

Crises (painful, infarctive)
Erection (priapism)
Limb effects (bone infarcts, marrow necrosis, osteomyelitis and aseptic necrosis)
Leg ulcers

OTHER ASPECTS OF SCA

(6 **H**s and 4 **A**s)

Haemolysis and anaemia (chronic)
Haemolytic crisis
Haemolysis due to transfusion
Hand–foot syndrome (dactylitis)
Hepatobiliary and abdominal involvement
Hyperviscosity due to transfusion
Aplastic crisis
Anaesthetic considerations
Alloimmunisation and autoimmunisation with transfusion
Accumulation of iron due to transfusion

INDICATIONS FOR HSCT IN SICKLE CELL DISEASE

Patients 16 years old or younger with SCD with an HLA-identical sibling bone marrow donor with 1 or more of the following.
(Mnemonic **STAR IS BORN**)

Stroke, central nervous system (CNS) haemorrhage or a neurological event lasting longer than 24 hours, or an abnormal cerebral magnetic resonance imaging (MRI) scan, cerebral arteriogram or MRI angiographic study and impaired neuropsychological testing

Transfusion requirement, but with red blood cell (RBC) alloimmunisation of more than two antibodies during long-term transfusion therapy

ACS, with a history of recurrent hospitalisations or exchange transfusions

Recurrent vaso-occlusive pain—three or more episodes per year for 3 years or more—or recurrent priapism

Impaired neuropsychological function and abnormal cerebral MRI scan

Stage I or II sickle lung disease

Bilateral proliferative retinopathy and major visual impairment in at least one eye

Osteonecrosis of multiple joints, with documented destructive changes

Respiratory disease—see **S** above

Nephropathy (moderate-severe proteinuria or GFR 30–50% of the predicted normal value)

COMPLICATIONS OF THALASSAEMIA

(Mnemonic **THALASSAEMIA**)

Tanner stage (pubertal delay)

Heart (cardiomyopathy)/**H**aematopoiesis (extramedullary)/**H**ypercoagulable

Anaemia

Liver/**L**ong tracts (neurological involvement)/**L**eg ulcers

Appearance (thalassaemic facies, pigmentation)

Sugar diabetes

Short stature

Arrhythmias

Eye/**E**ndocrine

Metabolic (hypocalcaemia)/**M**alocclusion

Iron overload/**I**cterus/**I**nfection/**I**atrogenic (DFS, DFO side effects)

Adenopathy and hepatosplenomegaly

ORDER FOR THE HAEMATOLOGICAL EXAMINATION

(Mnemonic 11 **S**s)

Sex, **S**yndrome, **S**ize, **S**tructure (hands), **S**cone (head), **S**ternum, **S**pine, **S**pleen (abdomen), **S**tand (gait and lower limbs), **S**BE (heart) and **S**tool

CAUSES OF CERVICAL LYMPHADENOPATHY
(Mnemonic **MATCHES**)

MAIS complex (*Mycobacterium Avium-Intracellulare-Scrofulaceum*)/**M**alignancy (lymphoma [non-Hodgkin], rhabdomyosarcoma)/**M**ucocutaneous lymph node syndrome (Kawasaki syndrome)
Atopic dermatitis
Tonsils: hypertrophy with upper respiratory tract infection (URTI)/**T**eeth: caries
Cat-scratch disease (*Bartonella henselae*)/**C**hlamydia trachomatis
HSV (gingivostomatitis)/**H**odgkin disease
EBV (Epstein-Barr virus)
Streptococcus A

CAUSES OF GENERALISED LYMPHADENOPATHY
(Mnemonic **MATCHES**)

Malignancy (neuroblastoma, leukaemia, lymphoma [non-Hodgkin])/**M**easles/**M**edications (e.g. phenytoin, isoniazid, allopurinol)
ALL/**A**ML/**A**denovirus/**A**utoimmune (JIA, SLE)
TB/**T**oxoplasma gondii/**T**yphoid (salmonella typhi)
CMV (cytomegalovirus)/**C**oxsackie virus/**C**occidioidomycosis
HIV/**H**erpes viruses: **H**HV-6 (roseola infantum); **H**VZ/**H**epatitis A, B, C/**H**odgkin disease/**H**istiocytosis X
EBV (Epstein-Barr virus)/**E**xanthemata (rubella, roseola, measles)/**E**nteroviruses/ **E**ndocrinopathies (Graves, Addison)/**E**ndocarditis
Staphylococcus/**S**ystemic viral infections (most common)/**S**arcoidosis/**S**torage diseases (Gaucher, Niemann-Pick)/**S**erum sickness/**S**epticaemia/**S**yphilis

LYMPHADENOPATHY (CERVICAL [Cx] OR GENERALISED *)
(Mnemonic **MATCHES**)

MAIS complex *[Cx]* (mycobacterium avium-intracellulare-scrofulaceum)/**M**alignancy* (neuroblastoma, leukaemia, lymphoma [non-Hodgkin's], rhabdomyosarcoma *[Cx]*)/**M**ucocutaneous lymph node syndrome (Kawasaki) *[Cx]*/**M**easles*/ **M**edications* (e.g. phenytoin, isoniazid, allopurinol)
ALL*/**A**ML*/**A**topic dermatitis *[Cx]*/**A**denovirus*/**A**utoimmune* (JIA, SLE)
TB* (tuberculosis, tubercle bacillus, mycobacteria tuberculosis)/**T**oxoplasma gondii*/**T**eeth: caries *[Cx]*/**T**yphoid* (salmonella typhi)
CMV* (cytomegalovirus)/**C**at-scratch disease *[Cx]* (*Bartonella henselae*)/**C**hlamydia trachomatis *[Cx]* **C**oxsackie virus*/**C**occidioidomycosis*
HIV*/**H**erpes viruses: **H**HV-6 (roseola infantum)*/**H**SV (gingivostomatitis) *[Cx]*/**H**VZ*/**H**epatitis A, B, C*/**H**odgkin's disease*/**H**istiocytosis*/**H**idradenitis suppurativa (axillary adenopathy in obese)
EBV* (Epstein-Barr virus; infectious mononucleosis)/**E**xanthemata* (rubella, roseola, measles)/**E**nteroviruses*/**E**ndocrinopathies* (Graves, Addison) **E**ndocarditis*
Streptococcus A *[Cx]*/**S**taphylococcus*/**S**ystemic viral infections* (most common)/**S**arcoidosis*/**S**torage diseases* (Gaucher, Niemann-Pick)/**S**erum sickness*/**S**epticaemia*/**S**yphilis*

A *very* abbreviated version
MAIS, **A**LL, **T**B, **C**MV, **H**IV, **E**BV, **S**trep

EXAMINATION/CHARACTERISTICS OF LUMP OR SWELLING (E.G. LYMPH NODE)
S and **T**

Inspection: **S**ite, **S**ize, **S**ides (edges), **S**hape, **S**ymmetry, **S**hine (colour), **S**urface, **S**urroundings

Palpation: **T**enderness, **T**emperature, **T**ethering (mobility), **T**ransmitted pulsation, **T**wo-finger separation (expansile pulsation with aneurysm), **T**hrill (from vascular lesion), **T**ension (consistency), **T**ap (for fluctuation), **T**ransfer contents (reducibility; disappears with pressure, but can reappear with opposing force applied), **T**ransient compressibility, **T**ongue attachment (moves with poking out tongue [thyroglossal cyst]), **T**racheal attachment (move up and down with swallowing: thyroid swellings); and finally, of occasional relevance:

Percussion (resonant means air present)

Auscultation (for bruits or bowel sounds [herniae])

The additional aspects to the examination of a lump are:
- *Associated pathology*. In the case of lymph nodes, indications of the primary pathology, whether it be indicating localised conditions (such as streptococcal pharyngitis) or generalised illnesses (such as EBV causing splenomegaly, hepatomegaly).
- The other aspects are local effects (such as a mass compressing and/or displacing the carotid sheath, or trachea or oesophagus) which includes: checking for contiguous disease (malignant masses in the lower cervical region can extend to the upper thorax); examining the lungs, particularly percussing (from behind) and auscultating the supraclavicular fossa (for upper lobe pathology).

PROMPT LYMPH NODE BIOPSY INDICATIONS
(Mnemonic **EXCISE**)

Enlarged beyond 1 cm neonatal, 2 cm (and growing), in older; enlarged in many sites
X-ray (CXR) abnormal: mediastinal nodes
Concerning (**C**ancer, **C**hronic inflammatory, **C**onnective tissue) symptoms: night sweats, loss of weight/**C**ervical (deep, lower) node/**C**RP persistently up despite treatment (like ESR)
Immobile (fixed)
Supraclavicular nodes
ENT symptoms and signs absent/**E**SR persistently up despite treatment (like CRP)

SPECTRUM OF DIFFERENTIAL DIAGNOSES OF LUMPS/SWELLING
(Mnemonic **SPECTRAL**)

Site (can describe with respect to fixed anatomical landmark, such as a bony prominence)/**S**ize (measure in cm)/**S**ides (edges)/**S**hape/**S**ymmetry (pathological nodes usually distributed asymmetrically)/**S**urface (smooth? irregular?)/**S**urroundings

Palpation (specific features of some swellings; e.g. collar-stud MAIS abscess has narrowing between lymph node and pus collection, prior to discharging)/**P**ercussion/**P**ulsatility (transmitted pulsation from a vascular lesion, or lesion on artery)

Edge/**E**xpansibility (specific form of pulsation, found by placing fingers on each side of a swelling, to see if they move away from each other, with each heartbeat, in three planes, as with an aneurysm)

Colour (e.g. red with acute pyogenic infection, cellulitis; purple over MAIS lymphadenitis)/**C**onsistency: soft (unlikely significant pathology), rubbery (classically lymphoma feels like this), firm or hard (possible malignancy or granulomatous disease)/**C**ompressibility

Tenderness/**T**emperature (using back of hand)/**T**ethering (mobility)/**T**hrill (from vascular lesion)/**T**ap (fluctuance is tested for by grasping the lump between the finger [usually either index or middle] and the thumb, and then tapping the central aspect of the lump with the other hand [usually with the index finger]; any resultant fluid thrill is perceived by the finger and thumb); fluctuance indicates fluid-filled swellings, such as lymphatic malformations (such as cystic hygromas), or liquid pus within an abscess/**T**ransfer contents (reducibility; disappears with pressure, but can reappear with opposing force applied)/**T**ransillumination (using pen torch, or auroscope light with attached ear speculum, applied to each side of swelling; lymphatic malformations [especially cystic hygromas] can transilluminate brilliantly)

Resonance (to percussion)/**R**elations (anatomical relations, which can be compressed by swelling)/**R**educibility (disappears with pressure, but can reappear withopposing force applied)

Auscultation/**A**ttachments: to underlying tissues (fixation); to tongue (moves upwards with protrusion of tongue [thyroglossal cyst]); to trachea (moves up and down with swallowing: thyroid swellings); so, attached to **t**issues, **t**ongue or **t**rachea

Local effects (e.g. torticollis, compression of neighbouring structures). Acute inflammation in a mass of inflamed nodes can cause reflex sternocleidomastoid muscle spasm, leading to torticollis with head tilt and restricted neck movement. Large masses can cause compression of local anatomical structures by swelling; this can include vascular malformations/hamartomatous swellings of lymph or blood vessels, enlarging secondary to bleeding, thrombosis or infection, which then can compress the trachea; or haemangiomata, which also can compress the trachea. Some lymphatic malformations can deform the expected configuration of the head and neck, to make the head appear displaced; cystic hygroma is the classic example of this

Lymph nodes draining the area

Chapter 11

Neonatology

3 AND 5: THE MOST USEFUL NUMBERS IN NEONATOLOGY

- **3.5 kg**: average **weight** of a term baby
- **35 cm**: average **head circumference** of a term baby
- **50 cm**: average **length** of a term baby
- **7.35–7.45**: normal range for **pH** in arterial blood
- **35–45 mmHg**: normal range **pCO$_2$** in arterial blood
- **135–145 mEq/L**: normal range for serum **sodium**
- **3.5–4.5 mEq/L**: normal range for serum **potassium**
- **3.5 mm**: size (internal diameter) of **endotracheal tube** used to intubate term baby
- **35–40 cm H$_2$O**: pressure at which **blow-off valve** operates **in most resuscitaire devices** (bag and mask) to prevent pressures above 35–40 cm H$_2$O being transmitted to baby causing pneumothorax
- **350 μmol/L: serum bilirubin level (SBR)** above which, historically, exchange transfusion was considered, to prevent kernicterus (actually it is 342 μmol/L, which is 20 mg/dL in the older pre-SI units, and led to the coining of the term **vigintiphobia** [fear of the number 20]; this pre-dated phototherapy)
- **35 weeks'** gestation: gestational age (really applies to 34–35 weeks, but close enough)
  - **under which** almost all babies will need (at least some) **nasogastric feeding**
  - **under which** excessive **oxygen** can still be **toxic to retinae**
  - **over which apnoea of prematurity stops** being a problem
- **35–60 breaths per minute**: range for normal **respiratory rate** (close enough; most references say around 40–60 breaths per minute)
- **135–160 beats per minute**: range for normal **heart rate** (close enough; most references say 140–160 beats per minute when awake, but can be 100–120 when asleep; some babies have a resting pulse rate below 100 when asleep, which is termed 'baseline bradycardia', being a normal variant)
- **30 WCC × 10^9**: highest white cell count in normal neonatal full blood count in first 24 hours of life

COMPLICATIONS OF PREMATURITY

(Mnemonic **PREMATURITY**)

Patent ductus arteriosus (PDA)
Respiratory distress syndrome (RDS; surfactant deficiency, hyaline membrane disease [HMD])
Encephalopathy: from bleed (periventricular, intraventricular, intracranial haemorrhage [PVH, IVH, ICH] or ischaemia [periventricular leukomalacia, PVL])
Metabolic immaturity (hypoglycaemia, hypocalcaemia, hypomagnesaemia)
Apnoea of prematurity
Thermoregulatory immaturity (importance of neutral thermal zone [NTZ])
Umbilical line requirement for those under 28 weeks
Retinopathy of prematurity
Infection/**I**mmunological immaturity
Transient anaemia (anaemia of prematurity)
Yellow (jaundice)

HAEMANGIOMATA
Associated conditions
PHACES association

Posterior fossa brain malformation (Dandy-Walker syndrome, cerebellar hypoplasia, developmental delay, seizures)
Haemangiomata of face/scalp (large, complex, segmented, > 5 cm diameter; can be subglottic)
Arterial malformations (aneurysms [including aorta {see below}, internal carotid, subclavian, cerebral arteries], moya-moya phenomenon, arterial stenoses)
Cardio-aortic anomalies (ventricular septal defect [VSD], patent ductus arteriosus [PDA], coarctation of the aorta, congenital aneurysms including ascending aorta and aortic arch, steal syndrome)
Eye anomalies (microphthalmia [ipsilateral to haemangioma], Horner syndrome, cataract, optic atrophy)/**E**ndocrine: lingual thyroid/hypothyroidism (congenital)
Sternal anomalies (clefts, pits)/**S**upraumbilical abdominal raphe (ventral developmental defects)

PELVIS association

Perineal segmented haemangioma
External genitalia anomalies
Lipomeningocele
Vesicorenal anomalies
Imperforate anus
Skin tag

Chapter 12

Nephrology
THE MANAGEMENT OF CKD
The management of CKD can be divided into over a dozen main areas, comprising the following, organised within the mnemonic **URAEMIA FACTS**.

Uraemic complications (includes monitoring for development of neuropathy, encephalopathy; measuring serum urea and creatinine)
Renal replacement therapy (dialysis, RTx)
Acid–base status
Electrolytes and fluids: this includes serum potassium; this is very important, but the candidate should not go directly to this unless the child is already on dialysis; it is usually not the most important problem in CKD; also includes salt and water balance (including hypertension)
Mineral and bone disease
Intake: nutrition/**I**mmunisation/**I**mmunosuppression
Anaemia

Family disruption/**F**inancial burden
ADHD/**A**nxiety/**A**ffective disorders (e.g. depression)
Cardiovascular/**C**ognitive effects/**C**ompliance (with treatment) issues
Therapeutic burden of care
Stature (growth)/**S**leep disturbance/**S**ocial/**S**chool

MYCOPHENOLATE MOFETIL (MMF) SIDE EFFECTS
(Mnemonic **MMG**)

Myelosuppression, increased risk of infection
Malignancy (haematological especially lymphoma, occurs in 0.6% versus 0.3% for AZA)
Gut effects (diarrhoea [30%], bleed [3%], perforation [rare])

SIROLIMUS (SLM) SIDE EFFECTS
(Mnemonic **HT LIMUS**)

Hyperlipidaemia/Hypercholesterolaemia/Hypertension/Hepatic necrosis (rare)
Thrombocytopaenia

Leucopenia and increased infection risk/**L**ymphoedema/**L**ung fibrosis (rare)
Intestinal: diarrhoea, abdominal pain/**I**nflammatory: stomatitis, pancreatitis
Malignancy (especially skin)/**M**uscle: rhabdomyolysis increased risk with statins
UV light: limit to avoid skin cancer
Slow wound healing

TACROLIMUS (TAC) SIDE EFFECTS
(Mnemonic **TACROLIMUS**)

Tremor/Tingling (neurotoxicity)
Alimentary (diarrhoea, constipation, nausea, vomiting, anorexia)/**A**naemia
Cancer risk increased
Renal toxicity (includes irreversible vasculopathy, interstitial fibrosis, tubular damage)
Osteoporosis
Lymphoproliferative disease/**L**ow Phosphate
Increased: blood pressure, [K$^+$], (creatinine)
Magnesium low
Urea high
Sugar diabetes

MAIN AGENTS THAT CAN CLAIM SUCCESS IN NS
(Mnemonic **CLAIM**)

CPA: 2 mg/kg/day for 8-12 weeks)/**C**alcineurin inhibitor: tacrolimus (TAC: 0.1 mg/kg/day in two divided doses)
Levamisole (2.5 mg/kg alternate daily for 12–24 months)
ACE inhibitors
Immunisation with pneumococcal vaccine
Mycophenolate mofetil (MMF: 25 mg/kg/day in divided doses for 12–24 months)/**M**onoclonal antibody: B-cell depleting: rituximab (RTX)

Chapter 13

Neurology
CP MIMICS

4 **M**s: **M**etabolic, **M**uscular dystrophies, **M**itochondrial disorders, **M**alformation syndromes

Metabolic: treatable (e.g. glutaric acidaemia 1); impersonates dyskinetic CP
Metabolic: treatment not available (e.g. Lesch–Nyhan; Sjögren–Larsson)
Muscular dystrophies (e.g. Becker muscular dystrophy)
Mitochondrial disorders (e.g. Leigh syndrome)
Malformation syndromes (e.g. Miller–Dieker [MDLS]); Rett syndrome

SEIZURES: ILAE GROUPINGS

Investigations: metabolic causes of seizures in neonates
(Mnemonic **BACCALAUREATES**)

Biotinidase (biotinidase deficiency)
Ammonia
Copper (low in Menkes)
Caeruloplasmin (low in Menkes)
Acylcarnitines (carnitine acylcarnitine translocase deficiency)
Lactate (elevated in mitochondrial disease)/**L**iver function tests
Amino acids
Urate (low in molybdenum cofactor deficiency)
Renal function tests
Electrolytes (includes calcium and magnesium)
Alpha amino-adipic semialdehyde (alpha ASA) (urine test; elevated levels in pyridoxine-dependent epilepsy, molybdenum cofactor deficiency and sulphite oxidase deficiency)
TORCH screen/**T**ogether (paired) tests: CSF/plasma amino acids (which include serine and glycine, to diagnose serine biosynthesis disorders, and glycine encephalopathy), CSF/plasma glucose and lactate (for glucose transporter type 1 deficiency syndrome)
EEG (burst suppression in various: [normal under 28 weeks], term asphyxia, meningoencephalitis, malformations, Ohtahara ARX mutation, pyridoxine-dependent epilepsy, pyridoxine 5′-phosphate responsive epilepsy, Menkes, mitochondrial glutamate SLC25A22 mutation, glycine encephalopathy, molybdenum cofactor deficiency, sulphite oxidase deficiency, purine synthesis disorder)
Sugar (glucose)/**S**ialotransferrin (congenital disorders of glycosylation [CDG])/**S**uccinylpurines (adenylosuccinate lyase deficiency [ASLD])/**S**ulphites (urine) (positive test in sulphite oxidase deficiency, and molybdenum cofactor deficiency)

STRUCTURAL CAUSES OF EPILEPSY

(Mnemonic **MTV-H**)

Malformations (malformations of cortical development [MCDs], focal cortical dysplasia [FCDs])
Tuberous sclerosis complex (TSC)/**T**umours/**T**rauma
Vascular malformation/**V**ascular accident (stroke, haemorrhagic or ischaemic)
Hippocampal sclerosis (HS)/**H**ypothalamic hamartoma (HH)/**H**ypoxic ischaemic encephalopathy (HIE)

SEIZURES: ILAE GROUPINGS

Neonatal period

(Mnemonic **OBE**)

Ohtahara syndrome (early infantile epileptic encephalopathy with suppression burst)
BFNS (benign familial neonatal seizures)
EME (early myoclonic encephalopathy)

SEIZURES: ILAE GROUPINGS

Infancy

Mnemonic to Dr West, who described the condition in his son (**MB**, **MB**, **MD**, **West**). Candidates should have knowledge of the asterisked conditions.

Malignant migrating partial seizures in infancy (MMPSI)
Benign familial infantile seizures (BFIS) and non-familial infantile seizures (Fukuyama-Watanabe-Vigevano syndrome)
Myoclonic epilepsy in infancy (MEI)
Benign familial neonatal–infantile seizures
Myoclonic encephalopathy in non-progressive disorders
Dravet syndrome (severe myoclonic epilepsy of infancy [SMEI])
West syndrome*

SEIZURES: ILAE GROUPINGS

Childhood

Candidates should have knowledge of the asterisked conditions.
(Mnemonic **FEEL BALANCE**)

Febrile seizures plus (FS+)* (can start in infancy): also called GEFS+ (generalised epilepsy with FS+)
Early onset childhood occipital epilepsy (Panayiotopoulos type); also called Panayiotopoulos syndrome
Epilepsy with myoclonic-atonic (previously astatic) seizures (EM-AS, also called Doose syndrome, or Myoclonic-Atonic Epilepsy [MAE])
EEG
Late-onset childhood occipital epilepsy (Gastaut type)
Benign epilepsy with centrotemporal spikes (BECTS)*
Absence, myoclonic—epilepsy with myoclonic absences (EMA)
Lennox-Gastaut syndrome (LGS)*
Absence—childhood absence epilepsy (CAE)*
Nocturnal—autosomal dominant nocturnal frontal lobe epilepsy (ADNFLE); also called epilepsy, nocturnal frontal lobe (ENFL)
CSWS—epileptic encephalopathy with continuous spike-and-wave during sleep (CSWS)
Epileptic encephalopathy, including Landau–Kleffner syndrome (LKS)*; also called acquired epileptic aphasia

SEIZURES: ILAE GROUPINGS

Adolescence
Candidates should have knowledge of the asterisked conditions
(Mnemonic **Juvenile TAPE**)

Juvenile absence epilepsy (JAE)
Juvenile myoclonic epilepsy (JME)*, also called Janz syndrome
Temporal lobe–other familial temporal lobe epilepsies
Autosomal dominant partial epilepsy with auditory features (ADPEAF). Also called autosomal dominant lateral temporal lobe epilepsy (ADLTLE) or epilepsy, familial temporal lobe (ETL)
Progressive myoclonus epilepsies (PME)
Epilepsy with generalised tonic–clonic seizures alone (EGTCSA)*

MYOCLONIC ENCEPHALOPATHY IN NON-PROGRESSIVE DISORDERS

Chromosomal syndromes
(Mnemonic **PAW**)

Prader–Willi
Angelman
Wolf-Hirschhorn

Wolf-Hirschhorn syndrome
(Mnemonic **WHirschhorns**)

Warrior
Helmet (facies)
Intellectual impairment
Restricted growth
Small head
Closure defects (**C**lefts [lip/palate], **C**oloboma of iris, **C**ardiac [ASD,VSD])
Hypertelorism
High forehead, **H**igh arched eyebrows
Ocular findings (protruding eyes, epicanthic folds)
Retrognathia
Nose: beaked, widened
Skeletal (scoliosis, kyphosis, dislocatable hips, talipes)

PANAYIOTOPOULOS SYNDROME
(Mnemonic **PaNayIOToPoULoSSS**)

Pallor
Nausea (**y**)
Incontinence
Ocular: mydriasis
Tone lost
Prolonged duration (**o**)
Unilateral eye deviation
Limited to under 14 years (**o**)
Salivation (hypersalivation), **S**yncope-like, **S**tatus common

ENCEPHALOPATHIC CONTINUUM
(Mnemonic **OWL**)

Ohtahara to **W**est to **L**GS

LENNOX GASTAUT SYNDROME (LGS)
Seizure semiology: three main types (**TAA**)

Tonic, **A**bsence (atypical), **A**tonic

LENNOX GASTAUT SYNDROME (LGS)
Treatment mnemonic

2 **V**s, 2 **C**s, 2 **R**s (2 VCRs), + 2 **L**s + **T**opiramate + **K**etogenic diet: **V**alproate, **V**agus nerve stimulation, **C**lonazepam, **C**orpus callosotomy, **R**ufinamide, **R**esection of focal cortex, **L**amotrigine, **L**evetiracetam, **T**opiramate, **K**etogenic

LENNOX GASTAUT SYNDROME (LGS)
Contraindicated AEDs in LGS
2 '**carb**'s and 3 with '**gab/a**' in name
Carbamazepine
Ox**carb**azepine
Gabapentin
Pre**gaba**lin
Tia**gab**ine

STATUS EPILEPTICUS MANAGEMENT
5 **P**s

Pams (benzodiazepines include diaze**pam**, loraze**pam** and midazolam)
Phenobarbitone
Phenytoin
Paraldehyde
Pentone (as in Thio-pentone) or **P**ropofol

SPECT SCANNING IN SEIZURE DISORDERS
(Mnemonic **SPECT**)

Seizure (area) **P**erfusion **E**valuated by **C**eretec with **T**echnetium

LEVETIRACETAM (LEV)
Advantages
(Mnemonic **LEV**)

Laboratory tests (e.g. drug levels) not needed
Excellent pharmacokinetics, excellent safety profile
Versatile (most types of epilepsy treated), very fast onset

WADA TEST

Anaesthetises each hemisphere to evaluate memory
(Mnemonic **WADA**)

Which hemisphere is dominant for language, to see if the other side can maintain
    memory function, after
Amytal sodium injection into internal carotid,
Dysfunctional hippocampus identified and
Amnesia avoided as complication

NEURAL TUBE DEFECTS

NTDs affecting incidence of NTDs

Known environmental influences implicated in the development of NTDs include the
following problems in the first-trimester pregnant mother.
(Mnemonic **NTDs causing NTDs**)

Nutritional causes (pregestational low folate [as above]; pregestational high BMI
    [> 29] increases risk 1.5- to 3.5-fold)
Temperature elevation (pregestational, from fevers or saunas; increases risk up to
    twofold)
Diabetes (pregestational high blood sugar levels; increases risk 2- to 10-fold) or **D**rugs
    (AEDs, particularly sodium valproate and carbamazepine; increase risk to 1–2%)

COMPLICATIONS OF SPINA BIFIDA

Cognitive, **C**ontinence plus 9 **S**s

Shunt (hydrocephalus)
Splints (and other aids: crutches, calipers, wheelchair)
Spine (scoliosis, kyphosis)
Skeleton (bone health: decreased bone mineral density; fracture propensity)
Sleep-disordered breathing
Skin: pressure ulcers, burns, latex allergy
Senses: sight and hearing
Size: growth and development—precocious puberty, growth hormone (GH)
    deficiency, short stature, obesity
Seizures

RECENT DETERIORATION IN SCOLIOSIS IN MMC PATIENT

Causes: **SC**, **SC**, **SC**
Scoliosis **C**auses: **S**hunt: **C**hiari, **S**yrinx, **C**ord (tethered)

DIAGNOSTIC CRITERIA FOR NF1

(Mnemonic **FIBROMA**)

Fibromatous tumours (plexiform neuromas)	occur in 30–50%
Iris hamartomas (Lisch nodules) > 2	occur in 90%
Bone lesions: tibial pseudoarthrosis; SWD	occur in 2%; 1%
Relative (first degree) with NF1	occur in 50%
Optic pathway glioma (OPG)	occur in 15–30%
Macules (CALM): 6 > 5 mm pre-, > 15 mm postpuberty	occurs in > 99%
Axillary and inguinal freckling	occurs in > 90%

LIST OF TUMOURS IN NF1

Alphabetic run: **LMNOP** + **DR G**:

Leukaemia (juvenile chronic myelogenous leukaemia, myelodysplastic syndromes)
Meningioma/**M**alignant peripheral nerve sheath tumours (MPNSTs)
Neurofibromas (dermal, diffuse plexiform, deep nodular plexiform)/
   Neurofibrosarcoma/**N**euroblastoma
Optic pathway glioma (OPG)
Phaeochromocytoma/**P**ilocytic astrocytoma/**P**arathyroid adenoma/**P**ancreatic
   somatostatinoma
+
Duodenal carcinoid/**D**uodenal somatostatinoma
Rhabdomyosarcoma/**R**etinal vasoproliferative tumours
Gliomas (hypothalamic-optochiasmatic, brainstem, cerebellar, second tumours after
   XRT of first tumours)/**G**astrointestinal stromal tumours (GIST)

PATHOLOGICAL PROCESSES IN SWS

(Mnemonic **HIT VIVAS**)

Hypoxia
Ischaemia
Thrombosis
Venous occlusion
Infarction
Vascular steal phenomena
Atrophy
Seizures

FEATURES OF SWS

(Mnemonic **STURGE**)

Seizures/**S**urgical resections for refractory epilepsy (callosotomy, lesionectomy,
   hemispherectomy)/**S**troke, **S**troke-like episodes/**S**tructural leptomeningeal
   involvement/**S**trabismus/**S**coliosis/**S**poradic/**S**omatic mutation
Trigeminal nerve distribution (V1, V2)/**T**rabeculectomy requirement for glaucoma
Uveal tract: choroidal vascular malformation/**U**nderactive thyroid/**U**nderproduction
   pituitary GH/**U**neven growth (body asymmetry)
Regional defects—hemiparesis, hemianopia/**R**estricted vision: field cuts
   (homonymous hemianopia)
Glaucoma/**G**oniotomy requirement/**G**lobal delay/**G**ene = **G**NAQ/**G**rowth hormone
   deficiency
Encephalotrigeminal angiomatosis (alternate name for SWS)/**E**ye enlargement/**E**ye
   pressure increased/**E**ducational opportunities limited (intellectual impairment)

TSC CLINICAL DIAGNOSTIC CRITERIA

Two major features, or one major feature and at least two minor features.

Major features (11):
- **Skin** (4). **SHAU**: **S**hagreen patch, **H**ypomelanotic macules (> 3, at least 5 mm diameter), **A**ngiofibromas (> 3) or fibrous cephalic plaque, **U**ngual fibromas (> 2).
- **Brain/eye** (4). **S**ub**e**pendymal **g**iant cell **a**strocytoma (**SEGA**), subependymal nodules (SEN), cortical dysplasias, multiple retinal hamartomas.
- **Others** (3). Heart, lung, kidney: cardiac rhabdomyoma, **l**ymph**a**ngioleio**m**yomatosis (LAM), angiomyolipomas (> 2) (of kidney).

Minor features (6):
- 'Confetti' hypomelanotic skin lesions, dental enamel pits (> 3), intraoral fibromas (> 2), retinal achromic patch, multiple renal cysts, non-renal hamartomas.

TSC DIAGNOSTIC CRITERIA

Major features

(Mnemonic **ASH CLUE**; old term for hypomelanotic macules: 'ash leaf' macules)

Ash leaf (hypomelanotic) macules (> 3, > 5 mm)/**A**ngiofibroma/**A**ngiomyolipoma
Subependymal nodules (SEN)/**S**ubependymal giant cell astrocytoma (SEGA)/
   Shagreen patches
Heart: rhabdomyoma, **H**amartomas (multiple retinal)
Cortical dysplasia
Lymphangioleiomyomatosis
Ungal fibromas
Establish genetic diagnosis: identifying TSC1/TSC2 pathogenic mutations sufficient

TSC DIAGNOSTIC CRITERIA

Minor features

(Mnemonic **MIND achromia**)

Multiple renal cysts
Intraoral fibromas (> 2)
Non-renal hamartomas
Dental enamel pits (> 3)
achromia: retina (achromic patch), skin ('confetti' hypomelanotic skin lesions)

TSC DIAGNOSTIC CRITERIA

Age-related manifestations of TSC

Age-related presentation can be represented approximately by three groups. There are four consistent aspects that occur across all ages. (Mnemonic **HEFS**)

Hypopigmented macules
Epilepsy
Facial angiofibromas
SEN

Age under 1 year (mnemonic **CHEFS**):

Cardiac rhabdomyoma
Hypomelanotic macules
Epilepsy
Facial angiofibroma
SEN

Age 5–15 (mnemonic **RHEFS**):

Renal angiomyolipoma
Hypopigmented macules
Epilepsy
Facial angiofibroma
SEN

Age 25–60 (mnemonic **LU-RHEFS**):

Liver hamartoma
Ungual hamartoma
RHEFS

INFANTILE NYSTAGMUS SYNDROME
(Mnemonic **INFANTILE**)

Idiopathic
Nutans (spasmus nutans syndrome [SNS])
Fusion maldevelopment nystagmus syndrome (also called latent nystagmus)/
  Foveal hypoplasia
Albinism
Nerve (Optic) hypoplasia (bilateral)
Transilluminate iris (to confirm albinism)
Iris absence (aniridia)
LEber's congenital amaurosis 1 (LCA1) or other retinal dystrophy/**LE**ns opacity
  (cataract)

UNILATERAL NYSTAGMUS
Importance is excluding tumours of **CHIASM**

Chiasmatic glioma
Hypothalamic glioma
Internuclear ophthalmoplegia (indicates brainstem disease)
Amblyopia/**A**bsent vision on one side (complete blindness—unilateral)
Spasmus nutans syndrome (SNS)
Maldevelopment fusion nystagmus (also called latent nystagmus)

PROPTOSIS
(Mnemonic **STARING CHILD**)

Sarcoma (metastatic Ewing's)/**S**arcoma (granulocytic [AML])/**S**arcoidosis
Thyroid eye disease (also called thyroid orbitopathy, thyroid-associated orbitopathy, Graves' orbitopathy, thyroid ophthalmopathy)/**T**hrombosis of cavernous sinus
Arachnoid cyst/**A**LL/**A**bscess
Rhabdomyosarcoma (orbital)/**R**etinoblastoma
Infection: orbital cellulitis/**I**nfiltrate: histiocytosis X
Neuroblastoma (metastatic)/**N**eurofibroma (orbital)
Glioma (optic nerve/chiasm)/**G**laucoma (includes in Sturge-Weber syndrome [SWS])
Chiasmal glioma/**C**raniosynostosis syndromes (Crouzon, Apert)
Haemangioma (orbital)/**H**istiocytosis X/**H**aemorrhage (orbital; e.g. trauma)
Inflammation: pseudotumour, paranasal sinuses (ethmoid, maxillary)
Lymphangioma (orbital)/**L**ymphoma (orbital)/**L**acrimal gland tumour
Dermoid cyst (orbital)/**D**istance in adult: protrusion of over 18 mm from the lateral rim of the orbit to corneal apex measured by exophthalmometer termed exophthalmos

PULSATILE PROPTOSIS
Causes: the 5 **A**s

Absent wing of sphenoid bone in NF1
Aortic incompetence
Arteriovenous malformation (carotid-cavernous sinus fistula)
Arachnoid cyst (intra-diploic in middle cranial fossa, expands bone, deforms posterolateral wall of orbit)
Accident (trauma): orbital roof fracture

THYROID EYE DISEASE (TED)
(Mnemonic **CHEMOSIS**)

Chemosis (conjunctival oedema)/**C**ornea: ulceration/**C**olour vision loss
Hyperthyroid signs: lid lag, lid retraction, infrequent blinking, wide palpebral fissure
Exophthalmos/**E**levated lid (lid retraction)
Muscles (extraocular) affected/**M**orning (transient) diplopia
Optic nerve compression if severe/**O**ptic atrophy (late)
Spasm of lids (blepharospasm) impersonates ptosis/**S**welling: periorbital
Impaired visual fields/**I**nflammation of conjunctivae
Sight threatened

   Alternate mnemonic for thyroid eye disease (**EXOPHT**)

Elevated lid (lid retraction)
Xtra-ocular muscles (EOMs) movements impaired: ophthalmoplegia
Optic nerve compression can cause visual failure/**O**ptic atrophy (late)
Proptosis
Hyperthyroid signs: lid lag, lid retraction, infrequent blinking, wide palpebral fissure
Tethering of EOMs/**T**ransient (morning) diplopia

DIFFERENTIAL DIAGNOSIS MNEMONIC FOR SEIZURES (ESPECIALLY AFEBRILE)
(Mnemonic **HEADSPACE**)

Hypo-glycaemia, calcaemia, magnesemia, natremia/**H**ypertension/**H**aemorrhage/
    Head injury
Encephalopathies/**E**ncephalitis
AV malformation/**A**neurysm
Developmental syndromes (e.g. NF1, TSC, SWS)/**D**rugs
Stroke—ischaemic or haemorrhagic/**S**hunt (VP shunt)/**S**OL/**S**torage disorders
Prolonged QT interval/**P**oisons (toxins)
Abscess + other CNS infections: meningitis/intrauterine TORCH infections
Cerebral palsy/**C**ancer (primary/secondary brain tumours)/**C**losed head injury (occult)
Epilepsy

HEMIPLEGIA CAUSES
Arterial ischaemic stroke (AIS)
(Mnemonic **SCA**)

Sickle cell anaemia/**S**epsis
Cardiac causes/**C**lotting tendency (thrombophilia)
Arteriopathies

HEMIPLEGIA CAUSES
Haemorrhagic stroke
(Mnemonic **CHAT**)

Cerebral vascular abnormalities/**C**oagulopathies
Hypertension/**H**aemophilia
AVM/**A**neurysm
Tumour (cerebral)/**T**hrombocytopaenia

SCOLIOSIS
Description of features of scoliosis
(Mnemonic, all starting with '**S**')

Scoliosis (site and convexity to which side)
Shoulders and hands (higher on side to which primary curve convex)
Scapulae (prominence on which side)
Skin (loin) crease symmetry
Superior iliac spine position
Spare ribs (rib cage rotation posteriorly or anteriorly)
Space between arms and body (asymmetry)

CAUSES OF ATAXIA

Acute, episodic and progressive
(Mnemonic **FLAMING SPINNER**)

FRDA (Friedreich ataxia) (MIM#229300)

Labyrinthitis (vertigo causing ataxia)/**L**ysosomal storage diseases

AT (ataxia-telangiectasia) (MIM#208900)/**A**betalipoproteinaemia (MIM#200100)/
   Argininosuccinic aciduria (MIM#207900)

Medulloblastoma/**M**etabolic: **M**SUD (maple syrup urine disease)
   (MIM#248600)/**M**LD (metachromatic leucodystrophy, also called arylsulfatase
   A [ARSA] deficiency) (MIM#250100)/**M**etal disease: Wilson disease
   (MIM#277900)/**M**igraine: basilar artery/**M**itochondrial disorders (Kearns-
   Sayre [MIM#530000], MERRF (*m*yoclonic *e*pilepsy with *r*agged *r*ed *f*ibres)
   [MIM#545000], NARP (*n*europathy, *a*taxia and *r*etinitis *p*igmentosa)
   [MIM#551500])/**M**ultiple sclerosis/**M**yxoedema (hypothyroidism)

Infection (e.g. cerebellitis, meningitis, mastoiditis)/**I**EMs (Inborn errors of
   metabolism e.g. OTC [*o*rnithine *t*rans*c*arbamylase deficiency] [MIM#311250])

Neuroblastoma (occult)

GBS (Guillain-Barré syndrome)/**G**enetic (hereditary) ataxias (many)

SCAs (spinocerebellar ataxias, autosomal dominant)/**S**CARs (spinocerebellar
   ataxias, autosomal recessive)/**S**PAX (spinocerebellar ataxias with prominent
   spasticity)/**S**upratentorial tumours

Post-infectious cerebellitis/**P**osterior fossa tumours/**P**aroxysmal vertigo/**P**ellagra
   (niacin deficiency; can cause the four Ds: dermatitis [photosensitive], diarrhoea,
   dementia and death)/**P**ellagra-like dermatosis (Hartnup disorder [HND])
   (MIM#234500)/**P**yruvate **C**arboxylase deficiency (MIM#266150)/**P**sychogenic
   (not real ataxia, but impersonating this)

Intoxication/**I**ngestion (drugs)/**I**nner ear pathology (e.g. labyrinthitis)

Nutritional deficiencies: deficiencies of vitamin B_1 (thiamine), B_3 (niacin/nicotinic
   acid), B_6 (pyridoxine), B_{12} (cobalamin), E

Neurodegenerative disorders

Ependymoma/**E**A (episodic ataxias)

Refsum disease (MIM#266500)/**R**ett syndrome (MIM#312750)

ATAXIA-TELANGIECTASIA (AT) FEATURES
(Mnemonic **ATAXIA CASE**)

ATM (ataxia-telangiectasia mutated) gene codes for serine-protein kinase ATM;
   only known cause/**A**ge: **a**taxia/cerebellar dysfunction (onset 1–4 years) **a**ntedates
   telangiectasia/Ig**A** (Immunoglobulin **A**) decreased

Telangiectasia of exposed areas (bulbar conjunctivae, nose [bridge], ears,
   neck, antecubital fossa): age 3 to 10 years/**T**en years of age often require
   wheelchair/**T**runcal ataxia/**T**one decreased/**T**hree out of ten develop malignancy
   (usually [85%] leukaemia or lymphoma)

Apraxia of eye movement (cannot follow object across field; vertical and horizontal
   saccadic movements affected) and nystagmus

X-ray of chest (CXR) for sinopulmonary infection (increased susceptibility)

Immune deficiency (cell mediated immunity decreased)/**I**onising radiation sensitivity

Absent reflexes

Choreoathetosis/**C**ancer risk 40–100 times normal; especially ALL, AML, lymphoma, brain tumours, adenocarcinoma of stomach, basal cell carcinoma, ovarian dysgerminoma

Alpha feto-protein (AFP) increased/**A**geing appears premature (grey hair)

Speech slurred (dysarthria)/**S**usceptibility to sinobronchopulmonary infections and serious neoplasia (as above)

Elevated carcinoembryonic antigen/**E**ndocrine: insulin resistant diabetes/**E**lasticity skin lost/**E**leven = chromosome locus (11q22.3)

FRIEDREICH ATAXIA (FRDA) FEATURES
(Mnemonic **FRIEDREICHS**)

FXN gene (at 9q13) codes for frataxin, a mitochondrial protein; only known cause/**F**ive–fifteen age group/**F**eet: pes cavus

Reduced sense of vibration, position/**R**omberg test positive/**R**ecessive

Impaired sense of vision

Eyes: optic atrophy/nystagmus

Dysarthria/**D**eafness

Reflexes in lower limb absent, but …

Extensor plantar/**E**quinovarus feet (plantar flexors, inverters affected)

Insulin requirement (T1DM)/**I**ron misdistribution in mitochondria allows oxidative damage, decreased ATP production

Cardiac disease; hypertrophic non-obstructive cardiomyopathy

Hyperglycaemia (diabetes in up to 30%)

Spastic lower limbs (pyramidal weakness)/**S**coliosis

MITOCHONDRIAL DISORDER FEATURES
(Mnemonic **MITOCHONDRIALS**)

Myopathy (proximal)/**M**yoclonus/**M**igraine

Inheritance recessive

Tubular (renal) defects

Optic atrophy

Cataract/**C**horea

Heart: cardiomyopathy/pre-excitation syndromes

Ophthalmoplegia

Neuropathy/**N**eurogenic weakness/**N**eurologic: encephalopathy

Deafness (sensorineural)/**D**iabetes/**D**ementia

Retinopathy (pigmentary)

Increased lactate: blood (fasting > 3.0 mmol/L); CSF > 1.5 mmol/L

Ataxia

Lid: ptosis

Seizure/**S**troke-like episodes/**S**pasticity

Chapter 14

Oncology
SYMPTOMS THAT MAY PRESENT IN CHILDREN
These include a mass, and the 8 Ps.

Pyrexia
Pain
Pallor
Purpura
Persistent squint
Personality change
Posterior fossa symptoms
Pretenders (i.e. ALL or neuroblastoma impersonating arthritis, or mediastinal lymph nodes impersonating asthma)

Chapter 15

The respiratory system
SIGNS OF LIFE-THREATENING ASTHMA
S and **C**

Silent child (can't speak)
Silent chest (poor air entry)
Cyanosis (or oxygen saturation < 90%)
Consciousness altered (due to hypoxia)
Collapse (exhausted)
Cardiac arrhythmia or **C**ardiac rate **s**low (pre-arrest)
Slow breathing (pre-arrest)

RESPIRATORY: CAUSES OF PROTRACTED NAUSEA IN CYSTIC FIBROSIS
When lung disease is stable, and not the cause, there is a wide range of pathologies for this not uncommon complaint. There are over a dozen common causes. (Mnemonic **FASTING**)

Fat maldigestion
Abdominal pain (functional; this is probably intestinal hypervigilance, where minor sensations become major)
Small bowel bacterial overgrowth/**S**plenic enlargement (portal hypertension)/**S**inusitis
Treatment: prescribed drug side effects; over-the-counter drug side effects
Inflammatory bowel disease, IBD (especially Crohn disease, which is 12 times more common in CF)/**I**ncreased intracranial pressure (ICP)
Non-prescribable (alternative/complementary) treatments
Gastrointestinal tract causes (5 **G**s): **G**astro-oesophageal reflux, **G**astritis, **G**astroparesis (diabetic), **G**allstones, **G**iardia—to sort out which is the case, investigations can involve endoscopy and imaging; treatment may involve treating CFRD, PERT tailoring and medications (depending on the likeliest diagnosis, the possibilities include high-dose proton pump inhibitors, metronidazole, domperidone, ondansetron or even antidepressants)

CAUSES OF ABDOMINAL PAIN IN CYSTIC FIBROSIS

This can be a diagnostic and management problem, not dissimilar, in scope, to protracted nausea as above. Constipation is a common cause. Other causes are many. (Mnemonic **GUARDING**)

Gastro-oesophageal reflux/oesophagitis
Underdosing PERT
Appendicitis
Renal stones/**R**espiratory disease related: lower-lobe pneumonia, muscle strain (rectus)
DIOS/**D**uodenal ulcer
Inflamed pancreas (pancreatitis)/**I**BD/**I**ntussusception
Non-organic/functional (e.g. grief reaction with death of friend with CF; recognising own mortality with deteriorating health—may be unrelated to CF)
Gallbladder/biliary related: cholelithiasis, common bile duct stricture, cholecystitis

SELECTED CAUSES OF OBSTRUCTIVE SLEEP APNOEA

(Mnemonic **COMPACTED BREATHING**)

Crouzon syndrome (FGFR 2 & 3)/**C**ervical fusion (Klippel–Feil syndrome)
Obesity/**O**verbite (and other dental anomalies)
Marfan syndrome (FBN 1)/**M**oebius sequence/**M**yelomeningocele
Pfeiffer syndrome (FGFR 1,2)/**P**rader–Willi (deletion at 15q11-q13)/**P**aralysed vocal cord
Adenotonsillar hypertrophy/**A**pert syndrome (FGFR 2)/**A**chondroplasia (FGFR 3)
CP/**C**HARGE (choanal stenosis/atresia; CHD7)/**C**hotzen (Saethre-Chotzen; TWIST)
Tracheal/subglottic stenosis/**T**racheomalacia/laryngomalacia
Extra tissue (fatty infiltration upper airway structures, storage disorders, airway papillomatosis, cystic hygroma [lymphatic malformation], nasal polyps in CF)
Down syndrome (normal-size tongue, small pharynx causing relative macroglossia)
Burns to head and neck/**B**eckwith-Wiedemann (11p15.5) (macroglossia)
Rhinitis (allergic)/**R**obin sequence (hypoplasia of mandibular area before 9 weeks in utero causes glossoptosis)/**R**epaired cleft lip/palate/pharyngeal flap
Endocrine disease: hypothyroidism/hypopituitarism (both cause decreased muscle tone)
Arthritis (JIA; TMJ involvement causing micrognathia)/**A**rnold–Chiari malformation (ACM) type II (including in spina bifida)
Treacher Collins syndrome (TCOF 1)
Haematological: SCA/**H**allermann–Streiff syndrome (malar hypoplasia, micrognathia with hypoplastic rami and anterior displacement of TMJ, high narrow palate)
Inborn errors of metabolism: mucopolysaccharidoses (MPSs)
Neuromuscular weakness (SMA, myasthenia gravis, myopathies)
Goldenhar syndrome (hemifacial microsomia: 1st and 2nd branchial arch syndrome [14q32])

PARAMETERS RECORDED ON POLYSOMNOGRAPHY (PSG)
This is the gold standard for diagnosis of OSA.
(Mnemonic **SLEEPING OVER**)

Submental EMG
Limb movements via EMG
EEG–AASM recommended
Eye movement
Position of body
Intensity of respiratory effort
Nasal airflow
Grade snoring (frequency and/or volume)
Oxygen saturation (detects brief drops in SpO_2 by lowering averaging time to 2 seconds)
Video recording
End-tidal CO_2 signal (reduced in hypopnea; absent in apnoea)
Rhythm ECG

Chapter 16

Rheumatology
SELECTED DIFFERENTIAL DIAGNOSES FOR SWOLLEN JOINTS
(Mnemonic **VIRAL JOINT**)

Viral (Parvo, EBV)/**V**asculitides (Henoch–Schönlein, Kawasaki)
Infective (bacterial: septic joint, osteomyelitis, discitis, sacroiliitis, Lyme)
Reactive (post-streptococcal, rheumatic fever, Reiter, serum sickness)
Autoimmune (SLE, dermatomyositis, systemic sclerosis, MCTD, psoriasis, Behçet's)
Leukaemia (ALL, AML)

JIA + other inflammatory disorders (inflammatory bowel disease, sarcoidosis)
Osteo: benign (osteoid osteoma/osteoblastoma)/malignant (osteosarcoma/Ewing)
Immunodeficiency (common variable immunodeficiency)
Neoplasia (neuroblastoma, rhabdomyosarcoma)
Trauma

JDM: DRUGS USED OTHER THAN STEROIDS
(Mnemonic **MB I CATCH MD**)

Methotrexate (MTX)
Biological disease-modifying anti-rheumatic drugs (bDMARDs)

Intravenous immunoglobulin (IVIG)

Cyclophosphamide (CPA)
Azathioprine (AZA)
Tacrolimus (TAC)
Cyclosporine (CSA)
Hydroxychloroquine (HCQ)

Mycophenolate mofetil (MMF)
Diltiazem (calcium channel blocker for calcinosis)

METHOTREXATE

(Mnemonic **MTX**)

Mucositis/**M**yelosuppression
Transaminase increase (i.e. hepatotoxicity)
X-rays warranted (*chest* X-ray for pneumonia [e.g. varicella pneumonia] or pneumonitis [exceedingly rare])/**X**tra folate recommended

AZATHIOPRINE

(Mnemonic **AZATHIOPS**)

Alimentary system effects (anorexia, nausea, vomiting, diarrhoea)
Zoster and other infections (especially opportunistic)
Aplastic anaemia (various forms of myelosuppression)/**A**lopecia
TPMT low means increased myelotoxicity
Haematological malignancy (AML, lymphoma)/**H**aemorrhage (low platelets)
Interstitial pneumonitis (rare)
Occlusive hepatic (hepatic veno-occlusive disease; rare)
PML (progressive multifocal leukoencephalopathy; rare)
Skin cancer/**S**teatorrhoea

CYCLOPHOSPHAMIDE

(Mnemonic **CPA**)

Cystitis (haemorrhagic)
Pancytopenia
Alopecia/**A**ctivation of latent/opportunistic infections (e.g. herpes zoster, TB, PCP)

TACROLMUS

(Mnemonic **TACROLIMUS**)

Tremor/**T**ingling (neurotoxicity)
Alimentary (diarrhoea, constipation, nausea, vomiting, anorexia)/**A**naemia
Cancer risk increased
Renal toxicity (includes irreversible vasculopathy, interstitial fibrosis, tubular damage)
Osteoporosis
Lymphoproliferative disease/**L**ow Phosphate
Increased: blood pressure, [K$^+$], (creatinine)
Magnesium low
Urea high
Sugar diabetes

CYCLOSPORINE
(Mnemonic **CSA**)

Compromised kidneys (nephrotoxicity includes irreversible vasculopathy, interstitial fibrosis, tubular damage)
Secondary malignancy potential (especially lymphoproliferative)
Anaemia/**A**ccelerated blood pressure (hypertension), hair growth (hypertrichosis) and gums (gingival hyperplasia)/**A**dditional myopathy (caused by CSA per se; this can contribute to osteoporosis)

pSLE: DIFFERENCES TO ADULT SLE
Compared to adults with SLE, there is a *change* (increase) in the frequency of several aspects of SLE in children.
(Mnemonic **CHANGE**)

Chorea
Hepatosplenomegaly
Avascular
Necrosis
Glomerulonephritis
Exclusively paediatric problems: growth abnormalities, neonatal lupus

Index

Page numbers followed by '*f*' indicate figures, and '*t*' indicate tables.